Basic Neurochemistry

Basic Neurochemistry

Molecular, Cellular, and Medical Aspects
Fifth Edition

Editor-in-Chief

George J. Siegel, M.D.

Chief, Neurology Service
Hines Veterans Affairs Hospital
Hines, Illinois, and
Professor of Neurology and Cellular
and Molecular Biochemistry,
Loyola University Chicago
School of Medicine,
Maywood, Illinois

Editors

Bernard W. Agranoff, M.D.

Ralph W. Gerard Professor of Neuroscience
Department of Psychiatry, and
Director of Mental Health Research Institute
Professor of Biological Chemistry
University of Michigan
Ann Arbor, Michigan

R. Wayne Albers, Ph.D.

Chief, Section on Enzyme Chemistry
Laboratory of Neurochemistry
National Institute of Neurological
Disorders and Stroke
National Institutes of Health
Bethesda, Maryland

Perry B. Molinoff, M.D.

Professor and Chairman
Department of Pharmacology
School of Medicine
University of Pennsylvania
Philadelphia, Pennsylvania

Raven Press 🐚 New York

Raven Press, Ltd., 1185 Avenue of the Americas, New York, New York 10036

Made in the United States of America

Library of Congress Cataloging-in-Publication Data

Basic neurochemistry : molecular, cellular, and medical aspects /
    editor-in-chief, George J. Siegel ; editors, Bernard W. Agranoff,
    R. Wayne Albers, Perry B. Molinoff.—5th ed.
        p.   cm.
    Includes bibliographical references and index.
    ISBN 0-7817-0104-X
    1. Neurochemistry.   I. Siegel, George J.
    [DNLM: 1. Neurochemistry.   WL 104 B311   1993]
    QP356.3.B27   1993
    612.8′042—dc20
    DNLM/DLC
    for Library of Congress   93-24375
                                                                  CIP

Great care has been taken to maintain the accuracy of the information contained in the volume. However, neither Raven Press nor the editors can be held responsible for errors or for any consequences arising from the use of the information contained herein.

Materials appearing in this book prepared by individuals as part of their official duties as U.S. Government employees are not covered by the above mentioned copyright.

9   8   7   6   5   4   3   2   1

Contents

Part Five   Medical Neurochemistry

Contributors

R. Wayne Albers, Ph.D.
Chief, Section on Enzyme Chemistry
Laboratory of Neurochemistry
National Institute of Neurological Disorders
  and Stroke
National Institutes of Health
9000 Rockville Pike
Bethesda, Maryland 20892

Bernard W. Agranoff, M.D.
Ralph W. Gerard Professor of Neurosciences
Department of Psychiatry, and
Director, Mental Health Research Institute
Professor of Biological Chemistry
University of Michigan
1103 E. Huron Street
Ann Arbor, Michigan 48104-1687

Alaric T. Arenander, Ph.D.
Assistant Research Biologist
Department of Anatomy and Cell Biology
UCLA School of Medicine
Los Angeles, California 90024

Jack D. Barchas, M.D.
Associate Dean
UCLA School of Medicine
12-138 Center for Health Sciences
10833 LeConte Avenue
Los Angeles, California 90024-1722

Robert L. Barchi, M.D., Ph.D.
David Mahoney Professor of Neurological Sciences
Chairman, Department of Neuroscience
Director, David Mahoney Institute of
  Neurological Sciences
Professor of Neurology
University of Pennsylvania School of Medicine
36th and Hamilton Walk
Philadelphia, Pennsylvania 19104

A. Lorris Betz, M.D., Ph.D.
Professor of Pediatrics, Surgery, and Neurology
D3227 Medical Professional Building
University of Michigan
1103 E. Huron Street
Ann Arbor, Michigan 48109-0718

John P. Blass, M.D., Ph.D.
Burke Professor of Neurology and Medicine
Director, Dementia Research Service
Department of Neurology
Cornell University Medical College, and
Burke Medical Research Institute
785 Mamaroneck Avenue
White Plains, New York 10605

Scott T. Brady, Ph.D.
Associate Professor, Department of Cell Biology
  and Neuroscience
University of Texas Southwestern Medical Center
5323 Harry Hines Blvd
Dallas, Texas 75236-9039

Joan Heller Brown, Ph.D.
Professor, Department of Pharmacology
University of California, San Diego
9500 Gilman Drive
La Jolla, California 92093

Michael J. Brownstein, M.D.
Chief, Laboratory of Cell Biology
National Institute of Mental Health
National Institutes of Health
9000 Rockville Pike
Bethesda, Maryland 20892

Linda B. Buck, Ph.D.
Assistant Professor, Department of Neurobiology
Harvard Medical School
Boston, Massachusetts

William A. Catterall, Ph.D.
Professor and Chairman, Department of Pharmacology
University of Washington School of Medicine
Seattle, Washington 98195

Donald D. Clarke, Ph.D.
Professor of Biochemistry
Chemistry Department
Fordham University
441 E. Fordham Road
Bronx, New York 10458

ix

Arthur J. L. Cooper, Ph.D.
Associate Professor
Department of Biochemistry and Neurology
Cornell University Medical College
1300 York Avenue
New York, New York 10021

Carl W. Cotman, Ph.D.
Director, Irvine Research Unit in Brain Aging
Department of Psychobiology and Neurology
University of California
Irvine, California 92717-4450

Janet L. Cyr, Ph.D.
Postdoctoral Fellow
Department of Cell Biology and Neuroscience
University of Texas Southwestern Medical Center
5323 Harry Hines Blvd
Dallas, Texas 75236-9039

Timothy M. DeLorey, Ph.D.
Postdoctoral Fellow
Department of Pharmacology and Mental
* Retardation Research Center*
UCLA School of Medicine
1300 LeConte Avenue
Los Angeles, California 90024-1735

Jean de Vellis, Ph.D.
Professor, Department of Anatomy and Cell Biology
UCLA School of Medicine
Los Angeles, California 90024

Darryl C. De Vivo, M.D.
Sidney Carter Professor of Neurology
Professor of Pediatrics
College of Physicians and Surgeons
Columbia University
630 West 168th Street
New York, New York 10032

Salvatore DiMauro, M.D.
Lucy G. Moses Professor of Neurology
Columbia-Presbyterian Medical Center
College of Physicians and Surgeons
Columbia University
630 West 168th Street
New York, New York 10032

Raymond Dingledine, Ph.D.
Professor and Chairman, Department of
* Pharmacology*
Emory University School of Medicine
1510 Clifton Road
Atlanta, Georgia 30322

Ronald S. Duman, Ph.D.
Associate Professor
Department of Psychiatry
Yale University School of Medicine
34 Park Street
New Haven, Connecticut 06508

Glen R. Elliott, M.D., Ph.D.
Associate Professor, Department of Psychiatry
Director, Child and Adolescent Psychiatry
Langley Porter Psychiatric Institute
University of California–San Francisco
401 Parnassus Avenue
San Francisco, California 94143–0984

S. D. Erulkar, Ph.D.
Professor, Department of Pharmacology
University of Pennsylvania School of Medicine
36th and Hamilton Walk
Philadelphia, Pennsylvania 19104-6084

Akhlaq A. Farooqui, Ph.D.
Research Scientist, Department of Medical
* Biochemistry*
1645 Neil Avenue
Ohio State University
Columbus, Ohio 43210

Kym F. Faull, Ph.D.
Assistant Professor
Departments of Psychiatry and Biobehavioral Sciences,
* and Chemistry and Biochemistry*
Director, Center for Molecular and Medical
* Sciences Mass Spectrometry*
University of California–Los Angeles
Los Angeles, California 90024

Caleb E. Finch, Ph.D.
ARCO and William F. Kieschnick Professor in the
* Neurobiology of Aging*
Neurogerontology Division
Andrus Gerontology Center
3715 McClintlock Avenue, and
Department of Biological Sciences
University of Southern California
Los Angeles, California 90089-0191

Stuart Firestein, Ph.D.
Assistant Professor
Section of Neurobiology
Yale University School of Medicine
New Haven, Connecticut 06510

Stephen K. Fisher, Ph.D.
Associate Professor of Pharmacology, and
Associate Research Scientist
Mental Health Research Institute
University of Michigan
1103 E. Huron Street
Ann Arbor, Michigan 48104-1687

Alan Frazer, Ph.D.
Professor and Chairman
Department of Pharmacology
University of Texas Health Science Center
at San Antonio
7703 Floyd Curl Drive
San Antonio, Texas 78284

Kirk A. Frey, M.D., Ph.D.
Assistant Professor of Internal Medicine
Departments of Internal Medicine and Neurology, and
Assistant Research Scientist
Mental Health Research Institute
University of Michigan Hospitals
1500 E. Medical Center Drive
Ann Arbor, Michigan 48109-0028

Gary W. Goldstein, M.D.
Professor of Neurology and Pediatrics
Johns Hopkins University School of Medicine
and President, Kennedy Krieger Research Institute
707 N. Broadway
Baltimore, Maryland 21205

Fernando Gómez-Pinilla, Ph.D.
Assistant Professor
Neurology/Irvine Research Institute in Brain Aging
University of California, Irvine
Irvine, California 92717-4550

Richard H. Goodman, M.D., Ph.D.
Director, Vollum Institute for Advanced
Biomedical Research
Oregon Health Sciences University
3181 SW Sam Jackson Park Road
Portland, Oregon 97201-3098

Jack Peter Green, M.D., Ph.D.
Professor and Chairman
Department of Pharmacology
Mount Sinai School of Medicine
City University of New York
One Gustave Levy Place
New York, New York 10029

Paul Greengard, Ph.D.
Vincent Astor Professor
Head, Laboratory of Molecular and Cellular
Neuroscience
Rockefeller University
1230 York Avenue
New York, New York 10021

Amiya K. Hajra, Ph.D.
Professor of Biological Chemistry, and
Associate Research Scientist
Mental Health Research Institute
University of Michigan
1103 E. Huron Street
Ann Arbor, Michigan 48104-1687

Mark W. Hamblin, M.D., Ph.D.
Assistant Professor, Dpeartment of Psychiatry and
Behavioral Science
University of Washington
Staff Psychiatrist, VA Medical Center
Seattle, Washington 98108

Richard Hammerschlag, Ph.D.
Research Scientist
Division of Neurosciences
Beckman Research Institute of the City of Hope
1450 E. Duarte Road
Duarte, California 91010

Steven E. Haun, M.D.
Assistant Professor, Department of
Medical Biochemistry
Ohio State University
Columbus, Ohio 43210

Julie G. Hensler, Ph.D.
Assistant Professor
Department of Pharmacology
University of Texas Health Science Center
at San Antonio
7703 Floyd Curl Drive
San Antonio, Texas 78284-7764

Bertil Hille, Ph.D.
Professor, Department of Physiology and Biophysics
G424 Health Sciences Bldg
University of Washington School of Medicine
Seattle, Washington 98195

Jacob M. Hiller, Ph.D.
Research Associate Professor, Department of Psychiatry
New York University Medical Center
550 First Avenue
New York, New York 10016

Lloyd A. Horrocks, Ph.D.
Professor Emeritus
Department of Medical Biochemistry
Ohio State University
1645 Neil Avenue
Columbus, Ohio 43210

Jennifer S. Kahle, Ph.D.
Postdoctoral Fellow
Irvine Research Unit in Brain Aging
University of California, Irvine
Irvine, California 92717-4550

Robert Katzman, M.D.
Professor, Department of Neurosciences
University of California, San Diego
9500 Gilman Drive
La Jolla, California 92093

Irwin J. Kopin, M.D.
Director, Intramural Research Program
National Institute of Neurological Disorders and Stroke
National Institutes of Health
9000 Rockville Pike
Bethesda, Maryland 20892

Malcolm J. Low, M.D., Ph.D.
Assistant Scientist
Vollum Institute of Advanced Biomedical Research
Oregon Health Science University
3181 SW Sam Jackson Park Road
Portland, Oregon 97201

Joel Linden, Ph.D.
Associate Professor, Department of Internal Medicine
and Physiology
University of Virginia
Box 158
Health Sciences Center
Charlottesville, Virginia 22908

Robert C. Malenka, M.D., Ph.D.
Assistant Professor, Psychiatry Department
Langley Porter Psychiatric Institute
University of California–San Francisco
401 Parnassus Avenue
San Francisco, California 94143–0984

Robert F. Margolskeem M.D., Ph.D.
Associate Member, Department of Neurosciences
Roche Institute of Molecular Biology
Nutley, New Jersey 07110

Chris J. McBain, Ph.D.
Senior Staff Fellow
NICHD-LCMN
National Institutes of Health
9000 Rockville Pike
Bethesda, Maryland 20892

Bruce S. McEwen, Ph.D.
Professor and Head, Laboratory of
Neuroendocrinology
Rockefeller University
1230 York Avenue
New York, New York 10021

Dale E. McFarlin, M.D. (Deceased)
Acting Chief, Neuroimmunology Branch
National Institute of Neurological Disorders
and Stroke
National Institutes of Health
9000 Rockville Pike
Bethesda, Maryland 20892

Paul McGonigle, Ph.D.
Research Associate Professor,
Department of Pharmacology
University of Pennsylvania School of Medicine
124 John Morgan Bldg
36th and Hamilton Walk
Philadelphia, Pennsylvania 19104-6084

Brian Meldrum, Ph.D.
Professor of Experimental Neurology
Institute of Psychiatry
Department of Neurology
De Crespigny Park
Denmark Hill
London SE5 8AF
UNITED KINGDOM

Perry B. Molinoff, M.D.
A. N. Richards Professor and Chairman
Department of Pharmacology
University of Pennsylvania School of Medicine
36th and Hamilton Walk
Philadelphia, Pennsylvania 19104-6084

Pierre Morell, Ph.D.
Department of Biochemistry
321 Brain and Development Research Center
University of North Carolina at Chapel Hill
Chapel Hill, North Carolina 27599-7250

Eric J. Nestler, M.D., Ph.D.
Elizabeth and House Jameson Associate Professor
of Psychiatry and Pharmacology
Yale University School of Medicine
34 Park Street
New Haven, Connecticut 06508

William T. Norton, Ph.D.
Professor, Department of Neurology (Neurochemistry)
Albert Einstein College of Medicine
Yeshiva University
1300 Morris Park Avenue
Bronx, New York 10461

Richard W. Olsen, Ph.D.
Professor, Department of Pharmacology
UCLA School of Medicine
Center for Health Sciences
10833 LeConte Avenue
Los Angeles, California 90024

David E. Pleasure, M.D.
Professor, Neurology and Pediatrics
University of Pennsylvania and Children's Hospital
of Philadelphia
34th and Civic Center Blvd
Philadelphia, Pennsylvania 19104

William A. Pulsinelli, M.D., Ph.D.
Professor and Chairman
Department of Neurology
University of Tennessee, Memphis
Health Sciences Center
855 Monroe Avenue
Memphis, Tennessee 38163

Richard H. Quarles, Ph.D.
Laboratory of Molecular and Cellular Neurobiology
National Institute of Neurological Disorders
and Stroke
National Institutes of Health
9000 Rockville Pike
Bethesda, Maryland 20892

Bruce Quinn, M.D., Ph.D.
Neuropathology Fellow, Department of Pathology
UCLA School of Medicine
1300 LeConte Avenue
Los Angeles, California 90024

Cedric S. Raine, Ph.D., D.Sc.
Professor of Pathology and Neuroscience
Department of Pathology
Albert Einstein College of Medicine
Yeshiva University
1300 Morris Park Avenue
Bronx, New York 10461

Dennis J. Selkoe, M.D.
Associate Professor, Department of Neurology
Program in Neuroscience
Harvard Medical School
and Center for Neurologic Diseases
Brigham and Women's Hospital
75 Francis Street
Boston, Massachusetts 02115

George J. Siegel, M.D.
Professor of Neurology and Cellular and Molecular
Biochemistry, and Vice-Chairman,
Department of Neurology
Loyola University Chicago
School of Medicine, and Chief Neurology Service
Hines Veterans Affairs Hospital
Hines, Illinois 60141

Eric J. Simon, Ph.D.
Professor, Departments of Psychiatry and Pharmacology
New York University Medical Center
550 First Avenue
New York, New York 10016

Hitoshi Shichi, Ph.D.
Professor, Department of Ophthalmology
Wayne State University School of Medicine
Kresge Eye Institute
4717 St. Antoine
Detroit, Michigan 48201

Louis Sokoloff, M.D.
Chief, Laboratory of Cerebral Metabolism
National Institute of Mental Health
National Institutes of Health
9000 Rockville Pike
Bethesda, Maryland 20850

William L. Stahl, Ph.D.
Professor, Departments of Physiology, Biophysics,
and Medicine (Neurology)
University of Washington School of Medicine
and Veterans Affairs Medical Center
1660 S. Columbian Way
Seattle, Washington 98108

Kunihiko Suzuki, M.D.
Director, Brain and Development Research Center
Professor, Departments of Neurology and Psychiatry
University of North Carolina School of Medicine
Chapel Hill, North Carolina 27599

Palmer Taylor, Ph.D.
Professor and Chairman, Department of
*   Pharmacology*
University of California, San Diego
9500 Gilman Drive
San Diego, California 92093

Allan J. Tobin, Ph.D.
Professor, Department of Biology, and
*   Chair for Interdepartmental Program for*
*   Neuroscience*
Molecular Biology Institute
and Brain Research Institute
UCLA School of Medicine
1300 LeConte Avenue
Los Angeles, California 90024-1606

Michael D. Uhler, Ph.D.
Associate Professor of Biological Chemistry, and
Associate Research Scientist
Mental Health Research Institute
University of Michigan
1103 E. Huron Street
Ann Arbor, Michigan 48104-1687

Ted B. Usdin, M.D., Ph.D.
Senior Staff Fellow
Laboratory of Cell Biology
National Institute of Mental Health
National Institutes of Health
Bethesda, Maryland 20892

Norman Weiner, M.D.
Professor of Pharmacology
University of Colorado School of Medicine
Health Sciences Center
Denver, Colorado 80262

Leonhard S. Wolfe, M.D., Ph.D.
Professor, Department of Neurochemistry
Montreal Neurological Institute
3801 University Street
Montreal, Quebec H3A 2B4
CANADA

Marc Yudkoff, M.D.
Professor of Pediatrics
University of Pennsylvania School of Medicine
Children's Hospital of Philadelphia
1 Children's Center
Philadelphia, Pennsylvania 19104

Acknowledgments

We are mindful of our debt to previous contributors to this evolving text and express our gratitude for their figures and information that are carried forward. We are sad to note the passing of Dale E. McFarlin, M.D., a foremost investigator in the field of neuroimmunology and contributor to the chapter on "Diseases Involving Myelin." We wish to express our gratitude to our many colleagues for generously sharing their expertise, and to the many investigators whose important work is not explicitly referenced. The skill and judgment of the University of Michigan Biomedical Communications group, including Chris Burke, Holly Fischer, and Lorie Manzardo, are also gratefully acknowledged.

We are specially indebted to Graham Lees and Jasna Markovac of Raven Press, who shared in the planning and implementation of the Fifth edition, and we appreciate the excellent production assistance from Raven Press, in particular the work of Kathleen Lyons and Nancy Kirkpatrick.

The opportunity for the Editors to organize and produce *Basic Neurochemistry* is due in large measure to the support we are fortunate to receive from our respective institutions, for which we are grateful.

George J. Siegel
Bernard W. Agranoff
R. Wayne Albers
Perry B. Molinoff

Excerpts from the Preface to the Fourth Edition

The addition of the phrase, "Molecular, Cellular, and Medical Aspects" to the title of this Fourth Edition of *Basic Neurochemistry* emphasizes our belief that the flourishing of neurochemistry derives from correlations among phenomena that are observed at multiple levels. As discussed in the Preface to the First Edition in 1972, integrating hypotheses are being developed to account for the functioning of the nervous system in terms of molecular events. The current growth of correlative power stems not only from increases in sensitivity and resolution of analytical biochemistry—more data from smaller samples—but equally from technology that permits observing and quantitating molecular events in functioning, complex, and relatively intact biological structures. Examples range from recording the conductance of single ion channels in patches of membrane, to measuring processes in transfected cells or transgenic animals, to imaging receptor-ligand binding, metabolism, and blood flow in brains of awake functioning humans.

Advances in molecular genetics have generated an enthusiastic sense of anticipation among neurobiologists over the past decade. The derivative applications are, on the one hand, revealing more about molecular structures and, on the other, elucidating nervous system development and the bases of genetic diseases affecting human behavior. We are encouraged to believe that increased knowledge of the molecular basis of neurobiology will ultimately lead to an understanding of the coding of experiences that comprise memory and are the substrate of behavior and mind.

Basic Neurochemistry had its origin in the Conference on Neurochemistry Curriculum initiated and organized by R. Wayne Albers, Robert Katzman, and George Siegel under the sponsorship of the National Institute for Neurological Diseases and Stroke, June 19 and 20, 1969, Bronx, New York. At this conference, a group of 30 neuroscientists constructed a syllabus outline delineating the scope of a neurochemistry curriculum appropriate for medical, graduate, and postgraduate neuroscience students. Out of this outline grew the first edition, edited by R. Wayne Albers, George Siegel, Robert Katzman, and Bernard Agranoff. It was anticipated that the book would evolve with the emergence of the field and would stimulate continuing reappraisal of the scientific and educational aspects of neurochemistry. The Editors elected to assign the copyright and all royalties to the American Society for Neurochemistry, the royalties to be used for educational purposes. These funds have been used to sponsor the Annual Basic Neurochemistry Lectureship. With the Fourth Edition, we welcome Perry Molinoff as a coeditor.

George J. Siegel
Bernard W. Agranoff
R. Wayne Albers
Perry B. Molinoff

Preface

In organizing the Fifth Edition, we have again considered that the subject matter of *Basic Neurochemistry* should encompass, as comprehensively as possible, research that elucidates brain function and dysfunction at the level of molecular and cellular biochemistry. Testament to the growing difficulty of this task is the recent proliferation of journals specializing not just in neurobiology but in particular cells, parts of cells, and classes of molecules. To accomplish this within a single volume has required editorial constraints on the authors to restrict references to reviews and articles that are key to entering the relevant literature. We acknowledge here that many important contributions have not been cited. It has also been necessary to restrict, more than we would like, the presentation of historical contexts. A treasury of such information may be found in the chapter by Donald B. Tower, "Neurochemistry in Historical Perspective" in the third edition of this text (Little, Brown, & Co., Boston, 1982, pp. 1–18). As the Fifth Edition goes to press, we are pleased to note that the American Society for Neurochemistry and the International Society for Neurochemistry are achieving their twenty-fifth years (see historical review by H. Bachelard in *J. Neurochem,* 61: S287–S307, 1993).

In the preface to the First Edition, the utility of "integrating hypotheses" was discussed primarily from the standpoint of obtaining an understanding of function and disease in molecular terms. Twenty years later we observe that the process works in both directions. Today, the tools of molecular biology permit rational strategies for elucidating altered gene structures that underly any genetic disease, and methods are available for creating experimental defects that are themselves tools for defining the physiological roles of genes and gene products in complex nervous system functions. Presently, investigations of most neurologic diseases are guided by plausible hypotheses. Interestingly, many "answers," whether identification of gene products (e.g., multitudinous K^+ channels or glutamate receptors) or of gene pathology (e.g., extended trinucleotide repeats), generate tantalizing vistas of unexplored molecular and cellular biochemistry. We hope to provide a taste of this feast of ideas and to whet the appetite of readers as much as was ours in the preparation of the Fifth Edition.

The pace of neurochemical research has made this Fifth Edition, more so than previous editions, a new book. This time, the explosion of information has come about mainly through the investigations of gene expression and mapping or applications of derivative technology. There are new chapters on the molecular basis for olfaction and taste, neurotransmitter and growth-factor receptor families and second messenger signaling systems, amino acid and purinergic neurotransmission, neurotransmitter uptake systems, and molecular targets of drugs of abuse. Portions of the book have been revised to expand coverage of amine transmitters, eicosanoids and neuronal function, developmental neurobiology, gene expression, aging, cytoskeletal development, and plasticity and cognitive functions. Other portions have been updated to account for evolving research in molecular genetics of neurologic diseases, disorders of cognition and basal ganglia, epilepsy, and prion diseases. Yet, the accelerating flow of information exchange stimulates the emergence of new concepts even as this edition goes to press.

While this book is designed to be a useful reference for investigators, its major goal of introducing neurochemistry to advanced students places a premium on clarity of presentation of data and concepts. To this end, we devoted attention in this edition to color graphics. A set of projection slides of the figures will also enhance the usefulness of the book.

George J. Siegel
Bernard W. Agranoff
R. Wayne Albers
Perry B. Molinoff

PART ONE

Neural Membranes

CHAPTER 1

Neurocellular Anatomy

CEDRIC S. RAINE

AN UNDERSTANDING OF NEUROANATOMY IS NECESSARY TO THE STUDY OF NEUROCHEMISTRY

Despite the advent of molecular genetics in neurobiology, our understanding of the functional relationships of the components of the central nervous system (CNS) remains in its infancy, particularly in the areas of cellular interaction and synaptic modulation. Nevertheless, the fine structural relationships of most elements of nervous system tissue have been well described [1–5]. (The excellent neuroanatomical atlases of Peters et al. [3] and Palay and Chan-Palay [1] should be consulted for detailed ultrastructural analyses of specific cell types, particularly of neurons with their diverse forms and con-

Basic Neurochemistry: Molecular, Cellular, and Medical Aspects, 5th Ed., edited by G. J. Siegel et al. Published by Raven Press, Ltd., New York, 1994. Correspondence to Cedric S. Raine, Department of Pathology, Albert Einstein College of Medicine, 1300 Morris Park Avenue, Bronx, New York 10461.

nections.) This chapter provides a concise description of the major cytoarchitectural features of the nervous system and gives an entrance into the relevant literature. Although the fine structure of the organelles of the CNS and peripheral nervous system (PNS) is not peculiar to these tissues, the interactions between cell types, such as synaptic contacts between neurons and myelin sheaths around axons, are unique. These specializations and those that allow for the sequestration of the CNS from the outside world, namely, the blood-brain barrier and the absence of lymphatics, become major issues in considerations of normal and disease processes in the nervous system. For the sake of simplicity, the present section is subdivided first into a section on general organization and then according to major cell types.

Diverse cell types are organized into assemblies and patterns such that specialized components are integrated into a physiology of the whole organ

Central nervous system parenchyma is made up of nerve cells and their afferent and efferent extensions (dendrites and axons), all closely enveloped by glial cells. Coronal section of the cerebral hemispheres of the brain reveals an outer convoluted rim of gray matter overlying the white matter (Fig. 1). Gray matter, which also exists as islands within the white matter, contains mainly nerve cell bodies and glia and lacks significant amounts of myelin, the lipid component responsible for the whiteness of white matter. More distally along the neuraxis in the spinal cord, the cerebral situation is reversed. White matter

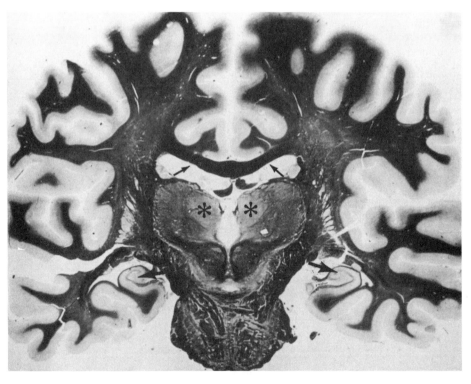

FIG. 1. Coronal section of the human brain at the thalamic level stained by the Heidenhain technique for myelin. Gray matter stains faintly; all myelinated regions are black. The thalamus (*) lies beneath the lateral ventricles and is separated at this level by the beginning of the third ventricle. The roof of the lateral ventricles is formed by the corpus callosum *(small arrows)*. The Ammon's horns are shown at the *large arrows*. Note the outline of gyri and sulci at the surface of the cerebral hemispheres, sectioned here near the junction of the frontal and parietal cortex.

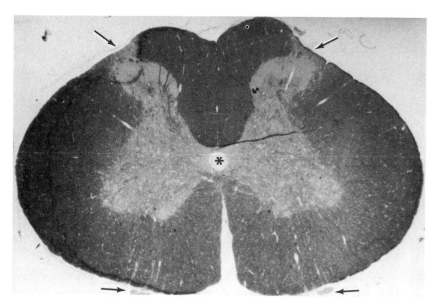

FIG. 2.   Transverse section of a rabbit lumbar spinal cord at L-1. Gray matter is seen as a paler staining area in an H configuration formed by the dorsal and ventral horns with the central canal in the center (*). The dorsal horns would meet the incoming dorsal spine nerve roots at the *upper arrows.* The anterior roots can be seen below *(arrows),* opposite the ventral horns from which they received their fibers. The white matter occupies a major part of the spinal cord and stains darker. Epon section, 1 μm, stained with toluidine blue.

surrounds gray matter, which is arranged in a characteristic H formation (Fig. 2).

A highly diagrammatic representation of the major CNS elements is shown in Fig. 3. The entire CNS is bathed both internally and externally by cerebrospinal fluid (CSF), which circulates throughout the ventricular and leptomeningeal spaces. This fluid, a type of plasma ultrafiltrate, plays a significant role in protecting the CNS from mechanical trauma, balancing electrolytes and protein, and maintaining ventricular pressure (see Chap. 32). The outer surface of the CNS is invested by the triple-membrane system of the meninges. The outermost is the dura mater (derived from the mesoderm), which is tightly adherent to the inner surfaces of the calvaria. The arachnoid membrane is closely applied to the inner surface of the dura mater. The innermost of the meninges, the pia mater, loosely covers the CNS surface. The pia and arachnoid together (derived from the ectoderm) are called the leptomeninges. CSF occupies the subarachnoid space (between the arachnoid and the pia) and the ventricles. The CNS parenchyma is overlaid by a layer of subpial astrocytes, which, in turn, is covered on its leptomeningeal aspect by a basal lamina (see Fig. 3). On the inner (ventricular) surface, the CNS parenchyma is separated from the CSF by a layer of ciliated ependymal cells, which are thought to facilitate the movement of CSF. The production and circulation of CSF are maintained by the choroid plexus, grape-like collections of vascular tissue and cells that protrude into the ventricles (see Chap. 32). Resorption of CSF is effected by vascular structures known as arachnoid villi, located in the leptomeninges over the surface of the brain (see Chap. 32).

Ependymal cells abut layers of astrocytes, which, in turn, envelop neurons, neurites, and vascular components. In addition to neurons and glial cells (astrocytes and oligodendrocytes), the CNS parenchyma contains blood vessels, macrophages (pericytes), and microglial cells.

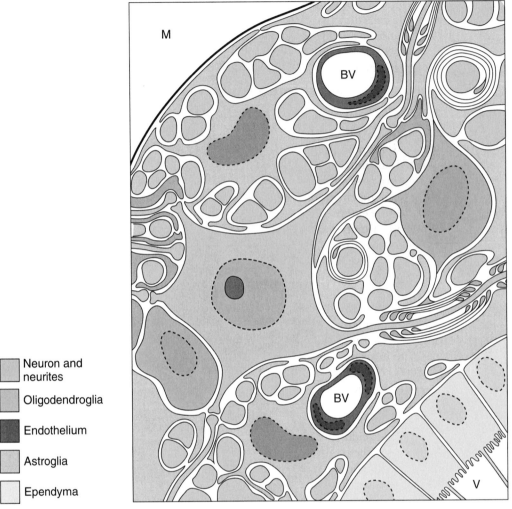

FIG. 3. The major components of the CNS and their interrelationships. Microglia are not depicted. In this simplified schema, the CNS extends from its meningeal surface (M); through the basal lamina *(solid black line)* overlying the subpial astrocyte layer of the CNS parenchyma; across the CNS parenchyma proper (containing neurons and glia) and subependymal astrocytes, to ciliated ependymal cells lining the ventricular space (V). Note how the astrocyte also invests blood vessels (BV), neurons, and cell processes. The pia-astroglia (glia limitans) provides the barrier between the exterior (dura and blood vessels) and the CNS parenchyma. One neuron is seen *(center)*, with synaptic contacts on its soma and dendrites. Its axon emerges to the right and is myelinated by an oligodendrocyte *(above)*. Other axons are shown in transverse section, some of which are myelinated. The oligodendrocyte to the lower left of the neuron is of the nonmyelinating satellite type. The subarachnoid space of the meninges (M) and the ventricles (V) contain cerebrospinal fluid.

The PNS and the autonomic nervous system consist of bundles of myelinated and nonmyelinated axons enveloped by Schwann cells, the PNS counterparts of oligodendrocytes. Nerve bundles are enclosed by the perineurium and the epineurium, which are tough, fibrous, elastic sheaths. Between individual nerve fibers are isolated connective tissue (endoneurial) cells and blood vessels. The ganglia (e.g., dorsal root and sympathetic ganglia), located peripherally to the CNS, are made up of large neurons, usually unipolar or bipolar, surrounded by satellite cells that are specialized Schwann cells. A dendrite and an axon, both of which can be of great length (up to several feet), arise from each neuron.

CHARACTERISTICS OF THE NEURON

From an historical standpoint, no other cell type has attracted as much attention or caused as much controversy as the nerve cell. It is impossible in a single chapter to delineate comprehensively the extensive structural, topographical, and functional variation achieved by this cell type. Consequently, despite an enormous literature, the neuron still defies precise definition, particularly with regard to function. It is known that the neuronal population is usually established shortly after birth, that mature neurons do not divide, and that in humans, there is a daily dropout of neurons amounting to approximately 20,000 cells. These facts alone make the neuron unique. (Development and maturation of neurons are discussed in Chap. 28.)

Neurons can be excitatory, inhibitory, or modulatory in their effect; motor, sensory, or secretory in their function. They can be influenced by a large repertoire of neurotransmitters and hormones (see Chap. 8). This enormous repertoire of functions, associated with different developmental influences on different neurons, is largely reflected in the variation of dendritic and axonal outgrowth. Specialization also occurs at axonal terminals, where a variety of junctional complexes (synapses) exist. The subtle synaptic modifications are best visualized ultrastructurally, although immunohistochemical staining also permits distinction among synapses on the basis of transmitter type.

General structural features of neurons are the perikarya, dendrites, and axons

The stereotypic image of a neuron is that of a stellate cell body (soma or perikaryon) with broad dendrites and a fine axon emerging from one pole—an impression gained from the older work of Purkinje, who first described the nerve cell in 1839, and of Deiters, Ramón y Cajal, and Golgi at the end of the nineteenth century and early twentieth century. However, this does not hold true for many neurons. The neuron is the most polymorphic cell in the body and defies formal classification on the basis of shape, location, function, fine structure, or transmitter substance. Although early workers described the neuron as a globular mass suspended between nerve fibers, the teased preparations of Deiters and his contemporaries soon proved this not to be the case. Later work using impregnation staining and culture techniques, elaborated on Deiters' findings. Before Deiters and Ramón y Cajal, neurons were believed to form a syncytium, with no intervening membranes—a postulate also proposed for neuroglia. Today, of course, we are familiar with the specialized membranes and the enormous variety of nerve cell shapes and sizes. They range from the small globular cerebellar granule cells, with a perikaryal diameter of approximately 6 to 8 μm, to the pear-shaped Purkinje cells and star-shaped anterior horn cells, both of which may reach diameters of 60 to 80 μm in humans. Perikaryal size is generally a poor index of total cell volume, however, and it is a general rule in neuroanatomy that neurites occupy a greater percentage of the cell surface area than does the soma. For example, the pyramidal cell of the somatosensory cortex has a cell body that accounts for only 4 percent of the total cell surface area, whereas from its dendritic tree, the dendritic spines alone claim 43 percent (Mungai, quoted by Peters et al. [3]). Hyden [2] quotes Scholl (1956), who calculated that the perikaryon of a ''cortical cell'' represents 10 percent of the neuronal surface area. In the feline reticular formation, some giant cells possess ratios between soma and dendrites of about 1:5. A single axon is the usual rule, but some cells, like the Golgi cells of the cerebellum, are endowed with several, some of which may show branching.

The extent of the branching displayed by the dendrites is a useful index of their functional importance. Dendritic trees represent the expression of the receptive fields, and large fields can receive inputs from multiple origins. A cell with a less developed dendritic ramification (e.g., the cerebellar granule cell), synapses with a more homogeneous population of afferent sources.

The axon emerges from a neuron as a slender thread and frequently does not branch until it nears its target. In contrast to the dendrite and the soma (with very few exceptions), the axon is frequently myelinated, thus increasing its efficiency as a conducting unit. Myelin, a spirally wrapped membrane (see Chap. 6), is laid down in segments (internodes) by oligodendrocytes in the CNS and by Schwann cells in the PNS. The naked regions of axon between adjacent myelin internodes are known as nodes of Ranvier (see Figs. 20 and 21).

Neurons contain the same intracellular components as do other cells

No unique cytoplasmic inclusions of the neuron serve to distinguish it from any other cell. Neurons have all the morphological counterparts of other cell types, the structures are similarly distributed, and some of the most common, the Golgi apparatus and mitochondria, for example, were first described in neurons (Fig. 4).

The Nucleus

A large, usually spherical nucleus containing a prominent nucleolus is typical of most neurons. The nucleochromatin is invariably pale, with little dense heterochromatin. In some neurons (e.g., cerebellar granule cells), the karyoplasm (nucleoplasm) may show more differentiation and dense heterochromatin. The nucleolus is vesiculated and clearly delineated from the rest of the karyoplasm. It usually contains two textures, the

pars fibrosa (fine bundles of filaments) and the pars granulosa, in which dense granules predominate. An additional juxtaposed structure, found in neurons of the female of some species, is the nucleolar satellite, or sex chromatin, which consists of dense, but loosely packed, coiled filaments. The nucleus is enclosed by the nuclear envelope, made up on the cytoplasmic side by the inner membrane of the perikaryon (sometimes seen in continuity with the endoplasmic reticulum; Fig. 5) and a more regular membrane on the inner, nuclear aspect. Between the two is a clear channel of between 20 and 40 nm. Periodically, the inner and outer membranes of the envelope come together to form a single diaphragm—a nuclear pore (Fig. 5). In tangential section, nuclear pores are seen as empty vesicular structures, approximately 70 nm in diameter. In some neurons, as in Purkinje cells, that segment of the nuclear envelope which faces the dendritic pole is deeply invaginated.

The Perikaryon

The body of the neuron, the perikaryon, is rich in organelles (Fig. 4). It often stands out poorly from a homogeneous background neuropil, most of which is composed of nonmyelinated neurites (axons and dendrites), synaptic complexes, and glial cell processes. Closer inspection shows that, like all cells, the neuron is delineated by a typical triple-layered unit membrane approximately 7.5 nm wide. Among the most prominent features of the perikaryal cytoplasm is a system of membranous cisternae, divisible into rough endoplasmic reticulum (ER), which forms part of the Nissl substance; smooth (agranular) ER; subsurface cisternae (the hypolemmal system); and the Golgi apparatus. Although these various components are structurally interconnected, each possesses distinct enzymologic properties. Also present within the cytoplasm are abundant lysosomes, lipofuscin granules (aging pigment), mitochondria, multivesicular bodies, neuro-

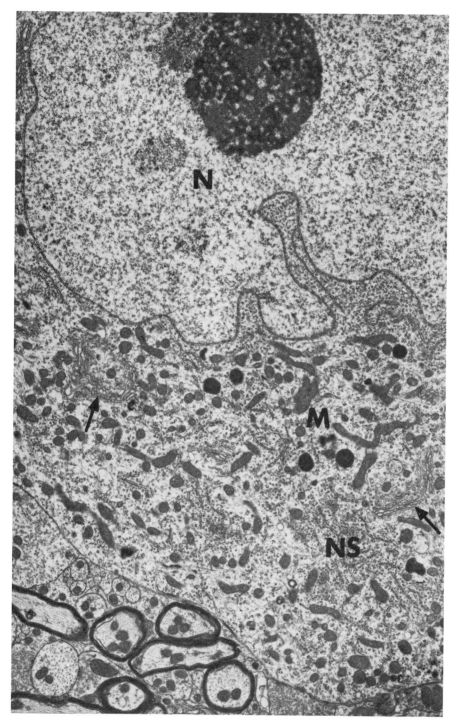

FIG. 4.   A motor neuron from the spinal cord of an adult rat shows a nucleus (N) containing a nucleolus, clearly divisible into a pars fibrosa and a pars granulosa, and a perikaryon filled with organelles. Among these, Golgi apparatus *(arrows)*, Nissl substance (S), mitochondria (M), and lysosomes (L) can be seen. An axosomatic synapse (S) occurs below, and two axodendritic synapses abut a dendrite (D). ×8,000.

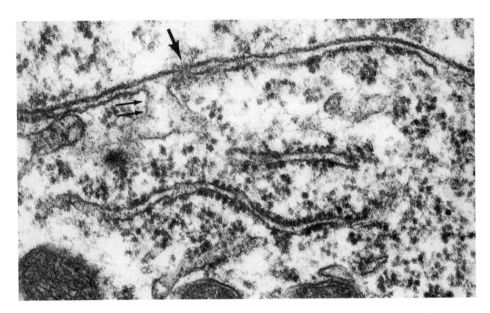

FIG. 5.   Detail of the nuclear envelope showing a nuclear pore *(single arrow)* and the outer leaflet connected to smooth ER *(double arrows)*. Two cisternae of rough ER with associated ribosomes are also present. ×80,000.

tubules, neurofilaments, and ribosomes. The major neuronal organelles are as follows.

Nissl Substance.   The intracytoplasmic basophilic masses that ramify loosely throughout the cytoplasm and that are typical of most neurons are known collectively as Nissl substance (Figs. 4 and 5). The distribution of Nissl substance in certain neurons is characteristic and used as a criterion for identification. By electron microscopy (EM), this substance is seen to comprise regular arrays or scattered portions of flattened cisternae of rough ER, surrounded by clouds of free polyribosomes. The membranes of rough ER are studded with rows of ribosomes. A space of 20 to 40 nm is maintained within cisternae. Sometimes, cisternal walls meet at fenestrations. Unlike the rough ER of glandular cells or other protein-secreting cells, such as plasma cells, the rough ER of neurons probably produces most of its proteins for the neuron's own use, a feature imposed by the extraordinary functional demands placed on the cell. Nissl substance does not penetrate axons but does extend along dendrites.

Smooth ER.   Most neurons contain at least a few cisternae of smooth (agranular) ER, sometimes difficult to differentiate from rough ER owing to disorderly arrangement of ribosomes. Ribosomes are not associated with these membranes and the cisternae usually assume a meandering, branching course throughout the cytoplasm. In some neurons, smooth ER is quite prominent, for example, in Purkinje cells. Individual cisterns of smooth ER extend along axons and dendrites. Smooth ER within axons has been implicated in protein transport.

Subsurface Cisternae.   Although not a constant feature, a system of smooth, membrane-bound, flattened cisternae can be found in many neurons. These structures, referred to as hypolemmal cisternae by Palay and Chan-Palay [1], abut the plasmalemma of the neuron and constitute a secondary membranous boundary within the cell. The distance between these cisternae and the plasmalemma is usually 10 to 12 nm, and on occasion, a mitochondrion may be found in close association with the innermost leaflet (e.g., in Purkinje cells). Similar cisternae have been described beneath synaptic complexes, but their functional significance is not known. Some authors have suggested that such a system may play a role in the uptake of metabolites.

Golgi Apparatus.   Undoubtedly the most impressive demonstration of the Golgi system, a highly specialized form of agranular reticulum, is achieved by using the metal impregnation techniques of Golgi. Ultrastructurally, the Golgi apparatus consists of aggregates of smooth-walled cisternae and a variety of vesicles. It is surrounded by a heterogeneous assemblage of organelles, including mitochondria, lysosomes, and multivesicular bodies. In most neurons, the Golgi apparatus encompasses the nucleus and extends into dendrites but is absent from axons. A three-dimensional analysis of the system reveals that the stacks of cisternae are pierced periodically by fenestrae. Tangential sections of these fenestrations show them to be circular profiles. A multitude of vesicles is associated with each segment of Golgi apparatus, in particular, "coated" vesicles, which proliferate from the lateral margins of flattened cisternae (Fig. 6). Such structures have been variously named, but the term alveolate vesicle seems to be generally accepted. Histochemical staining reveals that these bodies are rich in acid hydrolases, and they are believed to represent primary lysosomes [6]. Acid phosphatase is also found elsewhere in the cisternae but in lesser amounts than in alveolate vesicles.

Lysosomes.   The principal organelle responsible for the degradation of cellular waste is the lysosome. It is a common constituent of all cell types of the nervous system and is particularly prominent in neurons, where it can be seen at various stages of development

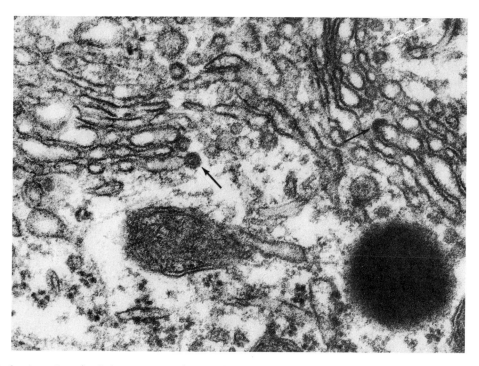

FIG. 6.   A portion of a Golgi apparatus. The smooth-membraned cisternae appear beaded. The many circular profiles represent tangentially sectioned fenestrae and alveolate vesicles (primary lysosomes). Two of the latter can be seen budding from Golgi saccules *(arrows)*. Mitochondria and a dense body (secondary lysosomes) are also present. ×60,000.

(Fig. 4). It ranges in size from 0.1 to 1 or 2 μm in diameter. The primary lysosome is elaborated from Golgi saccules as a small, vesicular structure (Fig. 6). Its function is to fuse with the membrane of waste-containing vacuoles (phagosomes), into which it releases hydrolytic enzymes. (This is discussed in Chap. 38). The sequestered material is then degraded within the vacuole, and the organelle becomes a secondary lysosome and is usually electron dense and large. The matrix of this organelle will give a positive reaction when tested histochemically for acid phosphatase. Residual bodies containing nondegradable material are considered to be tertiary lysosomes, and in the neuron, some are represented by lipofuscin granules (Fig. 7). These granules contain brown pigment and lamellar stacks of membrane material and are more common in the aged brain. (For more details on lysosomes, the inter-

ested reader is referred to Novikoff and Holtzman [6]).

Multivesicular Bodies.   Multivesicular bodies are usually found in association with the Golgi apparatus and are visualized by EM as small, single membrane-bound sacs approximately 0.5 μm in diameter. They contain several minute, spherical profiles, sometimes arranged about the periphery. They are believed to belong to the lysosome series (prior to secondary lysosomes) because they contain acid hydrolases and are apparently derived from primary lysosomes.

Neurotubules.   The neurotubule has been the subject of intense research in recent years [7]. Neurotubules are usually arranged haphazardly throughout the perikaryon of neurons but are aligned longitudinally in axons and dendrites. Each neurotubule consists of a dense-walled structure enclosing a

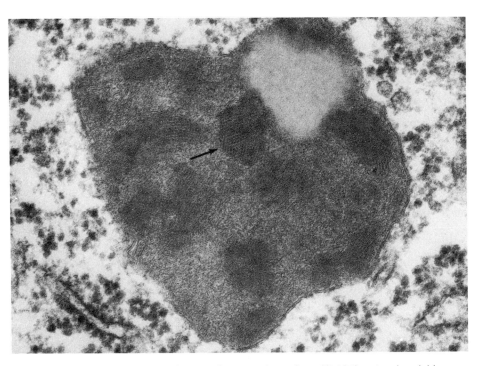

FIG. 7.   A lipofuscin granule from a cortical neuron shows membrane-bound lipid (dense) and a soluble component (gray). The denser component is lamellated. The lamellae appear as paracrystalline arrays of tubular profiles when sectioned transversely *(arrow).* The granule is surrounded by a single unit membrane. Free ribosomes can also be seen. ×96,000.

clear lumen, in the middle of which may be found an electron-dense dot. Sometimes, axonal neurotubules display 5-nm filamentous interconnecting side-arms. The diameter of neurotubules varies between 22 and 24 nm. High-resolution studies indicate that each neurotubule wall consists of 13 filamentous subunits arranged helically around a lumen (see also Chap. 27).

Neurofilaments. Neurofilaments belong to the family of intermediate filaments and are usually found in association with neurotubules. The function of these two organelles has been debated for some time and although it seems reasonable to assume that they play a role in the maintenance of form, their role in axoplasmic transport remains to be clarified [8] (see Chap. 27). Neurofilaments have a diameter of approximately 10 nm, are of indeterminate length, and frequently occur in bundles. They are constant components of axons but are rarer in dendrites. In the axon, individual filaments can be seen to possess a minute lumen and to be interconnected by proteinaceous side-arms, thereby forming a meshwork. Because of these cross-bridges, they do not form tightly packed bundles in the normal axon, in contrast to filaments within astrocytic processes (see Fig. 14), which lack cross-bridges. Neurofilaments within neuronal somata do not usually display cross-bridges and can be found in tight bundles. A form of filamentous structure finer than neurofilaments is seen at the tips of growing neurites, particularly in the growth cones of developing axons. These structures, known as microfilaments, are 5 nm in size and are composed of actin. They facilitate movement and growth, since it has been shown that axonal extension can be arrested pharmacologically by treatment with compounds that depolymerize these structures. The biochemistry of neurotubules and neurofilaments is dealt with in more detail in Soifer [7] and Wang et al. [8].

Mitochondria. Mitochondria are the centers for oxidative phosphorylation. These organelles occur ubiquitously in the neuron and

its processes (Figs. 4 and 6). Their overall shape may change from one type of neuron to another, but their basic morphology is identical to that in other cell types. Mitochondria consist morphologically of double-membraned sacs surrounded by protuberances, or cristae, extending from the inner membrane into the matrix space. (The review by Novikoff and Holtzman [6] discusses in more detail the ultrastructure and enzymatic properties of mitochondria and the above cellular components.)

The Axon

As the axon egresses, it becomes physiologically and structurally divisible into distinct regions: the axon hillock, the initial segment, the axon proper, and the axonal termination. (These segments are discussed in detail by Peters and co-workers [3].) Basically, the segments differ ultrastructurally in membrane morphology and the content of rough and smooth ER. The axon hillock may contain fragments of Nissl substance, including abundant ribosomes, which diminish as the hillock continues into the initial segment. Here, the various axoplasmic components begin to align longitudinally. A few ribosomes and smooth ER still persist, and some axoaxonic synapses occur. More interesting, however, is the axolemma of the initial segment, the region for the generation of the action potential, which is underlaid by a dense granular layer similar to that seen at the nodes of Ranvier. Also present in this region are neurotubules, neurofilaments, and mitochondria. The arrangement of the neurotubules in the initial segment, unlike their scattered pattern in the distal axon, is in fascicles; they are interconnected by side-arms [3,8]. Beyond the initial segment, the axon maintains a relatively uniform morphology. It contains the axolemma (without any structural modification, except at nodes and the termination, where submembranous densities are seen); microtubules, sometimes cross-linked; neurofilaments, connected by side-arms; mitochondria; and tubulovesicular profiles, probably derived from smooth ER. Myelinated axons show granular densifications beneath and axolemma at the nodes of Ranvier [9], and synaptic complexes may also occur in the same regions. In myelinated fibers, there is a concentration of sodium channels at the nodal axon, a feature underlying the rapid (saltatory) conduction of such fibers [10] (see Chaps. 4 and 9). The terminal portion of the axon arborizes and enlarges at its synaptic regions, where it might contain synaptic vesicles beneath the specialized presynaptic junction.

The Dendrite

The afferent components of neurons, dendrites are frequently arranged around the neuronal soma in stellate fashion. In some neurons, they may arise from a single trunk from which they branch into a dendritic tree. Unlike axons, they generally lack neurofilaments, although they may contain fragments of Nissl substance; however, large branches of dendrites in close proximity to neurons may contain small bundles of neurofilaments. Some difficulty may be encountered in distinguishing small unmyelinated axons, terminal segments of axons, and small dendrites. In the absence of synaptic data, they can often be assessed by the content of neurofilaments. The synaptic regions of dendrites occur either along the main stems (Fig. 8) or at small protuberances known as dendritic spines or thorns. Axon terminals abut these structures.

The Synapse

Axons and dendrites emerging from different neurons intercommunicate by means of specialized junctional complexes known as synapses. This was first proposed by Sherrington in 1897, who also proposed the term synapse. The existence of synapses was immediately demonstrable by EM and can be rec-

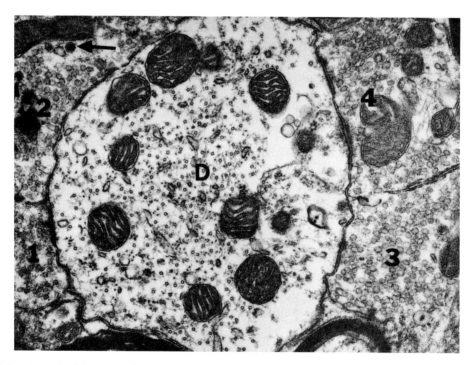

FIG. 8. A dendrite (D) emerging from a motor neuron in the anterior horn of a rat spinal cord is contacted by four axonal terminals. Terminal 1 contains clear spherical synaptic vesicles; terminals 2 and 3 contain both clear spherical and dense-core vesicles *(arrows)*; and terminal 4 contains many clear flattened (inhibitory) synaptic vesicles. Note also the synaptic thickenings and, within the dendrite, the mitochondria, neurofilaments, and neurotubules. ×33,000.

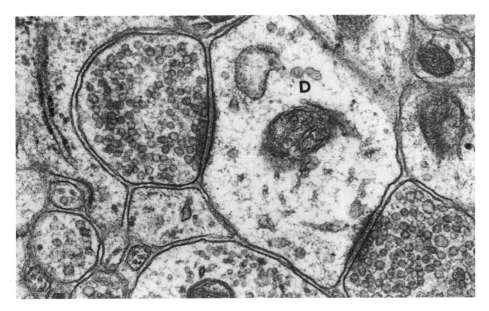

FIG. 9.   A dendrite (D) is flanked by two axon terminals packed with clear spherical synaptic vesicles. Details of the synaptic region are clearly shown. ×75,000.

ognized today in a dynamic fashion by Nomarski and confocal optics by light microscopy and by scanning EM. With the development of neurochemical approaches to neurobiology (see Chap. 9), an understanding of synaptic form and function becomes of fundamental importance. As was noted in the first ultrastructural study on synapses (Palade and Palay in 1954, quoted in Mugnaini and Walberg [4]), synapses display interface specialization and are frequently polarized or asymmetrical. The asymmetry is due to the unequal distribution of electron-dense (osmiophilic) material, or thickening, applied to the apposing membranes of the junctional complex and the heavier accumulation of organelles within the presynaptic (usually axonal) component. The closely applied membranes constituting the synaptic site are overlaid on the presynaptic and post-synaptic aspects by an osmiophilic material similar to that seen in desmosomes (see section on ependymal cells, below) and are separated by a gap (cleft) of between 15 and 20 nm. The presynaptic component usually contains a collection of clear, 40 to 50-nm

synaptic vesicles and several small mitochondria approximately 0.2 to 0.5 μm in diameter (Figs. 8–10). Occasionally 24-nm microtubules, coated vesicles, and cisternae of smooth ER are not uncommon in this region. On the postsynaptic side is a density referred to as the subsynaptic web, but apart from an infrequent, closely applied packet of smooth ER (subsurface cisterna) belonging to the hypolemmal system, there are no aggregations of organelles in the dendrite.

At the neuromuscular junction, the morphological organization is somewhat different. Here the axon terminal is greatly enlarged and it is ensheathed by Schwann cells; the postsynaptic (sarcolemmal) membrane displays less density and is extensively infolded.

Before elaborating further on synaptic diversity, it might be helpful to outline briefly other ways in which synapses have been classified in the past. Using the light microscope, Ramón y Cajal [11] was able to identify 11 distinct groups of synapses. Today, most neuroanatomists apply a more fundamental classification schema to syn-

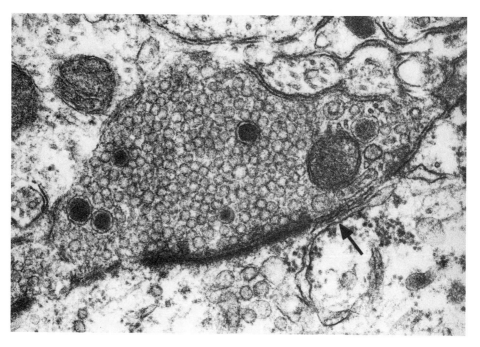

FIG. 10. An axonal terminal at the surface of a neuron from the dorsal horn of a rabbit spinal cord contains both dense-core and clear spherical synaptic vesicles lying above the membrane thickenings. A subsurface cisterna *(arrow)* is also seen. ×68,000.

apses, depending on the profiles between which the synapse is formed (i.e., axodendritic, axosomatic, axoaxonic, dendrodendritic, somatosomatic, and somatodendritic). Unfortunately, such a list totally disregards the type of transmission (chemical or electrical) and, in the case of chemical synapses, the neurotransmitter involved.

In terms of physiologic typing, three groups of synapses are recognized: excitatory, inhibitory, and modulatory. Some neuroanatomical studies [11] on excitatory and inhibitory synapses have claimed that excitatory synapses possess spherical synaptic vesicles, whereas inhibitory synapses contain a predominance of flattened vesicles (Fig. 8). Other studies (e.g., Gray [12]) have correlated this synaptic vesicular diversity with physiologic data. In his study on cerebellum. Gray showed that neurons, with a known predominance of excitatory input on dendrites and an inhibitory input on the cell body, possessed two corresponding types of synapses;

however, although this interpretation fits well in some loci of the CNS, it does not hold true for all regions. Furthermore, some workers feel that the differences between flat and spherical vesicles may reflect an artifact of aldehyde fixation or a difference in physiologic state at the time of sampling. In the light of these criticisms, it is clear that further confirmation as to the correlation between flattened vesicles and inhibitory synapses is required.

Another criterion for the classification of synapses by EM was introduced in 1959 by Gray [12]. Briefly, certain synapses in the cerebral cortex can be grouped into two types, depending on the length of the contact area between synaptic membranes and the amount of postsynaptic thickening. Relationships have been found between type 1—the membranes of which are closely apposed for long distances and have a large amount of associated postsynaptic thickening—and excitatory axodendritic synapses.

Type 2 synapses, conversely, are mainly axosomatic, show less close apposition and thickening at the junction, and are believed to be inhibitory. This broad grouping has been confirmed in the cerebral cortex by a number of workers, but it does not hold true for all regions of the CNS.

Most of the data from studies on synapse *in situ* or on synaptosomes (see Part II) have been on cholinergic transmission. Our understanding of the vast family of chemical synapses belonging to the autonomic nervous system that utilize biogenic amines (Chap. 12) as neurotransmitter substances is still in its infancy. Morphologically, catecholaminergic synapses are similar but possess, in addition to clear vesicles, slightly larger dense-core or granular vesicles of variable dimension (Figs. 8 and 10). These vesicles were first identified as synaptic vesicles by Grillo and Palay (see Bloom [13]), who segregated classes of granular vesicles based on vesicle and core size, but no relationship was made between granular vesicles and transmitter substances. About the same time, EM autoradiographic techniques were being employed and, using tritiated norepinephrine, Wolfe and co-workers [14] labeled granular vesicles within axonal terminals. Since this work, other labeling techniques for aminergic synapses have been developed. Several of the methods and requirements for detecting such transmitters have been reviewed by Bloom [13]. Catecholaminergic vesicles are generally classified on a size basis, and not all have dense cores. Another, still unclassified, category of synapses may be the so-called silent synapses observed in CNS tissue both *in vitro* and *in vivo*. These synapses are morphologically identical to functional synapses but are physiologically dormant.

Finally, with regard to synaptic type, there is the well-characterized electrical synapse [15], where current can pass from cell to cell across regions of membrane apposition that essentially lack the associated collections of organelles present at the chemical synapse. In the electrical synapse (Fig. 11),

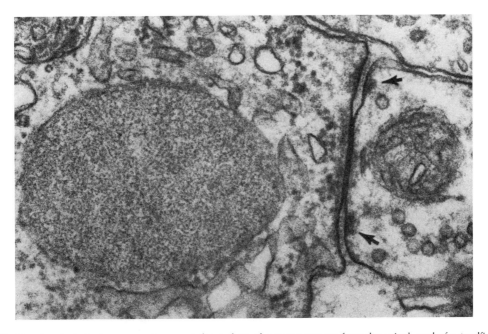

FIG. 11. An electrotonic synapse is seen at the surface of a motor neuron from the spinal cord of a toadfish. Between the neuronal soma *(left)* and the axonal termination *(right)*, a gap junction flanked by desmosomes *(arrows)* is visible. (Photography courtesy of Drs. G. D. Pappas and J. S. Keeter.) ×80,000.

the unit membranes are closely apposed, and, indeed, the outer leaflets sometimes fuse to form a pentalaminar structure; however, in most places, a gap of approximately 20 nm exists, producing a so-called gap junction. Not infrequently, such gap junctions are separated by desmosome-like regions [3]. Sometimes, electrical synapses exist at terminals that also display typical chemical synapses; in such cases, the structure is referred to as a mixed synapse. The comparative morphology of electrical and chemical synapses has been reviewed by Pappas and Waxman [15].

Molecular markers of neurons

The characterization of the vast array of neuron-specific cytoskeletal elements like intermediate filaments, microtubules and their associated proteins [16,17], and the neurotransmitters and their receptors [18] have led to the development of correspondingly large numbers of molecular and immunologic probes which are now routinely applied in neuroanatomical analyses. While the neuron is normally an immunologically-inert cell type, incapable of participating in T cell interactions via the expression of major histocompatibility complex (MHC) antigens or the production of soluble mediators (cytokines), its possessing unique proteins (some of which are antigenic) normally sequestered by the blood-brain barrier (BBB) from the circulating immune system, theoretically renders it vulnerable to immune-mediated damage should the BBB be breached. However, despite the multitude of conditions in which BBB leakage occurs, with the exception of a few types of neuronal degeneration associated with certain paraneoplastic and carcinomatous conditions and of nerve terminal destruction due to antibodies against neuronal receptors (the acetylcholine receptor in myasthenia gravis), neuronal damage due to specific immune-mediated mechanisms is an infrequent phenomenon.

CHARACTERISTICS OF NEUROGLIA

In 1846, Virchow first recognized the existence in the CNS of a fragile, nonnervous, interstitial component made up of stellate or spindle-shaped cells, morphologically distinct from neurons, which he named neuroglia ("nerve glue"). It was not until the early part of the twentieth century that this interstitial element was classified as distinct cell types [3,4]. Today, we recognize three broad groups of glial cells: (1) true glial cells (macroglia), such as astrocytes and oligodendrocytes, of ectodermal origin; (2) microglia, of mesodermal origin; and (3) ependymal cells, also of ectodermal origin and sharing the same stem cell as true glia (i.e., the spongioblast). Microglia invade the CNS at the time of vascularization via the pia mater, the walls of blood vessels, and the tela choroidea.

Glial cells differ from neurons in that they possess no synaptic contacts and retain the ability to divide throughout life, particularly in response to injury. The rough schema represented by Fig. 3 demonstrates the interrelationships between the macroglia and other CNS components.

Virtually nothing can enter or leave the CNS parenchyma without passing through an astrocytic interphase

The complex packing achieved by the processes and cell bodies of astrocytes underscores their involvement in brain metabolism. Although astrocytes have traditionally been subdivided into protoplasmic and fibrous astrocytes [4], these two forms probably represent the opposite ends of a spectrum of the same cell type. However, Raff et al. [19] have suggested that the two groups of astrocytes might derive from different progenitors and that the progenitor of the fibrous astrocyte is the same as that of the oligodendrocyte. The structural components of fibrous and protoplasmic astrocytes are identical; the differences are quantitative. In the early days of EM, differences between the two variants were more apparent owing to impre-

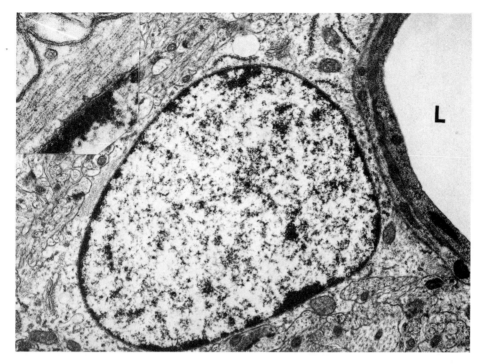

FIG. 12.   A protoplasmic astrocyte abuts a blood vessel (lumen at L) in rat cerebral cortex. The nucleus shows a rim of denser chromatin, and the cytoplasm contains many organelles, including Golgi and rough ER. ×10,000. **Inset:** Detail of perinuclear cytoplasm showing filaments. ×44,000.

cise techniques but with the development of better procedures, the differences became less apparent.

Protoplasmic astrocytes range in size from 10 to 40 μm, are frequently located in gray matter in relation to capillaries, and have a clearer cytoplasm than do fibrous astrocytes (Fig. 12). Within the perikaryon of both types of astrocytes are scattered 9-nm filaments and 24-nm microtubules (Fig. 13); glycogen granules; lysosomes and lipofuscin-like bodies; isolated cisternae of rough ER; a small Golgi apparatus opposite one pole of the nucleus; and small, elongated mitochondria, often extending together with loose bundles of filaments along cell processes. A centriole is not uncommon. Characteristically, the nucleus is ovoid and the nucleochromatin homogeneous, except for a narrow continuous rim of dense chromatin and one or two poorly defined nucleoli. The fibrous astrocyte occurs in white matter (Fig. 13). Its processes are twig-like, being composed of large numbers of 9-nm glial filaments arranged in tight bundles. The filaments within these cell processes can be distinguished from neurofilaments by their close packing and the absence of side-arms (Figs. 13 and 14). Desmosomes and gap junctions occur between adjacent astrocytic processes.

In addition to protoplasmic and fibrous forms, regional specialization occurs among astrocytes. The outer membranes of astrocytes located in subpial zones and adjacent to blood vessels possess a specialized thickening. Desmosomes and gap junctions are very common in these regions between astrocytic processes. In the cerebellar cortex, protoplasmic astrocytes can be segregated into three classes—the Golgi epithelial cell, the lamellar or velate astrocyte, and the smooth astrocyte [1]—each ultrastructurally distinct.

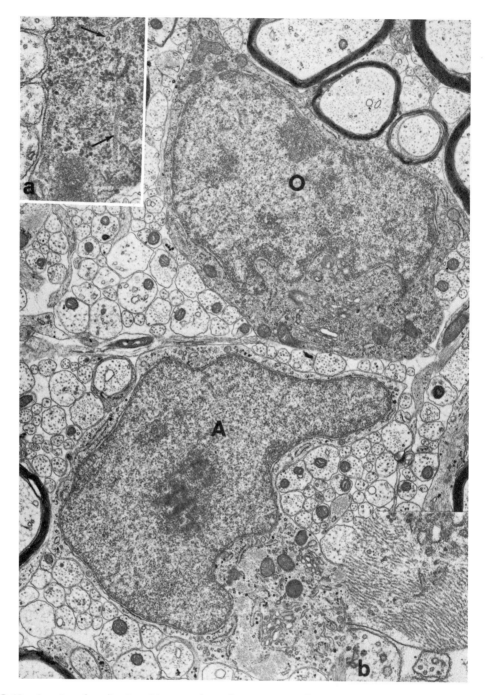

FIG. 13.   A section of myelinating white matter from a kitten contains a fibrous astrocyte (A) and an oligodendrocyte (O). The nucleus of the astrocyte (A) has homogeneous chromatin with a denser rim and a central nucleolus. That of the oligodendrocyte (O) is denser and more heterogeneous. Note the denser oligodendrocytic cytoplasm and the prominent filaments within the astrocyte. ×15,000. **Inset a:** Detail of the oligodendrocyte, showing microtubules *(arrows)* and absence of filaments. ×45,000. **Inset b:** Detail of astrocytic cytoplasm showing filaments, glycogen, rough ER, and Golgi apparatus. ×45,000.

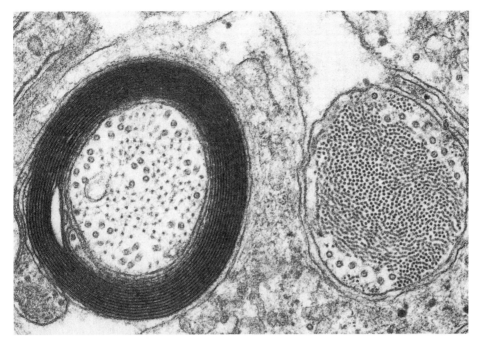

FIG. 14.   Transverse sections are shown of a myelinated axon *(left)* and the process of a fibrous astrocyte *(right)* in dog spinal cord. The axon contains scattered neurotubules and loosely-packed neurofilaments interconnected by side-arm material. The astrocytic process contains a bundle of closely-packed filaments with no cross-bridges, flanked by several microtubules. Sometimes, a lumen can be seen within a filament. ×60,000.

Astrocyte Function

The functions of astrocytes have long been debated. Their major role is related to a connective tissue or skeletal function, since they invest, possibly sustain, and provide a packing for other CNS components. In the case of astrocytic ensheathment around synaptic complexes and the bodies of some neurons (e.g., Purkinje cells), it may be speculated that the astrocyte serves to isolate these structures.

One well-known function of the astrocyte is concerned with repair. Subsequent to trauma, astrocytes invariably proliferate, swell, accumulate glycogen, and undergo fibrosis by the accumulation of filaments, expressed neurochemically as an increase in glial fibrillary acidic protein (GFAP). This state of gliosis may be total, in which case all other elements are lost, leaving a glial scar, or it may be a generalized response occur-ring against a background of regenerated or normal CNS parenchyma. Fibrous astrocytosis can occur in both the gray and white matter, thereby indicating common links between protoplasmic and fibrous astrocytes. With age, both fibrous and protoplasmic astrocytes accumulate filaments. In some diseases, astrocytes have been shown to become macrophages. It is interesting to note that the astrocyte is probably the most disease-resistant component in the CNS because very few diseases (one of them, alcoholism) cause depletion of astrocytes.

Another putative role of the astrocyte is its involvement in transport mechanisms and in the BBB system. It was believed for some time that transport of water and electrolytes was effected by the astrocyte, a fact never definitively demonstrated and largely inferred from pathological or experimental evidence. It is known, for example, that damage to the brain vasculature, local injury due to heat or cold, and inflammatory changes produce focal swelling of astrocytes, presumably owing to disturbances in fluid transport. The astrocytic investment of blood vessels might suggest a role in the BBB system, but the studies of Reese and Karnovsky [20] and Brightman [21] indicate that the astrocytic end-feet provide little resistance to the movement of molecules and that blockage of the passage of material into the brain occurs at the endothelial cell-lining blood vessels (see Chap. 30). Finally, it is believed that astrocytes are responsible for the regulation of local pH levels and local ionic balances.

Molecular markers

Although antigenically distinct from other cell types by virtue of its expressing GFAP [17], there is no documented evidence of astrocytic disease related to an immunologic response to GFAP on any other astroglial molecule. GFAP remains the singularly most used cytoplasmic marker of astrocytes. A reliable marker for astrocytic membranes remains to be described. Interestingly, there is increasing evidence demonstrating the ability of astrocytes to serve as accessory cells of the immune system in a number of immune-mediated conditions (e.g. [22,23]). In this regard, astrocytes are well known for their ability to express class II MHC antigens (molecules essential for the presentation of antigen to helper/inducer CD4+ T cells) as well as their ability to synthesize a number of cytokines (e.g., interleukin-1, tumor necrosis factor, and interferon γ). It appears therefore that in circumstances in which the BBB is interrupted, the astrocyte is a facultative phagocyte with the potential to interact with lymphocytes.

Oligodendrocytes are myelin-producing cells in the CNS

The ultrastructural studies of Schultz and co-workers (1957) and Farquhar and Hartman in 1957 (discussed in Mugnaini and Walberg [4]) were among the first to contrast the EM features of oligodendrocytes with astrocytes (Fig. 12). The study of Mugnaini and Walberg [4] more explicitly laid down the morphological criteria for identifying these cells and, apart from subsequent technical improvements, our EM understanding of these cells has changed little since that time [5,24].

As with the astrocytes, oligodendrocytes are highly variable, differing in location, morphology, and function, but definable by some morphological criteria. The cell soma ranges from 10 to 20 μm and is roughly globular and more dense than that of an astrocyte. The margin of the cell is irregular and compressed against the adjacent neuropil. Few cell processes are seen, in contrast to the astrocyte. Within the cytoplasm, many organelles are found. Parallel cisterns of rough ER and a widely dispersed Golgi apparatus are common. Free ribosomes occur, scattered amid occasional multivesicular bodies, mitochondria, and coated vesicles. Serving to distinguish the oligodendrocyte from the astrocyte is the apparent absence of glial filaments and the constant presence of 24-nm microtubules (Fig. 13), most common at the margins of the cell, in the occasional cell process, and in the cytoplasmic loops around myelin sheaths. Lamellar dense bodies typical of oligodendrocytes are also present [5]. The nucleus is usually ovoid, but slight lobation is not uncommon. The nucleochromatin stains heavily and contains clumps of denser heterochromatin; the whole structure is sometimes difficult to discern from the background cytoplasm. Desmosomes and gap junctions occur between interfascicular oligodendrocytes [5].

Ultrastructural studies on the developing nervous system and labeling studies have demonstrated variability in oligodendrocyte morphology and activity. Mori and Leblond (see Raine [5]) separated oligodendrocytes into three groups based on location, stainability, and DNA turnover. Their three classes correspond to satellite, intermediate, and interfascicular (myelinating) oligodendrocytes. Satellite oligodendrocytes are small

(~10 μm), restricted to gray matter, and closely applied to the surface of neurons. They are assumed to play a role in the maintenance of the neuron and are also known to be potential myelinating cells. Interfascicular oligodendrocytes are large (~20 μm) during myelination but, in the adult, range from 10 to 15 μm, with the nucleus occupying a large percentage of the cell volume. Intermediate oligodendrocytes are regarded as satellite or potential myelinating forms. The nucleus of these cells is small, the cytoplasm occupying the greater area of the soma.

Oligodendrocytes and Myelin

Myelinating oligodendrocytes have been studied extensively [5,25]. Examination of the CNS during myelinogenesis (Fig. 15) reveals connections between the cell body and the myelin sheath [26]; however, connections between these elements have never been demonstrated in a normal adult animal, unlike the PNS counterpart, the Schwann cell. In contrast to the Schwann cell (see below), the oligodendrocyte is capable of producing many internodes of myelin simultaneously. It is estimated that oligodendrocytes in the optic nerve might produce between 30 and 50 internodes of myelin [5]. In addition to this heavy structural commitment, the oligodendrocyte is known to possess a slow mitotic rate and a poor regenerative capacity. Damage to only a few oligodendrocytes can therefore be expected to produce an appreciable area of primary demyelination. In most CNS diseases in which myelin is a target, oligodendrocytes are known to be among the most vulnerable elements and the first to degenerate.

Somewhat analogous to the neuron, the relatively small oligodendrocyte soma produces and supports many more times it own volume of membrane and cytoplasm. For example, consider an average 12-μm oligodendrocyte producing 20 internodes of myelin (the lowest number quoted by Peters and Proskauer; see Raine [5]). Each axon has a diameter of 3 μm (small for CNS fibers) and is covered by six lamellae of myelin (a conservative estimate), each lamella representing two fused layers of unit membrane. By statistical analysis, taking into account the length of myelin internode (possibly 500 μm) and the length of the membranes of the cell processes connecting the sheaths to the cell body (~12 μm), the ratio between the surface area of the cell soma and the myelin it sustains is approximately 1:620. In most cases, however, this ratio is probably in the region of 1:3,000. In rare instances, oligodendrocytes have been shown to elaborate myelin around structures other than axons in that myelin has been documented around neuronal somata and nonaxonal profiles. (Myelin formation is discussed in Chap. 6.)

Molecular markers of oligodendrocytes

The oligodendrocyte is potentially highly vulnerable to immune-mediated damage since it shares with the myelin sheath many molecules with known affinities to elicit specific T and B cell responses which lead to its destruction. Many of these molecules (e.g., myelin basic protein, proteolipid protein, myelin-associated glycoprotein, galactocerebroside, etc.) have been used to generate specific antibodies which are routinely applied to anatomical analyses of oligodendrocytes *in vivo* and *in vitro*. However, unlike the astrocyte, the oligodendrocyte appears to be immunologically inert, expressing no molecules (e.g., class I or II MHC) suggestive of interactions with the immune system [27].

The microglial cell plays a role in phagocytosis and inflammatory responses

Of the few remaining types of CNS cells, the most interesting, and probably the most enigmatic, is the microglial cell, a cell of mesodermal origin, located in the normal brain in a resting state and purported to become a very mobile, active macrophage during disease. Microglia can be selectively stained and

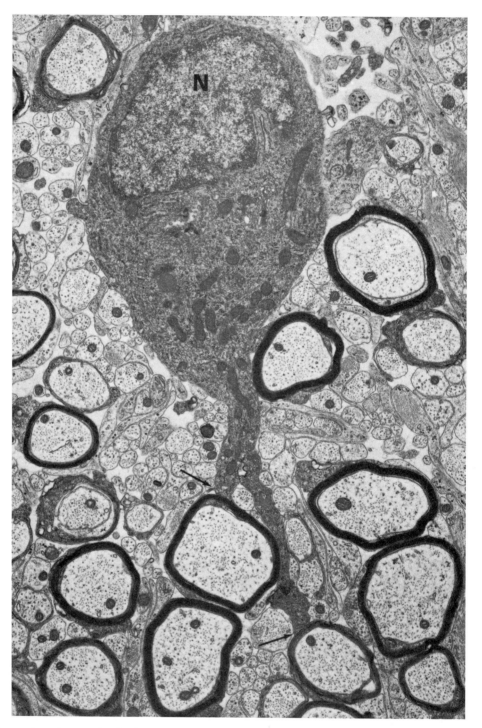

FIG. 15. A myelinating oligodendrocyte, nucleus (N), from the spinal cord of a 2-day-old kitten extends cytoplasmic connections to at least two myelin sheaths *(arrows)*. Other myelinated and unmyelinated fibers at various stages of development, as well as glial processes, are seen in the surrounding neuropil. ×12,750.

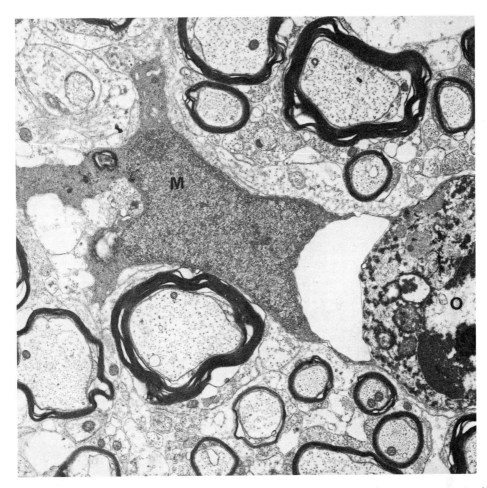

FIG. 16. A microglial cell (M) has elaborated two cytoplasmic arms to encompass a degenerating apoptotic oligodendrocyte (O) in the spinal cord of a 3-day-old kitten. The microglial cell nucleus is difficult to distinguish from the narrow rim of densely staining cytoplasm, which also contains some membranous debris. ×10,000.

demonstrated by light microscopy using Hortega's silver carbonate method, but no comparable technique exists for their ultrastructural demonstration. The cells have spindle-shaped bodies and a thin rim of densely staining cytoplasm difficult to distinguish from the nucleus. The nucleochromatin is homogeneously dense, and the cytoplasm does not contain an abundance of organelles, although representatives of the usual components can be found. During normal wear and tear, some CNS elements degenerate, and microglia phagocytose the debris (Fig. 16). Their identification and numbers (as determined by light micros-

copy) differ from species to species. The rabbit CNS is known to be richly endowed. In a number of disease instances (e.g., trauma), microglia are known to be stimulated and to migrate to the area of injury, where they phagocytose debris. The relatively brief mention of this cell type in the major EM textbooks [3] and the conflicting EM descriptions [27] are indicative of the uncertainty attached to their identification. Pericytes are believed by some to be a resting form of microglial cell. Perivascular macrophages have also been described which are of bone marrow origin and which are distinct from parenchymal microglia.

Molecular markers of microglial cells

In recent years, there has been a veritable explosion of activity in the field of microglial cell biology with the realization that this cell type is capable of functioning as a highly efficient accessory cell of the immune system. While no particularly microglial-specific molecule has been identified, a number of antibodies raised against monocytic markers and complement receptor molecules have proven to stain microglial cells *in situ* and *in vitro*. There is strong evidence that microglia express class II MHC upon activation [29–31] frequently in the absence of a T cell response. This suggests that class II MHC expression may represent a marker of activation or in some way elevate the cells to a state of immunologic awareness. Microglia are also well known producers of a number of cytokines with known effects upon T cells. Taken in concert, the increasing evidence of an immunologic role for microglia in a wide spectrum of conditions probably supports the putative monocytic origin of this cell type.

Ependymal cells line the ventricles and the central canal of the spinal cord

Ependymal cells are arranged in single-palisade arrays and line the ventricles of the brain and central canal of the spinal cord. They are usually ciliated, their cilia extending into the ventricular cavity. Their fine structure has been elucidated by Brightman and Palay [32]. They possess several features that clearly differentiate them from any other CNS cell. The cilia emerge from the apical pole of the cell, where they are attached to a blepharoplast, the basal body (Fig. 17), which is anchored in the cytoplasm by means of ciliary rootlets and a basal foot.

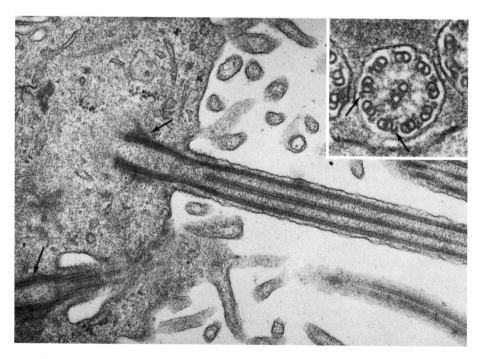

FIG. 17.   The surface of an ependymal cell contains basal bodies *(arrows)* connected to the microtubules of cilia, seen here in longitudinal section. Several microvilli are also present. ×37,000. **Inset:** Ependymal cilia in transverse section possess a central doublet of microtubules surrounded by nine pairs, one of each pair having a characteristic hook-like appendage *(arrows).* ×100,000.

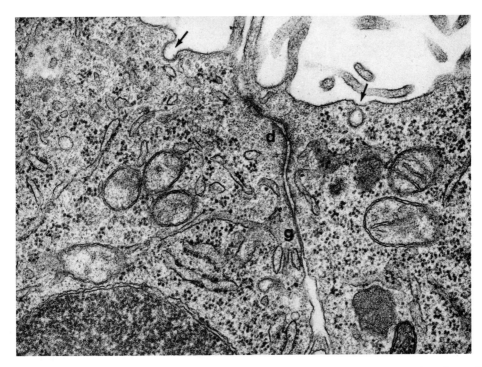

FIG. 18.   A typical desmosome (d) and gap junction (g) between two ependymal cells. Microvilli and coated pits *(arrows)* are seen along the cell surface. ×35,000.

The basal foot is the contractile component that determines the direction of the ciliary beat. Like all flagellar structures, the cilium contains the common microtubule arrangement of nine peripheral pairs around a central doublet (Fig. 17). In the vicinity of the basal body, the arrangement is one of nine triplets; at the tip of each cilium the pattern is one of haphazardly organized single tubules. Also extending from the free surface of the cell are numerous microvilli containing actin microfilaments (Fig. 17). The cytoplasm stains intensely, having an electron density about equal to that of the oligodendrocyte, whereas the nucleus is similar to that of the astrocyte. Microtubules, large whorls of filaments, coated vesicles, rough ER; Golgi apparatus; lysosomes, and abundant small, dense mitochondria are also present. The base of the cell is composed of involuted processes that interdigitate with the underlying neuropil. The lateral margins of each cell characteristically display long, compound, junctional complexes (Fig. 18) made up of desmosomes (zonula adherentes) and tight junctions (zonula occludentes).

The biochemical properties of these structures are well known. Desmosomes display protease sensitivity, divalent cation dependency, and osmotic insensitivity, whereas the membranes are mainly of the smooth type. In direct contrast to desmosomes, the tight junction (and also gap junctions and synapses) displays no protease sensitivity, divalent cation dependency, nor osmotic sensitivity, whereas the membranes are complex. These facts have been used in the development of techniques to isolate purified preparations of junctional complexes.

The Schwann cell is the myelin-producing cell of the PNS

When axons leave the CNS, they lose their neuroglial interrelationships and traverse a short transitional zone, where they are in-

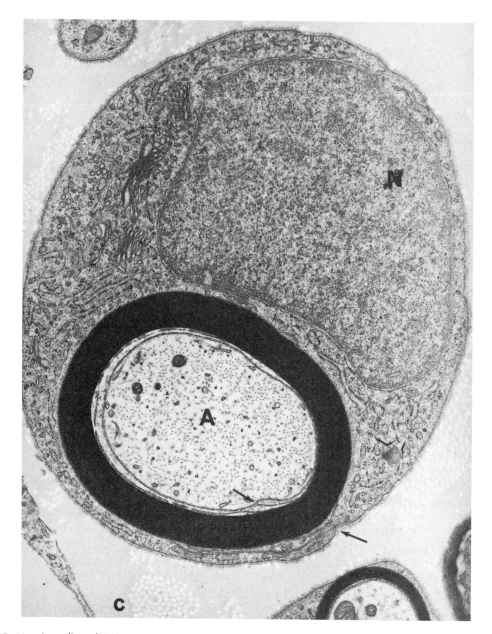

FIG. 19. A myelinated PNS axon (A) is surrounded by a Schwann cell, nucleus (N). Note the fuzzy basal lamina around the cell, the rich cytoplasm, the inner and outer mesaxons *(arrows)*, the close proximity of the cell to its myelin sheath, and the 1:1 (cell: myelin internode) relationship. A process of an endoneurial cell is seen *(lower left)*, and unstained collagen (c) lies in the endoneurial space *(white dots)*. ×20,000.

vested by an astroglial sheath enclosed in the basal lamina of the glia limitans. The basal lamina then becomes continuous with that of axon-investing Schwann cells, at which point the astroglial covering terminates. Schwann cells, therefore, are the axon-en-

sheathing cells of the PNS, equivalent functionally to the oligodendrocyte of the CNS. Along the myelinated fibers of the PNS, each internode of myelin is elaborated by one Schwann cell and each Schwann cell elaborates one internode. This ratio of one internode of myelin to one Schwann cell is a fundamental distinction between this cell type and its CNS analog, the oligodendrocyte, which is able to proliferate internodes in the ratio of 1:30 or greater. Another distinction is that the Schwann cell body always remains in intimate contact with its myelin internode (Fig. 19), whereas the oligodendrocyte extends processes toward its internodes. Periodically, myelin lamellae open up into ridges of Schwann cell cytoplasm, producing bands of cytoplasm around the fiber, Schmidt-Lanterman incisures, reputed to be the stretch points along PNS fibers. These incisures are usually not present in the CNS. The PNS myelin period is 11.9 nm in preserved specimens (some 30 percent less than in the fresh state), in contrast to the 10.6 nm of central myelin. In addition to these structural differences, PNS myelin is known to differ biochemically and antigenically from that of the CNS (see Chaps. 6 and 37). Not all PNS fibers are myelinated, but in contrast to nonmyelinated fibers in the CNS, nonmyelineated fibers in the PNS are suspended in groups within Schwann cell cytoplasm, each axon connected to the extracellular space by a short channel, the mesaxon, formed by the invaginated Schwann cell plasmalemma.

Ultrastructurally, the Schwann cell is unique and distinct from the oligodendrocyte. Each Schwann cell is surrounded by a basal lamina made up of mucopolysaccharide approximately 20 to 30 nm thick that does not extend into the mesaxon (Fig. 19). The basal laminae of adjacent myelinating Schwann cells at the nodes of Ranvier are continuous, and Schwann cell processes ("fingers") interdigitate so that the PNS myelinated axon is never in direct contact with the extracelllar space. These nodal Schwann cell fingers display intimate relationships with the axolemma (Figs. 20 and 21), suggesting that the entire nodal complex might serve as an electrogenic pump for the recycling of ions [9]. A similar arrangement between the nodal axon and the fingers of astroglial cells is seen in the CNS. The Schwann cells of nonmyelinated PNS fibers overlap, and there are no nodes of Ranvier.

The cytoplasm of the Schwann cell is

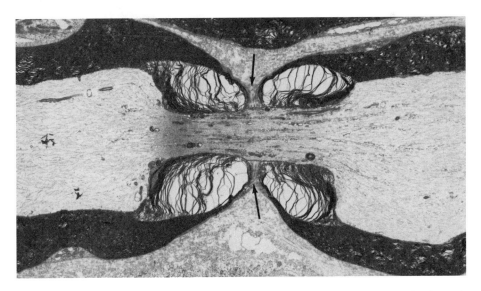

FIG. 20. Low-power electron micrograph of a node of Ranvier in longitudinal section. Note the abrupt decrease in internodal axon diameter where it becomes paranodal and the attendant condensation of axoplasmic constituents. Paranodal myelin is artifactually distorted, a common phenomenon in large-diameter fibers. The nodal gap substance (arrows) contains Schwann cell fingers; the nodal axon is bulbous; and lysosomes lie beneath the axolemma within the bulge. Beaded smooth ER sacs are also seen. ×5,000.

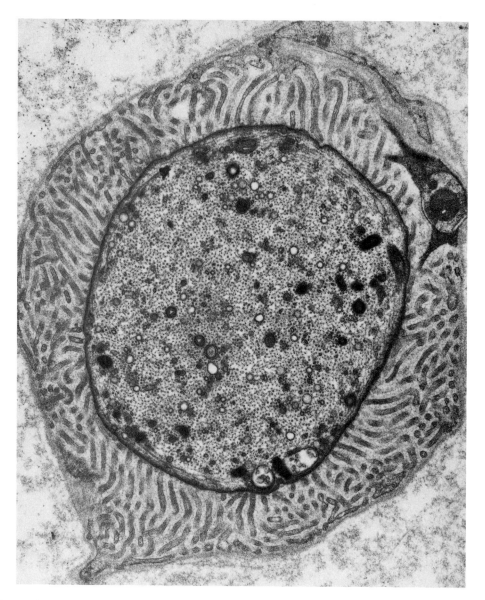

FIG. 21. A transverse section of the node of Ranvier (7–8 μm across) of a large fiber shows a prominent complex of Schwann cell fingers around an axon highlighted by its subaxolemmal densification and closely packed organelles. The Schwann cell fingers arise from an outer collar of flattened cytoplasm and abut the axon at regular intervals of approximately 80 nm. The basal lamina of the nerve fiber encircles the entire complex. The nodal gap substance is granular and sometimes linear. Within the axoplasm, note the transversely sectioned sacs of beaded smooth ER, mitochondria, dense lamellar bodies (which appear to maintain a peripheral location), flattened smooth ER sacs, dense-core vesicles, cross-bridged neurofilaments, and microtubules, which in places run parallel to the circumference of the axon *(above left* and *lower right),* perhaps in a spiral fashion. ×16,000.

rich in organelles. A Golgi apparatus is located near the nucleus, and cisternae of rough ER occur throughout the cell. Lysosomes, multivesicular bodies, glycogen granules, and lipid granules (*pi* granules) can also be seen. The cell is rich in filaments (in contrast to the oligodendrocyte) and microtubules. The plasmalemma frequently shows pinocytic vesicles. Small, round mitochondria are scattered throughout the soma. The nucleus, which stains intensely, is flattened, and oriented longitudinally along the nerve fiber. Aggregates of dense heterochromatin are arranged peripherally. (Additional details concerning the Schwann cells are outlined by Peters et al. [3].)

Schwann Cells During Disease

In sharp contrast to the oligodendrocyte, the Schwann cell responds vigorously to most forms of injury (see Chap. 37). An active phase of mitosis occurs following traumatic insult, and the cells are capable of local migration. Studies on their behavior after primary demyelination have shown that they are able to phagocytose damaged myelin. They possess remarkable reparatory properties and begin to lay down new myelin approximately 1 week after a fiber loses its myelin sheath. Studies on PNS and CNS remyelination [33] have shown that by 3 months after primary demyelination, PNS fibers are well remyelinated, whereas similarly affected areas in the CNS show relatively little proliferation of new myelin. Under circumstances of severe injury (e.g., transection), axons degenerate, and the Schwann cells form tubes (Büngner bands) containing cell bodies and processes surrounded by a single basal lamina. These structures provide channels along which regenerating axons might later grow. The presence and integrity of the Schwann cell basal lamina is essential for reinnervation.

Other PNS Elements

The extracellular space between PNS nerve fibers is occupied by bundles of collagen fibrils, blood vessels, and endoneurial cells [34]. Endoneurial cells are elongated spindle-shaped cells with tenuous processes relatively poor in organelles except for large cisternae of rough ER. There is some evidence that these cells proliferate collagen fibrils. Sometimes mast cells, the histamine producers of connective tissue, can be seen. Bundles of nerve fibers are arranged in fascicles emarginated by flattened connective tissue cells forming the perineurium, an essential component in the blood-nerve barrier system. Fascicles of nerve fibers are aggregated into nerves and invested by a tough elastic sheath of cells known as the epineurium.

ACKNOWLEDGMENTS

The excellent technical assistance of Everett Swanson, Howard Finch, and Miriam Pakingan is appreciated. I thank Michele Briggs for her secretarial assistance.

The work represented by this chapter was supported in part by USPHS Grants NS 08952 and NS 11920; and NMSS RG 1001-H-8 from the National Multiple Sclerosis Society.

REFERENCES

1. Palay, S. L., and Chan-Palay, V. *Cerebellar Cortex: Cytology and Organization*. New York: Springer, 1974.
2. Hyden, H. The neuron. In J. Brachet and A. E. Mirsky (eds.), *The Cell*. New York: Academic, 1960, Vol. 5, pp. 215–323.
3. Peters, A., Palay, S. L., and Webster, H. de F. *The Fine Structure of the Nervous System: The Cells and Their Processes*. New York: Oxford University Press, 1991.
4. Mugnaini, E., and Walberg, F. Ultrastructure of neuroglia. *Ergeb. Anat. Entwicklungsgesch.* 37:194–236, 1964.
5. Raine, S. C. Oligodendrocytes and central nervous system myelin. In R. L. Davis and D. M. Robertson (eds.), *Textbook of Neuropathology*, 2nd ed. Baltimore: Williams & Wilkins, 1990, pp. 115–140.
6. Novikoff, A. B., and Holtzman, E. *Cells and Organelles*. New York: Holt, Rinehart and Winston, 1976.
7. Soifer, D. (ed.), Dynamic Aspects of Microtubule Biology. *Ann. N. Y. Acad. Sci.* 466, 1986.

8. Wang, E., Fischman, B., Liem, R. L., and Sun, T.-T. (eds.), Intermediate Filaments. *Ann. N. Y. Acad. Sci.* 455, 1985.

9. Raine, C. S. Differences in the nodes of Ranvier of large and small diameter fibres in the PNS. *J. Neurocytol.* 11:935–947, 1982.

10. Ritchie, J. M. Physiological basis of conduction in myelinated nerve fibers. In P. Morell (ed.), *Myelin.* New York: Plenum, 1984, pp. 117–146.

11. Bodian, D. Synaptic diversity and characterization by electron microscopy. In G. D. Pappas and D. P. Purpura (eds.), *Structure and Function of Synapses.* New York: Raven, 1972, pp. 45–65.

12. Gray, E. G. Electron microscopy of excitatory and inhibitory synapses: A brief review. *Prog. Brain Res.* 31:141, 1969.

13. Bloom, F. E. Localization of neurotransmitters by electron microscopy. In *Neurotransmitters (Proc. ARNMD).* Baltimore: Williams & Wilkins, 1972, Vol. 50, pp. 25–57.

14. Wolfe, D. E., Potter, L. T., Richardson, K. C., and Axelrod, J. Localizing tritiated norepinephrine in sympathetic axons by electron microscopic autoradiography. *Science* 138: 440–442, 1962.

15. Pappas, G. D., and Waxman, S. Synaptic fine structure: Morphological correlates of chemical and electronic transmission. In G. D. Pappas and D. P. Purpura (eds.), *Structure and Function of Synapses.* New York: Raven, 1972, pp. 1–43.

16. Liem, R. K. H. Neuronal intermediate filaments. *Curr. Opin. Cell Biol.* 2:86–90, 1990.

17. Cleveland, D. W., and Hoffman, P. N. Neuronal and glial cytoskeletons. *Curr. Opin. Neurobiol.* 1:346–353, 1991.

18. McGeer, P. L., Eccles, J. C., and McGeer, E. G. (eds.), *Molecular Neurobiology of the Mammalian Brain.* New York: Plenum, 1987.

19. Raff, M. C., Miller, R. H., and Noble, M. A. Glial progenitor cell that develops in vitro into an astrocyte or an oligodendrocyte depending on culture medium. *Nature* 303: 390–396, 1983.

20. Reese, T. S., and Karnovsky, M. J. Fine structural localization of a blood-brain barrier to exogenous peroxidase. *J. Cell Biol.* 34: 207–217, 1967.

21. Brightman, M. The distribution within the brain of ferritin injected into cerebrospinal fluid compartments. II. Parenchymal distribution. *Am. J. Anat.* 117:193–220, 1965.

22. Yong, V. W., and Antel, J. P. Major histocompatibility complex molecules on glial cells. *Semin. Neurosci.* 4:231–240, 1992.

23. Benveniste, E. N. Cytokines: influence on glial cell gene expression and function. *Chem. Immunol.* 52:106–153, 1992.

24. Norton, W. T. (ed.), Oligodendroglia *(Advances in Neurochemistry, Vol 5).* New York: Plenum, 1984.

25. Raine, C. S. Morphology of myelin and myelination. In P. Morell (ed.), *Myelin,* 2nd ed. New York: Plenum, 1984, pp. 1–50.

26. Bunge, R. P. Glial cells and the central myelin sheath. *Physiol. Rev.* 48:197–248, 1968.

27. Fujita, S., and Kitamura, T. Origin of brain macrophages and the nature of the microglia. In Zimmerman, H. (ed.), *Progress in Neuropathology.* New York: Grune and Stratton, 1976, Vol. 2, pp. 1–50.

28. Lee, S. C., and Raine, C. S. Multiple sclerosis: oligodendrocytes in active lesions do not express class II MHC molecules. *J. Neuroimmunol.* 25:261–266, 1989.

29. Dickson, D. W., Mattiace, L. A., Kure, K., et al. Biology of disease. Microglia in human disease, with an emphasis on acquired immune deficiency syndrome. *Lab. Invest.* 64:135–156, 1991.

30. Matsumoto, Y., Ohmori, K., and Fujiwara, M. Microglial and astroglial reactions to inflammatory lesions of experimental autoimmune encephalomyelitis in the rat central nervous system. *J. Neuroimmunol.* 37:23–33, 1992.

31. Gehrmann, J., Gold, R., Linington, C., et al. Spinal cord microglia in experimental allergic neuritis. Evidence for fast and remote activation. *Lab. Invest.* 67:106–113, 1992.

32. Brightman, M., and Palay, S. L. The fine structure of ependyma in the brain of the rat. *J. Cell Biol.* 19:415–440, 1963.

33. Raine, C. S., Wisniewski, H., and Prineas, J. An ultrastructural study of experimental demyelination and remyelination. II. Chronic experimental allergic encephalomyelitis in the peripheral nervous system. *Lab Invest.* 21: 316–327, 1969.

34. Babel, J., Bischoff, A., and Spoendlin, H. Ultrastructure of the peripheral nervous system and sense organs. In *Atlas of Normal and Pathologic Anatomy.* St. Louis: Mosby, pp. 1–171, 1970.

CHAPTER 2

Cell Membrane Structure and Functions

R. WAYNE ALBERS

Basic Neurochemistry: Molecular, Cellular, and Medical Aspects, 5th Ed., edited by G. J. Siegel et al. Published by Raven Press, Ltd., New York, 1994. Correspondence to R. Wayne Albers; Laboratory of Neurochemistry; NINDS, LNC; National Institutes of Health; Bldg. 36; Rm. 4D-20; Bethesda, Maryland 20892.

PHOSPHOLIPID BILAYERS

Neurons are specialized to integrate environmental stimuli, both spatially and temporally. These processes generate signals that are rapidly transmitted along axonal plasma membranes to other cells. This chapter begins with a discussion of the physical chemistry underlying the structure of cell membranes. Subsequent sections describe the general organization of membranes and examples of different classes of membrane proteins (Fig. 1). Finally the biochemical processes that produce and maintain plasma membranes are summarized with attention to those that are important for neural functions.

Cells are separated from their environment by lipid bilayers

The fundamental importance of lipids in membrane structure was established early in this century by demonstrations that positive correlations exist between cell membrane permeabilities to small nonelectrolytes and the oil/water partition coefficients of these molecules. Contemporary measurements of the electrical impedance of cell suspensions suggested that cells are surrounded by a hydrocarbon barrier which was first estimated to be about 3.3 nm thick. It was originally thought that a membrane containing a lipid monolayer could account for these data. However a subsequent experiment compared the area of a monolayer formed from the total membrane lipids derived from erythrocytes with the surface area of these cells. A ratio of nearly 2 was found. These studies and other work on the physical chemistry of lipids fortified the concept of a continuous lipid bilayer in cell membranes. The reality of the bilayer structure as a principal and universal membrane component has received support from many other studies including the interpretation of X-ray diffraction data obtained from intact cell membranes.

Forces acting between lipids and also between lipids and proteins are primarily noncovalent: electrostatic, hydrogen bonding, and van der Waals interactions. Although these are all individually weak relative to covalent bonds, they sum to produce associations of considerable stability. Ionic and polar parts of molecules can interact with the dipoles of water to become hydrated. A substance is soluble if its molecules interact with water more strongly than with each other. Large molecules may have surface domains that differ in polarity. Their hydrophobic surfaces may aggregate forming *micelles,* which minimize the exposure of nonpolar domains to the aqueous phase. Molecules that have segregated polar and nonpolar surface domains are termed *amphipathic* and include most lipids and some proteins.

Amphipathic molecules that have comparable extents of polar and nonpolar surfaces tend to form bilayered lamellar structures [1]

Phospholipids, which are the major cell membrane lipids, have a polar head group

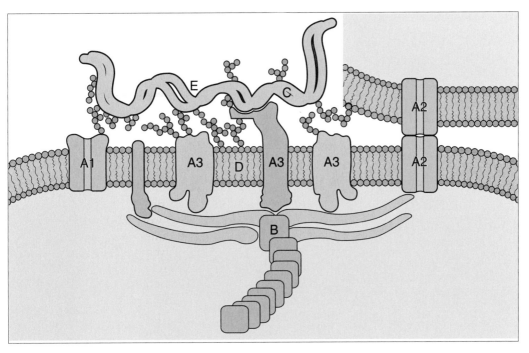

FIG. 1.   Overview of plasma membrane structure. Plasma membranes are distinguishable from other cellular membranes by the presence of both glycolipids and glycoproteins on their outer surfaces and the attachment of cytoskeletal proteins to their cytoplasmic surfaces. Interrelations among typical membrane components are depicted here. Proteins that are inserted through the lipid bilayer (A1–A3), termed "integral" membrane proteins, are often glycosylated (●), as are some bilayer lipids (D) and many components of the extracellular matrix (E). Many interactions at the extracellular surface are stabilized by hydrogen bonding among these glycosyl residues. Certain integral membrane proteins can interact by virtue of specific receptor sites with intracellular proteins (B), with extracellular components (C), and also to form specific junctions with other cells (A2). A host of integral membrane proteins mediate different signal transduction and active transport pathways.

consisting of a glycerophosphorylester moiety and a hydrocarbon tail, usually of two esterified fatty acids (see Chap. 5). The head groups can interact with water and aqueous phase solutes whereas the nonpolar tails form a separate phase.

Three principal phases of differing structure are formed by phospholipids in the presence of water (Fig. 2). Although only the lamellar structure is ordinarily found in cell membranes, hexagonal phases may occur during some membrane transformations. The importance of molecular geometry for bilayer stability is illustrated by the effects of phospholipase components of certain venoms which can hydrolyze one of the fatty acid moieties from membrane phospholipids.

The resultant lysophosphatides may transform bilayers into hexagonal phase structures (Fig. 2) which can disrupt membrane continuity sufficiently to produce cell lysis. The ability to form micelles is characteristic of detergent molecules, which commonly have polar and lipophilic domains that differ in volume. In contrast to the destabilizing effects of lysophosphatides and other detergents on membranes, cholesterol can stabilize phospholipid bilayers by inserting into the structure at the interfaces between the head and tail regions so as to satisfy the bulk requirements for a planar geometry.

Multilamellar structures may form spontaneously if small amounts of water are added to solid or liquid phase phospholip-

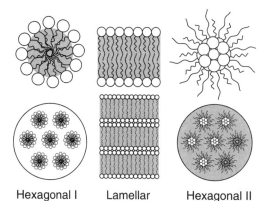

Hexagonal I   Lamellar   Hexagonal II

FIG. 2. Complex lipids interact with water and with each other to form different states of aggregation or "phases" shown here schematically. *Open circles or ellipses* represent the more polar "head groups" and the *dark lines and areas* represent the nonpolar hydrocarbon chains. The phase structures are generally classified as illustrated in the *lower row of the figure.* The hexagonal I and lamellar phases can be dispersed in aqueous media to form the micellar structures shown in the *top row.* Hexagonal II phase lipids will form "reverse micelles" in nonpolar solvents. The stability of lamellar structures relative to hexagonal structures depends upon fatty acid chain length, presence of double bonds, relative sizes of polar head and hydrocarbon tail groups, and temperature.

ids. Upon dilution, these can be dispersed to form vesicular structures called *liposomes.* Unilamellar liposomes are employed in studies of bilayer properties and often may be combined with membrane proteins to reconstitute functional membrane systems. There are two general ways to induce proteins to insert into liposomes: both phospholipids and membrane proteins may form micelles with detergents; as the detergent is removed by dialysis, the micelles transform into protein-containing vesicles. Alternatively, one may employ sonication to allow proteins to insert during the disruption of preformed phospholipid vesicles. Certain proteins may spontaneously insert into preformed vesicles. A valuable technique for studying the properties of proteins inserted into bilayers employs a single bilayer lamella *(black lipid membrane)* formed across a small aperture in a thin partition between two aqueous com-

partments. Because pristine lipid bilayers have very low ion conductivities, the modifications of ion conducting properties produced by membrane proteins can be measured with great sensitivity (see Chap. 4).

In aqueous systems, phospholipid structures may manifest either gel (rigid) or liquid-crystalline (two-dimensionally fluid) properties. In the case of pure phospholipids, these states interconvert at a well-defined transition temperature, T_c, that increases with alkyl chain length, and decreases with introduction of unsaturation. In cell membranes there is marked heterogeneity in both the polar and nonpolar domains of the bilayer. This, as well as the presence of cholesterol, maintains the fluid state over a broad temperature range. In the fluid state, membrane components are very mobile within the plane of each bilayer. However, spontaneous transverse movement of phospholipids between bilayer leaflets rarely occurs. Because of this, the two leaflets of a given membrane can maintain different lipid compositions. As examples, most plasma membranes contain substantially more phosphatidylethanolamine in the cytoplasmic leaflet than in the outer leaflet whereas glycolipids are almost exclusively confined to the extracytoplasmic leaflet.

Glycolipids also may segregate laterally to form microdomains that are stabilized by hydrogen bonding between carbohydrate residues. The glycolipids with more complex polar groups, such as the gangliosides (see Chap. 5), have a marked tendency to form micelles, rather than bilayers. Thus, they are potential participants in membrane destabilizing processes such as pore formation and vesicle fusion [2].

A major fraction of the bilayer phospholipids are physically constrained by their association with integral membrane protein [3]

In addition to interacting with each other to form the bilayer, membrane lipids may also interact in varying degrees with membrane proteins. Some physical measurements, such as electron spin resonance, have indicated that the acyl moieties of lipids immediately surrounding integral membrane proteins are motionally restricted and reoriented relative to the bilayer. This "annulus" fraction can comprise 20 to 90 percent of the total membrane phospholipid. Because the annulus lipids appear to equilibrate rapidly (within μsec) with the bulk membrane lipids in comparison with the time scale of most enzymes (within msec), the significance of such interactions has been questioned. However, some membrane proteins preferentially interact with certain lipid species and these interactions influence the protein structure. For example, the Na,K-ATPase preferentially binds negatively charged phospholipids, and this association promotes the catalytic activity.

Diffusional flow of water across cell membrane lipid bilayers is sufficient to account for the water permeability of most cells

Measurements of water permeability of lipid bilayers of varying composition have ranged from $2-1000 \times 10^{-5}$ cm/sec [4]. Corresponding measurements of cell membrane water permeabilities are in the same range.

Single channel conductances for ions tend to be around 10^{-11} S and the membrane conductances of most cells are of the order of 10^{-3} S/cm^2, which suggests an average of about 10^8 ion-conducting channels/cm^2. From measurements of channel-forming peptides, the water permeability of ion channels is about 10^{-14} cm^3/sec. This density of ion channels would provide about 10^{-6} cm/sec or only about 1 percent of the total cell water permeability. Therefore, ion channels make slight contribution to water permeability in most cells. Erythrocytes are a known exception, with a water permeability of about 2×10^{-2} cm^2. Their high content of band III anion exchanger has been proposed to

account for this phenomenon. However, high water permeability has now been linked to the presence of a specific membrane protein, designated CHIP28.

Proton conduction is facilitated in the headgroup regions of phospholipid monolayers [5]

In model systems, pH changes have been shown to be transmitted more rapidly along these interfaces than in bulk solution. This may have particular importance in mitochondrial ATP synthesis and other processes depending on transmembrane proton gradients. This high mobility may not be restricted to protons: nuclear magnetic resonance (NMR) studies have shown that the mean residence times of metal cations with phospholipid head groups are also very short.

MEMBRANE PROTEINS

Membrane proteins can be broadly classified as *integral*, if they have peptide domains that insert directly into the lipid bilayer, or *associated*, if they bind by other means

Integral membrane proteins have domains of nonpolar amino acid residues that traverse the bilayer lipids once or many times. Associations usually occur through interactions with specific binding domains of integral membrane proteins or by insertion of covalently bound lipids into the bilayer.

Although there is a rapidly expanding database of the primary sequences of integral membrane proteins, correspondingly detailed structural information is available for only a few, primarily because of the difficulty in obtaining membrane protein crystals adequate for X-ray diffraction studies. Consequently, the continuing efforts to develop techniques that predict structural information from combinations of sequence and

Average residue length: 5.1Å
Peptide backbone: 6.8Å

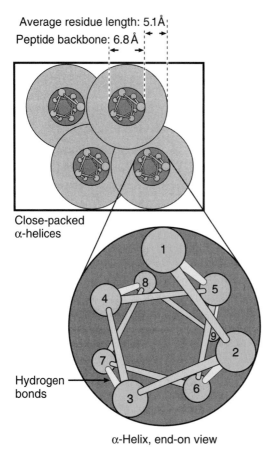

Close-packed
α-helices

Hydrogen
bonds

α-Helix, end-on view

FIG. 3. The transmembrane domains of integral membrane proteins are predominantly α helices. This structure causes the amino acid side chains to project radially. When several parallel α helices are closely packed, their side chains may intermesh as shown, or steric constraints may cause the formation of interchain channels. The outwardly directed residues must be predominantly hydrophobic to interact with the fatty acid chains of lipid bilayers. The bilayer is about 3 nm thick. Each peptide residue extends an α helix by 0.15 nm. Thus, although local modifications of the bilayer or interactions with other membrane polypeptides may alter this requirement, transmembrane segments usually require about 20 residues to span the bilayer. Integral membrane proteins are characterized by the presence of hydrophobic segments approximating this length (Fig. 4).

other structural data are particularly important when they are applicable to membrane proteins. Some generalizations about integral membrane protein structures have been proposed, but they are necessarily tentative.

Transmembrane domains of integral membranes are nearly always α helices

Peptide bonds are intrinsically polar and form hydrogen bonds either with water or internally between the carbonyl oxygen and the amide nitrogen. Within the lipid bilayer, where water is essentially not available, peptides adopt the configuration that maximizes their internal hydrogen bonding. This is usually an α helix. A length of α helix sufficient to span the usual bilayer requires 18–21 residues (Fig. 3). Because the surface properties of an α helix are determined by residue side chains, a single segment that serves merely to anchor the protein might be expected to consist largely of hydrophobic residues. This hypothesis is confirmed by many experimental observations. For this reason, derivation of "hydrophobicity profiles" from protein sequence data has become routine (Fig. 4).

Proteins that span the membrane only once are classified as monotopic or bitopic ([6], Fig. 5)

Cytochrome b_5 is considered to be monotopic: it has a single hydrophobic segment that forms a hairpin loop, which anchors the protein at the cytoplasmic surface, but is thought not to totally penetrate the bilayer. Bitopic proteins are more common, having a single transmembrane helix which may be

FIG. 4. Analysis of the distribution of hydrophobic residues within the amino acid sequence of an integral membrane protein may suggest the location of its transmembrane segments. **Bar graph:** "Hydrophobicity indices," which are based on physical properties of the amino acid residues, correlate reasonably well with the frequencies of occurrence of these residues in known transmembrane segments of integral membrane proteins. The consensus index used here (D. Eisenberg, *Annu. Rev. Biochem.* 53:595–623, 1984) assigns negative values to polar residues and positive values to hydrophobic residues in such a manner that the mean value is zero. The graph lists the one-letter codes of the

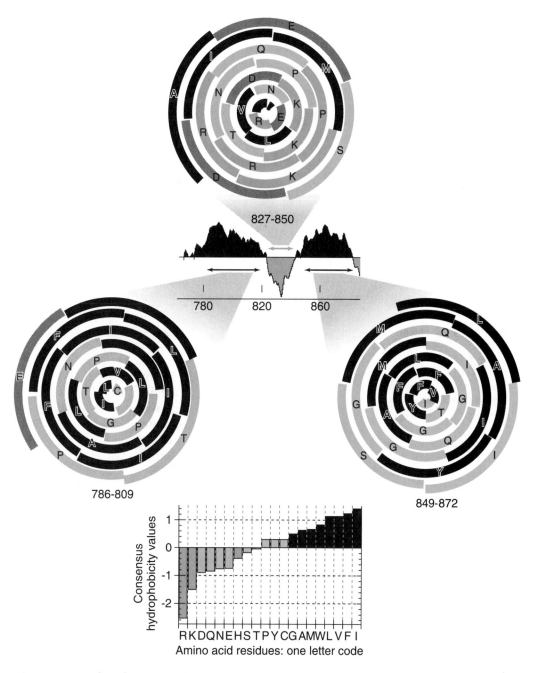

FIG. 4. *(continued)* residues in ascending rank order. The *colors of the bars* define the code employed for classes of amino acid residues in the helical wheel display. **Line graph:** Hydrophobicity plots of the catalytic subunit of the sodium pump suggest seven or more transmembrane segments. Two of these (5 and 6) are indicated by the *major black segments* of the plot. The *segments defined by the arrows* are displayed as **helical wheels:** These are diagrams of peptide sequences in α-helical configuration (as in Fig. 3). Each 100° arc is assigned a color: dark red for basic residues (HKR), gray for acidic residues (DE), light red for neutral polar residues (CGNPQSTY), and black for hydrophobic residues (AFILMVW). A characteristic of presumptive transmembrane segments is the occurrence of isolated polar residues in an otherwise hydrophobic environment. For example, presumptive transmembrane helix 5 of the sodium pump α-subunit contains one asparagine (N), one threonine (T), and two proline (P) residues within a run of 21 otherwise nonpolar residues. Such residues may participate in the formation of ionophoric pathways across the membrane, but they are also found in presumptive transmembrane segments that are unlikely to have transport functions.

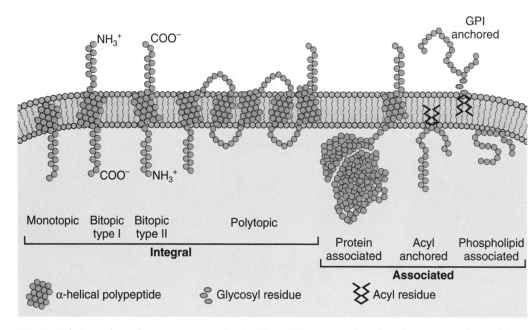

FIG. 5.   **Left:** Integral membrane proteins can be classified with respect to the orientation and complexity of their transmembrane segments. **Right:** Proteins may associate with membranes through several types of interactions with the bilayer lipids and also by interacting with integral membrane proteins.

oriented with the N-terminus either on the cytoplasmic surface (type II) or on the extracytoplasmic surface (type I). In many cases this single transmembrane helix may function only as a membrane anchor. Some of the receptor-activated tyrosine kinases are bitopic. Agonist-occupation of the extracytoplasmic receptor domain can activate the cytoplasmic kinase function despite their apparently tenuous interconnection. However, most integral membrane proteins with transducing functions are polytopic: single polypeptide chains that mediate such functions as voltage-dependent ion conductance are believed to traverse the bilayer as many as 16 times.

Transmembrane segments of integral membrane proteins are often intimately involved in the function as well as the structure of these proteins

In nearly all cases the peptides constituting ion channels, transport pumps, receptors-effector complexes, etc. have multiple trans-membrane segments that interact among themselves in addition to traversing the lipid bilayer. Transmembrane segments are seldom observed to contain only hydrophobic residues. Instead, polar and helix-destabilizing residues commonly occur within the predominantly hydrophobic segments (Fig. 4). Segments that both form transmembrane channels and participate in interior protein structure frequently are found to have polar and nonpolar residues on opposite sides, forming amphipathic helices.

The transmembrane helices of polytopic peptides are often closely packed so as to largely exclude interior phospholipids

Two examples for which there is substantial evidence are bacteriorhodopsin and the sarcoplasmic Ca^{2+}-pump. Peptide bonds have substantial dipole moments which are transmitted to the ends of α helices. This circumstance would be expected to favor close packing of anti-parallel helices and is, in fact, consistent with the observed disposition of helices in bacteriorhodopsin [7]. Inter-sub-unit packing in oligomeric proteins can also involve interactions of extramembranous protein domains and encompassed lipids.

The fluidity of the bilayer permits specific interactions among different integral membrane proteins [8]

For example, the interactions of neurotransmitters and hormones with their receptors often modulates the affinity of the receptor for transducer proteins, which in turn will interact with effector proteins (see Chap. 17). A given effector protein, such as adenylate cyclase, may respond to multiple receptors by means of associations with different transducers that affect its activity in different ways. These dynamic interactions require rapid diffusion within the plane of the membrane bilayer. Extensive redistribution of membrane proteins can result from the occupation of external receptor sites, as classically exemplified by the clustering of membrane antigens that occurs consequent to binding bivalent antibodies.

In contrast to these examples of lateral mobility, the distribution of integral membrane proteins on cell surfaces can be restricted to varying extents by specific interactions with other proteins. Examples are the localization of Na^+ pumps to the basolateral domains of epithelial cells, of Na^+ channels to nodes of Ranvier, and of nicotinic acetylcholine receptors to the postsynaptic membranes of neuromuscular junctions. Some membranes are partitioned into local domains by networks of cytoskeletal proteins. Membrane proteins may have their translational motion restricted by such a network and yet exhibit rapid rotational diffusion limited only by the bilayer viscosity.

Anchoring catalytic proteins to membranes may enhance reaction rates as a consequence of constraining diffusion pathways to two dimensions. Particularly dramatic effects may occur in reactions that occur among membrane proteins because of further constraints on their orientation relative to the bilayer plane. Realization of enhanced rates requires a highly fluid membrane bilayer and membrane fluidity can be subject to regulation [9,10].

Interactions between integral membrane proteins and other structural proteins are involved in most mechanical cell functions

These include cell motility, endo- and exocytosis, formation of cell junctions, and regulation of cell shape. Several peripheral membrane protein families are known that mediate specific interactions among integral membrane proteins, cytoskeletal proteins, and contractile proteins.

The association of cytoskeletal proteins membranes has been best studied in erythrocytes. In these cells, a major structural link of plasma membranes to cytoskeleton is mediated by an interaction between the anion antiporter (see Chap. 3) and *ankyrin*, a 215 kDa monomeric protein. Ankyrin links the anion antiporter with a rod-shaped 225 kDa subunit of the tetrameric protein, *spectrin*. Spectrin, in turn, self-associates to form a network parallel to the membrane. Spectrin has further links to actin polymers that form the principal microfilamentous component. Neurons contain spectrin and additional variants, termed *fodrins*. Fodrins are found throughout neurons whereas spectrin occurs only in soma and dendrites. These associations are undoubtedly subject to complex regulation. For example, phosphorylation of ankyrin can alter its affinity for spectrin. Brain fodrin has binding sites for spectrin, actin, and microtubules. Cytoskeletal interactions with neuronal membranes may occur in forming and modifying synaptic junctions (see Chap. 50). Neurotransmitter release probably also involves interactions of membrane and cytoskeletal components. In support of this concept, intracellular injection of an antibody to fodrin has been shown to interfere with catecholamine release from chromaffin cells.

Certain transmembrane glycoproteins can mediate interactions between the cytoskeleton and the extracellular matrix

These glycoproteins possess specific receptors both for sites found on extracellular matrix proteins or other cell surfaces and for sites on cytoskeletal proteins. In some cases, the extracellular binding specificity is for the Arg-Gly-Asp ("RGD") site found on matrix proteins such as fibronectin [11] while the intracellular specificity is for a cytoskeletal protein, such as *talin,* which may further interact with an intermediate filament protein (Fig. 5).

The "integrins" are major receptors that attach cells to extracellular matrix proteins [12]. They are heterodimers with 120–180 kDa α-subunits (14 identified types) and 90–110 kDa β-subunits (8 identified types). Different cell types express different combinations of the subunit types. These have varying selectivities for such extracellular components as collagens, laminins, and fibronectins.

Neural cell adhesion molecules (N-CAMs) belong to a family of cell surface glycoproteins of wide distribution that are structurally part of the immunoglobulin superfamily. Their roles in neural development have been studied intensively [13]. Differential splicing of mRNAs can result in the expression of at least three different polypeptides from a single N-CAM gene. Two of these (130 and 160 kDa) are transmembrane glycoproteins characterized by identical extracellular domains and differing "small" and "large" cytoplasmic domains. A third form is not a transmembrane peptide, but rather its extracellular domain is anchored to the membrane by a covalent attachment involving phosphatidylinositol (Fig. 5; see Chap. 5).

The N-terminal extracellular domains of N-CAMs are heavily glycosylated and contain long, unbranched polysialic acid chains. Increased sialylation suppresses the adhesive properties of the extracellular domains. Variations in polysialic acid content apparently influence cell and axon migrations (see Chap. 28). The extracellular binding sites of N-CAMs are homotypic, i.e., they can bind to each other. A heparin-binding site is also present.

Cadherins are a family of membrane proteins with Ca^{2+}-dependent homotypic adhesion receptors that may be largely responsible for the preferential adhesion of similar cell types [13]. Tissue-specific types have been characterized, including epithelial and neural varieties, termed E-cadherin and N-cadherin, respectively. Cadherins can also associate with cytoskeletal components, particularly at zonula adherens junctions, where underlying structures contain α-actinin and F-actin.

Covalently attached lipids frequently participate in binding proteins to membranes ([14], Fig. 5)

Myristate can be added cotranslationally to N-terminal glycines of a number of peripheral proteins, thus participating in their binding to the cytoplasmic surface of plasma membranes. These proteins include the catalytic subunit of cAMP-dependent protein kinase, calcineurin B, and NADH-cytochrome b_5 reductase.

Fatty acids, most commonly *palmitate,* can be linked as thioesters to a cysteine residue which is usually located near a membrane-binding domain of a protein. Both integral membrane proteins, such as rhodopsin and transferrin receptor, and membrane-associated proteins, such as ankyrin and vinculin, may become acylated posttranslationally.

Proteins can be anchored covalently to the external surface of plasma membranes via *complex glycosylated phosphoinositides* [15]. These can be converted from membrane-bound to water-soluble forms through the action of phosphoinositide-specific phospholipase C. Examples are alkaline phosphatase, 5'-nucleotidase, one form of acetylcholinesterase (see Chap. 10), and one form of N-CAM. The diacylglycerol moiety provided by single phosphoinositide appears to be sufficient to produce a stable membrane anchor (see Chap. 5).

A number of proteins can be post-translationally modified by the addition of isoprenyl derivatives [16]. One pathway for synthesis of these anchors involves precursor proteins possessing a C-terminal sequence, -CXXX. The precursors are modified by transfer of a C_{20} group from geranylgeranyl pyrophosphate to the cysteine sulfhydryl. The three terminal amino acids are then cleaved and finally a methyl group is added to the newly exposed α-carboxyl of the cysteine. Members of this group include many signal transduction proteins of the small G-protein class and the γ-subunits of heterotrimeric G proteins.

Electrostatic coupling of peripheral membrane proteins to the bilayer lipids may occur

One example is spectrin, which binds to phosphatidylserine [17]. Several proteins are characterized by a Ca^{2+}-dependent phospholipid-binding domain. These include several enzymes and structural proteins which become membrane-bound subsequent to Ca^{2+} activation: protein kinase C, phospholipase A_2, and synaptotagmin.

Allosteric regulation of the hydrophobicity of protein-binding surfaces frequently occurs

One of the best known cases is the Ca^{2+}-dependent binding of calmodulin to other proteins (see Chap. 3). A family of proteins that exhibit Ca^{2+}-dependent associations with cell membranes have lately been termed "annexins" [18,19]. Ca^{2+} binding increases the affinity of these proteins for direct interaction with phospholipids and, conversely, interactions with phospholipids increase their affinities for Ca^{2+}. Some can also interact with actin microfilaments and thus can link cytoskeletal components to the membrane.

Newly synthesized integral membrane proteins and secreted proteins are inserted into the endoplasmic reticulum (ER) bilayer by similar mechanisms

Although the same ribosomal machinery is used for synthesizing cytoplasmic, integral membrane, and secreted proteins, the latter two classes require additional mediators for targeting and insertion through the bilayer.

The information that targets a polypeptide to the ER membrane is contained in a segment near the N-terminus called a *signal sequence*. These sequences are highly variable but include a hydrophobic segment of nine or more residues bracketed by basic residues at the N-terminus and a mixture of acidic and basic residues at the C-terminus. Membrane proteins possess additional, predominantly hydrophobic segments ("topogenic sequences") that determine their primary membrane topologies, i.e., the number of times they traverse the bilayer.

In many cases, targeting to the endoplasmic reticulum begins with interaction of a *signal recognition particle* (SRP) with the nascent signal sequence as it emerges from the mRNA-ribosome complex (Fig. 6). SRP is an 11 S ribonucleoprotein consisting of six different peptides and one 7S RNA. Translation is arrested if SRP binds to the complex in the absence of ER membranes. Elongation of the nascent peptide can proceed after the ribosome-bound SRP interacts with a component of the ER membrane, the *SRP receptor* or *docking protein*. This interaction is followed by SRP dissociation from the ribosome and insertion of the signal sequence into the ER membrane, permitting the mRNA translation to continue. GTP binding and hydrolysis is required at this step. Both SRP and the SRP receptor have GTP-binding domains, but present evidence implicates the receptor in this stage [20]. Once a conjunction of the ribosomal complex with the ER membrane is effected, the growing peptide passes through the membrane. This mechanism is called *cotranslational insertion*.

Most secreted proteins are synthesized

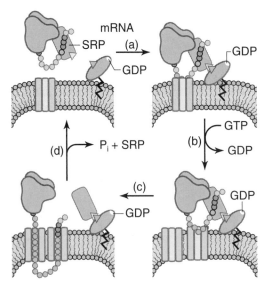

FIG. 6. Initiation of membrane protein insertion into the endoplasmic reticulum: (a) Signal-recognition particles (, SRP) associate with ribosomes ( ) and the signal sequences ( ) of nascent membrane proteins. (b) These complexes associate with SRP receptors in the ER membrane. The SRP receptors contain bound GDP. (c) Bound GDP is exchanged for cytoplasmic GTP and (d) translocation of peptides occurs as GTP is hydrolyzed. The peptides are oriented N → C outward as they insert through a membrane. (Adapted from [20] with permission.)

in this manner as ''pro-proteins'' with amino-terminal *signal sequences.* After the rest of the peptide has been exported, the signal sequence is cleaved from a secreted product by a *signal peptidase,* itself a membrane protein with its active site within the ER lumen. Some integral membrane proteins, having a single anchoring segment near the NH_2-terminal, may insert by a similar mechanism involving an *uncleaved signal sequence* (Fig. 6). However other proteins have a single anchor near their COOH-terminals, and their insertion requires, in addition, a *stop-transfer sequence* to form a permanent transmembrane segment, and cleavage of the initial signal peptide.

Polytopic membrane proteins contain two or more topogenic sequences. An example is opsin, which traverses the membrane seven times. Since it has four intraluminal domains, as many as four stop-transfer sequences may be required. By the use of selectively deleted cDNA and subsequent translation of the corresponding RNA transcripts, the experimental indications are that, in fact, the first and sixth transmembrane segments of opsin contain the stop-transfer sequences that are hypothesized to be necessary for proper membrane insertion [21].

However not all cases of membrane protein insertion seem to conform to this model. Ribosomal synthesis of some integral membrane proteins is not inhibited by SRP. For example, the Ca^{2+}-pump ATPase contains stop-transfer sequences, and although SRP is required for membrane insertion, the absence of membranes containing the docking protein does not arrest its synthesis [22]. Other integral membrane proteins, such as cytochrome b_5, can be synthesized on free ribosomes and subsequently insert into membranes in the absence of SRP. The *spontaneous insertion hypothesis* attempts to account for the occurrence of post-translational insertion by postulating that two hydrophobic peptide segments associate to form a hairpin configuration that can insert into a lipid bilayer independently of facilitating proteins. This model does not explain how hydrophilic sequences, which form the extra-cytoplasmic domains of many integral membrane proteins, are transported across a lipid bilayer that constitutes a large energy barrier.

To circumvent this problem and to account for all possible configurations of integral membrane proteins, a *unitary hypothesis* postulates *translocator proteins* in the ER membrane that can interact with topogenic sequences to form hydrophilic channels that traverse the bilayer. Combinations of stop-transfer sequences, cleaved signal sequences, and appropriate responses by the translocator proteins to these signals can account for most of the observed transmembrane dispositions of polypeptide segments [23].

The existence of channel-forming proteins in rough endoplasmic reticulum has been demonstrated: 250 pS conductance events are induced in these membranes when protein synthesis is aborted with puromycin [24]. Because puromycin causes nascent peptides to dissociate from ribosomes, a reasonable interpretation is that ribosomes lacking such peptides can combine with and open channels in ER translocator proteins, whereas these channels remain closed in the absence of ribosomes and are normally blocked by the nascent peptides. One candidate translocator subunit is a 34 kDa type I bitopic glycoprotein that associates with nascent polypeptides and constitutes >1 percent of microsomal protein [20].

"Molecular chaperones" are frequently required to mediate correct protein folding [25]

It has been widely held that nascent polypeptides assume their "native" conformations spontaneously as they emerge from the ribosome. In its strict form, this model implies that the genetic information that specifies a primary sequence completely defines the native protein conformation. This concept is undergoing revision because of the discovery of auxiliary proteins, "molecular chaperones," that regulate polypeptide folding. The signal recognition particle and other proteins that recognize topogenic sequences are examples of this functional class. Another molecular chaperone was originally identified as an immunoglobulin heavy chain binding protein, "BiP." It is a resident protein of the ER. BiP and other related proteins can bind to certain short peptide segments. This activates hydrolysis of a bound ATP, which in turn causes release of the peptide. This seems analogous to the GTPase activity of SRP. The peptide selectivity of BiP has been shown to involve binding to seven adjacent residues. The binding-site peptide specificity has been described as similar to the composition of the interior of folded proteins. It is also comparable to that of transmembrane sequences. BiP has been shown to interact with newly synthesized α-

subunits of nicotinic acetylcholine receptors [26]. It also binds to $\alpha\gamma$- and $\alpha\delta$-complexes but not to the mature receptor, which is a pentamer of four different subunits, $\alpha_2\beta\gamma\delta$, in which the two alphas are not adjacent (see Chap. 11). A role for BiP in assisting the correct assembly of these subunits is possible but not yet fully demonstrated.

Newly synthesized plasma membrane proteins move from the ER through a succession of Golgi compartments, finally entering into pre-existing plasma membrane from the trans-Golgi network ([27]; Fig. 7)

Each transit event is thought to be initiated by binding of "coat proteins" to a patch of the cytoplasmic surface of a Golgi membrane to form a "coated pit." The coated pit membrane is transformed into a vesicle. Scission of the vesicle is followed by its fusion with the membrane of the next compartment.

The set of coat proteins, termed "COPs," mediate vesicular transport of proteins through the internal Golgi compartments. Subunits of the intra-Golgi vesicle coat complex, termed α-, β-, γ- and δ-COP, have been identified. Among these, the α-COP has similarities to clathrin heavy chain and β-COP has similarities to adaptins *(vide infra)*. One hypothesis is that the process mediated by this complex consists of a non-selective "bulk flow" of most of the membrane proteins and soluble components through successive Golgi compartments. These proteins are progressively subjected to various covalent modifications by enzymes that reside in different Golgi compartments. Thus, both the endoplasmic reticulum and the various Golgi compartments contain characteristic resident proteins. Although the "default" mechanism of vesicular traffic outward from the ER is non-selective, there are "active" and selective mechanisms for retaining the resident proteins such as retrograde or "salvage" transport from Golgi to ER. ER-resident proteins have a C-terminal signature sequence, Lys-Asp-Glu-Leu or

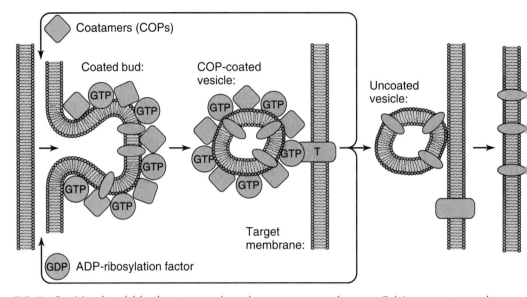

FIG. 7. Provisional model for the transport of membrane components from one Golgi compartment to the next. *On the left,* an area of a Golgi membrane containing the transiting proteins (red) that binds resident proteins, including "COPs" and the ADP-ribosylation factor. This initiates the formation of a coated vesicle. The detached vesicle binds to an unknown component, T, of the target membrane, which may be another Golgi compartment, the plasma membrane, or an intracellular organelle. The coat proteins are released and recycled as the vesicle and the transiting proteins fuse with the target membrane *(right).* (Adapted from [27] with permission.)

"KDEL," that is recognized by the salvage mechanism.

A different set of coat proteins, the clathrin complexes, function between the trans-Golgi network and its target membranes ([28]; Fig. 8). Clathrin consists of three molecules of clathrin heavy chain, which form a "triskelion" by joining together near their C-termini. Each heavy chain is divided into proximal and distal domains by a hinge region. Clathrin light chains associate with the proximal domains of the heavy chains. Clathrin triskelions self-assemble into extensive lattices by interacting at the heavy chain N-termini. However the interaction of these lattices with membrane proteins is mediated by another set of proteins termed *adaptins*. The combination of lattice-forming by clathrin and protein selection by adaptins produces a concentration of targeted integral membranes within "coated pits" in both trans-Golgi and plasma membranes. Different adaptins reside in dif-

ferent membranes. For example, the adaptin AP-2 is involved in the assembly of coated pits on the plasma membrane (endocytosis) whereas AP-1 participates in the corresponding assembly on the trans-Golgi network (secretion).

Fusion of vesicles with their target membranes involves disassembly of the coat proteins. In the case of clathrin, this is mediated by an "undercoating ATPase," hsc 70, now known to be a constitutive member of the heat-shock protein family which includes several other molecular chaperones. Each step of vesicular transit from the Golgi to the target membrane appears to involve both ATPase and GTPase activities.

Post-translational modifications play a role in the targeting of some membrane proteins. For example, proteins that acquire mannose-6-phosphate subsequently appear in lysosomes. In both epithelial cells and neurons, membrane proteins with glycosyl-phosphatidylinositol anchors move almost

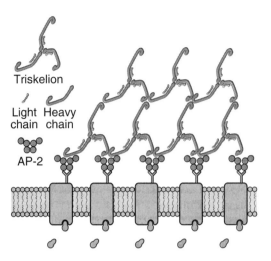

Triskelion

Light Heavy
chain chain

AP-2

FIG. 8. Endocytosis of membrane components. The scheme shown here is derived from studies of the recycling of membrane receptors for ligands such as transferrin and insulin. Recycling of synaptic vesicle membranes occurs by a similar process. Ligand binding to the receptor appears to induce a conformational change that permits a tyrosine-containing β turn in the cytoplasmic domain ("Y") to interact with one of the adaptins (AP-2). Clathrin binding to the adaptins then produces the "coated pits" that develop into endocytotic vesicles. Clathrin consists of three heavy chains (~190 kDa each) that join near their C-terminus to form a triskelion. Three light chains, of undetermined function, associate with the proximal segments of the heavy chains, possibly via an amphipathic α helix (heptad repeats) found in their central domains.

exclusively to the apical plasma membrane, the analog of which in neurons is the axon [29]. Some proteins that are retained in the basolateral membranes of epithelial cells and, correspondingly, in the soma and dendrites of neurons, contain a cytoplasmic tyrosine-containing β-turn similar to the endocytotic signal sequence (Fig. 8).

In the case of neurons, some of the vesicles released from the trans-Golgi network reach their targets by fast axoplasmic transport (see Chap. 27)

Voltage-dependent release of some of the classical neurotransmitters, triggered by the presynaptic influx of Ca^{2+}, may occur within 200 μsec of the stimulus. This is apparently achieved by a mechanism that keeps a population of these vesicles poised for rapid fusion with the presynaptic plasma membranes (see Chap. 9). Interactions with actin microfilaments and small G proteins appear to participate in this process. Just as it is advantageous to recover neurotransmitters or their metabolites locally by active transport in many instances (see Chap. 3), the maintenance of adequate supplies of the membrane constituents that package rapidly secreted neurotransmitters is facilitated by processes that recycle synaptic vesicle components from the presynaptic plasma membranes (see Chap. 9).

REFERENCES

1. Tanford, C. *The Hydrophobic Effect: Formation of micelles and biological membranes, 2nd ed.*, New York: Wiley Interscience, 1980.
2. Zeller, C., and R. Marchase. Gangliosides as modulators of cell function. *Am. J Physiol.* 262 (6 Pt 1): C1341–C1355, 1992.
3. Jost, P. C., and O. H. Griffith. The lipid-protein interface in biological membranes. *Ann. N. Y. Acad. Sci.* 348:391–407, 1980.
4. Finkelstein, A. Water movement through membrane channels. *Curr. Top. Membr. Transp.* 21:298–308, 1984.
5. Prats, M., Teissie, J., and Tocanne, J.-F. Lateral proton conduction at lipid-water interfaces and its implications for the chemiosmotic-coupling hypothesis. *Nature* 322: 756–758, 1986.
6. Jennings, M. L. Topography of membrane proteins. *Annu. Rev. Biochem.* 58:999–1027, 1989.
7. Henderson, R., Baldwin, J. M., Ceska, T. A., Zemlin, F., Beckman, E., and Downing, K. H. Model for the structure of bacteriorhodopsin based on high-resolution cryo-microscopy. *J. Mol. Biol.* 213(4):899–929, 1990.
8. Poo, M. Mobility and localization of proteins in excitable membranes. *Annu. Rev. Neurosci.* 8:369–406, 1985.
9. Grasberger, B., Minton, A. P., DeLisi, C., and Metzger, H. Interaction between proteins localized in membranes. *Proc. Natl. Acad. Sci. U.S.A.* 83(17):6258–6262, 1986.

10. Adam, G., and Delbruck, M. Reduction of dimensionality in biological diffusion processes. In *Structural Chemistry and Molecular Biology.* New York: W. H. Freeman, 1968.

11. Ruoslahti, E., and Pierscbacher, M. D. Arg-Gly-Asp: a versatile cell recognition signal. *Cell* 44:517–518, 1986.

12. Hynes, R. O. Integrins: versatility, modulation, and signaling in cell adhesion. *Cell* 69:11–25, 1992.

13. Hynes, R. O., and Lander, A. D. Contact and adhesive specificities in the associations, migrations, and targeting of cells and axons. *Cell* 68:303–322, 1992.

14. Sefton, B. M., and Buss, J. E. The covalent modification of eukaryotic proteins with lipid. *J. Cell Biol.* 104(6):1449–1453, 1987.

15. Low, M. G. The glycosyl-phosphatidylinositol anchor of membrane proteins. *Biomed. Biochem. Acta* 988:427–454, 1989.

16. Clarke, S. Protein isoperenylation and methylation at carboxyl-terminal cysteine residues. *Annu. Rev. Biochem.* 61:355–386, 1992.

17. Maksymiw, R., Sui, S. F., Gaub, H., and Sackman, E. Electrostatic coupling of spectrin dimers to phosphatidylserine-containing lipid lamellae. *Biochem.* 26(11):2983–2990, 1987.

18. Crompton, M. R., Moss, S. E., and Crumpton, M. J. Diversity in the lipocortin/calpactin family. *Cell* 55:1–3, 1988.

19. Creutz, C. E. The annexins and exocytosis. *Science* 258:924–930, 1992.

20. Rapoport, T. A. Protein transport across the ER membrane. *Trends Biochem. Sci.* 15:355–358, 1990.

21. Friedlander, M., and G. Blobel. Bovine opsin has more than one signal sequence. *Nature* 318:338, 1985.

22. Anderson, D. J., Mostov, K. E., and Blobel, G. Mechanisms of integration of de novo-synthesized polypeptides into membranes. *Proc. Natl. Acad. Sci. U.S.A.* 80:7249–7253, 1983.

23. Singer, S. J., Maher, P. A. A., and Yaffe, M. P. On the translocation of proteins across membranes. *Proc. Natl. Acad. Sci. U.S.A.* 84:1015–1019, 1987.

24. Simon, S. M., and Blobel, G. A protein-conducting channel in the endoplasmic reticulum. *Cell* 65:371–380, 1991.

25. Ellis, R. J., and van der Vies, S. M. Molecular chaperones. *Annu. Rev. Biochem.* 60:321–347, 1991.

26. Blount, P., and Merlie, J. P. BIP associates with newly synthesized subunits of the mouse muscle nicotinic receptor. *J. Cell Biol.* 113(5):1125–1132, 1991.

27. Rothman, J., and Orci, L. Molecular dissection of the secretory pathway. *Nature* 355:409–415, 1992.

28. Pryor, N. K., Wuestehube, L. J., and Schekman, R. Vesicle-mediated protein sorting. *Annu. Rev. Biochem.* 61:471–516, 1992.

29. Dotti, C., Parton, R., and Simons, K. Polarized sorting of glypiated proteins in hippocampal neurons. *Nature* 349:158–161, 1991.

CHAPTER 3

Membrane Transport

R. Wayne Albers, George J. Siegel, and William L. Stahl

Basic Neurochemistry: Molecular, Cellular, and Medical Aspects, 5th Ed., edited by G. J. Siegel et al. Published by Raven Press, Ltd., New York, 1994. Correspondence to R. Wayne Albers; Laboratory of Neurochemistry; NINDS, LNC, National Institutes of Health; Bldg. 36, Rm. 4D-20; Bethesda, Maryland 20892.

TRANSPORT PROCESSES

Ion gradients are generated across cell membranes by transport proteins and are required for some of the most basic neural functions

These ion gradients produce the voltages across plasma membranes that drive the propagated signaling functions of neurons. Other uses of the potential energy of ion gradients include

1. the synthesis of ATP in mitochondria,
2. concentrative acquisitions or recoveries of nutrients, metabolites, and neurotransmitters; and
3. regulation via control of intracellular ionic concentrations.

Some transporters are electrogenic, i.e., their operation can move electric charge across membranes [1]. Well-characterized examples of transport proteins in each category will be discussed. These are now sufficiently numerous to inspire analyses of their structural and evolutionary interrelations. One generalization permitted from present evidence is that most of the major families of transport proteins arose prior to the divergence of eukaryocytes from prokaryocytes [1].

Concentration gradients across membranes result from two opposing processes: diffusion and active transport

The Gibbs equation describes the free energy (ΔG) released by the diffusion of a solute or required for its transport in the opposite direction:

$$\Delta G_{diff} = RT \ln (C_2 / C_1) \qquad (1)$$

where $R = 1.99$ cal/deg Kelvin; $T =$ degrees Kelvin; C_1 and $C_2 =$ concentrations of the solute on opposite sides of a permeable membrane.

Because cell membranes are selective in their ion permeabilities, the active transport of charged solutes produces electrical as well as chemical potentials (see Chap. 4). The energy stored as electrical potential is given by:

$$\Delta G_{emf} = ZFV \qquad (2)$$

where Z is valence, F is the Faraday constant (23,500 cal/volt/mol), and V is the transmembrane potential difference in volts. The free energy change related to movement of one mol of a solute with respect to the combined electrochemical gradient is described by the sum of equations 1 and 2:

$$\Delta G_{total} = RT \ln(C_2/C_1) + ZFV \qquad (3)$$

The chemical and electrical diffusion components are equal and opposite only in an equilibrium state. When work occurs, ΔG is not equal to zero and a steady state can only be maintained if sufficient energy is supplied by some exergonic process.

In the case of neurons and certain other cells in which the ionic currents are carried primarily by Na^+ and K^+, the energy input to maintain a steady-state electrochemical gradient can be approximated by the application of Eq. 3 to just these species:

$$\Delta G_{total} = RT \ln([Na^+]_e/[Na^+]_i) + ZFV$$
$$+ RT \ln([K^+]_i/[K^+]_e) - ZFV \qquad (4)$$
$$= RT \ln([Na^+]_e[K^+]_i/[Na^+]_i[K^+]_e)$$

Assuming typical values for Na^+ and K^+ concentration gradients ($[Na^+]_e/[Na^+]_i = 12$, $[K^+]_i/[K^+]_e = 50$), ΔG is about 3.8 kcal/mol of Na^+ exchanged for K^+. The hydrolysis of a high energy phosphate bond of ATP may yield about 12 kcal/mol, thus permitting the exchange of about 3 mol of cation for each mol of ATP hydrolyzed. This is the ratio of Na^+ transported per mole of ATP that has been measured in various tissue preparations.

The processes mediated by transport proteins are generative and those mediated by channel proteins are dissipative

Channels permit diffusion of ions or molecules across membranes at a direction and rate determined by prevailing electrochemical gradients. They can apparently achieve adequate selectivity without strong interactions with ions. Typical ion channels conduct several thousand ions per millisecond (see Chap. 4). In contrast, transport proteins

form highly specific and relatively strong complexes with their substrates. These interactions initiate conformational transitions of the transport proteins culminating in release of the substrate ions on the opposite face of the membrane. Transport processes typically require several milliseconds per ion. Because of these strong interactions, the relationships between solute concentration and rate of transport can be described by saturation kinetics as in the case of enzyme-catalyzed reactions.

Selective transport of molecules or ions through membranes may occur without coupling to any other substrate. Such a process is termed *facilitative* or *uncoupled* transport. An example is the stereo-selective entrance of D-glucose into neurons. Binding of an appropriate transport substrate is sufficient to initiate an uncoupled transport cycle, in which the substrate is conveyed across the membrane and the unoccupied transport-binding site is restored to its original orientation (Fig. 1).

Secondary or *flux-coupled* transport processes obligatorily couple the transport of one molecular or ionic species to the transport of another. The coupled processes are termed *symport* or *antiport* according to the relative directions of the two transport events (Fig. 1). Many essential nutrients are accumulated by symport systems coupled to Na^+ or proton gradients. Neurotransmitter re-uptake systems are similarly coupled symporters and are described below. In coupled transport, both substrates must be available—either simultaneously or sequentially—on the same side of the membrane in the case of a symporter, and on opposite sides in the case of an antiporter. Substrate-velocity kinetics for these systems are analogous to those of multi-substrate enzymes. More than two substrates are involved in some secondary transport systems, as exemplified by the bumetanide-sensitive (Na^+, K^+, 2 Cl^-)-symporter (*vide infra*).

Primary active transport processes comprise those in which one or more substrates are transported in concert with a chemical

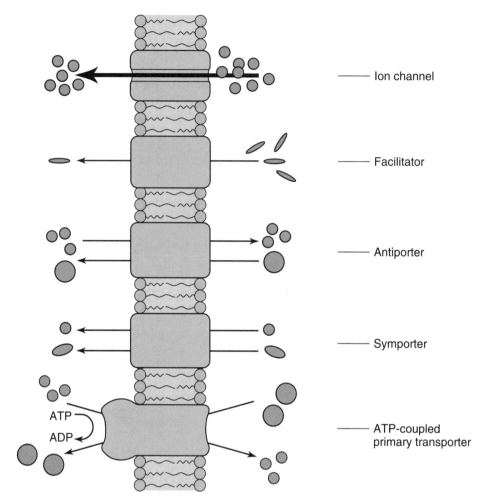

Ion channel

Facilitator

Antiporter

Symporter

ATP-coupled
primary transporter

FIG. 1. Types of membrane transport proteins. *Ion channels* provide diffusion paths across cell membranes that may be regulated by membrane voltage, interactions with ligands, and/or by phosphorylation (see Chap. 4). *Facilitators* provide highly selective pathways, e.g., for D-glucose, but are not coupled to energy sources, and therefore cannot concentrate their substrates. Transporters are coupled to energy sources and thus can alter the steady-state distribution of their substrate ions and/or molecules. *Secondary transporters* derive energy from existing ion gradients to transport a second ion or molecule in a direction that is either the same (symport) or opposite to (antiport) that of the energizing ion. *Primary transporters* couple a chemical reaction to protein conformational transitions which supply energy to generate concentration gradients of one or more substrates across cell membranes.

reaction that provides the free energy for concentrative substrate accumulation (Fig. 1). All of the known primary processes transport cations: H^+, Na^+, K^+, and Ca^{2+}. The principal function of primary Na^+ and K^+ transport in most cells is to store energy. In contrast, H^+ and Ca^{2+} pumps act as regulators of intracellular or intraorganellar concentrations of these ions, which in turn control the rates of other cell functions (*vide infra*).

Biochemical terminology is curiously inadequate to describe proteins that have energy-transducing functions. In addition to proteins that implement primary active transport, members of this group include proteins that produce contractile forces (myosins, dyneins), those that transport macromolecules and organelles intracellularly (kinesins, see Chap. 27), and some that transform the shapes or relative positions of other macromolecules (peptidyl transfer-ases, DNA helicases, topoisomerases). Most of these proteins catalyze ATP or GTP hydrolysis. However, these hydrolytic activities are only byproducts of their primary energy-transducing functions, which produce various forms of local ordering of cellular structure. These functions transcend the usual definition of an enzyme as a catalyst. For this reason, it is preferable to refer to primary active transport systems as pumps rather than as ATPases. On the other hand, the concept of "substrate" is usually restricted to molecules that are chemically transformed as a result of forming a transient complex with enzymes. In the case of membrane pumps, the bound molecules or ions are transported rather than transformed, but because in every other way they behave as substrates, the term will be so applied in the following discussion.

THE ATP-DEPENDENT Na$^+$, K$^+$-PUMP

The principal primary active transport system in neurons, as in most other animal cells, is a pump that concurrently extrudes Na$^+$ and accumulates K$^+$

The protein that constitutes this molecular machinery can be measured as an ATPase activity and, for brevity, is termed the Na,K-ATPase. Different tissues have vastly different requirements for pumping Na$^+$ and K$^+$, depending on their functions. That these fluxes are produced by the Na,K-ATPase has been established conclusively by experimentally reconstituting the pump activity in artificial vesicles composed only of lipids and the purified protein components of the ATPase [2]. In the reconstituted system, as in intact erythrocytes, the measured stoichiometry is 3 Na$^+$ ions and 2 K$^+$ ions pumped per molecule of ATP hydrolyzed. Transport by the Na,K-ATPase is specifically inhibited by cardiac glycosides such as ouabain.

The purified Na$^+$-pump consists of two different polypeptide subunits, α and β. The α-subunit contains the catalytic and ionophoric domains. It is polytopic with eight probable transmembrane domains (Fig. 2). The β-subunit is a monotopic glycoprotein. Its major domain is extracellular and exhibits some of the characteristics of adhesion molecules. Several studies have demonstrated that the α-subunit is not functional and is not inserted into plasma membranes when expressed in the absence of the β-subunit. The minimum functional oligomeric structure may be $\alpha\beta$, although $(\alpha\beta)_2$ and higher oligomers readily form. Phospholipid, 100–200 molecules per molecule of enzyme, is required to maintain activity. This is maximally promoted by negatively charged phospholipids such as phosphatidylserine.

The Na$^+$,K$^+$-pump exists in multiple forms

Different genes specify three different α-subunit isoforms. Two β-subunit genes have been identified in mammals and a third form was identified in frog. The mammalian β_2 isoform is identical with a glycoprotein first identified as an adhesion molecule, "AMOG," transiently expressed on the surface of cerebellar Bergman glia during the differentiation of granule cells. As the brain matures, β_2 is widely expressed on astrocytes.

The major form of the catalytic subunit that is expressed in kidney has been designated α_1 and all three forms appear to be expressed in rodent brains. The three forms show about 85 percent sequence similarity, with the most substantial differences occurring in the N-terminal region. The regions including the catalytic phosphorylation site are identical for a length of 85 residues and there are major hydrophobic domains with 94–96 percent similarity. The isoforms are expressed to varying extents at different stages of development and in different cell types (*vide infra*).

Na$^+$ and K$^+$ concentration gradients are controlled by the Na$^+$,K$^+$-pump

Transmembrane gradients for a number of ions are shown in Chap. 4, Table 1. Energy

Comparative membrane topology

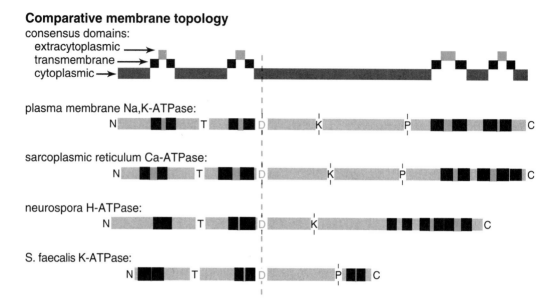

FIG. 2.   Conservation of structure and sequence in P-type transport ATPases. The probable topological distribution of peptide segments with respect to the plane of the membrane bilayer has been deduced from hydropathy plots, determinations of accessibility to proteases, and to other probe molecules. The candidate transmembrane segments are indicated by *black bar segments.* Loci of certain highly conserved sequences are indicated by *capital letters within the bars:* in terms of the single letter amino acid code, (T) TGES; (D) DKTGTLT; (K) KGAP; (P) PXL, where X is S or A. D is the active site aspartyl residue that is transiently phosphorylated in each catalytic cycle. The K and P sites probably participate in ATP binding. The functional role of the T site may relate to energy transduction. Note the apparent conservation of structure in the left half of the map across species and functional diversities.

for the work of producing the gradients for Na^+ and K^+ is provided by the hydrolysis of ATP. Wherever ions occur at concentrations removed from their electrochemical equilibria, their transport must be linked to metabolism, directly or indirectly.

The pump rate can be regulated experimentally by both the internal Na^+ and external K^+ concentrations. However, under physiological conditions, the $[Na^+]_i$ is usually less than saturating for the pump internal Na^+ sites, whereas $[K^+]_o$ is sufficient to saturate the external K^+ sites. Thus the pump rate is ordinarily more responsive to changes in internal Na^+ than to changes in external K^+.

A major fraction of cerebral energy production is required for Na^+ extrusion

Cation flux during action potentials is two to three orders of magnitude greater than in the resting state. For example, the Na^+ entry and K^+ efflux from a squid giant axon during a single action potential (duration ~1 msec) is about 3×10^{-12} mol cm^{-2} membrane. The resting membrane flux in this tissue is 12×10^{-12} mol cm^{-2} sec^{-1} (see Chap. 4). Therefore, it would take the pump about 0.25 seconds to regenerate the flux of one spike at the resting membrane pump rate. Based on these estimates, in order to maintain a steady-state at conduction frequencies ranging from 10 to 100 impulses/sec, the Na^+,K^+-pump rate would have to increase by 2.5 to 25 times its resting level.

Although the electrical currents associated with either excitatory or inhibitory postsynaptic membrane potentials (about 10 mV) may produce ion flux densities about one-tenth of those produced during an action potential, these postsynaptic depolarizations may last 10 to 1,000 times longer than action potentials and may occupy much larger membrane areas.

From measurements of ouabain-sensitive O_2 consumption in "depolarized" brain slices, it is estimated that 25 to 40 percent of brain energy utilization may be related to Na,K-ATPase activity. This estimate is similar to estimates based on the *in vitro* V_{max} and the total Na,K-ATPase activity expressed in brain.

The estimated total energy expenditure for the biosynthetic processes in mature brain (including osmotic work, protein and lipid synthesis, and turnover of neurotransmitters) is relatively small, probably less than 10 percent of total ATP utilization. The energy utilized by processes such as axoplasmic transport, Ca^{2+} transport, receptor-mediated P_i turnover, phosphorylation reactions, and vesicle recycling may be of significant proportions. However, it is evident that Na^+ transport is the single process that accounts for the largest share of energy flux.

Coupled active transport of Na^+ and K^+ results from a cycle of conformational transitions of the transport protein

The ATPase activity that is associated with the Na^+-pump is actually the sum of a Na^+-dependent phosphorylation of an aspartyl residue at the catalytic site of the pump protein and subsequent K^+-dependent hydrolysis of enzyme acylphosphate (Fig. 3). These molecular events direct metabolic energy into the pumping process. The initial phosphorylation of an enzyme molecule by ATP occurs only after 3 Na^+ have bound to sites accessible from the cytoplasmic side of the plasma membrane. In this "$E_1 \sim P$" conformation, the phosphorylation is readily reversible, i.e., the energy state of the protein acylphosphate is comparable to that of the ATP phosphate bond. However, the phosphorylation initiates a rapid transition of the pump to the E_2—P state, from which the Na^+ is discharged extracellularly. K^+ then binds to E_2—P, initiating hydrolysis of the acylphosphate. This destabilizes E_2, which sponta-

neously reverts to E_1, carrying K^+ into the cell. The cycle is completed as the K^+ dissociates in concert with initiation of the next cycle by ATP binding.

The Na^+,K^+-pump and the cell membrane potential are interactive

The ratio of Na^+ to K^+ exchanged is $3:2$ per mol ATP in almost all systems studied. The net outward flux of positive charge tends to hyperpolarize the membrane. Therefore, the pump is termed *electrogenic*.

Pump-related electrical potentials in excitable cells are usually less than 10 mV, but under certain conditions may be 30 percent of the resting membrane potential. The electrogenic potential of the pump may shorten the duration of the action potential, contribute to negative after-potentials, and, in heart cells, produce the hyperpolarization observed after sustained increases in firing rate. The latter is a possible cause of cardiac arrhythmias.

Because the pump produces net current and electrical potential, conversely, the membrane potential affects the pump rate. An increase in membrane potential (hyperpolarization) reduces the net positive charge efflux. Studies to determine the voltage-sensitive step have utilized the Na^+,K^+-pump reconstituted into liposomes or into black lipid membranes (see Chap. 4). Liposomes can be subjected to a membrane potential by filling them with KCl in the presence of valinomycin. The imposed potential (equivalent to cell depolarization) accelerates Na^+/K^+ exchange up to 30 percent at saturating cytoplasmic Na^+ and ATP concentrations, but not when ATP is rate-limiting. Under the latter condition, the rate-limiting enzyme reaction is $E_2(K^+)_e \rightarrow E_1(K^+)_i$, (Fig. 3, step 6). This step is excluded because voltage dependence is not seen when step 6 is rate-limiting. The accelerating effect of potential is relatively greater at low external ("cytoplasmic") Na^+ concentrations, indicating an increase in the apparent affinity for Na^+. Thus it is suggested that the membrane potential has an effect on

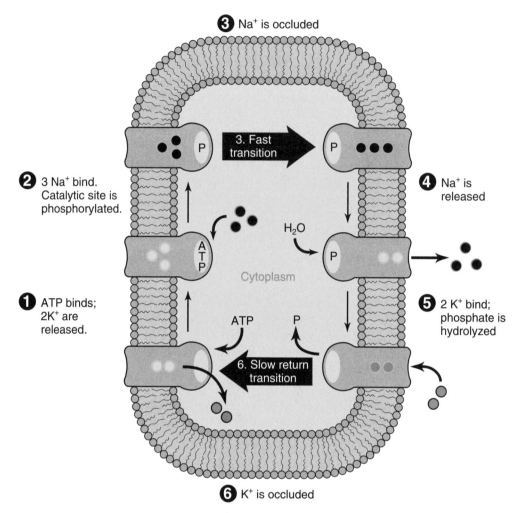

FIG. 3. The mechanism of the ATP-dependent Na$^+$ pump. The sequence of reaction steps is indicated by the *large arrows. On the left,* pump molecules are in the E$_1$ conformation, which has high affinity for Na$^+$ and ATP and low affinity for K$^+$. Ionophoric sites are accessible only from the cytoplasmic side; *step 1:* K$^+$ is discharged as metabolic energy is added to the system by ATP binding; *step 2:* 3 Na$^+$ bind and the enzyme is reversibly phosphorylated. *Step 3:* The conformational transition from E$_1 \sim$ P to E$_2$—P, shown at the top, is the "power stroke" of the pump during which the ionophoric sites with their three bound Na$^+$ ions become accessible to the extracellular side and decrease their affinity for Na$^+$. Part of the free energy of the enzyme acylphosphate has been dissipated in this process. *Step 4:* 3 Na$^+$ dissociate from E$_2$—P; *step 5:* 2 K$^+$ bind and more free energy is dissipated as the enzyme acylphosphate is hydrolyzed. At this point, the 2 K$^+$ become tightly bound ("occluded") and in *step 6:* E$_2$ reverts to E$_1$, carrying the K$^+$ to the cytoplasmic side.

a Na$^+$-dependent enzyme reaction in which there is net transport of one positive charge. A likely candidate is step 3:

$$(Na^+)_i E_1 \sim P \rightarrow (Na^+)_e E_2—P$$

However, recent direct measurements of the transient current induced by pump phosphorylation indicates that the current appears as the sodium ions are discharged [3].

REGULATION OF Na⁺-PUMP EXPRESSION

The activity of Na,K-ATPase increases dramatically during development

The activity of rat brain Na,K-ATPase per milligram of protein increases about ten times from fetal to adult stages [4]. The most rapid increase in Na,K-ATPase is just prior to rapid myelination. This stage, during which membranes become specialized for cation transport, corresponds to the time of glial cell proliferation, intricate elaboration of neuronal and glial processes, and increasing neuronal excitability.

Varying "loads" for Na⁺ secretion or K⁺ uptake can induce different levels of cellular expression

Elevated internal $[Na^+]$ can influence genomic expression either by a direct effect on a DNA-binding site, causing increased expression of the Fos and Jun gene regulatory proteins, or by virtue of an induced rise in $[Ca^{2+}]_i$ which can lead to activation of AP-1 gene regulatory sites [5]. In experimental hypokalemia, compensatory K^+ release from skeletal muscle appears to be achieved by selective down-regulation of the α_2 isoform in muscle [6] concomitant with increased pump activity in the kidneys, which express the α_1 isoform.

The genes for different Na⁺-pump isoforms have different regulatory binding sites. The α- and β-subunits appear to be translated independently in some cells and coordinately in others. However, assembly into heterodimers appears to be necessary prior to Golgi processing and integration into plasma membranes.

Corticosteroids and thyroid hormone participate in homeostatic Na⁺ pump responses to varying degrees in different cells

Thyroid hormone and insulin function in this context during development of the cen-tral nervous system. Thyroid hormone increases metabolic rate of various muscle and epithelial tissues but not of mature brain. An increased cation flux in target tissues is proposed to generate the thermogenic response to thyroid hormone. Thyroid hormone increases the level of pump expression in some tissues [7]. These include skeletal and heart muscle, tissues which can account for most of the thermogenic effect of thyroid. In neonatal, but not in adult, brain both α_1 and α_2 isoforms are increased by thyroid hormone.

Glucocorticosteroids increase Na,K-ATPase activity levels in a number of tissues, including kidney, intestine, and other osmoregulatory tissues, such as fish gills that mediate adaptive responses to maintain salt and water balance. In cardiocytes, aldosterone induces increased expression of α_1 and β_1 mRNAs and increased Na⁺-pump activity [8]. It has been suggested that aldosterone regulation in cardiocytes may involve a Na⁺-sensitive gene regulatory pathway, because the aldosterone-induced increase in mRNA is accompanied by a transient Na⁺ influx and both the mRNA increase and the Na⁺ current are suppressed by the channel-blocking agent, amiloride. Some neurons in adult brain express corticosteroid receptors at high levels (see Chap. 49) but their relationship to Na⁺-pump regulation has not been established.

The inductive effect of adrenal hormones on Na,K-ATPase is pronounced in the developing animal. Maternal adrenalectomy almost completely prevents the normal rise in kidney enzyme activity in the fetus. Significant stimulation of immature kitten and rat cerebral Na,K-ATPase (but not that of adult brain) has been produced by administration of cortisol, methylprednisolone, or ACTH to intact animals.

The Na⁺-pump must often be localized to certain plasma membrane domains to fulfill the requirements of cellular physiology

In almost all epithelial cells adapted for secretion or reabsorption, such as kidney tu-

A

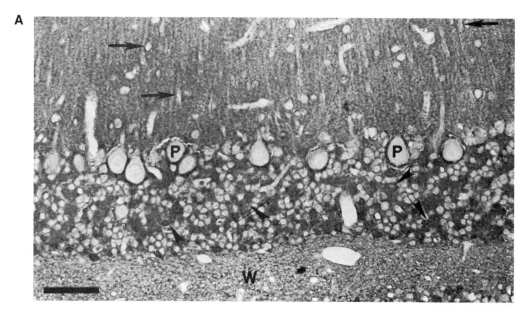

B

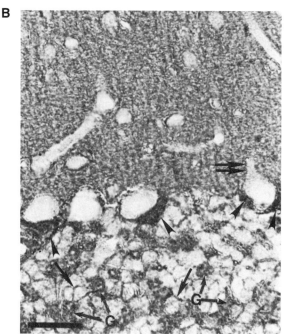

FIG. 4. Localization of the Na^+,K^+-pump in cerebellum and choroid plexus. These figures show immunocytochemical localization in mouse tissues with the peroxidase-conjugated antibody method. **A:** Cerebellum immunoreactivity is seen along the surfaces of Purkinje cell bodies (P) and within synaptic glomeruli of the granular layer *(arrowheads)*. The neuropil of the molecular layer is stained more diffusely and with distinct vertical striations *(arrows)* that extend to the cortical surface. White matter (W), although stained weakly, has punctate deposits throughout. Original magnification: ×315; bar, 50 μm. **B:** Cerebellar cortex has intensely stained basket regions adjacent to Purkinje cells and little staining along the apical dendrites *(double arrows)* of Purkinje cells. While reaction product is dense over glomeruli (G), a fine deposition outlines the plasmalemma of granule cell bodies *(arrows)*. Original magnification: ×620; bar, 50 μm. (From Siegel, Holm, Schreiber, Desmond, and Ernst, *J. Histochem. Cytochem.* 32: 1309, 1984).

bules and exocrine glands, Na,K-ATPase is concentrated asymmetrically on the basolateral or antiluminal surfaces. The two exceptions are the retinal pigment epithelium and choroid plexus ependyma where the enzyme is concentrated on the apical or luminal surface (Fig. 4). These localizations are consistent with the vectorial properties of the transport functions of these cells but the intracellular routing and membrane targeting processes are obscure.

In the nervous system, Na^+-pumps are concentrated in membrane regions associated with high ionic flux, including nodes of

C

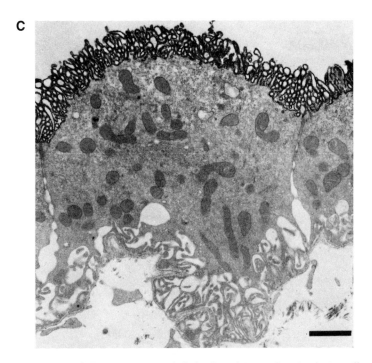

FIG. 4.   *(continued)*. **C.** Choroid plexus contains epithelial cells with intensely stained microvillar and intermicrovillar plasma membranes. The basal and lateral plasma membrane surfaces are not stained. Original magnification ×8,000; bar = 2 μm. (From Ernst, Palacios and Siegel, *J. Histochem. Cytochem* 34:189, 1986.)

Ranvier, axon terminals, synaptic membranes, dendrites, and glial membranes that comprise the neuropil of gray matter. Within the retina, heavy concentrations are found in the retinal photoreceptor inner segments [9].

Within the nervous system, all three α-subunit isoforms are expressed, but to different extents in different regions and cell types. For example, α_3 mRNA is much more abundant than α_1 mRNA in brainstem and subcortical nuclei, spinal anterior and posterior gray columns, and cerebellar Purkinje cells. In the spinal cord, α_1 is restricted to a set of laterally situated anterior horn cells (Fig. 5). The α_1 isoform appears in neurons, glia and Schwann cells, and choroid plexus epithelium. The α_2 isoform is found diffusely throughout the CNS, predominantly in glia, although neuronal localization has not been excluded. The α_3 isoform appears to be restricted to neurons. Different dorsal root ganglion cells can be shown to express α_3 alone or together with α_1.

POST-TRANSLATIONAL REGULATION OF THE Na$^+$-PUMP

Na,K-ATPase activity can be altered by protein kinase A or protein kinase C phosphorylation

Purified Na$^+$-pump can be partially inhibited by phosphorylation, *in vitro*, by cAMP-dependent protein kinase and by Ca^{2+}/diacylglycerol-dependent protein kinase. Addition of the protein phosphatase, calcineurin, can reverse this inhibition. In isolated kidney tubules, dopamine can acutely inhibit pump ATPase whereas α-adrenergic agonists can activate it. In isolated rat brain striatal neurons, substantial inhibition requires their simultaneous exposure to both D$_1$ and D$_2$ do-

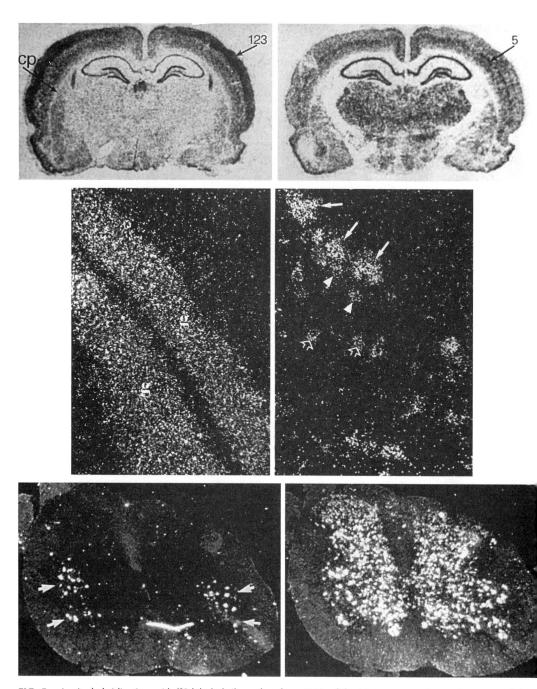

FIG. 5.   *In situ* hybridization with ^{35}S-labeled riboprobes for mRNA of the Na$^+$-pump catalytic subunits, α_1 *(left)* and α_3 *(right).* **Top:** Autoradiogram of rat cerebrum; CP, caudate-putamen; 1,2,3,5 identify cortical layers. **Middle:** Dark field microscopic view of rat cerebellar cortex; g, granule cell layer; *white arrows* indicate Purkinje cells; *arrowheads* indicate basket cells; *open arrows* indicate stellate cells. Magnification: left, ×312; right, ×500. (From Hieber et al. (1991) *Mol. Cell Neurobiol.* 11:253–262, with permission.) **Bottom:** Rat lumbar spinal cord, dark field view; *arrowheads* indicate anterior horn cells. (From Mata, et al., *Brain Res.,* 546:47–54, 1991, with permission.)

pamine agonists and a mechanism involving the kinase-regulated phosphatase inhibitor DARPP32 (see Chap. 22).

In some tissues there appears to be short-term regulation by glucocorticoids that may involve lipocortin and release of arachidonic acid. Clearly different regulatory mechanisms function in different cell types.

Insulin has the short-term effect of reducing K^+ efflux and $[Na^+]_i$ in muscle. Evidence for the existence of latent Na^+-pumps, i.e., intracellular vesicles which can insert rapidly into plasma membranes in response to insulin, has been obtained in skeletal muscle [10]. The α_2 isoform is selectively expressed in these vesicles. Although experimentally induced diabetes is accompanied by reduced Na,K-ATPase activity in sciatic nerve perineurium, dorsal root ganglia, and certain layers of rabbit retina, the genesis of this effect is not known.

The existence of endogenously synthesized Na^+-pump inhibitors is still controversial

Cardiotonic steroids are selective Na^+-pump inhibitors that bind to the α-subunit at a "receptor" of unknown physiological function. The critical requirement for activity of these molecules is that the C/D ring junction must have a *cis* configuration. Steroids of this configuration are produced by a variety of plants and some toads. However their biosynthesis has not been demonstrated in mammals. A variety of putative endogenous Na^+-pump inhibitors have been purified from mammalian tissues and fluids, based on various criteria of similarity to cardiotonic steroids [11].

OTHER ATP-DEPENDENT TRANSPORT SYSTEMS

There are several distinct types of ATP-dependent transport systems

Mitochondria, chloroplasts, and prokaryocyte plasma membranes contain "F type"

ATPases. These function as ATP synthetases by using energy derived from a proton gradient which, in the case of mitochondria, is generated by proton pumps such as cytochrome oxidase. The F-type pump proteins can bind ADP and orthophosphate in close proximity. Proton flow through these pumps induces further conformational transitions involving these binding sites that achieve ATP synthesis by the condensation of the bound ligands with elimination of water. F-type ATPases are complexes of five or more different subunits.

The principal generators of transmembrane cation gradients are members of a family of proteins generally designated "P-type" ATPases because a common feature of their transport mechanisms is the phosphorylation of an aspartyl residue in their major cytoplasmic domain. Structural similarities among the several P-type cation transport ATPases are shown in Fig. 2. In all cases that have been examined, the transport mechanism appears to be analogous to that of Fig. 3. The known functions of these pumps are confined to cation transport across plasma and endoplasmic reticulum membranes. A copper-transporting P-type ATPase is the product of the gene that is defective in Menke's disease ([12], see Chap. 37).

The "V-type" ATP-dependent proton transporters constitute a distinct class that occurs in membranes of Golgi-derived vesicles. V-type pumps occur in lysosomes, endosomes, endocrine secretory vesicles, presynaptic storage vesicles for neurotransmitters and peptide hormones, and in Golgi cisternae. In each case, protons are pumped out of the cytoplasm into the vesicle. Whether all Golgi-derived structures contain identical pumps has not been established. However, one investigation revealed only a single gene coding for the α-subunit of this pump. The multisubunit structures of these proton pumps bear similarities to the F-type ATPases but their sensitivities to inhibitors differ and the sequences of their major subunits are known to differ.

The "ATP-binding cassette" (ABC) proteins constitute a superfamily with members present in species from prokaryocytes to mammals [13]. They have two domains, consisting of six transmembrane segments, alternating with two cytoplasmic nucleotide-binding domains. Some members of this family appear to have dual functions as ATP-dependent peptide transporters and as ATP-regulated chloride channels *(vide infra)*.

The multidrug resistance P-glycoprotein (MDRG) is a member of this family that is expressed in both astrocytes and brain capillary endothelial cells. MDRG may account for some of the drug-exclusion properties of the blood-brain barrier (see Chap. 32; [14]). This protein clearly has the ability to transport a variety of organic compounds out of cells, notably a variety of anti-tumor agents including vinblastine and doxorubicin. Neuroblastomas express variable levels of P-glycoprotein that correlate with their resistance to drug treatment [15].

The P-glycoprotein appears to function both as an ATP-dependent transporter and as a volume-activated ATP-dependent Cl^- channel [16]. Its level of expression has been shown to correlate with the rate of efflux of ATP from cultured cells. This observation has prompted a proposal that some of the transport functions of P-glycoprotein may be energized by the electrochemical gradient of ATP rather than by its hydrolysis. The cystic fibrosis gene product is also a member of the ABC superfamily which displays volume-activated ATP-dependent Cl^- channel activity.

Studies of the patterns of expression of these two proteins suggest that their regulation is coordinately controlled and that both may function as volume-sensitive Cl^- channels in epithelial cells.

Other members of the ABC superfamily participate in transmembrane peptide transport, for example, in the presentation of class I major histocompatibility antigens to the cell surface. This has led to a suggestion that similar transporters may function as peptide hormone transporters [17].

REGULATION OF INTRACELLULAR Ca^{2+}

Low free Ca^{2+} concentrations are maintained in the cytosol by Ca-ATPases and Na^+/Ca^{2+} antiporters

The concentration of cytosolic free Ca^{2+}, $[Ca^{2+}]_i$, is between 10^{-8} and 10^{-7} M in unstimulated cells, which is several orders of magnitude lower than that of extracellular free Ca^{2+}. Cells also maintain stores of Ca^{2+} in the endoplasmic reticulum. Regulation of $[Ca^{2+}]_i$ is vital to the function of all cells, but is particularly important in the regulation of intraneuronal signals. $[Ca^{2+}]_i$ regulates certain plasma membrane cation channels (see Chap. 4), acts in second-messenger systems (see Chaps. 20–22), and participates in neurotransmitter release (see Chap. 9). Impairment of Ca^{2+} regulation can be catastrophic to the cell (see Chap. 42). Ca^{2+} enters the cytosol through both voltage- and ligand-gated channels in the plasma membrane (see Chap. 4) and through ligand-gated channels in the endoplasmic reticulum.

The endoplasmic reticulum contains two distinct, but structurally related Ca^{2+}-release channels

One of them, the IP_3 receptor, binds the second messenger, inositol 1,4,5-trisphosphate with high affinity. The other channel (ryanodine-sensitive) was first identified in muscle as the mediator of the phenomenon of Ca^{2+}-induced Ca^{2+} release. During excitation, extracellular Ca^{2+} enters through voltage-dependent channels in "transverse tubule" extensions of plasma membrane that are closely apposed to sarcoplasmic reticulum containing a high density of ryanodine-sensitive channels. The latter are opened in a highly cooperative manner by Ca^{2+} binding—a positive feedback activation of Ca^{2+} release from the sarcoplasmic store. Similar channels occur in brain and other tissues. The localizations of IP_3- and ryanodine-sensitive channels are distinct and both are expressed in multiple subtypes. In certain cells the Ca^{2+} sensitivity of the ryanodine-sensitive channels can be increased by cyclic adenosine diphosphate ribose (cADPR), which is derived from NAD^+ [18]. In the case of sea urchin eggs, NAD is rapidly converted to cADPR upon sperm-binding, which rapidly releases the ER Ca^{2+}, consistent with a second-messenger role for this molecule. cADPR functions in glucose-activated release of internal Ca^{2+} in pancreatic β cells, whereas IP_3 is ineffective. Both IP_3 and cADPR can activate Ca^{2+} release from cerebellar microsomes.

Regulation of the concentration of $[Ca^{2+}]_i$ is accomplished by an efficient but complex system that involves several different types of transport molecules located in the plasma membrane and in intracellular organelle membranes including mitochondria and endoplasmic reticulum (ER) (Fig. 6; [19]).

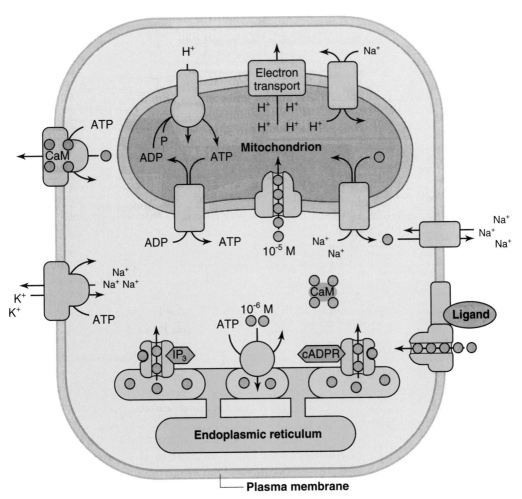

FIG. 6. Ca^{2+} homeostasis. Ca^{2+} ⬤ enters cells through a variety of ligand- and voltage-regulated channels, but intracellular free Ca^{2+} is normally maintained at less than micromolar levels. Intracellular Ca^{2+} is probably regulated coordinately by a Na^+/Ca^{2+} antiporter in plasma membranes and by several different Ca-ATPases in plasma membranes and endoplasmic reticulum. The driving force for Na^+/Ca^{2+} antiporter exchange is the inwardly directed Na^+ gradient which is maintained by the Na,K-ATPase. Mitochondria may participate transiently in Ca^{2+} homeostasis if the capacities of these other systems are exceeded. Internal stores of Ca^{2+} may be released from endoplasmic reticulum through the action of second messengers, such as IP_3 or Ca^{2+} itself, in response to various receptor systems.

TABLE 1.   Calcium homeostasis systems in rat brain

System	Location	M_r	Ca^{2+} affinity	Regulatory molecules	mRNA localizations
SERCA	ER	90–115,000	1 μM	phospholamban	SERCA2: high levels in hippocampus, cerebellar Purkinje neurons
PMCA	PM	130–140,000	100–200 nM	calmodulin	PMCA1: cerebral cortex; hippocampus PMCA2: cerebellar Purkinje neurons PMCA3: choroid plexus; habenula PMCA4: ?
Na^+-Ca^{2+} antiporter	PM	36,000[a]	1–3 μM	?	?
Ca^{2+}-binding proteins	cytoplasm	12–28,000	0.1–10 μM		widely distributed; some have unique localizations

[a] The brain antiporter has been partially purified, but not yet cloned [36].
ER, endoplasmic reticulum; PM, plasma membrane.

Several small (12–28 kDa) cytosolic Ca^{2+}-binding proteins (CBP) with differing distributions in CNS, have affinity constants in the appropriate range (0.1–10 μM) to contribute to Ca^{2+} buffering (Table 1). CBP include calmodulin, parvalbumin, calbindin, and calretinin [19–21]. Calmodulin, one of the most important high affinity CBP, is widely distributed in dendrites and cell bodies of many neurons at high concentrations (>1 mM), but not in presynaptic terminals or axons. It may buffer up to 120 μM cell Ca^{2+} in brain and its total buffering capacity is limited by its concentration in individual cells. The other three proteins appear to have more restricted distributions. For example, in hippocampus, CA1 and CA3 pyramidal neurons do not contain parvalbumin, but some cells of CA1 and CA2 contain calbindin. Granule cells of the dentate gyrus contain calbindin, but not parvalbumin. These interesting patterns of localization have not been explained. In some cases the more important functions of CBP may be as Ca^{2+}-dependent cofactors in signal transduction.

It has been difficult to draw conclusions about the relative contributions to Ca^{2+} regulation made by each of these systems under physiological conditions because selective inhibitors for each system have not been available. Their relative importance has been inferred from studies of the Ca^{2+} affinities of isolated membranes or vesicles. Recently thapsigargin, a sesquiterpene lactone, was found to selectively inhibit smooth endoplasmic reticulum Ca-ATPase (SERCA) activity [22]. It may provide a means to determine the contribution of the ER pump to regulation of Ca^{2+} homeostasis.

SERCA is the best understood regulator of intracellular Ca^{2+}[20]

This transporter, $M_r \sim 100,000$, has been purified from skeletal muscle where it brings about muscle relaxation by sequestering cytoplasmic calcium into the sarcoplasmic reticulum (see Chap. 33). It has a relatively low affinity for Ca^{2+} ($K_m \sim 1$ μM Ca^{2+}) and may be involved in fine-tuning the cytosolic Ca^{2+} levels in many cell types. Molecular cloning studies have demonstrated at least three separate genes for SERCA. Of these, SERCA-2 is the major form expressed in brain. *In situ* hybridization studies [23] have shown SERCA-2 to be widely distributed, and expressed at high levels in cerebellar Purkinje cells, hippocampus, cerebral cortex, thalamus, and other areas. SERCA contains a domain which interacts with phospholamban, a small protein which can be phosphorylated by cAMP-dependent protein kinase. Phosphorylation of phospholamban leads to increased pump activity [24]. Recent studies using the Ca^{2+}-pump inhibitor, thapsigargin [22], demonstrated that SERCA activity in brain is very low compared to that of skeletal and cardiac muscle.

Mitochondria contain Ca^{2+}-linked antiporters which participate in intracellular Ca^{2+} regulation [19,20]

They can accumulate large amounts of Ca^{2+}, but uptake appears to be an order of magnitude lower than that of ER. The affinity of mitochondria for Ca^{2+} ($K_m \sim 10$ μM) is probably insufficient for a role in regulation of reactions except under conditions when large influxes of Ca^{2+} occur and other homeostatic processes are unable to regulate Ca^{2+} levels. Ca^{2+} is transported into respiring mitochondria by a secondary transport process driven by the membrane potential. Ca^{2+} uptake is compensated by extrusion of 2 H^+ produced by the respiratory chain. Extrusion occurs primarily by a separate Na^+/Ca^{2+} antiporter, similar to that present in the plasma membrane.

Plasma membranes contain two types of Ca^{2+} transporters

The first is a low affinity, high transport capacity Na^+/Ca^{2+}-exchanger or antiporter. It is energetically driven by the Na^+ gradient (Fig. 6). Although its normal function is to transport Ca^{2+} out of cells, it has been found that either raising $[Na^+]_i$ or lowering $[Na^+]_o$ induces Ca^{2+} influx into cells. The exchange or antiport process is electrogenic since the stoichiometry is 3 Na^+ per Ca^2 in most tissues [25]. The antiporter has a low affinity for Ca^{2+} with $K_m \sim 10$-15 μM, but the presence of ATP reduces K_m values for Ca^{2+} to about

1–3 μM [25]. Since the antiporter may pump up to ten times as much Ca^{2+} as the Ca-ATPase in some tissues, it has been speculated that the antiporter could be the sole regulator of intracellular Ca^{2+} ions. The low Ca^{2+} affinity of the antiporter makes it an unlikely candidate for setting resting $[Ca^{2+}]_i$ which is approximately 50–200 nM. Also the voltage dependence of the system might lead to reversal of its transport mode from extrusion to influx during cell stimulation [25]. The role of the antiporter at different stages and levels of intracellular Ca^{2+} remains to be determined. Intracellular Na^+/Ca^{2+} antiporters present in both ER and mitochondria may also play a significant role in calcium regulation.

Plasma membranes also have Ca-ATPase (PMCA) activities which possess high affinity for Ca^{2+} ($K_m \sim 100$-200 nM), but relatively low transport capacity [24]. The stoichiometry of PMCA is one Ca^{2+} transported for each ATP hydrolyzed. These pumps probably do not carry out bulk movements of Ca^{2+}, but are most effective in maintaining very low levels of cytosolic Ca^{2+} in resting cells. PMCAs have structural as well as enzymatic similarities to SERCAs. A distinguishing characteristic of the PMCA is activation by calmodulin. In the absence of calmodulin the K_m for Ca^{2+} is 5–10 μM. Calmodulin is activated by Ca^{2+} and subsequently the activated calmodulin binds to the PMCA, decreasing its K_m for Ca^{2+} by 20–30 fold. This highly cooperative activation mechanism is very sensitive to small changes in $[Ca^{2+}]_i$.

The plasma membrane Ca^{2+}-pumps have $M_r \sim 130$-140,000, whereas the SERCAs have $M_r \sim 90$-115,000. The increased size of PMCA is due to a calmodulin-binding domain near the C-terminus. A family of at least five PMCAs have been described and form a multigene family [26]. Three isoforms (mRNA) found in rat brain were designated PMCA1, PMCA2, and PMCA3. A fourth, PMCA4, has been found in human teratoma cells and rat and bovine brain [27]. Complex distributions of isoforms are found in rat brain [28]. PMCA1 mRNA is widely distributed in rat tissues with highest levels in CA1 pyramidal cells of hippocampus. Cerebellar Purkinje neurons have the highest levels of PMCA2 mRNA and PMCA3 is highest in habenula and choroid plexus. The isoforms found in rat brain range in molecular weight from about 127,000 to 133,000 with 81 to 85 percent amino acid sequence homology. In addition several alternatively spliced variants accounting for a total of nine possible PMCA molecules have been described [27]. However, the biochemical and transport properties of the individual molecules are unknown and it has not been determined if all are transcribed into protein. Individual plasma membrane isoforms may differ in Ca^{2+} affinities or other functional characteristics.

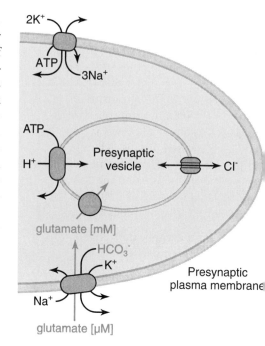

SECONDARY TRANSPORT SYSTEMS

Numerous secondary active transport systems are important mediators of neural functions

Active transport of a variety of molecules and ions occurs via specific carriers linked to the Na^+ gradient (Fig. 1). Symporters mediate neurotransmitter and amino acid uptake. Antiporters include systems that remove cytoplasmic calcium ions and protons. Several examples of each of these will be discussed in succeeding sections.

The uptake of amine and amino acid neurotransmitters from the synaptic cleft and their storage in vesicles is accomplished by the tandem action of two transport systems

These are localized, respectively, in the presynaptic plasmalemma and in the storage vesicle membranes (Fig. 7). Two different families of plasmalemma neurotransmitter transporters have been identified [29]. Both of these appear to be distinct from other identified families of Na^+-dependent cotransporters.

FIG. 7.　Processes involved in neurotransmitter uptake at nerve endings. Concentration into the cytoplasm is achieved by means of a Na^+ symporter with high affinity for the neurotransmitter. Synaptic vesicles membranes contain an ATP-dependent proton pump and Cl^- channels which acidify their internal space. These membranes also contain transporters that are selective for the neurotransmitter. Whether these operate as proton antiporters or as potential-driven facilitators has not been determined.

One family includes transporters specific respectively for GABA, glycine, choline, proline, taurine, norepinephrine, dopamine, and serotonin. These proteins consist of about 630 residues and, based upon hydropathy plots, are considered to have a topology that traverses the plasma membrane 12 or 13 times. There is 45 to 70 percent sequence similarity among the members of this group. Abolition of the transmembrane Na^+ gradient blocks the uptake of these neurotransmitters. Transport has been shown to be Cl^--dependent in the cases of GABA, glycine, and serotonin. Thus, amino acid or amine uptake by this family of transporters is energized by coupling to Na^+ and, in most ases, Cl^- symport and ultimately derives from the Na^+,K^+-pump.

The pharmacology of the plasmalemma transporters is under intense study with the object of designing drugs that can modulate the uptake of specific transmitters. Drugs that affect dopamine, norepinephrine, and serotonin uptake are known to alter mood and behavior (see Chaps. 41 and 48). Cocaine blocks norepinephrine, dopamine, and serotonin plasmalemma transporters with apparent K_i's of 10^{-7}, 10^{-6}, and 10^{-6} M, respectively. Transport blocking agents, such as GBR12909, have been found that have higher affinity for the dopamine transporter ($K_i \sim 10^{-9}$ M) and 100-fold less affinity for the norepinephrine transporter. The antidepressants, paroxetine, and chlorimipramine, are potent inhibitors of the serotonin transporter ($K_i \sim 10^{-9} - 10^{-10}$ M).

Members of the second identified family of plasma membrane transporters are specific for glutamate and aspartate. Two identified members of this family, designated GLAST-1 and GLT-1, appear to be specific to brain and are expressed predominantly in glia. GLAST-1 mRNA is expressed diffusely throughout the cerebrum, but is restricted to the Purkinje cell layer of cerebellar cortex. A third member, EAAC-1, is expressed abundantly in brain, intestine, and kidney and at lower levels in liver and heart. Within brain, EAAC-1 mRNA is found predominantly in neurons, especially in certain neuronal subsets of hippocampus, cerebellar cortex, and cerebral cortex. The neuronal uptake of glutamate and aspartate may be critical for regulating presynaptic transmitter supplies and receptor sensitivities in local networks where transmission rates may be high.

These three transporters have about 50 percent sequence similarity and an inferred topology of 6 to 10 transmembrane segments. They all energize amino acid uptake by Na^+ symport coupled to K^+ antiport and are Cl^--independent. While they are all specific for glutamate and aspartate, the details of glutamate transport may vary among them. GLT-1, expressed in HeLa cells, has an apparent K_m for L-glutamate of about 2 μM, whereas that for EAAC-1, expressed in *Xenopus* oocytes, is reported as 12 μM.

A study of glutamate uptake by salamander retinal glia suggests a stoichiometry of 1 $glu^- + 2\ Na^+$ taken into the cell in exchange for the extrusion of 1 K^+ and 1 HCO_3^- or OH^-. The net influx of 1 positive charge produces membrane depolarization. The anion efflux produces an internal acidification. With this stoichiometry and a "normal" membrane potential and ion concentrations, the transporter could theoretically reduce extracellular glutamate to 0.6 μM. However, under depolarizing or anoxic conditions, the membrane potential will fall and the Na^+ and K^+ gradients will be reduced to levels that theoretically allow extracellular accumulation of ~370 μM glutamate. Thus, under conditions such as seizure, anoxia, ischemia, and hypoglycemia, there may be an efflux of glutamate through the transporters, raising external glutamate to toxic levels (see Chaps. 17 and 42). In addition, sustained glutamatergic neuronal transmission may, because of the increased rate of glutamate uptake, be a cause of intracellular acidosis, reduced membrane potentials, and reduction of Na^+ and K^+ gradients such as are associated with seizures.

Operating in tandem with the plasmalemma transporters are the ATP-dependent systems that concentrate neurotransmitters in presynaptic vesicles (Fig. 7). Protons are transported into the vesicles by a vacuolar-type ATPase, as discussed above. The concentrative uptake of GABA, glutamate, glycine, acetylcholine, and the catecholamines are each mediated by specific transporters in the vesicle membranes. It appears that the import of neurotransmitters can be energized by either the proton gradient or the membrane potential, depending on pH and $[Cl^-]$ [30].

Monoamine vesicular transporters are characterized by a broad selectivity, encompassing dopamine, norepinephrine, seroto-nin, and also by reserpine inhibition. Two slightly different forms have been cloned and sequenced. One is expressed in mono-amine-containing cells of brain and the other is primarily expressed in adrenal chro-maffin cells. The brain form displays highest affinity for serotonin with an apparent K_m ~ 2 μM. Predictions from hydropathy plots predict 12 transmembrane segments in both cases.

Vesicle transporters for the amino acid neurotransmitters have been partially puri-fied and reconstituted into liposomes, but not yet cloned and sequenced. These trans-porters share several features. They have low affinity and high specificity for their particu-lar neurotransmitter. In general they do not transport or interact with the various analogs that bind to receptors. Thus neuronal neuro-transmitter specificity, in the case of amino acid neurotransmitters, is displayed by both the plasmalemma and synaptical vesicle transporters. The neuronal specificity for a particular monoamine may be characterized by its plasmalemma transporters and by the presence of key biosynthetic enzymes, rather than by synaptic vesicle transporters.

Uptake into vesicles can be blocked by nigericin, proton ionophores, or other agents which dissipate the proton gradient, and by *N*-ethylmaleimide which inhibits V-type ATPases. Uptake into synaptic vesicles is not affected by agents that act on other transport systems such as Na^+, Ca^{2+}, ouabain, vanadate, or oligomycin. A low concentra-tion of extravesicular Cl^- stimulates the up-take of glutamate and catecholamines into their respective vesicles but does not affect glycine or GABA vesicular uptake.

Regulation of extracellular K+, intracellular water, and pH

Rapid Clearance of K+ from the Extracellular Space is Critically Important Because Elevated Extracellular K+ Increases Neuronal Excitability

Normal neuronal activity can lead to eleva-tions of 1–3 mM in extracellular K^+ ($[K^+]_e$) and, during epileptogenesis, levels can be 3–4 times higher (see Chap. 43). Both neu-rons and astroglia are involved in K^+ uptake and both active and passive transport are probably important. The relative contribu-tions of the two cell types and of the two cell processes remains controversial. It is clear that neurons accumulate K^+ almost exclu-sively by means of active transport, but the Na^+,K^+-pump is slow relative to the channel-mediated K^+ release from neurons and to the rates of K^+ increase in the extracellular space. Moreover, the neuronal Na^+,K^+-pump is satu-rated at low $[K^+]_e$ making it a poor regulator for this purpose.

Astroglia can take up K^+ passively by a process termed spatial buffering (Fig. 8A). In this case the K^+ conductance of perineuro-nal glial processes is high relative to that of neurons. A high local $[K^+]_e$ can diffuse into the glial cytoplasm and an equal amount of K^+ can exit from distal processes of the same cell or from cells coupled to them by gap junctions, into regions where the $[K^+]_e$ is lower. K^+ is thereby transferred away from the site where the initial increase has oc-curred. K^+ can then be recovered by neurons at the slower pace consistent with normal Na^+,K^+-pump activity. The process of spatial buffering has received strong support in the case of Müller cells, glia that extend from the

---

FIG. 8.   **A:** Spatial buffering by astrocytes. This conceptual diagram indicates the pathways available for K^+ ions to diffuse through the glial syncytium ⬤ subsequent to their release from neuronal membranes ◯ during neural activity. **B:** Regulation of cell volume. The mechanisms of osmotic activation of ion pathways vary with cell type. Detection of volume changes may involve cytoskeletal proteins which interact with channels and/or transporters. Regulatory volume decrease (RVD) may be initiated by stretch-activated channels that permit efflux of KCl. Acute regulatory volume increase (RVI) produces Na^+ Cl^- influx, with or without coupling to K^+ influx. Chronic exposure to hypertonic media initiates adaptation mechanisms that include transcriptional activation of osmolyte symporters.

A

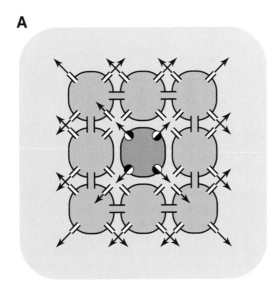

⬗ Voltage gated
potassium channels

∥ Inward-rectifying
potassium channels

▤ Gap junctions

B

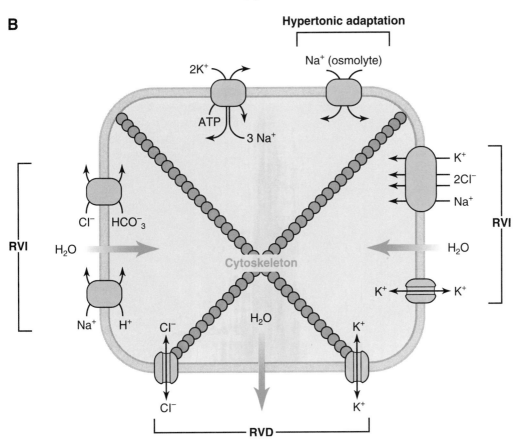

pigment epithelium to the vitreous surface of the retina. Most of the K^+-conductance channels of this cell are localized to the Müller cell end feet which contact the vitreous surface, so that high concentrations of K^+ at the basal surface lead to K^+ efflux at the end feet [31]. Another proposed mechanism to facilitate K^+ uptake into glia is based on the regulation of Cl^- channels *(vide infra)*.

Intracellular pH can be regulated by ATP-dependent proton pumps, by Na^+/H^+ antiporters and by anion antiporters

Cerebral metabolic energy is primarily derived from the oxidation of glucose to CO_2 which, in the steady-state, could enter the circulation without disturbing the ionic balance. However, to the extent that oxidation is incomplete, i.e., that there is lactate or ketoacid production (see Chap. 31) or that CO_2 equilibrates to $H^+ + HCO_3^-$, local pH will decrease. *In vivo* cerebral respiration is profoundly sensitive to pH, decreasing with decreasing pH, so that without adequate pH control, local metabolic deficits may be intensified and propagated [32].

Many epithelial cells can extrude protons via a transport ATPase in their plasma membranes. The best characterized mammalian enzyme of this type is the type-2 H,K-ATPase from gastric epithelia. Its occurrence in neural tissue has not been reported.

A Na^+/H^+ antiporter occurs in synaptosomes, in glia, and in neuroblastoma cells (Fig. 8B). It is relatively inactive at neutral pH. However, a decrease in intracellular pH produces an efflux of protons at the expense of the Na^+ gradient. Although the antiporter has a Na^+/H^+ stoichiometry of $1:1$, it is allosterically regulated by the internal pH: protonation of a cytoplasmic site increases the affinity of the proton ionophoric site, thus amplifying its sensitivity to changes in intracellular pH. The Na^+/H^+ antiporter is also regulated by receptor mechanisms in some cells. Several growth factors and hormones produce transient cytoplasmic alkalinization, perhaps by mediating a protein kinase phosphorylation of the antiporter to increase its internal proton affinity. Other mechanisms may also be important for local pH control. The combined activities of a HCO_3^-/Cl^- antiporter and carbonic anhydrase mediate CO_2 transport in erythrocytes. A similar system may play a role in pH regulation in brain.

The volume of a cell is determined by its content of osmotically active impermeant molecules and ions (Fig. 8B)

Cell volume will change because of an altered internal solute content (isotonic response) or because of altered extracellular solute content (hyper- or hypotonic responses). Impairment of brain energy metabolism, such as may ensue from ischemia, anoxia, or trauma, produces an isotonic cellular swelling called "cytotoxic edema" and produces further effects by the coincident release of glutamate (see Chaps. 40 and 42). Cellular swelling ensues from extracellular hypotonicity. This is most often manifest as hyponatremia, which may ensue acutely from post-surgical fluid therapies. Chronic hyponatremia can result from congestive heart failure, Addison's disease, or a "syndrome of inappropriate vasopressin release." A general reduction in brain size resulting from acute extracellular hypertonicity, may produce neurological disturbances. This condition may be a component of pathology such as kidney disease (uremia) and diabetes mellitus (hyperglycemia).

Cells have short-term mechanisms that tend to restore their volume toward "normal" primarily by shifting the distributions of Na^+, K^+, and Cl^-. The details of the mechanisms appear to vary with cell type. Subsequent to cell swelling, regulatory volume decrease (RVD) usually involves opening ion channels. Subsequent to hyperosmotic shrinking regulatory volume increase (RVI) frequently involves activation of (Na^+/H^+) antiporters and $(Na^+, K^+, 2 Cl^-)$ symporters. The primary detectors of volume and osmotic changes are presently unknown. Since cell membranes can readily change shape but do not stretch significantly, whereas cytoskeletal elements form tensile elements, the latter are more likely candidates. Cell shape is determined by the interactions of cytoskeletal elements, membranes, and components of the extracellular matrix (see Chaps. 2 and 27). Stretch-activated cation channels have been demonstrated in both neuroblastoma cells and astrocytes in culture. Activation of Cl^- channels by cellular swelling is an identified characteristic of both the MDR and CFTR proteins [13], at least one of which occurs in astrocytes.

Altered extracellular tonicity can induce compensatory changes in the concentrations of certain intracellular substances, termed osmolytes. These mechanisms involve gene regulation. Glioma cells in culture have been shown to respond within a few hours exposure to hypertonic medium by transcribing high levels of the Na^+/inositol symporter [33]. In brain, active osmolytes include taurine, glutamine, glutamate, *myo*-inositol, creatine, glycerophosphorylcholine, and choline. Na^+-dependent symporters for most of these compounds have been identified [33].

There may be multiple mechanisms of K^+ clearance by glia

Glial processes invest nearly all extrasynaptic neuronal processes. Thus, the extracellular space of neuropil consists primarily of the 150–250 Å clefts between glia and neurons. Neural activity discharges K^+ into this space which lowers the membrane potential of adjacent cells. Usually the upper limit of axonal impulse conduction frequency is set by a conduction block that occurs when extracellular K^+ accumulates to 25–30 mM. Depolarization by high levels of extracellular K^+ can have indirect effects on dendrites, soma, and nerve terminals, leading to repetitive firing and such phenomena as spreading depression.

Glial cells have higher K^+ permeability than most neurons. Because individual glial cells ramify among different neurons and are interconnected to other glial cells by gap junctions, the K^+ efflux of any given neuron can distribute into the local glial syncytium and compensatory K^+ efflux will occur through the more distal reaches of the syncytium where the external $[K^+]$ is lower. It should be noted that this process has no energy input. The glia simply provide an extensive pathway for K^+ to diffuse from a higher to a lower concentration. In retinal Müller cells, a form of glial cell that extends from the deep layers of the retina to the vitreous humor, this is an important clearance mechanism [34]. Glial swelling has been shown to accompany neural activity. This suggests a K^+ clearance mechanism resulting from activation of the $(Na^+, K^+, 2 Cl^-)$ symporter as in the RVI mechanism discussed above. This symporter does have an energy input, the Na^+ gradient coupled to the Na^+ pump, and could operate where a large K^+ sink is not present. As noted, the α_2 isoform of the Na^+ pump is expressed in glia. This isoform also occurs in muscle, in which case it resides in a latent pool of vesicles that insert into the plasma membrane upon hormonal activation.

Glucose crosses the blood-brain barrier and the plasma membranes of most cells via a facilitated diffusion process

It is noteworthy that, despite the vital dependence of brain on an adequate supply of glucose (see Chap. 31), it appears to have no cellular mechanism for active transport of glucose. Instead, local blood flow must be regulated to supply the local metabolic requirements (see Chaps. 31 and 46).

Five different isoforms (GLUT 1–5) of glucose facilitators have been identified in mammalian cells. They seem to vary chiefly in their responses to regulatory influences: GLUT 1 is negatively regulated by glucose; GLUT 4 can be held in an extracellular reserve of endocytotic vesicles that respond to insulin by fusion with the plasma membrane.

Although regulation of the other forms has not been defined, they are all differentially expressed. GLUT 3 is expressed by glia and certain neurons, whereas GLUT 1 is expressed in the brain epithelial and endothelial cells that comprise the blood-brain barrier and also in glia, Schwann cells, and perineurium of peripheral nerves. The other isoforms have not been conclusively identified in brain. The high rate of glucose utilization by neurons and the fact that GLUT 3 is not demonstrable in all neurons, suggest that there may be yet unidentified mediators of neuronal glucose transport [35].

REFERENCES

1. Laüger, P. *Electrogenic Ion Pumps.* Sunderland, MA: Sinauer Associates, 1991.
2. Stahl, W. L. The Na,K-ATPase of nervous tissue. *Neurochem. Int.* 8:449–476, 1986.
3. Fendler, K., Froehlich, J., Jaruschewski, S., et al. *Correlation of charge translocation with the reaction cycle of the Na,K-ATPase.* Woods Hole, MA: Rockefeller University Press, 1991.
4. Bertoni, J. M., and Siegel, G. J. Development of Na,K-ATPase in rat cerebrum: correlation with Na^+-dependent phosphorylation and K^+-p-nitrophenylphosphatase. *J. Neurochem.* 31:1501–1511, 1978.
5. Rayson, B. M. $[Ca^{2+}]_i$ regulates transcription rate of the Na^+/K^+-ATPase α_1 subunit. *J. Biol. Chem.* 266:21335–21338, 1991.
6. McDonough, A. A., Hensley, C. B., and Azuma, K. K. Differential regulation of sodium pump isoforms in heart. *Semin. Nephrol.* 12:49–55, 1992.
7. Ismail-Beigi, F. Regulation of Na^+,K^+-ATPase expression by thyroid hormone. *Semin. Nephrol.* 12:44–48, 1992.
8. Ikeda, U., Hyman, R., Smith, T. W., and Medford, R. M. Aldosterone-mediated regulation of Na^+,K^+-ATPase gene expression in adult and neonatal rat cardiocytes. *J. Biol. Chem.* 266:12058–12066, 1991.
9. McGrail, K. M., Phillips, J. M., and Sweadner, K. J. Immunofluorescent localization of three Na,K-ATPase isozymes in the rat central nervous system: both neurons and glia can express more than one Na,K-ATPase. *J. Neurosci.* 11:381–391, 1991.
10. Hundal, H. S., Marette, A., Mitsumoto, Y., Ramlal, T., Blostein, R., and Klip, A. Insulin induces translocation of the α_2- and β_1-subunits of the Na^+/K^+-ATPase from intracellular compartments to the plasma membrane in mammalian skeletal muscle. *J. Biol. Chem.* 267:5040–5043, 1992.
11. Kelly, R. A., and Smith, T. W. Is ouabain the endogenous digitalis? [Editorial]. *Circulation* 86:694–697, 1992.
12. Vulpe, C., Levinson, B., Whitney, S., Packman, S., and Gitschier, J. Isolation of a candidate gene for Menkes disease and evidence that it encodes a copper-transporting ATPase. *Nature Genetics* 3:7–13, 1993.
13. Hyde, S. C., Emsley, P., Hartshorn, M. J., et al. Structural model of ATP-binding proteins associated with cystic fibrosis, multidrug resistance and bacterial transport. *Nature* 346:362–365, 1990.
14. Tatsuta, T., Naito, M., Ohara, T., Sugawara, I., and Tsuruo, T. Functional involvement of P-glycoprotein in blood-brain barrier. *J. Biol. Chem.* 267(28):20383–20391, 1992.
15. Chan, H. S., Haddad, G., Thorner, P. S., et al. P-glycoprotein expression as a predictor of the outcome of therapy for neuroblastoma. *N. Engl. J. Med.* 325:1608–1614, 1991.
16. Gill, D. R., Hyde, S. C., Higgins, C. F., Valverde, M. A., Mintenig, G. M., and Sepulveda, F. V. Separation of drug transport and chloride channel functions of the human multidrug resistance P-glycoprotein. *Cell* 71:23–32, 1992.
17. Becker, K. F., Allmeier, H., and Hollt, V. New mechanisms of hormone secretion: MDR-like gene products as extrusion pumps for hormones? *Horm. Metab. Res.* 24:210–213, 1992.
18. Galione, A. Cyclic ADP-ribose: a new way to control calcium. *Science* 259:325–326, 1993.
19. Miller, R. The control of neuronal Ca^{2+} homeostasis. *Prog. Neurobiol.* 37:255–285, 1991.
20. Carafoli, E. Intracellular calcium homeostasis. *Annu. Rev. Biochem.* 56:395–433, 1987.
21. McBurney, R. N., and Neering, I. R. Neuronal calcium homeostasis. *Trends Neurosci.* 10:164–169, 1987.
22. Kijima, Y., Ogunbunmi, E., and Fleischer, S. Drug action of thapsigargin on the Ca^{2+} pump protein of sarcoplasmic reticulum. *J. Biol. Chem.* 266:22912–22918, 1991.
23. Miller, K. K., Verma, A., Snyder, S. H., and Ross, C. A. Localization of an endoplasmic

reticulum calcium ATPase mRNA in rat brain by in situ hybridization. *Neuroscience* 43:1–9, 1991.

24. Carafoli, E. The calcium pumping ATPase of the plasma membrane. *Annu. Rev. Physiol.* 53: 531–547, 1991.

25. Allen, T., Noble, D., and Reuter, H. *Sodium-Calcium Exchange.* New York: Oxford Press, 1989.

26. Strehler, E. Plasma membrane Ca^{2+} pumps and Na^+/Ca^{2+} exchangers. *Semins. Cell Biol.* 1: 283–295, 1990.

27. Brandt, P., and Neve, R. L. Expression of plasma membrane calcium-pumping ATPase mRNAs in developing rat brain and adult brain subregions: evidence for stage-specific expression. *J. Neurochem.* 59:1566–1569, 1992.

28. Stahl, W. L., Eakin, T. J., Owens, J. W. M., et al. Plasma membrane Ca^{2+}-ATPase isoforms: distribution of mRNAs in rat brain by in situ hybridization. *Brain Res. Mol. Brain Res.* 16(3–4):223–231, 1992.

29. Amara, S. A tale of two families. *Nature* 360: 420–421, 1992.

30. Tabb, J., FE, K., van Dyke, K., and Ueda, T. Glutamate transport into synaptic vesicles. *J. Biol. Chem.* 267:15412–15418, 1992.

31. Newman, E. A. Distribution of potassium conductance in mammalian Müller (glial) cells: a comparative study. *J. Neurosci.* 7:2423–2432, 1987.

32. Siejö, B. K., von Hanwehr, R., Nergelius, G., Nevander, G., and Ingvar, M. Extra- and intracellular pH in the brain during seizures and in the recovery period following the arrest of seizure activity. *J. Cereb. Blood Flow Metab.* 5(1): 47–57, 1985.

33. Strange, K. Regulation of solute and water balance and cell volume in the central nervous system [editorial]. *J. Am. Soc. Nephrol.* 3: 12–27, 1992.

34. Karwoski, C. J., Lu, H. K., and Newman, E. A. Spatial buffering of light-evoked potassium increases by retinal Müller (glial) cells. *Science* 244:578–580, 1989.

35. Mantych, G. J., James, D. E., Chung, H. D., and Devaskar, S. U. Cellular localization and characterization of Glut 3 glucose transporter isoform in human brain. *Endocrinology* 131: 1270–1278, 1992.

36. Michaelis, M. L., Nunley, E. W., Jayawickreme, C., Hurlbert, M., Schueler, S., and Guilly, C. *J. Neurochem.* 58:147–157, 1992.

CHAPTER 4

Electrical Excitability and Ion Channels

BERTIL HILLE AND WILLIAM A. CATTERALL

Basic Neurochemistry: Molecular, Cellular, and Medical Aspects, 5th Ed., edited by G. J. Siegel et al. Published by Raven Press, Ltd., New York, 1994. Correspondence to Bertil Hille, Department of Physiology and Biophysics (SJ-40), G424 Health Sciences Bldg, University of Washington School of Medicine, Seattle, Washington 98195.

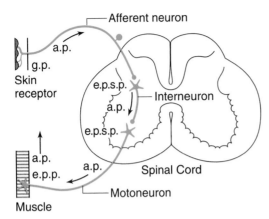

FIG. 1. Path of excitation in a simplified spinal reflex that mediates withdrawal of the arm from a painful stimulus. In each of the three neurons and in the muscle cell, excitation starts with a localized slow potential and is propagated via an action potential (a.p.). The slow potentials are generator potential (g.p.) at the skin; excitatory postsynaptic potentials (e.p.s.p.) at the interneuron and the motoneuron; and end-plate potential (e.p.p.) at the neuromuscular junction. Each neuron makes additional connections to other pathways that are not shown.

The nervous system enables animals to receive and act on internal and external stimuli with speed and in a coordinated manner. Activity of the nervous system is reflected in a variety of electrical and chemical signals that arise in the receptor organs, the nerve cells, and the effector organs, including the muscles and secretory glands. Consider, for example, a simple reflex arc mediating reflex withdrawal of the hand from a hot surface. Four cell types are involved in a network shown diagrammatically in Fig. 1. The message travels from skin receptors through the network as a volley of electrical disturbances, terminating in the contraction of some muscles. This chapter concerns the origin of electrical potentials in such excitable cells. As we shall see, potentials are generated by the passive diffusion of ions such as Na^+, K^+, Ca^{2+}, and Cl^-, through highly selective molecular pores in the cell surface membrane called ion channels. Over 100 genes coding for subunits of ion channels have been identified. Ion channels play a role in membrane excitation as central as the role of enzymes

in metabolism. The opening and closing of specific channels shape the membrane potential changes and give rise to characteristic electrical messages. (The interested reader is referred to Hodgkin [1], Armstrong [2], Nicholls et al. [3] and Hille [4,5] for more detailed treatment of this subject.)

ELECTRICAL PHENOMENA IN EXCITABLE CELLS

All excitable cells have a membrane potential

At rest, the entire cytoplasm is electrically more negative than the external bathing fluid by 30 to 100 mV. All of this potential drop appears across the extremely thin external cell membrane, as may be ascertained by recording with an electrolyte-filled glass pipette microelectrode. When such an electrode is used to probe potentials around an excitable cell, a sudden negative drop appears at the moment the thin tip of the pipette breaks through the cell surface. By convention, the membrane potential is always reported in terms of "inside" minus "outside," so the resting potential is a negative number; for example, -70 mV in a myelinated nerve fiber. Signals that make the cytoplasm more positive are said to depolarize the membrane, and those making it more negative are said to hyperpolarize the membrane.

Electrical signals recorded from cells are basically of two types: stereotyped action potentials characteristic of each cell type and a variety of slow potentials

The action potential of axons is a brief, spike-like depolarization that propagates regeneratively as an electrical wave without decrement and at a high, constant velocity from one end of the axon to the other [3]. It is used for all rapid signaling over a distance. For example, in the reflex arc of Fig. 1, action potentials in motor axons might carry the message from spinal cord to arm, telling the muscle fibers of the biceps to contract. In large mammalian axons at body temperature, the action potential at any one patch of membrane may last only 0.4 msec as it propagates at a speed of 100 m/sec. The action potential is normally elicited when the cell membrane is depolarized by some type of stimulus to beyond a threshold level; and it is said to be produced in an all-or-nothing manner because a subthreshold stimulus gives no propagated response, whereas every suprathreshold stimulus elicits the stereotyped propagating wave. Underlying the propagated action potential is a regenerative wave of opening and closing of voltage-gated ion channels that sweeps along the axon. Action potentials are also frequently referred to as spikes, or impulses. Most nerve cell and muscle cell membranes can make action potentials and are said to be electrically excitable, but a few cannot.

By contrast, slow potentials are localized membrane depolarizations and hyperpolarizations, with time courses ranging from several milliseconds to minutes. They are associated with a variety of transduction mechanisms. For example, slow potentials arise at the synaptic site of action of neurotransmitter molecules (see Chap. 10) and of some hormones, and also in sensory endings of chemosensors (see Chap. 8), mechanosensors, and photoreceptors (see Chap. 7). These electrical signals in sensory endings are frequently called generator, or receptor, potentials, and the signals arising postsynaptically at chemical synapses are called postsynaptic potentials. Slow potentials are graded in relation to their stimulus and sum with each other both spatially and temporally within the cell while decaying passively over a distance of no more than a few millimeters from their site of generation. Underlying the slow potential is a graded and local opening or closing of ion channels reflecting the intensity of the stimulus. These channels are gated by stimuli other than voltage. The natural stimulus for the initiation of propagated action potentials is a depolarizing slow potential exceeding the firing threshold. Thus, impulses in a wide variety of presynaptic cells often give rise to a barrage of excitatory (depolarizing) and inhibitory (hyperpolarizing) postsynaptic potentials in the dendrites of a postsynaptic neuron. These slow potentials sum within the dendrites and cell body to provide the drive stimulating or suppressing initiation of action potentials at the axon hillock, which then propagate down the axon. In each of the four cell populations involved in the reflex arc in Fig. 1, depolarizing slow potentials give rise to propagating action potentials as the message moves forward.

THE IONIC HYPOTHESIS AND THE MEMBRANE THEORY

In the late nineteenth century, such scientific giants as Kohlrausch, Arrhenius, Ostwald, Nernst, and Planck elucidated the nature of ionic dissociation and movement in aqueous solution, and physiologists realized that the currents and potentials in excitable cells might be due to the diffusion of ions. This view was put in a clear form as early as 1902 by Julius Bernstein in his "membrane theory." He postulated that

1. Electrical potentials arise across a semipermeable plasma membrane that completely envelops each cell.
2. The potential arises because of concentration gradients of ions such as K^+ across the membrane and because the membrane is not equally permeable to all ions.
3. The potentials change when some chemical alteration in the membrane changes the ion permeability.

Although 50 more years of electrophysiological work were required to complete the proof, the membrane theory is now fully tested and is no longer a hypothesis. Before we can discuss its consequences in further detail, we must review the physical chemistry of electrodiffusion.

RULES OF IONIC ELECTRICITY

How do membrane potentials arise?

Consider the electrolyte system represented in Fig. 2 (left), where a porous membrane separates aqueous solutions of unequal concentrations of a fictitious salt KA. Two electrodes permit the potential difference between the two solutions to be measured. Now, assume that the membrane pores are permeable exclusively to K^+ so that K^+ begins to diffuse across the membrane but A^- does not. For simple statistical reasons, the movement of K^+ from the concentrated side to the dilute side will initially exceed the movement in the reverse direction, and we expect a net flux of K^+ down the concentration gradient. However, this process does not continue long since K^+ carries a positive charge from one compartment to the other and leaves a net negative charge behind. The growing separation of charge creates an electrical potential difference (the membrane potential) between the two solutions, and a positive charge appears on the side into which the K^+ ions diffuse, thereby setting up an electrical force that tends to oppose further net movement of K^+.

Equilibrium potential is membrane potential at which there are no net ion movements

The membrane potential reached in a system with only one permeant ion and no perturbing forces is called the equilibrium, or Nernst, potential for that ion; thus, the final membrane potential for the system in Fig. 2 is the potassium equilibrium potential E_K. At that potential, there is no further net movement of K^+, and unless otherwise disturbed, the membrane potential and ion gradient will remain stable indefinitely. The value of the Nernst potential is derived from thermodynamics by recognizing that the change of electrochemical potential $\Delta\mu_j$ for moving the permeant ion j^{+z} across the membrane must be zero at equilibrium:

$$\Delta\mu_j = 0 = RT \ln \frac{[j]_o}{[j]_i} - zFE \qquad (1)$$

where R is the gas constant [8.31 joules (J)/deg/mol], T is absolute temperature in Kelvin (°C + 273.2), and F is Faraday's constant [96,500 coulombs (C)/mol]. Using terms appropriate to biology, $[j]_o$ and $[j]_i$ represent activities of ion j^{+z} outside and inside a cell; z is the ionic valence, and E the membrane potential defined as "inside minus outside." Solving for E and calling it E_j to denote the ion at equilibrium gives the Nernst equation for j:

$$E_j = \frac{RT}{zF} \ln \frac{[j]_o}{[j]_i} \qquad (2)$$

For practical use at 20°C, the Nernst equation can be rewritten

$$E_j = \frac{58 \text{ mV}}{z} \log \frac{[j]_o}{[j]_i} \qquad (3)$$

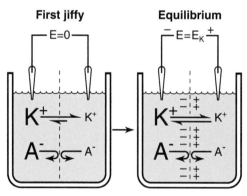

First jiffy

E=0

Equilibrium

$E=E_K$

FIG. 2.   Origin of the membrane potential in a purely K^+-permeable membrane. The porous membrane separates unequal concentrations of the dissociated salt K^+A^-. In the first "jiffy," the membrane potential E, recorded by the electrodes above, is zero, and K^+ diffuses to the right down the concentration gradient. The anion A^- cannot cross the membrane, so a net positive charge builds up on the right-hand side and a negative charge on the left. At equilibrium, the membrane potential, caused by the charge separation, has built up to the Nernst potential E_K, and the fluxes of K^+ become equal in the two directions.

TABLE 1. Approximate free ion concentrations in mammalian skeletal muscle

Ion	Extracellular concentration (mM)	Intracellular concentration (mM)	$\frac{[Ion]_o}{[Ion]_i}$	Nernst potential[a] (mV)
Na^+	145	12	12	+66
K^+	4	155	0.026	−97
Ca^{2+}	1.5	$<10^{-3}$	>1,500	>97
Cl^-	120	4^b	30^b	-90^b

[a] Equilibrium potentials calculated at 37°C from the Nernst equation.
[b] Calculated assuming a −90 mV resting potential for the muscle membrane and assuming that chloride ions are at equilibrium at rest.

showing that for a 10:1 transmembrane gradient, a monovalent ion can give 58 mV of membrane potential. Table 1 gives approximate intracellular and extracellular concentrations of the four electrically most important ions in a mammalian skeletal muscle cell and the Nernst potentials calculated from these numbers at 37°C (neglecting possible activity coefficient corrections). Experimentally, it is found that the resting muscle membrane is primarily permeable to K^+ and Cl^-, and therefore the resting potential in muscle is −90 mV, close to the equilibrium potentials E_K and E_{Cl}. During a propagated action potential, ion channels permeable to Na^+ open, some Na^+ enters the fiber, and the membrane potential swings transiently toward E_{Na}. When these pores close again, the membrane potential returns to near E_K and E_{Cl}. To summarize, membrane potentials arise by diffusion of a small number of ions down their concentration gradient across a permselective membrane.

Fluxes and nonequilibrium potentials are found in real cells

Although the concept of equilibrium potentials is essential to understand and predict the membrane potentials generated by ion permeability, real cells are actually never at equilibrium, because different ion channels open and close during excitation and, even at rest, several types of channels are open simultaneously. Under these circumstances, the ion gradients are dissipated constantly, albeit slowly, and ion pumps are always

needed in the long run to maintain a steady state (see Chap. 3). The net passive flux M_j of each ion is proportional to the permeability P_j for that ion and is often given, at least approximately, by an empirical formula called the Goldman-Hodgkin-Katz flux equation [3–6]:

$$M_j = P_j z_j \frac{EF}{RT} \frac{[j]_o - [j]_i \exp(z_j EF/RT)}{1 - \exp(z_j EF/RT)}$$

(4)

Experimentally, these fluxes may be measured as an electric current or by using radioactive tracers or with sensitive indicator substances responding to the ion in question by fluorescence or other optical changes. In most cases, the fluxes are too small to detect by the less sensitive classical method of chemical analysis for the total amount of an ion.

When the membrane is permeable to several ions, the steady-state potential is given by the sum of contributions of the permeant ions, weighted according to their relative permeabilities:

$$E = \frac{RT}{F} \ln \frac{P_{Na}[Na^+]_o + P_K[K^+]_o + P_{Cl}[Cl^-]_i}{P_{Na}[Na^+]_i + P_K[K^+]_i + P_{Cl}[Cl^-]_o}$$

(5)

This Goldman-Hodgkin-Katz voltage equation is often used to determine the relative permeabilities to ions from experiments where the bathing ion concentrations are varied and changes in the membrane potential are recorded. It has the same form as the equation usually used to describe the responses of ion-selective electrodes in analytical work in the laboratory.

During excitation, ion channels open or close, ions move, and the membrane potential changes

The extra ion fluxes during activity act as an extra load on the Na^+-K^+ and the Ca^{2+} pump, consuming ATP and stimulating an extra burst of cellular oxygen consumption until the original gradients are restored. How large are these fluxes? The physical minimum, calculated from the rules of electricity, is a very small number. Only 10^{-12} equivalents of charge need be moved to polarize 1 cm^2 of membrane by 100 mV, meaning that, ideally, the movement of 1 $pmol/cm^2$ of monovalent ion would be enough to depolarize the membrane more than fully. This quantity, related to the electrical capacitance of the membrane, is a constant throughout the animal and plant kingdoms, as would be the case were the effective thickness and dielectric constant of the insulating (hydrophobic) part of all cell plasma membranes similar. In practice, unmyelinated axons gain about 4 to 8 pmol of Na^+ and lose about the same amount of K^+ per square centimeter for one action potential. The figure is higher than the physical ideal because the oppositely directed fluxes of Na^+ and K^+ overlap considerably in time, working against each other. With this kind of Na^+ gain, a squid unmyelinated giant axon of 1 mm diameter could be stimulated 10^5 times, and a mammalian fiber of 0.2-μm diameter only 10 to 15 times before the internal Na^+ concentration would be doubled, assuming that the Na^+-K^+ pump had been blocked. In myelinated nerve, the Na^+ gain in one impulse is very small, amounting to only 2×10^{-7} mol/kg of nerve because of the special low-capacitance properties of myelin.

Transport systems may also produce membrane potentials

The equations just discussed are those for passive electrodiffusion in ion channels where the only motive forces on ions are thermal and electrical, and they do indeed explain almost all the potentials of excitable cells. However, there is another type of electric current source in cells that can generate potentials: the ion pumps and other membrane devices that couple ion movements to the movements of other molecules. In excitable cells, the most prominent is the Na^+-K^+ pump (see Chap. 3), which gives a net export of positive charge and hence tends to hyperpolarize the cell-surface membrane in proportion to the rate of pumping [3]; but hyperpolarization from this electrogenic pumping is typically only a modest few millivolts. By contrast, mitochondria (and plant, algal, and fungal cells) have powerful current sources in their proton transport system. Their membrane potentials are at times dominated by this electrogenic system and would then not be describable in terms of diffusion in simple passive channels.

ELECTRICALLY EXCITABLE CELLS

Permeability changes of the action potential

Given the rules of ionic electricity, the major biological problem in understanding action potentials is to describe and explain the ion permeability mechanisms in the membrane. The opening and closing of ion channels involves passive conformational changes driven by electric field changes or ligand binding but not by direct consumption of metabolic energy. The independence of immediate metabolic input can be demonstrated in studies with internally perfused cells and with channels reconstituted into lipid bilayers. For example, the great majority of the axoplasm can be squeezed from one cut end of a squid giant axon and the axon reinflated with a continuously flowing salt solution that enters at one end and leaves at the other, and excitability can still be preserved. A giant axon internally perfused with isotonic potassium sulfate can continue to fire several 100,000 impulses. Analogous experiments using dialysis techniques or excised patches of membrane have been done with many other excitable cells. These experiments prove that ATP and other intracellular, small molecules of metabolism are not required either for many cycles of opening and closing of Na⁺, K⁺, or Ca²⁺ channels or for the resulting depolarizing and repolarizing ionic current flows. They also show, however, that intracellular ATP, guanosine cyclic 3',5' phosphate (cGMP) and Ca²⁺, as well as phosphorylation by a variety of protein kinases, can be powerful modulators of channel activities. In the long term, ATP and other molecules are also needed to fuel the Na⁺-K⁺ and Ca²⁺ pumps and for synthesis and trafficking of membrane components. We must emphasize that channels differ from pumps in their structure, mechanism of ion flux, function, and regulation.

Gating mechanisms for Na⁺ and K⁺ channels in the axolemma are voltage dependent

In a classic series of experiments, Hodgkin, Huxley, and Katz [1,3–5,7] measured the kinetics of ion permeability changes in squid giant-axon membranes by a direct electrical method called the voltage clamp. As the name implies, the method controls the membrane voltage electrically (usually to follow step changes of potential) while ion movements are recorded directly as electric current flowing across the membrane. The recorded current may be resolved into individual ionic components by changing the ions in the solutions that bathe the membrane. The voltage clamp is a rapid and sensitive assay for studying the opening and closing of ion channels. A widely used miniature version of the voltage clamp is the patch clamp, a technique with sufficient sensitivity to study the current flow in a single ion channel [8]. A glass micropipette with a tip diameter <1 μm is a fire polished at the tip and then pressed against the membrane of a cell. Because the tip is smoothed rather than having sharp edges, it seals to the membrane in the annular contact zone, rather than piercing the membrane, and defines a tiny patch of the cell surface whose few ion channels can easily be detected by the currents flowing through them. The patch clamp can readily measure a flux of as little as 10^{-20} mol of ion in less than 1 msec.

With the voltage clamp, Hodgkin and Huxley [7] discovered that the processes underlying gating (the opening and closing conformational changes) of axonal Na⁺ and K⁺ channels are controlled by the membrane potential and therefore derive their energy from the work done by the electric field on charges or dipolar groups associated with the channel macromolecule. Hodgkin and Huxley [7] identified currents from two types of ion-selective channels—Na⁺ channels and K⁺ channels—which account for almost all of the current in axon membranes, and they made a kinetic model of the opening and closing steps, which may be simplified as shown in Fig. 3. Depolarization of the membrane is sensed by the voltage sensor of each channel and causes the conformational reactions to proceed to the right. Repolarization or hyperpolarization causes them to proceed to the left. We can understand the action potential in these terms. The action potential, caused by a depolarizing stimulus, begins with a transient, voltage-gated opening of

Na⁺ Channels

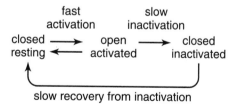

K⁺ Channels

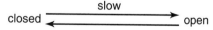

Simplified kinetic model for opening and closing steps of Na⁺ and K⁺ channels. (Adapted from Hodgkin and Huxley [7].)

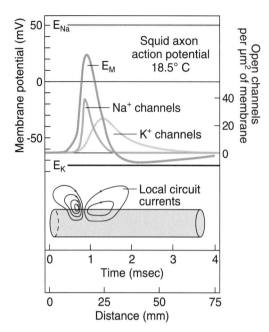

FIG. 4. Events of the propagated action potential calculated from the Hodgkin-Huxley [7] kinetic model. Because the action potential is a nondecrementing wave, the diagram shows equivalently the time course of events at one point in the axon, or the spatial distribution of events at one time as the excitation propagates to the left. **Upper:** Action potential (E_M) and the opening and closing of Na$^+$ and K$^+$ channels. The Nernst potentials for Na$^+$ and K$^+$ are indicated by E_{Na} and E_K. **Lower:** Local circuit currents. The intense loop on the left spreads the depolarization to the left into the unexcited membrane.

Na$^+$ channels that allows Na$^+$ to enter the fiber and depolarize the membrane fully, followed by a transient, voltage-gated opening of K$^+$ channels that allows K$^+$ to leave and repolarize the membrane. Figure 4 shows a calculation of the temporal relation between channel-opening and membrane-potential changes in an axon at 18.5°C, using the model of Hodgkin and Huxley [7].

The action potential is propagated by local spread of depolarization

If there are no chemical or mechanical signals for voltage-gated channels to open, how does the action potential propagate smoothly down an axon, bringing new channels into play ahead of it? Any electrical de-

polarization or hyperpolarization of a cell membrane spreads a small distance in either direction from its source by a purely passive process often called cable, or electrotonic, spread. The spread occurs because the intracellular and extracellular media are much better conductors than is the membrane, so any changes injected at one point across the membrane repel each other and disperse along the membrane surface. Electrophysiologists usually describe this process formally in terms of current flow in an electrical equivalent circuit, with resistors and capacitors representing the geometry of the cell and its membranes. One of the common resulting equations is called the cable equation in analogy to the similar description of how signals spread in electrical cables. The lower part of Fig. 4 shows diagrammatically the so-called local circuit currents that spread the depolarization forward. In this way, an excited depolarized membrane area smoothly depolarizes the next unexcited region ahead of the action potential, bringing it above firing threshold, opening Na$^+$ channels there, and advancing the wave of excitation. The action potential in the upper part of Fig. 4 is calculated by combining the known "cable properties" of the squid giant axon with the rules of ionic electricity and the kinetic equations (Hodgkin-Huxley equations) for the voltage-dependent gating of Na$^+$ and K$^+$ channels. The success of the calculations means that the factors described are sufficient to account for action-potential propagation.

Membranes at nodes of Ranvier are characterized by high concentrations of Na$^+$ channels

A wide variety of cells have now been studied by voltage-clamp methods, and quantitative descriptions of their permeability changes are available. All axons, whether vertebrate or invertebrate, operate on the same principles: They have a small background permeability, primarily to K^+, which sets the resting potential, and display brief, dramatic openings of Na^+ and K^+ channels in sequence to shape the action potentials. Chapter 6 describes myelin, a special adaptation of large (1-20-μm diameter) vertebrate nerve fibers for higher conduction speed. In myelinated nerves, like unmyelinated ones, the depolarization spreads from one excitable membrane patch to another by local circuit currents; but because of the insulating properties of the coating myelin, the excitable patches of axon membrane (the nodes of Ranvier) may be more than 1 mm apart, so the rate of progression of the impulse is faster. The wavelength of an action potential is such that 20 to 40 nodes of Ranvier are active at one time, and every 15 to 20 μsec, a new node in front begins to depolarize, and an old one behind finishes repolarizing. Nodes of Ranvier have Na^+ channels similar to those of other axon membranes, but nodal membranes have at least ten times as many channels per unit area to depolarize the long, passive, internodal myelin. The Na^+-K^+ pump may be distributed similarly (see Chap. 3). The internodal axon membrane has K^+ channels but far fewer Na^+ channels [9]; although hidden underneath the myelin, these K^+ channels may contribute to maintaining the resting potential. After experimental demyelination by diphtheria toxin (a process taking several days), and probably in the course of several demyelinating diseases (see Chap. 37), Na^+ channels and excitability can develop in a formerly inexcitable internodal section of axon [10].

A wide repertoire of voltage-sensitive channels are found among cell types

In seeking diversity among types of channels, we need not look to evolution, for channels seem to be conservative and quite similar among animals with nervous systems. Rather, diversity is found in the different cell types in any one organism, where the repertoire of functioning channels is adapted to the special role each cell plays in the body. All axons have only to transmit brief action potentials that code a message by their frequency, so their channels are similar. However, the action potential of a variety of muscles and secretory cells may serve instead to time the duration or fix the intensity of a contraction or a secretory response, and their action potentials are never as brief and rarely as invariant as those of axons. Their activities may require more than ten types of channels, several of which are subject to modulatory influences, often phosphorylation, that regulate the overall behavior of the cell. A neuron cell body also has many more channel types than does the axon coming from it. In all of these cell types, it is not uncommon to find several Ca^{2+} channels that open with depolarization, supplementing the depolarizing effect of Na^+ channels by adding a slower, depolarizing Ca^{2+} influx or sometimes even acting alone to depolarize the membrane without Na^+ channels [11,12]. Ca^{2+} channels have a special importance, because the entering Ca^{2+} often plays the role of a chemical messenger to activate exocytosis (secretion), contraction, gating of other channels, ciliary reorientation, metabolic pathways, etc. Indeed, whenever an electrical message activates any nonelectrical event, a change of the intracellular free Ca^{2+} concentration acts as an intermediary. Ca^{2+} channels are particularly concentrated in nerve terminals where a Ca^{2+} influx is required for release of chemical neurotransmitters. In addition, muscles, secretory cells, and neuron cell bodies usually have many types of K^+ channels, some opened by depolarization, as in axons, some also opened by raised intracellular free Ca^{2+}, and some turned off by depolarization. Several of these K^+ channels may be modulated by neurotransmitters and hormones. The electric eel electroplax has a high density of conventional Na^{2+} channels to generate the strong currents of the electric discharge and resting K^+ channels that turn off with depolarization to avoid opposing the effect of the Na^+ channels.

FUNCTIONAL PROPERTIES OF VOLTAGE-GATED ION CHANNELS

Ion channels are macromolecules or macromolecular complexes that form aqueous pores in the lipid membrane

Much of what we know about ion channel function comes from voltage-clamp and patch-clamp studies on channels still imbedded in the cell membrane [1–5]. Figure 5A summarizes the major functional properties of a voltage-gated macromolecular channel in terms of a fanciful cartoon. The pore is narrow enough in one place, the ionic selectivity filter, to "feel" each ion and to distinguish among Na^+, K^+, Ca^{2+}, and Cl^-. The channel also contains charged or dipolar components that sense the electric field in the membrane and drive conformational changes that, in effect, open and close gates controlling the permeability of the pore. In Na^+, K^+, and Ca^{2+} channels, the gates seem to close the axoplasmic mouth of the pore, and

the selectivity filter seems to be near the outer end of the pore.

How do we know that a channel is a pore? By far the most convincing evidence is the large ion flux a single channel can handle. It is not unusual in patch clamp work to measure ionic currents of 2 to 10 pA flowing each time one channel in the patch is open. This would correspond to 12 to 60×10^6 monovalent ions moving per second. Such a turnover number is several orders of magnitude faster than known carrier mechanisms and agrees well with the theoretical properties of a pore of atomic dimensions. Similar fluxes have been observed with pore-forming antibiotic peptides in model systems. These substances, including gramicidin A, alamethicin, and monazomycin, spontaneously form pores permeable to water and small ions in lipid bilayer membranes, as well as in biological membranes. Their antibiotic effect can be attributed to the collapsing of ion gradients across membranes. They are small

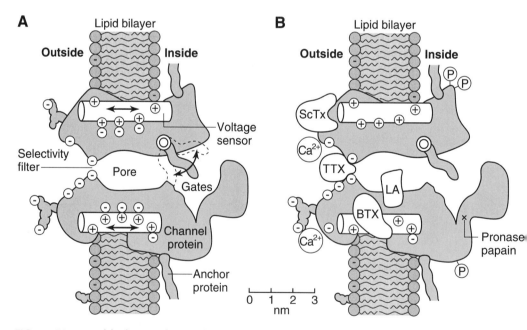

FIG. 5. Diagram of the functional units of an ion channel (**A**) and the hypothesized binding sites for several drugs and toxins affecting Na^+ channels (**B**). The drawing is fanciful, and the dimension and shapes of the parts are not known. Drug receptors: (TTX) tetrodotoxin and saxitonin; (ScTx) scorpion toxins and anemone toxins; (BTX) batrachotoxin, aconitine, veratridine, and grayanotoxin; (LA) local anesthetics; (Ca^{2+}) divalent ions screening and associating with surface negative charge.

enough to be synthesized in many variants in the laboratory and are an excellent model system for elucidating structure-function relations in ion pores. Several of the antibiotic substances even have very steeply voltage-dependent gating; however, none of the pore-forming agents characterized so far can discriminate between small cations to the degree that Na^+ channels or K^+ channels can.

Water molecules break and make hydrogen bonds with other waters 10^{11} to 10^{12} times per second, and alkali ions exchange water molecules or other oxygen ligands at least 10^9 times per second. In these terms, the progress of an ion across the membrane is not the movement of a fixed hydrated complex; rather it is a continual exchange of oxygen ligands as the ion dances through the sea of relatively free water molecules and polar groups that form the wall of the pore. It is generally assumed that polar and charged groups are in the pore to provide stabilization energy to the permeating ion, compensating for those water molecules that must be left behind as the ion enters into the pore. Evidence for important negative charges at the mouth or in the selectivity filter of Na^+, K^+, and Ca^{2+} channels comes from a block of their permeability as the pH of the external medium is lowered below pH 5.5 [5] as well as from site-directed mutagenesis of aspartate and glutamate residues in cloned channels (see below).

The minimum size of ion channels has been determined from the van der Waals dimensions of ions that will go through them [5]. For example, Na^+ channels will pass at least ten ions other than Na^+, many of them organic ions. The largest is aminoguanidinium, which requires an orifice of somewhat more than 3×5 Å in the selectivity filter of the channel. A sodium ion (ionic diameter 1.90 Å) crossing such a narrow region would have to be partly, but not fully, dehydrated. It might still be in contact with three water molecules (diameter 2.80 Å) at the moment of maximum dehydration.

Because channels are narrow and neither geometrically nor chemically uniform along their length, ion fluxes cannot be perfectly described by the equations of free diffusion already discussed, and models capable of describing temporary binding to attractive sites and jumps over energy barriers are frequently used instead. Formally, the kinetics of flux through channels are construed similarly to enzyme kinetics. It is assumed that the channel passes through a sequence of "channel-ion complexes" as it catalyzes the progression of an ion across the membrane. Such theories also can describe other properties of ion channels, such as selectivity, saturation, competition, and block by permeant ions [5].

Voltage-dependent gating requires voltage-dependent conformational changes in the protein component(s) of ion channels

On theoretical grounds, a membrane protein that responds to a change in membrane potential must have charged or dipolar amino acid residues, or both, located within the membrane electric field, acting as voltage sensors as illustrated in Fig. 5A. Changes in the membrane potential then exert a force on these protein-bound dipoles and charges. If the energy of the field-charge interactions is great enough, the protein may be induced to undergo a change to a new stable, conformational state in which the net charge or the location of charge within the membrane electric field has been altered. For such a voltage-driven change of state, the steepness of the state function versus membrane potential curve defines the equivalent number of charges that move according to a Boltzmann distribution. On this basis, Hodgkin and Huxley [7] predicted that activation of Na^+ channels would require the movement of six positive charges from the intracellular to the extracellular side of the membrane. The movement of a larger number of charges through a proportionately smaller fraction of the membrane electrical field would be equivalent. Good candidates for such gating charge have been identified in the amino acid sequences of voltage-gated channels.

Such a movement of membrane-bound charge gives rise to a "gating" current that can be detected electrophysiologically. Tiny gating currents associated with activation of Na^+ channels were first detected in studies of the squid giant axon [13]. Their voltage and time dependence are consistent with the multistep changes of channel state from resting to active. Inactivation of channels during a depolarizing prepulse blocks gating currents with the same time and voltage dependence as it blocks sodium currents. The moving charged groups are amino acids whose position in the protein structure is altered in the conformational change leading to activation.

In contrast to activation, fast inactivation from the open state of Na^+ channels and certain K^+ channels does not seem to be a strongly voltage-sensitive process [13,14]. This inactivation can be blocked irreversibly by proteolytic enzymes acting from the intracellular side of the channel. For some Ca^{2+} channels, intracellular calcium itself plays an important role in inactivation. It seems from these results and from site-directed mutagenesis experiments that regions of ion channels that are exposed at the intracellular surface of the membrane are important in mediating the process of inactivation.

Pharmacological agents acting on ion channels help define their functions

The Na^+ channel is so essential to successful body function that it has become the target in the evolution of several potent poisons. The pharmacology of such agents has provided important insights to the further definition of functional regions of the channel [2,4,5,15]. Figure 5B shows the supposed sites of action of the four most prominent classes of Na^+ channel agents. At the outer end of the channel is a site where the puffer fish poison, tetrodotoxin (TTX), a small, lipid-insoluble charged molecule binds with a K_i of 1 to 10 nM and blocks Na^+ permeability.

An analogous substance, saxitoxin (STX), also called paralytic shellfish poison, has the same action. Both of these molecules have been tritiated and are widely used to count the number of sodium channels in a tissue, as diagnostic tools in physiological experiments, and as markers for chemical isolation of the channels. For example, there are 200 to 500 toxin-binding sites per square micrometer of membrane in squid giant axons and in frog skeletal muscle. A second important class of Na^+ channel blockers includes such clinically useful local anesthetics as lidocaine and procaine and related antiarrhythmic agents. They are lipid-soluble amines with a hydrophobic end and a polar end, and they bind to a hydrophobic site on the channel protein where they also interact with the inactivation gating machinery. The relevant clinical actions of local anesthetics are fully explained by their mode of blocking Na^+ channels. Two other classes of toxins either open Na^+ channels spontaneously or prevent them from closing normally once they have opened. These are lipid-soluble steroids, such as the frog-skin poison, batrachotoxin (BTX), the plant alkaloids aconitine and veratridine, both acting at a site within the membrane, and peptide toxins from scorpion and anemone venoms, which act at two sites on the outer surface of the membrane. Most scorpion and anemone toxins block the inactivation gating step specifically. All of these reagents play an important role in studies of the molecular properties of Na^+ channels. It is interesting to note that the affinity of the channel for each of these classes of toxins depends on the gating conformational state of the channel.

Similarly specific agents are being sought that will affect K^+ channels or Ca^{2+} channels; most K^+ channels can be blocked by tetraethylammonium ion, Cs^{2+} and Ba^{2+}, and 4-aminopyridine. Except for 4-aminopyridine, there is good evidence that these ions become lodged within the channel at a narrow place from which they may be dislodged by K^+ coming from the other side [2]. In addition, certain K^+ channels can be distinguished by their ability to be blocked by polypeptide toxins from scorpion (charybdotoxin), bee (apamin), or snake (dendrotoxin) venoms [15]. Ca^{2+} channels can be blocked by externally applied divalent ions, including Mn^{2+}, Co^{2+}, Cd^{2+}, and Ni^{2+}. Different Ca^{2+} channel subtypes can be distinguished by their block by dihydropyridines (nifedipine), cone snail toxins (ω-conotoxin), and spider toxins (agatoxins) [12].

MOLECULAR COMPONENTS OF VOLTAGE-SENSITIVE ION CHANNELS

Why should we study the structural properties of the channel macromolecules themselves? Although biophysical techniques define the functional properties of voltage-sensitive ion channels clearly, it is important to relate those functional properties to the structure of the channel proteins. Understanding the structural basis for function should help to establish the basic physical and chemical principles underlying electrical excitation and signal transmission in excitable cells.

Although much is now known about the structure and function of Na^+, Ca^{2+}, and K^+ channels, we focus on the Na^+ channel as an example here because it was the first ion channel whose structure was characterized. Since the structural basis of selective ion conductance and voltage-dependent gating may be conserved among different channels, we anticipate that the information derived from studies of each channel type will be relevant for the others.

Radiolabeled neurotoxins that act on Na^+ channels are used as molecular probes to tag the channel proteins, allowing their identification

Photoreactive derivatives of the polypeptide toxins of scorpion venom have been covalently attached to Na^+ channels in intact cell membranes allowing direct identification of channel components without purification. Reversible binding of saxitoxin and tetrodotoxin to their common receptor has been used as a biochemical assay for the channel protein. Solubilization of excitable membranes with nonionic detergents releases the Na^+ channel in association with detergent in a form that retains the ability to bind saxitoxin and tetrodotoxin with high affinity. Once released from the membrane in this way, the channel can be purified by chromatographic techniques that separate glycoproteins by size, charge, and composition of covalently attached carbohydrate. Using this general strategy, Na^+ channels have been purified from the electric organ of the electric eel and from mammalian brain and skeletal muscle [17–19].

Covalent labeling of Na^+ channels in intact excitable cells or membranes and purification of channels solubilized by nonionic detergents result in identification of a large glycoprotein with a molecular weight of 260,000 as the principal component. In eel electroplax, it appears to be the only protein component, but in mammalian brain this large α-subunit is associated with two additional polypeptides: β_1 with a molecular weight of 36,000 and β_2 with a molecular weight of 33,000. In skeletal muscle, the α-subunit is associated with a single polypeptide with a molecular weight of 38,000 that is similar in properties to the β_1-subunit from brain.

Figure 6A illustrates the most probable arrangement of the subunits of the Na^+ channel from brain. The α-subunit is a transmembrane polypeptide since it has sites for attachment of several carbohydrate chains and for binding of neurotoxins on the external surface of the channel and sites for phosphorylation by cAMP-dependent protein kinase on the intracellular surface. Since this single polypeptide suffices to form a channel by itself (see below), a transmembrane orientation is essential to its function. The β_1- and β_2-subunits are also heavily glycosylated. The β_1-subunit is noncovalently attached to the α-subunit while the β_2-subunit is covalently

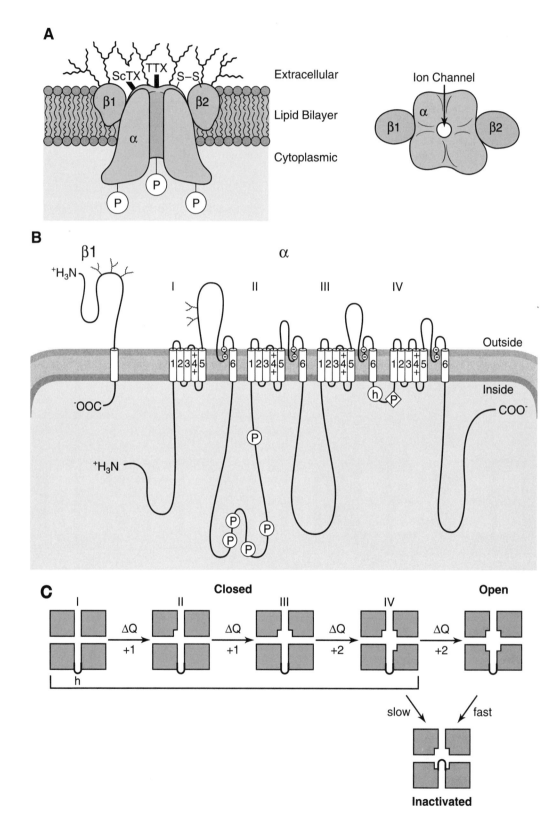

attached to the α-subunit via a disulfide bond. The β-subunits are integral membrane proteins that interact with the phospholipid bilayer. Approximately 25 percent of the mass of the α-subunit and approximately 30 percent of the mass of β_1- and β_2-subunits is carbohydrate. Much of this carbohydrate is sialic acid, which contributes to the strong net negative charge of the channel subunits. It is not known whether these extensive carbohydrate moieties play a physiological role in channel function. However, they are required for normal biosynthesis and assembly of the functional channel in neurons. If glycosylation is inhibited, newly synthesized α-subunits are rapidly degraded and are not inserted into the cell surface membrane.

Purified Na⁺ channels are functional after reconstitution

An important step in the study of a purified membrane transport protein is to reconstitute its transport function in the pure state. This has been accomplished in two ways for the Na⁺ channel. In the first approach, purified channels were incorporated into vesicles of pure phospholipid. Activation of the reconstituted channels by treatment with the neurotoxins veratridine or batrachotoxin markedly increased the permeability of the vesicles to Na⁺. The purified channels retain the ion selectivity and pharmacological properties of native channels. In the second approach, ion conductance mediated by single purified channels was measured electrically. Channels reconstituted in phospholipid vesicles were studied directly using patch-clamp methods or incorporated into planar, phospholipid bilayer membranes by fusion. The individual purified channels observed retained the single-channel conductance, ion selectivity, and voltage dependence of activation and inactivation that are characteristic of native channels. Hence purified Na⁺ channels seem to contain all the functional components necessary for electrical excitability.

Primary structures of Na⁺ channel subunits are determined by cDNA cloning

The amino acid sequences of the Na⁺ channel α- and β_1-subunits have been determined by cloning DNA complementary to the mRNA encoding them using antibodies and oligonucleotides developed form work on purified Na⁺ channels. The amino acid sequence of the subunits is then deduced from the nucleotide sequence of the mRNA encoding them [20,21]. The primary structures of these subunits are illustrated as transmembrane folding models in Fig. 6B. The large α-subunits are composed of 1,800 to 2,000 amino acids and contain four repeated domains having greater than 50 percent inter-

FIG. 6.   Structural model of the sodium channel. **A(Left):** A topological model of the rat brain sodium channel illustrating the probable transmembrane orientation of the three subunits, the binding sites for tetrodotoxin (TTX) and scorpion toxin (ScTX), oligosaccharide chains *(wavy lines)*, and cAMP-dependent phosphorylation sites (P). **Right:** An *enface* view of the protein from the extracellular side illustrating the formation of a transmembrane ion pore in the midst of a square array of four transmembrane domains of the α-subunit. **B:** A transmembrane folding model of the α- and β-subunits of the Na⁺ channel. The amino acid sequence is illustrated as a narrow line with each segment approximately proportional to its length in the molecule. Transmembrane α helices are illustrated as cylinders. The positions of amino acids required for specific functions of Na⁺ channels are also indicated: ++, positively charged voltage sensors in the S4 transmembrane segments; O, residues required for high affinity binding of tetrodotoxin with their charge characteristics indicated by −, +, or open field; h, residues required for fast inactivation; Ⓟ , sites for phosphorylation by cAMP-dependent protein kinase; and ⓟ , sites for phosphorylation by protein kinase C. **C:** Sequential gating of the sodium channel. A reaction pathway from closed to open sodium channels is depicted. Each square represents one homologous domain of the α-subunit. Each domain undergoes a conformational change initiated by a voltage-driven movement of its S4 segment leading eventually to an open channel. Inactivation of the channel occurs from the final closed state and the open state by folding of the intracellular loop connecting domains III and IV into the intracellular mouth of the transmembrane pore.

nal sequence identity. This sequence similarity implies similar secondary and tertiary structures for the four domains. Each domain contains six segments that are predicted to form transmembrane α helices and additional hydrophobic sequences that are thought to be membrane associated and to contribute to formation of the outer mouth of the transmembrane pore (see below). All of these predicted transmembrane segments are in the four homologous domains, which are connected by relatively hydrophilic intracellular amino acid sequences. In contrast, the smaller β_1-subunits of Na$^+$ channels consist of a large extracellular N-terminal segment, a single transmembrane segment, and a short intracellular segment (Fig. 6B).

K$^+$ channels have been identified by genetic means

Genes that harbor mutations causing an easily detectable altered phenotype in the fruit fly *Drosophila* can be cloned directly from genomic DNA without information about the protein they encode. The *Shaker* mutation in *Drosophila* causes flies to shake under ether anesthesia and is accompanied by a loss of a specific K$^+$ current in the nerve and muscle of the mutant flies. By cloning successive pieces of genomic DNA from the region of the chromosome that specifies this mutation, DNA clones were isolated that encoded a protein related in amino acid sequence to the α-subunit of Na$^+$ channels (22). The K$^+$ channel protein is analogous to one of the homologous domains of Na$^+$ or Ca^{2+} channels (22) and is thought to function as a tetramer of four separate subunits in analogy to the structure of Na$^+$ channels. K$^+$ channels may be the ancestral voltage-gated ion channels from which the larger Na$^+$ and Ca^{2+} channels evolved by two cycles of gene duplication (5).

How do the primary structures of the ion channel subunits serve to carry out their functions?

The cloning of the cDNA encoding the Na$^+$ channel subunits permits alternative tests of the functional properties of the polypeptides. cDNA clones can be used to synthesize mRNA encoding the subunits or to isolate the natural mRNA by specific hybridization. When injected into appropriate recipient cells such as frog oocytes, isolated mRNAs can be translated to yield functional proteins. In such experiments, mRNA encoding only the α-subunit of the channel is capable of directing the synthesis of functional channels in oocytes [23,24]. The α-subunits therefore seem sufficient to carry out the basic functions of the channel. However, coexpression of the β_1-subunit accelerates inactivation and shifts its voltage dependence toward more negative membrane potentials, conferring more physiologically correct functional properties on the expressed channel [21]. Similar experiments with K$^+$ channels also show that only the principal subunits are required for channel function (22). These results indicate that the principal subunits of the voltage-gated ion channels are functionally autonomous, but the auxiliary subunits may improve expression and modulate physiological properties.

How does the structure of the α-subunit of the Na$^+$ channel allow it to mediate selective ion transport and voltage-dependent gating? The answer remains unknown, but working hypotheses have been developed from extensive structure-function studies that help to guide current research on this problem. Both the gap junction channel and the nicotinic acetylcholine receptor (see Chap. 10) are high-conductance ion channels that form a transmembrane pore at the center of a pseudosymmetrical array of subunits. By analogy, it is believed that the transmembrane pore of the Na$^+$ channel may be formed at the center of a square array of its four homologous domains (Fig. 6A). Formation of a transmembrane pore in the center of a symmetric or pseudosymmetric array of homologous structural units may be a common theme in the structure of high conductance ion channels.

Which amino acid sequences are involved in forming the pore? For Na$^+$ channels, insight into this question has come from studies of the amino acid residues required for binding of tetrodotoxin, which is thought to block the outer mouth of the transmembrane pore (Fig. 5B). Site-directed mutagenesis experiments show that residues that are required for high affinity tetrodotoxin binding are located in analogous positions in all four domains near the carboxyl ends of the short hydrophobic segments between transmembrane α helices S5 and S6 [25] (Fig. 6B). Most of these are negatively charged glutamate and aspartate residues which may interact with permeant ions as they approach and move through the channel. In agreement with this idea, mutation of the only two of these residues that are not negatively charged (see domains III and IV, Fig. 6B) to glutamic acid residues, as present in the analogous positions in the Ca^{2+} channel, confers Ca^{2+} selectivity on the Na^+ channel [26]. Previous results also implicated these same regions of the K^+ channel in determining ion selectivity and conductance [27]. Evidently, these membrane-associated segments form the outer mouth and at least part of the walls of the transmembrane pore of the voltage-gated ion channels.

Structural models for voltage-dependent gating of ion channels must identify the voltage-sensors or gating charges (Fig. 4A) within the channel structure and suggest a plausible mechanism for transmembrane movement of gating charge and its coupling to the opening of a transmembrane pore. The S4 segments of the homologous domains have been proposed as voltage sensors [19,20,28]. These segments, which are highly conserved in structure in Na^+, Ca^{2+}, and K^+ channels, consist of repeated triplets of two hydrophobic amino acids followed by a positively charged residue. In the α-helical configuration, these segments would form a spiral staircase of positive charge across the membrane, a structure that is well suited for transmembrane movement of gating charge (Fig. 5). Each positive charge is proposed to be neutralized by a negative charge in one of the surrounding transmembrane seg-

ments to form a spiral array of ion pairs (Fig. 5). Direct evidence in favor of designating the S4 segments as voltage sensors comes from mutagenesis studies of Na^+ and K^+ channels [22,29]. Neutralization of positive charges results in progressive reduction of the steepness of voltage-dependent gating and of the apparent gating charge as expected if the S4 segments are indeed the voltage sensors. The mechanism by which they may serve to activate the channels is still unknown. At the resting membrane potential, the force of the electric field would pull the positive charges inward and push the negative charges outward to stabilize one set of ion pair interactions. Depolarization would abolish this force and allow an outward movement of the S4 helix to take up new ion pair partners. A simple spiral movement as suggested in a sliding helix model of gating [19] would have the net effect of transferring one positive charge across the membrane permeability barrier to yield a total of at least four gating charges transferred in the four homologous domains. A more complex propagating helix motion mediated by a β sheet-α helix transition [28] would also permit large gating-charge movements with more complex time courses. In either case, the movement of the S4 helix in each domain is proposed to initiate a more general conformational change in that domain. After conformational changes have occurred in all four domains, the transmembrane pore can open and conduct ions (Fig. 6C).

Shortly after opening, many voltage-gated ion channels inactivate. The inactivation process of Na^+ channels can be prevented by treatment of the intracellular surface of the channel with proteolytic enzymes, implicating protein structures at the intracellular surface of the membrane in the process of inactivation [2]. Antibodies directed against the intracellular segment connecting domains III and IV (h, Fig. 6B) can completely block inactivation [30], expression of the Na^+ channel as two pieces with a cut between domains III and IV greatly slows inactivation [29], and phosphorylation of a single serine residue in this segment by protein kinase C also slows inactivation [31]. This short, highly conserved segment contains clusters of charged and hydrophobic amino acid residues. The clusters of charged residues are not required for fast Na⁺ channel inactivation, but a single cluster of three hydrophobic residues is required [32]. Mutation of these three hydrophobic residues to the hydrophilic residue glutamine completely eliminates fast inactivation of Na⁺ channels. The phenylalanine at position 1,489 is the critical residue; mutation of this single amino acid to glutamine nearly completely blocks fast inactivation of the channel. The segment of the Na⁺ channel between domains III and IV is therefore proposed to serve as the inactivation gate by forming a hinged lid which folds over the intracellular mouth of the pore after activation (Fig. 7A). The cluster of hydrophobic residues including phenylalanine 1,489 is thought to enter the intracellular mouth of the pore and bind there as a latch to keep the channel inactivated.

A detailed model of K⁺ channel inactivation has also been derived from mutagenesis experiments [33,34]. The N-terminal of the K⁺ channel serves as an inactivation particle and both charged and hydrophobic residues are involved. A ball-and-chain mechanism [13,33,34] has been proposed in which the N-terminal segment serves as a loosely tethered ball and inactivates the channel by diffusion and binding to the intracellular mouth of the pore (Fig. 7B). Consistent with this mechanism, synthetic peptides whose amino acid sequences correspond to that of the inactivation particle region can restore inactivation to channel mutants whose N-terminus has been removed. The mechanisms of inactivation of Na⁺ and K⁺ channels are similar in that hydrophobic amino acid residues seem to mediate binding of an inactivation particle to the intracellular mouth of the transmembrane pore of the activated channel in each; they differ in that charged amino acid residues are important in the inactiva-

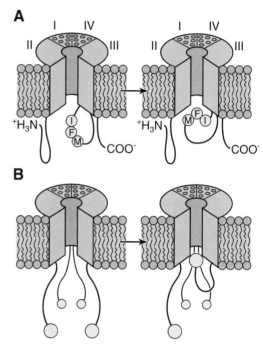

FIG. 7.   Mechanisms of inactivation of Na⁺ and K⁺ channels. **A:** A hinged-lid model for Na⁺ channel inactivation illustrating the inactivation gate formed by the intracellular segment connecting domains III and IV and the critical cluster of hydrophobic residues (IFM, isoleucine-phenylalanine-methionine) that forms a latch holding the inactivation gate closed **B:** A ball-and-chain model of K⁺ channel inactivation. Each of the four subunits of a K⁺ channel has a ball-and-chain structure at its N-terminal. Any one of the four can bind to the intracellular mouth of the open channel and inactivate it.

tion particle of K⁺ channels but not Na⁺ channels and that the inactivation particle is located over 200 residues from the membrane at the N-terminus of the K⁺ channel compared to only 12 residues from the membrane between domains III and IV of the Na⁺ channel. It is likely that the hinged-lid mechanism of Na⁺ channel inactivation evolved from the ball-and-chain mechanism of K⁺ channels.

These models for formation of a voltage-gated transmembrane pore by the Na⁺ and K⁺ channels are still speculative at this time. However, they illustrate a general scientific method: New data such as the amino-acid sequences of the ion channel subunits inevitably lead to the formulation of specific hypotheses. These hypotheses then spawn a new generation of experiments designed to test their merit. The next phase of research on the molecular properties of ion channels should give us clearer insight into the molecular basis for two of the critical functions of ion channels: selective ion conductance and voltage-dependent gating.

OTHER CHANNELS

The general experimental strategy used in studies of the Na^+ channel has now been applied to voltage-sensitive Ca^{2+} channels. Drugs and neurotoxins that act on Ca^{2+} channels have been used to identify their protein components, and experiments to restore their function in purified form and to determine their primary and secondary structures have been completed. As for Na^+ channels, Ca^{2+} channels have a principal subunit, designated α_1, which is functionally autonomous, but co-expression with the auxiliary α_2-, β-, γ-, and δ-subunits modulates the properties of the expressed channel and can greatly increase the level of expression. Since voltage-gated ion channels are likely to have evolved from common ancestor proteins, comparison of the conserved structural and functional features among the principal subunits of many different channels will sharpen our view of the molecular basis of their function as illustrated above by the comparison of the inactivation mechanisms of Na^+ and K^+ channels.

The channels used in the action potential contrast with those generating slow potentials at synapses and sensory receptors by having strongly voltage-dependent gating. The other channels have gates controlled by chemical transmitters, intracellular messengers or by other energies, such as mechanical deformations in touch and hearing. In general, less is known about these channels than about Na^+ and K^+ channels of action potentials, with the exception of the nicotinic ace-

tylcholine receptor channel of the neuromuscular junction (see Chap. 11). The ionic selectivity of these channels include a very broad, monovalent, anion permeability at inhibitory synapses, a cation permeability (about equal for Na^+ and K^+) at excitatory synapses, at the neuromuscular junction, and at many sensory transducers, and other more selective K^+ and Na^+ permeabilities in other synapses. The acetylcholine receptors of the neuromuscular junction and brain, the excitatory glutamate receptors, and the inhibitory GABA and glycine receptors have all been solubilized and chemically purified and the amino-acid sequences of their subunits have been determined by methods of molecular genetics (see Chap. 11). The structural features which are responsible for the function of these ligand-gated channels are being rapidly elucidated.

It should be emphasized that there is a great diversity of ion channels playing many roles in cells throughout the body. We can speculate that hundreds of genes code for structural components of channels. Beyond their functions in the nervous system, channel activity in endocrine cells regulates the episodes of secretion of insulin from the pancreas and epinephrine from the adrenal gland. Channels form part of the regulated pathway for the ion movements underlying absorption and secretion of electrolytes by epithelia. Channels also participate in cellular signaling pathways in many other electrically inexcitable cells. Thus while they are especially prominent in the function of the nervous system, ion channels are actually a basic component of all animal cells, indeed of all eukaryotic cells [5].

ACKNOWLEDGMENTS

The preparation of this chapter was supported by Grants NS-08174 and NS-15751 from the National Institutes of Health.

REFERENCES

1. Hodgkin, A. L. *The Conduction of the Nervous Impulse.* Springfield, IL: Charles C Thomas, 1964.
2. Armstrong, C. M. Ionic pores, gates, and gating currents. *Q. Rev. Biophys.* 7:179–210, 1975.
3. Nicholls, J. G., Martin, A. R., and Wallace, B. G. *From Neuron to Brain,* 3rd ed. Sunderland, MA: Sinauer Associates, 1992.
4. Hille, B. Ionic Basis of Resting and Action Potentials. In J. M. Brookhart, et al. (eds.), *Handbook of Physiology.* Washington, D.C.: American Physiological Society, 1977, Vol. 1, pp. 99–136.
5. Hille, B. *Ionic Channels of Excitable Membranes,* 2nd ed. Sunderland, MA: Sinauer Associates, 1992.
6. Hodgkin, A. L., and Katz, B. The effect of sodium ions on the electrical activity of the giant axon of the squid. *J. Physiol. (Lond.)* 108: 37–77, 1949.
7. Hodgkin, A. L., and Huxley, A. F. A quantitative description of membrane current and its application to conduction and excitation in nerve. *J. Physiol. (Lond.)* 117:500–544, 1952.
8. Hamill, O. P., Marty, A., Neher, E., Sakmann, B., and Sigworth, F. J. Improved patch-clamp techniques for high-resolution current recording from cells and cell-free membrane patches. *Pflugers Arch.* 391:85–100, 1981.
9. Chiu, S. Y., and Schwarz, W. Sodium and potassium currents in acutely demyelinated internodes of rabbit sciatic nerves. *J. Physiol. (Lond.)* 391:631–649, 1987.
10. Bostock, H., and Sears, T. A. The internodal axon membrane: Electrical excitability and continuous conduction in segmental demyelination. *J. Physiol. (Lond.)* 280:273–301, 1978.
11. Hagiwara, S., and Byerly, L. Calcium channel. *Annu. Rev. Neurosci.* 4:69–125, 1981.
12. Hess, P. Calcium channels in vertebrate cells. *Annu. Rev. Neurosci.* 13:337–356, 1990.
13. Armstrong, C. M. Sodium channels and gating currents. *Physiol. Rev.* 61:644–683, 1981.
14. Hoshi, T., Zagotta, W. N., and Aldrich, R. W. Biophysical and molecular mechanisms of *Shaker* potassium channel inactivation. *Science* 250:533–538, 1990.
15. Catterall, W. A. Neurotoxins acting on sodium channels. *Annu. Rev. Pharmacol. Toxicol.* 20:15–43, 1980.
16. Rudy, B. Diversity and ubiquity of K channels. *Neuroscience* 25:729–749, 1988.

17. Agnew, W. S. Voltage-regulated sodium channel molecules. *Annu. Rev. Biochem.* 46: 517–530, 1984.
18. Barchi, R. L. Voltage-sensitive sodium ion channels. Molecular properties and functional reconstitution. *Trends Biochem. Sci.* 9: 358–361, 1984.
19. Catterall, W. A. Molecular properties of voltage-sensitive sodium channels. *Annu. Rev. Biochem.* 55:953–985, 1986.
20. Noda, M., Ikeda, T., Kayano, T., Suzuki, H., Takeshima, H., Kurasaki, M., Takahashi, H., and Numa, S. Existence of distinct sodium channel messenger RNAs in rat brain. *Nature* 320:188–192, 1986.
21. Isom, L., De Jongh, K., Patton, D. E., Reber, B. F. X., Offord, J., Charbonneau, H., Walsh, K., Goldin, A. L., and Catterall, W. A. Primary structure and functional expression of the β_1 subunit of the rat brain sodium channel. *Science* 256:839–842, 1992.
22. Jan, L. Y., and Jan, Y. N. Structural elements involved in specific K^+ channel functions. *Annu. Rev. Physiol.* 54:537–555, 1992.
23. Noda, M., Ikeda, T., Suzuki, H., Takeshima, H., Takahashi, T., Kuno, M., and Numa, S. Expression of functional sodium channels from cloned cDNA. *Nature* 322:826–828, 1986.
24. Goldin, A. L., Snutch, T., Lubbert, H., Dowsett, A., Marshall, J., et al. Messenger RNA coding for only the alpha subunit of the rat brain Na channel is sufficient for expression of functional channels in *Xenopus oocytes. Proc. Natl. Acad. Sci. U.S.A.* 83:7503–7507, 1986.
25. Terlau, H., Heinemann, S. H., Stühmer, W., Pusch, M., Conti, F., Imoto, K., and Numa, S. Mapping the site of block by tetrodotoxin and saxitoxin of sodium channel II. *FEBS Lett.* 293: 93–96, 1991.
26. Heinemann, S. H., Terlau, H., Stühmer, W., Imoto, K., and Numa, S. Calcium channel characteristics conferred on the sodium channel by single mutations. *Nature* 356: 441–443, 1992.
27. Miller, C. Annus mirabilis for potassium channels. *Science* 252:1092–1096, 1990.
28. Guy, H. R., and Conti, F. Pursuing the structure and function of voltage-gated channels. *Trends Neurosci.* 13:201–206, 1990.
29. Stühmer, W., Conti, F., Suzuki, H., Wang, X., Noda, M., Yahadi, N., Kubo, H., and Numa,

S. Structural parts involved in activation and inactivation of the sodium channel. *Nature* 339:597–603, 1989.

30. Vassilev, P., Scheuer, T., and Catterall, W. A. Inhibition of inactivation of single sodium channels by a site-directed antibody. *Proc. Natl. Acad. Sci. U.S.A.* 86:8147–8151, 1989.

31. West, J. W., Numann, R., Murphy, B. J., Scheuer, T., and Catterall, W. A. A phosphorylation site in a conserved intracellular loop is required for modulation of sodium channels by protein kinase C. *Science* 254:866–868, 1991.

32. West, J. W., Patton, D. E., Scheuer, T., Wang, Y.-L., Goldin, A. L., and Catterall, W. A. A cluster of hydrophobic amino acid residues required for fast sodium channel inactivation. *Proc. Natl. Acad. U.S.A.* 89:10910–10914.

33. Hoshi, T., Zagotta, W., and Aldrich, R. W. Biophysical and molecular mechanisms of Shaker potassium channel inactivation. *Science* 250:533–538, 1990.

34. Zagotta, W., Hoshi, T., and Aldrich, R. W. Restoration of inactivation in mutants of *Shaker* potassium channels by a peptide derived from Sh B. *Science* 250:568–571, 1990.

Lipids

BERNARD W. AGRANOFF AND AMIYA K. HAJRA

Since lipids constitute about one half of brain tissue dry weight it is not surprising that lipid biochemistry and neurochemistry have evolved together. Brain contains many complex lipids, some of which (gangliosides, cerebrosides, sulfatides, phosphoinositides) were first discovered in brain, where they are highly enriched compared with other tissues. Phospholipids account for the high total phosphorus content of brain, which led to an alchemical mystique in the nineteenth century that associated phosphorescence

Basic Neurochemistry: Molecular, Cellular, and Medical Aspects, 5th Ed., edited by G. J. Siegel et al. Published by Raven Press, Ltd., New York, 1994. Correspondence to Bernard W. Agranoff, Neuroscience Laboratory, University of Michigan, 1103 E. Huron, Ann Arbor, Michigan 48104-1687.

with thought, and to the apocryphal claim that fish are good "brain food" since fish, too, are rich in phosphorus.

PROPERTIES OF BRAIN LIPIDS

Lipids have multiple functions in brain

Lipids serve two principal functions: as repositories of chemical energy (storage fat, primarily triglycerides), and as structural components of cell membranes. Brain contains virtually no triglyceride, so it is in their role as membrane components that brain lipids command the attention of neurochemists. Lipids have many additional physiological functions. The biomessenger function of non-membrane lipids (steroid hormones and eicosanoids) has long been known. However, in recent years some membrane lipids, such as inositides and phosphatidylcholine, which were previously believed to have only a structural role, have also been shown to have important functions in the signal transduction process across biological membranes. We now also know that lipids covalently coupled to proteins play a major role in anchoring some proteins within biomembranes. These discoveries establish that lipids participate in the function as well as the structure of membranes.

Membrane lipids are amphiphilic molecules

All membrane lipids have a small polar (hydrophilic) and a large nonpolar (hydrophobic) component. The hydrophilic regions of lipid molecules associate with water and water-soluble ionic compounds by hydrogen and electrostatic bonding. The hydrophobic regions cannot form such bonds, and thus associate with each other outside the aqueous phase. Depending on the relative dominance of the hydrophobic and hydrophilic regions of a given lipid molecule, the amphiphiles will form either aggregates (micelles) or bilayers. Lipid molecules containing comparatively large polar groups, such as lysolipids, gangliosides, as well as natural and synthetic detergents which are fairly soluble in water, tend to form micelles once the solubility limit (critical micellar concentration) is reached. Most membrane lipids have very low aqueous solubilities and tend to associate in a hydrophobic "tail-to-tail" fashion to form bilayers, which are the basic structure of all biomembranes. (See Chap. 2 for further details of membrane structure.)

The hydrophobic components of many lipids consist of either isoprenoids or fatty acids and their derivatives

Lipids were originally defined operationally, on the basis of their extractability from tissues with organic solvents such as a chloroform/methanol mixture, but this is no longer the sole criterion. For example, the myelin component proteolipid is extractable into the lipid solvents, but nevertheless is not considered to be a lipid, since its structure is that of a highly hydrophobic polypeptide. We now know that there are many integral membrane proteins which contain "hydrophobic" membrane-spanning regions. Conversely, gangliosides are considered to be lipids on the basis of their structure, even though they are more polar than apolar. It is apparent, then, that lipids are defined not only by their physical properties, but also on the basis of their chemical structure. Chemically, lipids can be defined as compounds containing long chain fatty acids (and their derivatives) or linked isoprenoid units. The fatty acids are either esterified to glycerol, a trihydroxy alcohol or as amides of sphingosine, a long chain dihydroxyamine. The isoprenoids are made up of branched chain units and include sterols, such as cholesterol.

Isoprenoids have the unit structure of a five carbon branched chain

Isoprenoid units have the formula C_5H_8 and the structure

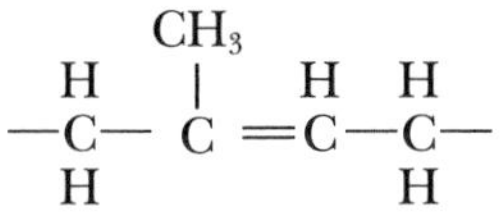

$$\begin{array}{ccc} & CH_3 & \\ H & | & H \quad H \\ -C- & C & =C-C- \\ H & & H \end{array}$$

The most abundant of these in brain is cholesterol. Unlike other tissues, normal adult brain contains virtually no cholesterol esters. Desmosterol, the immediate biosynthetic precursor of cholesterol, is found in developing brain and in some brain tumors but not in normal adult brain. Other isoprenoid substances present in brain are the dolichols, very long (up to C_{100}) branched chain alcohols which are cofactors for glycoprotein biosynthesis, squalene (the linear C_{30} precursor of all steroids), and the carotenoids, including retinal and retinoic acid. Some isoprene units such as farnesyl (C_{15}) and geraniol-geraniol (C_{20}) have been shown to be covalently linked via thioether bonds to membrane proteins. (See Fig. 7 for structures of some of these compounds and for the numbering system for cholesterol.)

Brain fatty acids are long chain carboxylic acids which may contain one or more double bonds

Brain contains a variety of straight chain monocarboxylic acids, usually with an even number of carbon atoms ranging from C_{12} to C_{26}. The hydrocarbon chain may be saturated or may contain one or more double bonds, all in *cis* (Z) configuration. When multiple double bonds are present, they are non-conjugated and generally three carbons apart. The unsaturated fatty acids are classified in three series, i.e., n − 3 (n minus 3:n = number of carbon atoms), n − 6 and n − 9 (or ω 3, ω 6, ω 9) indicating in each instance the position of the first double bond from the methyl (ω) end. The nomenclature convention is based on the fact that the fatty acids are elongated or degraded by C-2 units (see later) and in animals, the double bond in the fatty acyl chain can be introduced only in the first 9 carbons from the carboxylic end. The complete short hand notation for fatty acids consists of the number of carbon atoms, followed by the number of double bonds, and the position of the first double bond from the methyl end. Linoleic acid is 18:2, n − 6, i.e., it is an 18C essential fatty acid with two double bonds, and the first double bond from the methyl end is present at C_{12} (18 − 6 = 12). The brain contains some unusual fatty acids, such as odd-numbered fatty acids and 2-hydroxy fatty acids, prevalent in the cerebrosides. A list of major brain fatty acids with their common names and structures is given in Fig. 1.

COMPLEX LIPIDS

Glycerolipids are derivatives of glycerol and fatty acids

Most brain glycerolipids are derivatives of phosphatidic acid (PtdOH) which is diacylated *sn*-glycerol-3-phosphate. The notation *sn* refers to stereochemical numbering with the secondary hydroxyl group of glycerol at C-2 shown on the left (i.e., L-configuration of Fischer's projection) and the phosphate at C-3. This special nomenclature is employed because unlike the trioses (or other carbohydrates) glycerol does not have a reporter carbonyl group to assign an absolute D- or L-configuration. As shown in Fig. 2, the hydroxyl groups on C-1 and C-2 of glycerolipids are esterified with fatty acids. The substituent at *sn*-1 is usually saturated, whereas that at *sn*-2 is unsaturated. In addition, there are species in which *sn*-1 is either ether-linked to an aliphatic alcohol (alkyl) or to an α,β-unsaturated ether (alk-1′-enyl). The latter lipids are referred to as plasmalogens (Fig. 2). Although diacylglycerophospholipids are saponifiable (contain alkali-labile ester bonds) and acid-stable, the alkenyl ethers are alkali-stable and acid-labile. Alkyl ethers are stable to both acids and bases. A useful general term that includes all of these various aliphatic substituents—acyl, alkenyl, and alkyl—is "radyl," for example, 1,2-diradyl-*sn*-glycerol-3-phosphate.

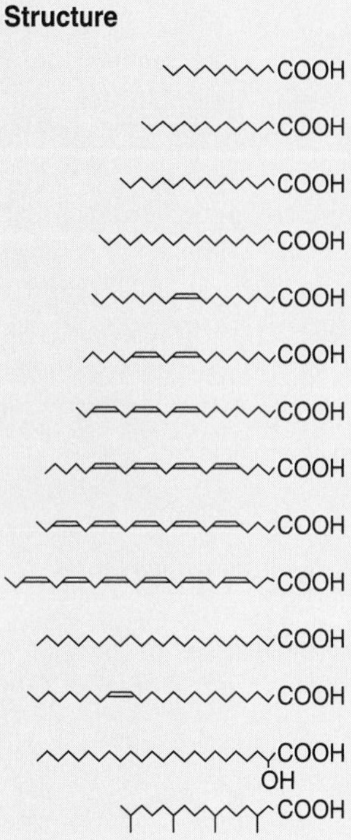

Structure	Chemical name	Trivial name	Abv.
～～～～COOH	Dodecanoic acid	Lauric acid	12:0
～～～～COOH	Tetradecanoic acid	Myristic acid	14:0
～～～～～COOH	Hexadecanoic acid	Palmitic acid	16:0
～～～～～COOH	Octadecanoic acid	Stearic acid	18:0
～～～=～～COOH	9-Octadecenoic acid	Oleic acid	18:1(n-9)
～～=～=～COOH	9,12-Octadecadienoic acid	Linoleic acid	18:2(n-6)
～=～=～～COOH	9,12,15-Octadecatrienoic acid	Linolenic acid	18:3(n-3)
～～=～=～=～COOH	5,8,11,14-Eicosatetraenoic acid	Arachidonic acid	20:4(n-6)
～=～=～=～=～COOH	5,8,11,14,17-Eicosapentenoic acid	EPA	20:5(n-3)
～=～=～=～=～=～COOH	4,7,10,13,16,19-Docosahexenoic acid		22:6(n-3)
～～～～～～COOH	Tetracosanoic acid	Lignoceric acid	24:0
～～～=～～～～COOH	15-Tetracosenoic acid	Nervonic acid	24:1(n-9)
～～～～～～COOH OH	2-Hydroxytetracosanoic acid	Cerebronic acid	24h:0
ＶＶＶＶＶ COOH	3,7,11,15-Tetramethylhexadecanoic acid	Phytanic acid	

FIG. 1.   Structures of some fatty acids of neurochemical interest (see also Fig. 7 and text). The "n − minus" nomenclature for the position of the double bond(s) is given here. Note that sometimes the position of the double bond from the carboxyl end is indicated by the symbol Δ, e.g., 18:2 (n − 6) as 18:2 $\Delta^{9,12}$.

If positions 1 and 2 are acylated and the *sn*-3 hydroxyl group is free, the lipid is 1,2-diacyl-*sn*-glycerol (DAG). The DAGs play both a biosynthetic (see later) and a cellular regulating role in that they activate protein kinase C (see Chap. 20). In addition, DAGs are known to be fusogenic and may play a role in altering cell morphology, for example, in fusion of synaptic vesicles. Other non-phosphorous-containing glycerides of interest are DAG-galactoside and its sulfate [1]. These minor glycolipids are found primarily in white matter and appear to be analogous to their sphingosine-containing counterparts, the cerebrosides, described below.

Glycerophospholipid classes are defined on the basis of the substituent base at *sn*-3 of the diacylglycerophosphoryl (phosphatidyl) function (Fig. 2). The bases are short chain polar alcohols phosphodiester-linked to PtdOH. The amount and distribution of these lipids vary with brain regions and also with age [2–4]. In quantitatively decreasing order in adult human brain they are phosphatidylethanolamine (PtdEtn) including plasmalogens, phosphatidylcholine (PtdCho), and phosphatidylserine (PtdSer). The phosphoinositides—phosphatidylinositol (PtdIns), phosphatidylinositol-4-phosphate, and phosphatidylinositol-4,5-bisphosphate—are quantitatively minor phospholipids but play an important role in signal transduction. (These lipids, also referred to as PI, PIP, PIP_2, respectively, are discussed in detail in Chap. 20). The phosphatidylglycerols in brain, as in other tissues, are present in mitochondrial membranes. Of these, cardiolipin (bisphosphatidylglycerol) is the most prevalent.

Each phospholipid class in a given tissue

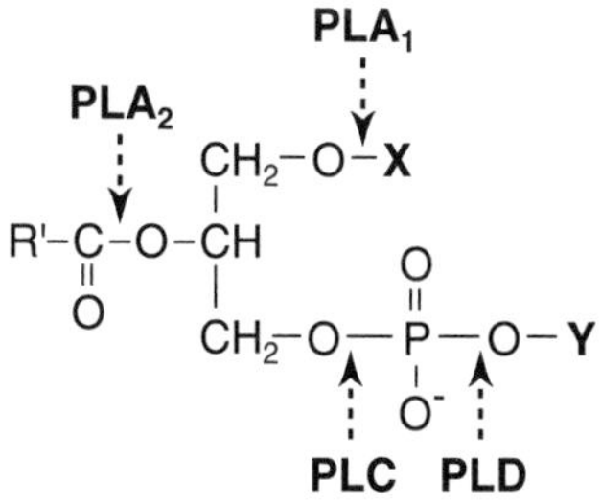

Y	Lipid	Abv.
H	Phosphatidate	PtdOH
$CH_2\text{-}CH_2\text{-}\overset{+}{N}H_3$	Phosphatidylethanolamine	PtdEtn
$CH_2\text{-}CH_2\text{-}\overset{+}{N}(CH_3)_3$	Phosphatidylcholine	PtdCho
$CH_2 - \overset{\overset{\displaystyle NH_3^+}{\textstyle\vert}}{\underset{\underset{\textstyle H}{\vert}}{C}} - COO^-$	Phosphatidylserine	PtdSer
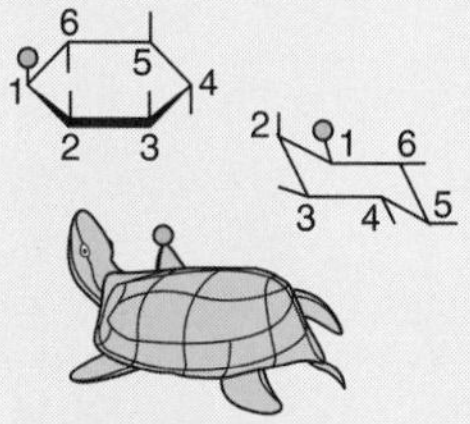	Phosphatidylinositol	PtdIns
$CH_2\text{-}CH(OH)\text{-}CH_2HO$	Phosphatidylglycerol	PtdGro
Phosphatidylglycerol	Cardiolipin	PtdGroPtd

FIG. 2.   The structure of phosphoglycerides. In most lipids, X is acyl, i.e., R—(C=O). In alkyl ethers, present mainly in brain ethanolamine phosphoglycerides (2–3%), X is a long chain hydrocarbon (C_{16}, C_{18}). For plasmalogens, which constitute about 60 percent of adult human brain PtdEtn, X is 1-alk-1′enyl (i.e., —CH=CH—R). Arrows indicate sites of enzymatic hydrolysis of the phosphoglycerides; PLA_1, phospholipase A_1; PLA_2, phospholipase A_2; PLC, phospholipase C; and PLD, phospholipase D. Note that myoinositol is written in the D-configuration where the 1′-position is linked to the PtdOH moiety. For polyphosphoinositides, additional phosphate groups are present in the 3, 4, or 5 positions (see Chap. 20 for further detail regarding the stereochemistry of inositol).

has a characteristic fatty acid composition. The composition of a given phospholipid class thus can be quite different in gray and white matter. This is exemplified by comparing an analysis of PtdEtn from both gray and white matter of human brain (Table 1). Though the same fatty acid may be present in a number of lipids, the quantitative fatty acid composition is different for each class of lipids, and remains fairly constant during the growth and development of the brain. The molecular species composition of different lipids in adult rat brain is shown in Table 2 [5]. This table illustrates the varieties of lipid present in neural membranes. They differ not only in the structure of the polar head groups (phospholipid classes), but within

each class there are a variety of combinations of pairs of fatty acid, giving rise to molecular species which differ in the nature and positional distribution of fatty acids esterified to the glycerol backbone. From this Table, we see for example, that the 1-stearoyl, 2-arachidonyl (18:0–20:4) species is predominant in inositides, whereas the species containing polyunsaturated (e.g., 22:6) acids are enriched in PtdEtn and PtdSer. As noted below, brain lipids contain some unusually long and polyunsaturated fatty acids from both the n − 3 and n − 6 families of essential fatty acids, which cannot be biosynthesized in the animal body de novo (see Chap. 23). This implies the existence of a mechanism for transporting essential fatty acids across the blood-

TABLE 1.   Fatty acid composition of phosphatidylethanolamine[a]

Fatty acid	Gray matter	White matter
14:0	0.2	0.5
16:0	6.7	6.7
16:1	0.4	1.4
18:0	26.0	9.0
18:1 n-9	11.9	42.4
18:2 n-6	Tr	Tr
20:1 n-9	1.5	7.9
20:2 n-9	Tr	2.4
20:3 n-9	0.5	1.6
20:3 n-6	Tr	Tr
20:4 n-6	13.8	6.4
22:4 n-6	Tr	Tr
22:5 n-6	14.3	13.7
22:5 n-3	Tr	0.5
22:6 n-3	24.3	3.4

Adapted from O'Brien and Sampson [4].
[a] PtdEtn was isolated from a 55-year-old human brain. Methyl esters were identified by GLC.

brain barrier. There is considerable interest in the role of the polyunsaturated fatty acids and their metabolites in brain following breakdown of their parent phospholipids in conditions such as ischemia and anoxia (see Chap. 42).

In sphingolipids, the long chain aminodiol sphingosine serves as the lipid backbone

Sphingosine resembles a monoradyl glycerol but has asymmetric carbons at both C-2 and C-3. The chiral configuration is like that of the tetrose D-erythrose, i.e., the amino group at C-2 and hydroxyl group at C-3 are in *cis* configuration (2S, 3R). Unlike unsaturated fatty acids, the double bond between C-4 and C-5 in sphingosine is in *trans* (E) configuration. In the IUPAC-IUB nomenclature, the saturated analog of sphingosine (dihydrosphingosine or D-erythro-2-amino-1,3-octadecanediol) is termed sphinganine, and sphingosine is named (E-4)sphingenine. While in most sphingolipids the sphingosine is 18C long, in brain gangliosides, there is a significant representation of the C_{20} homolog.

In sphingolipids the amino group of sphingosine is acylated with long chain fatty acids and the N-acylated product is termed a ceramide (Fig. 3). C-1 of ceramide is linked to different head groups to form various membrane lipids. For example sphingomyelin is the phosphodiester of ceramide and choline. The fatty acids in sphingomyelin have a bimodal distribution; in the white

TABLE 2.   Distribution profile of the major individual molecular species in the DAG moieties of rat brain phosphoglycerides[a]

Fatty Acid		PtdIns	PtdIns4,5P$_2$	PtdCho	PtdEtn	PtdSer
C-1	C-2	mol %	mol %	mol %	mol %	mol %
16:0	22:6	1.4	0.1	3.3	4.8	0.8
16:0	20:4	7.8	9.5	4.4	2.3	0.6
18:1	20:3	4.1	1.1	Tr	Tr	Tr
18:0	22:6	Tr	1.0	2.5	17.6	42.4
14:0	16:0	0.6	0.4	3.1	1.5	0.8
18:0	22:5	1.0	0.7	0.4	0.2	5.3
18:0	20:4	49.5	66.1	3.8	22.5	3.8
18:1	18:1	1.7	2.1	3.4	11.1	7.0
16:0	18:1	12.7	6.5	36.2	15.8	9.1
16:0	16:0	6.9	1.4	19.2	0.7	Tr
18:0	18:1	7.0	4.6	14.1	14.8	23.7

[a] Adapted from Lee and Hajra [5].
PtdIns, phosphatidylinositol; PtdIns4,5P$_2$, phosphatidylinositol-4,5-bisphosphate; PtdCho, phosphatidylcholine; PtdEtn, phosphatidylethanolamine; PtdSer, phosphatidylserine. PtdInsP was not measured.

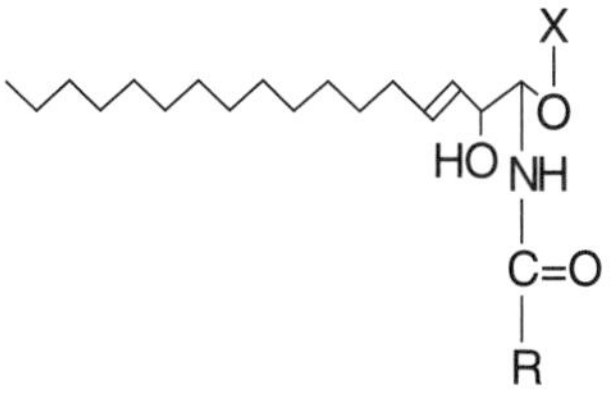

X	Lipid	Abv.
H	Ceramide	Cer
$\overset{O^-}{\underset{O}{\overset{\mid}{\underset{\parallel}{P}}}}$-O-CH$_2CH_2$$\overset{+}{N}$(CH$_3$)$_3$	Sphingomyelin	CerPCho
(CH$_2$OH galactose ring)	Galactocerebroside	CerGal
(CH$_2$OH glucose ring)	Glucocerebroside	CerGlc
Lactose (Glc-Gal)	Lactosylceramide	CerLac

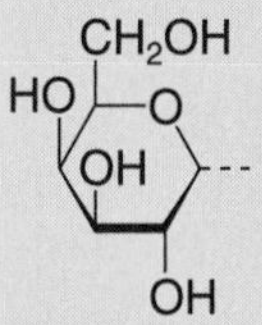

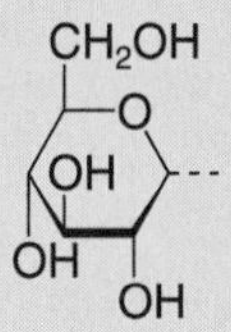

FIG. 3.   Structure of some simple sphingolipids. X may be a complex polysaccharide either containing sialic acid (gangliosides) or not (globosides). See also Figs. 4 and 9 for the structure of some of the complex brain sphingolipids.

matter they are mostly 24C long (i.e., lignoceric and nervonic, see Fig. 1) and in the gray matter stearic acid (18:0) is the predominant fatty acid. Most of the glycolipids in brain consist of ceramide glycosidically linked at C-1 with different mono- or polysaccharides. The major glycolipid of mammalian brain is galactocerebroside, i.e., galactose β-glycosidically linked to ceramide, which constitutes about 16 percent of total lipid in adult human brain. Galactocerebroside esterified to sulfate at the 3′ position of galactose (sulfatide) is also a major (~6 percent of total lipid) brain glycolipid. Cerebrosides are mainly present in brain white matter, especially in myelin, and they generally contain very long chain normal (lignoceric and nervonic), α-hydroxy (cerebronic), and odd number (23:0, 23h:0) fatty acids. Brain also contains a large number of other glycolipids which are polysaccharide derivatives of glucocerebroside (Cer-Glc). A number of monosaccharides, such as galactose (Gal), glucose (Glc), N-acetylglucosamine (GlcNAc), N-acetyl galactosamine (GalNAc), fucose etc., are present in various linkages in these carbohydrate head groups. One important carbohydrate is sialic acid, or N-acetyl (or N-glycolyl) neuraminic acid, an acetylated nine carbon compound (Fig. 4) containing a free carboxyl group which is enzymatically formed by condensation of N-acetyl (or N-glycolyl) manosamine with phosphoenolpyruvate. The sialic acid containing glycolipids are acidic in nature because of the presence of the free carboxylic group, and are termed gangliosides. A large number of gangliosides have been identified in neural and other tissues, making their classification and nomenclature somewhat complex. One popular nomenclature system is that of Svennerholm, who classified the gangliosides according to the number of sialic acid residues present in the molecule and its relative migration rate on thin-layer chromatograms [6]. IUPAC-IUB has proposed a different systematic nomenclature for both gangliosides and neutral glycolipids (globosides) [7]. The structure of a major brain ganglioside is shown in Fig. 4.

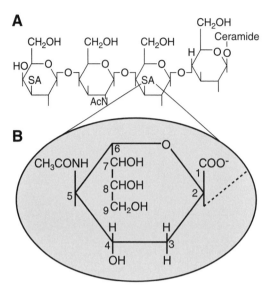

FIG. 4.   **A:** The structure of a major brain ganglioside which is termed GD$_{1a}$ according to the nomenclature of Svennerholm. G denotes ganglioside, D indicates disialo, 1 refers to the tetrasaccharide (Gal-GalNac-Gal-Glc-) backbone, and a distinguishes positional isomers in terms of the location of the sialic acid residues (see Fig. 9). In IUPAC-IUB nomenclature this ganglioside is termed as IV^{3}NeuAc,II^{3}NeuAc-Gg$_4$Cer where the roman numerals indicate the sugar moiety (from ceramide) to which the sialic acids (NeuAC) are attached, and the arabic numeral superscript denotes the position in the sugar moiety where NeuAC are attached; Gg refers to the ganglio (Gal-GalNAc-Gal-Glc) series and 4 to the four carbohydrate backbone for the "ganglio" series. **B:** The structure of sialic acid, also called N-acetyl (or N-glycolyl) neuraminic acid (NeuAc or NANA). Human brain gangliosides are all N-acetyl derivatives, however some other mammalian (e.g., bovine) brain may contain the N-glycolyl derivatives. The metabolic biosynthetic precursor for sialylation of glycoconjugates is CMP-sialic acid, which is a phosphodiester of the 5'OH of cytidine and the 2-position of neuraminic acid.

ANALYSIS OF BRAIN LIPIDS

Chromatographic methods are employed to analyze brain lipids

The lipids from brain are generally extracted by a mixture of chloroform and methanol, by methods which are variations of method originally described by Folch and coworkers [8]. In most common extraction procedures, the tissue or homogenate is treated with 19 volumes of a 2:1 (v/v) mixture of chloro-form-methanol. A single liquid phase is formed, leaving behind a residue of macro molecular material, primarily protein, with lesser amounts of DNA, RNA, and polysac charides. The subsequent addition of a small amount of water to the CHCl$_3$-methanol ex tract leads to separation of the chloroform rich and aqueous methanol phases; the lower (chloroform) phase contains the lip ids, whereas low-molecular-weight metabo lites are in the upper phase. If the lower phase is evaporated to dryness and taken back up in a lipid solvent such as chloroform proteolipid protein remains undissolved and can be removed at this point. Gangliosides can be extracted from the aqueous phase by repartitioning into an apolar solvent. The polyphosphoinositides and lysolipids are poorly extracted at neutral pH, so it is neces sary to acidify the initial chloroform/metha nol mixture for their recovery [9]. Unfortu nately, the acidity leads to cleavage of plasmalogens, primarily alkenyl-acyl PtdEtn There is thus no single procedure that result in quantitative recovery of all brain lipids Lipid classes are separated from a lipid ex tract by thin-layer chromatography (TLC or ion-exchange chromatography or by high-performance liquid chromatography (HPLC) using silicic acid as the stationary phase. To analyze individual fatty acids in a given lipid class, methyl esters can be pre pared directly by alkaline methanolysis of ex tracted lipid bands scraped from TLC plate following visualization, usually with a fluores cent spray. The amide-bound fatty acids of the sphingolipids require more vigorous conditions of methanolysis such as treatmen with hot HCl-methanol. The methyl esters are then separated by gas-liquid chromatog raphy (GLC). It is sometimes possible to sep arate subclasses of intact phospholipids on the basis of the number of fatty acid double bonds if Ag$^+$ is present in the silica gel of the TLC plates. This separation is based on π bonding between Ag$^+$ and the fatty acid dou ble bonds. The molecular species can also be separated by reverse-phase HPLC. For this purpose, a reporter group (e.g., UV-absorb ing benzoyl) can be attached either directly to the lipids (in the carbohydrate portion of glycolipids) or to the DAG backbone of lipid after the hydrolysis of the polar head group [5]. In this method, the separation of the derivatized DAGs is achieved on the basis of their differences in hydrophobicity. The gangliosides are separated from each other by high performance thin-layer chromatography (HPTLC; Fig. 5).

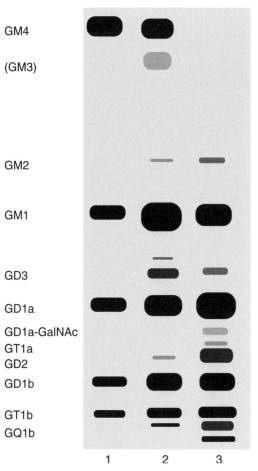

FIG. 5. Diagrammatic representation of thin-layer chromatograms of gangliosides from normal human white matter *(lane 2)* and gray matter *(lane 3)*. Lane 1 contains a mixture of isolated standards. Each lane contains about 7 μg sialic acid. Merck precoated HPTLC plates (silica gel 60, 200 μm thick) were used. The plate was developed with chloroform-methanol-water, 60:40:9 (containing 0.02% CaCl$_2$·2 H$_2$O). The bands were visualized with resorcinol-hydrochloric acid reagent. (Courtesy of R. K. Yu, see also Yu and Ando [6].)

The lipid composition of mammalian brain analyzed by these methods is found to change with age and is different from one region to another [2]. A typical lipid composition of gray and white matter of adult human brain is given in Table 3 [10].

BRAIN LIPID BIOSYNTHESIS

Acetyl coenzyme A is the precursor of both cholesterol and fatty acids

The hydrophobic chains of lipids (i.e., fatty acids and isoprenoids) are biosynthesized from the same 2 carbon starting unit, acetyl coenzyme A, with differences in condensation leading to different products. In cholesterol biosynthesis, two acetyl CoAs are condensed to form acetoacetyl CoA, which can be further condensed with a third acetyl CoA to form a C$_6$ branched chain dicarboxylic acyl CoA, i.e., β-hydroxy-β-methyl glutaryl (HMG) CoA. HMGCoA is reduced by 2 NADPH to form mevalonic acid, and this reduction is catalyzed by the enzyme HMGCoA reductase, the main regulatory enzyme for the biosynthesis of isoprenoids [11]. Mevalonic acid undergoes pyrophosphorylation by two consecutive reactions with ATP, and the product is decarboxylated to form isopentenyl pyrophosphate. This C$_5$H$_8$ isoprene unit is the building block of all isoprenoids. Two isoprene units (isopentenyl-PP and dimethyl allyl-PP) condense to form geranyl pyrophosphate (C$_{10}$) which then condenses with another C$_5$ unit to form farnesyl pyrophosphate (C$_{15}$), the precursor of many different isoprenoids such as dolichol, a very long chain (up to C$_{100}$) alcohol, ubiquinone (a redox coenzyme), and cholesterol. Farnesyl pyrophosphate also alkylates some proteins via a thioether bond which serves to attach them to biomembranes (see below). During cholesterol biosynthesis, two farnesyl pyrophosphate molecules reductively condense in a head-to-head manner to form squalene, a C$_{30}$ hydrocarbon. Squalene is oxidatively cyclized to form lanosterol, a C$_{30}$ hy-

TABLE 3.   Lipid composition of normal adult human brain[a]

Constituent	Gray matter (%)			White matter (%)		
	Fresh wt.	Dry wt.	Lipid	Fresh wt.	Dry wt.	Lipid
Water	81.9	—	—	71.6	—	—
Chloroform-methanol—insoluble residue	9.5	52.6	—	8.7	30.6	—
Proteolipid protein	0.5	2.7	—	2.4	8.4	—
Total lipid	5.9	32.7	100	15.6	54.9	100
Upper phase solids	2.2	12.1	—	1.7	6.0	—
Cholesterol	1.3	7.2	22.0	4.3	15.1	27.5
Phospholipid, total	4.1	22.7	69.5	7.2	25.2	45.9
PtdEtn	1.7	9.2	27.1	3.7	13.2	23.9
PtdCho	1.9	10.7	30.1	2.4	8.4	15.0
Sphingomyelin	0.4	2.3	6.9	1.2	4.2	7.7
Phosphoinositides	0.16	0.9	2.7	0.14	0.5	0.9
PtdSer	0.5	2.8	8.7	1.2	4.3	7.9
Galactocerebroside	0.3	1.8	5.4	3.1	10.9	19.8
Galactocerebroside sulfate	0.1	0.6	1.7	0.9	3.0	5.4
Ganglioside, total[b]	0.3	1.7	—	0.05	0.18	—

[a] Modified from Suzuki [10].
[b] Phospholipid fractions include plasmalogen, assuming that all plasmalogen is present as PtdEtn and PtdCho with a ratio of 4:1 in white matter, 1:1 in gray matter. In intact brain (based on microwaved rat brain), phosphoinositides are present in both white and gray matter in the ratio of 5:0.3:1 for PtdIns, PtdIns4P, PtdIns4,5P$_2$. Gangliosides are calculated on the basis of total sialic acid, assuming that sialic acid constitutes 30 percent of the weight of a typical ganglioside; G$_{D1a}$ is the major ganglioside of both gray and white matter.

droxysteroid. After three demethylations, lanosterol is converted to cholesterol (C$_{27}$). An outline of the pathway of biosynthesis of cholesterol is shown in Fig. 6. Once formed, brain cholesterol turns over very slowly, and there is both metabolic and analytic evidence to indicate an accretion of brain cholesterol with age.

Fatty acids are biosynthesized via elongation by C$_2$ units. Here acetyl CoA is carboxylated (by bicarbonate) to form malonyl CoA, which then condenses with an acyl CoA to form a β-ketoacyl CoA and CO$_2$. This release of CO$_2$ (HCO$_3^-$) drives the reaction forward and elongates the chain by acetyl units. The ketone group is then enzymatically reduced, dehydrated, and hydrogenated, ending up with an acyl CoA that is 2C longer than the parent acyl CoA. NADPH acts as the reducing agent for the reduction of both the ketone group and the double bond. All four reactions (condensation, reduction, dehydration, and hydrogenation) are carried out by the multifunctional fatty acid synthase, a large dimeric enzyme. This cycle is repeated until the proper chain length (>C$_{12}$) is attained, after which the fatty acid is hydrolyzed off from its thioester link with the enzyme. Preformed or exogenous fatty acids are chain lengthened by a similar mechanism, catalyzed by enzyme(s) present in the endoplasmic reticulum [12]. There is also a minor mitochondrial chain elongation system where acetyl CoA, instead of malonyl CoA, is utilized to lengthen the chain by C units. Fatty acids are also desaturated, mainly in the endoplasmic reticulum to form unsaturated fatty acids. Fatty acyl CoA desaturase of which Δ^9-desaturate is most active, removes two hydrogens from —CH$_2$—CH$_2$ groups of long chain (e.g., 18:0) acyl CoA by oxidizing them with molecular oxygen. The electrons are transferred via cytochrome b_5 which is in turn reduced by NADH (cytochrome b_5 reductase). As noted previously in animals a double bond can be introduced only within the first nine carbons from the carboxylic end of a fatty acid. For example

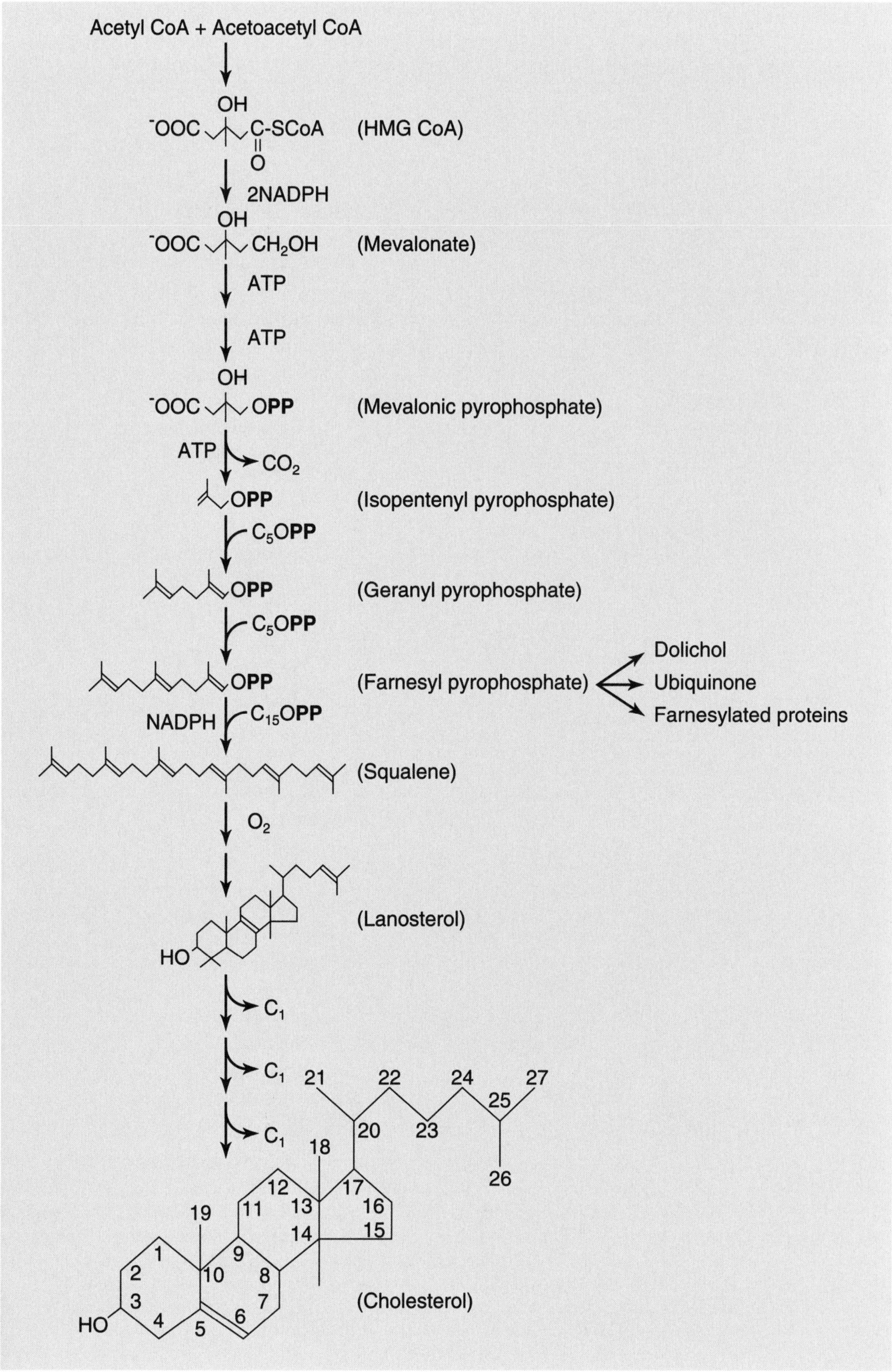

FIG. 6. Pathways of biosynthesis of isoprenoids.

stearic acid (18:0) is converted to oleic acid (18:1, n − 9) in brain but cannot be further converted to linoleic acid (18:2, n − 6). This means that, the fatty acids of the n − 3 and n − 6 series can only be obtained via dietary sources, mainly from plants, and so, are termed "essential fatty acids" (see also Chap. 23). They have important physiological roles, especially in the nervous system. In brain these fatty acids are chain elongated and further desaturated to form the major polyunsaturated fatty acids such as arachidonic (20:4, n − 6) and decosahexenoic acid (22:6, n − 3). A scheme for such chain elongation and desaturation is given in Fig. 7. It should be noted that the precursors of n − 3 and n − 6 series fatty acids are exoge-nous whereas those of the n − 9 series may be endogenous. If these exogenous precursors are not available in the diet (essential fatty acid deficiency) then n − 9 fatty acids are further chain elongated and desaturated to form abnormal fatty acids, as a compensatory response of the brain. One of these is 20:3, n − 9 (Fig. 7), which is termed "Mead acid" because it was discovered by James Mead in the tissues of animals which were fed a fat-free diet over extended periods [13]. The Mead acid substitutes for arachidonic acid, and like arachidonic acid in normal animals, it is enriched in inositides of essential fatty acid-deficient animals.

Fatty acids are degraded by C2 units in a manner similar to their biosynthesis. The

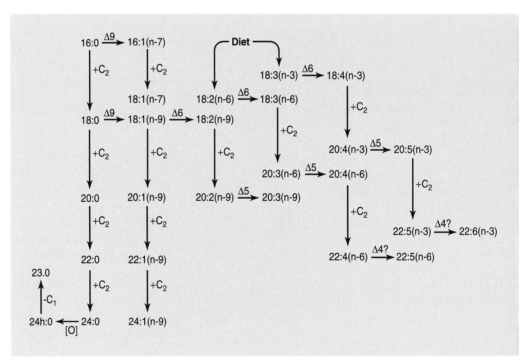

FIG. 7. Pathways of brain fatty acid synthesis. Palmitic acid (16:0) is the main end product of brain fatty acid synthase. It may then be elongated, desaturated, and/or β-oxidized to form different long chain fatty acids. The monoenes (18:1 Δ^9, 18:1 Δ^7, 24:1 Δ^{15}) are the main unsaturated fatty acids formed *de novo* by Δ^9 desaturation and chain elongation. As shown, the very long chain fatty acids are α-oxidized to form α-hydroxy and odd-numbered fatty acids. In severe essential fatty acid deficiency the abnormal polyenes (e.g., 20:3, n − 9) are also biosynthesized *de novo*. The polyunsaturated fatty acids are mainly formed from exogenous dietary fatty acids such as linoleic (n − 6) and linolenic (n − 3) acids by chain elongation and desaturation (Δ^5, Δ^6) as shown. It is doubtful whether there is a Δ^4 desaturase in brain. The Δ^4 desaturation is probably effected by first chain elongation (+C₂), then Δ^6 desaturation, followed by β-oxidation (−C₂) (i.e., by "retroconversion").

acyl CoAs are first dehydrogenated to α,β unsaturated acyl CoA, which are then hydrated to β-hydroxyacyl CoA, followed by oxidation to β-ketoacyl CoA. The C—C bond between C-2 and C-3 of the latter compound is broken by a free coenzyme A (thiolysis) to form an acyl CoA (2C shorter) and acetyl CoA. Unlike fatty acid biosynthesis, enzymes catalyzing β-oxidation of fatty acids are separate proteins, and these are present both in mitochondria and in peroxisomes. Though the biochemical steps are similar in the two cellular compartments, there are some differences between peroxisomal and mitochondrial β-oxidation pathways. In mitochondria the first dehydrogenation is carried out by an FAD-containing enzyme, which is coupled to oxidative phosphorylation thus generating ATP. In peroxisomes, however, this dehydrogenation is carried out by flavin-containing oxidase which reacts directly with molecular oxygen to form H_2O_2, which is further decomposed by peroxisomal catalase to H_2O and O_2, thus wasting the chemical energy [14]. Two separate mitochondrial enzymes (enoyl CoA hydratase and β-hydroxy acyl CoA dehydrogenase) catalyze the next two reaction steps, but in peroxisomes both the reactions are catalyzed by a multifunctional single enzyme protein. The peroxisomal β-oxidation pathway is probably responsible for the oxidation of very long chain fatty acids ($>C_{22}$) which are enriched in brain. Evidence for this is seen in a number of genetic diseases involving peroxisomal disorders, such as Zellweger cerebrohepatorenal syndrome and adrenoleukodystrophy, in which there is an accumulation of such very long chain fatty acids [15], especially in neural tissues (see Chap. 38).

In addition to the classical β-oxidation of fatty acids, known to occur in all tissues, significant α-oxidation, especially of the fatty acids of galactocerebroside, occurs in brain. In this reaction position 2 (α) of a long chain fatty acid is hydroxylated, then oxidized, and decarboxylated to form a fatty acid one carbon shorter than the parent fatty acid. This minor pathway may explain the origins of both the comparatively large amounts of odd carbon fatty acids and of 2-hydroxy fatty acids in brain galactocerebrosides. There is another α-oxidation pathway present in liver and other tissues which is defective in the genetic disorder Refsum disease. This results in the failure to metabolize the dietary branched chain fatty acid phytanic acid, which can be initially metabolized only by α-oxidation [16]. In Refsum disease this branched chain fatty acid accumulates in nervous tissues, resulting in severe neuropathy (see Chap. 38).

Phosphatidic acid is the precursor of all glycerolipids

sn-Glycerol-3-phosphate (G-3-P) formed by the enzymatic (glycerophosphate dehydrogenase) reduction of dihydroxyacetone phosphate (DHAP) by NADH, is consecutively acylated with two acyl CoAs to form phosphatidic acid (PtdOH). Alternatively, DHAP may be first acylated then reduced by NADPH to 1-acyl-GP (lysophosphatidate) which is further acylated to form PtdOH. Acyl DHAP is also the precursor of ether lipids. The ether bond is formed in a reaction where the acyl group of acyl DHAP is substituted by a long chain alcohol to form 1-0-alkyl DHAP. This is then reduced and converted to 1-alkyl, 2-acyl-*sn*-G-3-P, which is converted to the alkyl ether analog of PE, the precursor of PE plasmalogen (Fig. 8) [17].

Phosphatidate is hydrolyzed to 1,2-diacyl-*sn*-glycerol (DAG) which is the precursor of all zwitterionic membrane lipids, PtdCho, PtdEtn, and PtdSer. PtdCho is formed by the transfer of the phosphocholine group from CDP-choline to DAG, and PtdEtn is formed by a corresponding transfer of the head group from CDP-ethanolamine. The enzymes catalyzing the synthesis of CDP-choline and CDP-ethanolamine regulate the overall biosynthesis of PtdCho and PtdEtn. However, details of this regulatory mechanism are not known. In a minor alternative pathway PtdEtn is converted to PtdCho by sequential methylations, the methyl donor being *S*-adenosylmethionine. In animals

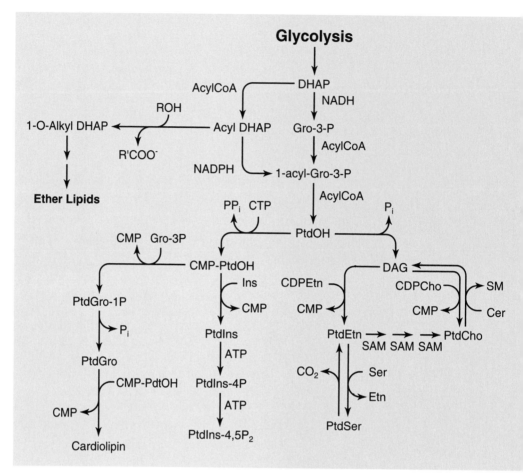

FIG. 8. Schematic representation of glycerophospholipid biosynthesis. Note that dihydroxyacetone phosphate (DHAP) may be reduced to glycerophosphate or may be first acylated and then serve as a precursor of ether lipid. The alkyl analog of phosphatidic acid (i.e., 1-0-alkyl,2-acyl-*sn*-glycerol-3-P) is converted to the alkyl analog of PtdEtn by the same DAG pathway as shown for the diacyl lipids and the alkyl analog of PtdEtn is dehydrogenated to form the 1-alk-1'enyl analog of PtdEtn, i.e., plasmalogen (not shown). As mentioned in the text PtdOH is converted to DAG which is converted to the major brain lipids PtdCho and PtdEtn. The acidic lipids are formed via the conversion of PtdOH to CDP-DAG (CMP-PtdOH). PtdCho and PtdEtn are interconverted either via methylation or via base-exchange reactions to PtdSer. Not only PtdEtn (as shown) but also PtdCho is converted to PtdSer by base exchange reaction. The exchange of PtdCho's head group with ceramide to form sphingomyelin is also shown.

there is no direct pathway for the formation of PtdSer. PtdSer is formed in brain by a base-exchange reaction between PtdEtn, or PtdCho and serine. PtdSer is in turn decarboxylated in mitochondria to form PtdEtn [18].

The acidic phospholipids are synthesized by a completely different pathway where the phosphate group in PtdOH is retained in the product. In this scheme,

PtdOH is converted to the liponucleotide CMP-PtdOH (CDP-DAG, Fig. 8). CDP-DAG reacts with inositol to form PtdIns, or with GroP to form phosphatidyl glycerophosphate, which is converted to cardiolipin (bisphosphatidylglycerol), a mitochondria-specific phospholipid. PtdIns is phosphorylated in the inositol moiety to form PIP and PIP₂ which are involved in the signal transduction process across membranes (see Chap. 20).

The newly biosynthesized phosphoglycerides undergo deacylation to the corresponding lysolipids which are reconverted to the parent lipids by reacylation often with a different fatty acyl substitute. The reacylation of lysolipids occurs either by transferring acyl groups from acyl CoAs or from other phospholipids (CoA-independent acyltransferase). The acyltransferase(s) catalyzing the reacylation reactions are very specific toward the acyl donor and lysolipid substrates. It is thought that the specific distribution of fatty acids in each individual class of membrane phosphoglycerides is regulated by these "deacylation-reacylation" mechanisms. Thus, the initial fatty acid composition of a biosynthetized lipid may not reflect its ultimate composition.

Most of the enzymes catalyzing the biosynthesis of glycerolipids are bound to membranes mainly in endoplasmic reticulum. The enzymes catalyzing the biosynthesis of cardiolipin, however are in mitochondria. The acyl DHAP pathway enzymes, obligatory for the synthesis of ether lipids, are in peroxisomes, a finding that explains the deficiency of ether lipids in patients suffering from genetic peroxisomal disorders, as noted above [19].

The phosphoglycerides are hydrolyzed by specific phospholipases as indicated in Fig. 2. The acyl groups at C-1 and C-2 are hydrolyzed by phospholipase A_1 and A_2, respectively. The presence of PLA_1 in brain is inferential. The head groups are hydrolyzed by class-specific phospholipases. Thus, PtdCho and PtdIns are cleaved by different phospholipases. The bond between DAG and phosphate is hydrolyzed by phospholipase C whereas that between the phosphate and the polar alcohol is hydrolyzed by phospholipase D. These enzymes can be important not only for the catabolism of these lipids but also for the generation of biological signal transduction messenger molecules, such as DAG or arachidonic acid, which are the products of lipid hydrolysis (see Chaps. 20 and 23). Many of these enzymes are regulated, indirectly or directly, by cell-surface receptors. Brain also contains specific hydrolases, plasmalogenase and lysoplasmalogenase, which catalyze the hydrolysis of the alkenyl ether bond to form long chain aldehydes and lysolipids or glycerophosphorylethanolamine, respectively.

Sphingolipids are biosynthesized by adding head groups on the ceramide moiety

Sphinganine (dihydrosphingosine) is biosynthesized by a decarboxylating condensation of serine with palmitoyl CoA to form a keto intermediate, which is then reduced by NADPH (Fig. 9). Sphinganine is dehydrogenated, probably after acylation, to sphingenine (sphingosine). Free sphingosine can be enzymatically acylated with acyl CoA to form ceramide (Fig. 9) [20].

Ceramide is the precursor of all sphingolipids. Sphingomyelin is formed by a reaction exchanging ceramide with PC to form sphingomyelin and DAG (Figs. 8 and 9). The sphingosine-containing glycolipids are formed by consecutive glycosylation of ceramide by different nucleotide derivatives of carbohydrates. For example, galactocerebroside is formed by glycosylation of ceramide with UDPGal, whereas glucocerebroside is formed by glycosylation of ceramide with UDPGlc. The latter (Cer-Glc) is the precursor of neutral glycolipids (globosides) and acidic glycolipids (gangliosides). The CMP-derivative of the N-acetyl (or N-glycolyl) neuraminic acid (NANA or NeuAc) is the donor of this moiety to form gangliosides. Some of the reactions forming these complex glycolipids are shown in Fig. 9. These reactions occur in Golgi bodies and the specificity of these membrane-bound glycosyl transferases toward the lipid substrate and to the water-soluble nucleotide derivatives determines the structure of the product.

These glycolipids are broken down by specific hydrolases present in lysosomes. This enzymatic hydrolysis is stimulated by non-catalytic proteins also present in lysosomes. A congenital deficiency of either one of the hydrolases or in the helper proteins results in the accumulation of lipid intermediates in lysosomes, causing lysosomal stor-

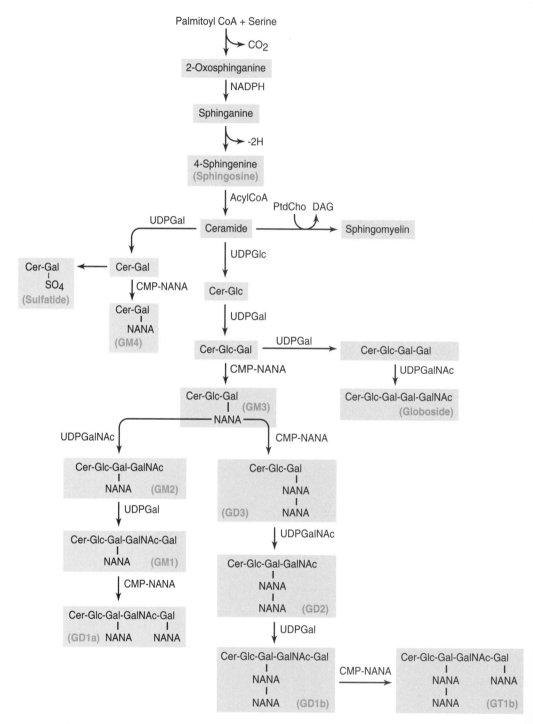

FIG. 9.   Pathways for biosynthesis of sphingolipids. Ceramide (Cer) is the precursor of all sphingolipids. Ceramide is converted to cerebroside (Cer-Gal), the main brain glycolipid, which is further converted to cerebroside sulfate (sulfatide) as shown. Cer-Gal is also converted to ganglioside (GM4) which is present in brain myelin. Most other gangliosides originate from Cer-Glc and the main pathways for formation of these lipids are shown. The abbreviations using Svennerholm nomenclature are shown in parenthesis. The main gangliosides of adult human brain are GM1, GD1a, GD1b and GT1b. NANA, *N*-acetyl neuraminic (sialic) acid.

age disease. For example, in Gaucher's disease Cer-Glc accumulates because of a defect in its hydrolysis, whereas in Tay-Sachs disease, the GM2 ganglioside concentration is increased because of a deficiency in the enzyme hydrolyzing off *N*-acetylgalactosamine [see Chap. 38].

LIPIDS IN THE CELLULAR MILIEU

Lipids are transported from one membrane to another by various means

As indicated above, lipids are often biosynthesized in one intracellular membrane and must be transported to other intracellular compartments for membrane biogenesis. Because lipids are insoluble in water, special mechanisms must exist for this inter- and intracellular transport of membrane lipids. The best understood of such mechanisms is vesicular transport, wherein the lipid particles are enclosed in membrane vesicles, which bud out from the donor membrane, travel to and then fuse with the receiving membrane. The well-characterized transport of blood cholesterol into cells via receptor-mediated endocytosis is a good example of this type of lipid intracellular transport. It is believed that the transport of cholesterol from endoplasmic reticulum to other membranes and the transport of glycolipids from Golgi bodies to plasma membrane are also mediated by similar transport mechanisms. The transport of phosphoglycerides is less clearly understood, but is believed to occur via a carrier-mediated mechanism, i.e., the lipids are complexed with a specific water-soluble protein carrier, which picks up lipids from one membrane and delivers them to another. A number of cellular proteins have been identified, which catalyze a rapid exchange of lipids from one membrane to another. Some of these proteins are specific for particular lipids such as PtdCho or PtdIns, where others are nonspecific. Such lipid-exchange proteins have been identified to be present in brain. Since they thus far have been shown only to exchange lipids however, it is not clear how they can effect a net transport of lipids from one membrane to another.

Lipids are asymmetrically oriented in some membranes

In the "fluid-mosaic" model of biomembranes, the lipids form a bimolecular leaflet in which proteins are embedded (see Chap. 2). This model, with some modifications, is very useful in explaining a number of membrane phenomena, but it does not take into account the complex arrangement (and function) of various polar head groups and different fatty acids present in biomembranes. In some biomembranes, such as those of red blood cells, the choline-containing phospholipids (PtdCho and sphingomyelin) are enriched in the outer leaflet while the amino lipids (PtdEtn and PtdSer) are concentrated in the inner leaflet of the plasma membrane. This arrangement probably also exists in the plasma membrane of most other cells. Similarly, the glycolipids (especially the gangliosides) are enriched in the extracellular side of the plasma membrane, where they may act as receptors for certain ligands (GM1 acts as a receptor for cholera toxin and GD1b for tetanus toxin) and function in intercellular communications. It is not clear how this asymmetric distribution of lipids in biomembranes is maintained. Lipids can move freely within the same plane of the bilayer but their movement from one leaflet of the bilayer to another is thermodynamically restricted. It is postulated that membrane may contain some proteins which catalyze a "flip-flop" transbilayer movements of lipids. Specificity of such "flippase" activity may be responsible for the asymmetric distribution of lipids between the inner and outer leaflets of the membrane bilayer.

Some proteins are anchored to the membranes by covalently linked lipids

In recent years, a number of membrane-bound proteins have been shown to be covalently linked with various lipids, which anchor the protein to the lipid bilayer. In brain proteolipid protein, fatty acids (14:0, 16:0) are attached to the protein via ester (to serine or threonine moiety) or thioester (to cysteine moiety) linkage. A number of cellular proteins are also acylated with myristic acid (14:0) to the free amino group of N-terminal amino acids. A class of proteins, including *ras* (an oncogene product), has been shown to form covalent links with C_{15} (farnesyl) or C_{20} isoprenes via a thioether linkage to cysteine [21]. Such hydrocarbon anchors are necessary for these proteins to exhibit their biological activities. A very novel lipo-

protein discovered as a variable surface antigen of trypanosomes, as well as for a number of mammalian proteins, were recently found to contain PtdIns. The PtdIns moiety is glycosidically linked to glucosamine which is further linked to a polymannan backbone. The polysaccharide chain is joined to the protein via ethanolamine phosphate, with an amide linkage to the carboxyl terminal of the protein [22]. A number of brain proteins attached to the outer surface of plasma membrane such as acetylcholine esterase and Thy-1 antigen have been shown to have such structures (Fig. 10). The phosphatidylinosi-

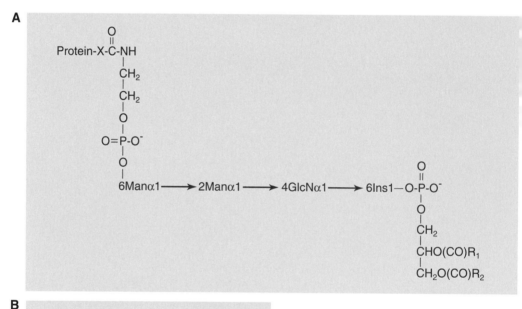

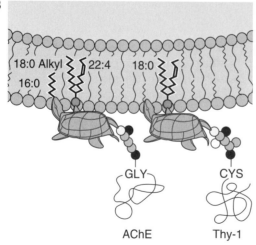

FIG. 10.   Structure of phosphatidylinositol anchors. **A:** The backbone structure of a GPI-anchor. Additional phosphoethanolamine (●), galactose (○), or GalNAc (◑) may be attached to one of the mannose moieties; (○, GlcNAc). **B:** The structure of GPI anchors of Thy-1 antigen and acetylcholine esterase. Acetylcholine esterase has an additional fatty acid moiety (16:0) attached to the 2-position of inositol. This third acyl group makes the PtdIns moiety refractory to the hydrolysis by PtdIns-specific PLC (see Chap. 20 for details of inositol stereochemistry.

tol moiety in these proteins may contain alkyl ether at C-1 of the glycerol, generally not found in free PtdIns. This lipid anchor is biosynthesized by sequential addition of the carbohydrate moiety to the PtdIns structure. PtdIns first reacts with UDPGlcNAc to form PtdIns6 → 1GlcNAc which is deacetylated to form free glucosamine linked to PtdIns. The D-mannose moieties are then transferred from dolichol-P-mannose to make the polysaccharide backbone which then forms a phosphodiester bond with 2-phosphoethanolamine, which is derived from PtdEtn. The whole structure is linked to the C-terminal amino acid of the protein, which is then exported to the outer surface of plasma membrane. The presence of a free-NH_2 group in the glucosamine residue makes the structure labile to nitrous acid. Bacterial PtdIns-specific phospholipase C hydrolyzes the bond between DAG and InsP, releasing the water-soluble protein polysaccharide-Ins-P moiety [22].

Lipids have multiple roles in cells

Recent discoveries show that the same lipid may have both structural and regulatory roles in the cell. For example, while arachidonic acid (20:4, n − 6) is a major constituent of brain inositides and PtdEtn, the free acid is also a precursor of a number of important biomessengers (eicosanoids) such as prostaglandins, prostacyclins, leukotrienes, and thromboxanes (see Chap. 23). Arachidonic acid itself acts as a biomessenger by activating certain isoforms of protein kinase C, or it is covalently linked to other groups such as forming an amide with ethanolamine, which (termed anandamide) recently has been shown to be the endogenous ligand for cannabinoid receptors in brain [23]. Similarly, DAG is an important precursor for lipid biosynthesis in endoplasmic reticulum, but in another cellular compartment (plasma membrane) it acts as a second messenger and activates protein kinase C. The major structural lipids such as PtdIns (and possibly also PtdCho) are also inti-

mately involved with the signal transduction process (see Chap. 20). A novel ether lipid 1-O-hexadecyl-2-acetyl-*sn*-glycero-3-phosphocholine termed platelet activating factor (PAF) has potent biomessenger activity in aggregating platelets and releasing eicosanoids. These recent discoveries point out the increasing importance of lipids not only in maintaining membrane structure, but also in the regulation of cellular metabolism and growth.

REFERENCES

1. Inoue, T., Deshmukh, D. S., and Pieringer, R. A. The association of the galactosyl diglycerides of brain with myelination. I. Changes in the concentration of monogalactosyl diglyceride in microsomal and myelin fractions of brain of rats during development. *J. Biol. Chem.* 246:5688–5694, 1971.
2. Sastry, P. S. Lipids of nervous tissue: Composition and metabolism. *Prog. Lipid Res.* 24:69–176, 1985.
3. Wells, M. A., and Dittmer, J. C. A comprehensive study of the postnatal changes in the concentration of the lipids of developing rat brain. *Biochemistry* 10:3169–3175, 1967.
4. O'Brien, J. S., and Sampson, E. L. Lipid composition of the normal human brain: Gray matter, white matter, and myelin. *J. Lipid Res.* 6:537–544, 1965.
5. Lee, C., and Hajra, A. K. Molecular species of diacylglycerols and phosphoglycerides and the postmortem changes in the molecular species of diacylglycerols in rat brain. *J. Neurochem.* 56:370–379, 1991.
6. Yu, R. K., and Ando, S. Structures of some new complex gangliosides. In L. Svennerholm, P. Mandel, H. Dreyfus, and P.-F. Urban (eds.), *Structure and Function of Gangliosides.* New York, Plenum, 1980, pp. 33–45.
7. Wiegandt, H. The gangliosides. In B. W. Agranoff and M. H. Aprison (eds.), *Advances in Neurochemistry,* New York: Plenum, 1982, Vol. 4, 149–223.
8. Folch, J., Lees, M., and Sloane-Stanley, G. H. A simple method for the isolation and purification of total lipids from animal tissues. *J. Biol. Chem.* 226:497–509, 1957.
9. Hajra, A. K., Fisher, S. K., and Agranoff, B.

W. Isolation, separation and analysis of phosphoinositides from biological sources. In A. A. Boulton, G. B. Baker, and L. A. Horrocks (eds.), *Neuromethods (Neurochemistry), Vol. 8: Lipids and Related Compounds.* Clifton, NJ: Humana Press, 1987.

10. Suzuki, K. Chemistry and metabolism of brain lipids. In G. J. Siegel, R. W. Albers, B. W. Agranoff, and R. Katzman (eds.). *Basic Neurochemistry,* 3rd ed., Little, Brown: Boston, 1981, pp. 355–370.

11. Brown, M. S., and Goldstein, J. L. A receptor-mediated pathway for cholesterol homeostasis. *Science* 232:34–47, 1986.

12. Cinti, D. L., Cook, L., Nagi, M. N., and Suneja, S. K. The fatty acid chain elongation system of mammalian endoplasmic reticulum. *Prog. Lipid Res.* 31:1–51, 1992.

13. Holman, R. T. Nutritional and biochemical evidences of acyl interaction with respect to essential polyunsaturated fatty acids. *Prog. Lipid Res.* 25:29–39, 1986.

14. deDuve, C. Microbodies in the living cell. *Sci. Am.* 248:74–84, 1983.

15. Moser, H. W., and Moser, A. B. Adrenoleukodystrophy (X-linked). In C. R. Scriver, A. L. Beaudet, W. S. Sly, and D. Valle (eds.), *The Metabolic Basis of Inherited Disease,* 6th ed. New York: McGraw Hill, 1989, pp. 1511–1532.

16. Steinberg, D. Refsum disease. In C. R. Scriver, A. L. Beaudet, W. S. Sly, and D. Valle (eds.), *The Metabolic Basis of Inherited Disease,* 6th ed. New York: McGraw Hill, 1989, pp. 1533–1550.

17. Hajra, A. K. Biosynthesis of *O*-alkylglycerol ether lipids. In H. K. Mangold, and F. Paultauf (eds.), *Ether Lipids: Biochemical and Biomedical Aspects.* New York: Academic, 1983, pp. 85–106.

18. Kennedy, E. P. The biosynthesis of phospholipids. In J. A. F. Op den Kamp, B. Roelofsen, and K. W. A. Wirtz (eds.), *Lipids and Membranes: Past, Present and Future,* Amsterdam: Elsevier, 1986, pp. 171–206.

19. Hajra, A. K., Horie, S., and Webber, K. O. The role of peroxisomes in glycerol ether metabolism. *Progr. Clin. Biol. Res.* 282:99–116, 1988.

20. Radin, N. S. Biosynthesis of the sphingoid bases: A provocation. *J. Lipid Res.* 25: 1536–1540, 1984.

21. Glomset, J. A., Gebb, M. H., and Farnsworth, C. C. Prenyl proteins in eukaryotic cells: a new type of membrane anchor. *Trends Biochem. Sci.* 15:139–142, 1990.

22. Low, M. G. The glycosyl-phosphatidylinositol anchor of membrane proteins. *Biochim. Biophys. Acta.* 988:427–454, 1989.

23. Devane, W. A., Hanus, L., Breuer, A., Pertwee, R. G., Stevenson, L. A., Griffin, G., Gibson, D., Mandelbaum, A., Etinger, A., and Mechoulam, R. *Science* 258:1946–1949, 1992.

GENERAL REFERENCES

Lajtha, A. (ed.). *Handbook of Neurochemistry, 2nd ed., Vol. 7: Structural Elements of the Nervous System.* New York: Plenum, 1985.

Svennerholm, L., Mandel, P., Dreyfus, H., and Urban, P.-F. (eds.). *Structure and Function of Gangliosides.* New York: Plenum, 1980.

Vance, D. E., and Vance, J. (eds.). *Biochemistry of Lipids, Lipoproteins and Membranes.* Amsterdam: Elsevier Science, 1991.

CHAPTER 6

Myelin Formation, Structure, and Biochemistry

PIERRE MORELL, RICHARD H. QUARLES, AND WILLIAM T. NORTON

The morphological distinction between white matter and gray matter is one that is useful for the neurochemist. White matter, so called for its glistening white appearance, is composed of myelinated axons, glial cells, and blood vessels. Gray matter contains, in addition, the nerve cell bodies with their extensive dendritic arborizations, and quite different ratios of the other elements. The predominant element of white matter is the myelin sheath, which comprises about 50 percent of the total dry weight. Myelin is mainly responsible for the gross chemical differences between white and gray matter.

Basic Neurochemistry: Molecular, Cellular, and Medical Aspects, 5th Ed., edited by G. J. Siegel et al. Published by Raven Press, Ltd., New York, 1994. Correspondence to Pierre Morell, Department of Biochemistry, 321 Brain and Development Research Center, CB# 7250, University of North Carolina, Chapel Hill, North Carolina 27599.

THE MYELIN SHEATH

The myelin sheath is a greatly extended and modified plasma membrane which is wrapped around the nerve axon in a spiral fashion (for review, see Raine [1]). The myelin membranes originate from, and are part of, the Schwann cell in the peripheral nervous system (PNS), and the oligodendroglial cells in the central nervous system (CNS) (see Chap. 1). Each myelin-generating cell furnishes myelin for only one segment of any given axon. The periodic interruptions where short portions of the axon are left uncovered by myelin are the *nodes of Ranvier*, and they are critical to the functioning of myelin.

Myelin facilitates conduction

Myelin is an electrical insulator, however, its function of facilitating conduction in axons has no exact analogy in electrical circuitry. In unmyelinated fibers, impulse conduction is propagated by local circuits of ion current that flow into the active region of the axonal membrane, through the axon, and out through adjacent sections of the membrane (Fig. 1). These local circuits depolarize the adjacent piece of membrane in a continuous sequential fashion. In myelinated axons, the excitable axonal membrane is exposed to the extracellular space only at the nodes of Ranvier; this is the location of sodium channels

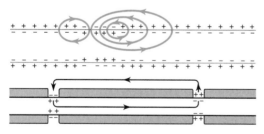

FIG. 1. Impulse conduction in unmyelinated *(top)* and myelinated *(bottom)* fibers. The *arrows* show the flow of action currents in local circuits into the active region of the membrane. In unmyelinated fibers the circuits flow through the adjacent piece of membrane, but in myelinated fibers the circuit flow jumps to the next node.

(see [2], for review). When the membrane at the node is excited, the local circuit generated cannot flow through the high-resistance sheath and therefore flows out through and depolarizes the membrane at the next node, which might be 1 mm or farther away (see Fig. 1). The low capacitance of the sheath means that little energy is required to depolarize the remaining membrane between the nodes, which results in an increased speed of local circuit spreading. Active excitation of the axonal membrane jumps from node to node; this form of impulse propagation is called *saltatory conduction* (Latin *saltare*, "to jump"). Such movement of the wave of depolarization is much more rapid than is the case in unmyelinated fibers. Furthermore, because only the nodes of Ranvier are excited during conduction in myelinated fibers, sodium flux into the nerve is much less than in unmyelinated fibers, where the entire membrane is involved. An example of the advantage of myelination is obtained by comparison of two different nerve fibers which both conduct at 25 m/sec at 20°C. The 500 μm diameter unmyelinated giant axon of the squid required 5,000 times as much energy and occupies about 1,500 times as much space as 12 μm diameter myelinated nerve in a frog.

Conduction velocity in myelinated fibers is proportional to the diameter, while in unmyelinated fibers it is proportional to the square root of the diameter. Thus, differences in energy and space requirements between the two types of fibers are exaggerated at higher conduction velocities. If nerves were not myelinated and equivalent conduction velocities were maintained, the human spinal cord would need to be as large as a good-sized tree trunk. Myelin, then, facilitates conduction while conserving space and energy. (For literature references and a more detailed treatment of this topic see Ritchie [3]).

Myelin has a characteristic ultrastructure

Myelin, as well as many of its morphological features, such as nodes of Ranvier and

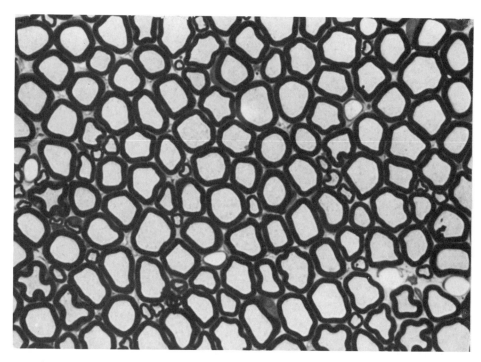

FIG. 2. Light micrograph of a 1 μm Epon section of rabbit peripheral nerve (anterior root), stained with toluidine blue. The myelin sheath appears as a thick black ring around the pale axon. ×600, before 30 percent reduction. (Courtesy of Dr. Cedric Raine.)

Schmidt-Lanterman clefts, can be seen readily in the light microscope (Fig. 2). However, much of our understanding of the organization of this structure has been derived from studies by three physical techniques: polarized light, X-ray diffraction, and electron microscopy. Structures with parallel axons, sciatic nerve as representative of the PNS and optic nerve or tract as representative of the CNS, have been studied. Myelin, when examined by polarized light, exhibits both a lipid-dependent and a protein-dependent birefringence. These results suggest that myelin is built up of layers; the lipid component of these layers is oriented radially to the axis of the nerve fiber, whereas the protein component is oriented tangentially to the nerve. Low-angle X-ray diffraction studies of myelin provide electron density plots of the repeating unit that show three peaks (each corresponding to protein plus lipid polar groups) and two troughs (lipid hydrocarbon chains).

The repeat distance varies somewhat depending on the species and whether the sample is from CNS or PNS. Thus, the results from these two techniques are consistent with a protein-lipid-protein-lipid-protein structure, in which the lipid portion is a bimolecular leaflet and adjacent protein layers are different in some way.

Figure 3 data for mammalian optic nerve shows a repeat distance of 80 Å. This spacing can accommodate one bimolecular layer of lipid (about 50 Å) and two protein layers (about 15 Å each). The main repeating unit of two such fused unit membranes is twice this figure, or 160 Å. (References to results obtained using this methodology, as well as to those obtained from more recent high-resolution studies, are reviewed in [5].) Although it is useful to think of myelin in terms of alternating protein and lipid layers, this concept has been modified somewhat in recent years to be compatible with the "fluid

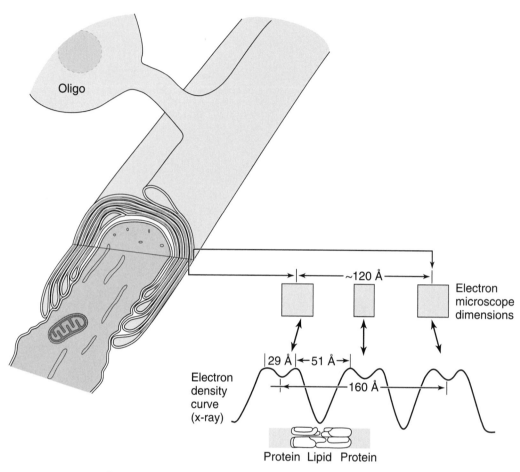

FIG. 3. A composite diagram summarizing some of the ultrastructural data on CNS myelin. At the top an oligo-dendroglial cell is shown connected to the sheath by a process. The cutaway view of the myelin and axon illustrates the relationship of these two structures at the nodal and paranodal regions. (Only a few myelin layers have been drawn for the sake of clarity.) At the internodal region, the cross section reveals the inner and outer mesaxons and their relationship to the inner cytoplasmic wedges and the outer loop of cytoplasm. Note that in contrast to PNS myelin, there is no full ring of cytoplasm surrounding the outside of the sheath. The lower part of the figure shows roughly the dimensions and appearance of one myelin repeating unit as seen with fixed and embedded preparations in the electron microscope. This is contrasted with the dimensions of the electron density curve of CNS myelin obtained by X-ray diffraction studies in fresh nerve. The components responsible for the peaks and troughs of the curve are sketched below. (From Norton [4]. Reprinted courtesy of Lea & Febiger, publishers.)

mosaic" model of membrane structure that includes intrinsic transmembrane proteins as well as extrinsic proteins.

The conclusions noted above are fully supported by electron microscope studies. This technique visualizes myelin as a series of alternating dark and less dark lines (protein layers) separated by unstained zones (the lipid hydrocarbon chains) (Figs. 4–7). The asymmetry in the staining of the protein layers results from the way the myelin sheath is generated from the cell plasma membrane (see next section and Figs. 8–10). The less dark, or intraperiod, line represents the closely apposed outer protein coats of the original cell membrane; the membranes are

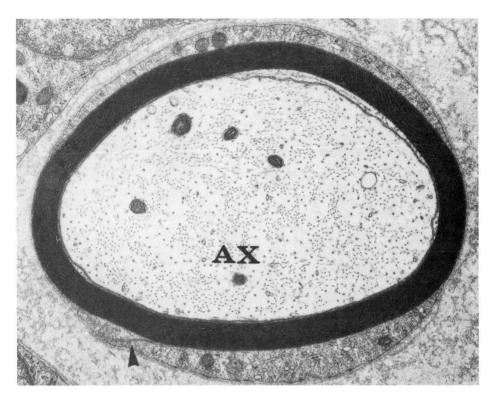

FIG. 4. Electron micrograph of a single peripheral nerve fiber from rabbit. Note that the myelin sheath has a lamellated structure and is surrounded by Schwann cell cytoplasm. The outer mesaxon *(arrowhead)* can be seen in lower left. (AX) axon ×18,000. (Courtesy of Dr. Cedric Raine.)

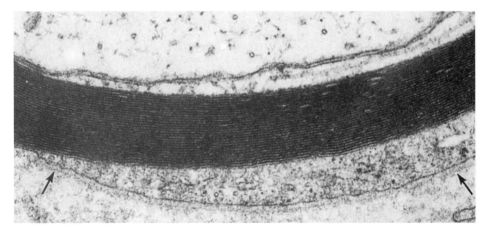

FIG. 5. Higher magnification of Fig. 4 to show the Schwann cell cytoplasm covered by basal lamina *(arrows)*. ×50,000.

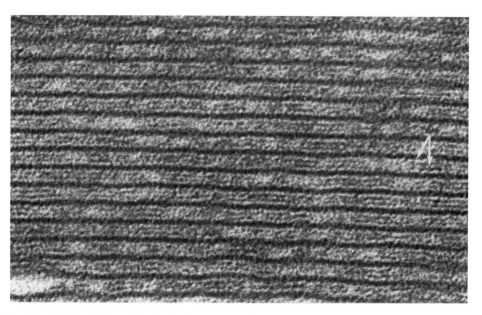

FIG. 6.   Magnification of the myelin sheath of Fig. 4. Note that the intraperiod line *(arrows)* at this high resolution is a double structure. ×350,000. (Courtesy of Dr. Cedric Raine.)

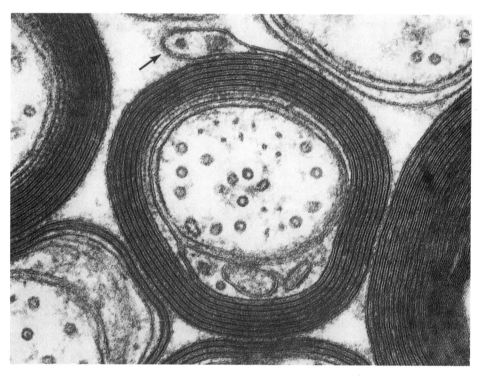

FIG. 7.   A typical CNS myelinated fiber from the spinal cord of an adult dog. Contrast this figure with the PNS fiber in Fig. 3. The course of the flattened oligodendrocytic process, beginning at the outer tongue *(arrow),* can be traced. Note that the fiber lacks investing cell cytoplasm and a basal lamina—as is the case in the PNS. The major dense line and the paler, double intraperiod line of the myelin sheath can be discerned. The axon contains neurotubules and neurofilaments. ×135,000.

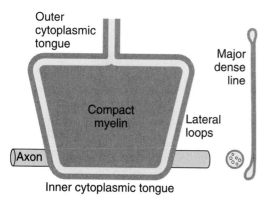

Outer cytoplasmic tongue

Major dense line

Compact myelin

Lateral loops

Axon

Inner cytoplasmic tongue

FIG. 8.   A diagram showing the appearance of CNS myelin if it were unrolled from the axon. One can visualize this structure arising from Fig. 3, if the glial cell process were pulled straight up and the myelin layers separated at the intermediate period line. The whole myelin internode forms a spade-shaped sheet surrounded by a continuous tube of oligodendroglial cell cytoplasm. This diagram shows that the lateral loops and inner and outer cytoplasmic tongues are parts of the same cytoplasmic tube. The drawing on the right shows the appearance of this sheet if it were sectioned along the vertical line, indicating that the compact myelin region is formed of two unit membranes fused at the cytoplasmic surfaces. (The drawing is not necessarily to scale.) (Adapted from [6].)

not actually fused as they can be resolved as a double line at high resolution (Figs. 6 and 7). The dark, or major period, line is the fused, inner protein coats of the cell membrane. Confirmation of this interpretation comes from examination of myelin of the PNS, which has been swollen in hypotonic solutions. Electron microscopy reveals splitting only at the intraperiod line, and the electron density plots show that the broadening occurs at the wider of the three peaks in the repeating unit. This approach shows the continuity of the membrane junction of the minor period with the extracellular space and proves that the wide electron density peak in peripheral nerve plots corresponds to the intraperiod lines seen in electron micrographs. The repeat distances observed by electron microscopy are less than those calculated from the low angle X-ray diffraction data, a consequence of the considerable shrinkage that takes place after fixation and dehydration. However, the difference in pe-

riodicity between the PNS myelin and CNS myelin is maintained; peripheral myelin has an average repeat distance of 119 Å and the central myelin of 107 Å.

Nodes of Ranvier

Two adjacents segments of myelin on one axon are separated by a node of Ranvier. In this region the axon is not covered by myelin. At the paranodal region and the Schmidt-Lanterman clefts, the cytoplasmic surfaces of myelin are not compacted, and Schwann or glial cell cytoplasm is included within the sheath. To visualize these structures one may refer to Figs. 8 and 9, adapted from those of Hirano and Dembitzer [6], which show that if myelin were unrolled from the axon it would be a flat, spade-shaped sheet surrounded by a tube of cytoplasm. Thus, as shown in electron micrographs of longitudinal sections of axon paranodal regions, the major dense line formed by apposition of the cytoplasmic faces opens up at the edges of the sheet, enclosing cytoplasm within a loop (see Figs. 3 and 9). These loop-shaped terminations of the sheath at the node are called *lateral loops*. The loops form membrane complexes with the axolemma called *transverse bands*, whereas myelin in the internodal region is separated from the axon by a gap of *periaxonal* space. The transverse bands are helical structures that seal the myelin to the axolemma but provide, by spaces between them, a tortuous path from the extracellular space to the periaxonal space.

Schmidt-Lanterman Clefts

The Schmidt-Lanterman clefts, structures common in peripheral, but rare in central, myelinated axons are regions where the cytoplasmic surfaces of the myelin sheath have not compacted to form the major dense line and therefore contain Schwann or glial cell cytoplasm (Fig. 9). These inclusions of cytoplasm are present in each layer of myelin. Therefore, the clefts can be visualized in the unrolled myelin sheet as tubes of cytoplasm similar to the tubes making up the lateral

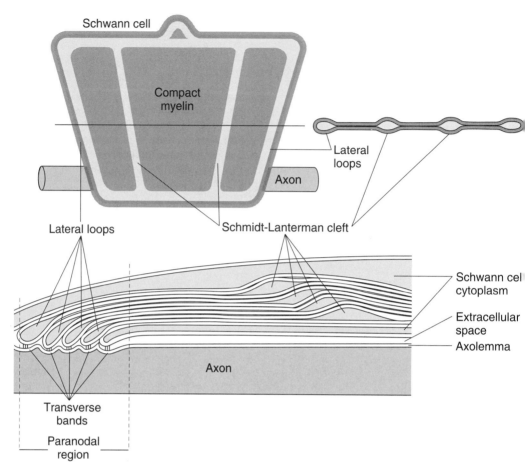

FIG. 9.   A diagram similar to Fig. 8, but showing one Schwann cell and its myelin sheath unrolled from a peripheral axon. The sheet of PNS myelin is, like CNS myelin, surrounded by a tube of cytoplasm and has additional tubes of cytoplasm, which make up the Schmidt-Lanterman clefts, running through the internodal regions. The horizontal section *(top right)* shows that these additional tubes of cytoplasm arise from regions where the cytoplasmic membrane surfaces have not fused. Diagram *(bottom)* is an enlarged view of a portion of *(top left)*, the Schwann cell and its membrane wrapped around the axon. The tube forming the lateral loops seals to the axolemma at the paranodal region, and the cytoplasmic tubes in the internodal region form the Schmidt-Lanterman clefts. (These drawings are not to scale.) (Adapted from [6].)

loops but in the middle regions of the sheet, rather than at the edges (Fig. 9).

Myelin is an extension of a cell membrane

Myelination in the PNS

Myelination in the PNS is preceded by invasion of the nerve bundle by Schwann cells, rapid multiplication of these cells, and segregation of the individual axons by Schwann cell processes. Smaller axons (≤ 1 μm), which will remain unmyelinated, are segregated; several may be enclosed in one cell, each within its own pocket, similar to the structure shown in Fig. 10A. Large axons (≥ 1 μm) destined for myelination are enclosed singly, one cell per axon per internode. These cells line up along the axons with intervals between them; the intervals become the nodes of Ranvier.

Before myelination the axon lies in an

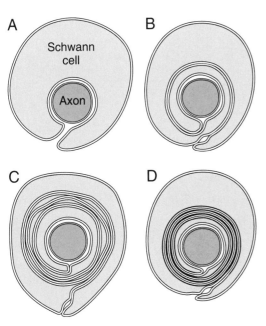

FIG. 10. Myelin formation in the peripheral nervous system. **A:** The Schwann cell has surrounded the axon but the external surfaces of the plasma membrane have not yet fused in the mesaxon. **B:** The mesaxon has fused into a five-layered structure and spiraled once around the axon. **C:** A few layers of myelin have formed but are not completely compacted. Note the cytoplasm trapped in zones where the cytoplasmic membrane surfaces have not yet fused. **D:** Compact myelin showing only a few layers for the sake of clarity. Note that Schwann cell cytoplasm forms a ring both inside and outside of the sheath. (From Norton [4]. Reprinted courtesy of Lea & Febiger, publishers.)

invagination of the Schwann cell (see Fig. 10A). The plasmalemma of the cell then surrounds the axon and joins to form a double membrane structure that communicates with the cell surface. This structure, called the *mesaxon,* then elongates around the axon in a spiral fashion (see Fig. 10). Thus, mature myelin is formed in this "jelly-roll" fashion; the mesaxon winds about the axon, and the cytoplasmic surfaces condense into a compact myelin sheath and form the major dense line. The two external surfaces form the myelin intraperiod line.

Myelination in the CNS

The structure of myelin in the CNS, formed by the oligodendroglial cell [7], has many similarities but also points of difference, with respect to the situation in the PNS. CNS nerve fibers are not separated by connective tissue, nor are they surrounded by cell cytoplasm, and specific glial nuclei are not obviously associated with particular myelinated fibers. CNS myelin is a spiral structure similar to PNS myelin; it has an inner mesaxon and an outer mesaxon that ends in a loop, or tongue, of glial cytoplasm (Fig. 3). Unlike peripheral nerve, where the sheath is surrounded by Schwann cell cytoplasm, the cytoplasmic tongue in the CNS is restricted to a small portion of the sheath. This glial tongue is continuous with the plasma membrane of the oligodendroglial cell through slender processes. One glial cell can myelinate many (40 or more) separate axons [8].

Myelin deposition in the PNS may result in a single axon having up to 100 myelin layers, and it is therefore improbable that myelin is laid down by a simple rotation of the Schwann cell nucleus around the axon. In the CNS, such a postulate is precluded by the fact that one glial cell can myelinate several axons. During myelination, there are increases in the length of the internode, the diameter of the axon, and the number of myelin layers. Myelin is therefore expanding in all planes at once. Any mechanism to account for this growth must assume the membrane system is able to expand and contract, and that layers slip over each other.

Myelin can be isolated in high yield and purity by conventional methods of subcellular fractionation

CNS Myelin Isolation

If CNS tissue is homogenized in media of low ionic strength, myelin peels off the axons and reforms in vesicles of the size range of nuclei and mitochondria. Because of their high lipid content, these myelin vesicles have the lowest intrinsic density of any membrane fraction of the nervous system. Procedures for isolation of myelin take advantage of both of these properties—large vesicle size and low density (see Norton and Cammer [9] for review.)

In a widely used method, a homogenate of nervous tissue in isotonic sucrose (0.3 M) is layered directly onto 0.85 M sucrose and centrifuged at high speed. Mitochondria and synaptosomes sediment through the denser sucrose and many of the smaller membrane fragments from other organelles remain in the 0.3 M sucrose layer. A crude myelin layer collects at the interface. The major impurities, microsomes, and axoplasm trapped in the vesicles during the homogenization procedure, are released by subjecting the myelin to osmotic shock in distilled water. The larger myelin particles can then be separated from the smaller, membranous material by low-speed centrifugation or by repeating the density gradient centrifugation on continuous or discontinuous gradients, usually of sucrose. On a continuous sucrose gradient, myelin forms a band centering at approximately 0.65 M sucrose, equivalent to a density of 1.08 g/ml. Thus, these preparations of purified myelin can be further subdivided arbitrarily into fractions of different densities by centrifugation on expanded continuous or discontinuous density gradients. These fractions differ somewhat in composition (described in a following section).

Demonstration of purity for a myelin preparation includes electron-microscopic appearance (the typical five-layered structure and repeat period of about 120 Å seen *in situ*); however, the difficulty of identifying small membrane vesicles of microsomes in a field of myelin membranes and the well-known sampling problems inherent in electron microscopy make this characterization unreliable after a certain purity level has been reached.

Markers characteristic of myelin include certain proteins, lipids, and enzymes described in following sections. Although such assays are useful, like electron microscopy they are not sensitive to small amounts of impurities. If purity of a myelin preparation is an issue, it is important to assay contamina-tion of myelin by other subcellular fractions using markers such as succinic dehydrogenase (mitochondria); (Na,K-ATPase and 5′-nucleotidase (plasma membranes); NADH-cytochrome-C reductase (microsomes); DNA (nuclei); RNA (nuclei, ribosomes, microsomes); lactate dehydrogenase (cytosol); β-glucosidase (lysosomes); and acetylcholinesterase (neuronal fragments). Although all of these markers are low in purified myelin, and set an outside limit for levels of contamination by other membranes, the actual contamination may be less than calculated by such methods since low levels of many different enzymes appear to be intrinsic to myelin (discussed in a following section).

PNS Myelin Isolation

Peripheral nerve myelin can be isolated by similar techniques, but especially vigorous homogenization conditions are required because of the large amounts of connective tissue and, sometimes, adipose tissue present in the nerve. The slightly lesser density of PNS myelin requires some adjustment of gradient composition to prevent loss of myelin.

CHARACTERISTIC COMPOSITION OF MYELIN

Myelin *in situ* has a water content of about 40 percent. The dry mass of both CNS and PNS myelin is characterized by a high proportion of lipid (70 to 85 percent) and, consequently, a low proportion of protein (15 to 30 percent). In contrast, most biological membranes have a higher ratio of proteins to lipids.

CNS myelin is enriched in certain lipids

Table 1 lists the composition of bovine, rat, and human myelin compared to bovine and human white matter, human gray matter, and rat whole brain. (The classification of brain lipids is discussed in Chap. 5.) All the lipids assayed in whole brain are also present

TABLE 1.   Composition of CNS myelin and brain[a]

Substance[b]	Myelin			White matter		Gray matter (human)	Whole brain (rat)
	Human	Bovine	Rat	Human	Bovine		
Protein	30.0	24.7	29.5	39.0	39.5	55.3	56.9
Lipid	70.0	75.3	70.5	54.9	55.0	32.7	37.0
Cholesterol	27.7	28.1	27.3	27.5	23.6	22.0	23.0
Cerebroside	22.7	24.0	23.7	19.8	22.5	5.4	14.6
Sulfatide	3.8	3.6	7.1	5.4	5.0	1.7	4.8
Total galactolipid	27.5	29.3	31.5	26.4	28.6	7.3	21.3
Ethanolamine phosphatides	15.6	17.4	16.7	14.9	13.6	22.7	19.8
Lecithin	11.2	10.9	11.3	12.8	12.9	26.7	22.0
Sphingomyelin	7.9	7.1	3.2	7.7	6.7	6.9	3.8
Phosphatidylserine	4.8	6.5	7.0	7.9	11.4	8.7	7.2
Phosphatidylinositol	0.6	0.8	1.2	0.9	0.9	2.7	2.4
Plasmalogens[c]	12.3	14.1	14.1	11.2	12.2	8.8	11.6
Total phospholipid	43.1	43.0	44.0	45.9	46.3	69.5	57.6

From W. Norton. In G. J. Siegel, R. W. Albers, B. W. Agranoff, and R. Katzman (eds.), Basic Neurochemistry, 3rd. ed. Boston: Little, Brown, 1981, p. 77.
[b] Protein and lipid figures in percent dry weight; all others in percent total lipid weight.
[c] Plasmalogens are primarily ethanolamine phosphatides.

in myelin; that is, there are no lipids localized exclusively in some "nonmyelin compartment" (with the exception of the mitochondrial specific lipid, diphosphatidylglycerol, not included in this table). We also know that the reverse is true; that is, there are no myelin lipids that are not also found in other subcellular fractions of the brain. Even though there are no "myelin-specific" lipids, cerebroside is the most typical of myelin. During development, the concentration of cerebroside in brain is directly proportional to the amount of myelin present.

In addition to cerebroside, the major lipids of myelin are cholesterol, and ethanolamine containing plasmalogens (glycerophospholipids containing an alkenyl ether bond—see Chap. 5). Lecithin is also a major myelin constituent, and sphingomyelin, a relatively minor one. Not only is the lipid class composition of myelin highly characteristic of this membrane, the fatty acid composition of many of the individual lipids is distinctive.

The data in Table 1 suggest that myelin accounts for much of the total lipid of white matter, and that the lipid composition of gray matter is quite different from that of myelin. It is of interest that the composition of brain myelin from all mammalian species studied is very much the same. However, there are some obvious species differences. For example, myelin of rat has less sphingomyelin than does that of bovine or human (Table 1). Although not shown in the table, there are also regional variations, for example, myelin isolated from the spinal cord has a higher lipid-to-protein ratio than brain myelin from the same species.

Besides the lipids listed in Table 1, there are several others of importance. If myelin is not extracted with acidified organic solvents, the polyphosphoinositides (see Chap. 20) remain tightly bound to the myelin protein, and therefore are not included in the lipid analysis. Triphosphoinositide accounts for between 4 and 6 percent of the total myelin phosphorus, and diphosphoinositide for 1 to 1.5 percent of the myelin phosphorus.

Several classes of lipids are minor components of myelin. These include at least three fatty acid esters of cerebroside and two glycerol-based lipids, diacylglyceryl-galacto-side and monoalkylmonoacylglycerylgalacto-side, collectively called galactosyldiglyceride. Some long chain alkanes also appear to be present. Myelin from mammals also contains 0.1 to 0.3 percent ganglioside (complex sialic acid-containing glycosphingolipids). The proportion of the different gangliosides to each other is different in myelin (greatly enriched in monosialoganglioside GM_1) relative to other brain membranes (enriched in the polysialo species). Myelin from certain species (including human) contains an additional unique ganglioside as a major component, sialosylgalactosylceramide, GM_4.

PNS myelin lipids are similar to those of CNS myelin

Myelin from the PNS has many of the same lipids as myelin of the CNS, although there are quantitative differences [10]. The analyses that have been made show that PNS myelin has less cerebroside and sulfatide and considerably more sphingomyelin than CNS myelin. Of interest is the presence of ganglioside LM_1 (sialosyl-lactoneotetraosylcera-mide) as a characteristic component of myelin in the PNS of some species. These differences in lipid composition between CNS and PNS myelin are not, however, as dramatic as the differences in protein composition discussed below.

CNS myelin contains unique proteins

The protein composition of CNS myelin is simpler than that of other brain membranes, with the proteolipid protein and basic protein(s), making up to 60 to 80 percent of the total in most species. Most other proteins and glycoproteins are present to lesser extents. With the exception of the basic proteins, myelin proteins are neither easily extractable nor soluble in aqueous media. However, like other membrane proteins, they may be solubilized in sodium dodecyl-sulfate solutions and, in this condition, can be separated readily by electrophoresis in polyacrylamide gels. This technique separates proteins primarily according to their molecular weight (a common notation is M for relative molecular mass, another is to state molecular weight in kiloDaltons, kDa). The presence of bound carbohydrates or unusual structural features disrupts somewhat the relationship between migration and molecular weight so that terminology for location of a protein in such a gel is taken to mean "apparent" molecular weight. Protein composition of human and rat brain myelin are illustrated in Fig. 11B and 11D, respectively. The quantitative predominance of two proteins, the positively charged myelin basic protein (MBP, $M_r = 18,500$) and proteolipid protein (PLP) in the gel pattern of human CNS myelin is clear. These proteins are major constituents of all mammalian CNS myelins and similar proteins are present in myelins of many lower species (for review and references see Benjamins et al. [11] and Lees and Brostoff [12].

Proteolipid Protein

Myelin PLP is the major component of the organic solvent extractable lipoprotein complexes of whole brain. This protein, also known as the Folch-Lees protein (see Lees and Brostoff [12] for review) has the unusual physical property of solubility in organic solvents. The molecular mass of PLP from sequence analysis is about 30,000, although it migrates anomalously fast on SDS gels and gives a lower apparent molecular mass. The amino acid sequence, strongly conserved during evolution, involves about 60 percent nonpolar amino acids and 40 percent polar amino acids. Proteolipid protein contains about 3 moles of fatty acids (primarily palmitate, oleate, or stearate) per mole protein in ester linkage to hydroxy amino acids. There is rapid turnover of the fatty acids independent of the peptide backbone [13]. The amino acid sequence suggests that there are several membrane spanning domains. Presumably, the properties of this protein promote the formation and stabilization of the characteristic compact, multilamellar structure of myelin (see Fig. 13).

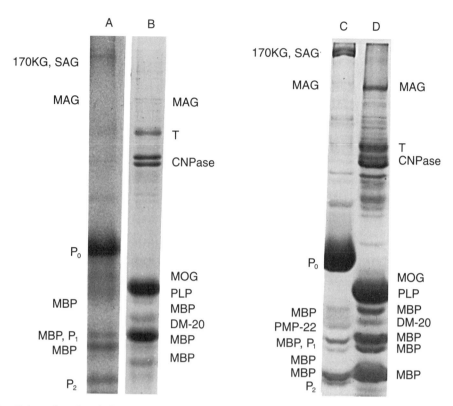

FIG. 11. Polyacrylamide gel electrophoresis of myelin proteins in the presence of sodium dodecyl sulfate (SDS). The proteins of human PNS myelin *(A)*, human CNS myelin *(B)*, rat PNS myelin *(C)* and rat CNS myelin *(D)* were solubilized with the detergent SDS, electrophoresed, and stained with Coomassie Brilliant Blue. The electrophoretic system separates proteins primarily according to their molecular size with the smallest proteins migrating the farthest toward the bottom of the gel. Abbreviations for the proteins are the same as in the text or defined below. The three MBP bands in *lanes A and B* are the 17.2, 18.5, and 21.5 kDa isoforms generated by alternative splicing of the mRNA in humans, and the four MBP bands in *lanes C and D* are the 14.0, 17.0, 18.5, and 21.5 kDa isoforms generated in rats (see Fig. 12). The 18.5 kDA MBP is also called P_1 in the terminology for the PNS. The 26 kDa MOG is probably the faint band just above PLP that is most apparent in *lane D*. CNPase electrophoreses as a tight doublet, and the lower and upper bands are sometimes referred to as CNP1 and CNP2, respectively. TU, tubulin. Note that the location shown for MAG (which stains too faintly to be seen well on the gels) is just above a discrete Coomassie blue-stained band in *lane D* which is probably the 96-kDa subunit of Na, K-ATPase. The 170-kDa glycoprotein in PNS myelin is labeled both as 170 kG and SAG for the recently proposed name of Schwann cell membrane glycoprotein (see text).

In addition to PLP, myelin of the CNS has lesser quantities of another protein, DM-20 (since $M_r = 20,000$), which has similar physical properties. This protein is coded by an alternative splicing of the RNA which gives rise to the major PLP. DNA and protein sequencing data both indicate that the structure of DM-20 is related to that of PLP by a deletion of 40 amino acids. DM-20 appears earlier than PLP during development (even before myelin formation in some cases) and it is thought that it might have a role in oligodendrocyte differentiation in addition to a structural role in myelin. The messages for PLP and DM-20 are each present in three sizes as a result of alternative usage of polyadenylation sites. (See [14,15] for entree into the literature).

Myelin Basic Proteins

The major basic protein (MBP) of myelin has long been of interest because it is the antigen that, when injected into an animal, elicits a cellular immune response that produces the CNS autoimmune disease called *experimental allergic encephalomyelitis* (see Chap. 37). MBP can be extracted from myelin as well as from white matter with either dilute acid or salt solutions; once extracted, it is very soluble in water. The amino acid sequences of the major basic protein for a number of species are similar (Lees and Brostoff [12]). These proteins have molecular weights of around 18,500; they are highly unfolded, with essentially no tertiary structure in solution. This basic protein shows microheterogeneity upon electrophoresis in alkaline conditions. This is due to a combination of phosphorylation, loss of the C-terminal arginine, and deamidation. There is also heterogeneity in the degree of methylation of an arginine at residue 106. MBP is located on the cytoplasmic face of the myelin membranes corresponding to the major dense line (see Fig. 13). The rapid turnover of the phosphate groups [16] present on about a quarter of the MBP molecules suggests this post-translational modification might influence the close apposition of the cytoplasmic bases of the membrane (whether phosphorylation modifies this process in a dynamic manner is a topic of speculation).

In addition to the major MBP, most species of mammals that have been studied contain various amounts of other basic proteins related to it in sequence. Mice and rats have a second smaller MBP, $M_r = 14,000$. The small MBP has the same N- and C-terminal sequences as the larger, but differs by a deletion of 40 residues. The ratio of these two basic proteins to each other changes during development; mature rats and mice have more of the $M_r = 14,000$ protein than of the $M_r = 18,000$ protein. Two other MBPs seen in many species have a molecular mass of 21,500 and 17,000, respectively. These two proteins are related structurally to the large and small basic proteins, respectively, by an addition near the amino-terminal end of a polypeptide sequence of M_r about 3,000. An-

other basic protein, present to some extent in humans, has $M_r = 17,200$ and is now known to be slightly different from $M_r = 17,000$ protein in other species. The different MBPs arise from alternative splicing of a common mRNA precursor. A diagrammatic representation of some of these alternative splicing schemes is presented (Fig. 12, see also Campagnoni [18]). The physiological significance of the heterogeneity of MBPs which results from alternative splicings is also an open question. Knowledge of the structure of the MBP gene has been much enhanced by the recent discovery that the exons which can be combined to make the various myelin basic proteins are part of a larger set of exons of a gene, GOLLI[MBP] Transcripts of this gene including various combinations of exons are expressed during early (pre-myelination) development [18]. If these mRNA products prove to be translated—and by implication involved in early development—it may give new insight into the evolution of myelin proteins.

CNPase

In addition to the PLP and MBP, there are many higher molecular weight proteins present in the gel electrophoretic pattern of myelin. These vary in amount depending on species (mouse and rat may have as much as 30 percent of the total myelin protein in this category) and degree of maturity (the younger the animal, the less myelin but the greater the proportion of higher molecular weight proteins). A number of proteins corresponding to bands visible in the high molecular weight region of the gel have been characterized. A double band with $M_r \approx 50,000$ is present in myelin from most species and has been identified with an enzyme activity, 2′,3′-cyclic nucleotide 3′ phosphodiesterase (CNP), which comprises several percent of myelin protein. Although there are low levels of this enzymatic activity associated with the surface membrane of many different types of cells, it is much enriched in my-

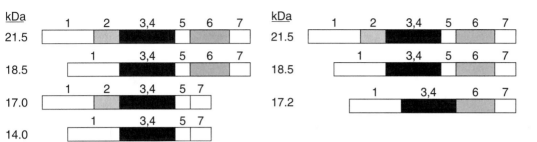

FIG. 12. The amino acid sequences corresponding to the various mouse MBPs are encoded in a gene containing at least seven exons (separated by introns—DNA regions whose base sequence does not code directly for proteins). The precursor RNA transcribed from this gene can be spliced to give a message containing all seven exons; this message codes for the $M_r = 21,500$ MBP. Alternative splicings result in messenger RNA species with deletions of exons 2 and/or 6 which code for the other MBPs. The exons forming the various mouse messenger species are indicated *above, left.* The corresponding gene in humans also contains seven exons which have minor base changes relative to the corresponding mouse sequences. Messenger RNA species derived from the human genome are indicated *above, right.* The messenger for $M_r = 21,500$ and $M_r = 18,500$ MBPs are formed in a manner analogous to the corresponding mouse proteins. Note, however, that the $M_r = 17,200$ human protein contains a slightly different exon complement than does the $M_r = 17,000$ mouse MBP. The figure is adapted from Kamholz et al. [17].

elin and in cells committed to formation of myelin. The enzyme is extremely active against the substrate of 2′,3′cAMP, as well as the cGMP, cCMP, and cUMP analogs, which are all hydrolyzed to the corresponding 2′-isomer. This is probably an artifactual activity; recall that the biologically active cyclic nucleotides are those with a 3′,5′ structure. The amino acid sequence deduced from available DNA clones is relatively conserved in different species. In mice, the two CNP polypeptides are generated by alternative splicing of the mRNA, with the larger polypeptide having an extra 20 amino acids at the N-terminus. The biological function of CNP is not known; it is of interest that it contains a consensus sequence found in G proteins, and it has also been proposed that it plays a role in a cytoskeletal network. In this connection it has been noted that CNP can be bound to membranes via an isoprenoid modification. See [19,20] for review of CNP biochemistry and molecular biology.

Myelin-Associated Glycoprotein (MAG) and Other Glycoproteins of CNS Myelin

The myelin-associated glycoprotein (MAG) is a quantitatively minor, 100 kDA glycopro-tein in purified myelin [21] that electrophoreses at the position shown in Fig. 11. However, because of the small amount (<1 percent of total protein) and its weak staining by Coomassie blue, it does not correspond to one of the discrete bands visible in the figure. Its presence can be demonstrated by staining with carbohydrate-specific stains, labeling with radioactive sugar precursors, or immunostaining of Western blots of gels. MAG is an integral membrane protein that is a member of the immunoglobulin (Ig) superfamily. This superfamily is composed of proteins in the immune system, nervous system, and other tissues that have amino acid sequence homologies and generally function in recognition and cell-cell interactions. MAG has a single transmembrane domain that separates the heavily glycosylated extracellular part of the molecule composed of 5 Ig-like domains from the intracellular, carboxy-terminal part of the molecule. About one third of the total mass of MAG is accounted for by carbohydrate, which consists primarily of N-linked oligosaccharides containing sialic acid, fucose, galactose, mannose, N-acetylglucosamine, and sulfate. MAG in rodents occurs in two developmentally regulated isoforms which differ in their cytoplasmic domains and are generated by alternative splicing of its mRNA. The isoform with a longer C-terminal tail (L-MAG) is predominant early in development during active myelination of the CNS, whereas the isoform with a shorter cytoplasmic tail (s-MAG) is predominant in the CNS of adult rodents. L-MAG is phosphorylated on serine, threonine, and tyrosine residues of its cytoplasmic domain.

MAG is not present in compact, multilamellar myelin, but is located exclusively in the periaxonal oligodendroglial membrane of CNS myelin sheaths [21]. This location next to the axon suggests that it functions in forming and maintaining contact between myelin-forming oligodendrocytes and the axolemma. Such a function in cell-cell interactions is also suggested by its membership in the Ig superfamily, members of which often function by binding to themselves (homophilic binding) or to other members of the family (heterophilic binding) on adjacent cells. The overall structure of MAG with five extracellular Ig-like domains is similar to that of neural cell adhesion molecule (N-CAM) which functions by homophilic binding (see Chap. 28). It is likely that MAG exhibits heterophilic binding to another member of the Ig superfamily on the axolemma, but its putative ligand has not yet been identified. Experiments providing direct evidence for a function of MAG in cell-cell interactions include:

1. Blocking oligodendrocyte-neuron interactions with an anti-MAG antibody;
2. Showing that MAG, containing liposomes bind to neurons; and
3. Demonstrations that transfection of MAG into cells promotes their interaction with neurons.

A relationship of MAG to the immune system and to other adhesion proteins is also demonstrated by the presence in most species of a sulfate-containing epitope in its oligosaccharide moieties that reacts with the HNK-1 monoclonal antibody [21]. HNK-1 was raised to a human lymphoblastoma and reacts with a subset of human lymphocytes as well as a number of neural adhesion proteins including N-CAM and MAG.

There are a large number of glycoproteins associated with white matter and myelin, many of which have not yet been well studied. However, there are a few others in addition to MAG that have now been cloned and partially characterized. One of these is a minor protein of $M_r = 26,000$ called the myelin-oligodendrocyte glycoprotein (abbreviated MOG; not to be confused with MAG) [22]. MOG is also in the Ig superfamily since it contains a single Ig-like domain. MOG has two potential transmembrane domains, a single site for N-linked glycosylation, and has been shown to be localized on the surface of myelin sheaths and oligodendrocytes. Although, the function of this glycoprotein is not yet known, it has been implicated as a target antigen in autoimmune aspects of demyelinating diseases of the CNS. There is also an $M_r = 105,000$ glycosylated protein in white matter called the oligodendrocyte-myelin glycoprotein (OMgp) [23] (the reader is pardoned for confusion concerning terminology). This glycoprotein is membrane bound through a phosphatidylinositol linkage and is characterized by a cysteine-rich motif at the N-terminus and a series of tandem leucine-rich repeats. Unlike MAG and MOG, it is not a member of the Ig superfamily, but, like many neural adhesion proteins, it does express the HNK-1 carbohydrate epitope. The $M_r = 120,000$ isoform of N-CAM that is attached to membranes by a phosphatidylinositol linkage is also present in oligodendrocytes and white matter.

Small amounts of proteins characteristic of membranes in general can also be identified on gels of myelin proteins. Noted in Fig. 11 is tubulin; although this may be present because of contamination of myelin preparation by other membranes, there is evidence suggesting it is an authentic myelin component. High resolution electrophoretic techniques demonstrate the presence of other minor protein bands; these may relate to the presence of numerous enzyme activities associated with the myelin sheath (discussed in a following section).

PNS myelin contains some unique proteins and some shared with the CNS

The Major PNS Myelin Protein is P_0, A Glycoprotein

The gel electrophoretic analysis (Fig. 11A,C) shows that a single protein, P_0, $M_r = 30,000$, accounts for more than half of the PNS myelin protein. The cloning and sequencing of the message for this protein by Lemke (see his review [24] and a more recent review by Uyemura [25]) led to derivation of amino acid sequences from several species. From this, it is deduced that the protein has about 220 amino acids with an intracellular domain; a hydrophobic transmembrane domain, and a single extracellular Ig-like domain. The amino-terminal extracellular domain includes a signal sequence for insertion of protein into the membrane and a glycosylation site. In addition to the well characterized carbohydrate chain, other post-translational modifications include sulfation, phosphorylation, and acylation. It is interesting to note that proteolipid protein and P_0 protein (so different in sequence, post-translational modifications, and structure) may have similar roles in formation of structures as closely related as myelins of the CNS and PNS. Transfection of HeLa cells with the P_0 gene and subsequent expression of this gene under the command of a viral promotor results in cell-cell interaction which can be demonstrated to be due to extracellular domains of P_0 [26].

Myelin Basic Protein in the PNS

MBP content in the PNS varies from approximately 5 to 18 percent of total protein, in contrast to the CNS where it is on the order of 30 percent. As in the CNS in most species, the $M_r = 18,500$ MBP is the most prominent component; it is often referred to as the P_1 protein in the nomenclature of peripheral myelin proteins. In rodents, the same four MBPs found in the CNS are present in the PNS with molecular weights of 21,000, 18,500, 17,000, and 14,000, respectively. In adult rodents, the $M_r = 14,000$ MBP is the most prominent component and is termed P_r in the PNS nomenclature. Another species-specific variation occurs in humans. In human PNS, the major basic protein is not the $M_r = 18,500$ form which is most prominent in the CNS, but rather a $M_r = 17,200$ form. (See [12] for review.) MBP may not play as critical a role in myelin structure in the PNS as it does in the CNS. The murine mutant, Shiverer, is lesioned with respect to MBP synthesis. That CNS myelin which is present has no dense line structure; this contrasts to the PNS which has almost normal myelin amount and structure although lacking MBP.

PNS myelin also contains another positively charged protein referred to as P_2 in the PNS terminology [12] and with M_r of about 15,000. It is unrelated in sequence to either P_1 or P_r but shows strong homology to a family of cytoplasmic lipid-binding proteins that are present in a variety of cell types (see [27] for review). The amount of P_2 protein is variable from species to species, accounting for about 15 percent of total protein in bovine PNS myelin, 5 percent in humans, and less than 1 percent in rodents. The P_2 protein is difficult to separate electrophoretically from the 14 kDA MBP of rodents (P_r), and this led to some confusion about the relative amounts of P_2 and MBP. P_2 protein is generally considered in the context of PNS myelin proteins since it was originally identified there and is quantitatively a prominent component in some species. Sensitive immunological techniques have, however, demonstrated that P_2 is expressed in small amounts of CNS myelin sheaths of some species. P_2 is an antigen for experimental allergic neuritis, the PNS counterpart of experimental allergic encephalomyelitis (EAE) (see Chap. 36). P_2 appears to be present in the major dense line of myelin sheaths where it may play a structural role similar to MBP, and there appears to be substantially more P_2 in large sheaths than small ones. The large variation in the amount and distribution of the protein from species to species and sheath to sheath raises so far unanswered questions about its function. Its similarities to cytoplasmic proteins whose functions appear to involve solubilization and transport of fatty acids and retinoids suggest that it might function similarly in myelination but there is currently no experimental evidence to support this hypothesis.

Other Glycoproteins of PNS Myelin

In addition to the major P_0 glycoprotein, PNS myelin contains several other glycoproteins. Both isoforms of MAG are present in the PNS [21], although s-MAG is the predominant isoform at all ages. Similarly to the CNS, MAG is present in the periaxonal membranes of the myelin-forming cells where it is believed to function in Schwann cell-axon interactions. However, in addition to the periaxonal location, MAG is also present in the Schwann cell membranes constituting the Schmidt-Lanterman incisures, paranodal loops, and the outer mesaxon. All of these locations are characterized by 12–14 nm spaces between the extracellular surfaces of adjacent membranes and the presence of cytoplasm on the inner side of the membranes. Correlative immunohistochemical data suggest that MAG is involved in maintaining the spacing of these membranes. A molecular model was proposed in which MAG functions to maintain this spacing by interacting with a component on the adjacent axolemma or Schwann cell membrane and with cytoskeletal elements inside the Schwann cell [21]. Furthermore, it was hypothesized that MAG might mediate chemomechanical forces transmitted between the cytoskeleton and the extracellular surfaces during generation of the myelin spiral. MAG interactions with the cytoskeleton could be modulated by phosphorylation of its cytoplasmic tail, and interactions with adjacent membranes could be affected by glycosylation. Clinical interest

in PNS MAG derives from the demonstration that human IgM monoclonal antibodies in patients with neuropathy react with a carbohydrate structure in MAG that is very similar to the adhesion-related, HNK-1 carbohydrate epitope (see Chap. 36).

PNS myelin also contains a glycoprotein of $M_r = 170,000$ (see Chap. 36) that accounts for about 5 percent of the total myelin protein and appears to be the same as a protein that was further characterized recently and called the Schwann cell membrane glycoprotein (SAG) [28]. In addition, a 22 kDa peripheral myelin protein (PMP-22) has recently been characterized [29] and is of particular interest because it appears to be the mutated protein in hypomyelinating trembler mice (see Chap. 37). Figure 11C shows that this protein is a quantitatively minor component of isolated PNS myelin of the rat. PMP-22 has a single site for N-linked glycosylation and four potential transmembrane domains. It is referred to as a "growth arrest protein" since its cDNA shows homology to that previously cloned from non-dividing fibroblasts, and the synthesis of PMP-22 and other myelin proteins ceases when Schwann cells begin to proliferate following nerve transection.

Myelin contains enzymes that function in metabolism (and ion transport?)

Several decades ago it was generally believed that myelin was an inert membrane that did not carry out any biochemical functions. Early studies of selected enzymes that showed little activity in myelin tended to confirm this belief. Recently, however, a large and growing number of enzymes have been discovered in myelin (for review and references, see Ledeen [30]). These findings imply that myelin is metabolically active in synthesis, processing, and metabolic turnover of some of its own components. Additionally, it may play an active role in ion transport not only with respect to maintenance of its own structure but also participation in buffering of ion levels in the vicinity of the axon.

A few enzymes are believed to be fairly myelin-specific (but probably also present in oligodendroglial membranes). This group includes CNP; isolated myelin contains about 60 percent of total brain CNP activity. The enzyme increases in brain and spinal cord during development in parallel with myelination, and low levels are present in the myelin-deficient jimpy and quaking mouse mutants. CNP is concentrated more in heavy myelin subfractions than in compact myelin, and is also high in oligodendroglial cells and their plasma membranes. CNP is very low in peripheral nerve and PNS myelin, suggesting some function more specialized to the CNS. A pH 7.2 cholesterol ester hydrolase may also be relatively myelin specific (although the enzyme is prominent in myelin, whether it is a different molecular species from that present in the extramyelin compartment is under debate). *N*-acetyl-L-aspartate aminohydroxylase, an enzyme operating on a substrate of unknown metabolic significance, is also enriched in myelin.

There are many enzymes that are not myelin-specific but appear to be intrinsic to myelin and not contaminants. Several proteolytic activities have been identified in purified myelin; well documented is the presence of neutral protease activity. The presence in myelin of cyclic AMP-stimulated kinase, calcium/calmodulin-dependent kinase, and protein kinase C activities has been reported. Phosphoprotein phosphatases are also present. The protein kinase C and phosphatase activities are presumed to be responsible for the rapid turnover of phosphate groups of myelin basic protein. Enzyme activity for acylation of proteolipid protein is also intrinsic to myelin.

Enzymes involved in metabolism of structural lipids include a number of steroid modifying enzymes and cholesterol esterifying enzyme, UDP-galactose:ceramide galactosyl-transferase and many enzymes of glycerophospholipid metabolism. The latter grouping includes CDP-choline:1,2-diradyl-*sn*-glycerol choline phosphotransferase; CDP-ethanolamine:1,2-diradyl-*sn*-glycerol

ethanolamine phosphotransferase; CTP:ethanolamine phosphate cytidyltransferase and choline and ethanolamine kinases; acyl-CoA:lysophospholipid acyltransferases and long chain acyl-CoA synthetase and others. Thus, all the enzymes necessary for phosphatidylethanolamine synthesis from diradyl-*sn*-glycerol and ethanolamine are present; it is likely that phospatidycholine can also be synthesized within myelin. Perhaps even more elemental building blocks can be assembled into lipids by myelin enzymes. Acyl-CoA synthetase is present in myelin, suggesting the capacity to integrate free fatty acids into myelin lipids. The extent of the contribution of these enzymes in myelin (relative to enzymes within the oligodendroglial perikaryon) to metabolism of myelin lipids is not known.

Other enzymes present in myelin include those involved in phosphoinositide metabolism; phosphatidylinositol kinase, diphosphoinositide kinase, the corresponding phosphatases, and diglyceride kinases. These are of interest because of the high concentration of polyphosphoinositides of myelin and the rapid turnover of their phosphate groups. This area of research has expanded toward characterization of signal transduction system(s). Evidence for the presence in myelin of muscarinic cholinergic receptors, G proteins, phospholipases C and D, and protein kinase C has appeared.

Certain enzymes shown to be present in myelin could be involved in ion transport. Carbonic anhydrase has generally been considered a soluble enzyme and a glial marker, but myelin accounts for a large part of the membrane-bound form in brain. This enzyme may play a role in removal of carbonic acid from metabolically active axons. The enzymes 5'-nucleotidase and Na,K-ATPase have long been considered specific markers for plasma membranes and are found in myelin at low levels. The 5'-nucleotidase activity may be related to a transport mechanism for adenosine, and Na,K-ATPase could well be involved in transport of monovalent cations. The presence of these enzymes suggests that myelin may have an active role in transport of material in and out of the axon. In connection with this hypothesis, it is of interest that proteolipid protein, when inserted into artificial bilayers, has proton ionophore properties. Potassium channels in myelin vesicles have also been described. An isoform of glutathione-5-transferase is present in myelin and may be involved in transport of certain larger molecules.

The protein kinases and carbonic anhydrase have also been shown to be present in PNS myelin, but relative to the situation for CNS myelin, less is known about enzymes in PNS myelin. The accessibility and relatively simple morphology of the PNS have made it a focus of detailed studies concerning interaction of the axon and the myelinating cell.

DEVELOPMENTAL BIOLOGY OF MYELIN

Myelination follows the order of phylogenetic development

As the nervous system matures, portions of the PNS myelinate first, then the spinal cord, and the brain last. In all parts of the nervous system there are many small fibers that never myelinate. Even within the brain, different areas myelinate at different rates, the intracortical association areas being the last to do so. In humans, the motor roots begin to myelinate in the fifth fetal month and the brain is almost completely myelinated by the end of the second year of life.

It is generally true that pathways in the nervous system become myelinated before they become completely functional. A relevant observation is that the CNS of rats and other nest-building animals myelinates largely postnatally, and the animals are quite helpless at birth. Grazing animals, such as horses, cows, and sheep, have considerably more myelin in the CNS at birth and a correspondingly much higher level of complex activity immediately postnatally. Despite the attractiveness of the hypothesis that myelination is the terminal step in preparing a nervous system pathway for function, it

should be noted that the period of maximum myelination also coincides with many other changes in the nervous system.

Although it is easy to ascertain when myelination begins, it is difficult to determine when the process of accumulation stops. In the rat, myelin is still being deposited in the brain well past a year of age and possibly longer. The rat, however, continues to grow in body size and brain weight for most of its life span, and such a prolonged period of myelination may not occur in all species. However, even in the human, myelination continues in the neocortex at least through the end of the second decade.

The composition of myelin changes during development

Nervous system development is marked by several overlapping periods, each defined by one major event in brain growth and structural maturation. In the rat, whose CNS undergoes considerable development postnatally, the maximal rate of cellular proliferation (much of this involving oligodendroglial precursor cells) occurs at 10 days. The rat brain begins to form myelin postnatally at about 10 to 12 days. Although the maximal rate of accumulation of myelin in the rat is at about 20 days of age, in this species myelin accumulation continues at a decreasing rate throughout adulthood. At 6 months of age, 60 mg of myelin can be isolated from one brain. This represents an increase of about 1,500 percent over the 4 mg of myelin content of the brains of 15-day-old animals. During the same $5\frac{1}{2}$-month period, the brain weight increases by only 50 to 60 percent.

Myelin that is first deposited has a different composition from that of the adult [9]. As the rat matures, the myelin galactolipids increase by about 50 percent and lecithin decreases by a similar amount. Similar changes are seen in human myelin. The very small amount of desmosterol declines, but the other lipids remain relatively constant. In addition, the polysialogangliosides decrease and the monosialoganglioside, GM_1, increases to become the predominant ganglioide. These changes are not complete until the rat is about 2 months old. There is also a change in the composition of the protein portion as well as that of the lipid portion. Both basic protein and proteolipid protein increase in the myelin sheath during development, whereas the amount of higher molecular weight protein decreases.

Myelin subfractions may represent transitional forms of myelin

The studies summarized above on the composition of myelin from immature brains are consistent with the idea that myelin first laid down by the oligodendroglial cell may represent a transitional form with properties intermediate between those of mature compact myelin and the oligodendroglial cell membrane. As mentioned earlier, in the section on isolation, myelin can be separated into subfractions of different densities; in young animals depositing myelin the dense fractions are prominent. The lighter fractions are enriched in multilamellar myelin, whereas the denser fractions contain a large proportion of single membrane vesicles that resemble microsomes or plasma membrane fragments. Generally speaking, as one goes from light myelin fractions to heavier, the lipid/protein ratio decreases, the amount of basic protein decreases, the amount of MAG and of unidentified high molecular weight proteins increases, the CNP, carbonic anhydrase, and other enzymes increase, and the amount of proteolipid protein stays relatively constant. Metabolic studies described later lend support to the view that the dense fractions represent transitional forms.

SYNTHESIS AND METABOLISM OF MYELIN

Synthesis of myelin components is rapid during deposition of myelin

A remarkable amount of synthetic work is done by the oligodendroglial cell during the period of maximum myelination. Myelin accumulates in a 20-day-old rat brain at a rate of about 3.5 mg/day. Rough calculations show that there are about 20×10^6 oligodendroglia in such a brain, with each cell body having a dry weight of about 50×10^{-9} mg. Thus, on average, each cell makes about 175×10^{-9} mg of myelin per day, an amount more than three times the weight of the perikaryon. The rates of myelin accumulation increase rapidly prior to this peak and decrease rapidly afterward.

Myelin synthesis can be measured by studying the activity, *in vitro,* of enzymes involved in the synthesis of specific myelin components, by measuring incorporation *in vivo* of labeled precursors into myelin components, and by carrying out similar studies using tissue slices. For example, the activity of UDP-galactose:ceramide galactosyltransferase (the enzyme that catalyzes the last step of cerebroside synthesis) in mouse brain microsomes increases four-fold from 10 days to a peak activity at 20 days, just preceding the age of maximal rate of myelin accumulation. It then gradually declines, paralleling the declining rate of myelination. The synthesis of glucocerebroside, which is not a myelin lipid, follows a completely different developmental pattern. Many other enzymes involved in synthesis of lipids represented in myelin show increases during the period of rapid myelination.

In vivo studies using radioactive precursors generally furnish results similar to those of the enzyme assays *in vitro.* Incorporation of precursor into myelin specific lipids is greatest if the injection of precursor is at the time of the greatest myelin accumulation (around 20 days in the rat) and decreases at earlier or later ages. Similar results are obtained when radioactive precursors (e.g., acetate for lipids or leucine for proteins) are presented to brain and spinal cord slices. Incorporation of radioactive precursors into myelin is greatest when slices are obtained from rats about 20 days of age.

Some lipids and proteins must be transported to the site of myelin assembly

After myelin components have been synthesized they have to be assembled to form the membrane. Following intracranial injection of a radioactive amino acid, or application of a labeled precursor to tissue slices, radioactive basic protein is synthesized and integrated into myelin very rapidly—a lag time of only a few minutes (see [31]). In contrast, substantial amounts of radioactive proteolipid proteins are not found in myelin until after about 45 minutes. Thus, following synthesis, proteolipid protein enters a pool that is on its way to being integrated into myelin; in contrast, basic protein is incorporated into myelin as soon as it is made. This interpretation is compatible with the demonstration that proteolipid protein is synthesized on bound polysomes in the perikaryon. Presumably, the "pool" of proteolipid protein consists of membranous vesicles (including those involving endoplasmic reticulum and Golgi membrane) on their way to the myelin being formed at the end of the oligodendroglial cell processes. In contrast, myelin basic protein is synthesized on free polysomes which are actually associated with or in very close proximity to, the myelin sheath. Another difference in the processing of the two proteins during myelin assembly is that, following a pulse of incorporation of radioactive amino acids into newly synthesized protein, radioactive myelin basic protein appears more or less simultaneously in myelin subfractions of different densities. In contrast, proteolipid protein appears first in the densest myelin fractions and later into lighter (more mature) myelin fractions in a manner which suggests a precursor-product relationship. Metabolic experiments suggest that myelin-associated glycoprotein resembles proteolipid protein, while other high molecular weight proteins resemble basic protein, with respect to their kinetics of entry into myelin.

Lipids show similar heterogeneity with respect to processing on the way to form myelin. Following a pulse label, ethanolamine phospholipids are first found in the heavier myelin fractions, and then they rapidly enter the lighter (more mature) myelin. In contrast, choline phospholipids also appear rapidly and simultaneously in myelin subfractions differing in density.

The available information is not yet sufficient to provide a detailed model of membrane assembly, but a general picture emerges. Many high molecular weight proteins are present in a lipid-poor precursor membrane (oligodendroglial cell membrane), with all of the proteolipid protein and some basic protein added during the early stages of myelin formation. More of the basic protein and other high molecular weight proteins are added at later states of transition. The addition of proteolipid protein might be a rate-limiting step in myelin formation. The bulk of the lipids are added at later stages of myelin assembly, and their entry is directed by the proteins already present.

Myelin components exhibit great heterogeneity of metabolic turnover

A standard type of experiment to determine lipid turnover is to inject into rat brains a radioactive metabolic precursor, and then following sufficient time to allow for incorporation, follow loss of radioactivity from individual lipids as a function of time. It is known that some structural lipid components of myelin, notably cholesterol, cerebroside, and sulfatide, are relatively stable metabolically with half-lives of the order of many months. It is also clear that any given phospholipid turns over more slowly in myelin than in total membrane fraction or microsomes from whole brain.

For many lipids the relationship between loss of radioactivity (usually referred to as apparent half-life) and the real rate of degradation of a lipid is complicated by reutilization. For example, radioactive acetate is incorporated into fatty acids which are further processed to become part of glycerolipid molecules. At some future time when these lipids are degraded, (broken down to their constituent moieties) the fatty acid can, to a large extent, be reutilized for synthesis of new lipids. In contrast, radioactive glycero is also incorporated into glycerolipids but, upon degradation, the glycerol moiety is preferentially metabolized rather than being reutilized for biosynthesis. The apparent half-life (time course of loss of radioactivity) from phosphatidylcholine varies depending upon whether the molecule is labeled with radioactive phosphate, acetate, choline, or glycerol (the last named precursor yielding the shortest and presumably most accurate estimate). Even within a phospholipid class turnover of the glycerol backbone is greatly influenced by the fatty acid composition of the lipid (for discussion of these points see [32] and a review [33]).

A further complication is that the metabolic turnover of individual myelin components is multiphasic—at least two turnover rates can be measured. When young animals incorporate radioactive precursors, a significant percentage of the total incorporated label is still present in phospholipids some months later. One of several possible interpretations of these data is on the basis of morphology, the stabler metabolic pool consisting of deeper layers of myelin (less accessible for metabolic turnover?). Much of the myelin deposited in young animals during the period of rapid myelin accumulation is quickly transferred to this compartment—the metabolically stable pool. Some of the newly formed myelin may remain in outer layers and stay accessible for whatever mechanisms are involved in catabolism—thus accounting for the rapidly turning over pool. In contrast, in older animals radioactive precursors are incorporated less efficiently (because less myelin is accumulating and that label which is incorporated into phospholipids turns over rapidly (because of the slow rate of myelin accumulation newly synthesized phospholipid remains for a longer time in the metabolically active compartment).

The overall picture appears that myelin glycerophospholipids have metabolic half-lives (glycerol backbone catabolism) of the order of a week or less for the "fast" phase of turnover and of the order of a month for

the slower phase of turnover. If radioactive precursors other than glycerol are utilized the "apparent half life" of a given lipid is longer, in the case of precursors which label the fatty acyl moieties up to several times longer. Plasmalogens are unusual in their metabolism in that the hydrophilic moieties (acyl chain and vinyl ether chain) are reutilized so efficiently that when these chains are labeled *in vivo* with acetate or glucose the plasmalogens appear metabolically stable.

Myelin proteins show the same type of biphasic turnover as the lipids. Whereas, in the fast phase, both basic and proteolipid proteins show half-lives of the order of 2 to 3 weeks, several studies show that both of these proteins are metabolically stable in the slow phase, showing half-lives too long to be calculated accurately. Again, as with the lipids, myelin protein decay curves vary with the precursor used and the age of the animals injected. Shorter half-lives are seen if adult animals are labeled.

Although the discussion above indicates a half-life of the order of days to months for most myelin components, it is now known that there are some aspects of myelin metabolism which have a half-life of the order of minutes. The phosphate group of myelin basic proteins is in this category. Measurements of its half-life are limited by the time taken for injected $[^{32}P]$ phosphate to equilibrate with ATP, but it is clear that much of the phosphate cycles on and off the peptide backbone with a half-life which is of the order of minutes or faster [16]. It is also known that the monoesterified phosphate groups of polyphosphatidylinositol (those at positions 3 and 4) are labeled very quickly even in mature animals and also presumably have a rapid half-life. There is recent evidence that a significant portion of the phosphatidylinositol of myelin rapidly incorporates phosphate, suggesting that degradation (at least to the extent of phospholipase C cleavage) and subsequent resynthesis of at least some phosphatidylinositol of myelin. Finally, evidence for the presence in myelin of signal transduction systems (see section on enzymes in myelin) suggest that myelin metabolism includes many rapid events.

MOLECULAR ARCHITECTURE OF MYELIN

The currently accepted view of membrane structure is that of a lipid bilayer with some integral membrane proteins embedded in the bilayer and other extrinsic proteins attached to one surface or the other by weaker linkages. Both proteins and lipids are asymmetrically distributed, with the asymmetry of lipids being partial. The molecular architecture of the layered membranes of compact myelin appears to be determined by similar principals. Molecular models of compact myelin are hypothesized based on data from electron microscopy, immunostaining, X-ray diffraction, surface probe studies, structural abnormalities in mutant mice, correlations between structure and composition in various species, and predictions of protein structure from sequencing information (for review see [5]).

Presumably, the glycolipids in myelin, as in other membranes, are preferentially at the extracellular surfaces in the intraperiod line. Diffraction studies demonstrate that cholesterol is also enriched in the extracellular face of the myelin membrane, whereas ethanolamine plasmalogen is asymmetrically localized to the cytoplasmic half of the bilayer.

A diagrammatic representation of current ideas about the molecular organization of proteins in compact myelin of the CNS and PNS is shown in Fig. 13. PLP is an integral membrane protein that has several hy-

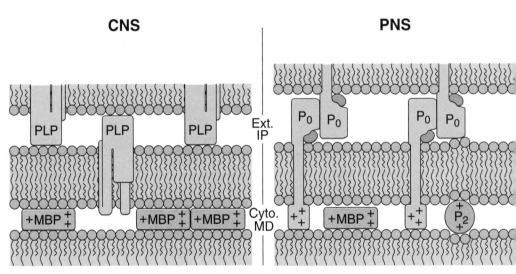

FIG. 13.   Diagrammatic representation of current concepts of the molecular organization of compact CNS and PNS myelin. The apposition of the extracellular (Ext.) surfaces of the oligodendrocyte or Schwann cell membranes to form the intraperiod (IP) line is shown in the upper part of the figure. The apposition of the cytoplasmic (Cyto.) surfaces of the membranes of the myelin-forming cells to form the major dense (MD) line is shown in the lower part of the figure. See the text for a detailed description of this model. The general shape of the external domain of P_0 and the position of the oligosaccharide (*dark structure at base of external domain*) are based on recent unpublished molecular modeling by Wells, Saavedra, Inouye, and Kirschner. These diagrams do not include CNP, MAG, or other quantitatively minor proteins of isolated myelin, because they probably do not play a major structural role in most of the compact myelin, and many of them are localized selectively in regions of myelin sheaths distinct from the compact myelin. These models for CNS and PNS myelin are similar in many ways to those proposed earlier by Braun [34], but have evolved as our knowledge of the primary, secondary, and tertiary structures of myelin proteins has increased. PLP, proteolipid protein; MBP, myelin basic protein; P_0, P_2—PNS myelin proteins. The authors are grateful to Allen Blaurock and Dan Kirschner for very helpful discussion and to Jeff Hammer for drafting and modifying the models on a Macintosh computer.

drophobic domains which may penetrate or pass entirely through the lipid bilayer, and several models for its orientation in the membrane have been proposed [13]. Although final consensus on the precise conformation of PLP has not been reached, most investigators agree that it plays a major role in stabilizing the intraperiod line of CNS myelin. By contrast MBP is an extrinsic protein localized exclusively at the cytoplasmic surface in the major dense line, a conclusion based on its amino acid sequence, inaccessibility to surface probes, and direct localization at the electron microscope level by immunocytochemistry. There is evidence to suggest that MBP forms dimers, and it is believed to be the principal protein stabilizing the major dense line, possibly by interacting with negatively charged lipids. The primary roles for PLP and MBP in stabilizing the intraperiod and major dense lines, respectively, are also supported by ultrastructural abnormalities observed in inherited dysmyelinating conditions in which very little PLP or MBP is made because their genes are mutated (see Chap. 37).

In the PNS, the major P_0 protein transverses the bilayer once and is believed to stabilize the intraperiod line by homophilic binding between Ig-like domains on adjacent layers (Fig. 13). The relatively large, glycosylated, extracellular Ig-like domain of P_0 probably accounts for the greater separation of extracellular surfaces in PNS myelin in comparison to CNS myelin where apposition of these surfaces is thought to be due to the very hydrophobic PLP (see [25]). It is also noteworthy that fish, the species in which compact myelin first appeared during evolution, do not have PLP, and P_0 is present in both PNS and CNS myelin [5]. The spacing of the intraperiod line in fish CNS myelin is greater than that in higher vertebrates and comparable to that of P_0-containing PNS myelin in other species. The P_0 protein also has a relatively large positively charged domain at the cytoplasmic side of the membrane, and it is believed that it also contributes significantly to stabilization of the major dense

line in the PNS. Although, MBP also probably plays a role at the major dense line, it does not appear to be as important as in the CNS, since there is less of it. Furthermore, murine mutants in which very little MBP is expressed have a relatively normal major dense line in the PNS although the CNS is severely affected (see Chap. 37). The P_2 protein may also contribute to the stability of the major dense line, although its amount varies drastically from species to species. Interestingly, larger amounts of P_2 protein in myelin of various species correlate with larger widths of the major dense lines as determined by X-ray diffraction [5].

Although the above model presents a static representation, the studies that demonstrate relatively rapid metabolism of certain myelin components suggest there may be some dynamic aspect of myelin structure such as occasional separation of the cytoplasmic faces of the membranes. More detailed analysis of both the static structural aspect and dynamic properties of the myelin sheath await conceptual and analytical advances.

ACKNOWLEDGMENT

We thank Dr. Cedric Raine for the elegant photomicrographs that illustrate this chapter.

REFERENCES

1. Raine, C. S. Morphology of myelin and myelination. In P. Morell (ed.), *Myelin,* 2nd ed. New York: Plenum, 1984, pp. 1–41.
2. Black, J. A., Kocsis, J. D., and Waxman, S. G. Ion channel organization of the myelinated fiber. *Trends Neurosci.* 13:48–54, 1991.
3. Ritchie, J. M. Physiological basis of conduction in myelinated nerve fibers. In P. Morell (ed.), *Myelin,* 2nd ed. New York: Plenum, 1984, pp. 117–141.
4. Norton, W. T. The myelin sheath. In E. S. Goldensohn and S. H. Appel (eds.). *Scientific*

Approaches to Clinical Neurology. Philadelphia: Lea & Febiger, 1977, pp. 259–298.

5. Kirchner, D. A., Blaurock, A. E. Organization, phylogenetic variations and dynamic transitions of myelin. R. E. Martenson (ed.), *Myelin: Biology and Chemistry.* Boca Raton, FL: CRC Press, 1991, pp. 413–448.

6. Hirano, A., and Dembitzer, H. M. A structural analysis of the myelin sheath in the central nervous system. *J. Cell Biol.* 34:555–567, 1967.

7. Bunge, R. P. Glial cells and the central myelin sheath. *Physiol. Rev.* 48:197–248, 1968.

8. Davison, A. N., and Peters, A. Myelination. Springfield, IL: Charles C Thomas, 1970.

9. Norton, W. T., and Cammer, W. Isolation and characterization of myelin. In P. Morell (ed.), *Myelin.* New York: Plenum, 1984, pp. 147–180.

10. Smith, M. E. Peripheral nervous system myelin properties and metabolism. In A. Lajtha (ed.), *Handbook of Neurochemistry,* 2nd ed. New York: Plenum, 1983, pp. 201–223.

11. Benjamins, J. A., Morell, P., Hartman, B. K., and Agrawal, H. C. CNS myelin. In A. Lajtha (ed.), *Handbook of Neurochemistry.* New York: Plenum, 1984, pp. 361–415.

12. Lees, M. B., and Brostoff, S. W. Proteins of myelin. In P. Morell (ed.), *Myelin,* 2nd ed. New York: Plenum, 1984, pp. 197–217.

13. Less, M. B., and Bizzozero, O. A. Structure and acylation of proteolipid protein. Martenson, R. E. (ed.), *Myelin: Biology and Chemistry.* Boca Raton, FL: CRC Press, 1991, pp. 237–255.

14. Macklin, W. B. The myelin proteolipid protein gene and its expression. Martenson, R. E. (ed.), *Myelin: Biology and Chemistry.* Boca Raton, FL: CRC Press, 1992, pp. 257–276.

15. Mikoshiba, K., Okano, H., Tamura, T., and Ikenaka, K. Structure and function of myelin protein genes. *Annu. Rev. Neurosci.* 140:201–217, 1991.

16. DesJardins, K. C., and Morell, P. The phosphate groups modifying myelin basic proteins are metabolically labile; the methyl groups are stable. *J. Cell Biol.* 97:438–446, 1983.

17. Kamholz, J., de Ferra, F., Puckett, C., and Lazzarini, R. Identification of three forms of human myelin basic protein by cDNA cloning. *Proc. Natl. Acad. Sci. U.S.A.* 83:4962–4966, 1986.

18. Campagnoni, A. T. Molecular biology of myelin proteins from the central nervous system. *J. Neurochem.* 51:1–14, 1988.

19. Sprinkle, T. J. 2′,3′-cyclic nucleotide 3′-phosphodiesterase, an oligodendrocyte-Schwann cell and myelin-associated enzyme of the nervous system. *Crit. Rev. Neurobiol.* 4(3):235–301, 1989.

20. Tsukada, Y., and Kurihara, T. 2′-3′-cyclic nucleotide 3′-phosphodiesterase: Molecular characterization and possible functional significance. Martenson, R. E., (ed.), *Myelin: Biology and Chemistry.* Boca Raton, FL: CRC Press, 1992, pp. 449–480.

21. Quarles, R. H., Colman, D. R., Salzer, J. L., and Trapp, B. D. Myelin-associated glycoprotein: Structure-function relationships and involvement in neurological diseases. Martenson, R. E. (ed.), *Myelin: Biology and Chemistry.* Boca Raton, FL: CRC Press, 1992, pp. 413–448.

22. Gardinier, M. V., Amiguet, P., Lingington, C., and Matthieu, J. M. Myelin/oligodendrocyte glycoprotein is a unique member of the immunoglobulin superfamily. *J. Neurosci. Res.* 33:177:187, 1992.

23. Mikol, D. D., Gulcher, J. R., and Stefansson, K. The oligodendrocyte-myelin glycoprotein belongs to a distinct family of proteins and contains the HNK-1 carbohydrate. *J. Cell. Biol.* 110:471–479, 1990.

24. Lemke, G. Molecular biology of the major myelin genes, *Trends Neurosci.* 9:266–269, 1986.

25. Uyemura, K., Kitamura, K., and Miura, M. Structure and molecular biology of P_0 protein. Martenson, R. E. (ed.), *Myelin: Biology and Chemistry.* Boca Raton, FL: CRC Press, 1991, pp. 413–448.

26. D'Urso, D., Brophy, P. J., Staugatis, S. M., Gillespie, C. S., Frey, A. B., Stempak, J. G., and Colman, D. R. Protein zero of peripheral nerve myelin: Biosynthesis, membrane insertion, and evidence for homotypic interaction. *Neuron* 2:449–460, 1990.

27. Martenson, R. E., and Uyemura, K. Myelin P_2, a neuritogenic member of the family of cytoplasmic lipid-binding proteins. Martenson, R. E. (ed.), *Myelin: Biology and Chemistry.* Boca Raton, FL: CRC Press, 1992, pp. 509–528.

28. Dieperink, M. K., O'Neill, A., Magnoni, G., Wollman, R. L., Heinrikson, R. L., Zucher-Neely, H. A., and Stefansson, K. SAG: A Schwann cell membrane glycoprotein. *J. Neurosci.* 12:2177–2185, 1992.

29. Snipes, G. J., Suter, U., Welcher, A. A., and

Shooter, E. M. Characterization of a novel peripheral nervous system myelin protein (PMP-22/SR13). *J. Cell. Biol.* 117:225–238, 1992.

30. Ledeen, R. W. Enzymes and receptors of myelin. Martenson, R. E. (ed.), *Myelin: Biology and Chemistry.* Boca Raton, FL: CRC Press, 1992, pp. 531–570.

31. Benjamins, J. A., and Smith, M. E. Metabolism of myelin. In P. Morell (ed.), *Myelin,* 2nd ed. New York: Plenum, 1984, pp. 225–249.

32. Ousley, A. H., and Morell, P. Individual molecular species of phosphatidylcholine and phosphatidylethanolamine in myelin turnover at different rates. *J. Biol. Chem.* 267:1992, pp. 10362–10369.

33. Dewille, J. W., and Horrocks, L. A. Synthesis and turnover of myelin phospholipids and cholesterol. Martenson, R. E. (ed.), *Myelin: Biology and Chemistry.* Boca Raton, FL: CRC Press, 1992, pp. 213–234.

34. Braun, P. E. Molecular organization of myelin. In P. Morell (ed.), *Myelin,* 2nd ed. New York: Plenum, 1984, pp. 97–113.

CHAPTER 7

Molecular Biology of Vision

HITOSHI SHICHI

PHYSIOLOGICAL BACKGROUND

Light-absorbing pigments differentiate rod cells for black-white vision, and three types of cone cells for color vision

The eye, a remarkable photosensor, can detect a single photon and transmit its signal to the brain. The receptors for light in the vertebrate eye are the visual (photoreceptor) cells of the retina. Each visual cell comprises two principal parts: the outer segment, which contains light-absorbing (visual) pigments; and the inner segment, which contains the nucleus, mitochondria, and other

Basic Neurochemistry: Molecular, Cellular, and Medical Aspects, 5th Ed., edited by G. J. Siegel et al. Published by Raven Press, Ltd., New York, 1994. Correspondence to Hitoshi Shichi, Department of Ophthalmology, Wayne State University School of Medicine, Detroit, Michigan 48201.

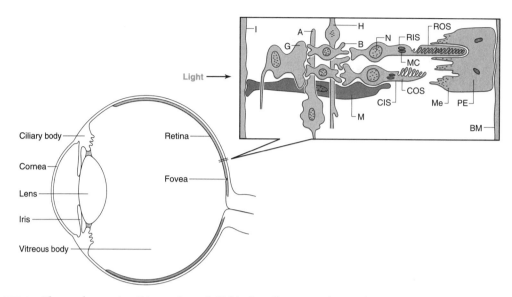

FIG. 1. The vertebrate retina: (A) amacrine cell; (B) bipolar cell; (BM) Bruch's membrane; (C) ciliary process (cilium); (CIS) cone inner segment; (COS) cone outer segment; (G) ganglion cell; (H) horizontal cell; (I) inner limiting membrane; (M) Müller cell (glial cell); (Me) melanine granule; (Mi) mitochondrion; (N) nucleus; (PE) retinal pigmented epithelium; (RIS) rod inner segment; (ROS) rod outer segment.

subcellular organelles and which metabolically supports the functions of the outer segment (Fig. 1). The segments are connected by the ciliary process, or cilium. The inner segments of visual cells have terminals that synapse with horizontal cells and bipolar cells. The bipolar cells, in turn, form synapses with ganglion and amacrine cells.

Visual cells are of two types. Rod cells, which have elongated outer segments, contain rhodopsin [light wavelength for maximum absorption (λ_{max}), ~500 nm], the visual pigment responsible for dim-light (black-and-white, or scotopic) vision. Cone cells, possessing cone-shaped outer segments, are the photoreceptors for daylight (color, or photopic) vision. In the human retina there are three types of cone cells, each containing one of three pigments: λ_{max} 420, 530, and 560 nm. According to one estimate, the human eye contains 120 million rod cells in the peripheral region of the retina and 6.5 million cone cells, concentrated mainly in the central, or foveal, region.

Absorption of light causes inhibition of vertebrate photoreceptor cells, which then initiate programs of responses among retinal neurons

The plasma membrane of each rod outer segment possesses several thousand Na^+ channels through which Na^+ enters the cell at a rate of about 2.6×10^4 Na^+ per channel per second. In contrast, the plasma membrane of the rod inner segment has ATP-dependent Na^+/K^+ pumps that pump Na^+ out of the cell. The Na^+ permeability of the outer segment is higher in the dark than in the light. Thus, the plasma membrane of the vertebrate rod cell shows a membrane potential of 35 to 45 mV (inside negative) and is depolarized in the dark. Light reduces the Na^+ permeability of the outer segment and hyperpolarizes the membrane. Therefore, "visual excitation" in the vertebrate photoreceptor means hyperpolarization, or inhibition, of the visual cell plasma membrane. The release of a chemical transmitter (glutamate or aspartate) at the synaptic terminal of a visual cell in the dark is also inhibited by light. The retina, which is part of the central nervous system, contains putative neurotransmitters, such as acetylcholine, dopamine, γ-amino-butyric acid (GABA), glycine, glutamate, aspartate, and neuropeptides [2]. For a given substance to be a neurotransmitter, it has to satisfy several criteria:

1. The substance is present in sufficient quantities in and synthesized by a specific neuron.
2. The substance is released in response to a stimulatory signal.
3. The released substance evokes a postsynaptic response.
4. The substance is rapidly inactivated.

By application of some of these criteria glutamate (or aspartate) has been identified as a neurotransmitter of the photoreceptors. GABA and dopamine are transmitters found in horizontal cells of fish retina. Amacrine cells are diverse and contain inhibitory transmitters such as GABA and glycine, as well as acetylcholine and dopamine. Amacrines also contain various neuropeptides (substance P, enkephalin, glucagon, somatostatin, neurotensin, neuropeptide Y, and cholecystokinin) which function as neuromodulators. The effects of neuromodulators are generally slower and last longer than those of neurotransmitters. The mechanism by which retinal neurons are regulated by neurotransmitters and modulators remains largely unknown.

Retinal responses to different light frequencies are encoded in the retina and conveyed to the thalamus and visual cortex

Absorption of photons by visual cells triggers a series of events that results in a particular pattern of stimulation of retinal and, eventually, cerebral neurons. In rod cell vision (dim light), the magnitude of neural response is directly related to the perception of brightness. In cone cell (color) vision, absorption of light by at least two cone cell pigments with different absorption maxima is essential to discriminate color. The ratio of magnitudes of the induced photoresponses determines the color perceived. The arrays of visual signals generated by the photoreceptor cells and programmed by retinal neurons, principally bipolar cells, are transmitted to the lateral geniculate bodies via ganglion cell axons, which make up the optic nerves and tracts. Impulses are conveyed by the geniculocalcarine radiations to the visual cortex of the brain, where the signals representing light intensity and wavelength are decoded separately by different neurons. The coding and decoding of visual signals, an important area of neurophysiology, is not covered here. This chapter deals primarily with the structure and function of photoreceptors and the molecular events that take place after photon absorption by the visual cells. (General reviews may be found in refs. 1–5).

PHOTORECEPTOR MEMBRANES AND VISUAL PIGMENTS

Rod outer segment membranes are arranged in stacks of disks containing rhodopsin

The outer segment of a rod cell consists of a stack of several hundred disks encased in a sack of plasma membrane. It is presumed that the disks are formed by evagination of the plasma membrane in the proximal region of the outer segment, followed by fusion of two adjacent evaginates, and detachment from the plasma membrane. This process is probably controlled by the ciliary process. The effect of this repeated evagination and disk formation is to increase greatly the area of rod cell membrane and, thus, the amount of visual pigment, a membrane-bound protein, that is exposed to light. As new disks are formed, older disks are pushed toward the apex of the outer segment. Disks that eventually reach the apex are shed from the tip and are phagocytized by the pigmented epithelial cells. In higher order animals, disk shedding follows a circadian rhythm; shedding is minimal in the dark and a burst of shedding occurs soon after the onset of light [6]. The life cycle of a single disk may last from a few days to months, depending on the species [7]. Disk membrane components, such as proteins, carbohydrates, and lipids, are synthesized in the inner segment and then transported to the basal region of the ciliary process, where membrane assembly occurs. In contrast to rod disks, cone disks generally remain continuous with the plasma membrane.

Rod outer segment membranes (>95 percent disk membranes, <5 percent plasma membrane) consist of 60 percent protein and 40 percent phospholipid. In vertebrate photoreceptors, phosphatidylethanolamine and phosphatidylcholine account for about 80 percent of the phospholipid. The most abundant polyunsaturated fatty acid is docosahexaenoic acid (22 carbons and six unsaturated bonds), linked to the middle carbon of the glycerol moiety of phospholipids. Their high levels of polyunsaturated fatty acids make rod membranes as fluid as olive oil, at physiological temperatures, allowing the integral membrane protein, rhodopsin, to rotate freely and diffuse within the membrane. This fluidity may be important in allowing photoactivated rhodopsin to collide quickly with so many molecules of the peripheral membrane proteins, such as guanine nucleotide-binding protein (G protein).

Rhodopsin is a transmembrane protein linked to 11-*cis*-retinal, which on photoabsorption, decomposes to opsin and all-*trans*-retinal

Rhodopsin has a molecular weight of about 40,000. Its C-terminus is exposed on the cytoplasmic surface of the disk, and its sugar-containing N-terminal sequence is exposed on the intraluminal surface. Half of the mass is embedded in the hydrophobic region of the membrane lipid bilayer, with the remaining half distributed equally on both surfaces of the membrane. The primary structures of visual pigment proteins are known so far for 20 visual pigments including human rhodopsin and cone pigments (Fig. 2) [4]. All visual pigments possess seven segments of hydrophobic sequences separated by segments of hydrophilic sequences. It has been hypothesized that the seven hydrophobic sequences, designated helices 1–7 (see bovine rhodopsin shown as an example in Fig. 3), are in α-helical conformation and form a bundle that spans the membrane from one side to the other. Two sugar moieties, each composed of three mannoses and three N-acetyl-glucosamines, are linked to asparagine-2 and asparagine-15 in bovine rhodopsin. Cysteine-322 and cysteine-323 carry palmitoyl groups which probably penetrate the membrane, thereby forming an additional polypeptide loop. The C-terminal sequence contains a cluster of serine and threonine residues that serve as phosphorylation sites.

The chromophore 11-*cis*-retinal is linked to the ϵ-amino group of lysine-296 by a protonated Schiff base. Protonated Schiff bases usually absorb light maximally at around 440 nm, but the λ_{max} of rhodopsin is near 500 nm. The 60-nm shift of λ_{max} toward the longer wavelength side (red shift) can be explained by the strength of interaction of the positive charge of the protonated Schiff base with a counter ion. The more the counter ion is removed from the Schiff base, the greater is the red shift. The counter ion is the carboxylate group of glutamic acid-113

FIG. 2.   The primary structures of visual pigments. The fly sequence is from drosophila. All other sequences are human. The lower three are the sequences of cone pigments deduced from cDNA sequences: (b) blue-sensitive, (r) red-sensitive, and (g) green-sensitive. The single-letter amino acid code used here is defined in the Glossary. Residues identical in all sequences are shown in boldface. Gaps necessary to maintain the alignment are connected by dashed lines. The transmembrane segments shown in Fig. 3 are indicated by the numbered arrows below the corresponding sequences. The lysine to which retinal is linked to form the chromophore is indicated as *K* near the center of transmembrane segment 7.

```
MESFAVAAQLGPHFAPLSNGSVVDKVTPMMAHLI---SPYWNQFPAMDPI  (fly)
MNGTEGPNFYVPFSNATGVV----------------RSPFEYPQYYLAEP  (rod)
MRKMSEEQFYLFKNISSV------------------GPWDGPQYHIAPV   (b)
MAQQWSLQRLAGRHPQDSYEDSTQSSIFTYTNSNSTRGPFEGPNYHIAPR  (r)
MAQQWSLQRLAGRHPQDSYEDSTQSSIFTYTNSNSTRGPFEGPNYHIAPR  (g)


W_AKILTAYMIMIGMISWCGNGVVIYIFATTKSLRTPANLLVINLAISDF  (fly)
WQFSMLAAYMFLLEVLGFPINFLTLYVTVQHKKLRTPLNYILLNLAVADL  (rod)
WAFYLQAAFMGTVFLIGFPLNAMVLVATLRYKKLRQPLNYILVNVSFGGF  (b)
WVYHLTSVWMIFVVTSAVFTNGLVLAATMKFKKLRHPLNWILVNLAVADL  (r)
WVYHLTSVWMIFVVISAVFTNGLVLAATMKFKKLRHPLNWILVNLAVADL  (g)
←―――――――1――――――――→        ←―――――――2―――――
GIMITNTPMMGINLYFETWVLGPMMCDIYAGLGSAFGCSSIWSMCMISLD  (fly)
FMVLGGFTSTLYTSLHGYFVFGPTGCNLEGFFATLGGFIALQSLVVLAIE  (rod)
LLCIFSVFPVFVASCNGYFVFGRHVCALEGFLGTVAGLVTGWSLAFLAFE  (b)
AETVIASTISIVNEVSGWFVLGHPMCVLEGYTVSLCGITGLWSLAIISWE  (r)
AETVIASTISVVNQVYGYFVLGHPMCVLEGYTVSLCGITGLWSLAIISWE  (g)
―――2――――→        ←――――――――3――――――――――
RYQVIVKGMAGRPMTIPLALGKIAYIWFMSSIWCLAPAFGWSRYVPEGNL  (fly)
RYVVVCKPMSNFRFGENHAIMGVAFTWVMALACAAPPLAGWSRYIPEGLQ  (rod)
RYIVICKPFGNFRFSSKHALTVVLATWTIGIGVSIPPFFGWSRFIPEGLQ  (b)
RWLVVCKPFGNVRFDAKLAIVGIAFSWIWSAVWTAPPIFGWSRYWPHGLK  (r)
RWMVVCKPFGNVRFDAKLAIVGIAFSWIWAAVWTAPPIFGWSRYWPHGLK  (g)
―3→        ←――――――――4――――――――→
TSCGIDYLERDWNPRSYLIFYSIFV--YYIPLFLICYSYWFIIAAVSAHE  (fly)
CSCGIDYYTLKPEVNNESFVIYMFVVHFTIPMIIIFFCYGQLVFTVKEAA  (rod)
CSCGPDWYTVGTKYRSESYTWFLFIFCFIVPLSLICFSYTQLLRALKAVA  (b)
TSCGPDVFSGSSYPGVQSYMIVLMVTCCIIPLAIIMLCYLQVWLAIRAVA  (r)
TSCGPDVFSGSSYPGVQSYMIVLMVTCCITPLSIIVLCYLQVWLAIRAVA  (g)
                    ←――――――――5―――――――――
KAMREQAKKMNV--------------------------------------  (fly)


KSLRSSEDAEKSAEGKLAKVALVTITLWFMAWTPYLVINCMGLFKFEG_LT  (fly)
AQQQESATTQKAEKEVTRMVIIMVIAFLI-CWVPYASVAFYIFTHQGSNFG  (rod)
AQQQQSQTTQKAEREVSRMVVVMVGSFCV_CYVPYAAFAMYMVNNRNHGLD  (b)
KQQKESESTQKAEKEVTRMVVVMIFAYCV_CWGPYTFFACFAAANPGYAFH  (r)
KQQKESESTQKAEKEVTRMVVVMVLAFCF_CWGPYAFFACFAAANPGYPFH  (g)
            ←――――――――6――――――――→
PLNTIWGACFAKSAACYNPIVYGISHPKYRLALKEKCPCCVFGKVDDGKS  (fly)
PIFMTIPAFFAKSAAIYNPVIYIMMNKQFRNCMLTTICCGKNPLGDDEAS  (rod)
LRLVTIPSFFSKSACIYNPIIYCFMNKQFQACIMKMVCEKAMTDESDTCS  (b)
PLMAALPAYFAKSATIYNPVIYVFMNRQFRNCILQLFGKKVDDGSELSSA  (r)
PLMAALPAFFAKSATIYNPVIYVFMNRQFRNCILQLFGKKVDDGSELSSA  (g)
←――――――7―――――――→
SDAQSEATASEAE---SKA  378                            (fly)
ATVSKTETS_____QVAPA  348                            (rod)
S__QKTEVSTVSSTQVGPN  348                            (b)
S___KTEVSSVSS__VSPA  364                            (r)
S___KTEVSSVSS__VSPA  364                            (g)
```

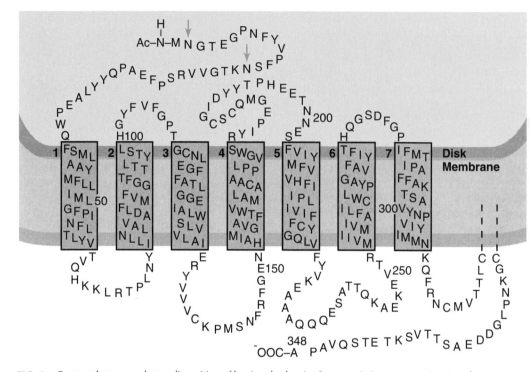

FIG. 3.   Proposed transmembrane disposition of bovine rhodopsin. Sugar moieties at asparagine-2 and asparagine-15 are shown with *red arrows*. Palmitoyl groups at cysteine-322 and cysteine-323 are indicated with broken lines. Hydroxyamino acid residues that may be phosphorylated by rhodopsin kinase are clustered in a C-terminal domain of the molecule.

(Fig. 3). When the helices are bundled together, the acidic residue may move in the vicinity of the chromophore and donates the necessary negative charge. On absorption of light, rhodopsin is decomposed to the opsin protein and all-*trans*-retinal. The reaction occurs through several spectrally distinct intermediates (Fig. 4). The formation of bathorhodopsin involves photoisomerization of the 11-*cis*-retinylidene chromophore to a constrained all-*trans* form and takes place within a few picoseconds after light absorption at physiological temperature. Bathorhodopsin then undergoes thermal relaxation, giving rise first to lumirhodopsin and then metarhodopsin I. The formation of metarhodopsin II is of particular importance, because it is presumably this intermediate that transmits the photosignal to a G protein.

Bleached rhodopsin must be regenerated to maintain normal vision

Regeneration of rhodopsin occurs by several mechanisms. The major mechanism involves isomerization of all-*trans*-retinal to the 11-*cis* form in the retinal pigmented epithelium, transport of 11-*cis*-retinal to the outer segment, and recombination with opsin. According to a current hypothesis [8], all-*trans* retinyl ester is isomerized to 11-*cis* form and quickly hydrolyzed. Thus, the free energy of hydrolysis of the ester coupled to isomerization drives the isomerization process. The shuttle of retinoids between the photoreceptor and pigmented epithelium may involve several retinoid-binding proteins. A second mechanism is photoconversion of thermal intermediates, such as metarhodopsins, to rhodopsin. For example, regeneration of squid rhodopsin occurs mainly by photo-

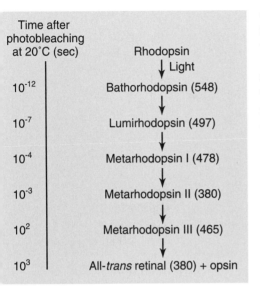

Time after photobleaching at 20°C (sec)	Rhodopsin
	↓ Light
10^{-12}	Bathorhodopsin (548)
	↓
10^{-7}	Lumirhodopsin (497)
	↓
10^{-4}	Metarhodopsin I (478)
	↓
10^{-3}	Metarhodopsin II (380)
	↓
10^{2}	Metarhodopsin III (465)
	↓
10^{3}	All-*trans* retinal (380) + opsin

FIG. 4.   Intermediates formed after photic bleaching of vertebrate rhodopsin. Numbers in parentheses are wavelengths of light (in nanometers) absorbed maximally by the individual intermediates.

isomerization of opsin-linked retinal at pH 10 and subsequent dark adaptation [9]. In a third mechanism, the photoisomerization of all-*trans*-retinal to the 11-*cis* form may take place within the rod outer segment. For example, all-*trans*-retinylidene phospholipid is photoisomerized to the 11-*cis* form within the disk membrane and reacts with opsin [10].

Cone cell pigments contain different opsins but with high sequence homology

The primary structures of the three human cone pigments were deduced from analysis of the genomic and complementary DNA clones encoding them [11] (Fig. 2). The sequences of cone pigments show 41 percent identity with rhodopsin. Red and green pigments show high sequence homology; only 15 of 364 residues are different. Genetic analysis locates the rhodopsin gene on chromosome 3 and the blue pigment gene on chromosome 7. Although none of the human cone pigments has been isolated, the

chicken cone pigment iodopsin has been purified and characterized. The primary structure of this pigment is known [12]. Iodopsin (λ_{max} 571 nm) forms bathoiodopsin on light absorption at -196°C. This intermediate reverts back to iodopsin on warming. If illuminated by 600-nm light at -183°C, iodopsin is converted to lumi-iodopsin which thermally decays to metaiodopsin I and metaiodopsin II.

PHOTOTRANSDUCTION

Light absorption by rhodopsin leads to closure of Na⁺-conductance channels via a chemical messenger system

Light is known to close the Na⁺ channels on outer segment plasma membrane and induce hyperpolarization of the membrane within 100 msec. The magnitude of light response reaches a maximum by absorption of several hundred photons per rod cell. Below the saturation light intensity, the relationship between the magnitude of light response (I) and energy of irradiating light (A) is given by

$$I = I_{max} \, A/(A + K)$$

where I_{max} is the magnitude of response at the saturation light intensity, and K is light energy required for 50 percent of the maximum response [13]. This equation has the same form as the Michaelis-Menten equation of enzyme kinetics. By analogy to enzyme kinetics, we may assume that rhodopsin reacts with light to form a complex, photoactivated rhodopsin (probably metarhodopsin II), which gives rise to an intracellular messenger X that links the photochemical reaction of rhodopsin to the plasma membrane. It is logical to postulate such a messenger because the disk membrane, where rhodopsin is localized, is not continuous with the plasma membrane that contains the Na⁺ channels.

The messenger compound must satisfy at least two properties. First, its concentration in the outer segment cytoplasm must change rapidly on light irradiation and return to the original level after light is turned off. Second, when the compound is introduced into the outer segment cytoplasm in the dark, it must mimic the effect of light. The first candidate proposed for messenger X is Ca^{2+} [14]. The Ca^{2+} hypothesis assumes that a large number of Ca^{2+} ions are sequestered within the disk in the dark and are released into cytoplasm when a single rhodopsin molecule in the disk membrane absorbs a photon. Ca^{2+} has been assumed to close the Na^+ channels in the plasma membrane. In support of the hypothesis, injection of Ca^{2+} into the outer segment in the dark suppresses Na^+ permeability and induces membrane hyperpolarization; however, several findings contradict this hypothesis. Cytoplasmic Ca^{2+} concentration in the outer segment does not increase on light illumination but decreases instead. There is no evidence that the disks can actively accumulate Ca^{2+} in the dark, and in patch-clamp experiments in which a small piece of outer segment plasma membrane is attached by suction to the tip of an electrode, exposure of the cytoplasmic surface of membrane to Ca^{2+} does not inhibit Na^{2+} conductance of the membrane fragment [15]. Thus, the Ca^{2+} hypothesis fails to explain the phototransduction process in vertebrate eyes.

A G-protein/cGMP system in outer segments is responsive to photoactivated rhodopsin

Another candidate for messenger X is related to guanosine cyclic 3′,5′-phosphate (cGMP). According to the cGMP hypothesis, the Na^+ channel is kept open by cGMP and closes when cGMP is hydrolyzed in light. The primary structure of the channel protein (a single polypeptide of 63,000 Da) was determined [16]. Exposure of an outer segment membrane fragment to cGMP in patch-clamp experiments increases its Na^+ conduc-

tance in the dark [15]. This effect is reversible. Concentration of cGMP in dark-adapted rod outer segments is high and decreases rapidly when the rod is irradiated at low Ca^{2+} concentrations. The decrease of cGMP is proportional to the log of light intensity. Hence, the amount of messenger X that is expected to "accumulate" in light is represented by the amount of cGMP hydrolyzed. cGMP phosphodiesterase (PDE), the enzyme that hydrolyzed cGMP to 5′-GMP, is indirectly activated by light. The activation is mediated by a G protein ($G_{\alpha\beta\gamma}$), called transducin, which is activated by photoactivated rhodopsin (R*) [17] (Fig. 5). According to the cGMP hypothesis, a single R* molecule may produce hundreds of active G-protein molecules. This is the rate-limiting step in rod vision. The polypeptide loops between helices 3 and 4 and helices 5 and 6 and a loop between helix 7 and the palmitoyl anchors of R* (Fig. 3) are probably involved in binding to G protein [5]. The G protein consists of three subunits, α, β, and γ, and has GDP bound to the α subunit in inactive form. The R* catalyzes exchange of GTP for GDP, and the G_α-GTP thus formed dissociates from the β- and γ-subunits. Two G_α-GTP molecules then activate one phosphodiesterase ($PDE_{\alpha\beta\gamma_2}$) molecule by dissociating the two γ-subunits (internal inhibitors) in succession. The G_β subunit is common to G proteins associated with various receptors, and G_α is specific to the individual receptors (see Chap. 21). Rod and cone outer segments have different G_α-subunits. The primary structure of rod G-protein subunits has been elucidated (references are found in Sugimoto et al. [18]).

The cGMP hypothesis can explain many aspects of phototransduction in vertebrate photoreceptors, including the effect of Ca^{2+}. The Ca^{2+} and cGMP concentrations in the photoreceptors are reciprocally related. Reduced Ca^{2+} concentration after irradiation is therefore expected to enhance cGMP level and open Na^+ channels. Thus, Ca^{2+} will play

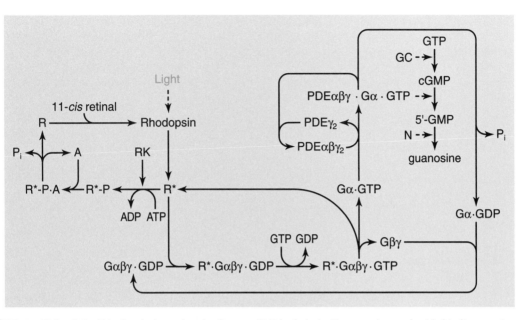

FIG. 5.   Light-elicited biochemical reactions leading to cGMP hydrolysis: $G_{\alpha\beta\gamma}$, guanine nucleotide-binding protein (transducin); $PGE_{\alpha\beta\gamma_2}$, phosphodiesterase; GC, guanylyl cyclase; N, 5'-nucleotidase; RK, rhodopsin kinase; R*, photo-activated rhodopsin; R, inactive form of rhodopsin; A, arrestin. cGMP binds to the cation channel protein of the plasma membrane and opens the channel.

an important role in the regulation of light adaptation [3,19]. Phototransduction for color vision proceeds very much like that for rod vision, involving cone pigments, GTP-binding protein, cGMP-phosphodiesterase, and cGMP-gated cation channels.

Although growing evidence supports the importance of the cGMP hypothesis for vertebrate vision, it remains unresolved whether cGMP plays a key role in invertebrate vision. Because invertebrate visual cells *depolarize* in light, a rise in cGMP is expected upon light absorption. However, light does not increase the cGMP level in invertebrate photoreceptors [20], and a different mechanism may exist. A mechanism proposed for invertebrate phototransduction involves light-stimulated hydrolysis of phosphatidyl-inositol-4,5-bisphosphate (PIP_2). Reception of an external signal by a variety of receptors is known to evoke hydrolysis of PIP_2 to diacylglycerol (DG) and inositol-1,4,5-triphos-

phate (IP_3) by activating phospholipase C (see Chap. 20). In this mechanism, both IP_3 and DG can serve as intracellular messengers; IP_3 increases intracellular Ca^{2+}, and DG stimulates protein kinase C. Injection of IP_3 into *Limulus* ventral photoreceptors in the dark mimics the light effect, evoking membrane depolarization without latency, and an increase in the intracellular Ca^{2+} level as well [22,23]. Injection of IP_3 into salamander rod outer segments induces membrane hyperpolarization in the dark.

Whatever mechanism is involved in phototransduction, the process must be regulated to reset the system. In the cGMP cascade mechanism, hydrolysis of G protein-bound GTP to GDP inactivates G protein. Thermal decay of R* (presumably metarhodopsin II) to opsin and all-*trans*-retinal terminates activation of G protein; R* is also inactivated by phosphorylation [24] and binding of arrestin (protein with a molecular weight of 48,000) to phosphorylated R* [25]. The mechanism of guanylate cyclase activation remains yet to be elucidated.

Regulation of G-protein-mediated membrane receptors by phosphorylation, as exemplified by phosphorylation of R*, may be of general importance. Different G-protein-mediated membrane receptors have structural similarities. For example, the mammalian β-adrenergic receptor and the muscarinic acetylcholine receptor show significant amino acid sequence homology with rhodopsin [26], and a β-receptor-specific protein kinase phosphorylates rhodopsin [27]. An arrestin-like protein modulates the β-receptor. Similarities between the photoreceptor system and other G protein-mediated membrane receptor systems suggest that they are evolutionarily related.

COLOR BLINDNESS

Red/green color blindness is explained by unequal intragenic recombination between a pair of the X-chromosomes

Amino acid sequences of the three cone pigments of human retina (Fig. 2) indicate that red and green pigments are very similar (96% homology) but blue pigment is different. The blue pigment gene is located on chromosome 7, whereas the red and green pigment genes reside on the X-chromosome [11]. Peculiarly, each X-chromosome has one red pigment gene and either one, two, or three green pigment genes in color normals. A hypothesis to explain the variability of the green pigment gene is that the red pigment gene occurs upstream of the 5′-end of the green pigment gene, and a pair of homologous red-green gene arrangements has undergone unequal recombinations during evolution. Red/green color blindness is explained by abnormalities in the unequal intragenic recombination as described below.

Approximately 8 percent of Caucasian males inherit a color abnormality: those who require only two primary wavelengths to match all colors (dichromats) and those who require three primary wavelengths but make color matches different from the normal (anomalous trichromats). Loss of one of the three color pigments (or systems) explains dichromats, while a shift in the spectral sensitivity of one of the three pigments (or systems) may be responsible for anomalous trichromacy. Blue cone abnormalities are inherited as autosomal traits and rare. Therefore, abnormalities in the red and green cone systems have been most extensively studied. From psychophysical studies, defects in the red and green cone systems are mapped to two tightly linked loci on the X-chromosome, and most likely to the loci of red and green pigment genes. What are the underlying genetic mechanisms that produce dichromats and anomalous trichromats? Nathans [28] hypothesizes that visual abnormalities are caused by alterations in red and green pigment genes by unequal intragenic recombination. Red and green pigment genes are similar and tightly linked on the X-chromosome as described above. If, during the development of ova and sperm cells, a pair of chromosomes join by crossing-over in the region encoding red and green pigments, and break between the two genes of one of the chromosomes, one chromosome may lose the green pigment gene and the other chromosome have two. On the other hand, breaking within a gene may result in a hybrid gene composed of part of the green pigment gene and part of the red pigment gene. If the X-chromosome lacking the green pigment gene is inherited, the carrier is a dichromat. Depending on the location of breakpoints, a variety of hybrid genes are generated; a man with a hybrid gene producing a pigment similar to the normal pigment will be a dichromat. However, the carriers of hybrid genes producing pigments with spectral sensitivities intermediate between those of red and green pigments will be anomalous trichromats.

RETINITIS PIGMENTOSA

Mutations in rhodopsin and other photoreceptor proteins are linked to retinitis pigmentosa

Retinitis pigmentosa (RP) is a group of human inherited retinopathies that affects about 1 in 3,000 [29]. RP may be classified into four types, autosomal dominant (10 percent), autosomal recessive (50 percent), sex-linked (15 percent), and allied diseases (25 percent). RP is characterized by loss of night vision in the early stage, followed by loss of peripheral vision.

The first gene suspected to be linked to dominant type RP was located on the long arm of chromosome 3 and its mutant product was found to be rhodopsin: replacement of proline 23 by histidine [30]. More than 30 point mutations within the rhodopsin gene have so far been reported. Another gene of dominant type RP, localized on the short arm of chromosome 6, was recently identified to be peripherin, a structural protein (35,000 Da) present in the rim of disks of rod outer segments [29]. A defect in the peripherin gene is involved in a hereditary retinopathy of the mouse (retinal degeneration slow or rds) [31]. In another form of mouse retinopathy (rd), a defect is in the beta subunit of cGMP-phosphodiesterase. These findings suggest that defects causing photoreceptor degenerations in different forms of RP could be in any structural and functional proteins associated with rod outer segments. Very little is known about how mutations in these proteins bring about degenerations of the rod cells. It is possible that various elements released into the subretinal space via retinal vasculature normally protect the photoreceptors and that mutations forfeit the protection. In RCS rats with inherited retinal dystrophy, in which the ability of the retinal pigmented epithelium to phagocytize photoreceptor outer segments is impaired, subretinal or intravitreal injection of basic fibroblast growth factor causes a significant delay in retinal degeneration [32].

Choroideremia can be classified, broadly, as an X-linked form of RP. A recent study of lymphoblasts from subjects with this disorder has disclosed deficient activity of geranylgeranyl transferase [33]. This enzyme catalyzes the transfer of geranylgeranyl groups to guanine nucleotide-binding proteins. This modification is necessary for these proteins to participate in membrane fusion processes (Figs. 2–5). Both the biogenesis of photoreceptor disks and their subsequent phagocytosis by the pigmented epithelial cells involve very active membrane fusion and turnover. Thus, it is quite possible that the pathology of RP may arise from an enzyme deficiency of this type.

REFERENCES

1. Shichi, H. *Biochemistry of Vision*. New York: Academic, 1983.
2. Berman, E. R. *Biochemistry of the Eye*. New York: Plenum, 1991.
3. Stryer, L. Visual excitation and recovery. *J. Biol. Chem.* 266:10711–10714, 1991.
4. Hargrave, P. A., and McDowell, J. H. Rhodopsin and phototransduction: a model system for G protein-linked receptors. *FASEB J.* 6: 2323–2331, 1992.
5. Khorana, H. G. Rhodopsin, photoreceptor of the rod cell. *J. Biol. Chem.* 267:1–4, 1992.
6. LaVail, M. M. Rod outer segment disk shedding in rat retina: Relationship to cyclic lighting. *Science* 194:1071–1074, 1976.
7. Young, R. W. Visual cells and the concept of renewal. *Invest. Ophthalmol.* 15:700–725, 1976.
8. Rando, R. R. Membrane phospholipids and the dark side of vision. *J. Bioenerg. Biomembr.* 23:133–146, 1991.
9. Suzuki, T., Sugahara, M., and Kito, Y. An intermediate in the photoregeneration of squid rhodopsin. *Biochim. Biophys. Acta.* 275: 260–270, 1972.
10. Shichi, H., and Somers, R. L. Possible involvement of retinylidene phospholipid in photoisomerization of all-*trans* to 11-*cis* retinal. *J. Biol. Chem.* 249:6570–6577, 1974.
11. Nathans, J., Thomas, D., and Hogness, D. S. Molecular genetics of human color vision: The genes encoding blue, green, and red pigments. *Science* 232:193–202, 1986.

12. Yoshizawa, T., and Kuwata, O. Iodopsin, a red-sensitive cone visual pigment in the chicken retina. *Photochem. Photobiol.* 54: 1061–1070, 1991.

13. Korenbrot, J. I. Signal mechanisms of phototransduction in retinal rod. *CRC Critical Rev. Biochem.* 17:223–256, 1985.

14. Hagins, W. A. The visual process: Excitatory mechanisms in the primary receptor cells. *Annu. Rev. Biophys. Bioeng.* 1:131–158, 1972.

15. Fesenko, E., Kolesnikov, S. S., and Lyubarsky, A. L. Induction by cyclic GMP of cationic conductance in plasma membrane of retinal rod outer segment. *Nature* 313:310–313, 1985.

16. Kaupp, U. B., Niidome, T., Tanabe, T., Terada, S., Boenigk, W., et al. Primary structure and functional expression from complementary DNA of the rod photoreceptor cyclic GMP-gated channel. *Nature* 342:762–766, 1989.

17. Stryer, L. Cyclic GMP cascade of vision. *Annu. Rev. Neurosci.* 9:87–119, 1986.

18. Sugimoto, K., Nukada, T., Tanabe, T., Takahashi, H., Noda, M., et al. Primary structure of the β-subunit of bovine transducin deduced from the cDNA sequence. *FEBS Lett.* 191: 235–240, 1985.

19. Torre, V., Matthews, H. R., and Lamb, T. D. Role of calcium in regulating the cyclic GMP cascade of phototransduction in retinal rods. *Proc. Natl. Acad. Sci. U.S.A.* 83:7109–7113, 1986.

20. Brown, J. E., Faddis, M., and Combs, A. Light does not induce an increase in cyclic-GMP content of squid or *Limulus* photoreceptors. *Exp. Eye Res.* 54:403–410, 1992.

21. Hokin, L. E. Receptors and phosphoinositide-generated second messengers. *Annu. Rev. Biochem.* 54:205–235, 1985.

22. Brown, J. E., Rubin, L. J., Ghalayini, A. J., Tarver, A. P., Irvine, R. F., et al. Myo-inositol polyphosphate may be a messenger for visual excitation in Limulus photoreceptors. *Nature* 311:160–163, 1984.

23. Fein, A. Excitation and adaptation of Limulus photoreceptors by light and inositol 1,4,5-triphosphate. *Trends Neurosci.* 9:110–114, 1986.

24. Liebman, P. A., Pugh, E. N. ATP mediates rapid reversal of cyclic GMP phosphodiesterase activation in visual receptor membranes. *Nature* 287:734–736, 1980.

25. Kuehn, H., Hall, S. W., Wilden, U. Light-induced binding of 48-KDa protein to photoreceptor membranes is highly enhanced by phosphorylation of rhodopsin. *FEBS Lett.* 176: 473–478, 1984.

26. Kubo, T., Fukuda, K., Mikami, A., Maeda, A., Takahashi, H., et al. Cloning, sequencing and expression of complementary DNA encoding the muscarinic acetylcholine receptor. *Nature* 232:411–416, 1986.

27. Benovic, J. L., Mayor, F., Somers, R. L., Caron, M. G., and Lefkowitz, R. J. Light-dependent phosphorylation of rhodopsin by β-adrenergic receptor kinase. *Nature* 321:869–872, 1986.

28. Nathans, J. Molecular biology of visual pigments. *Annu. Rev. Neurosci.* 10:163–194, 1987.

29. Humphries, P., Kenna, P., and Farrar, G. J. On the molecular genetics of retinitis pigmentosa. *Science* 256:804–808, 1992.

30. Dryja, T. P., McGee, T. L., Reichel, E., Hahn, L. B., et al. A potent mutation of the rhodopsin gene in one form of retinitis pigmentosa. *Nature* 343:364–366, 1990.

31. Arikawa, K., Molday, L. L., Molday, R. S., and Williams, D. S. Localization of peripherin/ rds in the disk membranes of cone and rod photoreceptors: Relationship to disk membrane morphogenesis and retinal degeneration. *J. Cell Biol.* 116:659–667, 1992.

32. Faktorovich, E. G., Steinberg, R. H., Yasumura, D., Matthes, M., and LaVail, M. M. Photoreceptor degeneration in inherited retinal dystrophy delayed by basic fibroblast growth factor. *Nature* 347:83–86, 1990.

33. Seabra, M. C., Brown, M. S., and Goldstein, J. L. Retinal degeneration in choroideremia: Deficiency of rat geranylgeranyl transferase. *Science* 259:377–381, 1993.

CHAPTER 8

Olfaction and Taste in Vertebrates: Molecular and Organizational Strategies Underlying Chemosensory Perception

LINDA B. BUCK, STUART FIRESTEIN, AND ROBERT F. MARGOLSKEE

In recent years, enormous strides have been made in the understanding of the molecular mechanisms which underlie olfaction and taste in vertebrates. The application of innovative physiological, biochemical, and molecular biological techniques has allowed for the identification and characterization of molecules involved in the initial events in perception in these two sensory systems and has provided fresh insight into the processes by which olfactory and gustatory discrimination are achieved.

OLFACTION

Olfactory discrimination

The mammalian olfactory system possesses enormous discriminatory power. It is claimed that humans can perceive many thousands of different odorous molecules (odorants) and that they can discriminate at least two to three thousand of these. It is also well known that even slight alterations in the structure of an odorant can lead to profound changes in perceived odor quality. One com-

Basic Neurochemistry: Molecular, Cellular, and Medical Aspects, 5th Ed., edited by G. J. Siegel et al. Published by Raven Press, Ltd., New York, 1994. Correspondence to Linda B. Buck, Department of Neurobiology, Harvard Medical School, Boston, Massachusetts 02115.

monly cited example is carvone whose L- and D- stereoisomers are perceived as spearmint and caraway, respectively. However, more subtle molecular alterations can also generate striking changes in perception.

Structural features underlying olfactory perception

The fine discriminatory power of the mammalian olfactory system is likely to derive from information processing events that occur at several distinct anatomical sites: the olfactory epithelium of the nasal cavity where odors are first sensed by olfactory sensory neurons, the olfactory bulb where information received from the sensory neurons is presumably processed, and the cortex where information received from the olfactory bulb is thought to be further refined to allow for the discrimination of thousands of different odors [1].

The initial events in olfaction occur in a specialized olfactory neuroepithelium which, in mammals, lines the posterior nasal cavity (Fig. 1). The olfactory epithelium contains three predominant cell types: the olfactory sensory neuron, the supporting (or sustentacular) cell, and the basal cell or stem cell. Olfactory neurons are the only mammalian neurons that are known to turn over throughout life. They are continuously replaced from the basal layer of stem cells. Two morphologically distinguishable types of dividing basal cell have been identified in mammals, the horizontal basal cell and the globose basal cell. At present, it is not clear what lineage relationship these two cell types bear to each other, but both have been proposed as stem cell precursors to the olfactory neuron.

The olfactory neuron is a bipolar cell that extends a single dendrite to the epithelial surface (Fig. 1). From the dendritic terminus, numerous fine cilia extend into the layer of mucus that lines the nasal lumen. It is thought that these cilia bear specific receptors for odorants. Evidence for the existence of specific odorant receptors on olfactory

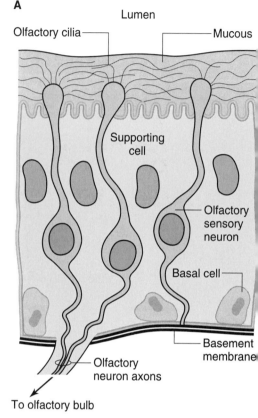

A

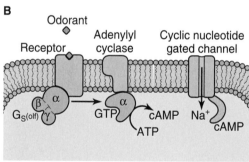

B

FIG. 1. A schematic diagram of the olfactory epithelium. The initial events in odor perception occur in the olfactory epithelium of the nasal cavity. Odorants interact with specific odorant receptors on the lumenal cilia of olfactory sensory neurons. The signals generated by these initial binding events are transmitted along olfactory neuron axons to the olfactory bulb of the brain.

cilia has come from the experiments of Rhein and Cagan, who showed that the olfactory cilia of fish, whose olfactory system senses amino acids as odors, specifically bind amino acids [2]. In addition, olfactory cilia isolated from a number of different species exhibit odorant-induced increases in adenylyl cyclase activity and cAMP as well as, in some cases, inositol trisphosphate [3–5]. This further suggests that the cilia are the site of olfactory signal transduction events. The activation of adenylyl cyclase is dependent on the presence of GTP and is therefore likely to be mediated by receptor-coupled GTP-binding proteins (G proteins), as will be discussed below.

Each olfactory neuron projects a single axon to the olfactory bulb where it forms synapses within specialized regions of neuropil, called glomeruli, with periglomerular interneurons and the two major output neurons of the bulb, the mitral and tufted cells. The bulbar neurons, in turn, project to the olfactory cortex.

Odorant receptors

Odor discrimination is likely to depend upon the ability of different olfactory sensory neurons to recognize different odorants. Indeed, electrophysiological studies of olfactory sensory neurons exposed to different odorants indicate that different neurons recognize different odorants or sets of odorants [6,7]. It is thought that the patterns of synapses formed in the olfactory bulb by olfactory neurons that recognize different odorants might constitute elementary 'odor codes.' It is not clear how many different types of odorant receptor would be required in such a coding scheme nor is it obvious how narrowly or broadly tuned they might be or how their expression might be organized to achieve a high level of sensory discrimination. Theoretically, odor discrimination could involve a very large number of different odorant receptors, each highly specific for one or a small set of odorants. At the other extreme, there could be a relatively

small number of different odorant receptors, each of low specificity and capable of interacting with a wide assortment of different odorous ligands. Individual olfactory neurons could each express only a single odorant receptor type or multiple different odorant receptors.

The recent identification and cloning of genes encoding odorant receptors [8] has made it possible to begin to address these questions. By assuming that odorant receptors would be encoded by a multigene family and that the odorant receptors would belong to a large superfamily of receptors that transduce signals via interaction with heterotrimeric G proteins, Buck and Axel were able to identify a novel multigene family in rat which appears to code for hundreds of diverse odorant receptors [8]. Northern blot analyses and cDNA library screens demonstrated that the members of this family are expressed in the olfactory epithelium, but not in a variety of other neural or non-neural tissues, and that, within the olfactory epithelium, they may be expressed exclusively by olfactory neurons. In a series of Southern blotting and genomic library screening experiments, they further showed that the odorant receptor multigene family contains many hundreds of genes, making this one of the largest, if not the largest, multigene family in the genome.

The amino acid sequences encoded by ten cDNAs sequenced in these initial experiments are shown in Fig. 2 [8]. As expected, the odorant receptors belong to the G protein-coupled receptor superfamily. Like other G protein-coupled receptors, the odorant receptors all display seven hydrophobic domains which are likely to serve as membrane spanning regions. This gives rise to a molecule that transverses the membrane seven times (Fig. 3). The odorant receptors also contain several limited sequence motifs which are commonly seen in members of the G protein-coupled superfamily, such as the NP pair in transmembrane domain 7 (TM7). However, the odorant receptors share extensive sequence motifs with one another that

```
                           I                                                                   II

F3    MDSSNRTRVSEFLLLGFVENKDLQPLIYGLFLFLSMYLVTVIGNISIIVAISDPCLHTPMYFFLSNLSFVDICFISTTVPKML    82
F5    MSSTNQSSVTEFLLLGLSRPQQQQLLFLLFLIMYLATVLGNLIILAIGTDSRLHTPMYFFLSNLSFVDVCFSSTTVPKXL      82
F6    MAWSTGQNLSTPGPFILLGFPGPRSMRIGLFLFLFIFALFLSMYLVVMYLLTVVGNLAIISLVGAHRCLQTPMYFFLCNLSFLEIWFTTACVPKTL  85
F12   MN--NQFITQFLLLGLPIPEEHQHLFYALFLVMYLTTILIGNLLIIIVLVQLDSQLHTPMYLFLSNLSFSDLCFSSVTMPKLL    83
I3    MERRNHSGRVSEFVLLGFPAPALRVLFFLSLLXYVLVLTENMLIIIAIRNHPTLHKPMYFLANMSFLEIWYVTVTIPKML      80
I7    MN--NKTVITHFLLLGLPIPPEHQQLFFALFLIMYLTTFIGNLLIIIVLVQLDSHLHTPMYFFLSNLSFSDLCFSSVTMKLL    83
I8    MTRRNQTAISQFFLLGLPPEYQHLFYALFLAMYLTTLLGNLIIIILILLDSHLHTPMYLFLSNLSFADLCFSSVTMPKLL      80
I9    MTGNNQTILIELFLLLGLPIPSEYHLFYALFLAMYLTIILGNLLIIVLVRLDSHLHHPMYLFLSNLSFSDLCFSSVTMPKLL    82
I14   MTRRNQTAISQFFLLGLPPEYQHLFYALFLAMYLTTLLGNLIIIILILLDSHLHTPMYLFLSNLSFSDLCFSSVTMPKLL      82
I15   MTEENQFVISQFLLLFLPIPSEHQHVFYALFLSMYLTTVLGNLIIILIHLDSHLHTPMYLFLSNLSFSDLCFSSVTMPKLL      82


                           III                                                                 IV

F3    ----VNIQTQNNVITYAGCITQIYFFLLFVELDNFLLTIMAYDRYVAICHPMHYTVIMNYKLCGFLVLVSWIVSVLHALFQSLMM    163
F5    ----ANHILGSQAISFSGCLTQLYFLLAVFGNMDHLLLAVMSYDRYVAICHPLHYTKMTRQLCVLLVVGSWVVANMNCLLHILLM    163
F6    ----ATFAPRGGVISLAGCATQMYFVFSLGCTEYFLLAVMAYDRYLAICLPLRYGGIMTPGLAMRLALGSWLCGFSAITVPATLI    166
F12   ----VNIYTQSKSITYEDCISQMCVFLVFAELGNFLLAVMAYDRYVAXCHPLCYTVIVNHRLCILLLLSWVISIFHAFIQSLIV    164
I3    ----QNMRSQDTSIPYGGCLAQIYFFMVFGDMESFLLVAMAYDRYVAICFPLHYTSIMSPKLCTCLVLLWMLTTSHAMMHTLLA    161
I7    AGFIGSKENHGQLISFEACMTQLYFFIGLGCTECVLLAVMAYDRYVAICHPLHYPVIVSSRLCVQMAAGSWAGGFGISMVKVFLI    168
I8    ----QNIQSQVPSISYAGCLTQIFFFLLFGYLGNLLLAVMAYDRYVAICFPLHYTNIMSHKLCTCLLLVFWIMTSSHAMMTLLA    161
I9    ----QNMQSQVPSIPYAGCLAQIYFFLFFGDLGNFLLVAMAYDRYVAICFPLHYMSIMSPKLCVSLVVLSWVLTTFHAMLHTLLM    163
I14   ----QNMQSQVPSISYTGCLTQLYFFMVFGDMESFLLVVMAYDRYVAICFPLRYTTIMSTKFCASLVLLWMLTMTHALLHTLLI    163
I15   ----QNMQSQVPSIFFAGCLTQLYFYIYFADLESFLLVAMAYDRYVAICHPLHYMSIMSPKLCVSLVVLSWVLTTFHAMLHTLLM    163


                           V                                                                   VI

F3    LALPFCTHLEIPHYFCEPNQVIQLTCSDAFLNDLVIYFTLVLLATVPLAGIFYSYFKIVSSICAISSVHGKYKAFSTCASHLSVV    248
F5    ARKSFCADNMIPHFFCDGTPLLKLSCSDTHLNELMILTEGAVVMVTPFVCILISYIHITCAVLRVSSPRGGWKSFSTCGSHLAVV    248
F6    ARLSFCGSRVINHFFCDISPWIVLSCTPTQVVELVSFGIAFCVILGSCGITLVSYAYIITTIKIPSARGRHRAFSTCSSHLTVV    251
F12   LQITFCGDVKIPHFFCELNQLSQLTCSDNFPSHLIMNLVPVMLAAISFSGILYSYFKIVSSIHSISTVQGKYKAFSTCASHLSIV    249
I3    ARLSFCENNVLNFFCDLFVLLKLACSDTYINELMIFIMSTLLIIIPFFLIVMSYARIISSILKVPSTQGICKVFSTCGSHLSVV    246
I7    SRLSYCGPNTINHFFCDVSPLLNLSCTDMSTAELTDFVLAIFILLGPLSVTGASYMATGAVMRIPSAAGRHKAFSTCASHLTVV    253
I8    ARLSFCENNVLLNFFCDLFVLLKLACSDTYVNELMIHIMGVIIIVIPFVLIIVISYAKIISSILKVPSTQSIHKVFSTCGSHLSVV    246
I9    ARLSFCEDSVIPHYFCDMSTLLKVACSDTHDNELAIFILGGPIVVILPFLLIVMSYARIVSSILKVPSSQSIHKAFSTCGSHLSVV    248
I14   ARLSFCEKNVILHFFCDISALLKLSCSDIYVNELMIYILGGLIIIIPFLLIVMSYVRIFFSILKFPSIQDIYKVFSTCGSHLSVV    248
I15   ARLSFCADNMIPHFFCDISPLLKLSCSDTHVNELVIFVMGGLVIVIPFVLIIVSYARVVASILKVPSVRGIHKIFSTCGSHLSVV    248


                           VII

F3    SLFYCTGLGVYLSSAANNSSQASATASVMYTVVTPMVNPFIYSLRNKDVKSVLKKTLCEEVIRSPPSLLHFFLVLCHLPCFIFCY    333
F5    CLFYGTVIAVYFNPSSSHLAGRDMAAAVMXAVVTPMLNPFIYSLRNSDMKAALRKVLAMRFPSKQ                        313
F6    LIWYGSTIFLHVRTSVESSLDLTKAITVLNTIVTPVLNPFIYTLRNKDVKEALRRTVKGK                             311
F12   SLFYSTGLGVYVSSAVVQSSHSAASASVMYTVVTPMLNPFIYSLRNKDVKRAJERLLEGNCKVHHWTG                     317
I3    SLFYGTIIGLYLCPAGNNSTVKEMVMAMMYTVVTPMLNPFIYSLRNRDMRALIRVICSMKITL                          310
I7    IIFYAASIFIYARPKALSAFDTNKLVSVLYAVIVPLFNPIIYCLRNQDVKRALRRTLHLAQDQEANTNKGSKIG               327
I8    SLFYGTIIGLYLCPSGDNFSLKGSAMAMMYTVVTPMLNPFIYSLRNRDMKQALIRVTCSKKISLPW                       312
I9    SLFYGTVIGLYLCPSANNSTVKETVMSLMYTMVTPMLNPFIYSLRNRDIKDALEKIMCKKQIPSFL                       312
I14   TLFYGTIFGIYLCPSGNNSTVKEIAMAMMYTVVTPMLNPFIYSLRNRDMKRALIRVICTKKISL                         314
I15   SLFYGTIIGLYLCPSANNSTVKETVMAMMYTVVTPMLNPFIYSLRNRDMKEALIRVLCKKKITFCL                       312
```

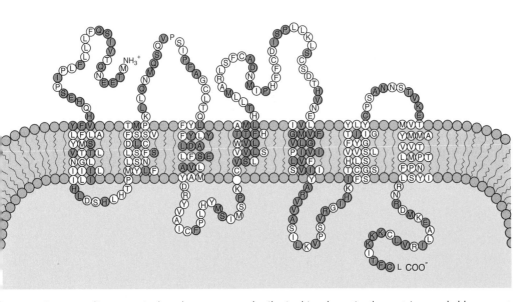

FIG. 3. Sequence divergence in the odorant receptor family. In this schematic, the protein encoded by one rat cDNA clone (I15) is shown traversing the plasma membrane seven times. The N-terminus is located extracellularly and the C-terminus intracellularly. The vertical cylinders indicate the seven putative membrane-spanning regions. Positions at which 60 percent or more of the ten receptors shown in Fig. 2 share the same residue as I15 are shown as white balls. More variable positions are shown as red balls. The extensive variability observed within several of the transmembrane domains is evident.

are not seen in other G protein-coupled receptors (Fig. 2).

There are two striking features of the odorant receptors that may be relevant to the role of these molecules in odor discrimination [8]. Although the odorant receptors, as a group, display a number of conserved sequence motifs, they also display an impressive degree of diversity in the non-conserved regions. Detailed studies involving *in vitro* mutagenesis and domain swapping have been performed with the β-adrenergic receptor and several other members of the G protein-coupled superfamily in order to ascertain what regions of these molecules are involved in ligand binding [9]. These studies indicate that many G protein-coupled receptors bind to ligand via a ligand-binding pocket which is formed in the plane of the membrane by a combination of the transmembrane domains. The importance of the transmembrane domains in ligand binding is further stressed in alignments of members of small families of G protein-coupled receptors that bind to the same ligand, such as the adrenergic receptor family and the muscarinic acetylcholine receptor family. These comparisons reveal that sequence conservation among receptors that bind the same ligand is highest in the transmembrane do-

FIG. 2. The protein sequences encoded by ten odorant receptor cDNA clones. Shaded residues are those conserved in 60 percent or more of the proteins. The presence of seven hydrophobic domains (I–VII), as well as short conserved motifs shared with other members of the superfamily, indicates that these molecules are members of the seven transmembrane domain, G protein-coupled receptor superfamily. The presence of extensive shared sequence motifs unique to the olfactory proteins indicates that these proteins are members of a novel receptor family within the superfamily. The pronounced sequence diversity evident in transmembrane domains III, IV, and V is likely to allow different members of the odorant receptor family to bind to structurally diverse odorous ligands. (Reproduced from *Cell* 65:175–187, by copyright permission of Cell Press.)

mains. In contrast, the odorant receptor family exhibits extensive sequence divergence in several transmembrane domains (TM3, TM4, and TM5) (Figs. 2 and 3). This diversity in potential ligand binding regions within the odorant receptor family is consistent with an ability of this family to interact with a large number of structurally diverse odorous ligands.

A second interesting feature of the odorant receptor family that may be important in odor discrimination is the presence of subfamilies with the family [8]. As already mentioned, transmembrane domain 5, which could be involved in ligand binding, is highly divergent in members of the odorant receptor family. However, as shown in Fig. 4, members of the odorant receptor family appear to fall into subfamilies whose members can be almost identical in this divergent region. It is likely that the members of divergent subfamilies recognize different structural classes of odorants. The highly related members of a subfamily might either recog-

A

F2	RYNE	VVIFIVVSLFLVLPFALIIMSYV	RIVSSILKVPSSQGIYK
F3	FLND	LVIYFTLVLLATVPLAGIFYSYF	KIVSSICAISSVHGKYK
F5	HLNE	LMILTEGAVVMVTPFVCILISYI	HITCAVLRVSSPRGGWK
F6	QVVE	LVSFGIAFCVILGSCGITLVSYA	YIITTIIKIPSARGRHR
F7	HVNE	LVIFVMGGIILVIPFVLIIVSYV	RIVSSILKVPSARGIRK
F8	FPSH	LTMHLVPVILAAISLSGILYSYF	KIVSSIRSMSSVQGKYK
F12	FPSH	LIMNLVPVMLAAISFSGILYSYF	KIVSSIHSISTVQGKYK
F13	FPSH	LIMNLVPVMLAAISFSGILYSYF	KIVSSIHSISSVKGKYK
F23	FLND	VIMYFALVLLAVVPLLGILYSYS	KIVSSIRAISTVQGKYK
F24	HEIE	MIILVLAAFNLISSLLVVLVSYL	FILIAILRMNSAEGRRK
I3	YINE	LMIFIMSTLLIIIPFFLIVMSYA	RIISSILKVPSTQGICK
I7	STAE	LTDFVLAIFILLGPLSVTGASYM	AITGAVMRIPSAAGRHK
I8	YVNE	LMIHIMGVIIIVIPFVLIVISYA	KIISSILKVPSTQSIHK
I9	HDNE	LAIFILGGPIVVLPFLLIIVSYA	RIVSSIFKVPSSQSIHK
I11	HLNE	LMILTEGAVVMVTPFVCILISYI	HITWAVLRVSSPRGGWK
I12	FPSH	LIMNLVPVMLGAISLSGILYSYF	KIVSSVRSISSVQGKHK
I14	YVNE	LMIYILGGLIIIIPFLLIVMSYV	RIFFSILKFPSIQDIYK
I15	HVNE	LVIFVMGGLVIVIPFVLIIVSYA	RVVASILKVPSVRGIHK

B

F12	FPSH	LIMNLVPVMLAAISFSGILYSYF	KIVSSIHSISTVQGKYK
F13	FPSH	LIMNLVPVMLAAISFSGILYSYF	KIVSSIRSVSSVKGKYK
F8	FPSH	LTMHLVPVILAAISLSGILYSYF	KIVSSIRSMSSVQGKYK
I12	FPSH	LIMNLVPVMLGAISLSGILYSYF	KIVSSVRSMSSVQGKHK
F23	FLND	VIMYFALVLLAVVPLLGILYSIS	KIVSSIRAISTVQGKYK
F3	FLND	LVIYFTLVLLATVPLAGIFYSYF	KIVSSICAISSVHGKYK

C

F7	HVNE	LVIFVMGGIILVIPFVLIIVSYV	RIVSSILKVPSARGIRK
I15	HVNE	LVIFVMGGLVIVIPFVLIIVSYA	RVVASILKVPSVRGIHK
I3	YINE	LMIFIMSTLLIIIPFFLIVMSYA	RIISSILKVPSTQGICK
I8	YVNE	LMIHIMGVIIIVIPFVLIVISYA	KIISSILKVPSTQSIHK
I9	HDNE	LAIFILGGPIVVLPFLLIIVSYA	RIVSSIFKVPSSQSIHK
I14	YVNE	LMIYILGGLIIIIPFLLIVMSYV	RIFFSILKFPSIQDIYK

D

F5	HLNE	LMILTEGAVVMVTPFVCILISYI	HITCAVLRVSSPRGGWK
I11	HLNE	LMILTEGAVVMVTPFVCILISYI	HITWAVLRVSSPRGGWK

FIG. 4.   Evidence for subfamilies within the odorant receptor family. The deduced protein sequences of 18 different cDNA clones in and around transmembrane domain V are shown. Residues shared by 60 percent or more of the proteins at a given position are *shaded* (**A**). Transmembrane domain V appears to be highly variable in members of the odorant receptor family (see Figs. 2 and 3). However, these proteins can be grouped into subfamilies (**B–D**) in which the individual subfamily members share considerable homology in this divergent region. (Reproduced from *Cell* 65:175–187, by copyright permission of Cell Press.)

nize the same odorants or detect subtle differences between structurally related odorants.

Interestingly, Southern blotting experiments indicate that subfamilies are a characteristic feature of the odorant receptor multigene family [8,10]. When different members of the multigene family are hybridized to Southern blots of restriction enzyme digested genomic DNA, distinct patterns of hybridizing species are seen, each of which is likely to represent a different member of the subfamily. The individual subfamilies appear to range in size from 1 to 20 members, but on average have about 7–10 members.

The remarkable size and diversity of the odorant receptor multigene family in mammals suggests that odor discrimination relies heavily on the initial event in olfactory perception, the interaction of odorant receptor with odorant. In this respect, olfaction contrasts sharply with color vision where signals derived from only three peripheral receptor types (the three color opsins) are processed to allow the perception of a multitude of different hues. The extremely large number of odorant receptor genes further suggests that individual receptors could be highly specific, each one recognizing only one odorant or a small set of structurally similar odorants.

Information coding

How might the information generated by hundreds of different receptor types be organized to achieve the high level of discrimination characteristic of the mammalian olfactory system? Most sensory systems localize environmental information in space and possess neural topographical maps of that spatial information. The olfactory system does not perceptually localize environmental information in external space. However, it could use spatial determinants within the nervous system to encode information. If so, topographical maps or spatial codes for odors might be evident within the olfactory epithelium or olfactory bulb. For example, olfactory neurons that express a particular

odorant receptor gene and therefore recognize the same odorants might be clustered in one region of the olfactory epithelium or might all form synapses at a discrete site in the olfactory bulb. On the other hand, neurons that express the same odorant receptor gene could be broadly distributed in the olfactory epithelium or form synapses at many different bulbar sites.

A Zonal Organization of Sensory Information in the Olfactory Epithelium

To address these questions, Ressler et al. analyzed the patterns of expression of different odorant receptor genes within the olfactory epithelium of the mouse [10]. They found that different odorant receptors are expressed in distinct topographical patterns within the nasal cavity. It appears that the olfactory epithelium is divided into a limited series of expression zones. These zones exhibit bilateral symmetry in the two nasal cavities and are virtually identical in different individuals. Within each zone, many different members of the odorant receptor gene family are expressed. Within a zone, an individual subfamily of related receptors is expressed in fewer than 1 percent of the resident olfactory neurons. However, each individual gene may be expressed only within a single zone. The zonal assignment of each gene appears to be strictly regulated. However, within each zone, neurons that express a particular receptor gene are broadly distributed. It thus appears that when an olfactory neuron or its progenitor chooses which odorant receptor gene(s) to express, it is restricted to a single zonal gene set, but may choose a receptor gene (or set of genes) to express from among the zonal set via a stochastic mechanism.

The odorant receptor expression zones in the olfactory epithelium exhibit a pronounced dorsal-ventral and medial-lateral organization [10]. Interestingly, the axonal projection from the olfactory epithelium to the olfactory bulb is also organized along the dorsal-ventral and medial-lateral axes [11].

Comparisons of the locations of the expression zones with the topographical patterning of projections between the olfactory epithelium and olfactory bulb indicate that the organization of odorant receptor gene expression in the epithelium is preserved in the axonal projection to the olfactory bulb [10]. Thus, it appears that all neurons that express a particular gene are found in one zone within the nasal cavity and that they all project axons to a particular broad region of the olfactory bulb. These results suggest that an initial organization of olfactory sensory information occurs in the olfactory epithelium and that this organization is maintained in the patterns of signals transmitted to the olfactory bulb [10]. This conclusion is consistent with the results of earlier electrophysiological studies which suggested that there might be regional differences in responsiveness to different odorants in the olfactory epithelium [1].

Sensory Organization in the Epithelium to Bulb Projection

Within the olfactory bulb, the axons of olfactory neurons are organized such that the axons of olfactory neurons that express the same receptor gene are localized to the same broad region [10]. It is possible that, within a bulbar region, a reassortment of axons occurs such that olfactory neurons that express the same receptor gene come to synapse at one or a few discrete sites within that bulbar region. Activity dependent mechanisms of synaptic refinement, similar to those that operate in the visual system, could conceivably produce such discrete foci of synapses within the bulb via a process of axonal reassortment and refinement [10]. For example, olfactory neurons whose axons have reached the bulb might only form permanent synapses when they and other neurons that have synapsed on the same bulbar neuron are simultaneously stimulated by an odorant. It is not presently known whether olfactory neurons that respond to the same odorant synapse at the same site in the olfactory bulb [1]. However,

there is evidence for the ability of different odorants to increase activity in different bulbar regions [1]. On the other hand, a finer pattern of synapses may not exist within the olfactory bulb. In this case, the cortex may interpret complex patterns of activity from bulbar output neurons as signifying different odors [10].

Sensitivity in odor perception

In recent years, significant advances have been made in the understanding of the signal transduction events that take place when an olfactory sensory neuron is exposed to an odorant. The reputed sensitivity of the olfactory system to extremely low concentrations of odorants and the fast recovery of this perceptual sensitivity are likely to derive from the capacity of the olfactory transduction apparatus to effectively amplify, and rapidly terminate, signals. Before discussing the biochemical events involved in the signal transduction process, it is instructive to consider the sensitivity of the olfactory system at the level of perception versus the individual neuron.

Although olfactory perception is believed to be extremely sensitive, the degree of sensitivity is controversial. Some reports, especially in insects, have suggested that odors involved in sexual attraction could be detected by male animals at the level of the single molecule, that is, concentrations as low as 10^{-14}M. Human olfactory thresholds of 10^{-11} M have been measured by psychophysical methods. In such studies, however, the actual concentration of odorant at the odorant receptor cannot be known definitively. Due to factors such as odor molecule interactions, diffusion, adsorption into mucus, and anatomical structures which may serve to trap and concentrate odor molecules these estimates could be as much as 2–4 orders of magnitude too low.

Physiological recordings from single receptor neurons suggest somewhat lower sensitivities, with $K_{1/2}$ values between 1 and 50 μM [7]. These values could allow for broad specificity and for rapid termination of odorant responses. For example, since $K_d = k_{off}/k_{on}$ and the on rate is ultimately limited by diffusional encounters between ligand and receptor (approximately $10^8 \text{ s}^{-1} \text{ M}^{-1}$) the K_d is limited by the range of acceptable off rates. A K_d of 10^{-6} would result in molecular encounters lasting a few hundred milliseconds, whereas a K_d of 10^{-11} would result in dwell times of more than 5 minutes.

It can be shown from the law of mass action that with significant amplification mechanisms, such that occupation of only a few receptors would be sufficient to elicit a response, thresholds as much as 5 or 6 orders of magnitude lower than the K_d can be attained. Thus K_d values of 10^{-6} could, in theory, produce threshold responses at odor concentrations as low as 10^{-11}, permitting the olfactory system to maintain the broad specificity seen in physiological recordings [7], and the high threshold sensitivity measured in psychophysical experiments. Several amplification mechanisms that could serve this purpose will be described below.

The signal transduction cascade

Odorant Recognition Initiates a Second Messenger System Leading to the Depolarization of the Neuron and the Generation of Action Potentials

Recordings of the electrical activity of single olfactory receptor neurons shows that exposure to odorants causes the membrane to depolarize leading to the generation of action potentials [12]. Underlying the initial depolarization is the influx of cations through a conductance in the specialized cilia extending from the distal end of the cell into the mucus lining of the nasal cavity (Fig. 5). The biochemical elements coupling odorant receptor binding to the opening of a cation channel are now understood in some detail [13]. A consensus view is presented in Fig. 6.

Early work in understanding the biochemistry of olfaction was stymied by the

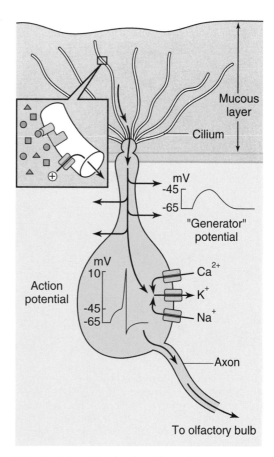

FIG. 5. Schematic drawing of an olfactory neuron showing the single bipolar morphology, with a single thick dendrite ending in a knob-like swelling and an unbranched axon projecting from the proximal soma centrally to the olfactory bulb. The cell is highly compartmentalized into transduction and signaling regions. Transduction occurs in the cilia which extend from the distal dendritic knob into the mucous layer. A receptor-coupled second messenger system (see Fig. 6) results in the opening of a cation selective channel in the ciliary membrane. The influx of cations depolarizes the cell membrane from its resting level near -65 mV to -45 mV in a graded manner. This depolarization spreads by passive current flow through the dendrite to the soma. A depolarization that reaches -45 mV is sufficient to activate voltage-gated Na^+ channels and initiate impulse generation. This Na^+ current, along with several varieties of voltage-dependent K^+ currents and a small Ca^{2+} current act to produce one or more action potentials that are propagated down the axon to the brain.

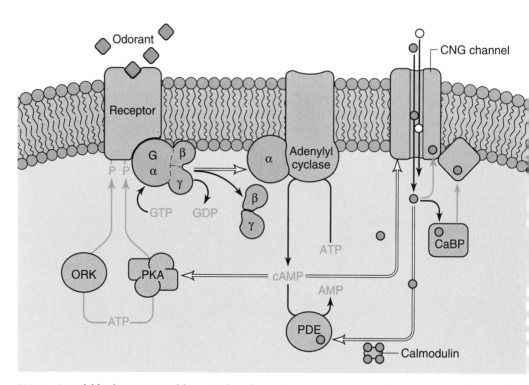

FIG. 6.　A model for the operation of the cAMP-based second messenger system in olfactory neurons. The individual steps are detailed in the text. Note that there are several feedback loops that act to modulate the response. These include inhibition of the channel by Ca^{2+} ions that permeate the channel, a cAMP-dependent protein kinase that may phosphorylate the receptor, and a receptor kinase that selectively phosphorylates occupied receptors. Sites of action are indicated by *open arrows* indicating stimulatory effects and *red arrows* indicating inhibitory effects. ORK, putative olfactory receptor kinase; PKA, protein kinase A; PDE, phosphodiesterase; CNG channel, cyclic nucleotide-gated channel; CaBP, putative calcium binding protein; ●, Ca^{2+}; ○, Na^{+}.

number and diversity of the stimuli. Lancet first pointed out, in 1985, that it might be possible to circumvent these difficulties by searching for a final common pathway, for example a second messenger system, utilized by all or at least a significant number of putative odorant receptors [3]. He and his coworkers first demonstrated the power of this approach by documenting an odor dependent increase in adenylate cyclase activity in an olfactory cilia enriched, cell-free preparation. These results implicated a G protein-coupled signal transduction system which generated the second messenger cyclic AMP and laid the groundwork for the subsequent biochemical and physiological identification of the components of this system.

A G protein that is likely to couple odor-ant receptors to other intracellular elements of the cascade (G_{olf}) was identified by Reed and his coworkers [13] and shown to be an isoform of G_s specific to olfactory neurons. It has been shown that high levels of G_{olf} are present in olfactory cilia. Since G_{olf} can interact with G protein-coupled receptors other than odorant receptors, it has been proposed that the existence of a separate gene for G_{olf} may, in some manner, permit the specific and high level of expression of this protein observed in olfactory neurons.

An adenylate cyclase has been identified in olfactory neurons which also appears to be specific to these cells and is biochemically distinct from other known isoforms of this enzyme. Also cloned and characterized by Reed and his coworkers it has been termed adenylate cyclase type III [13]. An important characteristic of this isozyme is that, when expressed in a mammalian cell line, its basal activity is extremely low, while in its stimulated state, it has a catalytic rate higher than other known cyclases. These properties could confer a high signal to noise ratio on the system, being quiescent in the absence of stimulus, but able to rapidly generate large amounts of cAMP upon odor exposure.

Consistent with this idea are the kinetics of cAMP accumulation which have been followed on a sub-second time scale by Breer and his colleagues using a rapid quench technique [5]. When odorants were added to an olfactory cilia preparation, cAMP increased linearly with odorant concentration up to a level four-fold greater than baseline. The increase peaked within 50 ms of exposure to the odor stimuli and returned to baseline levels within about 300 msec, suggesting that odorant stimulates the pulsatile production of cAMP.

In 1987 Nakamura and Gold [14] recorded ion currents from a ciliary conductance that was activated directly by cyclic AMP, without an intervening phosphorylation step. This was the final link between the biochemical cascade and the electrical signal. The channel was subsequently cloned and characterized in several species [13]. The channel is selective for cations, is curiously sensitive to both cAMP ($K_d = 20$ μM) and cGMP ($K_d = 5$ μM), and requires at least 3 molecules of cyclic nucleotide to bind for activation. It shares 65 percent homology with the cGMP activated channel found in photoreceptors, and, most interestingly, it also bears strong homology with voltage-sensitive channels such as K^+ and Ca^{2+} channels.

The activation of tens to hundreds of these channels and the subsequent influx of cations leads to depolarization of the cell membrane. Some of the important physiological characteristics of the odor response can be seen in recordings of the currents through the cyclic AMP sensitive channels in response to pulses of odor stimuli (Fig. 7)

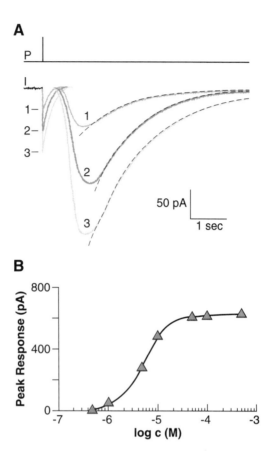

FIG. 7A: Three responses to 50 msec pulses of odor stimuli of low, intermediate, and saturating concentration. The initial fast, downward deflections are responses to KCl and provide a record of the time course and relative strength of the stimuli. The slower and larger downward deflections are the currents that flow in response to the odor pulses. Downward deflections of the current traces denote positive current flowing into the cell (i.e., a depolarizing current). Note the 100–200 msec latency between the arrival of the stimulus and the initiation of the current and also the continued activation of the current even after the stimulus has disappeared. These features are indicative of a second messenger process. The decay of the current is reasonably well fit by a single exponential time course *(dashed lines)*. **B:** Dose-response curve for a cell that responded to the odorant, cineole. The *solid line* is a fit of the Hill equation with a $K_{1/2}$ of 3×10^{-6} M and a Hill coefficient equal to 2. This curve shows the narrow operating range of the olfactory neuron.

[7]. There is a long (150–450 msec), concentration dependent latency between the binding of odor molecules and the activation of the current. The peak current amplitude is a sigmoidal function of the log odor concentration that can be fit by the Hill equation with a Hill coefficient of between 2–4. The suggested cooperativity in the response appears to emanate entirely from the channel's requirement for cooperative activation by cAMP.

This pathway provides several amplification steps between odorant binding and signal generation. Due to the electrically compact structure of the cell it is possible for the activation of only a few tens of channels to drive the membrane to threshold for action potential generation. Thus, it is theoretically possible that the limit of olfactory detection is the single molecule, although this has not yet been conclusively demonstrated.

Negative Feedback Processes Mediate Adaptation in the Odor-Induced Response

Upon application of a sustained odor stimulus to an olfactory neuron, the current response is transient, falling back to baseline within 4–5 seconds [12]. The termination of a response in the continued presence of agonist is characteristic of many signaling systems and is variously known as adaptation or desensitization, depending on the putative site of the off mechanism. Typically a negative feedback process is at work such that the accumulation of a product of the agonist response serves to turn off an upstream link in the signal generating cascade. In the olfactory neuron, two feedback messengers have been identified, and, as might be expected, they are Ca^{2+} ions and cAMP.

The ion channel activated by cAMP is permeable to cations, including Ca^{2+} [15]. Thus, increased channel activation results in influx of Ca^{2+} and a transient rise in the intracellular concentration of Ca^{2+}. Intracellular Ca^{2+} concentrations of 1–3 μM have been found to lead to a decrease in the open probability of the ion channel, even in the presence of high concentrations of cAMP [7]. The mechanism could involve a direct effect of Ca^{2+} ions on the channel or be mediated via an intermediate Ca^{2+} binding protein. In either case, this is an attractive mechanism for mediating a rapid, but short lasting form of adaptation, since it is dependent on the influx of Ca^{2+} ions during the response to an odor.

A second pathway, utilizing a phosphorylation step, resembles desensitization mechanisms described for the β-adrenergic receptor and rhodopsin [5,9,16]. Cyclic AMP, in addition to opening the ion channel appears to activate a form of cAMP dependent protein kinase (PKA) which inactivates some earlier step in the transduction process. Addition of a peptide fragment of the Walsh inhibitor protein (WIPTIDE), a PKA antagonist, prolongs the odorant-induced production of cAMP [5]. Studies of desensitization of the β-adrenergic receptor and rhodopsin have revealed two specialized, but closely related kinases (β-adrenergic receptor kinase (βARK) and rhodopsin kinase, respectively) that phosphorylate the activated receptor. Interestingly, a recently characterized isoform of βARK has been shown to be highly enriched in olfactory sensory neurons [16]. Odorant induced phosphorylation of ciliary proteins by both PKA and PKC (protein kinase C) has been demonstrated, but the phosphorylated proteins have not been conclusively identified. Thus, it is possible that cAMP that is generated in response to odor stimulation activates negative feedback pathways that act to truncate an ongoing response.

Alternative Second Messenger Pathways May Be at Work in Olfactory Transduction

The role of cAMP in olfactory transduction is now well established. Are there alternative pathways such as those involving phospholipids and Ca^{2+}? The suspicion that there might be multiple pathways first arose from a series of experiments by Sklar et al. [4] in which a large panel of different odorants were tested for their ability to generate cAMP production in a preparation of bullfrog olfactory cilia. Floral and herbal odorants produced large responses, whereas some others, such as several putrid odorants, failed to induce changes in cAMP.

Extending these experiments to mammals, Breer and his colleagues have assayed for IP_3 production in rat using the odorants that failed to produce cAMP in the study by Sklar et al. [5]. They found rapid and significant increases in IP_3, the data being almost identical to that they had earlier produced for cAMP generation. Additionally they found that a given odorant led to the production of either cAMP or IP_3, never both. More recently they have found evidence for two pathways for adaptation, one utilizing PKA and the other PKC, and have shown that the responses to odors using one or the other pathway are completely additive. Utilizing cultured mammalian olfactory neurons, Ronnett and her colleagues have found evidence that many odorants can stimulate both IP_3 and cAMP production, but that the ratio of IP3 to cAMP varies according to odorant [17].

In mammalian olfactory neurons, increases in IP_3 can induce membrane depolarization, but it is not clear if this is specifically related to sensory transduction. As there are no organelles in the cilia, the IP_3 must act directly on a plasma membrane channel. However, IP_3 channels are not normally found in the plasma membrane. One intriguing exception to this was recently demonstrated in cultured olfactory neurons from lobster [18]. In these cells, injection of IP_3 produced a current that appeared similar to the odor induced current, and IP_3-gated channels were found in patches of membrane pulled from the cell soma. In summary, evidence is building for an IP_3 pathway in olfactory transduction, but it is less conclusive than that for cAMP.

TASTE

Physiological background

Taste Perception Can Be Reduced to Primary Stimuli

Our total perception of food is a complex experience based upon multiple senses: taste *per se* (sweet, sour, salty, bitter), olfaction (aromas), touch ("mouth feel," i.e., texture and fat content), thermoreception, and nociception (e.g., pungent spices and irritants). Taste proper is commonly divided into four categories of primary stimuli, sweet, sour, salty, and bitter. One other primary taste umami (savory) is controversial. Mixtures of these primaries can mimic the tastes of more complex foods.

The chemical complexity of taste stimuli suggests that taste receptor cells utilize multiple molecular mechanisms to detect and distinguish amongst these compounds. Our sense of taste can detect and discriminate various ionic stimuli (e.g., Na^+ as salty and H^+ as sour), sugars (sweet), and alkaloids (bitter). Sweet and bitter compounds display great structural diversity, suggesting the presence of multiple discriminatory receptors.

Taste Receptor Cells Are Organized into Taste Buds

The chemical detection of taste agents resides in specialized epithelial cells, taste receptor cells, which in vertebrates are present as ovoid clusters (taste buds) (Fig. 8) containing 50–100 cells. The taste buds are embedded within the non-sensory lingual epithelium of the tongue, and they are organized into focal collections termed taste papillae (fungiform, foliate, and circumvallate). Taste buds are also found in the palate, pharynx, and upper portion of the esophagus.

The taste bud is a polarized structure with a narrow apical opening (the taste pore), and basolateral synapses with afferent nerve fibers. Solutes in the oral cavity make contact with the apical membranes of the taste receptor cells via the taste pore. There

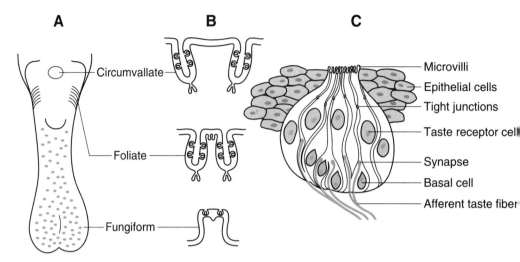

FIG. 8.   Rat tongue, taste papillae, and taste buds. **A:** Surface of the rat tongue showing location of the taste papillae. **B:** Cross section of the three main types of taste papillae: fungiform, foliate, and circumvallate. **C:** The taste bud contains 50–100 taste cells including receptor cells and basal cells.

is a significant amount of lateral connectedness between taste cells within a bud: both electrical (between taste receptor cells) and chemical synapses (between taste receptor cells and Merkel-like basal cells) have been demonstrated to occur [19]. Furthermore, there are also symmetrical synapses between taste receptor cells and Merkel-like basal cells [19]. In addition, Merkel-like basal cells also synapse with the afferent nerve fiber suggesting that they may function in effect as interneurons [19]. The extensive lateral interconnections within a bud, along with the branching of afferent fibers to synapse with several receptor cells within a given bud, suggest that much signal processing occurs peripherally within the taste bud itself [19].

Information coding

Sensory Afferents within Three Cranial Nerves Innervate the Taste Buds

The sensory fibers that innervate the taste buds travel in cranial nerves VII, IX, and X. The chorda tympani carries fibers from VII to innervate taste buds on the anterior portion of the tongue (buds within the fungi-form papillae and anterior portion of the foliate papillae). Buds within the circumvallate papillae and the posterior portion of the foliate papillae are innervated by the lingual branch of the glossopharyngeal nerve (IX). Taste buds of the epiglottis and the esophagus are innervated by the superior laryngeal branch of the vagus (X).

Projections from the afferent taste fiber synapse in the medulla within the gustatory portion of the nucleus of the solitary tract (Fig. 9). The more rostral portion of the nucleus of the solitary tract contains the gustatory nucleus, whereas the caudal portion receives afferent input from visceral organs (interoceptors of the carotid body and aortic arch; chemoreceptors of the digestive tract). The visceral inputs to the solitary tract relay their information to more rostral brain stem nuclei. Neurons from the gustatory nucleus project to the thalamus via the central tegmental tract and terminate in the small-cell (parvocellular) region of the ventral posterior media nucleus (VPMpc). The neurons of the VPMpc project to two regions of the cortex: the gustatory region of the postcentral gyrus and the inner face of the frontal operculum and insula.

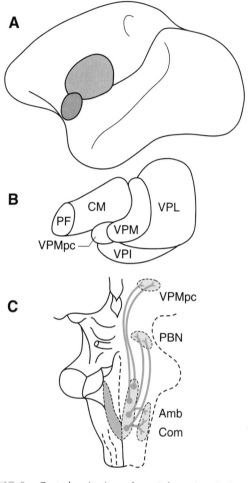

IG. 9. Central projections of taste information. **A:** Cortical taste projections. **B:** Thalamic taste projections. **C:** Medullary taste nuclei.

Information Coding of Taste Is Not Strictly According to a Labeled Line

Two current models for information coding within the gustatory system are: (a) labeled-line and (b) across-fiber pattern coding. The labeled line model proposes that each taste quality is transmitted via a separate pathway through the medulla, thalamus, and cortex [20]. Furthermore, this model predicts that individual gustatory fibers are narrowly tuned to a single taste quality and that the function of any one neuron would be to signal its particular encoded taste quality. The cross-fiber pattern coding model proposes that individual afferent fibers lack absolute specificity: populations of afferent fibers display relative preferences and thereby selectivity [21]. This model predicts broad, overlapping response spectra on the part of individual gustatory fibers.

Experimental results argue against a strict labeled-line model; however, gustatory information coding may utilize both types of mechanisms. For example, in the hamster, single chorda tympani fibers respond to multiple taste qualities (e.g., salt and sour, or sour and bitter). This implies that some type of pattern-recognition processing must occur, since multiple taste qualities are carried centrally by the same fiber. However, it is likely that some selectivity occurs within the fibers themselves with a preferential response to a given taste quality (e.g., salt > sour, or sour > bitter). Hence, an across-fiber pattern code could make use of several types of taste quality preferred fibers (e.g., salt best or sweet best).

Taste transduction

Taste Cells Have Multiple Types of Ion Channels

Taste receptor cells are electrically excitable cells capable of generating action potentials: voltage-dependent channels for Na^+, Ca^{2+} and K^+, similar to those in neurons, have been detected in vertebrate taste cells (for recent reviews see [19,22]). The surface distribution of these ion channels may reflect differences in their functional activities. The amphibian mudpuppy *(Necturus maculosus)* taste cell has a prominent voltage-gated K^+ conductance predominantly concentrated at its apical surface; Na^+ and Ca^{2+} channels are distributed throughout the surface of the mudpuppy taste cell [23]. However, mammalian taste cells do not display this prominent apical K^+ channel: no significant apical K^+ conductance could be found in the fungiform taste buds of the hamster [24]. Mammalian foliate and circumvallate-derived taste buds have not yet been tested for this apical K⁺ conductance. It has not been determined if the distribution of Na⁺ and Ca²⁺ channels in mammalian taste cells varies according to apical vs. basolateral surfaces. Multiple types of K⁺ channels have been found in vertebrate taste cells (reviewed in 22): (1) a voltage-independent K⁺ channel of ~40 pS conductance (frog); (2) a 90 pS delayed rectifier K⁺ conductance (rat) and; (3) a 225 pS Ca²⁺-dependent K⁺ channel (rat). In mammals, at least two types of Na⁺ conductances occur: (1) a tetrodotoxin blockable, voltage-dependent Na⁺ channel, similar to neuronal Na⁺ conductances and; (2) an amiloride blockable, voltage-independent Na⁺ channel, similar to epithelial Na⁺ conductances.

Sour and Salt Tastes Are Directly Mediated by Apical Ion Channels

Several lines of evidence suggest that salt taste in mammals is mediated via the voltage-independent, amiloride-blockable apical Na⁺ channel. These Na⁺ channels are of a type commonly found in epithelial cells involved in solute transport (e.g., renal epithelial cells). Micromolar concentrations of amiloride block this Na⁺ conductance in isolated taste cells and also block Na⁺ salt stimulation of gustatory nerve fibers [25]. Furthermore, psychophysical studies in man demonstrate that amiloride applied to the tongue can block the salt taste of Na⁺ salts [26]. The presumed mechanism for taste cell response to salt is direct inward conductance of Na⁺ ions through this amiloride-blockable channel leading to taste cell depolarization, action potential generation, and neurotransmitter release (Fig. 10). Other organisms may have significantly different mechanisms for salt perception: in the mud puppy, amiloride does not block nerve responses to NaCl, suggesting that this animal uses an alternative means of NaCl perception.

Sour taste is a function of the acidity of a solution, depending primarily on the proton concentration and to a lesser extent on the particular anion involved. As with salt, sour taste is perceived by direct action upon apical ion channels of taste cells (Fig. 10). In the mudpuppy, K⁺ channels are concentrated in the apical surface of the taste cell, and this apical K⁺ conductance dominates the resting potential of the mudpuppy taste cell [27]. Protons block voltage dependent Na⁺, Ca²⁺ and K⁺ currents in isolated taste cells, however, the major effect of protons in the mudpuppy taste cell is to block the apical K⁺ conductance (leading to taste cell depolarization) [23]. Patch-clamp recording of excised patches from the mudpuppy taste cell demonstrated H⁺ ion blockade of an 100 pS K⁺ channel.

Mammalian taste cells do not have a prominent apical K⁺ channel; they apparently detect protons via the amiloride-sensitive apical Na⁺ channel. In the hamster, protons block Na⁺ entry through the amiloride-sensitive Na⁺ channel, and protons enter the taste cell via the Na⁺ channel (amiloride also blocks H⁺-induced currents in the taste cell) [24]. In man, 200 mM NaCl tastes very salty, acid at pH 2.6 tastes very sour, however, 200 mM saline at pH 2.6 has neither sour nor salty taste (S. Kinnamon, *personal observations*). Presumably, in man, sour and salt are both transduced via the apical amiloride-sensitive Na⁺ channel.

Taste Cells Contain Receptors, G Proteins, and Second Messenger Effector Enzymes

Research on the biochemistry and molecular biology of taste has been hindered by the relative inaccessibility of taste receptor cells and the lack of high affinity ligands specific for taste receptors. Biochemical and histological analysis of mammalian taste tissue demonstrates high levels of adenylyl cyclase, phosphodiesterase, and IP₃ receptors. The catfish *(Ictalurus punctatus)* provides a very rich source of taste tissue: immunological and biochemical analysis demonstrates the presence of G_s-like and G_i-like guanine nucleotide binding regulatory proteins (G-proteins) in catfish taste membranes [28]. Recent work has used the polymerase chain

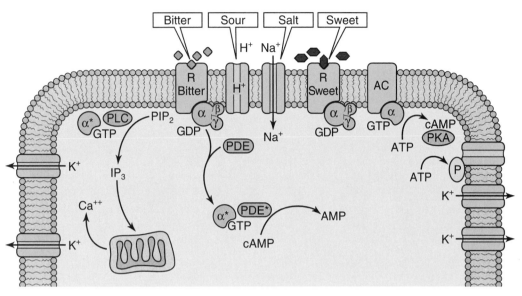

FIG. 10.   Proposed mechanisms for transduction of different taste stimuli. Salty stimuli (Na$^+$) enter taste cells via amiloride-sensitive Na$^+$ channels present in the apical membrane. Sour stimuli (H$^+$) block the amiloride-sensitive Na$^+$ channels (mammals) or block apical K$^+$ channels (mudpuppy). Sweet stimuli bind to specific receptors (R$_{sweet}$) coupled to G proteins ($\alpha\beta\gamma$): activation of this pathway leads to adenylyl cyclase (AC) generation of cAMP, which is proposed to activate protein kinase A (PKA) and lead to phosphorylation (P) and closure of basolateral K$^+$ channels. Closure of K$^+$ channels leads to taste cell depolarization. Bitter stimuli are thought to bind to specific receptors (R$_{bitter}$) coupled to G proteins. Two bitter transduction mechanisms are proposed. In one pathway a G$_q$-like G protein activates phospholipase C (PLC) leading to generation of 1,4,5-trisphosphate (IP$_3$). IP$_3$ causes Ca^{2+} release from internal stores which leads to neurotransmitter release onto gustatory afferents. A second pathway for bitter transduction is for gustducin to activate cAMP phosphodiesterase (PDE) and lead to decreased intracellular cAMP. This would lead to hyperpolarization of taste cells via decreased phosphorylation of basolateral K$^+$ channels.

reaction (PCR) on a rat taste cell specific cDNA library to molecularly clone the components of receptor/G-protein pathways (see below).

Sweet and Bitter Are Mediated by Receptor-Coupled Second Messenger Pathways

Sweet taste utilizes a G-protein dependent, receptor-mediated transduction pathway (Fig. 10). Sugars and artificial sweeteners bind to the taste cell surface and to taste cell membrane fractions. Biochemical studies with anterior tongue membranes (enriched for rat fungiform papillae) or intact taste buds (from rat circumvallate papillae) show that sweet compounds activate adenylyl cyclase which in turn elevates intracellular cAMP levels [29,30]. A competitive sugar antagonist inhibited sweet-induced elevation of cAMP [30], and in membrane extracts adenylyl cyclase activation by sucrose is GTP dependent [29]. These results argue for the presence of receptor(s) that upon activation by sweeteners activate G$_s$ (or a G$_s$-like protein), which in turn activates adenylyl cyclase to generate cAMP as the intracellular second messenger.

Electrophysiologic studies of rodent taste cells have shown that sucrose causes taste cell depolarization along with decreased K$^+$ conductance [31]. Injection of cAMP or cGMP into taste cells also elicits depolarization with decreased K$^+$ conductance [31]. These results argue for sweet pathway generated cyclic nucleotides as the mediator of taste cell depolarization via K$^+$ channel closure. There is no direct evidence for the existence in taste cells of a cyclic nucleotide responsive channel (such as is present in olfactory and photoreceptor cells). Rather, based on electrophysiology of frog taste receptor cells, it was proposed that cAMP activates protein kinase A to phosphorylate and thereby close the 40 pS basolateral K^+ channel; furthermore, it was proposed that sweet stimuli lead to taste cell depolarization via this mechanism [32].

Bitter agents are very structurally diverse, suggesting multiplicity of receptors and/or multiplicity of detection pathways (Fig. 10). Many bitter compounds are lipophilic and membrane permeant. It has been proposed that these compounds directly act on intracellular taste cell phosphodiesterases in either a stimulatory or inhibitory fashion. Other models for bitter have suggested nonreceptor mediated physical effects upon the lipid bilayer. However, it is unclear what specificity, if any, would be provided by taste cell membranes vs. any other type of membrane.

The intensely bitter compound denatonium chloride is membrane impermeant: using fura-2 imaging of intracellular Ca^{2+}, it was shown that denatonium causes a release of Ca^{2+} from internal stores [33]. Presumably, this effect is elicited by bitter receptor activation of a G_q-like G protein, which in turn activates phospholipase C to generate IP_3. Immunological and histochemical evidence demonstrates the presence of the IP_3 receptor in taste cells along with other components of the PI signaling pathway [34]. A recent study has demonstrated the presence of a G_q-like G protein in taste cells [35]; $G_{a_{14}}$ was shown to be specifically expressed in taste cells (see below).

Expression of Some G-Proteins Is Elevated in Taste Cells

Several known G-protein α subunits (α_s, α_{12}, α_{14}, α_{i-2}, and α_{i-3}) were cloned from a rat taste tissue specific cDNA library (Table 1) [35]. RNA expression of α_s, α_{14}, and α_{i-3} is elevated in taste buds versus the surrounding nonsensory epithelium (McLaughlin and Margolskee, *unpublished results*). G_s (or a G_s-like G protein) has been proposed to mediate sweet transduction; the elevated expression of G_s in taste buds is consistent with G_s itself playing a role in sweet transduction. Furthermore, the α-subunit of the G_s-like G_{olf} protein is not expressed in taste tissue (McLaughlin and Margolskee, *unpublished results*), ruling out any role for G_{olf} in taste transduction. G_{14} is a G_q-like G protein which can generate IP_3 via phospholipase C activation; G_{14} may play a role in denatonium (bitter) generation of IP_3 and subsequent Ca^{2+} release. G_{i-3} presumably inhibits adenylyl cyclase in taste cells; it may have a role in the termination of sweet responses or in bitter transduction via decreased levels of cAMP.

TABLE 1.   Isolates of G protein α-subunit clones from rat taste tissue

	5′KWIHCF 3′FLNKKD	5′DVGGQR 3′FLNKKD	5′HLFNSIC 3′VFDAVTD	5′TIVKQM 3′FLNKQD
α_{i-2}	4	—	—	—
$\alpha_{i-1,3}$	5	—	—	—
α_{q-1}	—	1	—	—
α_{q-2}	—	1	—	—
α_s	—	—	—	1
α_{gust}	5	—	4	1

Degenerate PCR primers corresponding to conserved amino acids of G proteins were made and used pairwise in the polymerase chain reaction to amplify DNA corresponding to G proteins. The G protein α-subunit isolates cloned from PCR amplified rat taste tissue cDNA are listed in the left hand column. The heading above each column lists the upstream (5′) and downstream (3′) primers.
The numbers in each column represent independent clonal isolates from the particular PCR amplification.
(From McLaughlin et al., *Nature* 357:563–569, 1992).

Gustducin Is a Taste Cell Specific G Protein Closely Related to the Transducins

A novel G protein α-subunit, α-gustducin, was recently cloned from rat taste tissue [35]. Gustducin mRNA and protein are expressed in taste buds of the circumvallate, foliate, and fungiform papillae. Gustducin is not expressed in non-sensory portions of the tongue, nor is it expressed in several other tissues (liver, heart, kidney, muscle, brain, retina, and olfactory epithelium). Gustducin is most closely related to the transducins (the rod and cone photoreceptor G proteins). At the amino acid level gustducin is 79 to 80 percent identical and 90 percent similar to the transducins. This is about the same level of relatedness as between rod and cone transducin (81 percent identical and 90 percent similar): α-gustducin is only 66 to 68 percent identical to α_i-subunits and only 46 percent identical to α_s. An alignment of the protein sequences of α-gustducin, and the α-transducins reveals that these three proteins are highly homologous throughout their entire length (Fig. 11). The carboxy-terminal 38 amino acids of α-gustducin and the α-transducins are identical. This C-terminal region of transducin has been implicated in its interaction with rhodopsin: suggesting that the taste receptor(s) which interacts with gustducin may have structural similarity to the opsins.

```
Gustducin   MGSGISSESK ESAKRSKELE KKLQEDAERD ARTVKLLLLG AGESGKSTIV KQMKIIHKNG  60
Bovinecone  MGSGASAEDK ELAKRSKELE KKLQEDADKE AKTVKLLLLG AGESGKSTIV KQMKIIHQDG  60
Bovinerod   MGAGASAEEK ....HSRELE KKLKEDAEKD ARTVKLLLLG AGESGKSTIV KQMKIIHQDG  56
Consensus   MGSGASAE-K E-AKRSKELE KKLQEDADKD ARTVKLLLLG AGESGKSTIV KQMKIIHQDG  60

Gustducin   YSKQECMEFK AVVYSNTLQS ILAIVKAMTT LGIDYVNPRS REDQQLLLSM ANTLEDGDMT 120
Bovinecone  YSPEECLEYK AIIYGNVLQS ILAIIRAMPT LGIDYAEVSC VDNGRQLNNL ANSIEEGTMP 120
Bovinerod   YSLEECLEFI AIIYGNTLQS ILAIVRAMTT LNIQYGDSAR QDDARKLMHM ANTIEEGTMP 116
Consensus   YS-EECLEFK AIIYGNTLQS ILAIVRAMTT LGIDY----- -DD-R-L--M ADTIEEGTMP 120

Gustducin   PQLAEIIKRL WGDPGIQACF ERASEYQLND SAAYYLNDLD RLTAPGYVPN EQDVLHSRVK 180
Bovinecone  PELVEVIRKL WKDGGVQACF DRAAEYQLND SASYYLNQLD RITAPDYLPN EQDVLRSRVK 180
Bovinerod   KEMSDIIQRL WKDSGIQACF DRASEYQLND SAGYYLSDLE RLVTPGYVPT EQDVLRSRVK 176
Consensus   PEL-EII-RL WKD-GIQACF DRASEYQLND SA-YYLNDLD RLTAPGYVPN EQDVLRSRVK 180

Gustducin   TTGIIETQFS FKDLNFRMFD VGGQRSERKK WIHCFEGVTC IIFCAALSAY DMVLVEDEEV 240
Bovinecone  TTGIIETKFS VKDLNFRMFD VGGQRSERKK WIHCFEGVTC IIFCAALSAY DMVLVEDDEV 240
Bovinerod   TTGIIETQFS FKDLNFRMFD VGGQRSERKK WIHCFEGVTC IIFIAALSAY DMVLVEDDEV 236
Consensus   TTGIIETQFS FKDLNFRMFD VGGQRSERKK WIHCFEGVTC IIFCAALSAY DMVLVEDDEV 240

Gustducin   NRMHESLHLF NSICNHKYFA TTSIVLFLNK KDLFQEKVTK VHLSICFPEY TGPNTFEDAG 300
Bovinecone  NRMHESLHLF NSICNHKYFA ATSIVLFLNK KDLFEEKIKK VHLSICFPEY DGNNSYEDAG 300
Bovinerod   NRMHESLHLF NSICNHRYFA TTSIVLFLNK KDVFSEKIKK AHLSICFPDY NGPNTYEDAG 296
Consensus   NRMHESLHLF NSICNHKYFA TTSIVLFLNK KDLF-EKIKK VHLSICFPEY -GPNTYEDAG 300

Gustducin   NYIKNQFLDL NLKKEDKEIY SHMTCATDTQ NVKFVFDAVT DIIIKENLKD CGLF 354
Bovinecone  NYIKSQFLDL NMRKDVKEIY SHMTCATDTQ NVKFVFDAVT DIIIKENLKD CGLF 354
Bovinerod   NYIKVQFLEL NMRRDVKEIY SHMTCATDTQ NVKFVFDAVT DIIIKENLKD CGLF 350
Consensus   NYIK-QFLDL NMRKDVKEIY SHMTCATDTQ NVKFVFDAVT DIIIKENLKD CGLF 354
```

FIG. 11.   Alignment of amino-acid sequences of α-subunits of rat gustducin, bovine rod transducin, and bovine cone transducin. Consensus sequence matches (i.e., at least 2 out of the 3 proteins match) are denoted by *shaded boxes*. Conservative changes are also within *shaded boxes*. Non-conservative changes are in *unshaded regions*. The *consensus line* shows positions where at least 2 of the 3 proteins match; *dashes in the consensus sequence* correspond to nonconserved positions. *Dots in the rod transducin sequence* correspond to gaps to align it with the other sequences. Note the high degree of conservation of the three sequences throughout their length. The last 38 amino acids of all three proteins are identical, this region has been implicated in receptor interaction. (From McLaughlin et al. *Nature* 357:563–569, 1992.)

It was proposed that gustducin's role in taste transduction would be similar to that of transducin in phototransduction [35]. In the retina, transducin relays activation of rhodopsin into activation of phosphodiesterase (PDE) by binding to the inhibitory γ subunit of PDE. A 22 amino acid long portion of rod transducin was recently shown to activate PDE [36]. This effector activation region is adjacent to transducin's C-terminal receptor interaction site: this region of rod and cone transducin is well conserved (86 percent identical, 95 percent similar) and closely related to the analogous region of gustducin (91 percent similar), consistent with gustducin's presumptive role as a PDE activator.

It was speculated that gustducin's role in taste is in the bitter pathway [35]. In this model, bitter receptor activation would lead to gustducin activation, which in turn would disinhibit taste cell cAMP PDE and lead to decreased levels of taste cell cAMP. This is consistent with the known high levels of taste cell PDE, and with the correlation between PDE activators and bitter compounds. That several PDE inhibitors enhance sweet perception may imply that there is cross-talk between bitter and sweet in the same taste cell or at least in the same taste bud, and explain the ability of sweeteners to partially mask bitter tastes in foods.

REFERENCES

1. Kauer, J. S. Coding in the olfactory system. In T. E. Finger and W. L. Silver (eds.), *Neurobiology of Taste and Smell.* New York: John Wiley, 1987, pp. 205–231.
2. Rhein, L. D., and Cagan, R. H. Biochemical studies of olfaction: binding specificity of odorants to a cilia preparation from rainbow trout olfactory rosettes. *J. Neurochem.* 41: 569–577, 1983.
3. Pace, U., Hanski, E., Salomon, Y., and Lancet, D. Odorant-sensitive adenylate cyclase may mediate olfactory reception. *Nature* 316: 255–258, 1985.
4. Sklar, P. B., Anholt, R. R. H., and Snyder, S. H. The odorant-sensitive adenylate cyclase of olfactory receptor cells: differential stimulation by distinct classes of odorants. *J. Biol. Chem.* 261:15538–15543, 1986.
5. Breer, H., Boekhoff, I., Krieger, J., Raming, K., Strotmann, J., and Tareilus, E. Molecular mechanisms of olfactory signal transduction. In D. P. Corey and S. D. Roper (eds.), *Sensory Transduction.* New York: The Rockefeller University Press, 1992, pp. 93–108.
6. Sicard, G., and Holley, A. Receptor cell responses to odorants: similarities and differences among odorants. *Bran Res.* 292: 283–296, 1984.
7. Firestein, S. Electrical signals in olfactory transduction. *Curr. Opin Neurobiology* 2: 444–448, 1992.
8. Buck, L., and Axel, R. A novel multigene family may encode odorant receptors: a molecular basis for odor recognition. *Cell* 65: 175–187, 1991.
9. Dohlman, H. G., Thorner, J., Caron, M. G., and Lefkowitz, R. J. Model systems for the study of seven-transmembrane-segment receptors. *Annu. Rev. Biochem.* 60:653–688, 1991.
10. Ressler, K. J., Sullivan, S. L., and Buck, L. B. A zonal organization of odorant receptor gene expression within the olfactory epithelium. *Cell* 73:597–609, 1993.
11. Astic, L., Saucier, D., and Holley, A. Topographical relationships between olfactory receptor cells and glomerular foci in the rat olfactory bulb. *Brain Res.* 424:144–152, 1987.
12. Firestein, S., Shepherd, G. M., and Werblin, F. S. Time course of the membrane current underlying sensory transduction in salamander olfactory receptor neurones. *J. Physiol. (Lond.)* 430:135–158, 1990.
13. Reed, R. R. Signaling pathways in odorant detection. *Neuron* 8:205–209, 1992.
14. Nakamura, T., and Gold, G. H. A cyclic-nucleotide gated conductance in olfactory receptor cilia. *Nature* 325:442–444, 1987.
15. Kurahashi, T., and Shibuya, T. Membrane responses and permeability changes to odorants in the solitary olfactory receptor cells of the newt. *Zoological Science* 6:19–30, 1989.
16. Dawson, T. M., Arriza, J. L., Jaworsky, D. E., Borisy, F. F., Attramadal, H., Lefkowitz, R. J., and Ronnett, G. V. Beta-adrenergic receptor kinase-2 and beta-arrestin-2 as mediators of odorant-induced desensitization. *Science* 259: 825–829, 1993.

17. Ronnett, G. V., and Snyder, S. H. Molecular messengers of olfaction. *Trends Neurosci.* 15: 508–513, 1992.

18. Fadool, D. A., Ache, B. W. Plasma membrane inositol 1,4,5-trisphosphate-activated channels mediate signal transduction in lobster olfactory receptor neurons. *Neuron.* 9:907–918, 1992.

19. Roper, S. D. The microphysiology of peripheral taste organs. *J. Neurosci.* 12:1127–1134, 1992.

20. Frank, M., and Pfaffmann, C. Taste nerve fibers: a random distribution of sensitivities to four tastes. *Science* 164:1183–1185, 1969.

21. Pfaffmann, C. Gustatory afferent impulses. *J. Cell Comp. Physiol.* 17:263–258, 1941.

22. Avenet, P., and Lindemann, B. Perspectives of taste reception. *J. Membr. Biol.* 112:1–8, 1989.

23. Kinnamon, S. C., Dionne, V. E., and Beam, K. G. Apical localization of K channels in taste cells provides the basis for sour taste transduction. *Proc. Natl. Acad. Sci. U. S. A.* 85: 7023–7027, 1988.

24. Gilbertson, T. A., Avenet, P., Kinnamon, S. C., and Roper, S. D. Proton currents through amiloride-sensitive Na channels in hamster taste cells: role in acid transduction. *J. Gen. Physiol.* 100:803–824, 1992.

25. Heck, G. L., Mierson, S., and DeSimone, J. A. Salt taste transduction occurs through an amiloride-sensitive sodium transport pathway. *Science* 223:403–405, 1984.

26. Schiffman, S. S., Lockhead, E., and Maes, F. W. Amiloride reduces the taste intensity of Na^+ and Li^+ salts and sweeteners. *Proc. Natl. Acad. Sci. U. S. A.* 80:6136–6140, 1983.

27. Kinnamon, S. C., and Roper, S. D. Membrane properties of isolated mud puppy taste cells. *J. Gen. Physiol.* 91:351–371, 1988.

28. Bruch, R. C., and Kalinoski, D. L. Interaction of GTP-binding regulatory proteins with chemosensory receptors. *J. Biol. Chem.* 262: 2401–2404, 1987.

29. Striem, B. J., Pace, U., Zehavi, U., Naim, M., and Lancet, D. Sweet tastants stimulate adenylate cyclase coupled to GTP binding protein in rat tongue membranes. *Biochem. J.* 260: 121–126, 1989.

30. Striem, B. J., Naim, M., and Lindemann, B. Generation of cyclic AMP in taste buds of the rat circumvallate papillae in response to sucrose. *Cell Physiol. Biochem.* 1:46–54, 1991.

31. Tonosaki, K., and Funakoshi, M. Cyclic nucleotides may mediate taste transduction. *Nature* 331:354–356, 1988.

32. Avenet, P., Hofmann, F., and Lindemann, B. Transduction in taste receptor cells requires cAMP-dependent protein kinase. *Nature* 331: 351–354, 1988.

33. Akabas, M. H., Dodd, J., and Al-Awqati, Q. A bitter substance induces a rise in intracellular calcium in a subpopulation of rat taste cells. *Science* 242:1047–1050, 1988.

34. Hwang, P. M., Verma, A., Bredt, D. S., and Snyder, S. Localization of phosphatidylinositol signaling components in rat taste cells: Role in bitter taste transduction. *Proc. Natl. Acad. Sci. U. S. A.* 87:7395–7399, 1990.

35. McLaughlin, S. K., McKinnon, P. J., Margolskee, R. F. Gustducin is a taste-cell-specific G protein closely related to the transducins. *Nature* 357:563–569, 1992.

36. Rarick, H., Artemyev, N. O., and Hamm, H. E. A site on rod G protein α subunit that mediates effector activation. *Science* 256: 1031–1033, 1992.

PART TWO

Synaptic Function

CHAPTER 9

Chemically Mediated Synaptic Transmission: An Overview

S. D. ERULKAR

Basic Neurochemistry: Molecular, Cellular, and Medical Aspects, 5th Ed., edited by G. J. Siegel et al. Published by Raven Press, Ltd., New York, 1994. Correspondence to Sol D. Erulkar, Department of Pharmacology, University of Pennsylvania School of Medicine, Philadelphia, Pennsylvania 19104.

CHARACTERISTICS OF CHEMICAL NEUROTRANSMISSION

Neurotransmitters are substances that, on release from nerve terminals, act on receptor sites at postsynaptic membranes to produce either excitation or inhibition of the target cell

These changes are brought about by changes in the distribution of ions across postsynaptic membranes of nerves, muscles, and glands. Chemically mediated transmission is one of the means by which an appropriate signal is transferred from one nerve cell to another, or from nerve fibers to muscle cells or even gland cells.

Elliott in 1904 [1] first suggested the possibility that information was transferred from one neuron to the next by the release of a chemical substance from nerve fibers; it was Loewi [2], however, who first showed the existence of a chemical substance in the perfusion fluid on stimulation of the vagus nerve. He and his collaborator Navratil later showed that this substance was acetylcholine.

Chemically mediated transmission involves the following processes:

1. Synthesis of the neurotransmitter at the presynaptic terminal.
2. Storage of the neurotransmitter or its precursor in the presynaptic terminal.
3. Release of the substance into the synaptic extracellular space.
4. Recognition and binding of the compound by postsynaptic receptors.
5. Inactivation and termination of the action of the neurotransmitter.

Some neurotransmitters such as acetylcholine (ACh), glycine, glutamate, and γ-aminobutyric acid (GABA), have an "inherent" biological activity such that the neurotransmitter directly causes an increase in conductance to certain ions by binding to ligand-activated ion channels at the postsynaptic membrane. Other neurotransmitters, such as norepinephrine, dopamine, and serotonin, have no direct activity but act indirectly via second messenger systems to bring about the postsynaptic response. These systems involve cAMP, cGMP, ITP, DAG, PGs, leukotrienes, epoxides, and Ca^{2+} (see [3]). These messengers act in the cytosol to activate target proteins, including protein kinases, which, in turn, act on substrates, such as ion channels, to produce the transmitter effects. These systems are described in detail in Chaps. 20–23.

Molecular mechanisms of synaptic transmission have been studied in a variety of preparations

The vertebrate neuromuscular junction, especially that of amphibia, provides convenient and available recording sites at which electrical activity resulting from transmitter release can be measured for long periods of time. The neurotransmitter is known to be ACh, and the structure is well defined. The disadvantage of this preparation is that electrodes cannot be placed within the presynaptic terminal to measure activity directly; rather, one relies on extracellular recording across a volume conductor. Studies using the squid giant synapse provide a means of circumventing this limitation. Electrodes can be placed intracellularly within the terminal as well as postsynaptically at the synaptic junction; however, the identity of the neurotransmitter is still unknown. Other preparations in which both pre- and postsynaptic nerve elements can be successfully impaled by microelectrodes have also been used and are becoming more popular. These include giant synapses in the lamprey, lobster, and cockroach; the photoreceptor of the barnacle; and the synapses of the Mauthner cells of fish.

In all these preparations, there is a close approximation of the nerve terminal and postsynaptic cell, with transmission occurring at discrete sites characterized by specializations of pre- and postsynaptic membranes. The released substance diffuses across the synaptic gap and interacts with postsynaptic receptors. The time delay from entry of action potentials into presynaptic nerve terminals to a response mediated by postsynaptic

receptors includes time required for the following events to occur:

1. Activation of presynaptic mechanisms related to release.
2. Diffusion across the synaptic gap (~50 μsec at the frog neuromuscular junction).
3. Response time of the postsynaptic receptor (~150 μsec at the frog neuromuscular junction).

The total time required varies from 0.5 to 3.5 msec. Most of this time (at least 350 μsec) must therefore be occupied by processes of release at the terminal, originally termed mobilization of neurotransmitter. It has now been suggested that this time is taken by the opening of Ca^{2+} gates to allow free ions to enter the terminal (see later).

This direct effect of a chemical substance crossing a short distance to act on its target site is thought of classically as neurotransmitter action: an effect that occurs rapidly but has limited duration. Our ideas have been somewhat modified, however, since it has been learned that certain substances can be released into the circulation to travel some distance before reaching their receptors. These substances were first called neurohormones to account for the effects of substances secreted into the bloodstream by neurosecretory cells in response to nerve impulses relayed via synapses. Although classical neurotransmitters are believed to act rapidly, some hypothalamic neuron terminals release peptides that cross a synaptic gap to act on other neurons where the action is slow and long-lasting. This is true also in the spinal cord, where the release of substance P (an undecapeptide) gives rise to a long-lasting depolarizing response.

In some tissues, such as the intestine, nerve terminals are not closely associated with specific smooth muscle cells, and transmitter is released into the extracellular space, where it diffuses locally to influence a number of cells. A particular transmitter may act locally at some synapses but may be released from other cells into the bloodstream to act at different receptors. Norepinephrine neurons in the central nervous system form contacts with close association to postsynaptic cells; chromaffin cells of the adrenal medulla release norepinephrine and epinephrine into the circulation from which they are carried to smooth muscle throughout the body.

The variety of synaptic systems and the many neurotransmitters involved make analysis difficult because of variations in the mechanisms underlying neurotransmitter release. However, as will be shown in this chapter, the principles underlying the mechanisms of release are strikingly similar from one synapse to the next regardless of the neurotransmitter released.

A single neurotransmitter may have different effects at receptors on different neurons, different effects at receptors on the same neuron, and similar effects at different receptors on the same neuron

In the abdominal ganglion of the mollusc *Aplysia californica*, ACh can elicit depolarization of the membranes of certain neurons, leading to increased frequency of action potential firing; in other neurons, the same neurotransmitter causes a hyperpolarization and depression of firing. Sometimes, both postsynaptic effects can be seen at the same neuron. The mechanisms underlying the responses involve a nonspecific increase in conductance to cations, causing membrane depolarization at some postsynaptic sites and an increase in Cl^- conductance, causing hyperpolarization, at others.

A recent review by MacDonald and Nowak (see [4]) points out that in glutamate excitation in vertebrate neurons, more than one receptor type mediates depolarizing responses. It is known that a single transmitter can have different effects at different neurons. It is also known that a single transmitter can activate more than one receptor on a given cell, but in vertebrate central neurons, Ascher and colleagues found three pharma-

cologically distinct receptor types (NMDA, quisqualate, and kainate) that lead to fast excitatory responses in the absence of extracellular Mg^{2+}. The co-existence of different receptor types with apparently similar functions is intriguing, particularly since the putative neurotransmitter L-glutamate activates the NMDA channel and the non-NMDA channels. However, the co-localized NMDA and non-NMDA glutamate-receptor subtypes have functionally distinct but coordinated roles regulated by the divalent cations present. When NMDA receptors are activated in neurons at resting membrane potential, they contribute minimally to postsynaptic excitation because the open NMDA channels are blocked by the rapid entry (and exit) of extracellular Mg^{2+} ions which effectively inhibits influx of Na^+ and Ca^{2+} ions. Sustained, but not transient, activation of non-NMDA receptors located at the same or nearby synapses by the release of L-glutamate during a synaptic volley depolarizes the neurons and significantly decreases the blockage of NMDA channels by Mg^{2+} ions because Mg^{2+} entry is dependent on the electrochemical gradient. With the Mg^{2+} block relieved, the activated NMDA channels permit an entry of Ca^{2+} ions sufficient to stimulate some biochemical processes speculated to underlie synaptic plasticity.

Several criteria must be satisfied before a substance can be defined as a neurotransmitter

The presynaptic neuron should be able to synthesize the substance or its precursor. The putative transmitter must be present in the terminal, usually in association with enzymes required for its synthesis; however, peptides are synthesized in the soma and transported via the axon to the terminal. The content of the terminal may be demonstrated by chemical measurement, histofluorescence, or immunological markers. The terminal should release the transmitter in a pharmacologically identifiable form. This is not to say that every substance released is necessarily a neurotransmitter. For instance, adrenal medullary cells release adenine, ATP, ADP, AMP, and dopamine-β-hydroxylase, together with catecholamines, yet the postsynaptic response is due to norepinephrine.

At the postsynaptic neuron, the putative neurotransmitter should faithfully reproduce the specific events of transmission resulting from stimulating the presynaptic neuron. This includes membrane changes, ionic conductances, and reversal potential. The effects should be seen at concentrations that are similar to those present after release of neurotransmitters by nerve stimulation. The effects of a putative transmitter should be blocked by known competitive antagonists in a dose-dependent manner similar to that seen with neuronal stimulation.

Finally, there should be some mechanism to terminate the action of the substance. This can include an enzyme capable of destroying the transmitter, such as acetylcholinesterase, which hydrolyzes ACh and thus makes it inactive. Catecholamines are either transported into nerve terminals or degraded; amino acids are either taken up into the nerve terminal or into glial cells that surround the synapse (or both); peptides are probably degraded by peptidases.

Acetylcholine was the first neurotransmitter to be identified in the central nervous system

The experimental evidence that led to this conclusion fulfilled the criteria described above. Basic to these studies was a statement by Sir Henry Dale to the effect that when a cholinergic or adrenergic neuron undergoes regeneration, the original transmitter is always restored and is "unchangeable." A corollary of Dale's principle applies to two different endings of the same neuron, one peripheral, the other central. In this case, identification of the peripheral transmitter may yield clues to the identity of the central transmitter. Eccles extended this concept to synapses at neurons in the ventral horn of the spinal cord. Spinal motoneurons of mammals have a main axon that innervates a specific skeletal muscle. This motor axon is known to release ACh at the neuromuscular junction (or end-plate region). There is, however, a motor axon collateral that branches from the main axon back into the spinal cord and projects to interneurons that in turn synapse on the original and other motoneurons. Eccles and his colleagues [5] showed by electrophysiological techniques that the neurotransmitter released from the terminals of the motor axon collateral was ACh. Inspection of Table 1 shows that concentrations of choline acetyltransferase, the enzyme responsible for ACh synthesis, acetylcholinesterase, the enzyme responsible for ACh hydrolysis, and ACh itself are high in the ventral region of the spinal cord. Finally, it was shown that ACh was present in the perfusate at the spinal cord after stimulation of the ventral root. The criteria for neurotransmitter identification have thus been satisfied.

It should be noted, however, that although application of Dale's principle has proved helpful, in certain cases, for neurotransmitter identification, the laws underlying it can no longer be thought of as inviolate. In fact, Dale never suggested that one neuron could only synthesize one neurotransmitter. There is convincing evidence that invertebrate neurons contain more than one neurotransmitter, although there is still no proof that all are released. In addition, there is morphological evidence that in certain mammalian neurons, peptide and nonpeptide neurotransmitters can coexist in the same terminal [6].

A large number of substances that may act as transmitters have been identified in nerve cells

In addition to ACh, the catecholamines dopamine, norepinephrine, and epinephrine have been shown convincingly to be neurotransmitters in the peripheral and central nervous systems. For dopamine, norepinephrine, and the indoleamine 5-hydroxy-

TABLE 1.   Distribution of components of ACh systems in dog tissues[a]

	ACh content (μg/g fresh tissue)	Choline acetylase activity (mg/ACh synthesized/ g wet wt/hr)	Acetylcholinesterase[b]
Sensory cortex	2.8	—	150
Motor cortex	4.5	3	178
Caudate nucleus	2.7	13.3	3936
Thalamus	3	3.1	409
Hypothalamus	1.8	2.0	323
Pons-medulla	—	—	—
Cerebellum	0.18	0.09	1075
Dorsal roots	0.04	<0.02	—
Ventral roots	15	11	149
Sympathetic ganglion	30	—	—

[a] From Paton [7].
[b] Rate of hydrolysis of methacholine, in μl CO_2 evolved/g wet wt/10 min, as an estimate of true cholinesterase activity.

tryptamine (serotonin), identification of neurons containing the transmitter has been facilitated by the development of fluorescent histochemical techniques (see Chaps. 12–14). Other primary amines, such as histamine, octopamine, phenylethylamine, and phenylethanolamine, and polyamines, such as putrecine, spermine, and spermidine, may also be transmitters. A number of amino acids also have well-documented effects on neurons. These include glutamic and aspartic acids, glycine, β-alanine, GABA, taurine, and possibly, proline (Chaps. 17,18). Evaluation of the physiological function of these substances is complicated by their ubiquitous distribution in cells. Other relatively small molecules have at times been suggested as neurotransmitters; these include Ca^{2+}, adenosine, ATP, cyclic AMP, GTP, cyclic GMP, CTP, estrogen, testosterone, corticosterone, and various prostaglandins.

A major development has been the appreciation of the role of small peptides as neurotransmitters

Substance P, an 11-amino acid peptide, was described as an active agent as early as 1931, but only recently has this peptide become widely recognized as an important neurotransmitter. A variety of peptides are present and distributed asymmetrically in nervous tissue. These range in size from carnosine and thyrotropin-releasing hormone (TRH), 2- and 3-amino acid peptides, respectively, to neurotensin and somatostatin, 13- and 14-amino acid peptides, respectively. Other putative peptide neurotransmitters include the enkephalins and endorphins, which may be the brain's natural morphine; agents known to be hormonally active, including insulin, angiotensin I and II, vasoactive intestinal polypeptide, cholecystokinin, prolactin, vasopressin, and oxytocin; and releasing factors, such as luteinizing hormone-releasing hormone (LHRH), melanocyte-stimulating hormone-release-inhibiting hormone, and somatostatin-release-inhibiting hormone. A number of other active peptides have been described in both vertebrates and invertebrates, but less is known about their structures and actions (see Chaps. 15 and 16).

The number of substances that must be considered putative neurotransmitters at present is at least 50 and is growing rapidly; however, rigorous proof of transmitter function has been obtained for only a very few of these substances. The realization that small peptides can be neurotransmitters increases the number of possible active agents, and the difficulties in chemical and physiological identification become enormous.

Fast and slow systems are involved in chemically mediated synaptic transmission

The first system involves fast, short-lived transmission resulting from relatively small molecules that bring about brief conductance changes at the postsynaptic membrane. These so-called classical neurotransmitters are synthesized in the nerve terminal and are classified by their chemical structure, e.g., ACh, catecholamines, indoleamines, and amino acids. A second system that involves neuroactive peptides may coexist in the terminals with the classical neurotransmitters; however, unlike the classical transmitters, they are synthesized in the cell bodies. The peptides can be grouped in families; each family is structurally related and contains long stretches of amino acid sequences that are homologous. Their actions are apparently long-lasting and are modulatory to those of the classical neurotransmitters.

STRUCTURAL, MOLECULAR, AND FUNCTIONAL CORRELATES OF TRANSMISSION

The model for studies on synaptic transmission is usually the amphibian neuromuscular junction

Certain structural features are seen universally at chemical synapses, even where the transmitter is unknown. Critical questions include: First, how does the structure of the presynaptic terminal correlate with its known function? Second, can the morphology provide clues to understanding the mechanisms of transmitter release? Several techniques have been used to study the morphology of the synapse. These include the use of transmission electron microscopy and freeze-fracture techniques. Specific receptors for neurotransmitters or peptides, especially at postsynaptic membranes, have been identified by immunocytochemical techniques that have proved to be particularly useful in the central nervous system.

The presynaptic terminal displays specific structural characteristics

Figure 1 shows an electron micrograph of longitudinal (Fig. 1A) and transverse (Fig. 1B) sections through a nerve terminal on frog sartorius muscle in the absence of nerve stimulation. The presynaptic terminal displays four characteristic features:

1. Synaptic vesicles, usually about 20 to 60 nm in diameter. At the neuromuscular junction they are spherical; in the central nervous system, they can also be ellipsoid or flattened in shape. A motor nerve terminal at a frog neuromuscular junction contains about 500,000 vesicles, and each vesicle is believed to contain a quantum of neurotransmitter that is released by exocytosis. The concept that each quantum of transmitter is contained in a vesicle is known as the vesicular hypothesis. Those vesicles that contain peptide neurotransmitters are synthesized in the rough endoplasmic reticulum of the cell body and transported to the nerve terminal in the axon after incorporation into the vesicle. On the other hand, vesicles such as those at the neuromuscular junction can certainly be filled with neurotransmitter at the terminal, but it is not known how the vesicles themselves reach the terminal.
2. Mitochondria that are usually located at some distance away from the synaptic surface.
3. Intramembranous specializations, including an endoplasmic reticulum.
4. Presynaptic densities.

Transmitter release is quantal at chemically mediated synapses

The vesicle, in which the neurotransmitter can be packaged, provides a structural choice for the quantal nature of the release; release itself is accomplished by means of exocytosis, whereby the vesicle membrane fuses

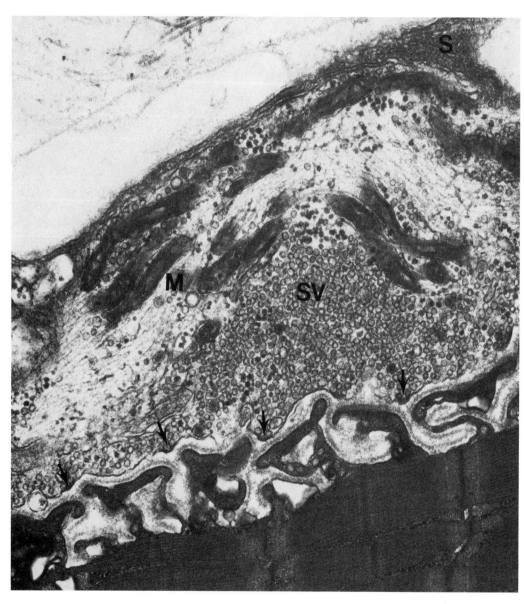

A

FIG. 1.   End-plate region of *Rana pipiens* sartorius muscle fiber **A:** Longitudinal thin section through a nerve terminal. *Arrows* denote active zones. Also shown are synaptic vesicles (SV), mitochondria (M), and Schwann cells (S). The postsynaptic component is represented by the thicker membrane at the top of the folds in the muscle surface (×30,400).

with the terminal membrane. Is there proof that this process actually occurs? Electron microscopy has been used to show the morphological events in real time by quick-freezing the synapse within a few milliseconds of eliciting release, so that the number of quanta released at a frog nerve muscle synapse could be compared to the number of exocytotic events that result from a single nerve stimulation. Over a wide range of transmitter release, augmented by K⁺-blocking agents such as 4-aminopyridine, one quantum accompanies one exocytotic event (Fig. 2) [8].

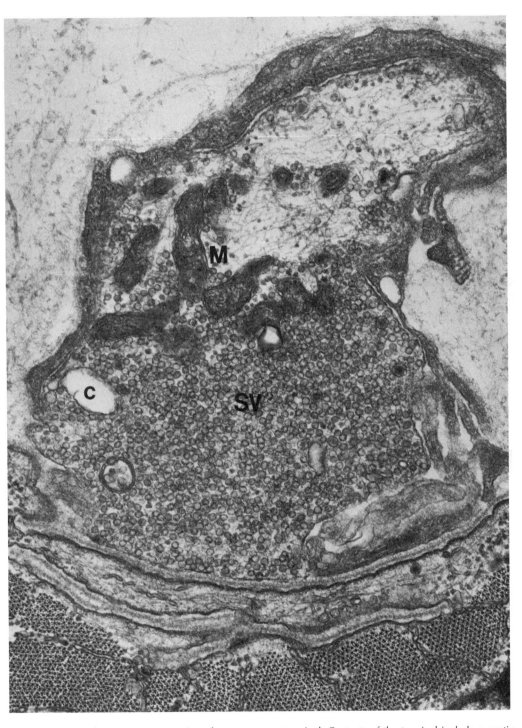

FIG. 1.   *(continued)*. **B:** Transverse section of a motor nerve terminal. Contents of the terminal include synaptic vesicles (SV), mitochondria (M), and cistern (C) (×36,800). (Courtesy of A. Stieber, N. D. Gonatas, and S. D. Erulkar.)

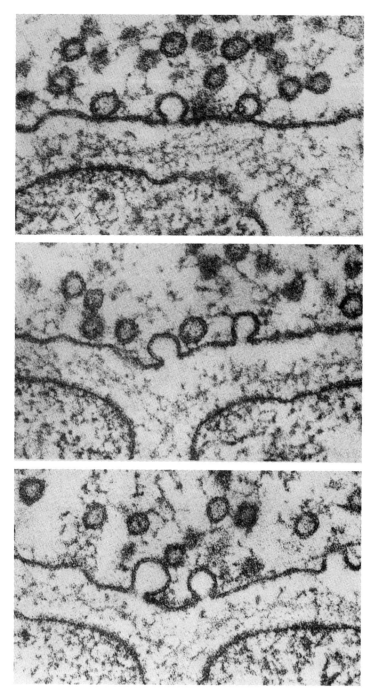

FIG. 2.   Three separate high-magnification (×145,000) views of freeze-substituted neuromuscular junctions in a muscle frozen during the abnormally large burst of ACh release that is provoked by a single nerve stimulus in 2 mM 4-aminopyridine, in this case delivered 5.1 msec before the muscle was frozen. These sections were cut unusually thin (~200 Å) to show the fine structure of the presynaptic membrane, which displayed many examples of synaptic vesicles apparently caught in the act of exocytosis. In all cases, these open vesicles were found just above the mouths of the postsynaptic folds, hence at the site of the presynaptic active zones. (From Heuser [8].)

Freeze-fracture technique permits visualization of synaptic vesicle openings during exocytosis

It is difficult to visualize exocytosis directly in conventional electron micrographs. This is in part because the exocytotic opening is usually smaller than the thickness of typical sections. The freeze-fracture technique is more suitable for this purpose because when tissue is fixed, frozen, and broken open, the fracture tends to split membranes and therefore to follow their hydrophobic interiors. While still frozen, this fractured surface can be replicated with platinum and examined with a resolution of 2 nm, which is high enough to see where intrinsic membrane proteins cross the lipid bilayer (Fig. 3) [9]. With this technique, it was possible to see the stomata of synaptic vesicles in the act of exocytosis during quantal release either during nerve stimulation or after application of a toxin such as black or brown widow spider venom. Furthermore, any agent that blocks release also blocks exocytosis. The process of exocytosis does not depend on action potentials in the nerve because it can be elicited by neurotoxins such as spider venom acting directly on the terminal.

Synaptic vesicles cluster over regions where neighboring membranes of two neurons appear thickened

Under transmission electron microscopy, it appears that these areas may represent sites of vesicle discharge, and they were named "synaptic complexes." Indeed, much evidence has accumulated to support the idea that these synaptic complexes adhere to each other. Even when the neurons are disrupted, thickened portions of the postsynaptic membranes cling to the presynaptic densities of the synaptosomes and can be separated only by strong proteolytic agents.

Couteaux and Pecot-Dechavassine [10] suggested in 1970 that a nerve has "active zones" for transmitter release, and evidence from freeze-fracture suggests that exocytosis is limited to these active zones of the synaptic membrane surface. However, it is known that the majority of individual active zones fail to release a quantum of neurotransmitter after a nerve impulse. There are approximately 500 active zones per nerve terminal at the frog nerve-muscle synapse, yet less than 250 quanta are released by action potentials after nerve stimulation.

The morphology of active zones suggests important questions for further investigation. Large (90 Å) intramembrane particles are present near the active zone, and consideration of their universal deployment and numbers at presynaptic active zones leads to the suggestion that they are the channels that admit Ca^{2+} to initiate transmitter release [11]. The cytoplasm of nerve terminals near active zones always contains a fuzzy material that makes contact with the releasable vesicles at the active zone. It is important to know the role of this material in inserting a new vesicle back into the active zone after it undergoes exocytosis, or for initiating the membrane interactions that lead to exocytosis. The active zones have a network of actin filaments that are linked with vesicles by a phosphoprotein called synapsin (see later, p. 200). It appears (see [11] for review) that the "tail of synapsin binds vesicles, whereas the globular head group binds actin or the head of another synapsin molecule, cross-linking the vesicles." The role of the synapsins in transmitter release is described later (p. 201). Finally, it remains to be determined whether all chemical synaptic transmission occurs at active zones [11].

Synaptic vesicles associated with presynaptic densities are in a favorable position to be discharged, and they contain an immediately available pool of transmitter

Prolonged stimulation would be expected to cause depletion of vesicles from the terminal. Experiments to show this have been frustrating, and some investigators have shown that the number of vesicles near the presyn-

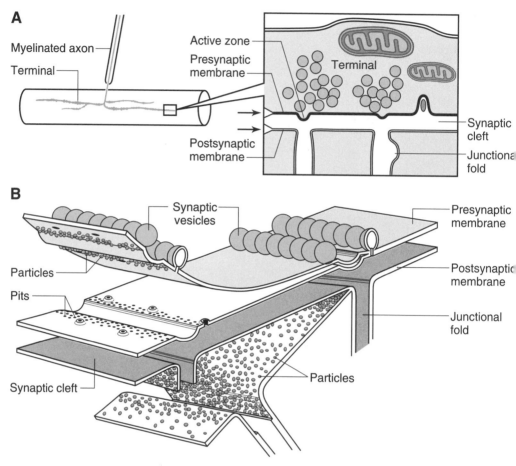

FIG. 3. Synaptic membrane structure. **A:** Entire frog neuromuscular junction *(left)* and longitudinal section through a portion of the nerve terminal *(right)*. *Arrows* indicate planes of cleavage during freeze-fracture. **B:** Three-dimensional view of presynaptic and postsynaptic membranes with active zones and immediately adjacent rows of synaptic vesicles. Plasma membranes are split along planes indicated by the *arrows* in **A** to illustrate structures observed on freeze-fracturing. The cytoplasmic half of the presynaptic membrane at the active zone shows on its fracture face protruding particles whose counterparts are seen as pits on the fracture face of the outer membrane leaflet. Vesicles that fuse with the presynaptic membrane give rise to characteristic protrusions and pores in the fracture faces. The fractured postsynaptic membrane in the region of the folds shows a high concentration of particles on the fracture face of the cytoplasmic leaflet; these are probably ACh receptors. (Courtesy of U. J. McMahan; from Nicholls et al. [9].)

aptic densities actually increases after a few minutes of nerve stimulation. In fact, although vesicles are in some way altered in number after repetitive nerve stimulation, they are not readily depleted. Stimulation of the frog neuromuscular junction can cause the release of millions of quanta with no resultant depletion of vesicles.

It appears that the vesicle membrane is somehow conserved during repetitive stimulation. The most detailed study on this topic was that of Heuser and Reese [12], who showed that during brief tetanic stimulation of frog motor nerve, horseradish peroxidase (HRP), which had been added to the extracellular space previously, appeared in the nerve terminal in coated vesicles and cisternae that became more evident with stimula-

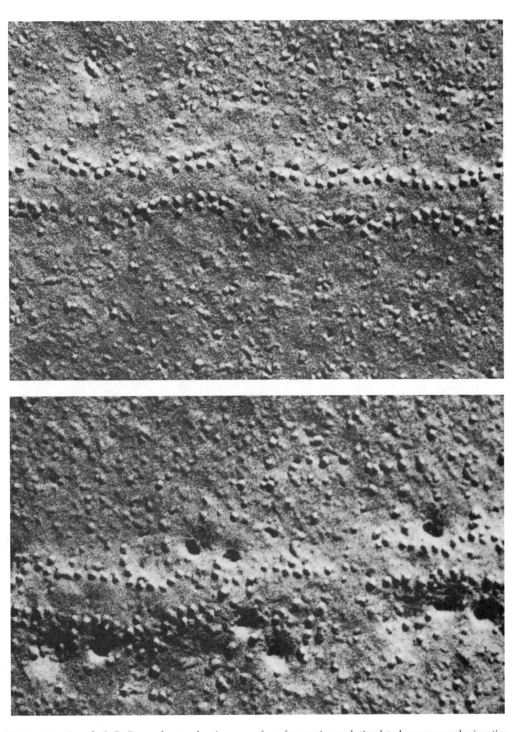

FIG. 3.   *(continued)*. **C, D:** Freeze-fractured active zones from frog resting and stimulated neuromuscular junction. The active zone is the region of presynaptic membrane surrounding double rows of intramembrane particles, which may be channels for Ca^{2+} entry that initiates transmitter release. Holes that appear in active zones during transmitter release *(lower picture)* are openings of synaptic vesicles engaged in exocytosis. This muscle was prepared by quick-freezing, and transmitter release was augmented with 4-aminopyridine, so that the morphological events (opening of synaptic vesicles) could be examined at the exact moment of transmitter release evoked by a single nerve shock. (×120,000.) (From Heuser and Reese [11], with permission.)

A   **B**

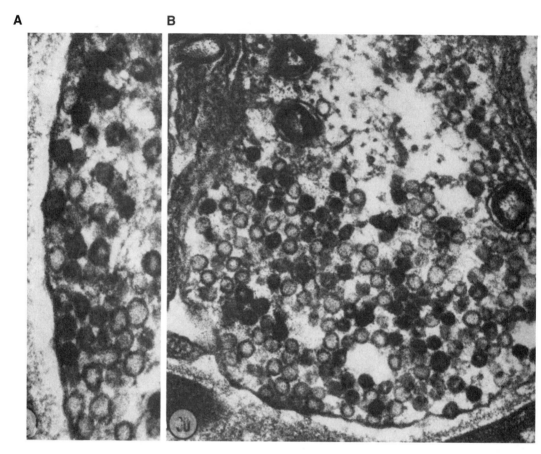

FIG. 4. Cross sections through normal regions of loaded terminals. Nearly 50% of the vesicles contain HRP, which corresponds to the number that should have been depleted by the stimulation and reformed from HRP-containing cisternae. **B:** The HRP-containing vesicles appear to be distributed randomly within the nerve terminal, including the area near the presynaptic surface, shown in more detail in **A** to illustrate that HRP-containing vesicles in contact with the plasma membrane do not discharge HRP, even though the tracer has been washed out of the synaptic cleft. (A, ×72,250; B, ×28,050.) (From Heuser and Reese [12], with permission.)

tion. When stimulation was stopped, the cisternae resolved, and HRP was then seen in vesicles (Fig. 4). The authors suggested that after fusion with the terminal membrane, synaptic vesicle membrane is retrieved by coated vesicles and cisternae and then recycled as new synaptic vesicles (Fig. 5). Whether this is the exclusive pathway for retrieval of vesicle membrane is still uncertain. Heuser and Reese themselves caution that HRP only marks the "fluid" phase, not the "adsorptive," or membrane, phase, so they have no direct proof that synaptic vesicle membrane is being recycled. More recent studies with the use of membrane markers, however, have shown that membranes from the terminal are incorporated in the formation of new synaptic vesicles (Fig. 6).

Stieber et al. [13] modified the experiment of Heuser and Reese [12] by examining, in double-labeling experiments, fluid and absorptive endocytosis with free HRP and wheat germ agglutinin (WGA) coupled to ferritin (WGA-ferritin), respectively (Fig. 6).

Immediately after nerve stimulation, both markers were taken up into cisternae and in tubular structures similar to the com-

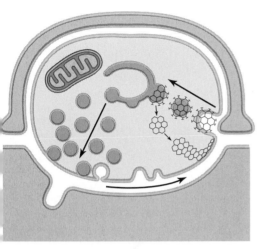

IG. 5. Synaptic vesicle recycling at the frog neuromus-
:ular junction. Diagram of cross-section of motor nerve
erminal, enclosed by Schwann sheath and by postsynap-
ic receptor membrane on striated muscle. A trough in
he postsynaptic membrane lies opposite an active zone
n the presynaptic terminal. Following an electrical shock
o the motor nerve, the synaptic vesicle membrane is
ncorporated into the terminal membrane and translo-
:ated as shown by the *arrows.* It is reincorporated by
ndocytosis into the terminal and transferred to the cister-
ae covered with a protein coat. At the cisternae, the
rotein coat is shed and a new "recycled" vesicle is
ormed. (Modified from Heuser and Reese [12] with per-
nission.)

artment for uncoupling of receptor from
igand (CURL). This early double-labeling
vas followed by the appearance of synaptic
esicles labeled with WGA-ferritin only
72–79 percent), HRP only (6–11 percent),
nd both labels (13–16 percent). The major-
ty of cisternae and putative CURL had both
abels throughout the duration of the experi-
nents (77–80 percent). Thus, two different
opulations of synaptic vesicles pinch off
rom the double-labeled cisternae, namely
hose enriched in "receptors" to WGA and
hose poor in receptors to WGA containing
nly HRP. The WGA-ferritin and HRP were
:o-localized in compartments involved in en-
locytosis and surface receptor recycling.
Furthermore, in the nerve terminal there
nay be a compartment involved in the recy-
:ling of surface receptors; certainly, the req-

uisite organelles for receptor recycling are
available.

Postsynaptic active zones are observed where synaptic terminals make contact with nerves or muscles

The position, but not necessarily the size, of
the postsynaptic active zone matches that of
the presynaptic active zone. The internal
membrane structure of the postsynaptic active zones varies with the type of transmitter
used. At most types of postsynaptic active
zones, intramembrane particles are more
concentrated than over the rest of the membrane. The concentration of intramembrane
particles varies up to $10,000/\mu m^2$ in cholinergic systems (a 100-fold increase over that
on the remaining membrane) (Fig. 7) and
down to aggregates barely discernible from
those in the rest of the membrane at certain
central nervous system synapses. The organization within the aggregate can also vary
from linear arrays to dispersed types of spacing, where distances between particles are
relatively constant.

For cholinergic nerve-muscle synapses,
there is good evidence that the intramembrane particles at the postsynaptic active
zones are the sites of ion channel-receptor
complexes. The heads of these particles protrude beyond the outer surface of the postsynaptic active zone into the synaptic cleft. The
synaptic cleft contains a basement membrane, or a similar, fuzzy material, concentrated in the center of the cleft at nerve-nerve
synapses, and side-arms periodically arise
from the central skein of cleft material to
make contact with the surface of the postsynaptic active zone. At nerve-muscle synapses,
the cytoplasmic side of this membrane is also
thickened by a coat of fuzzy material, 5 to 10
nm wide, and similar coats of material seem
to be a general feature of postsynaptic active
zones, regardless of the chemical nature of
the synapse.

The active zones of different types of
chemical synapses vary mainly in the concentration, size, and fracturing characteristics of

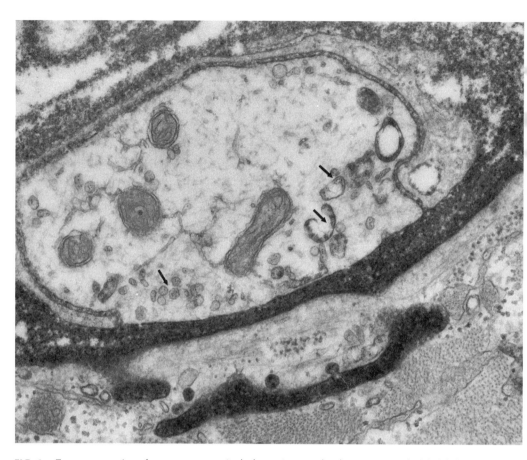

FIG. 6.   Transverse section of motor nerve terminal of sartorius muscle of *Rana pipiens* double-labeled with wheat germ-ferritin and free HRP. The protocol for this experiment was as follows: The frog, *Rana pipiens,* was anesthetized with tricaine methanesulfonate and the sartorius muscle exposed. Wheat germ-ferritin was then injected at many areas in the muscle, the skin sewn together, and the animal allowed to revive over a 2-hr period. It was then decapitated and a conventional nerve-muscle preparation of the sartorius made. The nerve-muscle preparation was then allowed to soak in HRP, D-tubocurarine, and Ringer's solution for 30 min, at the end of which the nerve was stimulated at 10 Hz for 15 min. When the stimulation was stopped, the muscle was left in the solution for a period of 30 min. It was then fixed in glutaraldehyde and prepared for electron microscopy. (×50,250.) (Courtesy of A. Stieber, N. D. Gonatas, and S. D. Erulkar.)

the intramembrane components and in the extent to which this and perhaps additional components extend into the cytoplasm. The postsynaptic active zone, therefore, is a membrane complex that involves both the cytoplasmic and external surfaces of the postsynaptic membrane. Its edges are very sharp, and the sharpness persists even at the edges of large postsynaptic active zones, where groups containing several hundred receptors separate into patches. These membrane

complexes are more stable than the rest of the membrane. Turnover of cholinergic receptors in the active zone has a time course of days, and active zones in general maintain their organization in the face of metabolic or mechanical damage that alters the rest of the surface membrane.

Two major integral proteins are known to be enriched at the postsynaptic membrane: the acetylcholine receptor (AChR), which is concentrated about 1,000-fold com-

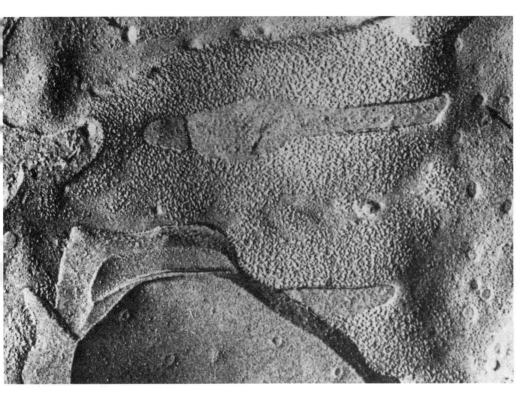

FIG. 7. In this freeze-fracture view the nerve terminal *(bottom)* has been ripped away, exposing the surface of muscle under it. The postsynaptic active zones clearly differ from the rest of the muscle membrane, which is marked by the caveolae characteristic of muscle cells *(arrow)*. More important are the numerous intramembrane particles at the active zones on the tops of the folds; these are thought to be ACh receptors. The vesicle openings on the outer leaflet of the nerve terminal *(bottom)* are formation sites of coated pits. These occur following transmitter release, but outside the active zones. (×75,000.) (From Heuser and Reese [11], with permission.)

pared to the extrajunctional membrane; and the voltage-activated sodium channel, which is concentrated about 20-fold at the receptor. Other proteins, including acetylcholinesterase, laminin, a heparin sulfate proteoglycan, and a cytoskeletal 43-kDa protein, have also been found (see [14]).

In terms of development, at the time of initial neurite-myotube contact, AChR clusters form on the myotubes, indicating that synaptogenesis is occurring. This suggested that some factor may be involved that induces these clusters. The best-known factor is a protein (or proteins) named agrin, which induces AChR clusters on myotubes and may also be involved in synaptogenesis throughout the nervous system [15].

THE NEUROMUSCULAR JUNCTION

The end-plate region also has been used to provide information on the nature of synaptic transmission with respect to its associated electrical activity

While the neuromuscular junction has the advantage of being a single synapse at which the neurotransmitter is known to be acetylcholine, it has the disadvantage that a microelectrode cannot penetrate the presynaptic terminal without causing damage.

Microelectrode recordings are used in two ways:

1. Intracellular recording, in which the electrode penetrates the muscle mem-

brane close to the end-plate region and records a transmembrane potential between the interior of the muscle and the outside.

2. Focal recording, in which the microelectrode records extracellularly from the surface of the muscle fiber. In this situation, the electrode records potentials from sites of the muscle membrane of approximately only 5 μm^2 compared to 500 μm^2 with intracellular recording. Furthermore, focal recording also allows the potential from the presynaptic nerve terminal to be recorded; while this is not as satisfactory as an electrode placed within the terminal, it does provide an indication of the time of the peak of the presynaptic current.

In the absence of motor nerve stimulation, intracellular recording at the end plate has revealed the presence of small subthreshold depolarizing potentials that appear to occur randomly

In 1952, Fatt and Katz [16] hypothesized that these events represented the release of packages or "quanta" of ACh from the nerve terminal. An interesting aspect of these potentials was their similarity in configuration, except for their amplitudes, to the end-plate potential (EPP) that is elicited when the motor nerve is stimulated. In view of the fact that the "miniature" end-plate potentials (MEPPs), as they were called, appeared to represent the basic unit of transmitter release, it was suggested that release was quantal and that the EPP itself reflected the release of many quanta of ACh. In fact, the rate of secretion of quanta is increased by the nerve impulse. Indeed, if the external Ca^{2+} concentration is reduced (see below), the evoked EPP becomes extremely small and its amplitude can become the same as those of the MEPPs. When the nerve terminal membrane is depolarized, the rate of spontaneous MEPPs is increased, provided that Ca^{2+} is present in the external medium. The amplitude of each MEPP is unchanged.

Similar events have been shown to occur a synapses of central neurons.

A histogram relating the amplitude o the MEPP with its frequency of occurrence can be constructed that shows that the MEPP amplitudes fall into peaks that are multiples of the mean MEPP amplitude. This experiment requires reduction of the external Ca^2 concentration and an increase in the concentration of Mg^{2+} (Fig. 8) [17]. This resul allowed the formulation of a statistical mode of the release process such that if there are n available release sites on nerve terminal and each has a probability p of releasing a quantum, then $m = np$, which is the mean number of quanta released per nerve im pulse, called *quantal content*.

Since this concept was first proposed a large literature has appeared concerning the interpretation of both n and p and the conditions under which they are valid. In particular, if n varies with time or p varies at different sites, these parameters will no longer be valid. Nevertheless, it is possible with these parameters under certain conditions to define the probability of x quanta being released by an impulse p_x. The probability will follow a binomial distribution such that

$$P_x = \frac{n_x}{N} = \frac{n!}{x!\,(n-x)!}\, p^x q^{(n-x)} \qquad (1)$$

where n_x is the number of trials in which x quanta are released; N is the total number of trials; p is the probability of release of a single quantum; and q is the probability that a quantum will not be released, $(1 - p)$. When p becomes small (<0.05) and n becomes large ($n > 100$), the Poisson distribution applies:

$$f(x) = \frac{n_x}{N} = \frac{e^{-m} m^x}{x!} \qquad (2)$$

This means that each event is not influenced by its previous history. Quantal content can also be measured by

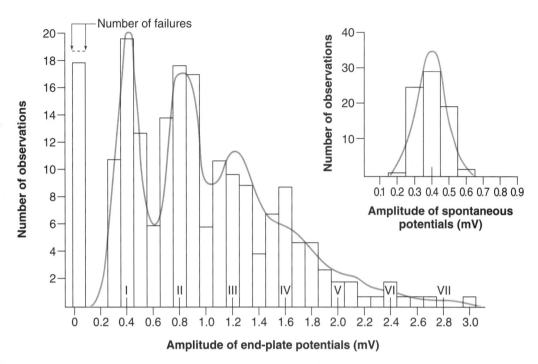

FIG. 8.   The distribution of amplitudes of evoked EPPs and of spontaneous MEPPs (**inset**), from a mammalian end-plate blocked with high concentrations of Mg^{2+}. Peaks of the EPP amplitude histogram occur at one, two, three, and four times the mean amplitude of the spontaneous potentials. A Gaussian curve is fitted to the latter and used to calculate the theoretical distribution of EPP amplitudes *(continuous curve); arrows* indicate expected number of failures. (From Boyd and Martin [17].)

$$m = \frac{\text{mean amplitude of EPP}}{\text{mean amplitude of MEPPs}} \quad (3)$$

or by the number of failures of transmission (n_0) that occur in N trials. If a Poisson distribution is followed, then

$$n_0/N = e^{-m} \quad \text{and} \quad m = \ln(N/n_0) \quad (4)$$

Calcium ions are necessary for transmission at synaptic junctions

In the nervous system, at the perfused superior cervical ganglion, when Ca^{2+} is withdrawn from the perfusing medium, there is no release of ACh from the preganglionic endings, either during stimulation of the sympathetic trunk or following the addition of K^+ to the external medium, thus causing

depolarization of the membrane. Katz and Miledi [18] provided the ultimate proof of the role of Ca^{2+} in transmitter release in an elegant series of experiments with the use of a Ca^{2+} pipette. They used a frog sartorius neuromuscular junction preparation and perfused it with a medium deficient in Ca^{2+} but with Mg^{2+} present. Stimulation of the motor nerve failed to elicit EPPs even though an action potential was conducted to the nerve terminal (Fig. 9A and D). When they used an electrode filled with 0.5 M $CaCl_2$, however, a small voltage applied to it either caused or prevented the release of Ca^{2+} from the pipette, depending on the polarity of the voltage. Release of Ca^{2+} before the stimulus caused an EPP to be elicited (Fig. 9B and C); after the stimulus, no EPP was elicited. What is clear is that for transmitter release to take place, Ca^{2+} must be present externally at the

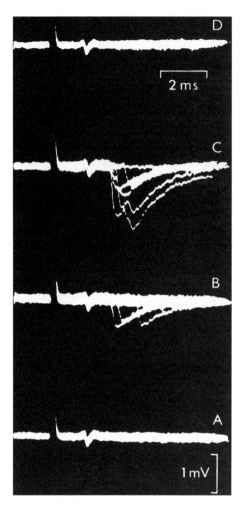

FIG. 9. The use of a Ca^{2+} pipette in exploring neuromuscular transmission. The frog sartorius muscle was immersed in Ca^{2+}-free solution containing 0.84 mM Mg^{2+}. A pipette filled with 0.5 M $CaCl_2$ was used to record focal external potentials from a junctional spot. Efflux of Ca^{2+} was controlled electrophoretically. In the four records, A–D, Ca^{2+} efflux was stopped initially by applying sufficient negative voltage to the pipette; the bias was then reduced in two steps, and finally reapplied. Several superimposed traces are shown at each stage. (From Katz and Miledi [18], with permission.)

terminal when the depolarization, in the form of the nerve impulse, arrives at the terminal.

At low external concentrations of Ca^{2+}, cooperativity is involved in neurotransmitter release. Either four Ca^{2+} are necessary for the release of one quantum or four Ca^{2+} sites have to be occupied for the release of one quantum of neurotransmitter. The value of four is not constant, and the observed value differs according to the site of the synapse.

The Ca^{2+} hypothesis thus suggested that with depolarization of the nerve terminal, Ca^{2+} attached to defined sites and entered the terminal, where by some unknown process it caused the release of neurotransmitter. There was, however, no direct proof of Ca^{2+} entry until Llinás and his colleagues [19] showed, by means of the luminescent dye aequorin, that at the squid giant synapse, Ca^{2+} entered the terminal during presynaptic depolarization. In the presence of tetraethylammonium (TEA), to block K^+ currents, and tetrodotoxin (TTX), to block Na^+ currents, an inwardly directed Ca^{2+} current could be recorded presynaptically in response to the depolarization. If the excitatory postsynaptic potential (EPSP) was recorded simultaneously, a delay of several milliseconds was obtained. On repolarization, the delay for the Ca^{2+} current was less than 0.2 msec. This shows that much of the time associated with the synaptic delay is due to the activation of Ca^{2+} conductance [19].

The so-called N-type Ca^{2+} channel that is irreversibly blocked by ω-conotoxin is responsible for voltage-activated release of neurotransmitters at the terminals of some neurons. This Ca^{2+} channel is dihydropyridine-insensitive and aligns precisely with active zones where vesicular exocytosis of neurotransmitters occurs. At the neuromuscular junction, ω-conotoxin blocks currents recorded from presynaptic terminals.

Calcium, once it enters a terminal, has numerous effects, including activation of protein kinases

Greengard and his colleagues [20] reported on the isolation of a protein, synapsin I, that acts as a substrate for cyclic AMP (cAMP)-dependent protein kinase, Ca^{2+}-calmodulin-dependent protein kinase, and protein kinase C in the brain (see Chap. 22). It is nteresting that synapsin I was found to be phosphorylated when nerve terminals were depolarized. There occurs an "actin-bunding" activity associated with synapsin I, such hat the activity only occurs with the dephosphorylated form of synapsin I. On phosphorylation, the bundling activity disappears and he significance of this bundling activity lies in the possibility that synapsin I may be involved in a mechanism whereby synaptic vesicles are held in a protein complex in the terminal with dephosphorylated synapsin I and not allowed to coalesce with the terminal membrane. Once depolarization occurs, phosphorylation takes place and the vesicles are freed to enable them to fuse with the terminal membrane, allowing exocytosis and neurotransmitter release to occur. Indeed, Llinás and his collaborators [20] have shown hat dephosphorylated synapsin I could block synaptic transmission when injected nto squid synapse preterminals. This occurred even when Ca^{2+} influx was unaffected. It appears that with depolarization, Ca^{2+} enters the terminal and activates a protein kinase that phosphorylates synapsin I, which allows the debundling of actin, which in turn allows synaptic vesicles to fuse with the terminal membrane. The fusion itself probably results through the action of another protein that can promote membrane-membrane fusion, and it may be that once the vesicle is freed, Ca^{2+} in the cytoplasm activates the protein, resulting in vesicular fusion and exocytosis. Calcium/calmodulin-dependent protein kinase II (CAM kinase II) injected presynaptically facilitated neurotransmitter release. The extent of the facilitation was related to the level along the presynaptic terminal penetrated by the CAM kinase II.

Thus the evidence suggests that in addition to releasing neurotransmitter, Ca^{2+} penetrates the presynaptic cytosol and activates CAM kinase II. This event, in turn, phosphorylates synapsin I, which reduces its binding to vesicles and/or cytoskeletal structures, allowing more vesicles to be released during a presynaptic depolarization.

The delay between the influx of Ca^{2+} into the presynaptic terminal and the postsynaptic response to the neurotransmitter consists of the initiation of release, diffusion of the transmitter across the cleft, and the response time of the postsynaptic receptor. The total time for this process is extremely small, yet it is clear that several reactions must take place at the terminal before release occurs. The rate constants of the reactions described must be extremely high, or the sites of Ca^{2+} entry must be very close to the location of the protein kinase that it activates, or both.

Finally, transmitter release can be elicited by some divalent cations other than Ca^{2+}; these include Sr^{2+} and Ba^{2+}. The release mechanism is most sensitive to Ca^{2+}, followed by Sr^{2+} and then Ba^{2+}, suggesting a higher affinity of Ca^{2+} for binding to the appropriate protein at the terminal.

EFFECTS OF TRANSMITTERS ON POSTSYNAPTIC NEURONAL EXCITABILITY

Neurotransmitters can alter the excitability of a postsynaptic cell by changing membrane potential and resistance

Although many common synaptic responses result in a change of both potential and resistance, this is not always the case. Furthermore, the effects of changing potential may either add to or oppose the effects of changing resistance.

In a typical electrically excitable neuron that has an axon projecting to some distant point, there is an integration of synaptic inputs from dendrites and soma at the axon hillock. If threshold depolarization is reached at this site, an action potential is initiated that will ultimately trigger transmitter release at the axon terminals. The level of depolarization that must be reached at the axon hillock for spike initiation is relatively constant, and thus the effect of membrane potential at the hillock is simple, in that depolarization brings the neuron closer to firing threshold, whereas hyperpolarization takes the neuron further from threshold.

Binding of a transmitter to a specific receptor causes a change in the transmembrane permeability to one or more ions

The effect on potential depends on which ionic permeabilities are changed. Because the ions in a tissue are not present in equal concentration on both sides of the cell membrane, there is a driving force, determined by the concentration gradient, for each ionic species (see Chap. 4). The asymmetrical ionic concentrations are maintained by the relative membrane impermeability to some ions and the activity of the Na^+-K^+ pump (see Chap. 3). By the Nernst equation (see Chap. 4), we can define an equilibrium potential (E) for any ion. The equilibrium potential is the one at which the electrical gradient is exactly equal to the chemical concentration gradient for that ion.

Figure 10 shows in diagrammatic form the equilibrium potentials for the major ionic species involved in determining potential shifts in neurons. To a first approximation, resting membrane potential (RMP) can be described by the Goldman-Hodgkin-Katz equation, which considers the contribution of Na^+, K^+, and Cl^- (see Chap. 4). Since the interior of cells is high in K^+ and low in Na^+ and Cl^-, RMP is determined by the balance of the electrical and chemical driving forces on all of these ions. Under resting conditions, K^+ permeability predominates and RMP is relatively near to E_{K^+}. The degree to which RMP deviates from E_{K^+} reflects active transport and the relative permeabilities to and the concentration gradients of the other ions. Ca^{2+} is not in electrochemical equilibrium, but its resting permeability is low enough so that the Ca^{2+} gradient does not contribute significantly to RMP.

Increased permeability to any ion can easily be detected by measuring transmembrane resistance. Permeability has an inverse relation to resistance, so the resistance falls during a response associated with an increased permeability to any ion. Resistance is usually measured by passing small pulses of current across the membrane and measuring the resulting voltage deflection. If the current is kept constant, the voltage produced will reflect changes in resistance according to Ohm's law.

When a neurotransmitter increases permeability to a single ion, the membrane potential will move in the direction of the equilibrium potential for that ion

If a neurotransmitter causes a specific decrease in the permeability to one ionic species, the membrane potential will move away from the equilibrium potential for that ion and toward that of the ion with the dominant permeability. Acetylcholine and glutamate regulate receptors that open ion channels allowing cations to flow through nonspecifically so that the equilibrium potentials will, under the right conditions, be at 0 mV. GABA and glycine increase Cl^- conductances, so that neuronal membranes become hyperpolarized as they strive to achieve the Cl^- equilibrium potential. The voltage-activated conductances for Na^{2+} (I_{Na}) and Ca^2 (I_{Ca}), which carry inward currents that depo

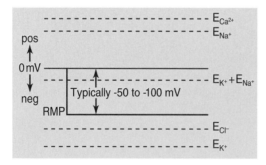

FIG. 10.   Typical ionic equilibrium potentials in excitable tissues. The resting membrane potential (RMP) is usually between -50 and -100 mV. The equilibrium potentials (E) for various ions are indicated. At the equilibrium potential, the electrical gradient for that ion is exactly equal to the concentration gradient, so that as many ions enter as leave the cell.

TABLE 2.   Transmitter-regulated ion channels in the vertebrate central nervous system[a]

Conductance	Transmitter	Receptor	Change	Cell effect
K$^+$ conductances				
I_A	Norepinephrine	α_1	Closes	Speeds
	Acetylcholine	M	Closes	Speeds
I_{AHP}	Acetylcholine	M_1	Reduces	Prolongs excitability
	Norepinephrine	β	Reduces	Decreases accommodation
	Norepinephrine	α_1	Reduces	Prolongs bursts
	Corticotropin-releasing factor		Reduces	Decreases accommodation
	Glutamate	KA	Reduces	Increases excitability
	Histamine	H_2	Reduces	Increases excitability
	Serotonin	1A	Reduces	Decreases accommodation
	Adenosine		Increases	Increases accommodation
	Bradykinin		Increases	Hyperpolarizes
I_{IR}	Glutamate	KA	Closes	Depolarizes
	Substance P		Closes	Depolarizes
	Dopamine	D2	Closes	Depolarizes
	Adenosine		Opens	Hyperpolarizes
	Norepinephrine	α_2?	Opens	Hyperpolarizes
	Opioids	μ, δ	Opens	Hyperpolarizes
	Dopamine	D1	Opens	Hyperpolarizes
	5-Hydroxytryptamine	1A	Opens	Hyperpolarizes
	GABA	B	Opens	Hyperpolarizes
I_M	Acetylcholine	M_1	Closes	Depolarizes
	Serotonin	1A	Closes	Depolarizes
	Substance P		Closes	Depolarizes
	Bradykinin		Closes	Depolarizes
	Somatostatin		Opens	Hyperpolarizes
Ca^{2+} conductances	Opioids	κ	Closes	Shortens action potential
	Opioids	$?\delta$	Closes	Shortens action potential
	GABA	B	Closes	Shortens action potential
	Norepinephrine	$?\alpha_1$	Closes	Shortens action potential
	Dopamine		Closes	Shortens action potential
	Acetylcholine	M	Closes	Shortens action potential

(I_A) Fast, transient, rapidly inactivating outward current; (I_{AHP}) Ca^{2+}-activated outward K$^+$ current responsible for hyperpolarization that follows a burst of action potentials; (I_{IR}) inward rectifier current whose K$^+$ channel conductance decreases with membrane depolarization and increases with membrane hyperpolarization; (I_M) current due to K$^+$ channels that are closed by ACh through its muscarinic receptor.
[a] This table offers a beginning formulation of transmitter-regulated ionic conductances based on recent articles and on the emerging criteria for characterizing specific forms of ion- and voltage-regulated channels and for assessing the specific receptor subtypes involved. Because most reports before 1985 could not utilize the full range of evaluative procedures now available, it is likely that these initial designations will require modification. (From Bloom [3].)

larize the membrane, do not appear to be affected by neurotransmitters. On the other hand, K$^+$ and some Ca^{2+} conductances are regulated by some transmitters. Table 2 lists the established transmitter-regulated ion channels in the vertebrate central nervous system. The best studied responses are the result of increased permeabilities to one or two ionic species.

Because E_{K^+} is more negative than RMP, an increase in K$^+$ permeability will hyperpolarize the cell whereas an increase in Na$^+$ permeability will depolarize the cell. In most neurons E_{Cl^-} is more negative than RMP, and, consequently, most specific Cl$^-$ permeability increases are hyperpolarizing. In some neurons, such as dorsal root ganglion cells, however, E_{Cl^-} is less negative than RMP, and an increase in Cl$^-$ permeability results in depolarization. At the vertebrate neuromuscular junction, and perhaps at most receptors mediating fast excitation in vertebrates, the transmitter acts to open a channel that allows nonspecific movement of cations. This is a different channel from those specific for cations such as Na^+ and K^+, which are turned on sequentially to generate and repolarize action potentials. In invertebrates, several transmitters have been found that activate a slower pharmacologically distinguishable increase in permeability to Na^+ and Ca^{2+}. Because Ca^{2+} has so many regulatory influences on a variety of neuronal functions, transmitter control of permeability to Ca^{2+} may have significant influences beyond the immediate voltage changes (see Chaps. 17 and 22).

Some responses to neurotransmitters are not associated with a decrease in resistance

These responses may be either hyperpolarizing, presumably the result of a specific decrease in Na^+ permeability [21], or depolarizing, a decreased K^+ permeability [21], and they tend to have a slower time course than those with increased permeability. The mechanisms that generate the potentials are unknown, but they are probably energy-requiring, in contrast to those where the permeability increases (which require no energy beyond that necessary to maintain concentration gradients), and may involve a second messenger. Although it has been suggested that cAMP and cyclic GMP (cGMP) are involved in several of these slow responses and although synthesis of both substances may be stimulated by neurotransmitters, it is not yet possible to correlate rigorously these biochemical changes with electrical changes. Some responses not accompanied by clear changes in conductance have been ascribed to activation of an electrogenic Na^+-K^+ pump, but this conclusion is controversial (see also Chap. 3). An elucidation of the mechanisms involved in responses not caused by permeability increases is one of the obvious challenges in neurobiology today.

In presynaptic inhibition, the effects of neurotransmitters on membrane resistance are of greater importance than is potential change

In some neurons, E_{Cl^-} is very near to RMP. I a transmitter increases permeability to Cl^- and E_{Cl^-} is equal to RMP, there would be no change in potential. Even so, any other input would be reduced in effectiveness. This is most easily understood by viewing the action of the second input as a current which, by Ohm's law, will produce less voltage when resistance has fallen. Since E_{Cl^-} is never very far from RMP, the short-circuiting effect of increasing Cl^- permeability may be very significant. An example is presynaptic inhibition, a process that has best been studied in the spinal cord, where it results from a synaptic ending on the presynaptic terminal of primary afferent fibers. The effect of activating this pathway onto the presynaptic terminal is to release GABA, which causes increased Cl^- permeability and a Cl^--dependent depolarization in the presynaptic terminal; in these fibers, E_{Cl^-} is less negative than RMP. In a manner not totally understood, there is a reduction in the amount of transmitter released from the presynaptic terminal when the afferent fiber discharges. The mechanism may be a short-circuiting of the terminal, due to increased Cl^- permeability, with blockade of impulse invasion into the terminal branches where transmitter release occurs. In a second type of transmitter action, the effects of neurotransmitters associated with a decrease, rather than an increase, in permeability may increase the responsiveness of neurons to other synaptic inputs. Also, in this type of synapse, the permeability decreases are often associated with only modest voltage shifts, and the alteration of membrane resistance may be the most significant result.

The patch-clamp technique allows measurement of currents resulting from ion transfer through single channels of the membrane

The principle of this technique is to establish a very high resistance seal between the rim of the micropipette and the membrane of the cell [22]. This large recording resistance (in the gigaohm range), plus special input amplifiers, allows measurement of currents of less than 1 pA.

Five configurations of the patch-clamp have been described (Fig. 11). In one configuration, currents from the whole cell can be conveniently obtained, provided that the cell is not too large and does not have many processes. In three other configurations, single-channel recordings are obtained. Unitary current values, conductance values for neurotransmitter-activated channels, and single-channel kinetics for durations of channel open and closed times can all be obtained using this technique. Horn and Marty [23] reported another technique whereby the membrane is permeabilized under the electrode tip with nystatin. This technique leaves the internal environment undisturbed.

Studies using the patch-clamp technique have measured the kinetics for opening and closing of ion channels in response to ACh. These studies were initiated by measurement of the end-plate current elicited in response to stimulation of the motor nerve. There occurs an initial delay, a rise of the end-plate current, and finally a decay, whose time course follows a single exponential with a rate constant α. This decay is voltage-dependent, being much faster at depolarizing voltages.

The decay is also temperature-dependent, with a Q_{10} of 2.8. Magleby and Stevens [24] therefore applied a kinetic model for the binding of the agonist A to the receptor R, leading to opening of the channel:

$$A + R \underset{k_{-1}}{\overset{k_{+1}}{\rightleftharpoons}} AR \underset{\alpha}{\overset{\beta}{\rightleftharpoons}} AR^* \qquad (5)$$

If the rate constants k_{+1} and k_{-1} are such that this reaction is very fast, AR is in equilibrium with A + R. If free ACh can no longer be detected in a short time period, the decay of the end-plate current can be thought of as the exponential closing of open channels AR* with rate constant α. The AR complex could then dissociate quickly to free receptor, and the agonist would be removed by hydrolysis, as in the case for ACh, or by uptake into the nerve terminals or glial cells. The voltage dependence of α could be explained by a gating process.

Studies of single-channel current kinetics show that the ACh receptor has several identifiable states whose transitions have known rate constants

Originally characterized electrophysiologically by Anderson and Stevens [25], these states were measured for current fluctuation and power spectra from resting and ACh-activated channels. The resulting curves showed a Lorentzian distribution such that:

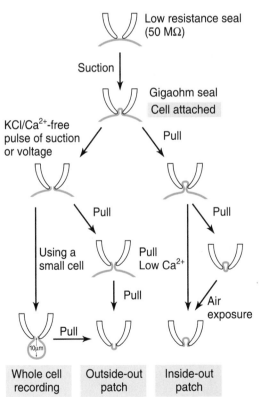

FIG. 11.   Configurations of the patch-clamp technique. (Modified from Hamill et al. [22].)

$$S(f) = \frac{s(0)}{1 + (f/f_c)^2} = \frac{s(0)}{1 + (2\pi f\tau)^2} \quad (6)$$

where f is frequency; $s(0)$ is the low-frequency intercept; f_c is the corner frequency; and $\tau = \frac{1}{2}f_c$ is the relaxation time constant. The relaxation time measured by these means lengthens with cooling and hyperpolarization as shown for the end-plate current. Experiments using different agonists have shown that the open-channel lifetime is much longer with suberyldicholine and much shorter with carbamylcholine than with ACh. It is interesting that this sequence is also true at snail neurons, where suberyldicholine acts as a hyperpolarizing agent.

The early studies on single-channel currents by patch-clamp techniques showed distributions for open times with a single exponential with time and a time constant that shortened with depolarization; however, it became clear that so-called single-channel openings were interrupted by extremely short closures, and this suggests a deviation from the kinetic scheme shown in Eq. 5. There had been some question with regard to the applicability of Eq. 5, for it was known that two molecules of ACh must combine with the receptor to cause the channel to open.

Once the two molecules are bound, the channel must be able to isomerize from the closed to the open state. The following scheme may then apply:

$$A + R \underset{k_{-1}}{\overset{k_{+1}}{\rightleftharpoons}} AR \underset{k_{-2}}{\overset{k_{+2}}{\rightleftharpoons}} A_2R \underset{\alpha}{\overset{\beta}{\rightleftharpoons}} A_2R^*$$

$$(7)$$

If, however, the binding reactions are much faster than the open-shut isomerization reaction, there may be many brief events resulting in this fast opening and closing. This would suggest that there are multiple openings and closings during a single occupancy by an agonist. With high concentrations of agonist, desensitization occurs, and the pattern of channel openings becomes typically one that progresses from bursts to clusters of bursts. The clusters are separated by long silent intervals.

At the present time, single-channel responses to ACh, glutamate, GABA, and serotonin have been obtained at various sites. Table 2 shows the changes in permeability to, and postsynaptic effects of, known transmitters. Although results of early studies showed that ACh-activated channels were permeable to Na^+ and K^+, it is now clear that these channels are permeant virtually nonselectively to cations. The same appears to be true insofar as selectivity is concerned for glutamate-activated channels, although GABA channels are selectively permeant to Cl^-.

The use of the patch-clamp technique has resulted in the finding that there are at least two populations of ACh receptor channels in muscle cells of many vertebrate species [26]: One type, located at the synapse of innervated adult muscle fibers, has a high (45 pS) single-channel conductance and fast kinetics; the other, found in nonsynaptic membrane of both embryonic and adult denervated muscle fibers, has a lower conductance (25 pS) and slower kinetics (Fig. 12). The separation into different channel populations is not confined to neurotransmitter-activated channels but has been described also for voltage-dependent channels.

A recent method for studying exocytosis and neurotransmitter secretion is the measurement of cell membrane capacitance. When the contents of secretory vesicles are exocytosed, the membrane area of the cell is increased by addition of vesicle membrane. Capacitance is proportional to membrane area and therefore exocytosis is accompanied by an increase in membrane capacitance. In 1982, Neher and Marty [27], using the whole-cell configuration of the patch-clamp and sinusoidal stimulation, measured a capacitance signal with a phase-sensitive detector from chromaffin cells. They correlated small changes in membrane capacitance in these cells with individual granule

A   **B**

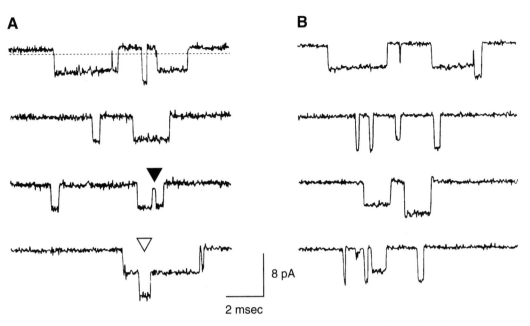

8 pA

2 msec

FIG. 12.   ACh receptor channel currents elicited by 0.2 μM ACh from "cell-attached" patches of **(A)** 1-day- and **(B)** 6-day-cultured myotomal muscle. In the top trace **(A)** the threshold for event discrimination is indicated by a *dashed line,* computed to be 2.5 times the standard deviation of base-line fluctuations. The data were digitized at 50-μsec intervals and redisplayed in analog fashion on a Hewlett-Packard monitor. The pipette potential was +40 mV, and the intracellular potential was approximately −85 mV in both recordings. This results in an estimated patch potential of −125 mV. (▼) An example of an opening to a subconductance state; (▽) coincident opening by two low-conductance channels. (From Brehm et al. [26].)

fusion and membrane retrieval events. This technique is now used to measure exocytosis, endocytosis, and stimulus-secretion coupling mechanisms in many secretory cells.

ACKNOWLEDGMENTS

I am grateful to Drs. David O. Carpenter and Thomas S. Reese for allowing me to use much of the chapter prepared for an earlier edition of this book. Support was provided by USPHS grant NS12211.

REFERENCES

1. Elliott, T. R. The action of adrenalin. *J. Physiol. (Lond.)* 32:401–467, 1905.
2. Loewi, O. Über humorole Übertragbarkeit der Herznervenwirkung. I. Mitteilung. *Pflugers Arch.* 189:239–242, 1921.
3. Bloom, F. E. Neurotransmitters: past, present, and future directions. *FASEB. J.* 2:32–41, 1988.
4. MacDonald, J. F., and Nowak, L. M. Mechanisms of blockade of excitatory amino acid receptor channels. *Trends Pharmacol. Sci.* 11:167–172, 1990.
5. Eccles, J. C., Fatt, P., and Koketsu, K. Cholinergic and inhibitory synapses in a pathway from motor-axon collaterals to motoneurones. *J. Physiol. (Lond.)* 126:524–562, 1954.
6. Chan-Palay, V., and Palay, S. L. (eds.). *Co-existence of Neuroactive Substances in Neurons.* New York: Wiley, 1984.
7. Paton, W. D. M. Central and synaptic transmission in the nervous system (pharmacological aspects). *Annu. Rev. Physiol.* 20:431–470, 1958.
8. Heuser, J. E. Synaptic vesicle exocytosis revealed in quick-frozen frog neuromuscular junction treated with 4-aminopyridine and

given a single electric shock. In W. M. Cowan, and J. Ferrendelli (eds.), *Approaches to the Cell Biology of Neurons.* Bethesda: Society for Neuroscience, 1976, pp. 215–239.

9. Nicholls, J. G., Martin, A. R., and Wallace, B. G. *From Neuron to Brain.* Sunderland, MA: Sinauer Associates, 1992.

10. Couteaux, R., and Pecot-Dechavassine, M. Vesicules synaptiques et poches au niveau des "zones actives" de la junction neuromusculaire. *C. R. Acad. Sci. Ser. C. Sci. Chem.* 271: 2346–2349, 1970.

11. Heuser, J. E., and Reese, T. S. Structure of the synapse. In E. R. Kandel (ed.), *Handbook of Physiology, The Nervous System I.* Bethesda: American Physiological Society, 1977, pp. 261–294.

12. Heuser, J. E., and Reese, T. S. Evidence for recycling of synaptic vesicle membrane during transmitter release at the frog neuromuscular junction. *J. Cell Biol.* 57:315–344, 1973.

13. Stieber, A., Erulkar, S. D., and Gonatas, N. K. A hypothesis for the superior sensitivity of wheat germ agglutinin as a neuroanatomical probe. *Brain Res.* 495:131–139, 1989.

14. Lupa, M. T., and Caldwell, J. H. Effect of agrin on the distribution of acetylcholine receptors and sodium channels on adult skeletal muscle fibers in culture. *J. Cell Biol.* 115:765–778, 1991.

15. McMahan, U. J., Horton, S. E., Werle, M. J., Honig, L. S., Kröger, S., Ruegg, M. A., and Escher, G. Agrin isoforms and their role in synaptogenesis. *Curr. Opin. Cell Biol.* 4: 869–874, 1992.

16. Fatt, P., and Katz, B. Spontaneous subthreshold activity at motor nerve endings. *J. Physiol. (Lond.)* 117:109–128, 1952.

17. Boyd, I. A., and Martin, A. R. The end-plate potential in mammalian muscle. *J. Physiol. (Lond.)* 132:74–91, 1956.

18. Katz, B., and Miledi, R. The effect of calcium on acetylcholine release from motor nerve terminals. *Proc. R. Soc. Lond. (Biol.)* 161: 496–503, 1965.

19. Llinás, R., Steinberg, I. Z., and Walton, K. Relationship between presynaptic calcium current and postsynaptic potential in squid giant synapse. *Biophys. J.* 33:323–351, 1981.

20. Llinás, R., Gruner, J. A., Sugimori, M., McGuinness, T. L., and Greengard, P. Regulation by synapsin I and Ca^{2+}-calmodulin-dependent protein kinase II of transmitter release in squid giant synapse. *J. Physiol. (Lond.)* 436: 257–282, 1991.

21. Weight, F. F. Synaptic mechanisms in amphibian sympathetic ganglia. In L. G. Elfvin (ed.), *Autonomic Ganglia.* New York: Wiley, 1983, pp. 309–344.

22. Hamill, O. P., Marty, A., Neher, E., Sakmann, B., and Sigworth, F. J. Improved patch-clamp techniques for high-resolution current recording from cells and cell-free membrane patches. *Pflugers Arch.* 391:85–100, 1981.

23. Horn, R., and Marty, A. Muscarinic activation of ionic currents measured by a new whole-cell recording method. *J. Gen. Physiol.* 92: 145–159, 1988.

24. Magleby, K. L., and Stevens, C. F. A quantitative description of end-plate currents. *J. Physiol. (Lond.)* 223:173–197, 1972.

25. Anderson, C. R., and Stevens, C. F. Voltage clamp analysis of acetylcholine produced end-plate current fluctuations at frog neuromuscular junction. *J. Physiol. (Lond.)* 235: 655–691, 1973.

26. Brehm, P., Kidokoro, Y., and Moody-Corbett, F. Acetylcholine receptor channel properties during development of *Xenopus* muscle cells in culture. *J. Physiol. (Lond)* 357:203–217, 1984.

27. Neher, E., and Marty, A. Discrete changes of cell membrane capacitance observed under conditions of enhanced secretion in bovine adrenal chromaffin cells. *Proc. Natl. Acad. Sci. U. S. A.* 79:6712–6716, 1982.

CHAPTER 10

Receptors and Signal Transduction: Classification and Quantitation

PAUL McGONIGLE AND PERRY B. MOLINOFF

Basic Neurochemistry: Molecular, Cellular, and Medical Aspects, 5th Ed., edited by G. J. Siegel et al. Published by Raven Press, Ltd., New York, 1994. Correspondence to Paul McGonigle, Department of Pharmacology, University of Pennsylvania School of Medicine, Philadelphia, Pennsylvania 19104-6084.

RECEPTORS AND TRANSMITTERS

Receptors are the constituents of a cell that have the ability to recognize a drug, hormone, or neurotransmitter

The idea that receptors exist dates to the turn of the century when Langley, Dale, and their colleagues suggested that receptive substances must exist on the surface membranes of excitable cells.

> First that two special substances at least (receptive substances) are present in the neural region of the muscle, and that nerve impulses can only cause contraction by acting on a receptive substance. Secondly that the receptive substances form more or less easily dissociable compounds. Thus nicotine in combining with these substances . . . [J.N. Langley, 1909].

In 1921, Loewi demonstrated the existence of the process of chemical neurotransmission. A variety of substances are now known or thought to be neurotransmitters. These include biogenic amines such as acetylcholine, norepinephrine, serotonin, amino acids such as glutamate and γ-aminobutyric acid (GABA), and numerous peptides (Table 1). Recent data suggesting that

Categories of synaptic transmission

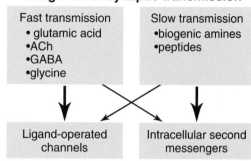

FIG. 1.   Categories of synaptic transmission. The primary mechanism of action of the amino acid neurotransmitters and of acetylcholine involves the opening of ligand-operated channels. Biogenic amines and peptides frequently function as neuromodulators requiring the production of intracellular second messengers. In some circumstances, however, glutamic acid and acetylcholine modulate intracellular second messengers while biogenic amines and peptides can be coupled to the activation of ion channels.

diffusable gases such as NO and CO may also function as neurotransmitters offer the probability of a further expansion of our concepts with regard to the molecules capable of functioning as neurotransmitters (see also Chaps. 21 and 50).

One approach to distinguishing classes of receptors is to identify molecules involved in fast as compared to slow transmission

Compounds usually thought of as interacting with ligand-gated ion channels and receptors for fast neurotransmission include glutamic acid, acetylcholine, and the inhibitory neurotransmitters GABA and glycine. Transmitters coupled to changes in intracellular second messengers such as cyclic AMP and inositol trisphosphate include serotonin and the catecholamines as well as many peptides. The transmitters that act through channels or second messenger systems can be associated with fast and slow transmission, respectively (Fig. 1). This simple categorization is a useful starting point but there are many notable exceptions. For example, although acetylcholine and glutamic acid are

TABLE 1.   Neurotransmitters known and putative

BIOGENIC AMINES	PEPTIDES
Catecholamines	Numerous:
Epinephrine	e.g., Substance P
Norepinephrine	Enkephalins
Dopamine	Somatostatin
Indoleamines	Neuropeptide Y
Serotonin (5-HT)	Vasoactive intestinal
Histamine	peptide (VIP)
Ester	
Acetylcholine	
	OTHER
AMINO ACIDS	Nitric oxide (NO)
	Carbon monoxide (CO)
Excitatory	Zinc
Glutamate	Arachidonic acid
Aspartate	Platelet-activating factor
Inhibitory	
γ-Aminobutyric acid	
(GABA)	
Glycine	

often coupled to (fast) ligand-gated ion channels, they may also act through (slow) metabotropic receptors to modulate levels of intracellular second messengers. Conversely, some of the effects of catecholamines appear to occur through modulation of the conductance of calcium and/or potassium channels.

The activity of neurotransmitters is mediated through interaction with members of a limited number of receptor families

These families include ligand-gated ion channels, G protein-coupled receptors, growth factors which have tyrosine kinase activity, and steroid receptors that are intracellular macromolecules that function to transport steroids into the nucleus, where they act to modulate transcriptional activity (Fig. 2).

The ligand-gated ion channels are heteromeric receptors containing multiple subunits. Hydrophobicity analysis suggests that each includes several transmembrane helices (Fig. 3). The prototypic member of this receptor family is the nicotinic cholinergic receptor. This receptor is composed of five subunits in a relative stoichiometry of $\alpha_2\beta\delta\gamma$.

The β-adrenergic receptor was the first member of what is now known as the G protein receptor-linked superfamily to be cloned and sequenced. The members of this family (Fig. 4) have sequence and presumed structural similarities to one another as well as to the visual pigment rhodopsin and to bacterial opsin. These proteins are thought to have seven membrane-spanning helices with an extracellular amino terminus and an intracellular carboxy terminus. Among other important structural features are sites for *N*-linked glycosylation on the amino terminus and sites for phosphorylation by protein kinases on the third intracellular loop and on the carboxy tail.

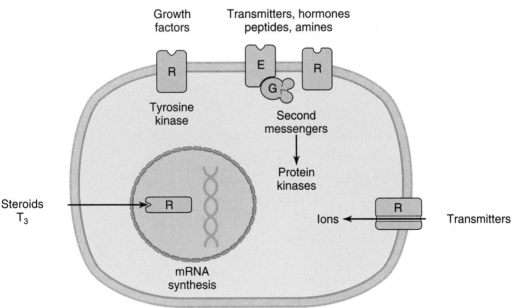

Classes of receptors

FIG. 2. Classes of receptors. Membrane-bound receptors may be coupled to ion flow, the generation of second messengers, or tyrosine phosphorylation mediated through tyrosine kinases. Steroid receptors, on the other hand, are intracellular molecules which serve to transport steroids into the cell nucleus.

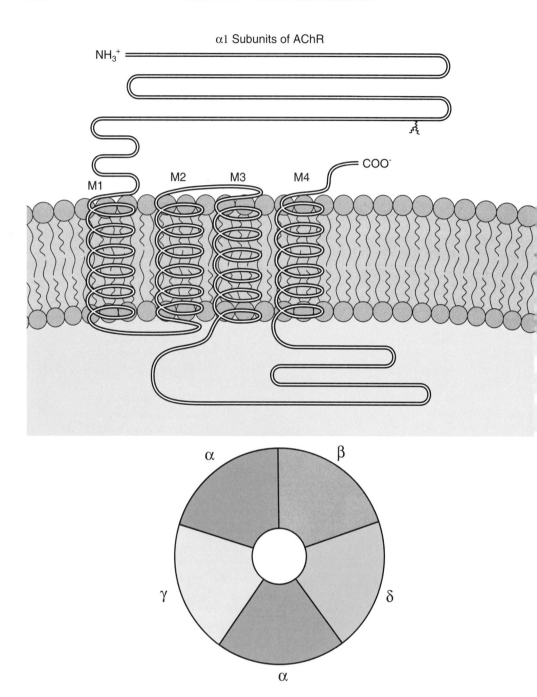

FIG. 3. Structural features of acetylcholine receptors. **Top:** The putative organization within the membrane of the α-subunit of the nicotinic acetylcholine receptor is shown. Major features include a large extracellular amino terminal segment of the receptor, four transmembrane helices, and a short carboxy terminus. A putative site for *N*-linked glycosylation is also shown. **Bottom:** Subunits of nicotinic receptors are organized to form a central cationic channel. The stoichiometry of the subunits is $\alpha_2\beta\delta\gamma$.

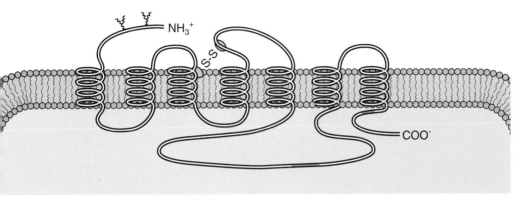

FIG. 4.   Generalized schematic diagram of a G protein-coupled receptor. Major structural features include an extracellular amino terminus containing sites for N-linked glycosylation and an intracellular carboxy terminus. The seven transmembrane helices represent the portions of the molecule with the highest conservation of amino acid residues across the members of this receptor family. Also indicated are the site of a conserved disulfide bond and sites for phosphorylation ——— on the third intracellular loop and/or the carboxyl tail.

The members of the G protein receptor-linked family act through a mechanism that involves the binding of GTP and displacement of GDP from a GTP-binding protein

There are now many members of the GTP-binding protein family. These proteins are usually distinguished by detecting differences in the structures of the α-subunits of $\alpha\beta\gamma$ heterotrimers. At least four families of G proteins have now been identified (Fig. 5).

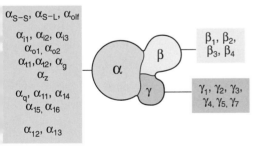

FIG. 5.   Structure and composition of G proteins. At least four families of G proteins exist. They have been identified on the basis of similarities in the sequences of their α-subunits. G proteins existing in cells are heterotrimers composed of α, β, and γ subunits.

Modulation of intracellular levels of cyclic AMP and changes in phosphoinositide hydrolysis are reactions mediated by G protein-coupled receptors

Stimulation and inhibition of adenylyl cyclase activity involve similar reactions in which GTP binds to the α-subunit of either G_s or G_i. The end result is a change in the activity of adenylyl cyclase and a change in intracellular levels of cyclic AMP (Fig. 6A,B). Cyclic AMP in turn binds to the regulatory subunit of protein kinase A, allowing phosphorylation mediated by the catalytic subunit of kinase A to occur. Termination of the signal involves enzymatic hydrolysis of cyclic AMP by phosphodiesterase and conversion of GTP to GDP by GTPase activity expressed by the α-subunits of various G proteins. The ternary complex composed of agonist, receptor, and G protein represents a high-affinity state of the receptor.

In other instances, transmitter-mediated activation of phospholipase C occurs. This results in the cleavage of phosphatidyl-inositol bisphosphate. Both diacylglycerol (DG) and inositol trisphosphate (IP_3) resulting from this reaction are biologically active. Diacylglycerol, which contains two molecules

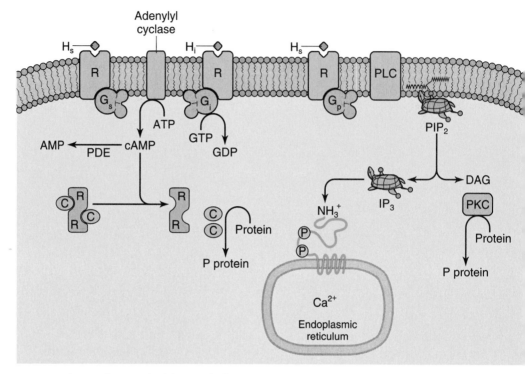

FIG. 6. **Left:** Stimulation and inhibition of adenylyl cyclase activity. Binding of a hormone or neurotransmitter linked to stimulation (H_s) or inhibition (H_i) of adenylyl cyclase activity leads to binding of GTP to a G protein and changes in the activity of adenylyl cyclase. These changes lead to increases or decreases in the formation of cyclic AMP which is in turn coupled to changes in the activity of protein kinase A (PKA). Cyclic AMP binds the regulatory subunit of protein kinase A, liberating the free active catalytic moiety which in turns catalyzes phosphorylation of a variety of protein substrates. **Right:** Stimulation of phospholipase C activity. Hormones coupled to changes in phospholipase C activity lead to activation of G proteins (G_p). Phospholipase C catalyzes the conversion of phosphotidylinositol bisphosphate (PIP_2) leading to release of inositol trisphosphate (IP_3) and diacylglycerol (DAG). Diacylglycerol is, in turn, an activator of protein kinase C, while IP_3 causes release of calcium from the endoplasmic reticulum.

of fatty acid, diffuses in the plane of the membrane and activates an enzyme, protein kinase C. Inositol trisphosphate, on the other hand, causes release of Ca^{2+} from stores in the endoplasmic reticulum (Fig. 6) (see Chap. 20).

inephrine and serotonin may act to stimulate or inhibit adenylyl cyclase activity, stimulate phospholipase C activity, and stimulate or inhibit potassium or calcium channels.

The specificity of receptor-mediated reactions depends on the nature of the transmitter, of the receptor, and of the associated messenger system

For example, acetylcholine can interact with different muscarinic receptors to inhibit adenylyl cyclase activity, or activate phospholipase C activity or potassium channels. Norep-

BINDING ASSAYS WITH RADIOLIGANDS TO STUDY RECEPTORS FOR NEUROTRANSMITTERS, HORMONES, AND DRUGS

In 1971, the first successful binding assays with radioligands made it possible to study nicotinic cholinergic receptors in the elecric organs of fish and eels. In 1973, the stereospecific binding of radiolabeled opiates to binding sites in mammalian brain was first described. Over the next ten years, quantitative radioligand binding assays were developed for receptors for a variety of drugs and transmitters, and ligands radiolabeled with ^3H or ^{125}I are now available for the study of many classes of receptors. This widespread availability of suitable ligands has led to a rapid expansion in the use of binding assays with radioligands to characterize receptors and receptor subtypes [1].

Before the widespread use of *in vitro* binding assays, the properties of receptors were inferred from the measurement of biological responses. This approach proved to be productive in the classification of receptors and even led to the identification of subtypes of receptors; however, measuring a biological response either *in vivo* or *in situ* can be very different from measuring receptor binding *in vitro*. For example, the tissue distribution of a drug administered *in vivo* may vary depending on its ability to cross diffusion barriers, such as the blood-brain barrier, or on the extent to which the drug binds to plasma proteins. The lipophilic or hydrophilic nature of a compound can determine whether or not it has equal access to all of the receptors in a given tissue. Also, drugs can be metabolized before they have an opportunity to interact with a receptor. These metabolic transformations can yield compounds that are either more or less active than the parent drug and thus can markedly alter the observed pharmacological specificity. Drugs not subject to structural alterations are often removed from the extracellular environment by neuronal and extraneuronal uptake mechanisms. Furthermore, *in vivo*, the response to a drug is frequently attenuated by compensatory feedback mechanisms. Interpretation of a measured biological response can also be difficult if the drug has multiple sites of action—a phenomenon that can also occur *in vitro* with tissues that contain multiple classes of receptor subtypes. In some cases, the receptor subtypes

mediate the same physiological response, and they may exert these effects through the same effector system. The observed pharmacological response will then be affected by the degree of selectivity of the drug and by the relative densities of the subtypes present in the tissue. In general, the most reliable characterization of receptors results from studies carried out with simple, isolated tissue preparations that exhibit reproducible, graded dose-response curves. Even with such preparations, it is often impossible to define accurately the kinetic characteristics of drug-receptor interactions.

Radioligand binding techniques supplement and overcome many limitations of studies of biological responses

Radioligands provide precise probes that permit specific examination of the initial interaction between a drug and its binding site. For example, the kinetics of association and dissociation of a receptor-radioligand complex can be accurately determined by using simple tissue homogenates. A pharmacological profile that is based on the equilibrium dissociation constants of a series of unlabeled ligands can be defined by measuring the inhibition of the binding of a radioligand by these unlabeled compounds. The use of radioligands also permits characterization of receptors in the absence of a measurable biological response. This may be important, for example, in the study of central nervous system receptors, where the effects of neurotransmitters are complex and isolated tissue preparations are difficult to obtain. The use of binding assays with radioligands can result in meaningful estimates of the number or density of receptors in a particular tissue. Consequently, changes in the density of receptors resulting from pathological conditions or pharmacological interventions can be monitored. Binding assays can also be used to discriminate multiple classes of receptors in a single tissue and to estimate their relative proportions. Moreover, binding assays with radioligands provide the only means by which receptors can be measured during solubilization, purification, and reconstitution—steps necessary for the complete understanding of receptor function.

Two basic types of assays utilize radioligands. The first, direct binding assays, measures the direct interaction of a radioligand with a receptor. Direct binding assays permit determination of both kinetic and equilibrium properties and provide estimates of the receptor density. They are also used to choose appropriate conditions and radioligands to determine the pharmacological properties of receptors. The second, indirect binding assays, measures the inhibition of the binding of a radioligand by an unlabeled ligand to deduce indirectly the affinity of receptors for the unlabeled ligand. This approach is particularly useful in the pharmacological characterization of receptors because studies can be carried out with compounds that would not be suitable radioligands, either because they are too lipophilic or because the receptor affinity for these compounds is too low.

DIRECT BINDING ASSAYS MEASURE BINDING OF A RADIOLIGAND TO A RECEPTOR

Equilibrium analysis

Analysis of Untransformed Data

The simplest model describing the interaction of a receptor, R, with a radioligand, L, to form a complex, RL, is the bimolecular reaction

$$[L] + [R] \underset{k_{-1}}{\overset{k_{+1}}{\rightleftharpoons}} [RL] \tag{1}$$

The concentration of the receptor-radioligand complex [RL] is frequently referred to as the amount bound [B]. According to the laws of mass action, at equilibrium,

$$K_d = \frac{[R][L]}{[B]} \tag{2}$$

where K_d is the equilibrium dissociation constant. The kinetic rate constants, k_{+1} and k_{-1}, and the equilibrium dissociation constant, K_d, are related such that

$$K_d = k_{-1}/k_{+1} \tag{3}$$

Since the total number of receptors $B_{max} = [R] + [B]$, substitution for [R] in Eq. 2 and rearrangement yields

$$[B] = \frac{B_{max}[L]}{[L] + K_d} \tag{4}$$

In a typical "saturation" experiment, increasing amounts of a radioligand are added to a fixed concentration of receptors, and the amount of radioligand bound to the receptor, [B], is measured as a function of the concentration of radioligand. The concentration of radioligand is increased until virtually all the receptors are occupied by the ligand (Fig. 7). Nonlinear regression analysis can be used to fit Eq. 4 to the data to provide estimates of both K_d and B_{max}.

In practice, the radioligand binds not only to the receptor, but also to other components of the assay system, including the walls of glass test tubes, filter paper, and constituents of the tissue. Although the exact nature of this nonspecific binding is usually unknown, it often occurs instantaneously. Nonspecific binding is generally nonsaturable and is proportional to the concentration of radioligand (Fig. 7). Misidentification of this nonspecific component is a common source of error in the analysis of radioligand binding data, resulting in an overestimate of the density of receptors and leading, in some cases, to the incorrect conclusion that multiple classes of receptors coexist in a given tissue [2]. Nonspecific binding can be quantified by adding high concentrations of an unlabeled competing ligand that is specific for the receptor of interest. The amount of radioligand that remains bound in the presence of the unlabeled ligand is defined as nonspecific binding. In a saturation experi-

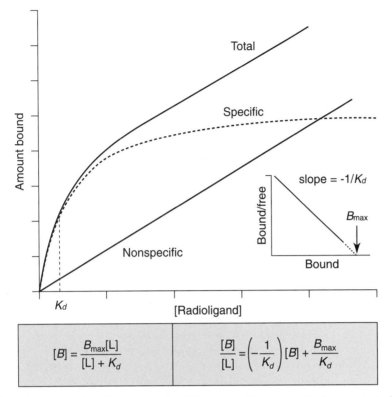

$$[B] = \frac{B_{max}[L]}{[L] + K_d}$$

$$\frac{[B]}{[L]} = \left(-\frac{1}{K_d}\right)[B] + \frac{B_{max}}{K_d}$$

FIG. 7. Analysis of saturation data. The amount of radioligand specifically bound to the receptor is determined by subtracting the amount of radioligand bound nonspecifically from the total amount bound. The left-hand equation describes the relationship between specific binding $[B]$ and the concentration of radioligand $[L]$ in terms of the total number of receptors B_{max} and the equilibrium dissociation constant K_d. **Inset:** Transformation of the saturation equation by the Scatchard method. The slope of this line is $-1/K_d$ and the intercept on the abscissa is B_{max}.

ment, the nonspecific component of binding at each concentration of radioligand is subtracted from the total amount of radioligand bound to yield the amount of radioligand specifically bound to the receptor (Fig. 7). The amount of nonspecific binding should be the same in experiments carried out with a variety of unlabeled ligands, including both agonists and antagonists. In general, the best results are obtained when the drug used to define specific binding is of a different chemical class from that of the radioligand and when the concentration of the competing ligand is approximately 100 times its K_d value. Higher concentrations of a competing ligand can inhibit nonspecific as well as specific binding.

Scatchard Analysis

A useful approach for analyzing binding data is to construct a Scatchard plot [3]. A plot of the ratio of bound $[B]$ to free $[L]$ ligand against the concentration of bound ligand is a straight line that has a slope equal to the negative reciprocal of the dissociation constant, $(-1/K_d)$, and an intercept on the abscissa equal to the total concentration of receptors (B_{max}) (Fig. 7, inset).

An advantage of using Scatchard analysis is that it provides an estimate of the total concentration of receptors without requiring saturating concentrations of radioligand. The concentration of receptors can be estimated by extrapolating a straight line to the abscissa. This is particularly important in systems with high levels of nonspecific binding. Estimates of B_{max} made by nonlinear regression analysis or Scatchard analysis are subject to significant error if the highest concentration of radioligand does not at least exceed the K_d value. Another advantage of the Scatchard plot is that visual inspection provides insight into whether or not a simple bimolecular reaction adequately describes the interaction between ligand and receptor. Curvature of a Scatchard plot implies that this interaction is complex. A Scatchard plot that is concave upward can result from a heterogeneous population of receptors, a multistep/multicomponent binding reaction, or from negative cooperativity between the binding sites. These possibilities can be distinguished by detailed kinetic analysis [4]. A Scatchard plot that is concave downward can result from positive cooperativity between the binding sites or from failure of the reaction to reach equilibrium at low concentrations of the ligand, since the time to reach equilibrium is a function of ligand concentration. These possibilities can also be distinguished by kinetic analysis.

Curvilinear Scatchard plots can be produced artifactually by a variety of factors (see below), such as an incorrect definition of nonspecific binding, incomplete separation of bound and free ligand, and dissociation of the receptor-ligand complex during the separation of bound and free ligand. If too high a concentration of competing ligand is used to define nonspecific binding (see above), a Scatchard plot that is concave upward will result. These factors are discussed in detail by Boeynaems and Dumont [5] and Weiland and Molinoff [6].

Kinetic analysis

Rate of Association

The rate of association of a radioligand with a receptor is determined by measuring the amount of bound ligand $[B]$ as a function of time. At time $t = 0$, a specific concentration of radioligand $[L]$ is added, and the amount of bound ligand $[B]$ is measured at various times until equilibrium is reached. The amount of radioligand bound at a given time depends on the simultaneously occurring processes of association and dissociation. In the simple bimolecular reaction described in Eq. 1, the rate of association of ligand-receptor complex is $k_{+1}[L][R]$, and the rate of dissociation of this complex is $k_{-1}[B]$. Thus, the measured rate of formation of $[B]$ is

$$\frac{d[B]}{dt} = k_{+1}[L][R] - k_{-1}[B] \qquad (5)$$

At equilibrium, $d[B]/dt = 0$, and

$$k_{+1}[L][R] = k_{-1}[B] \qquad (6)$$

Substitution for $[L]$, $[R]$ and k_{-1} in Eq. 5 yields a second-order rate equation that can be integrated to give

$$\ln \frac{[B_e]([L_t] - [B][B_e])/B_{max}}{[L_t]([B_e] - [B])}$$
$$= k_{+1}t \frac{[L_t](B_{max} - [B_e])}{[B_e]} \qquad (7)$$

where L_t is the total amount of radioligand added at the start of the reaction and B_e is the amount of radioligand bound at equilibrium (see [6] for derivation). The rate constant of association can be determined from the slope of a plot of the expression on the left-hand side of Eq. 7 against time (Fig. 8). If the reaction obeys simple bimolecular kinetics, this plot will result in a straight line. The only parameter in Eq. 7 that varies as a function of time is $[B]$. One disadvantage of this analysis is that the association rate constant is not independent of the equilibrium dissociation constant K_d because the term B_{max} appears in Eq. 7; however, the advantage of using the full second-order equation is that no assumptions are made about the relative concentrations of radioligand or receptor.

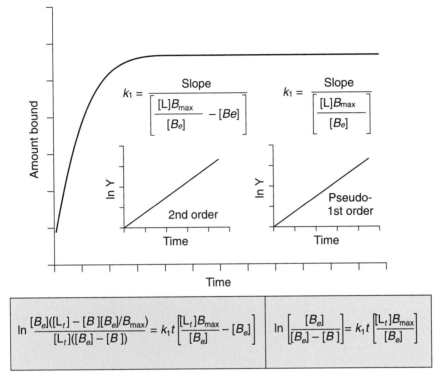

$$\ln \frac{[B_e]([L_t] - [B][B_e]/B_{max})}{[L_t]([B_e] - [B])} = k_1 t \left[\frac{[L_t]B_{max}}{[B_e]} - [B_e] \right] \qquad \ln \left[\frac{[B_e]}{[B_e] - [B]} \right] = k_1 t \left[\frac{[L_t]B_{max}}{[B_e]} \right]$$

FIG. 8.   Determination of association rate. The amount of radioligand bound is measured at various times. **Left inset:** Association is plotted according to the integrated form of the second-order rate equation, where $[B_e]$ is the amount of radioligand bound at equilibrium; k_{+1} is the association rate constant; and $Y = [B_e]([L] - [B]\cdot[B_e])/B_{max}/[L]([B_e] - [B])$. This plot is linear, and k_{+1} is directly related to the slope. **Right inset:** Association is plotted according to the integrated form of the pseudo-first-order rate equation, where $Y = [B_e]/([B_e] - [B])$. This equation assumes that the concentration of radioligand [L] is much greater than the total concentration of receptors B_{max}. This plot is linear, and k_{+1} is directly related to the slope.

In many studies of the binding of radioligands, the total concentration of radioligand $[L_t]$ is much greater than the total concentration of receptors $[B_{max}]$. Under these conditions there is little or no change in the concentration of free ligand [L] as the reaction proceeds to equilibrium. Even at equilibrium, only a small fraction of the total concentration of ligand $[L_t]$ is bound to the receptor. For all practical purposes, [L] is a constant, and the reaction can be considered a "pseudo-first-order" reaction. Thus, Eq. 7 can be simplified to [8]:

$$\ln \frac{[B_e]}{[B_e] + [B]} = k_{+1} t \frac{[L_t] B_{max}}{[B_e]} \qquad (8)$$

The association rate constant, k_{+1}, can be determined from the slope of a plot of the left-hand side of Eq. 8 versus time (Fig. 8). In addition to the assumption that $[L_t] \gg [B_e]$, the determination of k_{+1} again depends on the equilibrium measurement of B_{max}.

One method of analyzing the pseudo-first-order time course eliminates the need for an independent determination of B_{max}. This method requires measurement of the slopes of pseudo-first-order plots over a range of ligand concentrations. The slope of the pseudo-first-order plot is called k_{obs}. It can be shown that k_{obs} is related to the ligand concentration [L] such that a plot of k_{obs} versus ligand concentration results in a straight line

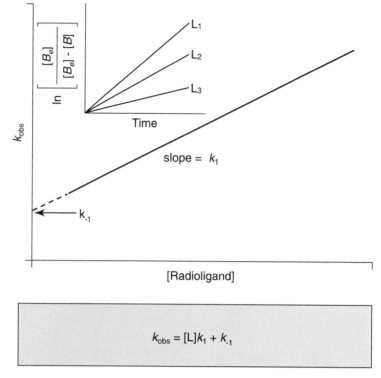

FIG. 9. Effect of radioligand concentration on k_{obs}. A plot of the slopes of the pseudo-first-order rate plots (k_{obs}) versus the concentrations of radioligand at which the association rates were measured is linear. The equation describes the relationship of k_{obs} to the rates of association (k_{+1}) and dissociation (k_{-1}). Use of this method to determine the association rate constant k_{+1} does not require independent determination of the total number of receptors. **Inset:** Pseudo-first-order rate plots measured at different concentrations of radioligand.

with a slope equal to k_{+1} and an intercept on the ordinate equal to k_{-1} (Fig. 9).

The association and dissociation rate constants determined by this method can be compared to the rate constants determined at a single concentration of ligand to confirm their accuracy. Curvilinear second-order plots and pseudo-first-order plots imply that a simple bimolecular reaction is not adequate to describe the interaction between the ligand and the receptor. More complex kinetics may result from the same factors that yield curvilinear Scatchard plots [2,6–8]. Moreover, under certain conditions, the use of radioligands that are racemic mixtures will result in multiple rate constants for association and dissociation [6]. Even when second-order or pseudo-first-order plots are linear, a more complex interaction is suggested if

the relationship between k_{obs} and concentration of the ligand is nonlinear. A ligand-induced conformational change in the receptor would cause such a relationship; however, detailed kinetics and equilibrium analysis are required to verify this model [6].

Rate of Dissociation

The rate of dissociation is determined by stopping the association of the ligand and receptor and measuring the amount of radioligand that remains bound as a function of time. In practice, the reaction between receptor and ligand is allowed to reach equilibrium, and the forward reaction is stopped by infinite dilution or by the addition of a high concentration of an unlabeled competing ligand. The rate of change of the concentra-

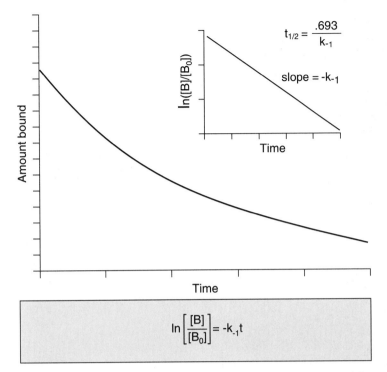

FIG. 10. Determination of dissociation rate. The amount of radioligand that remains bound following the termination of association is measured at various times. **Inset:** Dissociation is plotted according to the integrated form of the first-order rate equation, where $[B]/[B_0]$ is the ratio of the amount of ligand bound at a given time to the amount of radioligand bound just prior to the termination of association. The slope of this linear plot is the negative of the dissociation rate constant k_{-1}.

tion of the receptor-ligand complex is defined by

$$d[B]/dt = -k_{-1}[B] \qquad (9)$$

Integration of Eq. 9 yields

$$\ln[B]/[B_0] = -k_{-1}t \qquad (10)$$

where $[B_0]$ is the concentration of receptor-ligand complex just prior to dilution or the addition of a competing ligand. The dissociation rate constant, k_{-1}, a simple first-order rate constant, is the negative of the slope of a plot of $\ln[B]/[B_0]$ versus time (Fig. 10). A simple bimolecular reaction should be completely reversible; therefore, if the experiment is carried out for a sufficiently long time, the ligand should completely dissociate from the receptor.

Determining the dissociation rate constant has important methodological implications for the study of receptors. The most common technique used to study the binding of radioligands utilizes vacuum filtration to separate bound from free ligand. This process typically involves a 15-sec exposure to buffer during dilution, filtration, and rinsing of the filter. If the dissociation rate is too rapid, as indicated by a high rate constant, there will be a measurable loss of bound ligand during the filtration. This can sometimes be prevented by stopping the reaction and measuring bound ligand at a low temperature.

Nonlinear first-order dissociation plots may result from the same factors that can account for curvilinear second-order and pseudo-first-order association plots. In addition, if k_{-1} is dependent on the method of displacement, then cooperativity in binding should be suspected [9]. A more rapid dissociation by dilution than by competitive displacement suggests positive cooperativity, whereas a more rapid dissociation by displacement than by dilution indicates negative cooperativity. A two-step binding reaction that involves a third component can also cause the dissociation rate to vary with the method of displacement [7,8]. When using competitive displacement, it is sometimes useful to examine effects of both agonists and antagonists.

Once the association and dissociation rate constants have been determined, their ratio can be calculated to provide a kinetically determined estimate of the dissociation constant ($K_d = k_{-1}/k_{+1}$). This value can be compared to the dissociation constant derived from saturation experiments carried out under equilibrium conditions to verify its accuracy and to validate the assumptions made during the analysis. A significant discrepancy between the K_d value determined kinetically and at equilibrium implies that a simple bimolecular reaction is an inadequate model for the system and a more detailed kinetic analysis is required.

INDIRECT BINDING ASSAYS MEASURE INHIBITION OF RADIOLIGAND BINDING TO A RECEPTOR

Equilibrium analysis

The interactions of unlabeled ligands with a receptor can be characterized by studying their ability to inhibit the binding of a radioligand. Since unlabeled ligands are far more numerous than radioligands, indirect binding assays are essential to characterize a population of receptors completely. Traditionally, receptors have been classified in terms of the order of potency of various compounds that either cause or antagonize a functional response. Indirect binding assays make it possible to define the pharmacologi-

cal specificity of a receptor based on the dissociation constants for a variety of compounds determined from inhibition of the binding of a radioligand. Another important use of indirect binding assays is to define the level of nonspecific binding. An accurate definition of nonspecific binding is required for the analysis of both direct and indirect binding data and should be established prior to determining the kinetic and equilibrium properties of the radioligand.

Analysis of Untransformed Data

The simplest model describing the interaction of a radioligand [L] and a competitive inhibitor [I] with a receptor is

$$[L] + [R] \underset{k_{-1}}{\overset{k_{+1}}{\rightleftharpoons}} [B] \tag{11}$$

$$[I] + [R] \underset{k_{-1_i}}{\overset{k_{+1_i}}{\rightleftharpoons}} [B_i] \tag{12}$$

where $[B_i]$ is the concentration of receptor occupied by inhibitor. At equilibrium,

$$[B_i] = \frac{B_{\max}[I]}{[I] + K_i(1 + [L]/K_d)} \tag{13}$$

where K_i is the equilibrium dissociation constant of the competitive inhibitor. If K_d is much greater than the concentration of receptors in the assay, the fraction of receptors occupied by inhibitor f is

$$f = \frac{[B_i]}{B_{\max}} = \frac{[I]}{[I] + IC_{50}} \tag{14}$$

In this equation, IC_{50} is the concentration of inhibitor that blocks 50 percent of the binding measured in the absence of inhibitor.

In a typical competition experiment, the binding of a fixed concentration of radioligand is inhibited by increasing concentrations of an unlabeled ligand. The amount of radioligand that is bound to the receptor, $[B]$, is

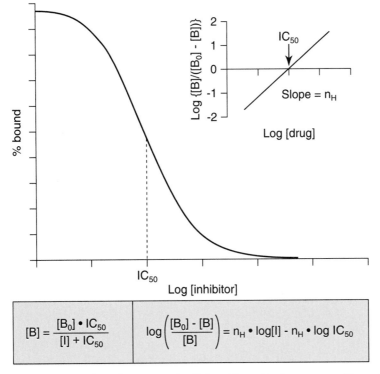

$$[B] = \frac{[B_0] \cdot IC_{50}}{[I] + IC_{50}} \qquad \log\left(\frac{[B_0] - [B]}{[B]}\right) = n_H \cdot \log[I] - n_H \cdot \log IC_{50}$$

FIG. 11.   Analysis of competition data. The amount of radioligand bound in the presence of increasing concentrations of an unlabeled competing ligand is measured. The *left-hand equation* describes the relationship between the amount of radioligand bound [B] and the concentration of inhibitor [I] in terms of the amount of radioligand bound in the absence of inhibitor [B_0] and the concentration of inhibitor that inhibits 50 percent of the binding of the radioligand (IC_{50}). **Inset:** A Hill plot is constructed according to the transformation described by the *right-hand equation.* The slope of this linear plot is equal to the Hill coefficient (n_H) and the intercept is log IC_{50}. The Hill plot deviates from linearity when the amount bound is greater than 90 percent or less than 10 percent of [B_0].

$$[B] = [B_0] - f[B_0] = \frac{[B_0]}{1 + [I]/IC_{50}} \quad (15)$$

$$K_i = \frac{IC_{50}}{1 + [L]/K_d} \quad (16)$$

where [B_0] is the amount of radioligand bound in the absence of inhibitor and $f[B_0]$ is the amount of bound radioligand displaced by inhibitor. Nonlinear regression analysis can be used to fit Eq. 15 to experimental data to provide an estimate of the IC_{50} value (Fig. 11).

Cheng and Prusoff Correction

The equilibrium dissociation constant K_i of an unlabeled competing ligand, [I], is related to the IC_{50} value, as described by Cheng and Prusoff [10]:

Since the concentration of free unlabeled ligand is difficult to determine experimentally, it is approximated by the total concentration of unlabeled ligand in the assay. This calculation is valid if the concentration of receptors is much lower than the dissociation constant of the unlabeled ligand. Furthermore, the amount of radioligand bound should be much less than the total concentration of radioligand; otherwise, a significant change in the concentration of free radioligand will occur in the presence of high concentrations of unlabeled competing ligand. If assay conditions are such that $[L]/K_d \ll 1$, then $K_i \approx IC_{50}$.

Hill Plot

Another useful method for analyzing indirect binding data is the construction of an indirect Hill plot [11]. A plot of $\log(([B_0] - [B])/[B])$ versus $\log[I]$ has a slope value of n_H, which is the apparent Hill coefficient, and an intercept on the abscissa of $\log IC_{50}$ (Fig. 11). Only those concentrations of unlabeled ligand that inhibit between 10 and 90 percent of specific binding are included, since the Hill plot deviates from linearity at the extremes [12]. If the reaction follows mass action principles at equilibrium, the apparent Hill coefficient will be equal to 1. A Hill coefficient significantly different from 1 indicates a more complex interaction between ligand and receptor. This may result from a heterogeneous population of binding sites, a two-step three-component binding system, negative or positive cooperativity between sites, or an incorrect definition of nonspecific binding [12].

It is important to note that addition of a competing ligand increases the time required for a binding reaction to reach equilibrium. Thus the incubation time of a binding assay carried out in the presence of a competing ligand should be greater than the time required for the binding of a radioligand to reach equilibrium in a direct binding assay. Under pseudo-first-order conditions, the time to equilibrium will be increased at most by a factor of $1 + [L]/K_d$ in the presence of a competing ligand [6].

Kinetic analysis

The rates of association and dissociation of an unlabeled competing ligand with a receptor can be determined by measuring the time course of the binding of a radioligand in the presence of a competing ligand. The concentration of receptors that can interact with a radioligand at any given time in the presence of a competing ligand will be reduced by an amount dependent on the rate of approach to equilibrium and the concentration of the competitor. Thus, the presence of competing ligand alters the time course of binding of radioligand. One of two approaches may be taken to determine the rates of association and dissociation of the unlabeled ligand. The kinetic rate constants for the radioligand may be determined in a separate experiment and substituted in the equation for the time course of the binding of the radioligand in the presence of a competing ligand [14]. Nonlinear regression analysis of data obtained in the presence of a competing ligand is used to derive estimates of the kinetic rate constant for the competing ligand. Alternatively, the time course for the binding of the radioligand can be measured in the absence and presence of the competing ligand. Simultaneous nonlinear regression analysis of both sets of data will provide estimates of the kinetic rate constants for both the radioligand and the competing ligand. The validity of this indirect method of determination of kinetic rate constants has been verified for several ligands that bind to β-adrenergic receptors [15].

There are two important limitations to the application of this method. Derivation of the equations assumes that pseudo-first-order conditions prevail, and violation of this assumption will invalidate the results of the analysis [14]. Thus assays should be carried out under conditions where less than 5 percent of the radioligand is bound to receptor at equilibrium. In addition, if binding of the competing ligand reaches equilibrium before the radioligand is bound to an appreciable extent, the kinetic rate constants cannot be resolved statistically [15].

RECEPTOR SUBTYPES

Subtypes of receptors for a variety of neurotransmitters exist in the central nervous system and peripheral tissues

Radioligand binding assays are routinely used to characterize the properties of receptor subtypes in a wide variety of tissues. This characterization is independent of the functional responses elicited by the receptors. The ligand-binding properties are particularly important in the study of the central nervous system because the effects mediated by neurotransmitter receptors are often complex behaviors that are not easily quantified. Under these circumstances, it is difficult to employ classical pharmacological techniques to characterize the relevant receptors. Studies of the binding of radioligands make it possible to discriminate subtypes of receptors that coexist in the same tissue, such as β_1- and β_2-adrenergic receptors. Both subtypes stimulate the enzyme adenylyl cyclase and both contribute to the chronotropic effects of catecholamines on the heart [16]. Characterization of β-adrenergic receptor subtypes based on studies of the chronotropic effects of various drugs would be likely to yield ambiguous results, whereas radioligand binding studies can provide a pharmacological profile for each subtype in a tissue and a measure of the relative proportion of each. Two approaches, based on direct and indirect assays, have been developed to study receptors in tissues that contain multiple receptor subtypes.

Direct binding assays utilize a radioligand selective for one subtype

If a radioligand is completely selective, the density of a single receptor subtype can be determined from a saturation experiment, and its pharmacological profile can be determined from studies of the inhibition of the binding of this radioligand by various competing ligands. Many radioligands have been shown to be highly selective. These include prazosin at the α_1-adrenergic receptor, clonidine at the α_2-adrenergic receptor, α-bungarotoxin at the nicotinic cholinergic receptor, and various benzamides and SCH 23390 at D_2 and D_1 receptors, respectively. If, as is more common, multiple classes of receptors bind a given radioligand with different affinities, nonlinear regression analysis of saturation data provides estimates of the relative densities of the subtypes and their affinities for the radioligand.

Nonlinear Regression Analysis

In addition to the existence of receptor subtypes, it is possible for a radioligand to have a high affinity for receptors of more than one neurotransmitter. For example, both dopamine and serotonin receptors in mammalian brain have a high affinity for [^{3}H]spiroperidol. Multiple populations of receptors or receptor subtypes can be detected in a saturation experiment if the radioligand is selective, i.e., has a significantly lower dissociation constant for its interaction with one class of receptors than for its interaction with another. The interaction of a radioligand with two types of receptors is modeled as the sum of two independent bimolecular reactions. Nonlinear least-squares regression analysis can be used to fit this model to saturation data (Fig. 12) to provide estimates of the dissociation constants and the densities of each receptor population. Results must be interpreted with caution, since all of the factors identified above that lead to curvilinear Scatchard plots also lead to complex saturation curves. The statistical validity of the two-site model is tested by comparing the goodness of fit of the one-site and two-site models. The improvement of fit is estimated from an F-test on the sum of squares of the residuals [19].

Scatchard Transformation

Scatchard transformation of saturation data for the interaction of a selective radioligand with multiple subtypes of receptor will result in a curvilinear plot (Fig. 12, inset). The degree of curvature will be determined by the selectivity of the radioligand and the relative proportions of binding sites with high and low affinities for the radioligand. The greater the selectivity of the radioligand, the more marked will be the curvature observed in the Scatchard plot. Transformed data of this kind can be used to obtain estimates of the parameters of the two subtypes. The depen-

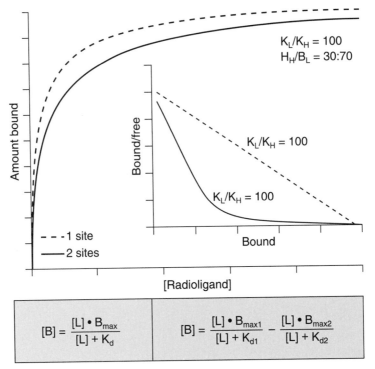

$$[B] = \frac{[L] \cdot B_{max}}{[L] + K_d}$$

$$[B] = \frac{[L] \cdot B_{max1}}{[L] + K_{d1}} - \frac{[L] \cdot B_{max2}}{[L] + K_{d2}}$$

FIG. 12.   Analysis of saturation data obtained with a nonselective and a selective radioligand: (- - -) binding of a nonselective ligand according to the one-site equation *(left)*, (——) binding of a 100-fold selective ($K_L/K_H = 100$) radioligand according to the two-site equation *(right)*, assuming that 30 percent of the receptors have a high affinity for the radioligand. **Inset:** Scatchard transformation of the saturation data results in a linear plot for the nonselective radioligand and a markedly curvilinear plot for the selective ligand.

dent variable, amount of ligand bound, appears, however, on both the abscissa and the ordinate, and therefore individual Scatchard equations cannot be simply added together. Moreover, any error in the measurement of the amount of radioligand bound is propagated from the abscissa to the ordinate. The ratio of bound to free ligand also demonstrates nonuniformity of variance, thus violating a basic assumption of regression analysis [4]. In the presence of multiple classes of receptors, the Scatchard plot is most effectively used to provide visual confirmation of the existence of a heterogeneous population of binding sites.

Indirect binding assays utilize a selective competing unlabeled ligand

Since selective radioligands are not available for most receptor subtypes, an approach has been developed that takes advantage of the availability of numerous selective unlabeled ligands. This method involves studies of the inhibition of the binding of a nonselective radioligand by unlabeled competing selective ligands. The relative proportions of the subtypes and their affinities for each ligand can be determined by nonlinear regression analysis of inhibition curves. Regardless of the ligand used for the determination, the number and relative proportions of the subtypes in a specific tissue should always be the same. In practice, it is usually impossible to discriminate more than two or at most three receptor subtypes on the basis of nonlinear regression analysis. The limits of resolution of nonlinear regression analysis depend on the relative proportions of the subtypes present and on the selectivity of the ligands. These limits have been experimentally evaluated in studies of β-adrenergic receptors by combining various proportions of previously characterized preparations of β₁- and β₂-adrenergic receptors [17]. A mixture of receptor subtypes present in a ratio of 9:1 or 1:9 required ligands that were at least 70-fold selective to resolve the properties of each subtype. Alternatively, a competing ligand that was only six-fold selective could discriminate a 50:50 mixture of receptor subtypes [17].

It is also important to verify that all the ligands are interacting with the receptors according to the principles of mass action. This is accomplished by performing indirect binding assays in tissues that contain only one receptor subtype. Analysis of inhibition data from these tissues should yield Hill coefficients equal to 1. This has been demonstrated for subtypes of the β-adrenergic receptor in studies of the binding of [^{125}I]iodohydroxypindolol in rat cortex, rat liver, and guinea pig ventricle. The rat cortex contains both β₁- and β₂-adrenergic receptors, and studies carried out with selective unlabeled antagonists resulted in markedly biphasic inhibition curves. In contrast, in the guinea pig ventricle, which contains only β₁ receptors, and in the rat liver, which contains only β₂ receptors, each antagonist produced monophasic inhibition curves and Hill coefficients of 1 [18].

If the concept of a receptor is to be meaningful, the properties of the receptor should be conserved in different tissues. Thus, the pharmacological profile of a receptor subtype should be the same, regardless of whether it is derived from tissues that contain a single subtype or those that contain multiple subtypes. This has been demonstrated in the β-adrenergic system where the dissociation constants for seven selective drugs measured in heterogeneous and homogeneous tissues were compared. The correlation coefficient for both β₁ and β₂ receptors for heterogeneous, compared to homogeneous, tissues was found to be 0.99 [18].

Nonlinear Regression Analysis

A Hill coefficient less than 1 often results from the presence of multiple classes of receptors. If an unlabeled competing ligand is selective for one of the subtypes—if it has a measurably lower dissociation constant for one population of sites than for the other—then inhibition curves will be shallow and Hill coefficients will be less than 1. Inhibition of the binding of a nonselective radioligand to two subtypes of receptor is modeled as the sum of two independent competition reactions. Nonlinear regression analysis is used to provide estimates of [B_0] and IC$_{50}$ for each subtype of receptor (Fig. 13). This analysis assumes that the interaction of both the radioligand and the competing ligand with each receptor subtype follows the principles of mass action. The improvement in fit with the two-site model compared to the one-site model is determined from the F value calculated from the residual sum of squares [20].

Accurate estimates of the proportion of each class of receptors and the affinity of each class of site for a selective competing ligand will be obtained only if the radioligand is entirely nonselective. Selectivity of only two- to threefold can markedly influence the results of subtype analysis [21]. The conclusion that a radioligand is nonselective is usually based on analysis of a saturation binding curve, as discussed above; however, the ability of these analytical methods to determine the selectivity of a radioligand is limited. Even under ideal conditions, selectivity is unlikely to be detected reliably unless the two classes of binding sites differ in their affinity for the radioligand by at least five- to sevenfold. Such slight selectivity can be detected and quantitated by the simultaneous analysis of multiple inhibition curves. This approach requires that a series of inhibition curves with a highly selective competing ligand be generated in the presence of increasing concentrations of radioligand. Simultaneous nonlinear regression analysis of these multiple inhibition curves provides ac-

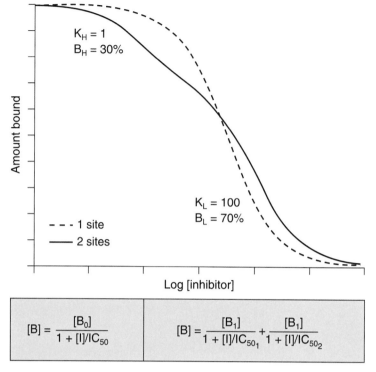

FIG. 13. Analysis of untransformed competition data. The inhibition of the binding of a nonselective radioligand by a selective and a nonselective competing ligand is illustrated: (- - -) inhibition resulting from a nonselective ligand *(left-hand equation)*; (——) inhibition by a 100-fold selective (K_L/K_H) competing ligand, assuming that 30 percent of the receptors have a high affinity for the competing ligand *(right-hand equation)*.

curate estimates of the density of each class of binding sites and the affinity of each class of sites for the labeled and unlabeled ligand. This method has been used to detect a three-fold selectivity of [^{125}I]iodopindolol for β_2-adrenergic receptors [21].

Interpretations of curvilinear Scatchard or Hofstee plots alternative to receptor heterogeneity

Ternary Complex Formation

A Hill coefficient less than 1 for the interaction of an agonist with a receptor can result from a two-step reaction that involves three components and leads to the formation of a ternary complex [8,22]. According to this reaction scheme, an agonist [H] binds to the receptor [R]:

$$[H] + [R] \rightleftharpoons [HR] \qquad (17)$$

The agonist occupies the receptor according to the principles of mass action as described above. The low-affinity receptor-agonist complex [HR] then interacts with a third component in the membrane, [N], to form a high-affinity ternary complex [HRN]:

$$(HR) + (N) \rightleftharpoons [HRN] \qquad (18)$$

Only one class of receptors is required in this two-step model. The receptors can exist in two different states, however, with distinct affinities for agonists. The extent of formation of the ternary complex is limited by the concentration of [N] in the membrane relative to that of [R] and by the affinity of [HR] for [N]. These factors also affect the apparent affinity of the receptor for the agonist and the shape of the agonist competition curve.

This ternary complex model appears to describe interactions of agonists with receptors in a number of systems in which receptors are linked to the stimulation or inhibition of adenylyl cyclase activity (see Chap. 21) or to the turnover of phosphoinositides (see Chap. 20). For example, the interaction of agonists with β-adrenergic receptors results in the formation of a high-affinity ternary complex composed of agonist, β receptor, and guanine nucleotide-binding protein [13]. The formation of this ternary complex appears to be a required step in the stimulation of adenylyl cyclase activity. Addition of a guanine nucleotide like GTP or $G_{pp}NH_p$ appears to destabilize the ternary complex so that only the initial interaction of the agonist with the receptor can be detected. In the presence of GTP, the affinity of the receptor for the agonist is decreased, and the slope of the inhibition curve is increased. Such effects of guanine nucleotides on the interactions of agonists with receptors have been reported for many receptors including β-adrenergic receptors, dopamine receptors, and α-adrenergic receptors. Thus, in systems coupled to the enzyme adenylyl cyclase, addition of GTP in radioligand binding assays appears to prevent the accumulation of ternary complex and permits characterization of the initial reaction between agonist and receptor.

Incorrect Definition of Nonspecific Binding

One of the most common errors in the interpretation of binding data is an incorrect definition of nonspecific binding, as discussed above. Such errors can be avoided by careful examination of the displacement curve of the competing ligand used to define nonspecific binding. The binding of the radioligand should decrease to a plateau at high concentrations of competing ligand, and this plateau should be the same for several different agonists and antagonists. A correct definition of nonspecific binding is an absolute re-

quirement for the quantitative measurement of receptor subtypes.

ACKNOWLEDGMENTS

During the preparation of this manuscript, the authors were supported by USPHS grants NS 18591, NS 18479, and GM 34781.

REFERENCES

1. Snyder, S. Drug and neurotransmitter receptors in the brain. *Science* 224:22–31, 1984.
2. Molinoff, P. B., Wolfe, B. B., and Weiland, G. A. Quantitative analysis of drug-receptor interactions. II. Determination of the properties of receptor subtypes. *Life Sci.* 29:427–443, 1981.
3. Scatchard, G. The attractions of proteins for small molecules and ions. *Ann. N. Y. Acad. Sci.* 51:660–672, 1949.
4. Munson, P. J., and Rodbard, D. LIGAND: A versatile computerized approach for characterization of ligand-binding systems. *Anal. Biochem.* 107:220–239, 1980.
5. Boeynaems, J. M., and Dumont, J. E. Quantitative analysis of the binding of ligands to their receptors. *J. Cyclic Nucleotide Res.* 1: 123–142, 1976.
6. Weiland, G. A., and Molinoff, P. B. Quantitative analysis of drug-receptor interactions. I. Determination of kinetic and equilibrium properties. *Life Sci.* 29:313–330, 1981.
7. Boeynaems, J. M., and Dumont, J. E. The two step model of ligand-receptor interaction. *Mol. Cell. Endocrinol.* 7:33–47, 1977.
8. Jacobs, S., and Cuatrecasas, P. The mobile receptor hypothesis and "cooperativity" of hormone binding. Application to insulin. *Biochem. Biophys. Acta* 433:482–495, 1976.
9. DeLean, A., and Rodbard, D. Kinetics of cooperative binding. In R. D. O'Brien (ed.), *The Receptors, A Comprehensive Treatise.* New York: Plenum, 1979, pp. 143–192.
10. Cheng, Y. C., and Prusoff, W. H. Relationship between the inhibition constant (K_i) and the concentration of inhibitor which causes 50% inhibition (I_{50}) of an enzymatic reaction. *Biochem. Pharmacol.* 22:3099–3108, 1973.

11. Hill, A. V. The possible effects of the aggregation of the molecules of haemoglobin on its dissociation curves. *J. Physiol. (Lond.)* 40: iv–vii, 1910.

12. Cornish-Bowden, A., and Koshland, D. E. Diagnostic uses of the Hill (Logit and Nernst) plots. *J. Mol. Biol.* 95:201–212, 1975.

13. Limbird, L. E. *Cell Surface Receptors: A Short Course on Theory and Methods.* Boston: Martinus Nijhoff, 1985, pp. 51–96.

14. Motulsky, H. J., and Mahan, L. C. The kinetics of competitive radioligand binding predicted by the laws of mass action. *Mol. Pharmacol.* 25: 1–9, 1984.

15. Contreras, M. L., Wolfe, B. B., and Molinoff, P. B. Kinetic analysis of the interactions of agonists and antagonists with beta adrenergic receptors. *J. Pharmacol. Exp. Ther.* 239: 136–143, 1986.

16. Liang, B. T., Frame, L. H., and Molinoff, P. B. β_2-Adrenergic receptors contribute to catecholamine-stimulated shortening of action potential duration in dog atrial muscle. *Proc. Natl. Acad. Sci. U. S. A.* 82:4521–4525, 1985.

17. DeLean, A., Hancock, A. A., and Lefkowitz R. J. Validation and statistical analysis of a computer modelling method for quantitative analysis of radioligand binding data for mixtures of pharmacological receptor subtypes. *Mol. Pharmacol.* 21:5–16, 1982.

18. Minneman, K. P., Hedberg, A., and Molinoff, P. B. Comparison of *beta* adrenergic receptor subtypes in mammalian tissues. *J. Pharmacol. Exp. Ther.* 211:502–508, 1979.

19. McGonigle, P., Huff, R. M., and Molinoff, P. B. A comprehensive method for the quantitative determination of dopamine receptor subtypes. *Ann. N. Y. Acad. Sci.* 430:77–90, 1984.

20. Snedecor, G. W., and Cochran, W. G. *Statistical Methods.* Ames, IA: Iowa State University Press, 1967.

21. McGonigle, P., Neve, K. A., and Molinoff, P. B. A quantitative method of analyzing the interaction of slightly selective radioligands with multiple receptor subtypes. *Mol. Pharmacol.* 30:329–337, 1986.

22. De Haën, C. The non-stoichiometric floating receptor model for hormone sensitive adenylyl cyclase. *J. Theor. Biol.* 58:383–400, 1976.

CHAPTER 11

Acetylcholine

PALMER TAYLOR AND JOAN HELLER BROWN

Basic Neurochemistry: Molecular, Cellular, and Medical Aspects, 5th Ed., edited by G. J. Siegel et al. Published by Raven Press, Ltd., New York, 1994. Correspondence to Palmer Taylor and Joan Heller Brown, Department of Pharmacology, 0636, University of California, San Diego, La Jolla, California 92093.

231

There is considerable evidence that acetylcholine (ACh) arrived within the evolutionary scheme long before the design of the nervous system and functional synapses. Bacteria, fungi, protozoa, and plants store ACh and possess biosynthetic and degradative capacities for turnover of the molecule. Even in higher systems, ACh distribution is far wider than the nervous system. For example, ACh is found in the cornea, certain ciliated epithelia, the spleen of ungulates, and in the human placenta [1]. Although definitive evidence is lacking, ACh has been proposed to play a role in development and tissue differentiation.

Acetylcholine was first proposed as a mediator of cellular function by Hunt in 1907, and in 1914 Dale [2] pointed out that its action closely mimicked the response of parasympathetic nerve stimulation (see also Chap. 9). Loewi, in 1921, provided clear evidence for ACh release by nerve stimulation. Separate receptors that explained the variety of actions of ACh became apparent in Dale's early experiments [2]. The nicotinic ACh receptor was the first transmitter receptor to be purified and to have its primary structure determined [3,4]. Over the past decade the primary structures of several subtypes of both nicotinic and muscarinic receptors have been ascertained as have the structures of cholinesterases, choline transporters, and choline acetyltransferase.

CHEMISTRY OF ACETYLCHOLINE

Torsional rotation in the ACh molecule can occur around bonds τ_1, τ_2, and τ_3 (Fig. 1). Since the methyl groups are symmetrically disposed around τ_3, and constraints may be placed on τ_1 by the planar acetoxy group, the most important torsion angle determining ACh conformation in solution is τ_2. A view from the β-methylene carbon of the molecule (Fig. 1) shows the lowest energy configurations around τ_2. Nuclear magnetic resonance (NMR) studies indicate that the *gauche* conformation is predominant in solution [5,6]. Studies of the activities of rigid analogs of ACh suggest that the *trans* conformation may be the active conformation at muscarinic receptors [7], while recent results of studies with NMR show that the acetoxy and quaternary nitrogens in the bound state of ACh are too close together for this conformation to exist when ACh is bound to the nicotinic receptor [6]. Hence the bound conformations of this flexible molecule appear to differ substantially with receptor subtype. This finding should not emerge as a great surprise, since it has been known for years that the structural modifications that enhance or diminish activity on muscarinic receptors are very different from those modifications that influence activity on nicotinic receptors [8].

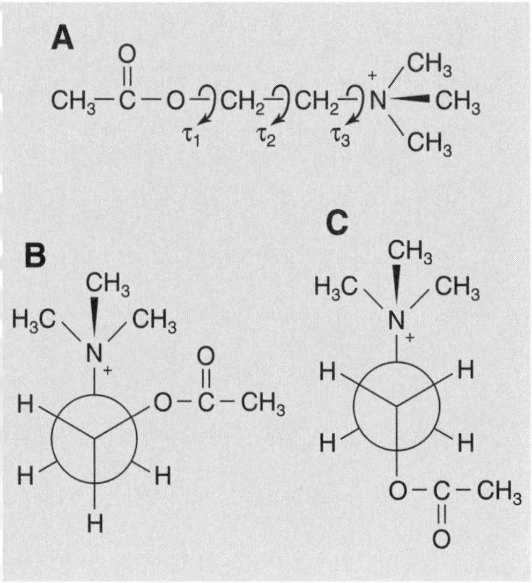

ORGANIZATION OF THE CHOLINERGIC NERVOUS SYSTEM

Chemical specificity of acetylcholine receptors

The subtyping of the receptors in the cholinergic nervous system was initially based on the pharmacological activity of two alkaloids: nicotine and muscarine (Fig. 2). This classification occurred long before the structures of these naturally occurring agonists were determined (Fig. 3). The greatly different activities of the antagonists atropine on muscarinic receptors and *d*-tubocurarine on nicotinic receptors further supported the argument that multiple classes of receptors exist for ACh. It was subsequently found that all nicotinic receptors are not identical. Those nicotinic receptors found in the neuromuscular junction, sometimes denoted as N_1 receptors, show selectivity for phenyltrimethylammonium as an agonist; elicit membrane depolarization in the presence of bisquaternary agents, with decamethonium being the most potent; are preferentially blocked by the competitive antagonist *d*-tubocurarine; and are irreversibly blocked by the snake α-toxins. Nicotinic receptors in ganglia, N_2 receptors, are preferentially stimulated by 1,1-dimethyl-4-phenylpiperazinium; competitively blocked by trimethaphan; blocked by bisquaternary agents, with hexamethonium being most potent; and are resistant to the snake α-toxins [9]. Not only do the ganglionic and neuromuscular types of the nicotinic receptors differ in primary structure, but each of these receptors also presents several subtypes.

FIG. 1.   Structure of acetylcholine. **A:** The three torsion angles τ_1, τ_2, τ_3. **B:** Newman projection of the *gauche* conformation. **C:** Newman projection of the *trans* conformation. The molecule is viewed in the plane of the paper from the left side and the bond angles around τ_2 compared.

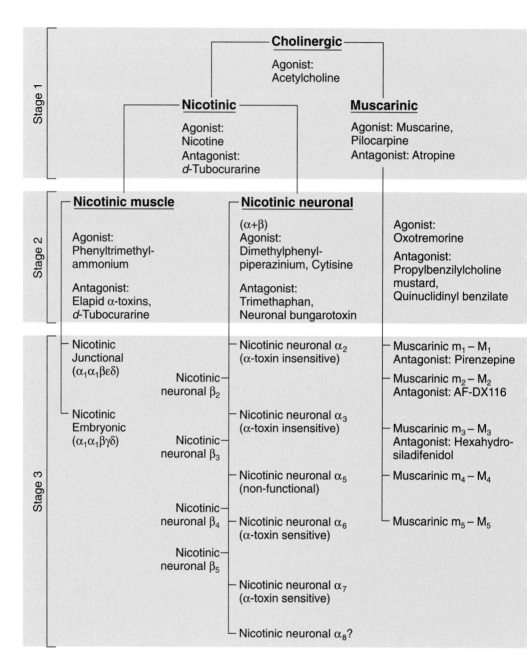

FIG. 2. Classification of cholinergic receptors. The diagram shows a historical classification of receptors analyzed on the basis of (stage 1) distinct responses with crude alkaloids, (stage 2) the partial resolution of receptor subtypes with chemically synthesized agonists and antagonists, and (stage 3) the distinction of primary structures of the receptors primarily through recombinant DNA techniques.

FIG. 3. Structure of compounds important to the classification of receptor subtypes at cholinergic synapses. Compounds are subdivided as nicotinic (N) and muscarinic (M). The compounds interacting with nicotinic receptors are further subdivided according to whether they are neuromuscular (N_1) or ganglionic selective (N_2). Those compounds with muscarinic subtype selectivity (M_1, M_2, M_3) are also noted.

Nicotinic and muscarinic agonists

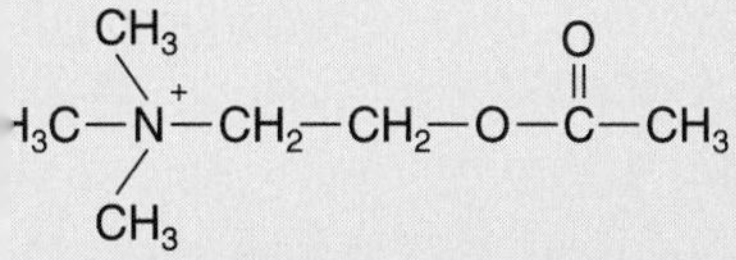

Acetylcholine (N + M)

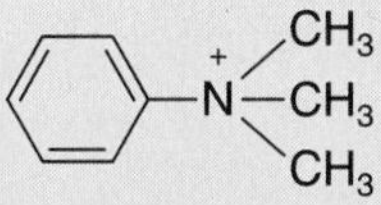

Phenyltrimethylammonium (N_1)

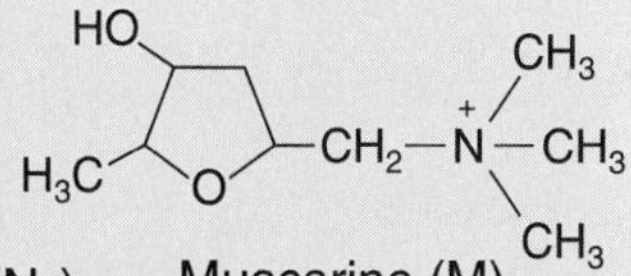

Muscarine (M)

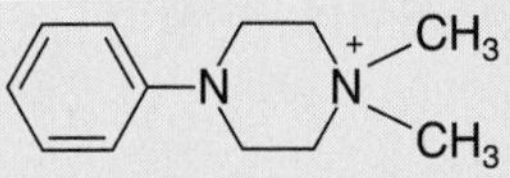

1,1-Dimethyl-4-phenylpiperazinium (N_2)

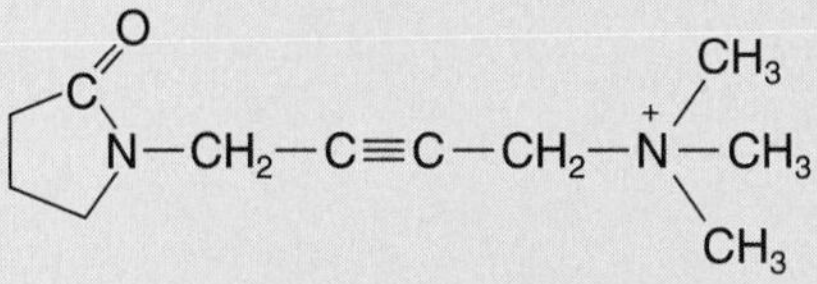

Oxotremorine-M (M)

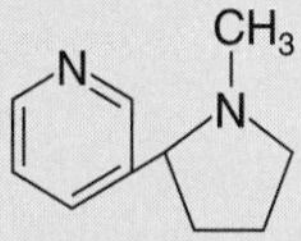

Nicotine ($N_1 + N_2$)

Nicotinic antagonists

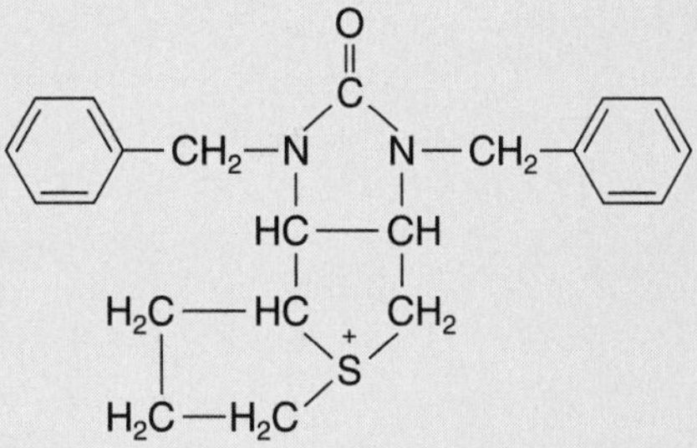

Trimethaphan (N_2)

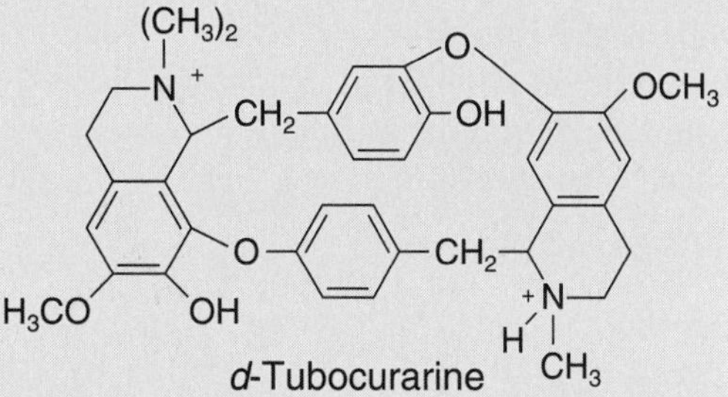

d-Tubocurarine

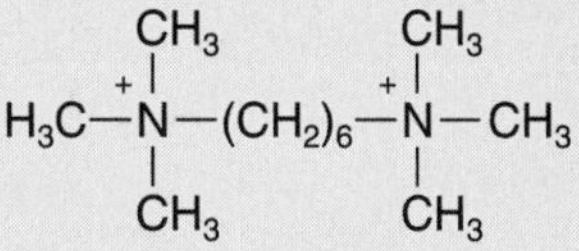

Hexamethonium (N_2)

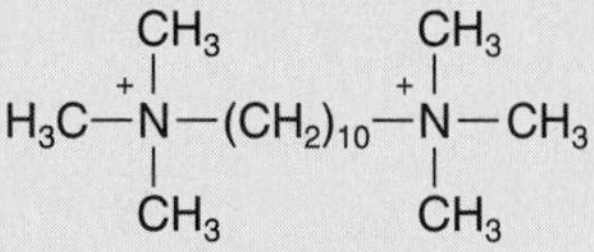

Decamethonium (N_1)

Muscarinic antagonists

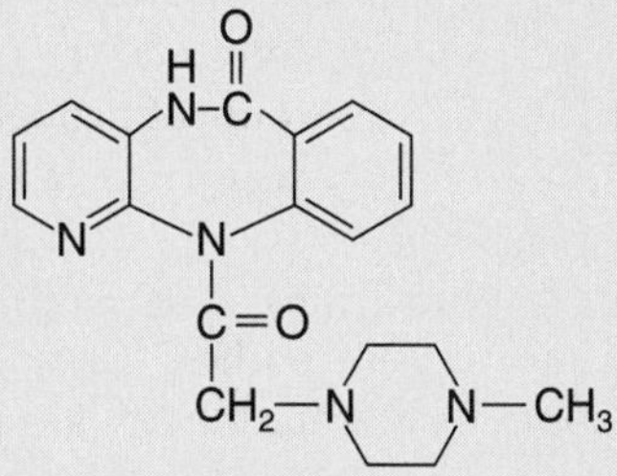

Pirenzepine (M_1)

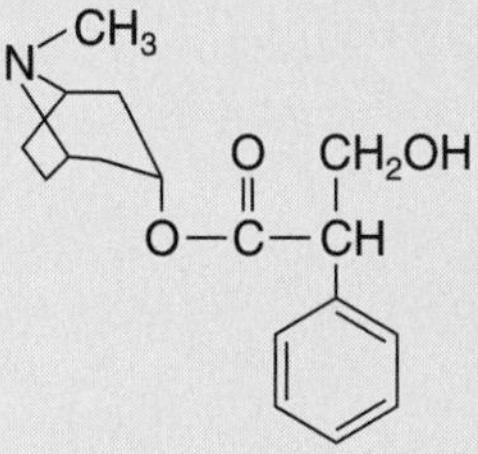

Atropine (M)

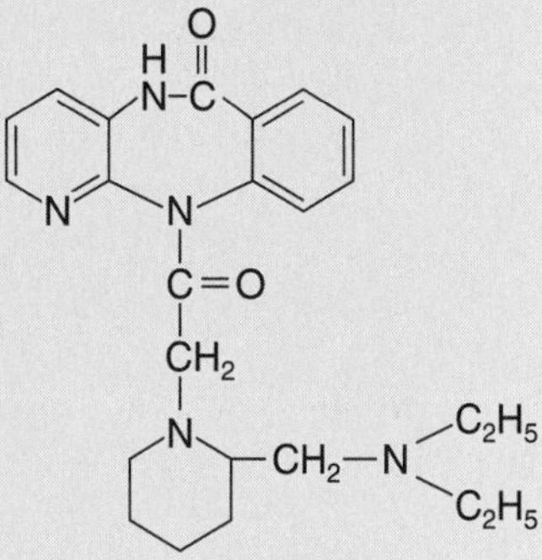

AF-DX116 (M_2)

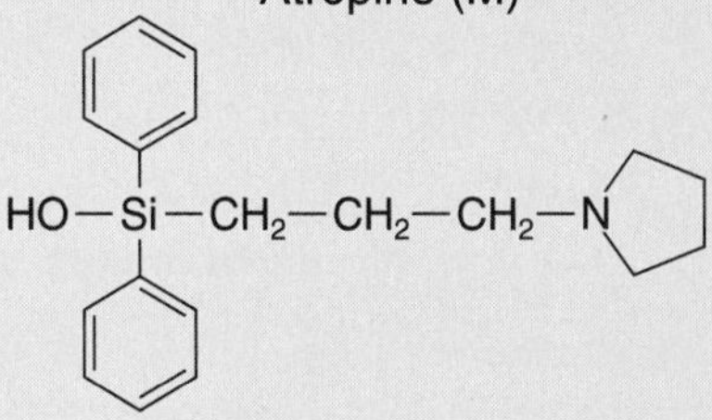

Hexahydrosiladifenidol (M_3)

Muscarinic receptors also exhibit distinct subtypes. The antagonist pirenzepine (PZ) has the highest affinity for one subtype, termed M_1, which is found mainly in neuronal tissues. Another antagonist, AF-DX116, has the highest affinity for M_2 receptors, the predominant muscarinic receptor subtype in mammalian heart. Two antagonists, 2-(4,4'-diacetoxydiphenylmethyl)pyridine (4-DAMP) and hexahydrosiladifenidol, are relatively selective for M_3 receptors present in smooth muscle and glands, whereas himbacine exhibits high affinity for M_4 receptors.

The intrinsic complexity and the multiplicity of cholinergic receptors became evident after elucidation of their primary structures

In the central nervous system, at least six different sequences of α-subunits of the nicotinic receptor have been identified [10]. Expression of the cloned genes encoding the individual α-subunits shows a different sensitivity toward various toxins and agonists.

At least five distinct muscarinic receptor genes have been cloned and sequenced. The genes are called m_1 to m_5. The m_1 to m_4 clones correlate with the m_1 to m_4 receptors identified pharmacologically. The subtypes differ in their ability to couple to different G proteins and hence elicit distinct cellular signaling events. The muscarinic and nicotinic receptor subtypes exhibit distinct regional locations of their mRNAs based on *in situ* hybridization. (The subtypes of receptors and gene families are discussed later in this chapter.)

From these considerations, the first two stages of cholinergic receptor classification are evident. Dale [2] was able to distinguish nicotinic and muscarinic receptor subtypes with crude alkaloids. Chemical synthesis and structure-activity relationships clearly revealed that nicotinic and muscarinic receptors were heterogeneous, but could not come close to uncovering the true diversity of receptor subtypes. Analysis of subtypes now comes from molecular cloning making possible the classification of receptors on the basis of primary structure (Fig. 2).

FUNCTIONAL ASPECTS OF CHOLINERGIC NEUROTRANSMISSION

The individual subtypes of receptors often show discrete anatomical locations in the peripheral nervous system, and this has further facilitated their classification. Nicotinic receptors are found in peripheral ganglia and skeletal muscle. Upon innervation of skeletal muscle, receptors congregate in the junctional or postsynaptic end-plate area. Upon denervation or in noninnervated embryonic muscle, the receptors are distributed across the surface of the muscle, and these extrajunctional receptors are synthesized and degraded rapidly. Junctional receptors exhibit far slower rates of turnover. Small differences in the binding of *d*-tubocurarine have been distinguished in studies of junctional and extrajunctional receptors. The basis for this difference appears to be a distinct subunit composition.

Ganglionic nicotinic receptors are found on postsynaptic neurons in both parasympathetic and sympathetic ganglia and in the adrenal gland. Ganglionic nicotinic receptors appear in tissues of neural crest embryonic origin and exhibit identical properties in sympathetic and parasympathetic ganglia.

Muscarinic receptors are responsible for postganglionic parasympathetic neurotransmission. Some sympathetic responses, such as sweating and piloerection, are also mediated through muscarinic receptors.

Both muscarinic and nicotinic responses are found in cortical and subcortical areas of the brain

A few specific central cholinergic pathways have been characterized. For example, Renshaw cells in the spinal cord play a role in modulating motoneuron activity by a feedback mechanism. Stimulation of Renshaw cells occurs through branches of the motoneuron, and the transmitter is ACh acting on nicotinic receptors. Both nicotinic and muscarinic receptors are widespread in the central nervous system. Some areas of the brain such as the optic tectum rely primarily on nicotinic responses. Muscarinic receptors with a high affinity for PZ appear to predominate in the hippocampus and cerebral cortex, whereas receptors with a low affinity for PZ predominate in the cerebellum and brainstem. The mapping of cholinergic pathways in the brain continues to be actively pursued and relies on several techniques [11]. Histochemical studies that employ antibodies selective for choline acetyltransferase and receptor autoradiography with labeled ligands have produced detailed maps of the central nervous system. In addition, the nerve cell bodies containing the mRNA encoding these proteins have also been defined through *in situ* hybridization with a cDNA or antisense mRNA. Studies involving iontophoretic application of transmitter, local stimulation, and intracellular or cell surface measurements of responses establish appropriate functional correlates.

Neurotransmission in autonomic ganglia is more complex than depolarization mediated by a single transmitter

The primary electrophysiological event following preganglionic nerve stimulation is the rapid depolarization of postsynaptic sites by released ACh acting on nicotinic receptors. Their activation gives rise to an initial excitatory postsynaptic potential (EPSP), which is due to an inward current through a cation channel (see Chaps. 4 and 9). This mechanism is virtually identical to that in the neuromuscular junction, with an immediate onset of the depolarization and decay over a few milliseconds. Nicotinic antagonists such as trimethaphan competitively block ganglionic transmission, whereas agents

such as hexamethonium produce blockade by occluding the channel. An action potential is generated in the postganglionic nerve when the initial EPSP attains a critical amplitude.

Several secondary events amplify or suppress this signal. These include the slow EPSP; the late, slow EPSP; and an inhibitory postsynaptic potential (IPSP). The slow EPSP is generated by ACh acting on muscarinic receptors and is blocked by atropine or the more selective antagonist PZ. It has a latency of approximately 1 sec and a duration of 30 to 60 sec. The late, slow EPSP can last for several minutes and is mediated by peptides found in ganglia, including substance P, angiotensin, leutinizing hormone-releasing hormone (LHRH), and the enkephalins. The slow EPSP and late, slow EPSP result from decreased K^+ conductance and are believed to regulate the sensitivity of the postsynaptic neuron to repetitive depolarization [12]. The IPSP seems to be mediated by the catecholamines, dopamine, and/or norepinephrine. The IPSP is blocked by α-adrenergic antagonists and atropine. Acetylcholine released from presynaptic terminals may act on a catecholamine-containing interneuron to stimulate the release of norepinephrine or dopamine. As in the case of the slow EPSP, the IPSP has a longer latency and duration of action than the fast EPSP. These secondary events vary with the individual ganglia and are believed to modulate the sensitivity to the primary event. Hence, drugs that selectively block the slow EPSP, such as atropine, will diminish the efficiency of ganglionic transmission rather than completely eliminating it. Similarly, drugs such as muscarine and the ganglion-selective muscarinic agonist McN-A–343 are not thought of as primary ganglionic stimulants. Rather, they enhance the initial EPSP under conditions of repetitive stimulation.

Since parasympathetic and sympathetic ganglia exhibit comparable sensitivities to nicotine and ACh in producing the initial EPSP, the pharmacological action of ganglionic stimulants depends on the profile of in-

TABLE 1.   Predominance of sympathetic or parasympathetic tone at effector sites; effects of autonomic ganglionic blockade

Site	Predominant tone	Primary effects of ganglionic blockade
Arterioles	Sympathetic (adrenergic)	Vasodilation; increased peripheral blood flow; hypotension
Veins	Sympathetic (adrenergic)	Dilation; pooling of blood; decreased venous return; decreased cardiac output
Heart	Parasympathetic (cholinergic)	Tachycardia
Iris	Parasympathetic (cholinergic)	Mydriasis
Ciliary muscle	Parasympathetic (cholinergic)	Cycloplegia (focus to far vision)
Gastrointestinal tract	Parasympathetic (cholinergic)	Reduced tone and motility of smooth muscle; constipation; decreased gastric and pancreatic secretions
Urinary bladder	Parasympathetic (cholinergic)	Urinary retention
Salivary glands	Parasympathetic (cholinergic)	Xerostomia
Sweat glands	Sympathetic (cholinergic)	Anhidrosis

nervation to particular organs or tissues (Table 1). For example, blood vessels are only innervated by the sympathetic nervous system; thus, ganglionic stimulation should only produce vasoconstriction. Similarly, the pharmacological effects of ganglionic blockade will depend on which component of the autonomic nervous system is exerting predominant tone at the effector organ. The response of systematically administered ACh is characteristic of stimulation of postganglionic effector sites rather than of the ganglia. Only when muscarinic receptors are blocked with atropine or an M_2 antagonist are the effects of stimulation of ganglia by administered ACh observed. This is a consequence of the greater abundance of muscarinic receptors at effector sites in innervated tissues and the relatively poor blood flow to ganglia.

In addition to their presence in the central nervous system and ganglia, muscarinic receptors are widely distributed at postsynaptic parasympathetic effector sites

Muscarinic receptors are found in visceral smooth muscle, in cardiac muscle, in secretory glands, and in the endothelial cells of the vasculature. Except for endothelial cells, each of these sites receives cholinergic innervation. Responses can be excitatory or inhibitory, depending on the tissue. Even within

a single tissue the responses may vary. For example, muscarinic stimulation causes gastrointestinal smooth muscle to depolarize and contract, except at sphincters, where hyperpolarization and relaxation are seen (Table 2). Smooth muscle in many tissues that are innervated by the cholinergic nervous system exhibits intrinsic electrical and/or mechanical activity. This activity is modified rather than initiated by cholinergic nerve stimulation. Cardiac muscle and smooth muscle exhibit spikes of electrical activity that are propagated between cells. These spikes are initiated by rhythmic fluctuations in resting membrane potential. In intestinal smooth muscle, cholinergic stimulation will cause a partial depolarization and increase the frequency by spike production. In contrast, cholinergic stimulation of atria will decrease the generation of spikes through hyperpolarization of the membrane.

Membrane depolarization typically results from an increase in Na^+ conductance. In addition, Ca^{2+} fluxes across the cell membrane, and the mobilization of intracellular Ca^{2+} from the endoplasmic or sarcoplasmic reticulum appear to be elicited by ACh acting on muscarinic receptors (see Chap. 20). The increase in intracellular free Ca^{2+} is involved in activation of contractile, metabolic, and secretory events. Stimulation of muscar-

TABLE 2.   Effects of ACh stimulation on peripheral tissues

Tissue	*Effects of ACh*
Vasculature (endothelial cells)	Release of endothelium-derived relaxing factor (nitric oxide) and vasodilation
Eye iris (pupillae sphincter muscle)	Contraction and miosis
Ciliary muscle	Contraction and accommodation of lens to near vision
Salivary glands and lacrimal glands	Secretion—thin and watery
Bronchi	Constriction; increased secretions
Heart	Bradycardia, decreased conduction (atrioventricular block at high doses)–small negative inotropic action
Gastrointestinal tract	Increased tone; increased gastrointestinal secretions; relaxation at sphincters
Urinary bladder	Contraction of detrusor muscle; relaxation of the sphincter
Sweat glands	Diaphoresis
Reproductive tract, male	Erection
Uterus	Variable, dependent on hormone influence

inic receptors has also been linked to changes in cyclic nucleotide concentrations. Reductions in cyclic AMP (cAMP) concentrations and increases in cyclic GMP (cGMP) concentrations are typical responses (see Chap. 21). The cyclic nucleotides may facilitate contraction or relaxation, depending on the particular tissue. Inhibitory responses also are associated with hyperpolarization, and this is a consequence of an increased K^+ conductance. Increases in K^+ conductance may be mediated by a direct receptor linkage to a K^+ channel or by increases in intracellular Ca^{2+}, which in turn activate K^+ channels. The mechanisms through which muscarinic receptors might couple to multiple cellular responses are considered later.

Stimulation of the motoneuron for skeletal muscle results in the release of acetylcholine and contraction of the skeletal muscle fibers

Contraction and associated electrical events can be produced by the intra-arterial injection of ACh close to the muscle. Since skeletal muscle does not possess inherent myogenic tone, the tone of apparently resting muscle is maintained by spontaneous and intermittent release of ACh. The consequences of spontaneous release at the motor end-plate of skeletal muscle are small depolarizations from the quantized release of ACh—miniature end-plate potentials (MEPPs) [13] (see Chaps. 9 and 32). Decay times for the MEPPs range between 1 and 2 msec, a value of about the same magnitude as the mean channel open time seen with ACh stimulation of the receptor. Stimulation of the motoneuron results in the release of several hundred quanta of ACh. The summation of MEPPs gives rise to a postsynaptic excitatory potential (PSEP), also termed *motor end-plate potential.* A sufficiently large and abrupt potential change at the end-plate will elicit an action potential by activating voltage-sensitive Na^+ channels. The action potential propagates in two-dimensional space across the surface of the muscle to release Ca^{2+} and elicit contraction. The PSEP may therefore be thought of as a generator potential. It is found only in junctional regions and arises from the opening of the receptor channel. Normal resting potentials in end-plates are about -70 mV. The PSEP causes the end-plate to depolarize partially to about -55 mV. It is the rapid and transient change from -70 to -55 mV in localized areas of the end-plate that triggers action potential generation [13].

Competitive blocking agents such as *d*-tubocurarine cause muscle paralysis by preventing access of acetylcholine to its binding site on the receptor

The end-plate potential with competitive blockade is maintained at −70 mV. Without frequent PSEPs, action potentials are not triggered, and there is flaccid paralysis of the muscle. The actions of competitive blocking agents can be surmounted by excess ACh. Depolarizing neuromuscular blocking agents, such as decamethonium or succinylcholine, produce depolarization of the end-plate such that the end-plate potential is found to reside at −55 mV. The high concentrations of depolarizing agent that are maintained in this synapse do not allow regions of the end-plate to repolarize, as would occur with a labile transmitter such as ACh. Since it is the transition between −70 and −55 mV that triggers the action potential, flaccid paralysis will also occur with a depolarizing block [9]. Excess ACh will not reverse the paralysis by depolarizing blocking agents. As might be expected if depolarization occurs in a nonuniform manner in microscopic areas within individual end-plates and in individual motor units, the onset of depolarization blockade is characterized by muscle twitching and fasciculations that are not evident in competitive block. Once paralysis occurs, the overall pharmacological actions of competitive and depolarizing blocking agents are similar, yet intracellular measurements of end-plate potential can distinguish these two classes of agents.

SYNTHESIS, STORAGE, AND RELEASE OF ACETYLCHOLINE

Acetylcholine is synthesized from its two immediate precursors, choline and acetyl coenzyme A

This reaction is a single step catalyzed by the enzyme choline acetyltransferase (ChAT) (EC 2.3.1.6):

$$\text{Choline} + \text{Acetyl coenzyme A} \rightleftharpoons$$

$$\text{Acetylcholine} + \text{Coenzyme A}$$

This enzymatic activity was first assayed in a cell-free preparation by Nachmansohn and Machado in 1943. ChAT has subsequently been purified and cloned from several sources [14]. The purification of ChAT has allowed production of specific antibodies, and it is now possible to carry out immunohistochemical mapping of cholinergic pathways using this enzyme as a specific marker. Whereas acetylcholinesterase, the enzyme responsible for degradation of ACh, is produced by cells containing cholinoreceptive sites as well as in cholinergic neurons, ChAT is found in the nervous system specifically at sites where ACh synthesis takes place. For example, the enzyme is found in relatively high concentration in the caudate nucleus but in relatively low amounts in the cerebellum. Within cholinergic neurons, ChAT is concentrated in nerve terminals, although it is also present in axons, where it is transported from its site of synthesis in the soma. When subcellular fractionation studies are carried out, ChAT is recovered in the synaptosomal fraction, and within synaptosomes it is primarily cytoplasmic. It has been suggested that ChAT is also bound to the outside of the storage vesicle under physiological conditions and that ACh synthesized in that location may be favorably situated to enter the vesicle.

Brain ChAT has a K_D for choline of approximately 1 mM and a K_D for acetyl coenzyme A (CoA) of approximately 10 μM. The activity of the isolated enzyme, assayed in the presence of optimal concentrations of cofactors and substrates, appears far greater than that reflected by the rate at which choline is converted to ACh *in vivo*. This suggests that the full activity of ChAT is not expressed *in vivo*. Inhibitors of ChAT do not decrease ACh synthesis when used *in vivo*; this may reflect a failure to achieve a sufficient local concentration of inhibitor but also suggests that this step is not rate limiting in the synthesis of ACh.

The acetyl CoA used for ACh synthesis in mammalian brain comes from pyruvate formed from glucose. It is uncertain how the acetyl CoA, generally thought to be formed at the inner membrane of the mitochondria, accesses the cytoplasmic ChAT, and it is possible that this is a rate-limiting step.

Acetylcholine formation is limited by the intracellular concentration of choline, which is determined by uptake of choline into the nerve ending

Choline is present in the plasma at a concentration of about 10 μM. A "low-affinity" choline uptake system with a K_m of 10 to 100 μM is present in all tissues, but cholinergic neurons also have an Na$^+$-dependent "high-affinity" choline uptake system with a K_m for choline of 1 to 5 μM [15]. The gene for a high-affinity choline transporter has recently been cloned from the rat central nervous system [16]. Its mRNA is found primarily in brain and spinal cord, with smaller amounts in heart. Although its amino acid sequence is indicative of 12 candidate membrane-spanning regions, a feature of other neurotransmitter transporter molecules, expression of the cDNA has not yielded the same kinetic parameters as the neuronal transporter. This high-affinity choline uptake system appears linked, in a still undefined way, to both ACh synthesis and release. The high-affinity uptake mechanisms would be saturated at 10 μM choline, so the plasma choline concentration is probably adequate for sustained ACh synthesis even under conditions of high demand, as observed in ganglia. Furthermore, since the plasma concentration of choline is above the K_m of the high-affinity choline transport system, one would not expect to increase choline in the nerve ending by increasing the plasma concentration of choline or by changing the K_m of the uptake system. One might, however, change neuronal choline content by altering the capacity of the high-affinity choline uptake mechanism,

i.e., changing the V_{max} for transport, and this has been reported to occur in some brain regions in response to increased or decreased neuronal activity. There is some dispute about whether the capacity of the uptake system is increased or whether choline influx is regulated by changes in the intraterminal concentration of choline; it is agreed, however, that some event associated with neuronal activity serves to enhance choline entry into neurons [15]. If the K_m of ChAT for choline *in vivo* is as high as that seen with the purified enzyme, one would expect ACh synthesis to increase in proportion to the greater availability of choline. Conversely, ACh synthesis should be diminished when high-affinity choline uptake is blocked. Hemicholinium-3 is a potent inhibitor of the high-affinity choline uptake system, with a K_I in the submicromolar range (Fig. 4). Treatment with this drug decreases ACh synthesis and leads to a reduction in ACh release during prolonged stimulation; these findings lend support to the notion that choline uptake is the rate-limiting factor in the biosynthesis of ACh. Surprisingly, the recently cloned Na$^+$-dependent high-affinity choline transporter is not sensitive to inhibition by hemicholinium [16], raising the question of whether it is indeed the physiological transporter.

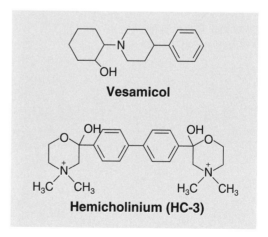

Vesamicol

Hemicholinium (HC-3)

FIG. 4.   Structures of hemicholinium (HC-3) and vesacimol.

Neurons cannot synthesize choline *de novo*; **it is therefore supplied either from plasma or by metabolism of choline-containing compounds**

At least half of the choline used in ACh synthesis is thought to come directly from recycling of released ACh, hydrolyzed to choline by cholinesterase. Presumably, the uptake of this metabolically derived choline occurs rapidly, before the choline diffuses away from the synaptic cleft. Another source of choline is from the breakdown of phosphatidylcholine, which may be increased in response to locally released ACh. Choline derived from these two sources becomes available in the extracellular space and is then subject to high-affinity uptake into the nerve ending. In the central nervous system these metabolic sources of choline may be particularly important, because choline in the plasma cannot pass the blood-brain barrier. Thus in the central nervous system, the high-affinity uptake of choline into cholinergic neurons might not be saturated, and ACh synthesis could be limited by the supply of choline, at least during sustained activity. This would be consistent with the finding that ACh stores in the brain are subject to variation, whereas ACh stores in ganglia and muscles remain relatively constant.

A slow release of acetylcholine from neurons at rest probably occurs at all cholinergic synapses

This was first described by Fatt and Katz, who recorded small, spontaneous depolarizations at frog neuromuscular junctions that were subthreshold for triggering action potentials. These MEPPs were shown to be due to the release of ACh. When the nerve was then stimulated and end-plate potentials recorded and analyzed, the magnitude of these potentials was always found to be some multiple of the magnitude of the MEPPs. It was suggested that each MEPP resulted from a finite quantity or quantum of released ACh and that the end-plate potentials resulted

from release of greater numbers of quanta during nerve stimulation (see also Chap. 9).

A possible structural basis for these discrete units of transmitter was discovered shortly thereafter when independent electron microscopic and subcellular fractionation studies by de Robertis and Whittaker revealed the presence of vesicles in cholinergic nerve endings. Subcellular fractionation of mammalian brain and *Torpedo* electric organs yields resealed nerve endings, or synaptosomes, that can be lysed to release a fraction enriched in vesicles. More than half of the ACh in the synaptosome is found associated with particles that look like the vesicles seen by electron microscopy. It is therefore clear that ACh is associated with a vesicle fraction, and it is likely that it is contained within the vesicle. The origin of the ACh that is free within the synaptosome is less clear. It may be ACh that is normally in the cytosol of the nerve ending, or it may be an artifact of release from the vesicles during their preparation (see Chap. 9).

The relationship between the amount of acetylcholine in a vesicle and the quanta of acetylcholine released can only be estimated

Estimates of the amount of ACh contained within cholinergic vesicles vary, and there is obviously some subjectivity in correcting the values obtained, e.g., for the percent of vesicles that are cholinergic or how much ACh would be lost during their preparation. Whittaker estimated that there are about 2,000 molecules of ACh in a cholinergic vesicle from the central nervous system. A similar estimate of about 1,600 molecules of ACh per vesicle was made using sympathetic ganglia. The most abundant source of cholinergic synaptic vesicles is the electric organ of *Torpedo*. Vesicles from *Torpedo* are far larger than those from mammalian species and are estimated to contain up to 100 times more ACh, i.e., 200,000 molecules per vesicle. The *Torpedo* vesicle has also been shown to contain ATP and, in its core, a proteoglycan of the heparin sulfate type. Both of these constituents may serve as counter-ions for ACh, which would otherwise be at a hyperosmotic concentration.

The amount of ACh in a quantum has been estimated by comparing the potential changes associated with MEPPs to those obtained by iontophoresis of known quantities of ACh. Based on such analysis, the amount of ACh per quantum at the snake neuromuscular junction was estimated to be something less than 10,000 molecules [17]. Given the possible error in these calculations, this would be within the range of that estimated to be contained in a vesicle. It is therefore likely that quanta are defined by the amount of releasable ACh in the vesicle. An alternative favored by some investigators is that ACh is released directly from the cytoplasm. In this model definable quanta are evident because channels in the membrane are open for finite periods of time when Ca^{2+} is elevated. A presynaptic membrane protein suggested to mediate Ca^{2+}-dependent translocation of ACh has recently been isolated by Israel and colleagues. Although there are some compelling arguments in support of this model, most investigators favor the notion that the vesicle serves not only as a unit of storage but as a unit of release. (The vesicle hypothesis and release of neurotransmitters in general are discussed also in Chap. 9.)

Depolarization of the nerve terminal by an action potential increases the number of quanta released per unit time

Release of ACh requires the presence of extracellular Ca^{2+}, which enters the neuron when it is depolarized. Most investigators feel that a voltage-dependent Ca^{2+} current is the initial event responsible for transmitter release, which occurs about 200 μsec later. The mechanism through which elevated Ca^{2+} increases the probability of ACh release is not yet known; phosphorylation or activation of proteins that causes the vesicle to fuse with the neuronal membrane are among the possibilities. Dependence on Ca^{2+} is a common feature of all exocytotic release mechanisms, and it is likely that exocytosis is a conserved mechanism for transmitter release. There is good evidence that adrenergic vesicles empty their contents into the synaptic cleft, because norepinephrine and epinephrine are released along with other contents of the storage vesicle. Although less rigorous data are available for cholinergic systems, cholinergic vesicles contain ATP, and release of ATP has been shown to accompany ACh secretion from these vesicles. Furthermore, as discussed in Chap. 9, Heuser and Reese demonstrated in electron microscopic studies at frog nerve terminals that vesicles fuse with the nerve membrane and that vesicular contents appear to be released by exocytosis; it has been difficult to ascertain, however, whether the fusions are sufficiently frequent to account for release on stimulation. The nerve ending also appears to endocytose the outer vesicle membrane to form vesicles that are subsequently refilled with ACh [17].

Torpedo synaptic vesicles have also been used to study mechanisms through which ACh, formed in the cytoplasm by ChAT, is concentrated in storage vesicles [18]. It appears that there is a specific ACh transporter and that ACh uptake is driven by an ATPase that pumps protons so that the inside of the vesicle is acidified and positively charged. There is evidence for a coupled mechanism for the counter transport of ACh and H^+ such that the vesicle remains iso-osmotic and electroneutral. An inhibitor of ACh transport into the vesicle has been studied in detail by Parsons and colleagues [18,19]. The inhibitor vesamicol (Fig. 4) inhibits ACh uptake, with an IC_{50} of about 40 nM. Inhibition is noncompetitive, suggesting that the drug does not act at the ACh-binding site on the transporter but rather another site on the same protein. Significantly, vesamicol blocks the evoked release of newly synthesized ACh from a number of preparations without significantly affecting high-affinity choline uptake, ACh synthesis, or Ca^{2+} influx. That ACh release is lost secondary to blockade of its uptake by the vesicle is powerful evidence that the vesicle is the site of ACh release.

All of the acetylcholine contained within the cholinergic neuron does not behave as if in a single compartment

Results of a variety of neurophysiological and biochemical experiments suggest that there are at least two distinguishable pools of ACh, only one of which is readily available for release. These have been referred to as the "readily available" or "depot" pool and as the "reserve" or "stationary" pool. The reserve pool serves to refill the readily available pool as it is utilized. Unless the rate of mobilization of ACh into the readily available pool is adequate, the amount of ACh that can be released may be limited. It is also likely that newly synthesized ACh is used to fill the readily available pool of ACh, because it is the newly synthesized ACh that is preferentially released during nerve stimulation. The relationship between these functionally defined pools and ACh storage vesicles is not known with certainty. It is possible that the readily available pool resides in vesicles poised for release near the nerve ending membrane, whereas the reserve pool is in more distant vesicles. Although cholinergic vesicles appear to be homogeneous, there may be subpopulations of vesicles that differ in size and density.

ACETYLCHOLINESTERASE AND THE TERMINATION OF ACETYLCHOLINE ACTION

Cholinesterases are widely distributed throughout the body in both neuronal and non-neuronal tissues

Based largely on substrate specificity, the cholinesterases are subdivided into the acetylcholinesterases (AChEs) (EC 3.1.1.7) and the butyryl or pseudocholinesterases (BuChE) (EC 3.1.1.8) [20,21]. Acetylcholines with an acyl group of the size of butyric acid or larger are very slowly hydrolyzed by the former enzyme; selective inhibitors for each enzyme have been identified. Butyrylcholinesterase is made primarily in the liver and appears in plasma; however, it is highly unlikely that appreciable concentrations of ACh diffuse from the locality of the synapse and elicit a systemic response. The distribution of BuChE mutations showing resistance to naturally occurring inhibitors suggests that this enzyme functions to hydrolyze dietary esters of potential toxicity. Although BuChE is localized in the nervous system during development, the existence of nonexpressing BuChE mutations in the human population demonstrates that this enzyme is not essential for nervous system function. In general, AChE distribution correlates with innervation and development in the nervous system. The AChEs also exhibit synaptic localization upon synapse formation. Acetyl- and butyrylcholinesterases are encoded by single, but distinct, genes.

Acetylcholinesterase exists in several molecular forms that differ in solubility and mode of membrane attachment rather than in catalytic activity

One class of molecular forms exists as a homomeric assembly of catalytic subunits that appear as monomers, dimers, or tetramers (Fig. 5). These forms also differ in their degree of hydrophobicity, and their amphiphilic character arises from a post-translational addition of a glycophospholipid on the carboxy-terminal amino acid. The glycophospholipid allows the enzyme to be tethered on the external surface of the cell membrane. Soluble globular forms of the enzyme have been identified in brain. In certain dopamine-containing neurons, AChE is co-released in a soluble form with dopamine on nerve stimulation; however, the function of the released enzyme is unknown.

The second class of AChEs exists as heteromeric assemblies of catalytic and structural subunits. One form consists of catalytic subunits (up to 12) linked by a disulfide bond to filamentous, collagen-containing structural subunits. These forms are often

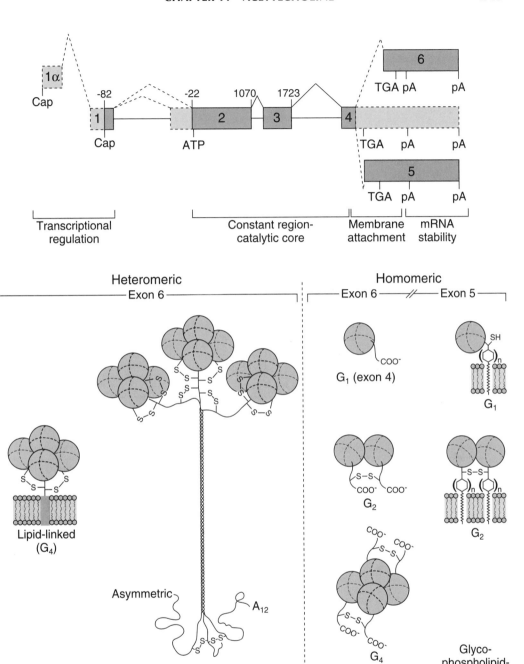

FIG. 5. Gene structure of AChE. Alternative cap sites in the 5' end of the gene allow for alternative promoter usage in different tissues. Alternative splice acceptor sites are also found in the nontranslated region. Exons 2, 3, and 4 encode an invariant core of the molecule that contains the essential catalytic residues. Just prior to the stop codon three splicing alternatives are evident: **1,** a continuation of exon 4; **2,** the 4–5 splice; and **3,** the 4–6 splice. The catalytic subunits produced are shown in the lower panel (Modified from ref. 20 with permission).

termed *asymmetric*, since the tail unit imparts substantial dimensional asymmetry to the molecule. The asymmetric species are localized to synaptic areas. The collagenous tail unit is responsible for this molecular form being associated with the basal lamina of the synapse rather than the plasma membrane. Asymmetric forms are particularly abundant in the neuromuscular junction. A second type of structural subunit, to which a tetramer of catalytic subunits is linked by disulfide bonds, has been characterized in brain. This subunit contains covalently attached lipid, enabling this form of the enzyme to associate with the plasma membrane. The different subunit assemblies and post-translational modifications lead to distinct localizations of AChE on the cell surface but appear not to affect their intrinsic catalytic activity.

The primary and tertiary structures of the cholinesterases are known

Cholinesterase genes encode a leader peptide, but the cholinesterases do not have obvious membrane-spanning regions in their primary structure [20]. Hence they are designed for secretion from the cell. It is interesting that the cholinesterases do not show sequence identity with the chymotrypsin and subtilisin families of serine hydrolases despite having virtually identical catalytic mechanisms. Rather, the cholinesterases have defined a new family of secreted proteins. Within this growing family of proteins are several non-neuronal esterases and proteins such as thyroglobulin and the tactins, which lack an intrinsic catalytic function.

The open reading frame in mammalian AChE genes is encoded by three invariant exons (exons 2, 3, and 4) followed by three splicing alternatives. Continuation through exon 4 gives rise to a monomeric species. Splicing to exon 5 gives rise to the carboxyl-terminal sequence signal for addition of glycophospholipid, while splicing to exon 6 encodes a sequence containing a cysteine that links to other catalytic or structural subunits. These species of AChE only differ in the last 40 residues in their carboxyl-termini.

The catalytic mechanism for acetylcholine hydrolysis involves formation of an acyl enzyme, followed by deacylation

The acylation step proceeds through the formation of a tetrahedral transition state. Alkylphosphate inhibitors such as diisopropylfluorophosphate are tetrahedral in configuration, and this geometric resemblance to the transition state, in part, accounts for their effectiveness as inhibitors of AChE. Acylation occurs on the active-site serine, which is rendered nucleophilic by proton withdrawal by glutamate 327 through histidine 440. The acetyl enzyme that is formed is short lived, which accounts for the high catalytic efficiency of the enzyme (Fig. 6). The availability of a crystal structure of AChE has enabled investigators to assign residues and domains in the cholinesterase responsible for catalysis and inhibitor specificity [22].

Inhibition of acetylcholinesterase occurs by several distinct mechanisms

Some AChE inhibitors are useful therapeutically, whereas others have proven useful as insecticides. Still others have been manufactured for a more insidious use in chemical warfare. Inhibitors such as edrophonium bind reversibly to the active site of the enzyme and prevent access of the substrate. Other reversible inhibitors, such as gallamine and propidium, bind to a peripheral site on the enzyme. The carbamoylating agents, such as neostigmine and physostigmine, form a carbamoyl enzyme by reacting with the active-site serine. The carbamoyl enzymes are more stable than the acetyl enzyme; their deacylation occurs over several minutes. Since the carbamoyl enzyme will not hydrolyze ACh, the carbamoylating agents are alternative substrates that are effective inhibitors of ACh hydrolysis. The alkylphosphates, such as diisopropylfluorophosphate or echothiophate, act in a similar manner; however, the alkylphosphorates and alkylphosphonates form extremely stable bonds with the active-site serine on the

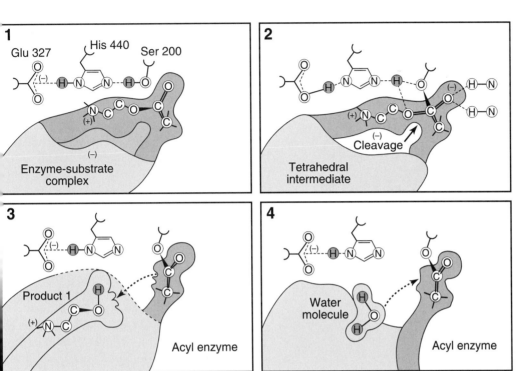

FIG. 6. Catalytic sequence in ACh hydrolysis. The active-site serine (position 200 in the *Torpedo* sequence) is rendered nucleophilic by a dicarboxylic amino acid (glutamate 327) serving as a proton sink and an imidazole group of histidine 440. The serine attacks the carbonyl carbon (**1**), forming a tetrahedral intermediate (**2**). The carbonyl oxygen is likely stabilized through hydrogen bonding in an oxyanion hole. Removal of the choline-leaving group forms an acyl enzyme (**3**). Attack by water is rapid and generates the free enzyme (**4**).

enzyme. The time required for their hydrolysis often exceeds that for biosynthesis and turnover of the enzyme. Accordingly, inhibition with the alkylphosphates is typically irreversible.

The consequences of acetylcholinesterase inhibition differ between synapses

At postganglionic parasympathetic effector sites, AChE inhibition enhances or potentiates the action of administered ACh or ACh released by nerve stimulation. This, in part, is a consequence of stimulation of receptors extending over a larger area from the point of transmitter release. Similarly, ganglionic transmission is enhanced by cholinesterase inhibitors. Since atropine and other muscarinic antagonists are effective antidotes of the toxicity of inhibitors of AChE, at least some central nervous system manifestations result largely from excessive muscarinic stimulation.

By prolonging the residence time of ACh in the synapse, AChE inhibition in the neuromuscular junction promotes a persistent depolarization of the motor end-plate. The decay of end-plate currents or potentials resulting from spontaneous release of ACh is prolonged from 1 to 2 msec to 5 to 30 msec. This indicates that the transmitter activates multiple receptors before diffusing from the synapse. Excessive depolarization of the end-plate resulting from slowly decaying end-plate potentials and a diminished capacity to initiate coordinated action potentials ensue. In a fashion similar to depolarizing blocking agents, fasciculations and muscle twitching are initially observed with AChE inhibition, followed by flaccid paralysis.

NICOTINIC RECEPTORS

The nicotinic acetylcholine receptor is the best characterized neurotransmitter receptor

Investigators were able to purify the nicotinic receptor about a decade before purification of other neurotransmitter receptors. Electric organs of the *Torpedo* species are a rich source of nicotinic receptors and consist of stacks of electrocytes that have differentiated from tissue of whose embryonic origin is similar to that of skeletal muscle. Upon differentiation, the electrogenic bud in the electrocyte proliferates, but the contractile elements atrophy. The excitable membrane encompasses the entire ventral surface of the electrocyte rather than being localized to small, focal junctional areas, as occurs in skeletal muscle. The electrical discharge in *Torpedo* relies solely on a PSEP resulting from depolarization of the postsynaptic membrane. Depolarization arises directly from the opening of receptor channels; in skeletal muscle and in the fresh water electric eel *Electrophorus electricus,* depolarization at the endplate activates a voltage-sensitive Na^+ channel that, in turn, causes the depolarization to spread across the surface of the muscle or electric organ. The density of receptors in *Torpedo* electric organs approaches 100 pmol/mg protein, which may be compared with 0.1 pmol/mg protein in skeletal muscle.

Studies of C. Y. Lee and his colleagues in the early 1960s established that snake α-toxins, such as α-bungarotoxin, irreversibly inactivate receptor function in intact skeletal muscle, and this finding led directly to the identification and subsequent isolation of the nicotinic ACh receptor from *Torpedo* [3] By virtue of their high affinity and very slow rates of dissociation, labeled α-toxins serve as markers of the receptor during solubilization and purification.

Purification of the nicotinic acetylcholine receptor facilitated examination of its overall structure

Antibodies were raised to the purified protein, and sufficient amino acid sequence of the receptor itself became available to permit the cloning and sequencing of the genes encoding the individual subunits of the receptor [4]. As a consequence of the high density of nicotinic ACh receptors in the postsynaptic membranes of *Torpedo*, sufficient order of the receptor is achieved in isolated membrane fragments that image reconstructions from electron microscopy have allowed a more detailed analysis of structure [23]. Finally, labeling of functional sites and determination of subunit composition contributed to our understanding of the structure of nicotinic receptors.

The nicotinic acetylcholine receptor consists of five subunits arranged around a pseudoaxis of symmetry

The subunits display homologous amino acid sequences with 30 to 40 percent identity of amino acid residues [3]. One of the subunits, designated α, is expressed in two copies; the other three, β, γ, and δ, are present as single copies (Fig. 7). Thus the receptor

FIG. 7.   **A:** Model of the nicotinic acetylcholine receptor showing the ligand binding site (neurotransmitter binding pocket), membrane bilayer, and the position of the channel gate. (Adapted from [23]). **B:** Image reconstruction of electron micrographs yielding a structure at 9 Å resolution. Shown are side and synaptic views. (Adapted from [23].) **C:** Electron density images of a section of the receptor molecule on the synaptic side taken 30 Å above the plane of the membrane and normal to the pseudo fivefold axis of symmetry. Arrows show route of entry of the neurotransmitter. The labels and stars indicate the respective positions of the two α-subunits and the bungarotoxin binding site. The pentameric structure of the receptor is evident with a presumed clockwise orientation of subunits α_1, γ, α_2, β, δ. (Adapted from [23].) **D:** Longitudinal view of the electron density of the receptor. The transmembrane area is shown between the dots. The visible transmembrane-spanning-helixes are shown by the V-shaped solid lines. This helix is believed to be the M2 region the sequence of which is shown. The area inside the rectangle is the transmembrane-spanning region. The cross denotes the conserved leucine (see Fig. 8C). The additional density in the cytoplasmic region arises from the 43-kDa subunit. The shaded area to the right indicates the zone of narrowest constriction.

A

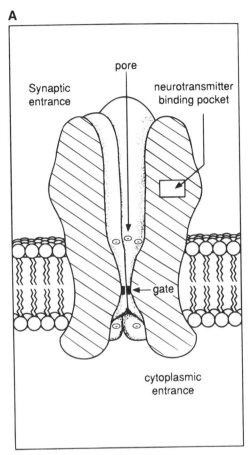

pore

Synaptic
entrance

neurotransmitter
binding pocket

gate

cytoplasmic
entrance

B

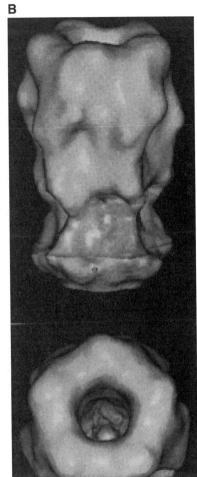

D

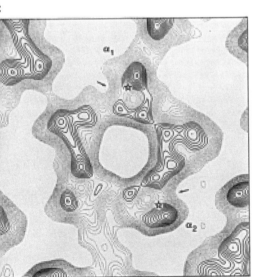

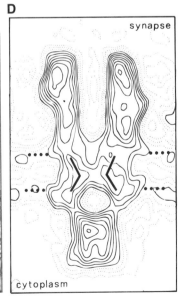

synapse

cytoplasm

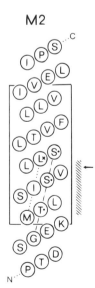

M2

is a pentamer of molecular mass of approximately 280 kDa. Structural studies show the subunits to be arranged around a central cavity, with the largest portion of the protein exposed toward the extracellular surface. The central cavity is believed to be the ion channel, which in the resting state is impermeable to ions; on activation, however, it opens to a diameter of 6.5 Å. The open channel is selective for cations; permeation of the channel by particular cations appears to be limited primarily by the diameter of the open channel. The α-subunits form the site for binding of agonists and competitive antagonists and provide the primary surface with which the larger snake α-toxins associate. A site for ligand binding exists toward the external perimeter on each of the α-subunits; occupation of both sites is necessary for receptor activation. Electrophysiological and ligand-binding measurements, together with analysis of the functional states of the receptor, indicate positive cooperativity in the association of agonists; Hill coefficients greater than unity have been described for agonist-elicited channel opening, agonist binding, and agonist-induced desensitization of the receptor [24]. Noncompetitive inhibitor sites within various depths of the internal channel have also been defined and are the sites of local anesthetic inhibition of receptor function.

Sequence identity among the subunits appears to be greatest in the hydrophobic regions. Various models for the disposition of the peptide chains have been proposed on the basis of hydropathy and reactivity of various residues to modifying agents and antibodies (Fig. 8). Four candidate membrane-spanning regions have been proposed, though only one clear α-helical segment is evident in the structure reconstructed from electron microscopy. All of these potential membrane-spanning domains appear after residue 200, with the amino-terminal portion of the molecule on the extracellular surface. The homology among the four subunits strongly suggests that the same pattern is found in all subunits. Further refinement of the structure of the receptor is likely to emerge from analysis of mutant receptors, reactivity of particular residues, and high resolution structural methods.

Aspartate 141 in the α-subunit is glycosylated and hence on the outside surface. After reduction of the receptor by dithiothreitol to convert disulfide bonds to free thiols, bromoacetylcholine and N-maleimidobenzyltrimethyl ammonium react with cysteine 192 or 193. Since the adjacent cysteines at residues 192 to 193 are unique to the α-subunit, this region is believed to play a role in the binding of agonists and α-toxins. Cysteines 192 and 193 appear to be linked by a disulfide bond, as are cysteines 128 and 142.

FIG. 8.   Features of the sequence of the ACh receptor. **A:** Schematic drawing of the sequence showing candidate regions for spanning the membrane. The region M2 is believed to be an α-helical segment and lines the internal pore of the receptor. M1, M3, and M4 contain hydrophobic sequences, but it is not known whether they traverse the membrane as α-helices. The nicotinic β-, γ-, and δ-subunits contain homologous M1–M4 hydrophobic domains at similar positions in the linear sequence. Two disulfide loops, 128–142 and 192–193, in the α-subunits are shown. While the other subunits contain the larger disulfide loop, they lack cysteines 192 and 193 and tyrosine 190. Sequences of other homologous subunits in ligand-gated channels (5-hydroxytryptamine, γ-aminobutyric acid, glycine, glutamate-A, kainic acid, and N-methyl-D-aspartic acid receptors are shown. The N-terminal portion is found on the extracellular (synaptic) surface. (Modified from [23] with permission.) **B:** Amino acid sequence between residues 179 and 207 in the α-subunit of various nicotinic receptors. Cysteines 192 and 193 and tyrosines 190 and 198 have been shown by chemical labeling and site-specific mutagenesis to be in the vicinity of the ligand-binding site. **C:** Amino acid sequence of the M2-spanning domain for the homologous series of ligand-gated ion channels. The conformation is believed to be α-helical, with the N-terminal portion (left-hand side) entering from the cytoplasmic side. The membrane-spanning region is largely hydrophobic, but with hydroxylated residues positioned at strategic positions in the α-helical wheel. Charged residues are found bordering the hydrophobic membrane-spanning region. The helices from each of the five subunits form the internal perimeter outlining the channel (see Fig. 7) and are believed to assume a bowed, hour-glass shape with the boxed leucine being near the constriction point (cf. [23]).

A

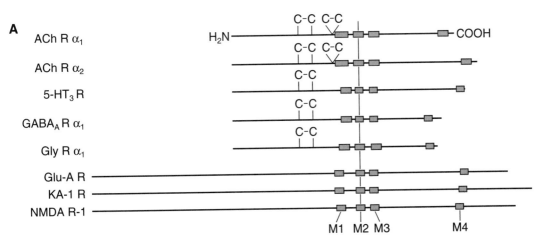

ACh R α₁

ACh R α₂

5-HT₃ R

GABA_A R α₁

Gly R α₁

Glu-A R

KA-1 R

NMDA R-1

B
Sequence in the α subunit of various acetylcholine receptors of muscle (α1) and neuronal origin (α2-α4)[a] between residues 179 and 207

		179																									207	
Torpedo c.	α1	K	D	Y	R	G	W	K	H	W	V	Y	Y	T	C	C	P	D	T	P	Y	L	D	I	T	Y	H	F	I	M
Torpedo m.	α1	K	D	Y	R	G	W	K	H	W	V	Y	Y	T	C	C	P	D	T	P	Y	L	D	I	T	Y	H	F	I	M
Xenopus l.	α1α	K	D	Y	R	G	W	K	H	W	V	Y	Y	D	C	C	P	E	T	P	Y	L	D	I	T	Y	H	F	L	L
Xenopus l.	α1β	K	D	Y	R	G	W	K	H	W	V	Y	Y	T	C	C	P	D	K	P	Y	L	D	I	T	Y	H	F	V	L
Chicken	α1	K	D	Y	R	G	W	K	H	W	V	Y	Y	A	C	C	P	D	T	P	Y	L	D	I	T	Y	H	F	L	M
Calf	α1	K	E	S	R	G	W	K	H	W	V	F	Y	A	C	C	P	S	T	P	Y	L	D	I	T	Y	H	F	V	M
Mouse	α1	K	E	A	R	G	W	K	H	W	V	F	Y	S	C	C	P	T	T	P	Y	L	D	I	T	Y	H	F	V	M
Human	α1	K	E	S	R	G	W	K	H	S	V	T	Y	S	C	C	P	D	T	P	Y	L	D	I	T	Y	H	F	V	M
Cobra	α	K	D	Y	R	G	F	W	H	S	V	N	Y	S	C	C	L	D	T	P·	Y	L	D	I	T	Y	H	F	I	L
Natrix t.	α	K	D	Y	R	G	F	W	H	S	V	N	Y	S	C	C	L	D	T	P	Y	L	D	I	T	Y	H	F	I	L
Drosophila	α	M	R	V	P	A	V	R	N	E	K	F	Y	S	C	C	-	E	E	P	Y	L	D	I	T	Y	N	L	T	L
Chicken	α2	I	N	A	I	G	R	Y	N	S	K	K	Y	D	C	C	-	T	E	I	Y	P	D	I	V	F	Y	F	V	I
Chicken	α3	I	K	A	P	G	Y	K	H	D	I	K	Y	N	C	C	-	E	E	I	Y	T	D	I	T	F	S	L	Y	I
Chicken	α4	I	N	S	V	G	N	Y	N	S	K	K	Y	E	C	C	-	T	E	I	Y	P	D	I	T	Y	S	F	I	I
Rat	α2	I	N	A	T	G	T	Y	N	S	K	K	Y	D	C	C	-	E	E	I	Y	Q	D	I	T	Y	S	L	Y	I
Rat	α3	I	K	A	P	G	Y	K	H	E	I	K	Y	N	C	C	-	E	E	I	Y	Q	D	I	T	Y	S	L	Y	I
Rat	α4	V	D	A	V	G	T	Y	M	T	R	K	Y	E	C	C	-	A	E	I	Y	P	D	I	T	Y	A	F	I	I
Rat	α5	M	S	A	M	G	S	K	G	N	R	T	D	S	C	C	W	Y			P	Y	I	T	Y	S	F	V	I	K	R

[a] The asterisks denote conserved residues. To date, no activity has been observed with rat α5 when expressed with other subunits of muscle or neuronal origin.

C
Charged amino acids (circled) and conserved leucine (boxed) on M2 are shown in relation to estimated position of bilayer

Torpedo, α (1)	G	Ⓔ	Ⓚ	M	T	L	S	I	S	V	L	L̄	S	L	T	V	F	L	L	V	I	V	Ⓔ	L
Torpedo, β (2)	G	Ⓔ	Ⓚ	M	S	L	S	I	S	A	L	L̄	A	T	V	V	F	L	L	L	L	A	Ⓓ	Ⓚ
Torpedo, γ (3)	G	Q	Ⓚ	C	T	L	S	I	S	V	L	L̄	A	Q	T	I	F	L	F	L	I	A	Q	Ⓚ
Torpedo, δ (2)	G	Ⓔ	Ⓚ	M	S	T	A	I	S	V	L	L̄	A	Q	A	V	F	L	L	L	T	S	Q	Ⓡ
N. AChR, α2 (4)	G	Ⓔ	Ⓚ	I	T	L	C	I	S	V	L	L̄	S	L	T	V	F	L	L	L	I	T	Ⓔ	I
N. AChR, β2 (5)	G	Ⓔ	Ⓚ	M	T	L	C	I	S	V	L	L̄	A	L	T	V	F	L	L	L	I	S	Ⓚ	I
GABA_A R, α1 (6)	P	A	Ⓡ	T	V	F	G	V	T	T	V	L̄	T	M	T	T	L	S	I	S	A	Ⓡ	N	S
GABA_A R, β1 (6)	A	A	Ⓡ	V	A	L	G	I	T	T	V	L̄	T	M	T	T	I	S	T	H	L	Ⓡ	Ⓔ	T
Glycine R, α1 (7)	P	A	Ⓡ	V	G	L	G	I	T	T	V	L̄	T	M	T	T	Q	S	S	G	S	Ⓡ	A	S
Glycine R, β1 (8)	A	A	Ⓡ	V	P	L	G	I	F	S	V	L̄	S	L	A	S	Ⓔ	C	T	T	L	A	A	Ⓔ
5-HT₃ R (9)	G	Ⓔ	Ⓡ	V	S	F	Ⓚ	I	T	L	L	L̄	G	Y	S	V	F	L	I	V	S	Ⓓ	T	L

Bilayer

Lophotoxin, a cyclic diterpinoid toxin, reacts covalently with tyrosine 190. A comparison of the structures and reactive sites of bromoacetylcholine and lophotoxin indicates that the acyl chain of ACh binds in a fashion antiparallel to the acyl chain between residues 190 and 192. Labeling studies with photoactive reagents and site-specific mutagenesis have suggested that aromatic residues in the first 200 amino acids participate in the formation of a binding site that is close to a subunit interface. Moreover, interfacing of particular α,γ and α,δ amino acid residues is critical to agonist and antagonist specificity and to eliciting cooperativity in the response [24]. Residues in the β- and δ-chain (serine 254 and 262) in the second candidate membrane-spanning domain have been labeled with the noncompetitive inhibitors chlorpromazine and tetraphenylphosphonium. These residues may define a sequence lining the channel. Conformational changes in this region could prove critical to channel opening. The cobra α-toxins and α-bungarotoxin form three disulfide loops in a leaf-life structure and bind to an extended surface area that is mainly encompassed by the α-subunit. Fluorescence energy-transfer measurements and electron microscopic imaging indicate that the α-toxin and agonist-binding sites are closer to the outer perimeter of the receptor than a central pseudo axis of symmetry. These sites also appear close to the membrane surface.

events for ACh achieve a conductance of 25 pS across the membrane and have an opening duration that is exponentially distributed around a value of about 1 msec. The duration of channel opening is dependent on the particular agonist, whereas the conductance of the open-channel state is usually agonist independent. Analyses of the frequencies of opening events have permitted an estimation of the kinetic constants for channel opening and ligand binding, and these numbers are in reasonable agreement with estimates of ligand binding and activation from rapid kinetic, or stopped-flow, studies. Overall, activation events can be described by Scheme 1. Two ligands (L) associate with the receptor (R) prior to the isomerization step to form the open-channel state L_2R^*. For ACh, the forward rate constant for binding, k_{+1}, is $1-2 \times 10^8\ \mathrm{M}^{-1}\ \mathrm{sec}^{-1}$; k_{+2} and k_{-2}, forward and reverse rate constants for isomerization, yield rates of isomerization consistent with opening events in the millisecond time frame. Since k_{+2} and k_{-2} are greater than k_{-1}, the rate constant for ligand dissociation, several opening and closing events with the fully liganded receptor occur prior to the

$$2L + R \underset{k_{-1}}{\overset{2k_{+1}}{\rightleftharpoons}} LR \underset{2k_{-1}}{\overset{k_{+1}}{\rightleftharpoons}} L_2R \underset{k_{-2}}{\overset{k_{+2}}{\rightleftharpoons}} L_2R^*$$

(Closed)   (Closed)   (Closed)   (Open)

Scheme 1

The events associated with ligand binding and activation of the receptor have been studied by the analysis of opening and closing events of individual channels

Electrophysiological studies use high-resistance patch electrodes of 1 to 2 μm diameter that form tight seals on the membrane surface. They have the capacity to record conductance changes of individual channels within the lumen of the electrode (see Chap. 9). The patch of membrane affixed to the electrode may be excised, inverted, or studied on the intact cell. The individual opening

dissociation of the first ligand. Binding of the first and second ligands appears not to be identical, even allowing for the statistical differences arising from the two sites. Such a conclusion is consistent with receptor structure, since different subunits are adjacent to the α-subunits in the pentamer.

Desensitization of receptors

Continued exposure of nicotinic receptors to agonist leads to a diminution of the response, even though the concentration of agonist available to the receptor has not changed. The loss of response from prior agonist exposure is called *desensitization*. Katz and Thesleff examined the kinetics of desensitization with microelectrodes and found that a cyclic scheme in which the receptor existed in two states, R and R′, prior to exposure to the ligand best described the process.

To achieve receptor desensitization and activation by a single ligand, multiple conformational states of the receptor are required. The binding steps represented in horizontal equilibria are rapid; vertical steps reflect the slow, unimolecular isomerizations involved in desensitization (Scheme 2). Rapid isomerization for channel opening should be added. To accommodate the additional complexities of the observed fast and slow steps of desensitization, additional states have to be included.

A simplified scheme, in which only one desensitized and one open-channel state of the receptor exist, is represented in Scheme 2, where R is the resting (activatible) state, R* the active (open channel) state, and R′ the desensitized state of the receptor; M is an allosteric constant defined by R′/R, and K and $K′$ are equilibrium constants for the indicated reactions.

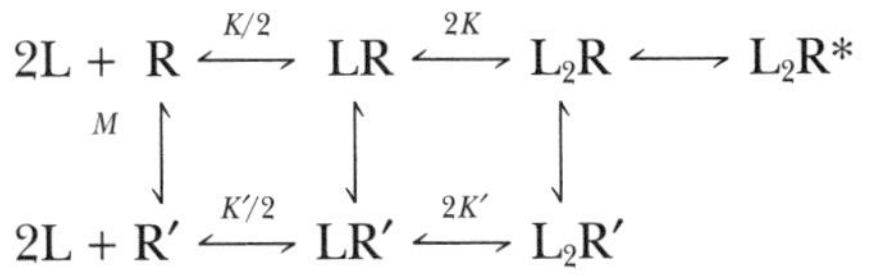

$$2L + R \xrightleftharpoons{K/2} LR \xrightleftharpoons{2K} L_2R \longleftrightarrow L_2R^*$$
$$\left\downarrow M \right. \quad\quad \left\downarrow\right. \quad\quad \left\downarrow\right.$$
$$2L + R' \xrightleftharpoons{K'/2} LR' \xrightleftharpoons{2K'} L_2R'$$

Scheme 2

In this scheme, $M < 1$ and $K′ < K$. Addition of ligand will eventually result in an increased fraction of R′ species due to the values dictated by the equilibrium constants. Direct binding experiments have confirmed the generality of this scheme for nicotinic receptors. Thus, distinct conformational states dictate the different temporal responses that ensue on addition of a ligand to the nicotinic receptor. No direct energy input or covalent modification of the receptor channel is required.

Nicotinic receptor subunits are part of a large superfamily of ligand-gated channels

Nicotinic receptors on neurons (i.e., those originating in the central nervous system or neural crest) show ligand specificities distinct from the nicotinic receptor in the neuromuscular junction. One of the most remarkable differences is the resistance of most nicotinic neuronal receptors to α-bungarotoxin and other snake α-toxins. This fact and the lack of an abundant source of neuronal central nervous system receptors limited initial progress in their isolation and characterization. However, low stringency hybridization with cDNAs encoding electric organ and muscle receptors provided a means to clone neuronal nicotinic receptor genes. Isolation of the candidate cDNA clones, their expression in cell systems to yield functional receptors, and the discrete regional localizations of the endogenous mRNAs encoding these receptor subunits revealed that the nicotinic receptor subunits are part of a large and widely distributed gene family. They are related in structure and sequence to inhibitory amino acids (γ-aminobutyric acid and glycine), to 5-hydroxytryptamine (5HT$_3$), and somewhat more distantly to the excitatory amino acid (glutamate) receptors.

At least ten neuronal nicotinic receptor subunit genes (α$_2$–α$_8$ and β$_2$–β$_4$) have been identified (Fig. 2). The α-subtypes are similar to the muscle α-subunit (α$_1$) and contain the ligand-binding site. The β-subunits fulfill a structural role and are analogous to β$_1$, γ, and δ in the muscle receptor. When pairs of α- and β-cDNAs are cotransfected into cells or their corresponding mRNAs are injected into oocytes, channel function gated by ACh or other nicotinic agonists can be achieved. In contrast to α$_2$, α$_3$, and α$_4$, α$_5$ does not appear to carry a ligand-binding site and may be β-like in character. The α$_7$- and α$_8$-subunits may function efficiently as a pentamer of a single subunit. Receptors containing α$_7$ may gate Ca^{2+} as the primary permeating ion. While not all combinations of α- and β-sub units can assemble as functional receptors, the number of permutations is large and leads to great diversity in receptor subtypes. A challenge relates to assigning biophysical and pharmacological signatures to all of the subunit combinations found *in vivo*.

Both nicotinic receptors and acetylcholinesterase are tightly regulated during differentiation and synapse formation

At present, we understand more about tissue-specific gene expression in muscle than nerve [25,26]. Both of these proteins show enhanced expression during myogenesis upon differentiating from a mononucleated myoblast to a multinucleated myotube. Curiously, enhanced receptor expression occurs largely by transcriptional activation, while the increase in cholinesterase expression arises from stabilization of the mRNA [26,27]. The receptor appears to cluster spontaneously, which involves a protein on the cytoplasmic side of the membrane (43K or Rapsyn) [28]. This protein links the receptor to cytoskeletal elements and restricts its diffusional mobility. Following innervation and synaptic activity, expression of the receptor and AChE persists in end-plate (junctional) regions and disappears in extrajunctional regions. The collagen-tail-containing species of AChE is localized to the basal lamina in the neuromuscular synapse.

With innervation and the development of electrically excitable synapses, the γ-subunit of the receptor is replaced by an ε-subunit; small changes in the biophysical properties of the receptor occur concomitantly. Upon denervation many of the developmental changes associated with innervation are reversed, and there is again an increase in expression of extrajunctional receptors containing the γ-subunit. In multinucleated muscle cells, particular subsynaptic nuclei drive the expression of these synapse-specific proteins. The factors controlling these regulatory events are incompletely understood, but calcitonin gene-related peptide (CGRP) and the protein, ACh receptor-inducing activity (ARIA), may be extracellular mediators of expression. In addition, intracellular Ca^{2+}, membrane depolarization, and protein kinase C play distinct roles in maintaining junctional, but inhibiting extrajunctional, expression of these two proteins. Extracellular proteins localized in the basal lamina, such as agrin, also influence synapse formation and maintenance.

MUSCARINIC RECEPTORS

Muscarinic and nicotinic receptors are structurally and functionally closer to other receptors in their respective families than to one another

The nicotinic receptor is far more similar to other ligand-gated ion channels (e.g., the γ-aminobutyric acid receptor) than to the muscarinic receptor. The muscarinic receptor in turn belongs to the same family as a number of other cell surface receptors (e.g., the adrenergic receptors) [29], which transduce their signals across membranes by interacting with GTP-binding proteins (G proteins described in Chap. 21). The involvement of several macromolecular interactions in activation of the muscarinic receptor contributes to the 100 to 250 msec latency characteristic of muscarinic responses, which are slow compared with those mediated by nicotinic receptors.

Cellular responses to muscarinic receptor stimulation include inhibition of adenylyl cyclase, stimulation of phospholipase C, and regulation of ion channels

A variety of types of effector cells in brain and periphery receive cholinergic innervation, and they respond in different ways to muscarinic receptor stimulation. Muscarinic receptors are also located on presynaptic neurons, where they regulate transmitter release. Despite this obvious functional diversity, the initial event that follows ligand binding to the muscarinic receptor may be in all cases the interaction of the receptor with a

G protein. Depending on the nature of the G protein, the receptor–G protein interaction can initiate any of several early biochemical events seen with muscarinic receptor occupation: inhibition of adenylyl cyclase, stimulation of phosphoinositide hydrolysis, or regulation of an ion channel (Fig. 9) [30].

Inhibition of Adenylyl Cyclase

Muscarinic inhibition of cAMP formation is most apparent when adenylyl cyclase is stimulated, for example, by activation of adrenergic receptors with catecholamines or forskolin. Simultaneous addition of cholinergic agonists decreases the amount of cAMP formed in response to the catecholamine, in some tissues almost completely. The result is diminished activation of cAMP-dependent protein kinase and decreased substrate phosphorylation catalyzed by this kinase. The mechanism by which the muscarinic receptor inhibits adenylyl cyclase is through activation of an inhibitory GTP-binding protein, G_i. This molecule competes with the G protein activated by stimulatory agonists (G_s) for regulation of adenylyl cyclase (see also Chaps. 10 and 21).

Stimulation of Phospholipase C

Muscarinic agonists stimulate phosphoinositide hydrolysis by activating a phosphoinositide-specific phospholipase C. Activation of the β-isoform of phospholipase C can be mediated through a GTP-binding protein that has been shown to be $G_{q/11}$ [31]. The hydrolysis of phosphatidylinositol bisphosphate yields two potential second messengers, inositol trisphosphate ($InsP_3$) and diacylglycerol (see Chap. 20). Diacylglycerol increases the activity of the Ca^{2+} and phospholipid-dependent protein kinase (protein kinase C). Inositol trisphosphate mobilizes Ca^{2+} from intracellular stores in the endoplasmic reticulum and thereby elevates cytosolic free Ca^{2+}. Subsequent responses are triggered by direct effects of Ca^{2+} on Ca^{2+}-regulated proteins and by phosphorylation mediated through Ca^{2+} calmodulin-dependent kinases and protein kinase C. Stimulation of a phospholipase D that hydrolyzes phosphatidylcholine also occurs in response to muscarinic receptor activation. This appears to be secondary to activation of protein kinase C and contributes to a secondary rise in diacylglycerol.

Regulation of Ion Channels

Muscarinic agonists also increase specific K^+ conductance and thereby hyperpolarize cardiac and other cell membranes. This muscarinic effect can be mimicked by GTP analogs in whole-cell clamp experiments, and the response is sensitive to pertussis toxin, which ribosylates and inactivates G_i and a related protein, G_o (see Chap. 9). The likelihood that a G protein links the muscarinic receptor to the K^+ channel is supported by recent data showing that purified G protein subunits regulate K^+ conductance and by evidence that other receptor-activated channels are likewise coupled to their receptors in a GTP-dependent fashion [32].

Intracellular Mediators of Muscarinic Receptor Action

The three events described above—inhibition of adenylyl cyclase, stimulation of phosphoinositide hydrolysis, and regulation of ion channels—all occur within the plasma membrane. They can be triggered directly by muscarinic receptor occupation independent of changes in cytosolic mediators. However, these primary events in turn affect the generation of cytosolic mediators such as cAMP, diacylglycerol, $InsP_3$, and Ca^{2+}, which generate other metabolic sequelae. For example, an increase in cytosolic free Ca^{2+} probably contributes to activation of phospholipase A_2, generating arachidonic acid, prostaglandins, and related eicosanoids (see Chap. 23). These products in turn can stimulate cGMP formation and can regulate ion channel activity. Increased Ca^{2+} can also activate Ca^{2+}-dependent ion channels (K^+, Cl^-), regulate cAMP phosphodiesterase, and activate Ca^{2+}-calmodulin-kinase-dependent protein phosphorylation. Protein kinase C is activated by DAG, generally in concert with Ca^{2+} and has effects on ion-channel activity, as well as on cholinergic secretory and con-

Primary biochemical responses
mediated by muscarinic acetylcholine receptors

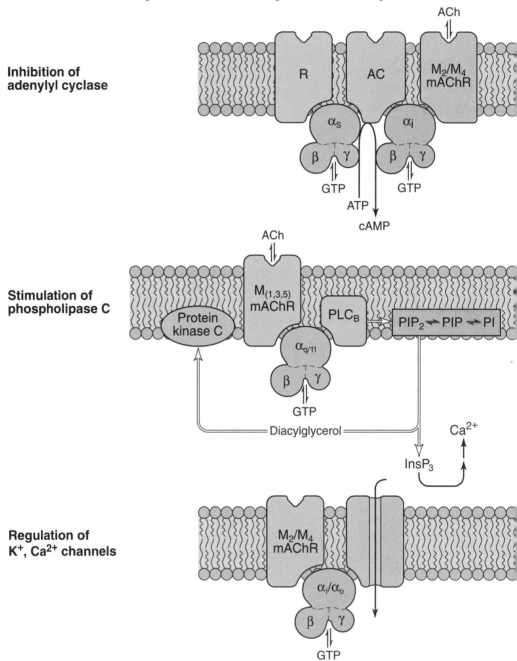

FIG. 9. Primary biochemical responses mediated by muscarinic ACh receptor. ACh interacts with a muscarinic receptor of the subtypes indicated to induce various responses. The M_2 and M_4 mAChR interact with the α-subunit of GTP-binding protein, G_i, known to inhibit adenylyl cyclase (AC). The M_1, M_3, and M_5 mAChR interact with GTP-binding proteins in the Gq family to activate phospholipase C (PLC) and K^+ channels, respectively. The M_2 and M_4 mAChR regulate certain ion channels through G_i and G_o. Mediators formed within the cell include cAMP, inositol trisphosphate ($InsP_3$), and diacylglycerol (DAG). The inositol phosphates are generated from phosphatidylinositol bisphosphate (PIP_2), phosphatidylinositol monophosphate (PIP), and phosphatidylinositol (PI).

tractile responses. Given the obviously complex set of possible interactions between the intracellular mediators, it is easy to explain how diverse cellular responses can be mediated through a single receptor activating relatively few primary responses (see Chap. 10).

Radioligand-binding studies using antagonists such as quinuclidinylbenzilate and N-methylscopolamine have been used to characterize muscarinic receptors

In membranes or homogenates from heart, brain, and other tissues, muscarinic agonists compete for antagonist-binding sites with Hill slopes of less than unity, i.e., agonists appear to interact with more than a single population of muscarinic receptors [29]. Direct binding experiments with radiolabeled agonists also show multiple binding sites for agonists. The competition curves are best fit by a model in which there are sites with low, high, and, in some cases, superhigh affinity for agonists. The addition of GTP to the binding assay can have a dramatic effect on the agonist competition curve or on direct agonist binding. The effect of GTP is to decrease the apparent affinity of the receptor for agonists. This results from a change in the interaction of the receptor with the GTP-binding protein that transduces its effects.

Agonists vary in the amount of heterogeneity in their binding. Some, like ACh, carbamylcholine, and methacholine, bind with high affinity to a large percentage of the total sites. Others, like oxotremorine and pilocarpine, bind to a single class of sites, and may show relatively little high-affinity binding. The capacity of an agonist to induce high-affinity binding correlates with the efficacy of that agonist for eliciting contractile responses or for stimulating phosphoinositide breakdown. It therefore appears that interaction of the receptor and G protein is critical to production of the cellular response.

Unlike agonists, most muscarinic antagonists such as quinuclidinylbenzilate, N-methylscopolamine, and atropine bind to

the receptor with Hill slopes of unity, as expected for a mass action interaction with a single receptor type. There is little difference in affinity for these ligands in various tissues. Similar findings with other antagonists initially suggested that all muscarinic receptors were the same. On the other hand, a number of functional studies suggested that muscarinic receptors were heterogeneous, and several atypical antagonists had been described throughout the years. Sequencing and expression studies of muscarinic receptors have now confirmed that there are at least five distinct subtypes of muscarinic receptors.

The selectivity of the antagonist pirenzepine forms the cornerstone for the classification of muscarinic receptors into pharmacologically defined subtypes

Pirenzepine binds to muscarinic receptors in cortex, hippocampus, and ganglia with relatively high affinity, and these sites have been termed M_1, as mentioned earlier. Heart, gland, and smooth muscle muscarinic receptors, as well as those in brainstem, cerebellum, and thalamus, show 30- to 50-fold lower affinity [29]. The affinity for classic antagonists like N-methylscopolamine is the same in all of these regions, emphasizing the unique selectivity of PZ. Direct binding studies using [³H]PZ confirm that only certain tissues and brain regions have receptors with high affinity for this antagonist. Results of pharmacological studies also indicate that PZ blocks muscarinic responses in ganglia better than responses in heart. Another antagonist, AF-DX 116, discriminates between the cardiac and glandular receptors that have low affinity for PZ and thereby allows further pharmacological classification of the cardiac muscarinic receptor as M_2.

Muscarinic receptors corresponding to the M_1 and M_2 subtypes have been purified from brain and atria and subsequently cloned

The cDNAs for the muscarinic receptors encode apparent glycoproteins of 55 to 70 kDa, which contain seven predicted transmembrane-spanning regions, similar to what is seen for the β-adrenergic receptor and other receptors that couple to G proteins (Fig. 10). There is only 38 percent homology between the proteins cloned from porcine brain and heart, and most of this is in the transmembrane domains [29]. The long cytoplasmic loop between the sixth and seventh transmembrane domains is markedly different for the two receptors. The cDNA encoding the receptor initially cloned from the brain has been termed m_1, whereas that cloned from the heart has been termed m_2.

The human and rat homologs of these receptor genes, as well as three additional subtypes termed m_3, m_4, and m_5, have subsequently been cloned and expressed

Comparison of the amino acid sequences of the five muscarinic receptor subtypes sug-

gests that they are members of a highly conserved gene family. The greatest sequence homology is in the transmembrane-spanning regions, whereas the third intracellular loop varies greatly among the receptor subtypes [29,33]. The cloned receptors, expressed in mammalian cells, show differences in antagonist affinity similar to those of the pharmacologically defined receptors. Thus the M_1 receptor is selectively blocked by PZ, the M_2 receptor by AFDX-116 and methoctramine, and the M_3 receptor by hexahydrosiladifenidol [29]. The regions in the receptor responsible for differences in antagonist affinity have not yet been clearly identified. Ligands are believed to bind to the receptor in a pocket deep within the transmembrane bundle formed by the seven transmembrane-spanning regions. The binding site for the covalent antagonist propylbenzilylcholine

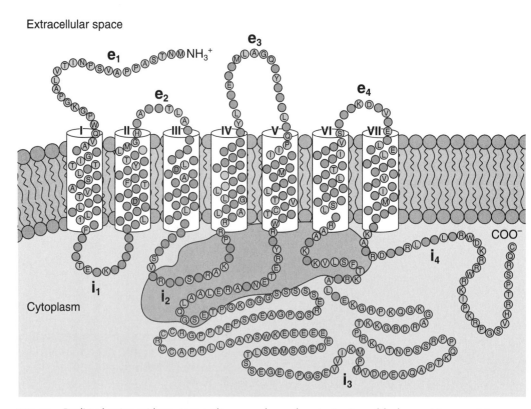

FIG. 10. Predicted amino acid sequence and transmembrane domain structure of the human M_1 muscarinic receptor. Amino acids that are identical among the M_1, M_2, M_3, and M_4 receptors are darkened. The shaded cloud represents the approximate region that determines receptor–G-protein coupling.

mustard has been mapped to a particular aspartic acid in the third transmembrane region, and mutagenesis of this amino acid profoundly affects ligand binding. It is hypothesized that this and perhaps other aspartates participate in ionic bonding with the ammonium headgroup of the cholinergic ligand [29].

Expression of the cloned receptors in Chinese hamster ovary cells, other mammalian cells, and *Xenopus* oocytes has demonstrated differential coupling of these receptors to cellular responses. In general the M_1, M_3, and M_5 receptors regulate phosphoinositide hydrolysis by stimulating phospholipase C. This occurs through selective coupling of the receptor to a pertussis toxin-insensitive G protein, probably $G_{q/11}$, which can activate the β-isoform of phospholipase C [31]. The same receptor subtypes also activate Ca^{2+}-dependent K^+ and Cl^- channels, secondary to the phospholipase C–mediated increase in intracellular Ca^{2+}. In contrast, the M_2 and M_4 receptors couple through a pertussis toxin–sensitive G protein (G_i) to inhibition of adenylyl cyclase. Regulation of K^+ and Ca^{2+} channels is also mediated through M_2 or M_4 receptor interaction with specific pertussis toxin–sensitive G proteins [32,34].

Chimeric receptors have been used to determine the regions critical for specifying coupling to particular responses. These studies demonstrate that it is the third intracellular (i_3) loop that defines functional specificity [29,33]. In particular, the amino acids proximal to the transmembrane domain (i.e., at the N-terminal and probably also the C-terminal ends of the i_3 loop) carry most of this information. These particular regions are similar in the M_1, M_3, and M_5 receptor and are also similar in the M_2 and M_4 receptors but distinguish these two groups from one another. There is also evidence that a portion of the second intracellular loop is required to specify G protein coupling correctly.

The selectivity in coupling is not absolute. Overexpression of receptors or of particular GTP-binding proteins supports interactions that may differ from those described above. For example, M_2 receptors expressed in Chinese hamster ovary cells not only inhibit adenylyl cyclase but can also stimulate phosphoinositide hydrolysis through a pertussis toxin–sensitive G protein [35]; this is not seen, however, when M_2 receptors are expressed in Y1 cells. These findings indicate that caution must be exercised in interpreting data obtained when receptors are expressed, often at high levels, in cells in which they do not normally function. Nonetheless, on the basis of current evidence it appears likely that biological responses to M_1, M_3, and M_5 receptors are mediated via receptor coupling to phospholipase C and the subsequent effects of Ca^{2+} mobilization and protein kinase C activation, whereas M_2 and M_4 receptors function via inhibition of adenylyl cyclase or direct ion-channel regulation.

REFERENCES

1. Rama-Sastry, B. V., and Sadavongvivad, C. Non-neuronal acetylcholine. *Pharmacol. Rev.* 30:65–132, 1979.
2. Dale, H. H. The action of certain esters and ethers of choline and their relation to muscarine. *J. Pharmacol.* 6:147–190, 1914.
3. Changeux, J. P. *The Acetylcholine Receptor, Fidia Research Foundation, Neuroscience Award Lectures (Vol. 4)*. In Changeux, J. P., Llinas, R. R., Purves, D. and Bloom, F. E., (eds.), New York: Raven Press, 1990, pp. 21–168.
4. Numa, S., Noda, M., Takahashi, H., Tanabe, T., Toyosoto, M., et al. Molecular structure of the acetylcholine receptor. *Cold Spring Harbor Symp. Quant. Biol.* 48:57–69, 1983.
5. Partington, P., Feeney, J., and Burgen, A. S. V. The conformation of acetylcholine and related compounds in aqueous solutions as studied by nuclear magnetic resonance spectroscopy. *Mol. Pharmacol.* 8:269–277, 1972.
6. Behling, R. W., Yamane, T., Navon, G., and Jelinski, L. W. Conformation of acetylcholine bound to the nicotinic acetylcholine receptor. *Proc. Natl. Acad. Sci. U.S.A.* 85:6721–6724, 1988.
7. Portoghese, P. S. Relationships between stereostructure and pharmacological activity. *Annu. Rev. Pharmacol.* 10:51–76, 1970.
8. Baker, R. W., Pauling, P., and Petcher, T. J.

Structure and activity of muscarinic stimulants. *Nature* 230:439–445, 1971.

9. Lefkowitz, R. J., Hoffman, B. B., and Taylor, P. Neurohumoral transmission: the autonomic and somatic motor nervous systems. In A. G. Gilman, T. W. Rall, A. S. Nies, and P. Taylor (eds.), *Goodman & Gilman's Pharmacological Basic of Therapeutics.* New York: Macmillan, 1990, pp. 84–121.

10. Deneris, E. S., Connolly, J., Rogers, S. W., and Duvoisin, R. Pharmacological and functional diversity of neuronal nicotinic acetylcholine receptors. *Trends Pharmacol. Sci.* 12:34–40, 1991.

11. Kasa, P. The cholinergic systems in brain and spinal cord. *Prog. Neurobiol.* 26:211–272, 1986.

12. Adams, P. R., Brown, D. A., and Constitini, A. Pharmacological inhibition of the M-current. *J. Physiol. (Lond.)* 332:223–262, 1982.

13. Llinás, R., and Precht, W. (eds.), *Neurobiology of the Frog.* Berlin: Springer-Verlag, 1976.

14. Berrard, S., Brice, A., Lottspeich, F., Bran, A., Barde, Y.-A., and Mallet, J. cDNA cloning and complete sequence of porcine choline acetyltransferase. *Proc. Natl. Acad. Sci. U.S.A.* 84: 9280–9284, 1987.

15. Jope, R. High affinity choline uptake and acetylcholine production in brain. Role in regulation of ACh synthesis. *Brain Res. Rev.* 1: 313–344, 1979.

16. Mayser, W., Schloss, P., and Betz, H. Primary structure and functional expression of a choline transporter expressed in the rat nervous system. *FEBS Lett.* 305:31–36, 1992.

17. Kuffler, S. W., Nicholls, J., and Martin, R. A. *From Neuron to Brain: A Cellular Approach to the Function of the Nervous System.* Sunderland, MA: Sinauer Associates Inc., 1984.

18. Parsons, S. M., Bahr, B.A., Gracz, M., Kaufman, R., Kornreich, W. D., et al. Acetylcholine transport: Fundamental properties and effects of pharmacologic agents. *Ann. N.Y. Acad. Sci.* 493:220–233, 1987.

19. Parsons, S. M., Prior, C., and Marshall, I. G. Acetylcholine transport, storage and release. *Int. Rev. Neurobiol.* 35:280–390, 1993.

20. Taylor, P. The cholinesterases. *J. Biol. Chem.* 266:4025–4028, 1991.

21. Massoulié, J., Pezzementi, L., Bon, S., Krejci, E., and Vallette, F.-M. Molecular and cellular biology of cholinesterases. *Prog. Neurobiol.* 41: 31–91, 1993.

22. Sussman, J. L., Harel, M., Frolow, F., Oefner, C., Goldman, A., Toker, L., and Silman, I. Atomic structure of acetylcholinesterase from *Torpedo californica.* A prototypic acetylcholine-binding protein. *Science* 253:872–878, 1992.

23. Unwin, N. Nicotinic acetylcholine receptor at 9 Å resolution. *J. Mol. Biol.* 229:1101–1124, 1993.

24. Sine, S. M., and Claudio, T. α- and δ-subunits regulate the affinity and cooperativity of ligand binding to the acetylcholine receptor. *J. Biol. Chem.* 266:19369–19377, 1991.

25. Hall, Z. W., and Sanes, J. R. Synaptic structure and development: The neuromuscular junction. *Cell/Neuron* 10(Suppl.):99–122, 1993.

26. Changeux, J. P. Compartmentalized transcription of acetylcholine receptor genes during motor end-plate epigenesis. *New Biologist* 3:413–429, 1991.

27. Fuentes, M. E., and Taylor, P. Control of acetylcholinesterase gene expression during myogenesis. *Neuron* 10:679–687, 1993.

28. Phillips, W. D., and Merlie, J. P. Recombinant neuromuscular synapses. *Bioessays* 14: 671–679, 1992.

29. Hulme, E., Birdsall, N., and Buckley, N. Muscarinic receptor subtypes. *Annu. Rev. Pharmacol. Toxicol.* 30:633–673, 1990.

30. Nathanson, N. Molecular properties of the muscarinic acetylcholine receptor. *Annu. Rev. Neurosci.* 10:195–236, 1987.

31. Berstein, G., Blank, J. L., Smrcka, A. V., Higashijima, T., Sternweis, P. C., Exton, J. H., and Ross, E. M. Reconstitution of agonist stimulated phosphatidylinositol 4–5 bisphosphate hydrolysis using purified m1 muscarinic receptor, $G_{q/11}$, and phospholipase C-β1. *J. Biol. Chem.* 267:8081–8088, 1992.

32. Brown, A. M., and Birnbaumer, L. Ionic channels and their regulation by G protein subunits. *Annu. Rev. Physiol.* 52:197–213, 1990.

33. Bonner, T. I. Domains of muscarinic acetylcholine receptors that confer specificity of G-protein coupling. *Trends Pharmacol. Sci.* 13: 48–50, 1992.

34. Kleuss, C., Heschelo, J., Ewel, C., Rosenthal, W., Schultz, G., and Wittig, B. Assignment of G-protein subtypes to specific receptors inducing inhibition of calcium currents. *Nature* 353:43–48, 1991.

35. Ashkenazi, A., Winslow, J. W., Peralta, E. G., Peterson, G. L., Schimerlik, M. I., Capon, D., and Ramachandran, J. An M_2 muscarinic receptor subtype coupled to both adenyl cyclase and phosphoinositide turnover. *Science* 238:672–675, 1987.

CHAPTER 12

Catecholamines

Norman Weiner and Perry B. Molinoff

Basic Neurochemistry: Molecular, Cellular, and Medical Aspects, 5th Ed., edited by G. J. Siegel et al. Published by Raven Press, Ltd., New York, 1994. Correspondence to Perry B. Molinoff, Department of Pharmacology, University of Pennsylvania School of Medicine, Philadelphia, Pennsylvania 19104-6084.

The catecholamines dopamine, norepinephrine, and epinephrine are neurotransmitters and/or hormones in the periphery and in the central nervous system. Norepinephrine is the principal postganglionic, sympathetic neurotransmitter. Dopamine, the precursor of norepinephrine, has biological activity in the periphery, most particularly in the kidney, and serves as a neurotransmitter in several important pathways in the central nervous system. Epinephrine, formed by the *N*-methylation of norepinephrine, is a hormone released from the adrenal gland, and it stimulates catecholamine receptors in a variety of organs. Small amounts of epinephrine are also found in the central nervous system, particularly in the brainstem (for review, see [1]).

BIOSYNTHESIS OF CATECHOLAMINES

The enzymatic processes involved in the formation of catecholamines have been more completely characterized than those for other neurotransmitters

The component enzymes in the pathway have been purified to homogeneity, which has allowed for detailed analysis of their kinetics, substrate specificity, and cofactor requirements and for the development of inhibitors (Fig. 1). The use of antibodies raised against the purified enzymes has permitted precise localization of the enzymes through immunocytochemical techniques.

Tyrosine hydroxylase is found in all cells that synthesize catecholamines and is the rate-limiting enzyme in their biosynthetic pathway

Tyrosine hydroxylase (TH) is a mixed-function oxidase that uses molecular oxygen and tyrosine as its substrates and biopterin as its cofactor [2]. Tyrosine hydroxylase is a homotetramer each of whose subunits has a molecular weight of approximately 60 kDa. It catalyzes the addition of a hydroxyl group to the meta position of tyrosine, thus forming 3,4-dihydroxy-L-phenylalanine (L-dopa). Tyrosine hydroxylase can also hydroxylate phenylalanine to form tyrosine, which is then converted to L-dopa; this alternative synthetic route may be of significance in patients affected with phenylketonuria, in which phenylalanine hydroxylase activity is

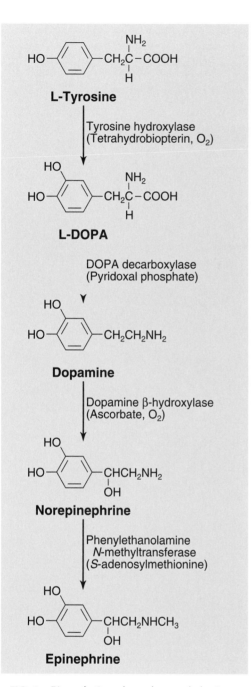

L-Tyrosine

Tyrosine hydroxylase
(Tetrahydrobiopterin, O$_2$)

L-DOPA

DOPA decarboxylase
(Pyridoxal phosphate)

Dopamine

Dopamine β-hydroxylase
(Ascorbate, O$_2$)

Norepinephrine

Phenylethanolamine
N-methyltransferase
(*S*-adenosylmethionine)

Epinephrine

FIG. 1. Biosynthetic pathway for catecholamines.

depressed (see Chap. 39). Tyrosine hydroxylase has a K_m for tyrosine in the micromolar range. As a result, it is virtually saturated by the high tissue concentrations of endogenous tyrosine. Although the availability of tyrosine does not ordinarily limit the rate of amine synthesis, the cofactor, biopterin, may be at subsaturating concentrations within catecholamine-containing neurons and thus may play an important role in regulating norepinephrine biosynthesis. Tyrosine hydroxylase is primarily a soluble enzyme, localized in the cytosol of catecholamine-containing neuronal processes; however, interactions with membrane constituents, such as phosphatidylserine, or with polyanions, such as heparin sulfate, have been shown to alter its kinetic characteristics. Analogs of tyrosine, such as α-methyl-*p*-tyrosine, are competitive inhibitors of TH. Sequence analysis [3] reveals consensus sequences for phosphorylation primarily in the N-terminal portion of the molecule (Fig. 2). The gene reveals considerable sequence homology with phenylalanine hydroxylase and tryptophan hydroxylase.

Dopa decarboxylase is a pyridoxine-dependent enzyme that catalyzes the removal of the carboxyl group from dopa to form dopamine

Dopa decarboxylase (DDC) has a low K_m and a high V_m with respect to L-dopa; thus, endogenous L-dopa is efficiently converted to dopamine, and negligible amounts of L-dopa are found in catecholamine-containing tissues [4]. Dopa decarboxylase can also decarboxylate 5-hydroxytryptophan, the precursor of serotonin, as well as other aromatic amino acids; accordingly, it has also been called aromatic amino acid decarboxylase. Dopa decarboxylase is widely distributed throughout the body, where it is found both in catecholamine- and serotonin-containing neurons and in non-neuronal tissues, such as kidney and blood vessels. In dopamine-containing neurons, this is the final step in the pathway. α-Methyldopa inhibits DDC *in vitro* and leads

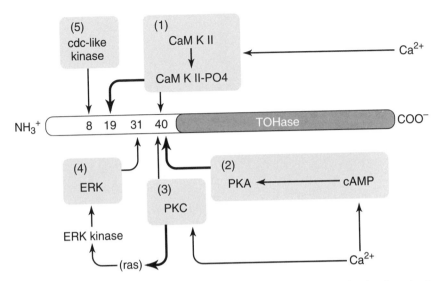

FIG. 2.   Schematic diagram of the phosphorylation sites on each of the four 60-kDa subunits of tyrosine hydroxylase (TOHase). Serine residues at the N-terminal end of each of four subunits of TOHase can be phosphorylated by at least five protein kinases. (1) Calcium/calmodulin-dependent protein kinase II (CaM K II) phosphorylates serine residue 19 and to a lesser extent serine 40. (2) cAMP-dependent protein kinase (PKA) phosphorylates serine residue 40. (3) Calcium/phosphatidylserine-activated protein kinase (PKC) phosphorylates serine 40. (4) Extracellular receptor-activated protein kinase (ERK) phosphorylates serine 31. (5) A *cdc*-like protein kinase phosphorylates serine 8. Phosphorylation on either serine 19 or 40 increases the activity of TOHase. Serine 19 phosphorylation requires the presence of an "activator protein" (also known as 14-3-3 protein) for the expression of increased activity. Phosphorylation of serines 8 and 31 has little effect on catalytic activity. The model shown includes the activation of ERK by an ERK-kinase. The ERK-kinase is activated by phosphorylation by PKC. (From Waymire, J. C., and Craviso, G. L., *Adv. Prot. Phosphatases* 7:495–506, 1993.)

to a reduction in blood pressure after being converted to the false transmitter α-methyl-norepinephrine.

For neurons that synthesize epinephrine or norepinephrine, dopamine-β-hydroxylase is the next step in the biosynthetic pathway

Like TH, dopamine-β-hydroxylase (DBH) is a mixed-function oxidase that uses molecular oxygen to form the hydroxyl group added to the β-carbon on the side chain of dopamine [5]. Ascorbate, reduced to dihydroascorbate during the reaction, provides a source of electrons. Dopamine-β-hydroxylase contains Cu^{2+}, which is involved in electron transfer in the reaction; accordingly, copper chelators, such as diethyldithiocarbamate, are potent inhibitors of DBH. Dopamine-β-hydroxylase is a tetrameric glycoprotein containing subunits of 77 and 73 kDa as determined by SDS gel electrophoresis. A full-length clone was isolated from a λgt11 library and shown to encode a polypeptide chain of 578 amino acids [6]. The enzyme is concentrated within the vesicles that store catecholamines; most of the DBH is bound to the inner vesicular membrane, but some is free within the vesicles. Dopamine-β-hydroxylase is released along with catecholamines from nerves and from the adrenal gland and is found in plasma.

In chromaffin cells that synthesize epinephrine, the final step in the pathway is catalyzed by the enzyme phenylethanolamine *N*-methyltransferase

These cells include a small group of neurons in the brainstem that utilize epinephrine as their neurotransmitter and the adrenal medullary cells for which epinephrine is the primary neurohormone. Phenylethanolamine *N*-methyltransferase (PNMT) transfers a methyl group from *S*-adenosylmethionine to the nitrogen of norepinephrine, forming a secondary amine [7]. The coding sequence of bovine PNMT is contained in a single open reading frame encoding a protein of 284 amino acids [8]. PNMT activity is regulated by corticosteroids. The high activity of PNMT in the adrenal medulla reflects the high concentrations of corticosteroids released into the venous sinuses that drain the adrenal cortex. Hypophysectomy, which causes a decrease in corticosteroid levels, results in marked reductions in the amount of this enzyme in adrenergic tissues; conversely, administration of large amounts of corticosteroids, particularly during the neonatal period, results in the synthesis of PNMT in sympathetic neurons that do not ordinarily express the enzyme.

STORAGE AND RELEASE OF CATECHOLAMINES

Catecholamines are concentrated in storage vesicles that are present in high density within nerve terminals

Ordinarily, low concentrations of catecholamines are free in the cytosol where they may be metabolized by enzymes including monoamine oxidase (MAO). Thus, conversion of tyrosine to L-dopa and L-dopa to dopamine occurs in the cytosol; dopamine then is taken up into the storage vesicles. In norepinephrine-containing neurons, the final β-hydroxylation occurs within the vesicles. In the adrenal gland, norepinephrine is *N*-methylated by PNMT in the cytoplasm. Epinephrine is then transported back into chromaffin granules for storage. cDNA clones encoding vesicular amine transporters have been obtained. The sequence suggests that the proteins have 12 transmembrane domains and are homologous to a family of bacterial drug resistance transporters. The expressed

protein has a high affinity for reserpine, which blocks vesicular uptake *in vivo* [9]. The mechanism that concentrates catecholamines within the vesicles is an adenosine triphosphate (ATP)-dependent process linked to a proton pump. The intravesicular concentration of catecholamines is approximately 0.5 M, and they exist in a complex with ATP and acidic proteins known as chromogranins. The vesicular uptake process has broad substrate specificity and can transport a variety of biogenic amines, including tryptamine, tyramine, and amphetamines; these amines may compete with endogenous catecholamines for vesicular storage sites. Reserpine is a specific, irreversible inhibitor of the vesicular amine pump that terminates the ability of the vesicles to concentrate the amines. Treatment with reserpine causes a profound depletion of endogenous catecholamines in neurons. The effect of reserpine is to inhibit the uptake of dopamine and other catecholamines into vesicles.

The vesicles play a dual role: They maintain a ready supply of catecholamines at the terminal available for release, and they mediate the process of release. When an action potential reaches the nerve terminal, Ca^{2+} channels open, allowing an influx of the cation into the terminal; increased intracellular Ca^{2+} promotes the fusion of vesicles with the neuronal membrane (see Chap. 9). The vesicles then discharge their soluble contents, including norepinephrine, ATP, and DBH, into the extraneuronal space [10]. The demonstration that DBH is released concurrently and proportionately with norepinephrine established that release occurs by the process of exocytosis, since proteins would not be expected to diffuse across cell membranes. Exocytotic release from sympathetic neurons may be the source of some of the DBH found in the plasma and cerebrospinal fluid of animals and humans. Indirectly acting sympathomimetics, like tyramine and amphetamine, release catecholamines by a mechanism that is neither dependent on Ca^{2+} nor associated with release of DBH. These drugs displace catecholamines from storage vesicles, resulting in leakage of neurotransmitter from the nerve terminals.

Despite marked fluctuations in the activity of catecholamine-containing neurons, the level of catecholamines within nerve terminals remains relatively constant

Efficient regulatory mechanisms operate to modulate the rate of synthesis of catecholamines [11]. A long-term process affecting catecholamine synthesis involves alterations in the amounts of TH and DBH present in nerve terminals [1]. When the level of neuronal activity of sympathetic neurons is increased for a prolonged period of time, the amounts of mRNA coding for TH and DBH are increased in the neuronal perikarya. Dopa decarboxylase does not appear to be modulated by this process. The newly synthesized enzyme molecules are then transported down the axon to the nerve terminals.

Alteration in the rate of synthesis of TH and DBH provides a mechanism to modulate synthesis of catecholamines in response to persistent changes in neuronal activity. In addition, two mechanisms operative at the level of the nerve terminal play important roles in the short-term modulation of catecholamine synthesis and are responsive to momentary changes in neuronal activity. Tyrosine hydroxylase, the rate-limiting enzyme in the synthesis pathway, is modulated by end-product inhibition [11]. Thus, free intraneuronal catecholamines inhibit the further activity of TH by competing at the site that binds the pterin cofactor; conversely, neuronal activity results in the release of catecholamines, a decrease in cytoplasmic levels, and disinhibition of the enzyme. An additional and probably more important effect of depolarization of catecholaminergic terminals is activation of TH. The kinetic characteristics of the enzyme change so that it has a higher affinity for the pterin cofactor and is less sensitive to end-product inhibition. Activation of the enzyme is associated with reversible phosphorylation of the enzyme [12]. Protein kinase C and cAMP-dependent and Ca^{2+}-calmodulin-dependent protein kinases are all capable of inducing phosphorylation of the enzyme, leading to an increase in activity (see Chap. 22).

Two enzymes are primarily responsible for the inactivation of catecholamines: monoamine oxidase and catechol-*O*-methyltransferase

Monoamine oxidase and catechol-*O*-methyltransferase (COMT) are widely distributed throughout the body (Fig. 3). Monoamine oxidase is a flavin-containing enzyme located on the outer membrane of the mitochondria [13]. This enzyme oxidatively deaminates catecholamines to their corresponding aldehydes; these can be converted, in turn, by aldehyde dehydrogenase to acids or by aldehyde reductase to form glycols. Because of its intracellular localization, MAO plays a strategic role in inactivating catecholamines that are free within the nerve terminal and not protected by storage vesicles. Accordingly, drugs that interfere with vesicular storage, such as reserpine, or indirectly acting sympathomimetics, such as amphetamines, which displace catecholamines from vesicles, cause a marked increase in deaminated metabolites. Isozymes of MAO with differential substrate specificities have been identified. MAO-A preferentially deaminates norepinephrine and serotonin, and it is selectively inhibited by clorgyline, whereas MAO-B acts on a broad spectrum of phenylethylamines including β-phenylethylamine. Monoamine oxidase B is selectively inhibited by deprenyl. Monoamine oxidase in the gastrointestinal tract and liver plays an important protective role by preventing access to the general circulation of ingested, indirectly acting amines, such as tyramine and phenylethylamine, that are contained in food; however, patients being treated for depression or hypertension with MAO inhibitors are not afforded this protection and can suffer severe hypertensive crises after ingesting foods that contain large amounts of tyramine. Such

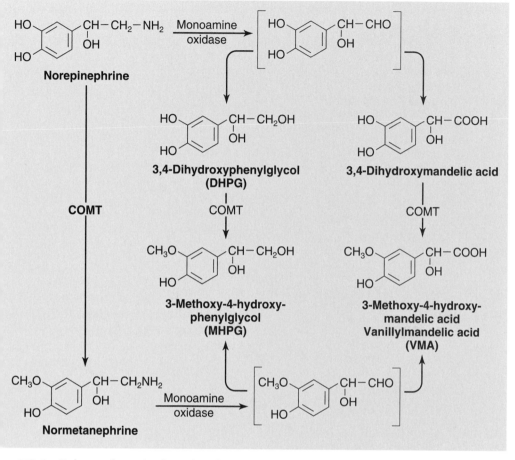

FIG. 3. Pathways of norepinephrine degradation. Unstable glycol aldehydes are shown in parentheses.

oods include port wine, Stilton cheese, and herring. A methyl substituent on the α-carbon of the phenylethylamine side chain protects against deamination by MAO; the prolonged action of amphetamine and related indirectly acting stimulants is in part a consequence of the presence of an α-methyl group, which prevents their inactivation by MAO.

Catechol-*O*-methyltransferase is found in nearly all cells, including erythrocytes [14]; thus, COMT acts on extraneuronal catecholamines. Most studies of COMT are carried out with enzyme purified from homogenates of liver. The enzyme, which requires Mg^{2+}, transfers a methyl group from the cosubstrate *S*-adenosylmethionine to the 3-hydroxy group on the catecholamine ring. This enzyme has broad substrate specificity, methylating virtually any catechol regardless of the side chain constituents; for this reason, competitive inhibitors of the enzyme that are of pharmacological significance have not been developed.

Measurement of catecholamine metabolites can provide insight into the rate of release or turnover of catecholamines in the brain. In clinical studies, metabolites of catecholamines are generally assayed in the cerebrospinal fluid, because the large quantities derived from the peripheral sympathomedullary system obscure the small contribution from the brain to urinary levels. However, acid metabolites are actively excreted from the cerebrospinal fluid; more reliable estimates of turnover in the brain are obtained when this transport process is blocked by pretreatment with the drug probenecid.

4-Hydroxy-3-methoxy-phenylacetic acid, more commonly known as homovanillic acid (HVA), is a major metabolite of dopamine. Spinal fluid levels of HVA provide insight into the turnover of dopamine in the striatum. Levels of HVA are decreased, for example, in cerebrospinal fluid of patients with Parkinson's disease (see Chap. 44). A metabolite of norepinephrine formed relatively selectively in the brain is 3-methoxy-4-hydroxy-phenylglycol (MHPG). Because this is a minor metabolite of the much larger amounts of norepinephrine metabolized in the periphery, it is estimated that between 30 and 50 percent of the MHPG excreted in urine is derived from brain. Levels of MHPG have been measured in cerebrospinal fluid and in urine to provide an index of norepinephrine turnover in the brain, and levels have been shown to be decreased in certain forms of depression (see Chap. 8).

The action of catecholamines released at the synapse is terminated by re-uptake into presynaptic nerve terminals

Catecholamines that have not been effectively removed from the synaptic cleft by the transport process diffuse into the extracellular space, where they may be catabolized by MAO and COMT in the liver and kidney. The catecholamine re-uptake process was originally described by Axelrod [15]. He observed that when radioactive norepinephrine was injected intravenously, it accumulated in tissues in direct proportion to the density of the sympathetic innervation in the tissue. The amine taken up into the tissues was protected from catabolic degradation, and studies of the subcellular distribution of catecholamines showed that they are localized in synaptic vesicles. Ablation of the sympathetic input to organs abolished the ability of vesicles to accumulate and store radioactive norepinephrine. Subsequent studies

demonstrated that this Na^+-dependent uptake process is a characteristic feature of catecholamine-containing neurons in both the periphery and the brain; the transport process has been extensively studied in sheared off nerve terminals or synaptosomes isolated from brain.

The uptake process is mediated by a carrier located on the outer membrane of the catecholaminergic neurons. It is saturable and obeys Michaelis-Menten kinetics. A transport process selective for norepinephrine is found only in noradrenergic neurons whereas a carrier with different specificity is found on dopamine-containing neurons. Cloning of genes encoding proteins responsible for uptake of norepinephrine and for dopamine has been accomplished, revealing proteins with conserved structural features [16]. The presence of 11-13 transmembrane domains is a recurrent theme. Transmembrane domains 1-2 and 4-8 show the highest degree of sequence identity. The uptake process is energy dependent, since it can be inhibited by incubation at a low temperature or by metabolic inhibitors. The energy requirements reflect a coupling of the uptake process with the Na^+ gradient across the neuronal membrane; drugs such as ouabain which inhibits Na,K-ATPase, or drugs like veratridine, which opens Na^+ channels, inhibit the uptake process. The linkage of uptake to the Na^+ gradient may be of physiological significance, since transport temporarily ceases at the time of depolarization-induced release of catecholamines. The uptake of catecholamines can be inhibited selectively by such drugs as tricyclic antidepressants and cocaine. In addition, a variety of phenylethylamines, such as amphetamine, bind to the carrier; thus, they can be concentrated within catecholamine-containing neurons and can compete with the catecholamines for transport.

Once an amine has been taken up across the neuronal membrane, it can be sequestered within adrenergic storage vesicles. Neuronal uptake is Na^+ dependent and is not affected by drugs like reserpine; uptake across the vesicle membrane requires Mg^{2+} and is inhibited by reserpine. Once a compound is taken up into the vesicles, it can be released in place of norepinephrine. Such substances are called false transmitters. Active uptake is also the mechanism whereby the neurotoxin 6-hydroxydopamine is accumulated in catecholamine-containing neurons, destroying them through the auto-oxidative liberation of hydrogen peroxide or through formation of a quinone.

ANATOMY OF CATECHOLAMINERGIC SYSTEMS

Our understanding of the function of catecholamine-containing neurons has been aided by neuroanatomical methods of visualizing these neurons

Nearly two decades ago, Falck and Hillarp took advantage of the fact that, in the presence of formaldehyde, catecholamines cyclize to form intensely fluorescent products [17]. With a fluorescence microscope, neurons containing catecholamines could be visualized in thin sections obtained from tissue previously exposed to formaldehyde vapor. Numerous investigators have used this technique to map the distribution of catecholamine-containing cell bodies and axonal pathways in the brain. A modification of the method uses glyoxylic acid and has resulted in enhanced sensitivity and a more stable fluorophor for even better visualization of the fine axons and terminals.

Once the enzymes that synthesize catecholamines were purified, it was possible to elicit antiserum against each enzyme. Thin sections of tissue can be incubated with antibody against a particular enzyme, e.g., rabbit anti-DBH. The section is then incubated with a second antibody linked to a marker, such as fluorescein (fluorescein-labeled goat anti-rabbit IgG) or horseradish peroxidase. The neurons containing these enzymes are thus stained specifically. By using this technique, the PNMT-containing neurons that synthesize epinephrine can be distinguished from noradrenergic neurons that are devoid of PNMT; similarly, noradrenergic neurons that contain DBH can be separated from the dopamine-containing neurons that do not possess this enzyme. Cloning the genes that encode for catecholaminergic biosynthetic enzymes makes it possible to use *in situ* hybridization to localize mRNAs within particular neurons (see Chaps. 24 and 25).

Finally, experimental advantage has been taken of the highly selective uptake process for catecholamines. Thus, after incubation with radioactive norepinephrine, noradrenergic axons can be demonstrated at the ultrastructural level by autoradiographic techniques. Alternatively, after administration of the congener 5-hydroxydopamine, which is taken up actively and stored within the vesicles, catecholamine-containing terminals can be distinguished by the presence of dense precipitates of 5-hydroxydopamine within their vesicles.

Cell bodies of noradrenergic neurons are clustered in the medulla oblongata, pons, and midbrain and are considered to be anatomically part of the reticular formation

On the basis of their major axonal projections, noradrenergic fibers can be divided into two major pathways: the dorsal and ventral bundles (Fig. 4). The cell bodies of origin for the dorsal bundle are contained in a dense nucleus known as the locus coeruleus, located on the lateral aspect of the fourth ventricle. Axons of neurons in the locus coeruleus have endings in the spinal cord and cerebellum and course anteriorly through the medial forebrain bundle to innervate the entire cerebral cortex and hippocampus. The ventrally located cell bodies send fibers that innervate the brainstem and hypothalamus. As demonstrated by immunocytochemical techniques, in the ventral portion of the pons and medulla there are a small number of neurons that contain PNMT; the axons of these epinephrine-containing neurons terminate primarily in the brainstem and hypothalamus.

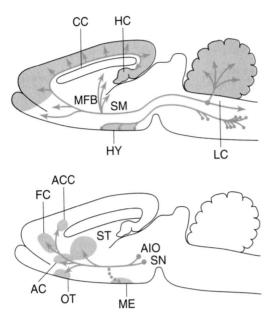

FIG. 4. Catecholaminergic neuronal pathways in the rat brain. *Upper:* Noradrenergic neuronal pathways. *Lower:* Dopaminergic neuronal pathways. (AC) nucleus accumbens; (ACC) anterior cingulate cortex; (CC) corpus callosum; (FC) frontal cortex; (HC) hippocampus; (HY) hypothalamus; (LC) locus coeruleus; (ME) median eminence; (MFB) median forebrain bundle; (OT) olfactory tubercle; (SM) stria medullaris; (SN) substantia nigra; (ST) striatum. (Courtesy of J. T. Coyle and S. H. Snyder.)

Cell bodies of dopamine-containing neurons are located primarily in the midbrain

Dopamine-containing neurons can be divided into three main groups: nigrostriatal, mesocortical, and tuberohypophysial. The major dopaminergic tract in brain originates in the zona compacta of the substantia nigra and sends axons that provide a dense innervation to the caudate nucleus and putamen of the corpus striatum; nearly 80 percent of all the dopamine in the brain is found in the corpus striatum. In Parkinson's disease, the nigrostriatal tract degenerates. This accounts for a profound depletion of dopamine from the striatum and for the symptoms of this disorder. The compound MPTP may be formed as a side product in the synthesis of an analog of the synthetic opiate meperidine. Ingestion or administration of small amounts of MPTP causes biochemical and clinical changes identical to those seen in Parkinson's disease (see also Chap. 44).

Dopamine-containing cell bodies that lie medial to the substantia nigra provide a diffuse, but modest, innervation to the forebrain, including the frontal and cingulate cortex, septum, nucleus accumbens, and olfactory tubercle. It has been hypothesized that antipsychotic neuroleptic drugs exert their therapeutic action through blockade of the effects of dopamine released by this system (see Chap. 47).

Dopamine-containing cell bodies in the arcuate and periventricular nuclei of the hypothalamus send axons that innervate the intermediate lobe of the pituitary and the median eminence. These neurons play an important role in regulating the release of pituitary hormones, especially prolactin (see Chap. 15). In addition to these major pathways, dopamine-containing interneurons have been found in the olfactory bulb and in the neural retina.

CATECHOLAMINE RECEPTORS

The brain contains multiple classes of receptors for catecholamines

Effects of dopamine are mediated through interaction with D_1-like (D_1 and D_5) and D_2-like (D_2, D_3, and D_4) receptors, while effects of norepinephrine and epinephrine are mediated through α_1- and α_2-adrenergic receptors and through β-adrenergic receptors. As of the present time, three subtypes of α_1-, three subtypes of α_2-, and three subtypes of β-adrenergic receptors have been identified (Table 1).

Autoreceptors

The postsynaptic receptors on any given neuron receive information from transmitters released by another neuron. Typically, postsynaptic receptors are located on dendrites or cell bodies of neurons, but they also may occur on axons or nerve terminals; in the latter case, an axoaxonic synaptic relation-

TABLE 1. Distinguishing features of multiple classes of catecholamine receptors

---

DOPAMINE RECEPTORS

Dopamine 1 (D_1) receptor family
Includes D_1 and D_5 receptors
Linked to stimulation of adenylyl cyclase
Ergot alkaloids (e.g., bromocryptine) are antagonists
SKF-38393 is a specific agonist
Butyrophenone neuroleptics are weak antagonists
Largely absent in pituitary, but present in parathyroid gland
Present in corpus striatum on intrinsic neurons sensitive to kainic acid
Studied with [^{3}H]SCH-23390 or [^{125}I]SCH-23982

Dopamine 2 (D_2) receptor family
Includes D_2, D_3, and D_4 receptors
D_2 receptors are linked to inhibition of adenylyl cyclase
The second messenger for D_3 and D_4 receptors remains unknown
Ergot alkaloids are agonists
N-propylnorapomorphine and aminotetralines are selective agonists
Butyrophenone neuroleptics are potent antagonists
Present in pituitary
Present in corpus striatum on axons and terminals of corticostriate neurons
Studied with [^{3}H]spiroperidol or [^{125}I]iodobenzamide

NOREPINEPHRINE AND EPINEPHRINE RECEPTORS

β Receptors
Linked to stimulation of adenylyl cyclase
No selective radioligands. Studied with [^{125}I]iodopindolol, [^{3}H]dihydroalprenolol, or [^{3}H]CGP-12177 (hydrophilic)

β_1 Receptors
Found in high density in the heart and cerebral cortex
Epinephrine and norepinephrine are equally potent agonists
Practolol and ICI 89,406 are selective antagonists
Marked regional variations in brain

β_2 Receptors
Linked to stimulation of adenylyl cyclase
Found in high density in the lung and cerebellum
Epinephrine is more potent than norepinephrine
Terbutaline and salbutamol are selective agonists
ICI 118,551 is a selective antagonist

β_3 Receptors
Associated with nonshivering thermogenesis in rodents
mRNA selectively expressed in brown adipose tissue
BRL 37344 is a selective agonist

α_1 RECEPTORS

Three subtypes, α_{1A}, α_{1B}, and α_{1C}, are known to exist
Located postsynaptically on blood vessels and in the spleen and peripheral tissues
Effects mediated through activation of phospholipase C and increases in intracellular Ca^{2+}
Prazosin, indoramin, and WB-4101 are selective antagonists of receptors localized in heart and vas deferens
Studied with [^{3}H]WB-4101, [^{3}H]prazosin, or [^{125}I]BE-2254

α_2 RECEPTORS

Three subtypes, α_{2A}, α_{2B}, and α_{2C}, are known to exist
Located on presynaptic nerve terminals in the periphery
Piperoxan and yohimbine are relatively selective antagonists
Clonidine and other imidazolines are selective agonists
Effects mediated through inhibition of adenylyl cyclase activity
Studied with [^{3}H]clonidine, [^{3}H]yohimbine, or [^{3}H]idazoxan

ship may cause presynaptic inhibition or excitation. In contrast, autoreceptors are situated on a given neuron and respond to transmitter molecules released from the same neuron. Autoreceptors may be widely distributed on the surface of the neuron. At the nerve terminal, they respond to transmitter molecules released into the synaptic cleft; on the cell body, they may respond to transmitter molecules released by dendrites. Functionally, most autoreceptors appear to regulate transmitter release in such a way that the released transmitter, acting on autoreceptors, regulates additional release. Autoreceptors have been identified for norepinephrine-, dopamine-, serotonin-, and GABA-containing neurons; however, the most detailed information is available from studies of norepinephrine-containing neurons. The major types of inhibitory autoreceptor described in both the peripheral sympathetic nervous system and the brain has

pharmacological properties resembling those of the α_2-adrenergic receptor [18].

In the peripheral sympathetic nervous system, autoreceptors of the β-adrenergic type have also been described. These differ from most other known autoreceptors in that norepinephrine acting on these receptors facilitates transmitter release and thus amplifies the effects of neuronal firing. This effect contrasts with the inhibitory action of α-adrenergic and dopamine autoreceptors, which exert negative feedback control on transmitter release.

DOPAMINE RECEPTORS

Two subtypes of dopamine receptor were initially identified on the basis of pharmacological and biochemical criteria [19]. D_1 receptors were shown to couple to stimulation of adenylyl cyclase activity, while D_2 receptors inhibited enzyme activity (Fig. 5). Multiple D_1-

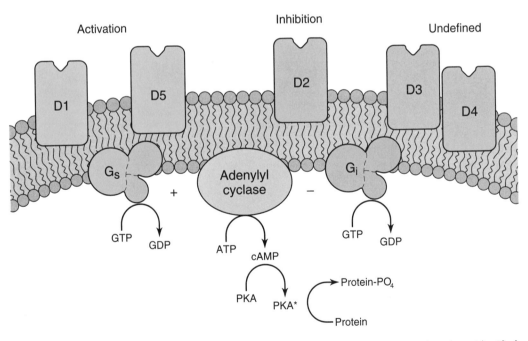

FIG. 5.   Effect of dopamine on adenylyl cyclase activity. Five subtypes of dopamine receptor have been identified. The D_1 and the D_5 receptors are coupled to stimulation of adenylyl cyclase. The D_2 receptor is coupled to inhibition of enzyme activity. Biochemical second messengers have not yet been identified for the D_3 and D_4 receptors. Adenylyl cyclase catalyzes the conversion of ATP into cAMP, which in turn causes dissociation of the regulatory and catalytic subunits of protein kinase A. The activated catalytic subunit catalyzes conversion of protein substrates into phosphoproteins.

TABLE 2. Properties of cloned dopamine receptor subtypes

	D_1	D_5	D_{2S}/D_{2L}	D_3	D_4
Amino acids					
Human	446	477	414/443	400	387
Chromosome	5	4	11	3	11
Effector pathways	↑cAMP	↑cAMP	↓cAMP ↑K^+ channel ↓Ca^{2+} channel	?	?
mRNA distribution	CPu nucleus accumbens olfactory tubercle	hippocampus hypothalamus	CPu nucleus accumbens olfactory tubercle	olfactory tubercle hypothalamus nucleus accumbens	frontal cortex medulla midbrain

like and D_2-like receptors have now been identified, and deduced amino acid sequences have been determined (Table 2). The known subtypes of dopamine receptor are members of the G protein-linked receptor family with seven hydrophobic domains, an extracellular N terminus, and an intracellular C terminus (Fig. 6). Consensus sequences for phosphorylation are found in the third intracellular (i_3) loop and the C-terminal tail. The D_1-like receptors have relatively small i_3 loops and long C-terminal tails, while the D_2-like receptors have large i_3 loops and short C-terminal tails.

The D_1-like receptors include the D_1 and D_5 receptors [20]. The recently cloned D_{1B} receptor is believed to be the rat homolog of the human D_5 receptor. The D_1-like receptors have a high affinity for benzazepines like SCH-23390 and a low affinity for benzamides and are coupled to stimulation of adenylyl cyclase activity. The most striking pharmacological difference among them is the high affinity of D_5 receptors for dopamine.

Molecular genetic studies have demonstrated the presence of two forms of mRNA coding for D_2 receptors, designated D_{2L} and D_{2S}

These two forms differ by 87 bases, corresponding to a 29-amino acid insert in the i_3 loop of the receptor (Fig. 6). The two species of D_2 receptor mRNA appear to arise through alternative splicing. Thus far, no dif-

ferences in pharmacological properties or in interaction with second-messenger systems have been reported. Both D_{2L} and D_{2S} receptors are coupled to inhibition of adenylyl cyclase activity. The D_3 receptor, a second member of the D_2-like receptor family, has been cloned and expressed in COS-7 cells. D_3 receptor mRNA is found in limbic areas of the brain as well as the nucleus accumbens. Comparison of the properties of D_2 and D_3 receptors shows that the D_3 receptor has a relatively high affinity for atypical neuroleptics and for dopamine autoreceptor inhibitors including (+)-UH232 and (+)-AJ76. The cloning of the D_4 receptor has introduced an additional level of complexity to the study of dopamine receptors. Of particular interest is the high affinity of D_4 receptors for the atypical neuroleptic clozapine. D_4 receptor mRNA has been detected in the frontal cortex, midbrain, amygdala, and medulla, with lower levels detected in the basal ganglia. The use of molecular approaches to the study of the D_4 receptor has been hampered by the high G/C content of its coding sequences. At present it is unclear which second-messenger system is linked to stimulation of D_3 or D_4 receptors.

The density of D_2 receptors in rat striatum is increased following lesions with 6-hydroxydopamine or administration of antagonists

Similar results for D_1 receptors were obtained following chronic administration of

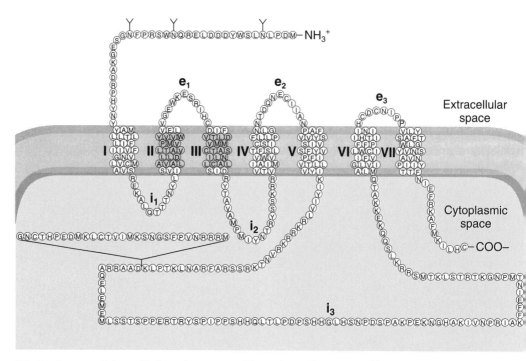

FIG. 6. Structure of the rat D_2 dopamine receptor. The amino acid sequence of the receptor is deduced from that of the cDNA. The D_2 receptor is a member of the G protein-linked receptor family with seven putative transmembrane helices, an extracellular N terminus containing possible sites for *N*-linked glycosylation (Y), and an intracellular C terminus. Transmembrane-spanning sequences (I to VII) are separated by extracellular (e_1 to e_3) and intracellular (i_1 to i_3) loops. An unusual feature of the D_2 receptor is the existence of a splice variant such that there are long and short isoforms that differ by the inclusion or exclusion of a 29-amino acid insert in the i_3 loop.

the D_1-selective antagonist SCH-23390. Subtypes of dopamine receptor may be co-regulated, since the D_2 antagonist sulpiride attenuated the ability of SCH-23390 to increase the density of D_1 receptors. The increase in the density of D_2 receptors following chronic administration of antagonists may be responsible for the development of a movement disorder called tardive dyskinesia (see Chap. 47).

Available behavioral data suggest that either acute or repeated administration of agonists acting at dopamine receptors results in augmentation of the behavioral effects of the drugs. This phenomenon, known as reverse tolerance or sensitization, is characterized by a selective increase in the intensity or duration or a shift to an earlier time of onset of stereotypical behaviors such as locomotion, sniffing, rearing, licking, or gnawing. Sensitization to indirect dopamine agonists like amphetamine or cocaine may involve an increase in the release of dopamine from presynaptic terminals. This mechanism is unlikely to be involved in the sensitization produced by apomorphine since this drug acts as a direct dopamine receptor agonist. The mechanisms underlying behavioral sensitization are likely to be complex. It is known, for example, that stereotypical behavior and locomotor hyperactivity are critically dependent on activation of both D_1 and D_2 receptors.

Agonists at dopamine receptors, including amphetamine, bromocriptine, and lisuride, have been shown to induce psychotic episodes

A strong correlation exists between the clinical doses of neuroleptics and their affinity for brain D_2 receptors. This has led to the hypothesis that psychotic disorders result from overstimulation of D_2 receptors. Long-term administration of neuroleptics to humans or experimental animals can result in an increase in the density of striatal D_2 receptors and in the appearance of extrapyramidal side effects, including parkinsonian movement disorders and tardive dyskinesia. A panel of antipsychotic drugs referred to as atypical neuroleptics, including clozapine, melperone, and fluperlapine, have been reported to produce fewer extrapyramidal side effects and have been useful in the treatment of patients with schizophrenia who respond poorly to typical antipsychotics such as haloperidol. The relative affinities of D_2, D_3, and D_4 receptors for typical and atypical neuroleptics, together with the selective expression of D_3 receptor mRNA in limbic areas of the brain, has led to the hypothesis that the clinical utility of neuroleptics in the treatment of psychiatric illness may be due, at least in part, to their ability to antagonize stimulation of D_3 or D_4 receptors, while the motor dysfunction observed following chronic treatment with typical neuroleptics could be due to alterations in the density of D_2 receptors in the striatum.

α- AND β-ADRENERGIC RECEPTORS

The pharmacological responses to catecholamines were ascribed to effects of α-adrenergic and β-adrenergic receptors in the late 1940s

Norepinephrine and epinephrine act at both α and β receptors, but isoproterenol, a synthetic agonist, acts only at β receptors. Numerous antagonists also differentiate between α and β receptors. The prototypic β-adrenergic receptor antagonist propranolol is essentially inactive at α receptors; the α-adrenergic receptor antagonist phentolamine is very weak at β receptors.

Physically distinct subtypes of β-adrenergic receptors exist and have important pharmacological consequences

Of the β receptors, those known as $β_1$-adrenergic receptors predominate in the heart and in the cerebral cortex whereas $β_2$-adrenergic receptors predominate in the lung and cerebellum (Table 3). However, in many cases, $β_1$- and $β_2$-adrenergic receptors coexist in the same tissue, sometimes mediating the same physiological effect. A major side effect of $β_2$-selective agonists like metaproterenol, used to treat bronchial asthma, is cardiac acceleration. This is due to the coexistence of $β_1$- and $β_2$-adrenergic receptors in the heart. Both classes of receptor are coupled to the electrophysiological effects of catecholamines in the heart.

The brain contains both $β_1$ and $β_2$ receptors, which cannot be differentiated in terms of their physiological functions. Moreover, radioactive drugs that bind exclusively to one or the other type of β receptor are not yet available. However, one can label all of the β-adrenergic receptors in a given tissue with a nonselective radioligand and then selectively inhibit the binding to one of the subtypes of β receptors with increasing concentrations of $β_1$- or $β_2$-selective agents [21]. ICI 89,406 and ICI 118,551 are highly selective antagonists at $β_1$- and $β_2$-adrenergic receptors, respectively. A similar approach can be used to define the anatomical localization of $β_1$- and $β_2$-adrenergic receptors using the technique of quantitative autoradiography. The density of $β_1$ receptors varies in different brain areas to a greater extent than does that of $β_2$ receptors. It has been suggested that this is due to the presence of $β_2$-adrenergic receptors on glia or blood vessels.

A third subtype of β-adrenergic receptor has recently been identified. This receptor has pharmacological properties distinct from those of $β_1$- or $β_2$-adrenergic receptors. Agonists that are selective for $β_3$ receptors exist and cause nonshivering thermogenesis in rodents. The role of the receptor in humans remains to be defined. mRNA for $β_3$-

TABLE 3. Subtypes of β-adrenergic receptors

Type	Potency (antagonist)	Characteristics	No. of amino acids	Second messenger	Introns
β₁	ISO > EPI = NE (Practolol) (ICI 89,406)	Fatty acid mobilization from adipose tissue, cardiac stimulation	477-C10 (human)	↑cAMP	No
β₂	ISO > EPI > NE (Butoxamine) (ICI 118,551)	Bronchodilation, vasodepression, inhibition of uterine contraction, glycogenolysis.	410-C5 (human)	↑cAMP	No
β₃	ISO > EPI BRL-37344 (Pindolol)	Lipolysis	402 (human)	↑cAMP	Yes

adrenergic receptors is selectively expressed in brown adipose tissue present in rodents and in newborn humans. Message can be detected in white adipose tissue, but the level of expression is very low.

Using the tools of molecular biology, the amino acid sequences of β-adrenergic receptors in brain and various tissues have been determined

A striking structural feature of the β-adrenergic receptors that have been cloned and sequenced (from turkey erythrocytes, hamster lung, and human placenta and brain) and of the other members of the G protein-linked receptor family is their topographical orientation with respect to the membrane [22] (see Fig. 6). Hydropathicity analysis suggests that there are seven hydrophobic regions, each of 20 to 25 amino acids. These are potentially membrane spanning. Other structural features of β-adrenergic receptors include a long C-terminal hydrophilic sequence thought to be intracellular, a somewhat shorter N-terminal hydrophilic sequence thought to be extracellular, and a long cytoplasmic loop between presumptive transmembrane segments V and VI. Sites for N-linked glycosylation are found in the N-terminal extracellular portion of the molecule, while numerous sites that may be phosphorylated are found in the C-terminal portion of the molecule and on the i_3 loop (see Chap. 22). Evidence from studies involving limited proteolysis and site-directed mutagenesis have led to the conclusion that the hydrophobic transmembrane helices are involved in the formation of the binding site for catecholamines, and the i_3 loop together with the C terminus may play a role in the interaction of the receptor with GTP-binding proteins (see Chap. 21). A conserved aspartate residue in transmembrane 3 and a pair of serines in transmembrane 5 are thought to provide counter ions for the amino and catechol hydroxyl groups, respectively [22].

Multiple serine and threonine residues on the i_3 loop and C terminus and consensus sequences for cAMP-dependent phosphorylation may be important in explaining processes including agonist-induced receptor sequestration and desensitization. cAMP- and non-cAMP-dependent phosphorylation of β-adrenergic receptors has been observed. β-Receptor-stimulated synthesis of cAMP results in activation of protein kinase A. The phosphorylated receptor is functionally uncoupled. Other receptors coupled to activation of adenylyl cyclase can also cause what is known as heterologous desensitization. In addition, occupancy of β-adrenergic receptors by agonists results in the activation of β-adrenergic receptor kinase, which leads to phosphorylation of the receptor. Although all of the residues phosphorylated by β-adrenergic receptor kinase have not been specifically identified, this reaction appears to contribute to a decrease in the ability of the receptor to activate G_s and thus adenylyl cyclase (see Chap. 22). The uncoupling of the receptor from G_s also appears to involve a protein called β-arrestin that is similar to 48K protein in the retina (see Chap. 7).

The proposed structure of the β-adrenergic receptor is strikingly similar in sequence and topography to that of bacterial rhodopsin (see Chap. 7) and the other members of the G protein-linked receptor family whose cDNAs have recently been cloned (see Chap. 10). Although these proteins mediate widely disparate biological effects, they show a high degree of homology. This is almost certainly related to the fact that, in each case, the immediate consequence of receptor activation is to promote an interaction between the receptor and a GTP-binding protein. The homologies between the members of the extended family of proteins are most evident within the presumed membrane-spanning helices.

Two families of α-adrenergic receptors exist

Radiolabeled agonists and antagonists have been used to label α receptors in both the brain and the peripheral tissues. As with β receptors, the binding properties of α receptors are essentially the same in the brain and the periphery. Some tissues possess only postsynaptic α_1 receptors, others postsynaptic α_2 receptors, and some organs have a mixture of both. Results of pharmacological and physiological studies have led to the suggestion that there are multiple types of α_1 and α_2 receptors. Of particular clinical importance are differences in the properties of junctional and extrajunctional α receptors. The proportions of α_1 and α_2 receptors also vary in different brain regions [23]. The physiological consequences of the two types of α receptors in the brain are unclear at the present time. It is striking that the drug specificity of postsynaptic α_2 receptors closely resembles that of adrenergic autoreceptors, which are therefore also referred to as α_2 receptors. Studies involving the binding of ra-

dioligands are also consistent with the suggestion that there are subtypes of both α_1- and α_2-adrenergic receptors (Tables 4 and 5). The suggestion that there are subtypes of α_1-adrenergic receptors was initially based on a comparison of the properties of [³H]prazosin and [³H]WB4-101 binding to α_1-adrenergic receptors in rat brain and uterus. Heterogeneity of α_2-adrenergic receptors was initially based on a comparison between the binding of [³H]clonidine and [³H]yohimbine in a variety of tissues and species. The observation that prazosin is more potent in neonatal rat lung [23] and cerebral cortex than in the human platelet, the prototypic tissue for the study of α_2 receptors, was interpreted as indicating a heterogeneity in the pharmacological characteristics of α_2-adrenergic receptors. Cloning and sequence analysis suggest that there are three subtypes of α_1-adrenergic receptor and three subtypes of α_2-adrenergic receptor [24]. In some instances the α_{1A} receptor has been linked to activation of Ca^{2+} channels, while the α_{1B} receptor has been shown to activate phospholipase C, resulting in liberation of diacylglycerol and inositoltrisphosphate (see Chap. 20). Prototypic tissues expressing each of the subtypes of α_2 receptor have been identified. All three of the known subtypes of α_2-adrenergic receptor are linked to inhibition of adenylyl cyclase activity. As is seen with other receptors linked to inhibition of adenylyl cyclase activity, the α_2-adrenergic receptors have long i_3 loops and relatively short C-terminal tails.

Not surprisingly, the known subtypes of α-adrenergic receptor share structural features with dopamine receptors (Fig. 6) and the other members of the G protein-linked receptor family. The degree of sequence identity is greater when the subtypes of α_1 or α_2 receptors are compared with each other than when α_1 and α_2 receptors are compared. The sequences of α_1 and α_2 receptors are not more closely related to each other than either is to the three known members of the β-adrenergic receptor family. Nomenclature

TABLE 4.   Subtypes of α_1-adrenergic receptors

	α_{1A}	α_{1B}	α_{1C}
PHARMACOLOGY			
Affinity for agonists[a]			
Affinity for antagonists			
WB-4101	High	Low	High
Phentolamine	High	Low	High
DISTRIBUTION	Renal artery	Liver, spleen, DDT$_1$ cells, MF-2 cells	Not yet identified in tissues
MECHANISM	Ca^{2+} channel	IP$_3$	?
STRUCTURE (CLONING-HUMAN)			
Number of amino acids	560	515	466
Human gene chromosome number	C5	C5	C8
N-linked glycosylation sites	2	4	3
Residues in N terminus	91	46	26
Residues in third cytoplasmic loop	73	71	67
Residues in C terminus	160	164	143
Number of introns	?	1	1

Modified from [24] with permission.
[a] No agonists have been identified that consistently show selectivity for one of the subtypes.

TABLE 5.   Subtypes of α_2-adrenergic receptors

	α_{2A}	α_{2B}	α_{2C}
PHARMACOLOGY			
Affinity for agonists[a]			
Affinity for antagonists (selective compounds)	Oxymetazoline BAM 1303	ARC 239 Prazosin Spiroxatrine	BAM 1303 WB-4101
PROTOTYPIC TISSUES AND CELL LINES	Human platelet HT29 cells	Neonatal rat lung NG108 cells	Opossum kidney OK cells
MECHANISM	All three subtypes have been shown to inhibit adenylyl cyclase		
STRUCTURE (CLONING-HUMAN)			
Number of amino acids	450	450	461
Human gene chromosome number	10	2	4
N-linked glycosylation sites	2	0	2
Residues in N terminus	33	13	51
Residues in third cytoplasmic loop	156	177	149
Residues in C terminus	20	20	22
Number of introns	0	0	?

Modified from [24] with permission.
[a] Norepinephrine and epinephrine appear to have similar affinities at the three subtypes.

notwithstanding, it is appropriate to think of three families of adrenergic receptor called α_1, α_2, and β. Sequence similarities both within and between families of adrenergic receptors are greater when the sequences of the putative transmembrane helices are compared than when one looks at overall sequence identity. It is sometimes difficult to distinguish between receptor subtypes and species homologs of the same receptor. Small differences in amino acid sequence can sometimes lead to large changes in the pharmacological specificity of an expressed receptor.

The possibility that additional catecholamine receptors remain to be identified clearly exists. Additional subtypes that have been characterized to a greater or lesser extent include the α_{2D} receptor in bovine pineal and subtypes of β-adrenergic receptor and dopamine receptor coupled to activation of phospholipase C. The β-adrenergic receptor in turkey erythrocytes probably represents a distinct subtype of β-adrenergic receptor but it can also be thought of as a species homolog of the mammalian β_1-adrenergic receptor.

DYNAMICS OF CATECHOLAMINE RECEPTORS

Neurotransmitter receptors are not static entities; changes in the number of receptors appear to be associated with altered synaptic activity

In both the peripheral sympathetic nervous system and the brain, destruction of catecholamine-containing nerves is associated with functional supersensitivity of postsynaptic sites. Conversely, administration of tricyclic antidepressants or inhibitors of MAO lead to functional subsensitivity. These changes appear to be a compensatory response involving changes in the density of β-adrenergic receptors (see below). Destruction of the dopamine-containing nigrostriatal pathway also has well-described behav-

ioral consequences. Because this pathway is uncrossed, a unilateral nigrostriatal lesion causes asymmetry in dopamine innervation between the two cerebral hemispheres. Behavioral studies demonstrate that the dopamine receptors in the denervated corpus striatum are supersensitive. Apomorphine, a dopamine agonist that stimulates dopamine receptors selectively, causes rotational behavior in rats with unilateral lesions. The extent of receptor supersensitivity can be quantified by measuring the amount of rotational behavior.

After selective nigrostriatal lesions have been produced in rats by injections of 6-hydroxydopamine in the substantia nigra, the number of dopamine receptors in the ipsilateral corpus striatum increases markedly, and the increase in the number of receptors may correlate with the extent of behavioral supersensitivity as monitored by rotational behavior [25]. Thus, the increase in receptor density appears to play a role in the behavioral supersensitivity of these animals.

Changes in the number of dopamine receptors may also be involved in pharmacological actions of neuroleptic drugs

One of the most serious side effects of the neuroleptic drugs is tardive dyskinesia, a disfiguring, excessive motor activity of the tongue, face, arms, and legs in patients treated chronically with large doses of the drugs (see Chap. 47). Paradoxically, reduction of the dosage worsens the symptoms, whereas increasing the dosage alleviates the symptoms. It has been suggested that tardive dyskinesia reflects supersensitivity of dopamine receptors that have been chronically blocked. This hypothesis gains support from direct demonstration that chronic treatment with neuroleptics leads to an increase in the number of dopamine receptors in the corpus striatum. Moreover, the ability of neuroleptics to elicit this increase correlates with their ability to block dopamine receptors.

The number of α_1 and α_2 receptors increases after the noradrenergic neurons in the brain have been destroyed by injections of 6-hydroxydopamine. It is interesting that after this induced destruction of norepinephrine-containing neurons, the number of β_1 receptors increases markedly, but no changes occur in the number of β_2 receptors [21]. This may be a consequence of the fact that β_2 receptors have a low affinity for norepinephrine and that the concentration of epinephrine in the brain is relatively low. Similarly, the chronic administration of tricyclic antidepressants, which blocks the reuptake of norepinephrine, leads to a selective decrease in the density of β_1-adrenergic receptors in the cerebral cortex. This suggests that the β_1-adrenergic receptors in the cortex are functionally innervated.

Exposure to agonists results in diminished responsiveness

Despite intensive efforts, the mechanisms underlying the decrease in the density of receptors on exposure to agonists remain to be determined. Mechanisms of receptor regulation have been most thoroughly investigated on transformed and transfected cell lines expressing subtypes of β-adrenergic receptor. Transcriptional, post-transcriptional, and post-translational regulatory phenomena have been described. Exposure of such cells to an agonist like isoproterenol results in an unexpected increase in mRNA levels. This is thought to be a consequence of the presence of a cAMP-response element (CRE) located approximately 50 bases upstream from the initiation codon. Exposure of cells to isoproterenol results in increases in cAMP and activation of protein kinase A. A CRE-binding protein is then phosphorylated, resulting in activation of the CRE. The resulting increase in mRNA levels is transient and does not have an obvious effect on the synthesis of receptor protein. Over a somewhat longer time scale, post-transcriptional regulatory mechanisms are activated. In particular, mRNA levels decline, apparently as a consequence of a decrease in mRNA stability. The mechanism underlying this change in message stability has not been elucidated. Transcriptional and post-transcriptional regulation of β-adrenergic receptor synthesis is superimposed on post-translational phenomena that have been described above (see also Chap. 22). Phosphorylation of the receptor by either protein kinase A or β-adrenergic receptor kinase leads to an uncoupling of the receptor from G_S and is probably responsible for much of the decreased responsiveness that is seen as a consequence of exposure of cells to an agonist. The role of receptor phosphorylation in down-regulation remains to be defined. Similarly, relatively little has been done to define mechanisms of regulation of other members of the catecholamine receptor family.

ACKNOWLEDGMENTS

Support was provided by NIH grants NS18479 and NS18591.

REFERENCES

1. Molinoff, P. B., and Axelrod, J. Biochemistry of catecholamines. *Annu. Rev. Biochem.* 40: 465–500, 1971.
2. Shiman, R., Akino, M., and Kaufman, S. Solubilization and partial purification of tyrosine hydroxylase from bovine adrenal medulla. *J. Biol. Chem.* 246:1330–1340, 1971.
3. Grima, B., Lamouroux, A., Blanot, F., Biguet, N. F., and Mallet, J. Complete coding sequence of rat tyrosine hydroxylase mRNA. *Proc. Natl. Acad. Sci. U.S.A.* 82:617–621, 1985.
4. Christenson, J. G., Dairman, W., and Udenfried, S. Preparation and properties of homogeneous aromatic L-amino acid decarboxylase from hog kidney. *Arch. Biochem. Biophys.* 141:356–367, 1970.
5. Craine, J. E., Daniels, G., and Kaufman, S. Dopamine-β-hydroxylase: The subunit structure and anion activation of the bovine adrenal enzyme. *J. Biol. Chem.* 248:7838–7844, 1973.

6. Lamouroux, A., Vigny, A., Biguet, N. F., Darmon, M. C., Franck, R., Henry, J.-P., and Mallet, J. The primary structure of human dopamine-β-hydroxylase: insights into the relationship between the soluble and the membrane-bound forms of the enzyme. *EMBO J.* 6:3931–3937, 1987.

7. Connett, R. J., and Kirshner, N. Purification and properties of bovine phenylethanolamine-*N*-methyltransferase. *J. Biol. Chem.* 245: 329–334, 1970.

8. Baetge, E. E., Suh, Y. H., and Joh, T. H. Complete nucleotide and deduced amino acid sequence of bovine phenylethanolamine *N*-methyltransferase: Partial amino acid homology with rat tyrosine hydroxylase. *Proc. Natl. Acad. Sci. U.S.A.* 83:5454–5458, 1986.

9. Liu, Y., Peter, D., Roghani, A., Schuldiner, S., Privé, G. G., Eisenberg, D., Brecha, N., and Edwards, R. H. A cDNA that suppresses MPP[+] toxicity encodes a vesicular amine transporter. *Cell* 70:539–551, 1992.

10. Weinshilboum, R. M., Thoa, N. B., Johnson, D. G., Kopin, I. J., and Axelrod, J. Proportional release of norepinephrine and dopamine-β-hydroxylase from sympathetic nerves. *Science* 174:1349–1351, 1971.

11. Alousi, A., and Weiner, N. The regulation of norepinephrine synthesis in sympathetic nerves: Effect of nerve stimulation, cocaine and catecholamine-releasing agents. *Proc. Natl. Acad. Sci. U.S.A.* 56:1491–1496, 1966.

12. Zigmond, R. E., Schwarzschild, M. A., and Rittenhouse, A. R. Acute regulation of tyrosine hydroxylase by nerve activity and by neurotransmitters via phosphorylation. *Annu. Rev. Neurosci.* 12:415–461, 1989.

13. Costa, E., and Sandler, M. *Monoamine Oxidase: New Vistas.* New York: Raven, 1972.

14. Nikodejevic, B., Sinoh, S., Daly, J. W., and Creveling, C. R. Catechol-*O*-methyltransferase II: A new class of inhibitors of catechol-*O*-methyl-transferase; 3,5-dihydroxy-4-methoxybenzoic acid and related compounds. *J. Pharmacol. Exp. Ther.* 174:83–93, 1970.

15. Axelrod, J. Noradrenaline: Fate and control of its biosynthesis. *Science* 173:598–606, 1971.

16. Amara, S. G., and Kuhar, M. J. Neurotransmitter transporters: Recent progress. *Annu. Rev. Neurosci.* 16:73–93, 1993.

17. Lindvall, O., and Björklund, A. Organization of catecholamine neurons in the rat central nervous system. In L. L. Iversen, S. D. Iversen, and S. H. Snyder (eds.), *Handbook of Psychopharmacology.* New York: Plenum, 1978, Vol. 9, pp. 139–231.

18. Langer, S. Z. Presynaptic regulation of catecholamine release. *Biochem. Pharmacol.* 23: 1793–1800, 1974.

19. Kebabian, J. W., and Calne, D. B. Multiple receptors for dopamine. *Nature* 277:93–96, 1979.

20. Sibley, D. R., and Monsma, F. J., Jr. Molecular biology of dopamine receptors. *Trends Pharmacol. Sci.* 13:61–68, 1992.

21. Minneman, K. P., Dibner, M. D., Wolfe, B. B., and Molinoff, P. B. β₁- and β₂-adrenergic receptors in rat cerebral cortex are independently regulated. *Science* 204:866–868, 1979.

22. Kobilka, B. Adrenergic receptors as models for G protein-coupled receptors. *Annu. Rev. Neurosci.* 15:87–114, 1992.

23. U'Prichard, D. C., and Snyder, S. H. Distinct α-noradrenergic receptors differentiated by binding and physiological relationships. *Life Sci.* 24:79–88, 1979.

24. Bylund, D. B. Subtypes of α₁- and α₂-adrenergic receptors. *FASEB J.* 6:832–839, 1992.

25. Creese, I., Burt, D. R., and Snyder, S. H. Biochemical actions of neuroleptic drugs: Focus on the dopamine receptor. In L. L. Iversen, S. D. Iversen, and S. H. Snyder (eds.), *Handbook of Psychopharmacology.* New York: Plenum, 1978, Vol. 10, pp. 37–90.

Serotonin

ALAN FRAZER AND JULIE G. HENSLER

Basic Neurochemistry: Molecular, Cellular, and Medical Aspects, 5th Ed., edited by G. J. Siegel et al. Published by Raven Press, Ltd., New York, 1994. Correspondence to Alan Frazer, Department of Pharmacology, University of Texas Health Science Center at San Antonio, San Antonio, Texas 78284.

THE NEUROTRANSMITTER
SEROTONIN

**The indolealkylamine 5-hydroxytryptamine
(5-HT; serotonin) was initially identified
because of interest in its cardiovascular
effects**

It has been known since the mid-nineteenth
century that, after blood clots, the serum possesses a substance that constricts vascular
smooth muscle so as to increase vascular
tone. Around the turn of the twentieth century, platelets were identified as the source
of this substance, and then, in the late 1940s,
Page and his collaborators isolated and characterized this "tonic" substance in "serum"
(hence, serotonin) [1].

The structures of serotonin and related
compounds are shown in Fig. 1. The combination of the hydroxyl group in the 5 position of the indole nucleus and a primary
amine nitrogen serving as a proton acceptor
at physiological pH makes 5-HT a hydrophilic substance. As such, it does not pass the
lipophilic blood-brain barrier readily. Thus,
its discovery in brain in 1953 by Twarog and
Page indicated that 5-HT was being synthesized in brain, where it might play an important role in brain function. The observation
about the same time that the psychedelic
drug (+)lysergic acid diethylamide (LSD) antagonized a response produced by 5-HT
(even though the response was contraction
of gastrointestinal smooth muscle) further
substantiated the idea that 5-HT had important behavioral effects. Subsequently, various
theories arose linking abnormalities of 5-HT
function to the development of a number of
psychiatric disorders, particularly schizophrenia and depression. Psychotherapeutic
drugs are now available that are effective in
depression, anxiety disorders, and schizophrenia; some of these drugs have potent,
and in some cases selective, effects on serotonin neurons in brain.

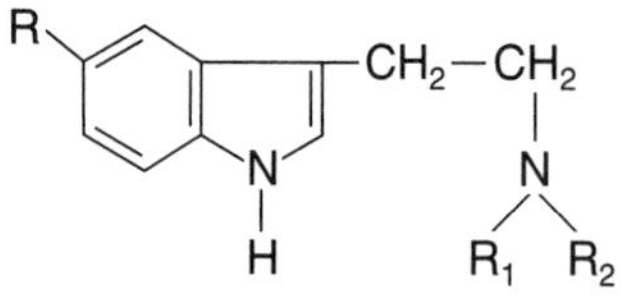

Compound	Position		
	R	R_1	R_2
Tryptamine	H	H	H
Serotonin	OH	H	H
Melatonin	OCH_3	$COCH_3$	H
Diethyltryptamine (DET)*	H	CH_3CH_2	CH_3CH_2
Dimethyltryptamine (DMT)*	H	CH_3	CH_3
Bufotenine*	OH	CH_3	CH_3

*Psychotropic (modifies mental activity)

FIG. 1.   Chemical structure of 5-hydroxytryptamine (5-HT; serotonin) and related indolealkylamines. The indole
ring structure consists of the benzene ring and the attached five-member ring structure containing nitrogen.

The amino acid L-tryptophan serves as the precursor for the synthesis of 5-HT

Not all cells that contain 5-HT synthesize it. For example, platelets do not synthesize 5-HT; rather, they accumulate 5-HT from plasma by an active transport mechanism found on the platelet membrane. Certain brain cells do synthesize 5-HT. The synthesis and primary metabolic pathways of 5-HT are shown in Fig. 2. The initial step in the synthesis of serotonin is the facilitated transport of the amino acid L-tryptophan from blood into brain. The primary source of tryptophan is dietary protein. Certain other neutral amino acids (e.g., phenylalanine, leucine, methionine) are transported into brain by the same carrier. The entry of tryptophan into brain is not only related to its concentration in blood, but is also a function of its concentration in relation to the concentrations of other neutral amino acids. Consequently, lowering the dietary intake of tryptophan while raising the intake of the amino acids with which it competes for transport into brain lowers the content of 5-HT in brain and changes certain behaviors associated with 5-HT function. This strategy for lowering the brain content of 5-HT has been used clinically to evaluate the importance of brain 5-HT in the mechanism of action of psychotherapeutic drugs [2].

Serotonergic neurons contain the enzyme L-tryptophan-5-monooxygenase (EC 1.14.16.4), more commonly termed tryptophan hydroxylase, that converts tryptophan to 5-hydroxytryptophan (5-HTP) (Fig. 2). This enzyme is found only in cells that synthesize 5-HT; its distribution in brain is similar to that of 5-HT itself. The enzyme requires both molecular oxygen and a reduced pteridine cofactor (such as L-erythro-tetrahydro-biopterin [BH$_4$]) for activity. In the enzymatic reaction, one atom of oxygen is used to form 5-HTP and the other is reduced to water. The pteridine cofactor donates electrons, and the unstable quinonoid dihydrobiopterin that results is regenerated immedi-

ately to the tetrahydrobiopterin form by an NADPH-linked enzymatic reaction.

The reaction can be represented as

$$\text{L-Tryptophan} + \text{BH}_4 + \text{O}_2 \rightarrow$$
$$\text{L-5-hydroxytryptophan}$$
$$+ \text{quinonoid BH}_4 + \text{H}_2\text{O}$$

The K_m of partially purified tryptophan hydroxylase for tryptophan is approximately 30 to 60 µM, a concentration comparable to that of tryptophan in brain. If the concentration of tryptophan in serotonergic neurons is assumed to be comparable to that in whole brain, the enzyme would not be saturated with its substrate. If this is so, then the formation of 5-HT in brain would be expected to rise as the brain concentration of tryptophan increases. This has been found to occur in response to raising the dietary intake of tryptophan.

The cloning and sequencing of cDNAs encoding tryptophan hydroxylase have been reported recently from both brain and pineal gland [3]. Some differences in biochemical properties, such as molecular weights, substrate specificity, and isoelectric points, had been reported previously between the enzyme(s) obtained from brain and those from pineal gland. However, the cDNAs isolated from both tissue sources appear to have identical nucleotide sequences, making it likely that tissue-specific differences in the properties of tryptophan hydroxylase result from differential post-translational processing. Tryptophan hydroxylase contains 444 amino acids, corresponding to a molecular weight of about 51 kDa and is 50 percent homologous with tyrosine hydroxylase, the rate-limiting enzyme in catecholamine biosynthesis (see Chap. 12). The greatest homology resides in the central and C-terminal regions of these enzymes, making it likely that these areas contain the catalytic site. Substrate specificity may reside in those amino acids nearer the N terminus.

The other enzyme involved in the synthesis of serotonin is aromatic L-amino acid

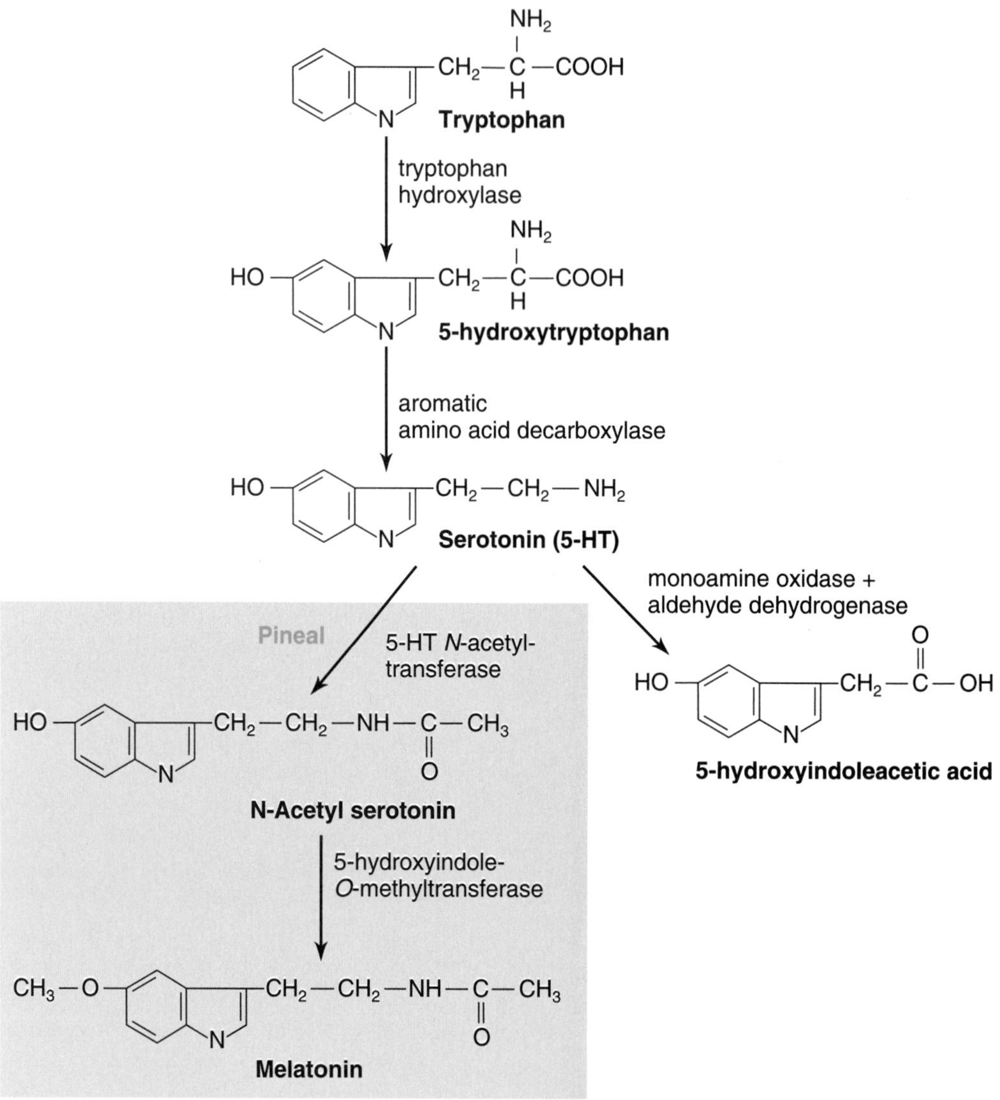

FIG. 2.   The biosynthesis and catabolism of serotonin. Note that in the pineal gland serotonin is converted enzymatically to melatonin.

decarboxylase (AADC), which converts 5-HTP to 5-HT (Fig. 2). This enzyme is present not only in serotonergic neurons but also in catecholaminergic neurons, where it converts 3,4-dihydroxyphenylalanine (DOPA) to dopamine (see Chap. 12). However, different conditions of pH or concentrations of substrate or cofactor are required for optimum activity of the enzyme(s) in brain homogenates when using either 5-HTP or DOPA as the substrate. Recently, cDNAs encoding AADC have been cloned [4]. The encoded protein contains 480 amino acids and has a molecular weight of 54 kDa. Characterization of the protein expressed in cells transfected with the cDNA shows that it decarboxylates either DOPA or 5-HTP. Also, *in situ* hybridization of the mRNA for the enzyme revealed its presence both in serotonergic cells in the dorsal raphe nucleus and in catecholaminergic cells in brain regions containing dopaminergic soma [5]. Taken together, these results support the idea that the enzymatic decarboxylation of both DOPA and 5-HTP is catalyzed by the same enzyme.

Because the decarboxylase enzyme is not saturated with 5-HTP under physiological conditions, it is possible to raise the content of 5-HT in brain not only by increasing the dietary intake of tryptophan but also by raising the intake of 5-HTP. This procedure, though, results in the formation of 5-HT in cells that would not normally contain it (e.g., catecholaminergic neurons) because of the nonselective nature of AADC.

The initial hydroxylation of tryptophan rather than the decarboxylation of 5-HTP appears to be the rate-limiting step in serotonin synthesis. Evidence in support of this view includes the fact that 5-HTP is found only in trace amounts in brain, presumably because it is decarboxylated about as rapidly as it is formed. As might be expected if the hydroxylation reaction is rate limiting, inhibition of this reaction results in a marked depletion of the content of 5-HT in brain. The enzyme inhibitor most widely used in experiments is *p*-chlorophenylalanine (PCPA). PCPA inhibits tryptophan hydroxylase irreversibly to cause a long-lasting reduction in 5-HT levels. Recovery of enzyme activity, and 5-HT biosynthesis, requires the synthesis of new enzyme.

Understanding the neuroanatomical organization of serotonergic cells in brain provides insight into the functions of this neurotransmitter, as well as its possible roles in mental processes and psychiatric disorders

Serotonin-containing neuronal cell bodies are restricted to discrete clusters or groups of cells located along the midline of the brainstem. Their axons, however, innervate nearly every area of the central nervous system (Fig. 3). In 1964, Dahlstrom and Fuxe, using the Falck-Hillarp technique of histofluorescence, observed that the majority of serotonergic soma were found in cell body groups previously designated by Taber, Brodal, and Walberg as the raphe nuclei. This earlier description of the raphe nuclei was based on cytoarchitectural criteria, i.e., on cell body structural characteristics and organization. Dahlstrom and Fuxe described nine groups of serotonin-containing cell bodies, which they designated B_1 through B_9, and which correspond for the most part with the raphe nuclei. Some serotonergic neuronal cell bodies, however, are found outside the raphe nuclei, and not all raphe neurons are serotonergic.

Over the course of the last three decades, a variety of techniques have been used to characterize the neuronal circuitry of serotonin cells in the central nervous system. The density of serotonergic innervation in the forebrain was initially underestimated because the original histofluorescence method was limited in sensitivity and did not permit the detection of many fine axons and terminals. Subsequent anatomical techniques (immunohistochemistry of 5-HT or tryptophan hydroxylase; retrograde and anterograde axonal transport studies) have allowed a more complete and accurate characterization of the serotonergic innervation of forebrain areas.

The largest group of serotonergic cells is group B_7 of Dahlstrom and Fuxe. Group B_7 is contiguous with a smaller group of serotonergic cells, B_6. Groups B_6 and B_7 are often considered together as the dorsal raphe nucleus, with B_6 being its caudal extension. Another prominent serotonergic cell body group is B_8, which corresponds to the median raphe nucleus, also termed the nucleus central superior (Fig. 4). Group B_9, part of the ventrolateral tegmentum of the pons and midbrain, forms a lateral extension of the median raphe and therefore is not considered one of the midline raphe nuclei. Ascending serotonergic projections innervat-

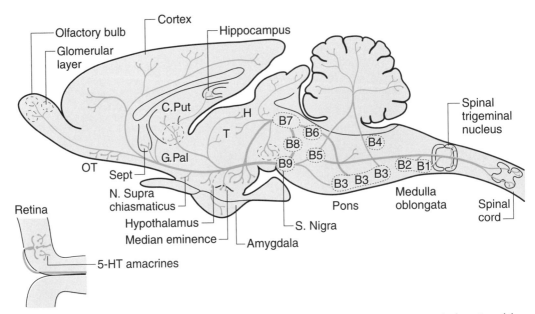

FIG. 3. Schematic drawing depicting the location of the serotonergic cell body groups in a sagittal section of the rat central nervous system and their major projections. (OT) olfactory tuberculum; (Sept) septum; (C. Put) nucleus caudate-putamen; (G. Pal) globus pallidus; (T) thalamus; (H) habenula; (S. Nigra) substantia nigra. (From Consolazione and Cuello [31].)

ing the cerebral cortex and other regions of the forebrain come from the dorsal raphe, median raphe, and B_9 cell group. The other raphe nuclei, B_1 to B_5, are more caudally situated (mid-pons to caudal medulla) and contain a smaller number of serotonergic cells. These cell body groups give rise to serotonergic axons that project within the brainstem and to the spinal cord (Fig. 3).

Afferent connections of the raphe nuclei begin with connections between the dorsal and median raphe nuclei, B_9, B_1, and B_3. The raphe nuclei receive input from other cell body groups in the brainstem such as the substantia nigra and ventral tegmental area (dopamine), superior vestibular nucleus (acetylcholine), locus coeruleus (norepinephrine), and nucleus prepositus hypoglossi and nucleus of the solitary tract (epinephrine). Other afferents include neurons from the hypothalamus, thalamus, and limbic forebrain structures.

Two main ascending serotonergic pathways emerge from the midbrain raphe nuclei

to the forebrain—the dorsal periventricular path and the ventral tegmental radiations. Both pathways converge in the caudal hypothalamus where they join the medial forebrain bundle (MFB).

A question of current interest is whether certain raphe nuclei send axons to innervate specific forebrain areas. Specific innervation could imply independent functions of sets of serotonergic neurons, dependent on their origin and terminal projections. Alternatively, if the serotonergic innervation of the forebrain arising from these raphe nuclei is nonselective and widespread, this would imply that serotonin is acting in a more general manner. There are data to support the idea of specificity of projections and perhaps function.

The dorsal and median raphe nuclei give rise to multiple, distinct sets of axons that form separate pathways to different brain regions. Functionally related structures in the brain are innervated by the same group of serotonergic neurons. For exam-

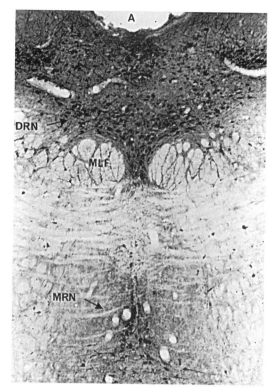

FIG. 4.   Serotonergic cell bodies in the midbrain raphe nuclei of the rat. Photomicrograph showing 5-HT neurons in the dorsal and median raphe nuclei. The dorsal raphe nucleus (DRN) lies in the central gray matter just beneath the cerebral aqueduct (A). The median raphe nucleus (MRN) lies in the central core of the midbrain, below the medial longitudinal fasciculus (MLF).

ple, the hippocampus and the septum (limbic structures) appear to be innervated predominantly by neurons of the median raphe, whereas the striatum and substantia nigra (basal ganglia-motor systems) are innervated by the dorsal raphe (Fig. 5). The two raphe nuclei send overlapping neuronal projections to the neocortex. In addition, cells within the dorsal and median raphe are organized in particular zones or groups that send axons to specific areas of brain such as the cortex or hippocampus. For example, the frontal cortex receives heavy innervation from the rostral and lateral subregions of the dorsal raphe nucleus. Functionally related structures in the brain can also be innervated by the same individual neurons. Serotoner-

gic neurons send collateral axons to more than one brain region, often terminal areas that are related in function such as the entorhinal cortex and hippocampus.

Serotonergic axon terminals, labeled by

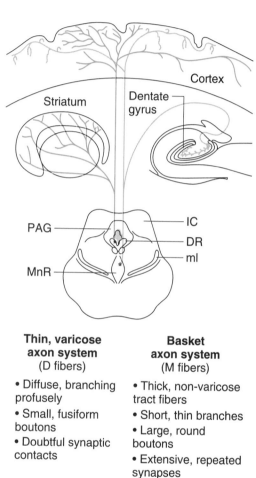

Thin, varicose axon system
(D fibers)

- Diffuse, branching profusely
- Small, fusiform boutons
- Doubtful synaptic contacts

Basket axon system
(M fibers)

- Thick, non-varicose tract fibers
- Short, thin branches
- Large, round boutons
- Extensive, repeated synapses

FIG. 5.   Simplified diagram of the main features of the dual serotonergic system innervating the forebrain. The fine varicose axon system (D fibers) arises from the dorsal raphe nucleus with fibers that branch profusely in their target areas. It is difficult to demonstrate the synaptic connections of these fibers, and therefore the incidence of synapses on these fibers is still being debated. The basket axon system (M fibers) arises from the median raphe nucleus with thick nonvaricose axons, giving rise to branches with characteristic axons that appear beaded, with round or oval varicosities. These large terminals make well-defined synapses with target cells. (DR) dorsal raphe nucleus; (IC) interior colliculus; (ml) medial lemniscus; (MnR) median raphe nucleus; (PAG) periaqueductal gray matter. (From Tork [32].)

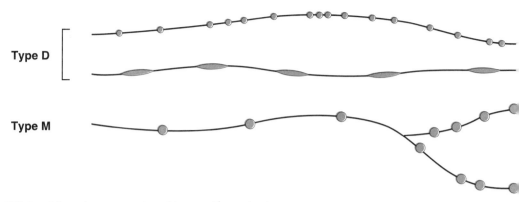

FIG. 6.   Schematic representation of the two classes of raphe-cortical axon terminals. Axons that arise in the dorsal raphe nucleus (type D) have heterogeneous varicosities that range in size. Axons from the median raphe nucleus (type M) have large spherical varicosities. (From Kosofsky and Molliver [33].)

uptake of tritiated serotonin or studied with immunohistochemical techniques, exhibit morphological differences related to the raphe nucleus of origin. Serotonergic axons from the median raphe nucleus (type M) look relatively coarse with large spherical varicosities. In contrast, axons from the dorsal raphe (type D) are very fine and typically have small, pleomorphic varicosities (Fig. 6). Dorsal raphe axons appear to be more vulnerable to certain neurotoxic amphetamine derivatives, e.g., 3,4-methylenedioxy-methamphetamine (MDMA; commonly termed ECSTASY) or *p*-chloroamphetamine (PCA). Median raphe axons appear to be more resistant to the neurotoxic effects of these drugs (see Molliver [6] or Jacobs and Azmitia [7] for a comprehensive review of serotonergic neuroanatomy).

The synthesis of 5-HT can increase markedly under conditions requiring a continuous supply of the neurotransmitter

Plasticity is an important concept in neurobiology. In general, this refers to the ability of neuronal systems to conform to either short- or long-term demands placed upon their activity or functioning. Many processes contribute to neuronal plasticity. One is the ability to increase the rate of neurotransmitter synthesis and release in response to increased neuronal activity. Serotonergic neurons have

this capability; the synthesis of 5-HT from tryptophan is increased in a frequency-dependent manner in response to electrical stimulation of serotonergic soma. The increase in synthesis results from the enhanced conversion of tryptophan to 5-HTP and has an absolute dependence on extracellular Ca^{2+}. It is likely that the increased synthesis results in part from alterations in the kinetic properties of tryptophan hydroxylase, perhaps due to Ca^{2+}-dependent phosphorylation of the enzyme. The increased activity of tryptophan hydroxylase does not result from the removal of enzyme inhibition caused by either 5-HT or 5-HTP. First, very high concentrations of these substances are needed to inhibit enzyme activity *in vitro*. Second, if rats are treated with monoamine oxidase inhibitors, which block the catabolism of 5-HT (see below), the brain concentration of 5-HT rises to well above control levels; *in vivo*, then, it appears that there is little end-product inhibition of serotonin synthesis.

Short-term requirements for increases in the synthesis of 5-HT can be met by processes that change the kinetic properties of tryptophan hydroxylase without necessitating the synthesis of more molecules of tryptophan hydroxylase. By contrast, situations requiring long-term increases in the synthesis and release of 5-HT result in the synthesis of tryptophan hydroxylase protein. For example, partial but substantial destruction (more han 60 percent) of central serotonergic neurons results in an increase in the synthesis of 5-HT in residual terminals. The increase in synthesis initially results from activation of existing tryptophan hydroxylase molecules, but the increased synthesis of 5-HT seen weeks after the lesion results from more tryptophan hydroxylase being present in the residual terminals. Recently, an increase in tryptophan hydroxylase mRNA has been reported in residual raphe serotonergic neurons after partial lesioning, consistent with the idea of an increase in the synthesis of tryptophan hydroxylase molecules in residual neurons.

As with other biogenic amine transmitters, 5-HT is stored primarily in vesicles and is released by an exocytotic mechanism

Peripheral sources of monoamine-containing cells have been utilized to study the properties of storage vesicles, e.g., chromaffin cells of the adrenal medulla for catecholamines (CAs) and parafollicular cells of the thyroid gland for 5-HT [8]. In some respects, the vesicles that store 5-HT resemble those that store CAs. For example, drugs such as reserpine and tetrabenazine, which inhibit the activity of the transporter localized to the vesicular membrane, deplete the brain content of 5-HT as well as CAs. This drug-induced reduction of 5-HT content shows that vesicular storage of 5-HT is needed to protect the indolealkylamine from intraneuronal degradation by monoamine oxidase.

In other respects, vesicles storing 5-HT are different from those storing CAs. In contrast to CA-containing vesicles, there is virtually no ATP in serotonergic vesicles. Also, serotonergic synaptic vesicles, but not chromaffin granules, contain a specific protein that binds 5-HT with high affinity. This serotonin-binding protein (SPB) disappears from forebrain following lesioning of the raphe nucleus, indicating that SPB is contained in serotonergic neurons. SPB is released along with serotonin by a Ca^{2+}-dependent process.

There is considerable evidence that the release of 5-HT occurs by exocytosis, i.e., by the discharge from the cell of the entire content of individual storage vessels [9]. First, 5-HT is sufficiently ionized at physiological pH so that it does not cross plasma membranes by simple diffusion. Second, most intraneuronal 5-HT is contained in storage vesicles, and other contents of the vesicle, including SPB, are released together with serotonin. In contrast, cytosolic proteins do not accompany electrical stimulation-elicited release of 5-HT. Third, the depolarization-induced release of 5-HT occurs by a Ca^{2+}-dependent process; indeed, it appears that the influx of Ca^{2+} with or without membrane depolarization can increase the release of 5-HT. Ca^{2+} has been reported to stimulate the fusion of vesicular membranes with the plasma membrane.

As expected, serotonergic terminals make the usual specialized synaptic contacts with target neurons and release serotonin following nerve stimulation. In most areas of the mammalian central nervous system, there are at least some sites where 5-HT is released and no evidence for synaptic specialization can be found (see Fig. 5). In this case neurotransmitter is released and then diffuses over some distance (as great as several hundred microns) [7]. The percentage of 5-HT terminals associated with synaptic specializations apparently varies in particular brain regions. This may have important implications for the type of information processing in which 5-HT is involved in these brain areas. The appearance of specialized synaptic contacts suggests relatively stable and strong associations between a presynaptic neuron and its target. Conversely, the lack of synaptic specialization implies a dynamic and perhaps less specific interaction with target neurons. In this case, 5-HT may act as a neuromodulator, i.e., adjusting or tuning ongoing synaptic activity. Typically, neuromodulatory effects involve a second messenger.

The rate of serotonin release is dependent on the firing rate of serotonergic soma in the raphe nuclei. Numerous studies utilizing a variety of techniques have revealed that procedures that increase raphe cell firing increase the release of 5-HT in terminal fields, whereas the opposite effect is observed when raphe cell firing decreases. This means that drugs that change the firing rate of serotonergic soma modify the release of serotonin as well. An important target for such drugs are somatodendritic autoreceptors, which, as is discussed later, are the $5\text{-}HT_{1A}$ receptor subtype. Administration of $5\text{-}HT_{1A}$ agonists such as 8-hydroxy-2-(di-*n*-propylamino)-tetralin (8-OH-DPAT) into the dorsal raphe nucleus slows the rate of firing of serotonergic soma. Using the newly developed technique of *in vivo* microdialysis, application of 8-OH-DPAT in the dorsal raphe nucleus was shown to decrease the release of 5-HT in the striatum [10]. Depending on the species, serotonergic autoreceptors in terminal fields appear to be either the $5\text{-}HT_{1B}$ or $5\text{-}HT_{1D}$ subtype. Administration of agonists of these receptors into areas receiving serotonergic innervation decreases the release of 5-HT measured *in vitro* or *in situ* using the technique of microdialysis [11].

The activity of 5-HT in the synapse is terminated primarily by its re-uptake into serotonergic terminals

Synaptic effects of many amino acid and monoaminergic neurotransmitters, including 5-HT, are terminated by binding of these molecules to specific transporter proteins. The transporter system for 5-HT is located on serotonergic neurons. Evidence for this comes from studies showing that the selective lesioning of serotonergic neurons in brain markedly reduces both the high-affinity uptake of [^{3}H]5-HT in areas of brain receiving serotonergic innervation and the specific binding of radioligands to the serotonin transporter. Glial cells also appear to be able to take up 5-HT by a high-affinity transport system.

The uptake system for 5-HT is saturable and of high affinity, with a K_m value for 5-HT of approximately 0.1 to 0.5 μM. The uptake of 5-HT is an active process that is temperature dependent and has an absolute requirement for external Na^+ and Cl^-; it is inhibited by metabolic inhibitors as well as by inhibitors of $Na^+,K^+\text{-}ATPase$ activity. From these and other data, it has been inferred that the energy requirement for 5-HT uptake is not directly used to transport 5-HT but rather is necessary to maintain the gradient of Na^+ across the plasma membrane upon which 5-HT uptake is dependent.

A recent advance that will aid considerably in understanding structure-function relationships of transporter proteins is the cloning, sequencing, and expression of several transporter proteins including that for 5-HT [12,13]. The cDNA isolated from rat brain predicts a protein containing 630 amino acids with a molecular weight of about 69 kDa. The putative structure has 12 transmembrane domains, with both the N and C termini being intracellular, and a large extracellular loop connecting transmembrane domains 3 and 4 containing potential glycosylation sites (Fig. 7). The predicted structure of the serotonin transporter is similar to the predicted structure of other cloned neurotransmitter transporters and quite distinct, for example, from the structure of G protein-linked receptors (see Fig. 8). The serotonin transporter exhibits about 50 percent absolute homology with the transporters for norepinephrine (NE) and dopamine, with the greatest homology being found in the first seven or eight transmembrane domains and the least conserved regions being the intracellular N- and C-terminal tails (Fig. 7).

As is discussed below, drugs that are selective inhibitors of the uptake of 5-HT, such as fluoxetine or sertraline, are widely used as antidepressants. Clomipramine, which has modest selectivity *in vivo* for inhibiting the uptake of 5-HT versus that of NE, is used for the treatment of an anxiety disorder termed obsessive-compulsive disorder. These drugs produce competitive inhibition of the uptake of 5-HT, and a single protein seems to be responsible for both the binding of these drugs and the uptake of 5-HT. It is likely that the serotonin transport inhibitors occupy

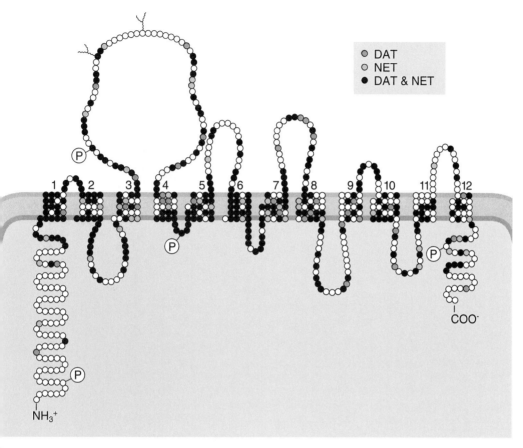

FIG. 7.   Putative structure of the rat serotonin transporter showing homologous amino acids with the rat dopamine transporter (DAT), human norepinephrine transporter (NET), or both. Possible phosphorylation (P) sites are shown, as are possible glycosylation sites on the large second extracellular loop. Note the considerable degree of homology in the twelve transmembrane-spanning regions. (Diagram courtesy of Dr. Beth J. Hoffman, Laboratory of Cell Biology, NIMH, Bethesda, MD.)

sites on the transporter protein that overlap the site that binds 5-HT.

The primary catabolic pathway for 5-HT is oxidative deamination by the enzyme monoamine oxidase

Monoamine oxidase (MAO) (EC 1.4.3.4.) converts serotonin to 5-hydroxyindoleacetaldehyde, and this product is oxidized by an NAD$^+$-dependent aldehyde dehydrogenase to form 5-hydroxyindoleacetic acid (5-HIAA) (see Fig. 2). The intermediate acetaldehyde can also be reduced by an NADH-dependent aldehyde reductase to form the alcohol 5-hydroxytryptophol. Whether oxidation or reduction takes place depends on the ratio of NAD$^+$/NADH in the tissue. In brain, 5-HIAA is the primary metabolite of serotonin.

There are at least two isoenzymes of MAO, referred to as type A and type B. These isoenzymes are integral flavoproteins of outer mitochondrial membranes in neurons, glia, and other cells. Evidence for the existence of isoenzymes was based initially on differing substrate specificities and sensitivities to inhibitors of MAO. For example, 5-HT

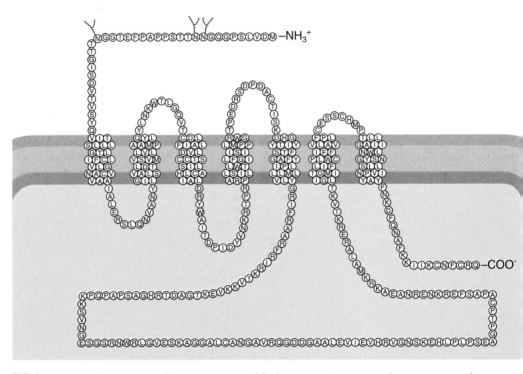

FIG. 8.   Amino acid sequence and putative structure of the human 5-HT$_{1A}$ receptor. The seven proposed transmembrane-spanning regions of the receptor protein, characteristic of the G protein-receptor family, are shown.

(and NE) is metabolized preferentially by type A MAO. Selective inhibitors of each form of MAO exist, e.g., clorgyline or moclobemide for type A or deprenyl for type B. Definitive proof of the existence of these two forms of MAO comes from the cloning of cDNAs encoding subunits of type A and type B MAO from human liver [14]. The deduced amino acid sequences of type A and type B MAOs show about 70 percent homology and have masses of 59.7 and 58 kDa, respectively. When each cDNA was cloned into an expression vector and transfected independently into a cell line, the activity of the proteins expressed resembled that of the endogenous enzymes from human brain, e.g., the expressed type A MAO preferred 5-HT as a substrate and was preferentially inhibited by clorgyline. From such data it was inferred that the functional differences between these two enzymes exist in their primary structures.

Several different techniques have been used to study the neuroanatomical localization of the two forms of MAO in brain. Originally, both histochemical and immunohistochemical techniques were used. More recently, *in situ* hybridization histochemistry has been used to demonstrate the location of the mRNAs for the two isoenzymes of MAO, and the development of radioligands selective for each form of MAO has enabled their distribution to be revealed by quantitative autoradiography. In general, the results from the use of these different techniques are similar. It is of some interest that there is more type A enzyme than type B enzyme throughout rat brain, whereas human brain contains more type B MAO than type A. Interestingly, serotonergic cell bodies contain predominantly type B MAO [15], so that serotonergic nerves (at least the soma) contain the form of MAO (type B) that does not preferentially metabolize 5-HT. This has led to the hypothesis that type B MAO in serotonergic neurons prevents the cell from accumulating various natural substrates (e.g., dopamine) that could interfere with the storage, release, and uptake of 5-HT. Furthermore, treatment of rats with clorgyline, a selective inhibitor of type A MAO, raises the brain content of 5-HT and reduces the conversion of 5-HT to 5-HIAA in brain [16]. Thus, 5-HT may well be oxidized preferentially by type A MAO *in vivo*, as it is *in vitro*, even though serotonergic neurons do not contain much of this form of the enzyme.

RECEPTORS FOR SEROTONIN

Pharmacological and physiological studies have contributed to the definition of the many receptor subtypes for serotonin

The initial suggestion that there might be more than one type of receptor for serotonin came from experiments of Gaddum and Picarrelli in 1957. Using the isolated guinea pig ileum, they demonstrated that only a portion of its contractile response to serotonin could be blocked by high concentrations of morphine, whereas the remainder of the response could be blocked by low concentrations of dibenzyline (phenoxybenzamine). Similarly, when maximally effective concentrations of dibenzyline were present, the remaining contractile response elicited by serotonin was blocked by low concentrations of morphine. They speculated that there were two different receptors of 5-HT in the ileum, termed D (blocked by dibenzyline) and M (blocked by morphine) receptors. The D receptor was thought to be on the smooth muscle of the ileum whereas the M receptor was considered to be on ganglia or nerves within the muscle.

In the 1970s, the development of radioligand binding assays (see Chap. 10) furthered our understanding of subtypes of receptors for serotonin. Initially, a number of radioligands, such as [^{3}H]5-HT, [^{3}H]LSD, and [^{3}H]spiperone, were used to label sites related to serotonin receptors. These radioligands were originally proposed by Per-

outka and Snyder in 1979 to label two classes of serotonin receptors in brain. Binding sites that were labeled with high affinity by [^{3}H]5-HT were designated the 5-HT$_1$ receptor; binding sites labeled with high affinity by [^{3}H]spiperone were termed the 5-HT$_2$ receptor. Many experiments have subsequently shown that the D receptor and the 5-HT$_2$ receptor are pharmacologically indistinguishable.

The binding of [^{3}H]5-HT to 5-HT$_1$ receptors was displaced by spiperone in a biphasic manner, suggesting that what was termed the 5-HT$_1$ receptor might be a heterogeneous population of receptors. The [^{3}H]5-HT binding site that showed high affinity for spiperone was termed the 5-HT$_{1A}$ subtype, whereas the component of [^{3}H]5-HT binding that showed low affinity for spiperone was called the 5-HT$_{1B}$ subtype. A high density of binding sites for [^{3}H]5-HT was found in the choroid plexus. These [^{3}H]5-HT binding sites were termed the 5-HT$_{1C}$ subtype, as they did not show the pharmacological characteristics used to classify the 5-HT$_{1A}$ or 5-HT$_{1B}$ binding site or the 5-HT$_2$ binding site. Subsequently, a fourth binding site for [^{3}H]5-HT was identified in bovine brain and was called the 5-HT$_{1D}$ receptor. The 5-HT$_{1D}$ receptor was identified by pharmacological criteria only in brains of species devoid of the 5-HT$_{1B}$ receptor such as pig, cow, guinea pig, and human [17].

Bradley and associates in 1986 proposed a classification scheme with three major types of receptors for serotonin, based on functional responses primarily in peripheral tissues as well as on pharmacological criteria [17]. The receptors were called 5-HT$_1$-like, 5-HT$_2$, and 5-HT$_3$. The term 5-HT$_1$-like was proposed for that heterogeneous group of receptors whose activation by 5-HT elicits functional responses that are (a) mimicked by 5-carboxamidotryptamine, a selective 5-HT$_1$ agonist; (b) potently antagonized by methiothepin and/or methysergide (two drugs that show high affinity to the 5-HT$_1$-binding site); and (c) not antagonized by compounds with high affinity and selectivity for other 5-HT receptor sites. For 5-HT$_2$ receptors, Bradley et al. proposed that responses elicited by their activation be potently antagonized by compounds with high affinity for the 5-HT$_2$ binding site and not inhibited by antagonists with selectivity for other serotonin receptor subtypes. The development of potent and selective antagonists of the 5-HT$_2$ receptor, such as ketanserin, has facilitated the assignment of certain effects mediated by 5-HT to the 5-HT$_2$ receptor. The M receptor of Gaddum and Picarrelli, originally described in guinea pig ileum, is pharmacologically distinct from all of the binding sites associated with serotonin receptors just described. Bradley and associates have renamed this receptor the 5-HT$_3$ receptor. The development of potent selective antagonists and an agonist, 2-methyl-5-HT, has provided useful tools for the pharmacological characterization of 5-HT$_3$ receptors.

Subsequently, an additional subtype of serotonin receptor has been described, the 5-HT$_4$ receptor. The 5-HT$_4$ receptor was originally described as a receptor in the central nervous system that could be stimulated by 5-HT to increase the activity of adenylyl cyclase. The pharmacological characteristics of the 5-HT$_4$ receptor do not resemble those of 5-HT$_1$-like, 5-HT$_2$, or 5-HT$_3$ receptors. 5-HT$_4$ receptors are also present in the periphery (gastrointestinal tract and heart) [18]. Studies of the 5-HT$_4$ receptor, which has not yet been cloned, have been hampered by the lack of a high-affinity radioligand.

In addition to these receptors, Gershon and associates [19] have shown in a series of investigations that the enteric nervous system has at least one additional receptor for 5-HT that does not belong to either the 5-HT$_3$ or the 5-HT$_2$ receptor class. This receptor has a high affinity for [^{3}H]5-HT and mediates a slow depolarization of a particular myenteric neuron. This response is not blocked by selective 5-HT$_3$ antagonists. The receptor has been termed the 5-HT$_{1P}$ receptor, as it has a high affinity for 5-HT and is found in the periphery [19].

The subtypes of serotonin receptors are coupled to a variety of signal transduction mechanisms

In both the hippocampus and the raphe nucleus, 5-HT$_{1A}$ receptors are coupled to the opening of K$^+$ channels, presumably directly through a G protein (see Chap. 9). In terminal field areas such as the hippocampus, 5-HT$_{1A}$ receptors are also coupled via a G protein to the inhibition of adenylyl cyclase activity (Table 1). The coupling of 5-HT$_{1A}$ receptors to the inhibition of adenylyl cyclase has *not* been observed in the dorsal raphe nucleus. In hippocampus, the stimulation of cAMP formation by 5-HT$_{1A}$ receptors has also been reported. Thus, the 5-HT$_{1A}$ receptor has been classified as being coupled to both the stimulation and the inhibition of adenylyl cyclase, even in the same brain region.

The 5-HT$_{1B}$ and 5-HT$_{1D}$ receptor subtypes are also linked to inhibition of adenylyl cyclase activity (Table 1). Binding sites that have been pharmacologically defined as 5-HT$_{1B}$ receptors have been characterized in certain rodents (rat, mouse, hamster), whereas the 5-HT$_{1D}$ receptor has been characterized using pharmacological criteria in species such as guinea pig, pig, cow, and human. In the substantia nigra, where a high density of 5-HT$_{1B}$ or 5-HT$_{1D}$ receptors has been demonstrated by radioligand binding studies, these serotonin receptors are linked to the inhibition of adenylyl cyclase through a G protein.

The 5-HT$_{1C}$ and 5-HT$_2$ receptors are coupled through a G protein to the stimulation of phosphoinositide (PI) hydrolysis (Table 1). 5-HT$_2$ receptor-mediated stimulation of PI hydrolysis has been well characterized in cerebral cortex. 5-HT$_{1C}$ receptor-mediated stimulation of PI hydrolysis has been studied in the choroid plexus. The stimulation of PI turnover by 5-HT in these tissues is not dependent on the activity of lipoxygenase or cyclooxygenase pathways, nor is it blocked by agents that inhibit neuronal firing, suggesting that coupling of the 5-HT$_2$ or 5-HT$_{1C}$ receptor to the enzyme phospholipase C mediates the PI response [17].

TABLE 1.   Subtypes of 5-HT receptors in brain

Receptor	Effector mechanism	Clone	Radioligands
5-HT$_1$			
1A	cAMP ↑↓; K$^+$ channels ↑	+	[^{3}H]DPAT
1B	cAMP ↓	+	[^{125}I]ICYP
1C	PI hydrolysis	+	[^{3}H]mesulergine
1D	cAMP ↓	+	[^{3}H]serotonin
5-HT$_2$ (D)	PI hydrolysis; K$^+$ channels ↓	+	[^{3}H]ketanserin
5-HT$_3$ (M)	Ligand-gated cation channel	+	[^{3}H]zacopride
5-HT$_4$	cAMP ↑	−	None

In addition to stimulation of PI hydrolysis, 5-HT$_2$ receptor activation results in a slow inward current and neuronal depolarization. This has been studied primarily in cortical regions as well as in the facial motor nucleus, where 5-HT$_2$ receptors are present in high density. 5-HT$_2$ receptors appear to be coupled through a G protein to the closing of K$^+$ channels, which results in this facilitory effect on neurons. Thus, as with the 5-HT$_{1A}$ receptor, which couples via G proteins to both an enzyme (adenylyl cyclase) and a K$^+$ channel, the 5-HT$_2$ receptor also couples via G proteins to an enzyme (phospholipase C) and to a K$^+$ channel.

The 5-HT$_3$ receptor is a ligand-gated ion channel (Table 1), i.e., it is an ion channel such that the response produced by its activation is not mediated by a second messenger or through G proteins. The depolarization mediated by 5-HT$_3$ receptors is caused by a transient inward current, specifically the opening of a channel for cations.

The 5-HT$_4$ receptor in colliculi neurons and hippocampus is coupled to the stimulation of adenylyl cyclase activity and to the inhibition of K$^+$ channels (Table 1). The inhibition of K$^+$ channels in colliculi neurons has been shown to involve cAMP production and the activation of cAMP-dependent protein kinase A. Although the second-messenger system associated with the 5-HT$_4$ receptor is cAMP, it remains to be seen whether other transduction mechanisms also couple to 5-HT$_4$ receptors.

The many subtypes of receptors for serotonin are not only differentiated by their pharmacology and second-messenger systems but also by their localization in the central nervous system

5-HT$_{1A}$ receptors are present in high density in the hippocampus, septum, amygdala, hypothalamus, and neocortex (Table 2). Destruction of serotonergic neurons with the neurotoxin 5,7-dihydroxytryptamine (5,7-DHT) does not reduce 5-HT$_{1A}$ receptor number in forebrain areas, indicating that 5-HT$_{1A}$ receptors are located postsynaptically in these brain regions. Many of these serotonergic terminal field areas are components of the limbic system, the pathway thought to be involved in the modulation of emotion. The presence of 5-HT$_{1A}$ receptors in high density in the limbic system indicates that the reported effects of 5-HT or serotonergic drugs on emotional states could be mediated by 5-HT$_{1A}$ receptors. The presence of 5-HT$_{1A}$ receptors in the neocortex suggests that this receptor may also be involved in cognitive or integrative functions of the cortex. 5-HT$_{1A}$ receptors are also present in high density in serotonergic cell body areas, in particular the dorsal and median raphe nuclei, where they function as somatodendritic autoreceptors, modulating the activity of serotonergic neurons. Neurotoxin-induced destruction of serotonergic cell bodies dramatically reduces the number of 5-HT$_{1A}$ receptors in these areas, consistent with their location on serotonergic soma.

The 5-HT$_{1B}$ receptor in rats and mice

TABLE 2. Distribution of subtypes of 5-HT receptors in brain[a]

	$5\text{-}HT_{1A}$	$5\text{-}HT_{1B}$	$5\text{-}HT_{1C}$	$5\text{-}HT_{1D}$	$5\text{-}HT_2$	$5\text{-}HT_3$
Neocortex	+++	++	+	++	+++	
Hippocampus	+++	+	+	+	+	+
Septum	+++	+	+	+	+	+
Amygdala	++	++	+	++	+	+
Hypothalamus	++	++	++	++	+	
Striatum		++	+	++	++	
Pallidum		+++	++	+++	+	
Substanta nigra		+++	++	+++		
Raphe	+++	+		+		
Area postrema						+++
Choroid plexus			+++			
Substantia gelatinosa	++					+++

Adapted from Palacios et al. [34].
[a] Greater amount of receptor in a particular area is indicated by an increased number of "pluses."

and the $5\text{-}HT_{1D}$ receptor in bovine and human brain are located in high density in the basal ganglia, particularly in the globus pallidus and the substantia nigra (Table 2). Functional studies indicate that the $5\text{-}HT_{1B}$ and $5\text{-}HT_{1D}$ receptors are located on presynaptic terminals of serotonergic neurons and modulate the release of serotonin. In addition to functioning as terminal autoreceptors, the $5\text{-}HT_{1B}$ and $5\text{-}HT_{1D}$ receptors are located postsynaptically where they may modulate the release of other neurotransmitters, such as acetylcholine. Thus, $5\text{-}HT_{1B}$ and $5\text{-}HT_{1D}$ receptors, although capable of being differentiated pharmacologically, appear to serve the same type of function and are localized in the same areas in the mammalian brain. The presence of these receptors in high density in the basal ganglia raises the interesting possibility that these receptors may be involved in diseases of the brain that involve the basal ganglia, such as Parkinson's disease.

$5\text{-}HT_{1C}$ receptors are present in high density in the choroid plexus. High-resolution autoradiography has shown that they are enriched on the epithelial cells of the choroid plexus. It has been proposed that 5-HT-induced activation of $5\text{-}HT_{1C}$ receptors could regulate the composition and volume of the cerebrospinal fluid. $5\text{-}HT_{1C}$ receptors are also found throughout the brain, in particular areas of the limbic system (hypothalamus, hippocampus, septum, neocortex) and those associated with motor behavior (substantia nigra, globus pallidus). However, $5\text{-}HT_{1C}$ receptors are present in these areas in much lower concentrations than in the choroid plexus (Table 2).

A high density of $5\text{-}HT_2$ receptors is found in many areas of the cortex. In the neocortex, these receptors are concentrated in layers I and V. $5\text{-}HT_2$ receptors are also found in particularly high density in the claustrum, a region that is connected to the visual cortex, in parts of the limbic system, and in the basal ganglia and the olfactory nuclei (Table 2). $5\text{-}HT_2$ receptors in the cortex are thought to be located postsynaptically on intrinsic cortical neurons, as destruction of projections to the cortex does not reduce the density of $5\text{-}HT_2$ receptors.

$5\text{-}HT_3$ receptors initially appeared to be confined to peripheral neurons, where they mediate depolarizing actions of 5-HT and modulate neurotransmitter release. $5\text{-}HT_3$ receptors are found in high density in peripheral ganglia and nerves (superior cervical ganglion and vagus nerve) as well as in the substantia gelatinosa of the spinal cord

Their localization in spinal cord and medulla suggests that 5-HT could modulate nociceptive mechanisms via the 5-HT$_3$ receptor. Using radioligand binding procedures, 5-HT$_3$ receptors have been demonstrated in brain, where they also modulate the release of neurotransmitters such as acetylcholine or dopamine. In the brain they are present in relatively high density in cortical and limbic areas. The highest density of 5-HT$_3$ receptor sites in the brain is in the area postrema, the site of the chemoreceptor trigger zone (Table 2). The antiemetic properties of 5-HT$_3$ receptor antagonists in chemotherapy-induced nausea and vomiting are now well established (see below).

The 5-HT$_4$ receptor, originally characterized by measuring cAMP production in cultured mouse collicular neurons, has also been localized in brain to the hippocampus. A more complete characterization of the distribution of this receptor in the brain, as well as its location postsynaptically and/or presynaptically, awaits the development of a selective radioligand for this receptor.

With the application of molecular biological techniques to the study of neurotransmitter receptors and the subsequent cloning of many of the 5-HT receptor subtypes, advances have been made in our understanding of the structure and function of these receptors

The first 5-HT receptor to be cloned was the 5-HT$_{1C}$ receptor, by Lubbert and co-workers in 1987. Over the course of the next five years, the 5-HT$_{1A}$, 5-HT$_{1B}$, 5-HT$_{1D}$, 5-HT$_2$, and 5-HT$_3$ receptors have also been cloned. The 5-HT$_{1A}$, 5-HT$_{1B}$, 5-HT$_{1C}$, 5-HT$_{1D}$, and 5-HT$_2$ receptors are single subunit proteins that are members of the G protein-receptor superfamily (Table 1). This receptor family is characterized by the presence of seven membrane-spanning regions in each receptor (Fig. 8) and by the ability to activate G protein-dependent processes, including activation or inhibition of adenylyl cyclase activity, activation of phosphoinositide turnover, and

opening or closing of ion channels. The transmembrane domains of G protein-coupled receptors are the most highly conserved regions of these proteins.

As discussed above, the 5-HT$_3$ receptor is a member of the ligand-gated ion channel family. Generally, receptors that are ligand-gated ion channels are composed of multiple subunits. Recently, a subunit of the 5-HT$_3$ receptor has been cloned by Julius and co-workers [20]. This protein has four hydrophobic transmembrane regions, a large NH$_2$-terminal extracellular domain, and a long cytoplasmic loop connecting transmembrane regions 3 and 4. This cloned receptor subunit exhibits sequence similarity to the α-subunit of the nicotinic acetylcholine receptor and the β$_1$-subunit of the GABA$_A$ receptor. Although single subunits of members of the ligand-gated ion channel receptor family can form functional homomeric receptors (receptors composed of subunits of a single type), they generally lack some of the properties of the native, multisubunit receptor. The cloned subunit of the 5-HT$_3$ receptor has been studied in *Xenopus* oocytes injected with mRNA encoding this receptor. Although the expressed receptor has the pharmacological and electrophysiological characteristics consistent with the native 5-HT$_3$ receptor, it is likely that the native 5-HT$_3$ receptor is composed of several subunits.

Molecular biological information has been used to propose alternative classifications for subtypes of 5-HT receptors. It has been suggested that the 5-HT$_{1C}$ receptor more properly belongs in the 5-HT$_2$ receptor classification. There is a greater structural sequence similarity between the 5-HT$_2$ and the 5-HT$_{1C}$ receptors than between the 5-HT$_{1C}$ and 5-HT$_{1A}$ receptors. Also, both the 5-HT$_{1C}$ and 5-HT$_2$ receptors are linked to the same second-messenger system, activation of the phospholipase C cascade. Finally, the pharmacological profiles of these two receptors are similar. A classification scheme based on the type of signal transducing process with subclassifications determined by the degree of structural homology among subtypes of receptor within each class has been proposed by several investigators [17].

Another issue has been raised by the use of molecular biological techniques for the study of neurotransmitter receptors: When is a receptor a subtype and when is it a species homolog (equivalent receptor in different species)? For example, the 5-HT$_{1B}$ and 5-HT$_{1D}$ receptors were originally considered to be species variants of the same receptor, with the 5-HT$_{1B}$ subtype being found in rats, mice, and opossum and the 5-HT$_{1D}$ subtype in cat, guinea pig, bovine, pig, and human brain. This conclusion was based on the observation that both the 5-HT$_{1B}$ and 5-HT$_{1D}$ receptors are coupled to the inhibition of adenylyl cyclase and on the finding that the distribution of these two receptors in brain are very similar. The pharmacological properties of these two receptors are also very similar. Recently, genes encoding a human 5-HT$_{1D}$ (5-HT$_{1D\alpha}$) receptor and a human 5-HT$_{1B}$ (5-HT$_{1D\beta}$) receptor have been cloned and characterized [21]. The human 5-HT$_{1D\alpha}$ receptor inhibits adenylyl cyclase activity and exhibits pharmacological properties that closely resemble those of the 5-HT$_{1D}$ receptor of cow and guinea pig brain. The human 5-HT$_{1D\beta}$ receptor is only slightly different from the rat 5-HT$_{1B}$ receptor in structure (4 percent of the transmembrane amino acids), although it is pharmacologically distinguishable from the rat 5-HT$_{1B}$ receptor. In contrast, the human 5-HT$_{1D\beta}$ receptor differs substantially from the human 5-HT$_{1D\alpha}$ receptor in the transmembrane regions (23 percent of the transmembrane amino acids), yet is essentially indistinguishable pharmacologically from the 5-HT$_{1D\alpha}$ receptor. Recently, a rat gene highly homologous to the human 5-HT$_{1D\alpha}$ sequence has been cloned and expressed and found to encode a receptor with a 5-HT$_{1D}$ pharmacological profile [21]. Thus, with molecular biological criteria and techniques, the 5-HT$_{1D}$ and 5-HT$_{1B}$ receptors have been identified in both human and rat and therefore appear not to be species variants or homologs, but are indeed receptor subtypes.

The cloned 5-HT$_2$ receptor has been used to gain insight into a controversy over the nature of agonist binding to the 5-HT$_2$ receptor. The hallucinogenic amphetamine derivative [^{3}H]DOB, an agonist, has been shown to bind to a small number of binding sites with properties very similar to those of the receptor labeled with the antagonist [^{3}H]ketanserin. Agonists, though, have higher affinities for the receptor labeled with [^{3}H]DOB than with [^{3}H]ketanserin. Some investigators interpreted these and other data as evidence for the existence of a new subtype of 5-HT$_2$ receptor, 5-HT$_{2A}$, whereas others interpreted these data as indicative of agonist high-affinity- and agonist low-affinity-preferring states of the 5-HT$_2$ receptor. In experiments in which the cDNA encoding the 5-HT$_2$ receptor was transfected into clonal cells binding sites for both the 5-HT$_2$ receptor antagonist ketanserin and the 5-HT$_2$ receptor agonist DOB were found, and, furthermore, agonists had higher affinities for [^{3}H]DOB binding than for [^{3}H]ketanserin binding. Thus, a single gene produces a protein with both binding sites, substantiating the view that agonist binding and antagonist binding are to different states of the 5-HT$_2$ receptor rather than to two different subtypes of the 5-HT$_2$ receptor.

Cloning of the various subtypes of receptors for serotonin has identified receptor sequences that can be used to generate radioactive probes for mRNAs encoding individual serotonin receptor subtypes. Using the technique of *in situ* hybridization, the localization of these mRNAs and thus the distribution of cells expressing the mRNAs for serotonin receptors can be established in brain. The anatomical distributions of 5-HT$_2$ receptors, visualized by quantitative autoradiography of radioligand binding, and the localization of 5-HT$_2$ receptor mRNA in brain are in very good agreement. A complementary distribution of 5-HT$_{1A}$ receptors and cells expressing 5-HT$_{1A}$ receptor mRNA has also been demonstrated, further supporting both a presynaptic autoregulatory and a postsynaptic modulatory role for this receptor in serotonergic transmission. The distribution of 5-HT$_{1C}$ receptor mRNA also corresponds to that of the 5-HT_{1C} receptor. The combination of *in situ* hybridization histochemistry with receptor autoradiography makes possible experiments examining the regulation of receptor synthesis after pharmacological manipulations.

Many of the serotonin receptor subtypes do not appear to undergo compensatory regulatory changes, as originally described by Cannon and Rosenblueth in 1949 for nicotinic cholinergic receptors in the periphery

Classically, a decrease in exposure of a tissue to its endogenous transmitter leads to a supersensitive or exaggerated response to exogenous agonist, which may be accounted for by an increase in the density of postsynaptic receptors for the transmitter (up-regulation). Conversely, increased exposure of a tissue to agonists will, over time, result in a decreased responsiveness to the agonist (desensitization), which may be due to a decrease in receptor density (down-regulation). Central β_1-noradrenergic and D_2-dopaminergic receptors undergo such regulatory processes.

Chronic or repeated administration of antidepressant drugs (e.g., MAO inhibitors or inhibitors of serotonin uptake) or 5-HT_{1A} receptor agonists to laboratory rats results in a desensitization of behavioral and electrophysiological responses believed to be mediated by 5-HT_{1A} receptors. Lesioning serotonergic neurons results in increased behavioral and electrophysiological responses. However, these treatments do not result in changes in 5-HT_{1A} receptors as measured with binding assays. Some investigators have reported diminished 5-HT_{1A} receptor-mediated inhibition of adenylyl cyclase following repeated administration of some antidepressant drugs to rats. However, desensitization of second-messenger function has not been observed consistently after chronic antidepressant or agonist treatments.

Lesions of serotonergic neurons do not cause detectable changes in 5-HT_{1B} receptors in forebrain areas and have been reported to cause up-regulation or down-regulation or not to affect the density of 5-HT_{1B} receptors in substantia nigra. Interpretation of these reports may be complicated by the fact that the 5-HT_{1B} receptor is located both pre- and postsynaptically. Cells maintained in culture represent an alternative to *in vivo* systems (i.e., the rat). The 5-HT_{1B} receptor is found on an epithelial cell line from opossum kidney (OK cells). Exposure of OK cells to 5-HT results in a time- and dose-dependent decrease in the density of 5-HT_{1B} receptors and in a desensitization of the 5-HT_{1B} receptor-mediated inhibition of forskolin-stimulated cAMP accumulation [22]. It seems, then, that the 5-HT_{1B} receptor can down-regulate in response to prolonged exposure to an agonist.

Following the lesioning of serotonergic neurons with neurotoxin, 5-HT_{1C} receptor-mediated PI hydrolysis in choroid plexus is increased, and these receptors undergo denervation supersensitivity. However, radioligand binding studies fail to show an increase in 5-HT_{1C} receptor number or in receptor up-regulation. Paradoxically, chronic administration of the antagonist mianserin to rats results in the down-regulation of the 5-HT_{1C} receptor.

5-HT_2 receptors also do not respond to changes in agonist exposure in the classic manner. Specifically, no change in 5-HT_2 receptor density is observed after lesioning serotonergic neurons or after depletion of serotonin stores. 5-HT_2 receptor-mediated PI hydrolysis is also unchanged after such treatments, suggesting that denervation supersensitivity does not occur. Thus, it appears that neither the 5-HT_2 receptor nor its second-messenger pathway is regulated by a decrease in neurotransmitter exposure. After the administration of hallucinogenic 5-HT_2 receptor agonists, chronic administration of selective inhibitors of serotonin uptake, or 5-HT_2 receptor antagonists, 5-HT_2 receptor-mediated PI hydrolysis becomes desensitized and 5-HT_2 receptors down-regulate. Given that agonist exposure causes desensitization of $5\text{-}HT_2$ receptors, it has been proposed by Leysen and Pauwels that the absence of supersensitivity after denervation may reflect low tonic activity at synapses innervating $5\text{-}HT_2$ receptors [23]. A cell line maintained in culture has proven useful in the study of $5\text{-}HT_2$ receptor regulation. P11 cells, isolated from the rat pituitary tumor 7315a, express $5\text{-}HT_2$ receptors coupled to PI hydrolysis. $5\text{-}HT_2$ receptors on P11 cells have been shown to down-regulate and to desensitize upon exposure to 5-HT, but not in response to antagonists. Such results might indicate that the antagonist-induced down-regulation of $5\text{-}HT_2$ receptors *in vivo* may be due to some indirect effect of the antagonists.

$5\text{-}HT_3$ receptors, located on neurons in the periphery and in the central nervous system, mediate fast, excitatory responses (membrane depolarization) to serotonin. Like many other receptors that are directly coupled to an ion channel, the $5\text{-}HT_3$ receptor exhibits rapid desensitization after sustained agonist exposure. In addition to preparations of peripheral neurons, cultured hippocampal cells and neuroblastoma cells have been used to study this phenomenon.

INVOLVEMENT OF SEROTONIN IN PHYSIOLOGICAL FUNCTIONS AND BEHAVIORS

In the central nervous system serotonin is involved in eating, sleep, sexual behavior, circadian rhythmicity, and neuroendocrine function

The hypothalamus secretes several releasing factors and release-inhibiting factors to control the secretion of anterior pituitary hormones. Serotonin is among the many neurotransmitters that participate in the hypothalamic control of pituitary secretion, particularly in the regulation of prolactin, adrenocorticotrophin (ACTH), and growth hormone. Measurement of these endocrine responses after administration of drugs that increase brain serotonin function provide one of the few methods currently available for assessing such function in humans. For example, administration of the serotonin precursor L-tryptophan increases plasma concentrations of prolactin and growth hormone. When administered to humans, serotonin agonists that stimulate $5\text{-}HT_{1A}$, $5\text{-}HT_{1C}$, and $5\text{-}HT_2$ receptors also increase plasma ACTH, prolactin, and growth homone levels. The neuroendocrine response in humans to the nonselective serotonergic receptor agonist *m*-CPP (*m*-chlorophenylpiperazine) or to L-tryptophan has been used clinically to assess the functioning of the central serotonergic system in patients with psychiatric disorders [24].

Research in cats has implicated serotonin in sleep and arousal states. Serotonergic neurons in the dorsal raphe nucleus show a dramatic change in activity across the sleep-wake-arousal cycle. Under quiet waking conditions, serotonergic neurons display a slow, clock-like activity, which shows a gradual decline as the animal becomes drowsy and enters slow wave sleep. A decrease in the regularity of firing accompanies this overall slowing of neuronal activity. During REM (rapid eye movement) sleep, the activity of these neurons ceases. In response to arousing stimuli, the firing rate of these serotonergic neurons increases. Auditory (click) or visual (flash) stimuli produce an excitation of dorsal raphe serotonergic neurons followed by an inhibition. However, exposing a cat to environmental stressors such as a loud noise or seeing a dog, although producing strong sympathetic activation and typical behavioral responses, does not alter the firing rate of these serotonergic neurons [7]. Because the tonic activity of serotonergic neurons appears to vary in a general manner in association with behavioral state and not in association with any specific behavioral response, Jacobs and co-workers have proposed that the role of central serotonergic neurons is to coordinate the activity of the nervous system, to set the tone of activity in conjunction with the organism's level of arousal.

Serotonin also appears to be involved in the regulation of circadian rhythms. The suprachiasmic nuclei (SCN) of the hypothalamus generate electrophysiological and metabolic cycles that repeat approximately every 24 hours. Ordinarily, this rhythm is synchronized or entrained to the environmental photoperiod, also about 24 hours. A serotonergic contribution to circadian rhythm regulation has been postulated because the SCN receive very dense serotonergic innervation from the midbrain raphe nuclei. Very little is known, however, about the function of this dense serotonergic input. Lesions of serotonergic neurons in laboratory animals have been reported by some, but not all, investigators to disrupt locomotor rhythms or to result in the loss of the daily rhythm of corticosterone. When isolated *in vitro*, the SCN continue to produce 24 hour rhythms in metabolism, vasopressin secretion, and spontaneous electrical activity, indicating that circadian time-keeping functions or pacemaker activity are endogenous characteristics of the SCN. The nonselective 5-HT agonist quipazine has been shown to reset or shift the rhythm of spontaneous electrical activity of single cells recorded extracellularly in SCN isolated in brain slices [25]. These results suggest that the SCN circadian pacemaker or clock is modulated by stimulation of serotonergic receptors in the SCN and that serotonergic projections to the SCN may modulate the phase of the SCN in intact animals.

Neurochemical research has focused on how feeding affects brain tryptophan concentrations and serotonin synthesis and availability, whereas pharmacological research has been carried out on the control of appetite by serotonergic drugs. In laboratory rats, administration of nonselective indirect-acting serotonergic agonists, such as fenfluramine, which acts to release serotonin, or 5-hydroxytryptophan, a precursor to serotonin synthesis, decreases feeding. From such data it has been inferred that serotonin inhibits food intake. Serotonin agonists activat-

ing postsynaptic 5-HT_{1C} and 5-HT_{1B} receptors also decrease feeding. Selective inhibitors of serotonin uptake have anorectic effects as well, presumably by enhancing physiological actions of endogenous serotonin. By contrast, small doses of selective 5-HT_{1A} agonists increase food intake in rats. The increased food consumption may be due to agonist activity at serotonin autoreceptors in the raphe nuclei. The activation of somatodendritic 5-HT_{1A} receptors would be expected to inhibit serotonergic neuronal firing and serotonin release. The hypophagic effects of fenfluramine or 5-HT_1 agonists are more pronounced in female rats, an effect of potential relevance to human eating disorders such as anorexia nervosa and bulimia nervosa, which have a higher rate of incidence in young women than in young men.

Not only does 5-HT have important physiological effects of its own, but it is also the precursor of the hormone melatonin

The human pineal gland weights about 150 mg and occupies the depression between the superior colliculi at the posterior border of the corpus callosum. Although there are physical connections between the pineal gland and brain, the pineal gland lies "outside" the blood-brain barrier (see Chap. 32) and is innervated primarily by sympathetic nerves arising from the superior cervical ganglia.

Extracts of the pineal gland were reported as early as 1917 to lighten frog skin *in vitro;* in the late 1950s, Lerner and associates isolated the pineal hormone that produced this effect and described its chemical structure, 5-methoxy-*N*-acetyltryptamine (melatonin) (Fig. 2). Melatonin is synthesized from serotonin, and the pineal gland contains all the enzymes necessary to synthesize serotonin from tryptophan, as well as two additional enzymes required to convert serotonin to melatonin (Fig. 2). The rate-limiting enzyme, serotonin *N*-acetyltransferase (NAT), converts serotonin to *N*-acetylserotonin, and this product is converted to melatonin by the enzyme 5-hydroxyindole-*O*-methyltransferase (HIOMT), which uses *S*-adenosyl methionine as the methyl donor.

A unique feature of pineal gland physiology is that the synthesis and secretion of melatonin are markedly influenced by the light-dark cycle. During daylight, the synthesis and secretion of melatonin are reduced, as is impulse flow along the sympathetic nerves innervating the pineal gland. At the onset of darkness, there is activation of these nerves, and the increased release of norepinephrine from them activates β-adrenoceptors on the pineal to increase the formation of cAMP, with activation of α_1-adrenoceptors further amplifying the response. This second messenger causes activation of NAT (and the increase in enzyme activity can be as much as 50- to 100-fold in the rat) so as to increase the synthesis of melatonin. Thus, the pineal gland functions as a neuroendocrine transducer. In mammals, photosensory information impinging on the retina influences the activity of its neuronal projections, which serves ultimately to inhibit or to stimulate the secretion of melatonin. A circadian rhythm of melatonin secretion persists in animals housed in continuous darkness. Thus, melatonin synthesis is turned on by an endogenous "clock," probably located within the suprachiasmatic nucleus of the hypothalamus, with the daily rhythm normally being entrained to the day-night, light-dark cycle [26].

The exact physiological and behavioral effects of melatonin in humans are unclear. Perhaps the strongest case can be made for melatonin playing a role in reproduction, particularly in seasonally breeding mammals such as hamsters or sheep that time their reproductive cycles via changes in the photoperiod. Information on day length may be relayed to the hypothalamic-pituitary-gonadal axis by the pattern of melatonin production. Although the effects of melatonin on reproduction were believed to be solely antigonadotropic, melatonin has now been shown to be capable of causing progonadotropic effects. The type of effect caused by melatonin is dependent on the time point in the photoperiod when it is administered, the length of the photoperiod, the species, and the dose administered.

SEROTONIN NEURONS AND RECEPTORS AS TARGETS FOR A WIDE VARIETY OF THERAPEUTIC DRUGS

The most widely used class of antidepressant drugs is commonly referred to as the tricyclic antidepressants (TCAs). It has been known for about 25 years that many of these drugs, e.g., imipramine and amitriptyline, are potent inhibitors of the uptake of NE and 5-HT. Some TCAs, e.g., desipramine, and protriptyline, inhibit the uptake of NE much more potently than the uptake of 5-HT. Thus, it was unclear whether the inhibition of serotonin uptake played any role in the antidepressant action of those tricyclic drugs that possessed this pharmacological property. Recently, though, effective antidepressants such as fluoxetine and sertraline have been marketed, and these drugs, referred to as selective serotonin re-uptake inhibitors (SRIs), are much more potent inhibitors of the uptake of 5-HT than that of NE [27]. Thus, selective inhibition of the uptake of either NE or 5-HT can result in an antidepressant effect (Fig. 9).

Another class of antidepressant drug is the monoamine oxidase inhibitors (MAOIs), e.g., phenelzine, isocarboxazid, or tranylcypromine. These drugs irreversibly inhibit the activity of the enzyme MAO (Fig. 9). MAO catabolizes biogenic amines such as 5-HT, dopamine, and NE, which implicates these neurotransmitters in the mechanisms of action of these drugs. Interestingly, studies have been carried out recently from which it was inferred that serotonin is needed for SRIs or MAOIs to produce a beneficial clini-

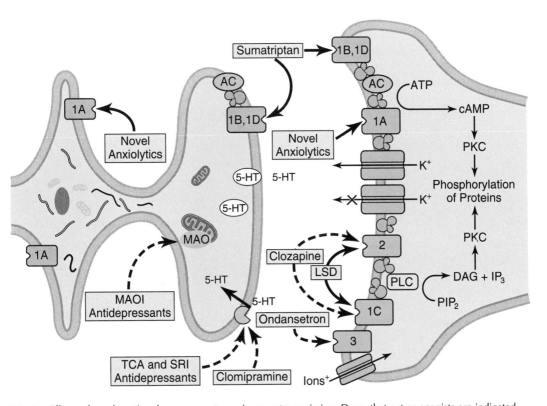

FIG. 9. Effects of psychoactive drugs on serotonergic neurotransmission. Drugs that act as agonists are indicated by **solid-line arrows,** whereas antagonists or inhibitors are shown with **broken-line arrows.** The 5-HT$_{1A}$ (1A) receptor acts as both a somatodendritic autoreceptor and a postsynaptic receptor; anxiolytic drugs such as buspirone are agonists at this receptor. In terminal fields, the autoreceptor is either the 5-HT$_{1B}$ (1B) or 5-HT$_{1D}$ (1D) subtype; these receptors also function as postsynaptic receptors. The antimigraine drug sumatriptan is an agonist at these receptors. There are both structural similarity and similarity in the second-messenger coupling of 5-HT$_2$ (2) and 5-HT$_{1C}$ (1C) receptors. Hallucinogenic drugs such as LSD are agonists at 5-HT$_2$ and 5-HT$_{1C}$ receptors, whereas novel antipsychotic drugs such as clozapine are antagonists. The 5-HT$_3$ (3) receptor, a ligand-gated ion channel, is blocked by drugs such as ondansetron effective in the treatment of chemotherapy-induced nausea and emesis. Another important target for psychotherapeutic drugs is the serotonin transporter, which is blocked by drugs effective in the treatment of depression or obsessive-compulsive disorder (clomipramine). The enzyme responsible for the catabolism of serotonin, MAO, is inhibited by another class of antidepressants. (AC) adenylyl cyclase; (PKC) protein kinase C; (DAG) diacyl-glycerol; (IP$_3$) inositol trisphosphate; (PIP$_2$) phosphatidylinositol bisphosphate. (This figure was kindly prepared by Dr. William Clarke, Department of Pharmacology, Mt. Sinai School of Medicine, New York, NY.)

cal response in depressed patients [2]. Such data are consistent with the idea that drug-induced enhancement of serotonergic transmission can produce amelioration of depressive symptomatology.

Inhibition of 5-HT uptake can cause not only an antidepressant effect but also may reduce the symptoms of an anxiety disorder termed obsessive-compulsive disorder. A TCA, clomipramine, which is somewhat se-lective *in vivo* as an inhibitor of 5-HT uptake, does produce clinically significant ameliora-tion of the symptoms associated with obses-sive-compulsive disorder. This clinical effect is also produced by many SRIs but is not found with drugs such as desipramine that selectively inhibit the uptake of NE.

The drugs most widely used for the treatment of generalized anxiety disorder (GAD) are benzodiazepines such as diazepam or lorazepam. These drugs act by enhancing the activity of the inhibitory amino acid transmitter GABA. In the past 10 years, novel anxiolytics have become available that seem to act initially through serotonergic mechanisms. These newer drugs, e.g., substituted azapirones such as buspirone or gepirone, share the common pharmacological property of agonism at the 5-HT$_{1A}$ receptor. This receptor functions as both the somatodendritic autoreceptor and a postsynaptic receptor, and research is currently under way to determine which anatomical locus is primarily involved in the anxiolytic activity of these drugs (Fig. 9).

Antipsychotic drugs effective in the treatment of schizophrenia are believed to act primarily by inhibiting central dopaminergic transmission by virtue of their being dopamine receptor antagonists. More recently available atypical antipsychotic drugs, such as clozapine, share this property but are more potent antagonists at 5-HT$_2$ and 5-HT$_{1C}$ receptors than classic or typical antipsychotic drugs such as chlorpromazine or haloperidol [28]. The balance between effects of antipsychotic drugs on dopaminergic and serotonergic function has been hypothesized to be important in their clinical effects. The relatively greater potency of atypical antipsychotic drugs on 5-HT$_2$/5-HT$_{1C}$ receptors may play some role in the ability of the atypical drugs to produce less extrapyramidal side effects than the more typical compounds or to be more effective for some symptoms of schizophrenia such as anergia (loss of energy) or anhedonia (inability to experience pleasure). The hallucinogenic activities of drugs such as LSD appear to be related to their agonist activity at 5-HT$_2$ or 5-HT$_{1C}$ receptors (Fig. 9) [29].

Drugs acting at 5-HT$_{1D}$ and 5-HT$_3$ receptors also have important therapeutic properties. For example, agonists at 5-HT$_{1D}$ receptors, such as the drug sumatriptan, are effective in the acute treatment of migraine headaches (Fig. 9). Whether the beneficial clinical effect of sumatriptan is related to its ability to cause cerebral vasoconstriction or

to block neurogenic extravasation from blood vessels within dura mater or to some other mechanism remains to be determined.

Finally, antagonists at 5-HT$_3$ receptors, such as ondansetron or granisetron (Fig. 9), are an important new class of drugs for the treatment of nausea and emesis in cancer patients receiving chemotherapy [30]. The site of action of these drugs appears to be 5-HT$_3$ receptors in the gastrointestinal (GI) tract even though the central area regulating emesis, i.e., the chemoreceptor trigger zone, possesses a high density of 5-HT$_3$ receptors. Large amounts of 5-HT are found in the enterochromaffin cells of the GI tract, and the enteric nerves innervating the smooth muscle of the GI tract contain 5-HT$_3$ receptors. It has been hypothesized that chemotherapy or radiation therapy causes the release of 5-HT from enterochromaffin cells; the 5-HT released activates 5-HT$_3$ receptors, causing depolarization of visceral afferent nerves and increasing their rate of firing. The enhanced afferent input leads to stimulation of the chemoreceptor trigger zone that produces nausea and vomiting. Antagonism of 5-HT$_3$ receptors would prevent or reduce this chain of events.

REFERENCES

1. Rapport, M. M., Green, A. A., and Page, I. H. Serum vasoconstrictor (serotonin). IV. Isolation and characterization. *J. Biol. Chem.* 176: 1243–1251, 1948.
2. Delgado, P. L., Charney, D. S., Price, L. H., Aghajanian, G. K., Landis, H., and Heninger, G. R. Serotonin function and the mechanism of antidepressant action. *Arch. Gen. Psychiatry* 47:411–418, 1990.
3. Kim, K. S., Wessel, T. C., Stone, D. M., Carver, C. H., Joh, T. H., and Park, D. H. Molecular cloning and characterization of cDNA encoding tryptophan hydroxylase from rat central serotonergic neurons. *Mol. Brain Res.* 9: 277–283, 1991.
4. Tanaka, T., Horio, Y., Taketoshi, M., Imamura, I., Ando-Yamamoto, M., Kangawa, K., Matsuo, H., Kuroda, M., and Wada, H. Molec-

ular cloning and sequencing of a cDNA of rat dopa decarboxylase: Partial amino acid homologies with other enzymes synthesizing catecholamines. *Proc. Natl. Acad. Sci. U.S.A.* 86:8142–8146, 1989.

5. Tison, F., Normand, E., Jaber, M., Aubert, I., and Bloch, B. Aromatic L-amino-acid decarboxylase (DOPA decarboxylase) gene expression in dopaminergic and serotonergic cells of the rat brainstem. *Neurosci. Lett.* 127: 203–206, 1991.

6. Molliver, M. E. Serotonergic neuronal systems: What their anatomic organization tells us about function. *J. Clin Psychopharmacol.* 7(6 Suppl.):3s–23s, 1987.

7. Jacobs, B. L., and Azmitia, E. C. Structure and function of the brain serotonin system. *Physiol. Rev.* 72:165–229, 1992.

8. Tamir, H., and Gershon, M. D. Serotonin-storing secretory vesicles. *Ann. N.Y. Acad. Sci.* 600:53–66, 1990.

9. Sanders-Bush, E., and Martin, L. L. Storage and release of serotonin. In N. N. Osborne (ed.), *Biology of Serotonin Transmission.* New York: Wiley, 95–118, 1982.

10. Bonvento, G., Scatton, B., Claustre, Y., and Rouquier, L. Effect of local injection of 8-OH-DPAT into the dorsal or median raphe nuclei on extracellular levels of serotonin in serotonergic projection areas in the rat brain. *Neurosci. Lett.* 137:101–104, 1992.

11. Hjorth, S., and Tao, R. The putative 5-HT$_{1B}$ receptor agonist CP-93, 129 suppresses rat hippocampal 5-HT release *in vivo*: Comparison with RU 24969. *Eur. J. Pharmacol.* 209: 249–252, 1991.

12. Blakely, R. D., Berson, H. E., Fremeau, R. T., Jr., Caron, M. G., Peek, M. M., Prince, H. K., and Bradley, C. C. Cloning and expression of a functional serotonin transporter from rat brain. *Nature* 354:66–70, 1991.

13. Hoffman, B. J., Mezey, E., and Brownstein, M. J. Cloning of a serotonin transporter affected by antidepressants. *Science* 254:579–580, 1991.

14. Shih, J. C. Molecular basis of human MAO A and B. *Neuropsychopharmacology* 4:1–3, 1991.

15. Richards, J. G., Saura, J., Ulrich, J., and Da Prada, M. Molecular neuroanatomy of monoamine oxidases in human brainstem. *Psychopharmacology* 106:S21–S23, 1992.

16. Cespuglio, R., Sarda, N., Gharib, H., Chas-

trette, N., Houdouin, F., Rampin, C., and Jouvet, M. Voltammetric detection of the release of 5-hydroxyindole compounds throughout the sleep-waking cycle of the rat. *Exp. Brain. Res.* 80:121–128, 1990.

17. Frazer, A., Maayani, S., and Wolfe, B. B. Subtypes of receptors for serotonin. *Annu. Rev. Pharmacol. Toxicol.* 30:307–348, 1990.

18. Bockaert, J., Fozard, J. R., Dumuis, A., and Clarke, D. E. The 5-HT$_4$ receptor: A place in the sun. *Trends Pharmacol. Sci.* 13:141–145, 1992.

19. Gershon, M. D., Wade, P. R., Kirchgessner, A. L., and Tamir, H. 5-HT receptor subtypes outside the central nervous system. Roles in the physiology of the gut. *Neuropsychopharmacology* 3:385–395, 1990.

20. Maricq, A. V., Peterson, A. S., Brake, A. J., Myers, R. M., and Julius, D. Primary structure and functional expression of the 5-HT$_3$ receptor, a serotonin-gated ion channel. *Science* 254:432–437, 1991.

21. Hartig, P. R., Branchek, T. A., and Weinshank, R. L. A subfamily of 5-HT$_{1D}$ receptor genes. *Trends Pharmacol. Sci.* 13:152–159, 1992.

22. Unsworth, C. D., and Molinoff, P. B. Regulation of the 5-hydroxytryptamine$_{1B}$ receptor in opossum kidney cells after exposure to agonists. *Mol. Pharmacol.* 42:464–470, 1992.

23. Sanders-Bush, E. Adaptive regulation of central serotonin receptors linked to phosphoinositide hydrolysis. *Neuropsychopharmacology* 3:411–416, 1990.

24. Murphy, D. L. Neuropsychiatric disorders and the multiple human brain serotonin receptor subtypes and subsystems. *Neuropsychopharmacology* 3:457–471, 1990.

25. Prosser, R. A., Miller, J. D., and Heller, C. A. A serotonin agonist phase-shifts the circadian clock in the suprachiasmatic nuclei *in vitro*. *Brain Res.* 534:336–339, 1990.

26. Reiter, R. J. Melatonin: The chemical expression of darkness. *Mol. Cell. Endocrinol.* 79: C153–C158, 1991.

27. Bauer, M. S., and Frazer, A. Mood disorders. In A. Frazer, P. B. Molinoff, and A. Winokur (eds.), *Biological Basis of Brain Function and Disease.* New York: Raven, 1994.

28. Meltzer, H. Y., Matsubara, S., and Lee, J.-C. Classification of typical and atypical antipsy-

chotic drugs on the basis of dopamine D_1, D_2 and serotonin$_2$ pK_i values. *J. Pharmacol. Exp. Ther.* 251:238–246, 1989.

29. Glennon R. A. Do classical hallucinogens act as 5-HT$_2$ agonists or antagonists? *Neuropsychopharmacology* 3:509–517, 1990.

30. Cubeddu, L. X., Hoffman, I. S., Fuenmayor, N. T., and Finn, A. L. Antagonism of serotonin S3 receptors with ondansetron prevents nausea and emesis induced by cyclophosphamide-containing chemotherapy regimens. *J. Clin. Oncol.* 8:1721–1727, 1990.

31. Consolazione, A., and Cuello, A. C. CNS serotonin pathways. In N. N. Osborne (ed.), *Biology of Serotonergic Transmission.* New York Wiley, 1982, pp. 29–61.

32. Tork, I. Anatomy of the serotonergic system. *Ann. N.Y. Acad. Sci.* 600:9–34, 1990.

33. Kosofsky, B. E., and Molliver, M. E. The serotoninergic innervation of cerebral cortex: Different classes of axon terminals arise from dorsal and median raphe nuclei. *Synapse* 1 153–168, 1987.

34. Palacios, J. M., Waeber, C., Hoyer, D., and Mengod, G. Distribution of serotonin receptors. *Ann. N.Y. Acad. Sci.* 600:36–52, 1990.

Histamine

JACK PETER GREEN

Basic Neurochemistry: Molecular, Cellular, and Medical Aspects, 5th Ed., edited by G. J. Siegel et al. Published by Raven Press, Ltd., New York, 1994. Correspondence to Jack Peter Green, Department of Pharmacology, Box 1215, Mount Sinai School of Medicine, City University of New York, One Gustave L. Levy Place, New York, New York 10029.

HISTAMINE HAS POWERFUL EFFECTS IN PERIPHERAL TISSUES AS WELL AS IN THE NERVOUS SYSTEM

The presence of histamine was described in brain and peripheral nerves of seven mammalian species 50 years ago [1]. During the next 20 years, evidence slowly accumulated that histamine may function in brain [2], but only in the past 10 years has the evidence become persuasive [3–7]. The delay in searching for a histaminergic neuronal system, in contrast to the exploration of other putative neurotransmitter systems, may rest on how research on histamine began. Soon after its discovery in ergot and before it was found in nearly all animal tissues, Dale and his associates [8] emphasized the similarities of the pharmacological effects of histamine to those of the anaphylactic reaction. Later work focused on the role of histamine in acid secretion and peptic ulcer disease, attention being paid to the "mainly pathological aspect of its significance" [8].

Yet, despite the sparse studies of histamine in the brain, histamine adventitiously led to the development of psychotropic drugs [9]. The phenothiazines were developed as antihistamines, and one of them, chlorpromazine, was observed to produce an unusual effect on mood, a "euphoric quietude," which led to its use in treating schizophrenia (see Chap. 47). Chemical modifications produced imipramine, which proved disappointing in treating schizophrenia but was effective in treating depression (see Chap. 48). Curiously, until about 15 years ago, no attention was given to histamine receptors as sites of action for these drugs. Now it is clear that many of the psychotropic drugs react with histamine receptors [9]. Which of the numerous pharmacological effects of these drugs are attributable to interactions with histamine receptors remains to be learned.

HISTAMINE, FOUND IN FOOD AND FORMED BY INTESTINAL BACTERIA, IS TAKEN UP FROM BLOOD BY MANY PERIPHERAL TISSUES BUT NOT READILY BY BRAIN

Histidine decarboxylase is a determinant of brain histamine levels

Histamine in brain [3–7] is formed from L-histidine which is taken up by an active process (see Chap. 32). Histidine is decarboxylated mainly by a specific histidine decarboxylase (EC 4.1.1.22), which has no other naturally occurring substrate, and, less efficiently, by aromatic-L-amino-acid decarboxylase (EC 4.1.1.28). The enzymes differ in their pH optima, K_m for histidine, response to inhibitors, antigenicities, and distribution in brain. (S)-α-fluoromethylhistidine irreversibly inactivates histidine decarboxylase, lowering levels of histamine, without influencing the activity of aromatic-L-amino-acid decarboxylase. Administration of L-histidine raises brain histamine levels, reflective of the affinity of histidine decarboxylase for histidine ($K_m = 120$ μM for the rat brain enzyme) and the relatively low concentration of histidine normally present in brain and blood. Since both mammalian decarboxylases can form histamine, injection of large amounts of histidine could influence not only neuronal histaminergic activity, but also histamine content at other sites containing aromatic-L-amino-acid decarboxylase (see also Chap. 39).

Several histidine decarboxylases have been sequenced

Histidine decarboxylase was purified from fetal rat liver [6], which has high histidine decarboxylase activity with properties similar to those of the brain enzyme. Antibody to the purified liver enzyme cross reacts with the enzyme from brain [6]. Activity of the enzyme appears to be dependent on pyridoxal-5'-phosphate (see Chap. 35). The purified enzyme consists of two 55-kDa subunits

[6]. As the cDNA clone of histidine decarboxylase from fetal rat liver encodes a protein of M_r 73,450, the enzyme is almost certainly processed post-translationally [10]. The amino acid sequence shows about 50 percent similarity to the sequence of rat dopa decarboxylase (EC 4.1.1.26) (see Chap. 12). There is greater similarity at the binding site for pyridoxal phosphate. The similarities in sequence, especially at the N-terminal part of histidine decarboxylase, account for cross-reactivities of antibodies of some histidine decarboxylases and dopa decarboxylases. The molecular weight of histidine decarboxylase from mouse mastocytoma is 74 kDa, and the cDNA-derived amino acid sequence shows 86 percent similarity to that of fetal rat liver [11]. Isozymes of histidine decarboxylase could also be due to potential sites of glycosylation, two in the fetal rat liver enzyme [10] and four in the mouse mastocytoma enzyme [11]. Two potential sites of phosphorylation that fit the recognition sequence of cAMP-dependent protein kinase may account for modulation of histidine decarboxylase by phosphorylation by cAMP-dependent protein kinase [10,11].

More than one pool of histamine exists in brain

In addition to its dominant presence in synaptosomal portions, about 20 percent of the histamine is found in the denser P_1 fraction that contains few synaptosomes [3–7]. Acute treatment with α-fluoromethylhistidine about halves the content of histamine; chronic treatment is needed to eliminate most of the histamine from brain. These data indicate that one pool is metabolized rapidly and another, slowly. The pool of histamine that turns over slowly may be non-neuronal, since lesioning histaminergic fibers reduces histamine content in the fraction containing nerve endings without influencing the content in the P_1 fraction [7]. This non-neuronal pool may be in mast cells, vascular cells, or both since histamine turns over slowly in both types of cells. The prevalence and regional distribution of mast cells in brain differ among species, but mast cells are not abundant and probably make slight contribution to histamine in brain. However, tissues associated with peripheral nerves are rich in mast cells [4].

Histaminergic cell bodies are found only in the tuberomammillary nucleus of the posterior hypothalamus

The histaminergic cell bodies and their projections are visualized by antibodies to histidine decarboxylase and to histamine coupled to protein [6]. The two approaches yield similar results (Fig. 1). The large bipolar or multipolar cell bodies (20 to 30 μm in diameter) are confined to the tuberomammillary nucleus in all species examined. In confirmation of the single source of the histaminergic system, only the tuberomammillary nucleus showed the mRNA for histidine decarboxylase [12]. Efferent fibers project predominantly ipsilaterally to almost all regions of the brain and to the spinal cord. Fibers also appear to penetrate the ependymal layer and to contact cerebrospinal fluid.

Some of the histaminergic neurons also contain glutamate decarboxylase and adenosine deaminase, a coexistence that could

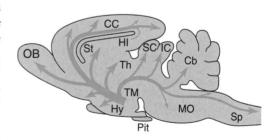

FIG. 1. A sagittal diagram of the histaminergic system in the rat brain. Arrows indicate fiber projections from the cell bodies. (Cb) cerebellum; (CC) cerebral cortex; (Hi) hippocampus; (Hy) hypothalamus; (IC) inferior colliculus; (MO) medulla oblongata; (OB) olfactory bulb; (Pit) pituitary; (SC) superior colliculus; (Sp) spinal cord; (St) striatum; (Th) thalamus; (TM) tuberomammillary nucleus.

imply a functional relationship among histamine, γ-aminobutyrate, and adenosine [12]. In addition, some of the tuberomammillary neurons also contain substance P, galanin, and a met-enkephalin [6].

Some of the histaminergic neurons receive synaptic input, through the ascending reticular system of adrenergic, noradrenergic, and serotonergic cell groups, respectively, C1 to C3, A1 and A2, and B5 to B9. These form synapses with dendrites. Neuropeptide Y and substance P terminals make contact with the somata and dendrites of the histamine neurons [6].

Histaminergic systems have been described in nonmammalian vertebrates too. In brains of birds, reptiles, amphibia, and fish, histamine has a nonuniform distribution, the diencephalon showing highest concentrations as in mammalian brain.

Histamine in mammalian brain is metabolized by histamine methyltransferase

Consistent failure to demonstrate a high-affinity uptake system for histamine in mammalian brain distinguishes histamine [3–5] from other aromatic biogenic amines that serves as neurotransmitters and whose synaptic activities are ended by re-uptake. Some invertebrate nerves may contain a high-affinity uptake system. Histamine released from mammalian nerve endings is thus inactivated solely by metabolism [3–5]. The major pathway of histamine metabolism in mammalian brain is methylation.

Histamine Methyltransferase

Histamine is methylated on the *tele*-nitrogen (or N^τ-nitrogen) by histamine methyltransferase (HMT) (EC 2.1.1.8). The methyl group is transferred from *S*-adenosyl-L-methionine to form *tele*-methylhistamine (*t*-MH) (Fig. 2) and *S*-adenosyl-L-homocysteine. Since histamine is tautomeric (Fig. 3), the other nitrogen in the ring, the *pros*-nitrogen (or N^π-nitrogen), could theoretically be

methylated. Efforts to show methylation of the *pros*-nitrogen by HMT have failed, and *pros*-methylhistamine cannot be found in brain by a gas chromatographic-mass spectrometric method that easily quantifies *t*-MH [13].

HMT is found in postsynaptic sites in neurons, glia, and cerebrospinal fluid [3–5]. The enzyme is selective for histamine, acting on no other known endogenous substance. The purified enzymes from guinea pig [14] and bovine [15,16] brain have similar K_m values for histamine (13 μM) and for *S*-adenosyl-L-methionine (6 μM). The guinea pig enzyme shows optima at pH 7.5 and 9, whereas the bovine enzyme shows no clear pH optimum [15]. The isoelectric point of the guinea pig enzyme (5.3) is lower than that of the bovine enzyme (5.9), which may reflect a relatively higher content of aspartate and/or glutamate of the guinea pig enzyme [14,16]. The apparent molecular weight of the enzyme from guinea pig, rat or mouse brain is 29 kDa compared with the 34 kDa of the enzyme from bovine brain. Another difference is that high concentrations of histamine (ten times the K_m value) inhibit the enzyme from guinea pig, rat, and mouse brain but not the enzyme from bovine brain[15,16].

Metoprine competitively inhibits all HMTs with a K_i of 58 nM [16]. The enzymes are inhibited by both the reaction products, *t*-MH and *S*-adenosyl-L-homocysteine. *t*-MH shows both noncompetitive and competitive inhibition of the bovine enzyme [16]. Kinetic and product inhibition studies of the enzyme from bovine brain are consistent with the formation of a ternary complex, with *S*-adenosyl-L-methionine binding before histamine, and *t*-MH dissociating first [15].

Tele-Methylhistamine in Mammalian Brain is Oxidatively Deaminated by Monoamine Oxidase B

t-MH can be oxidatively deaminated by monoamine oxidase B and by diamine oxidase, but diamine oxidase is lacking in brain [4]. Monoamine oxidase B in brain has a

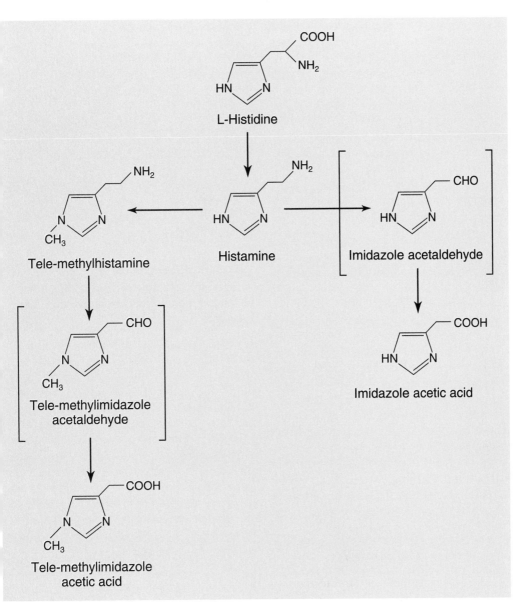

FIG. 2. Formation of histamine and its main metabolic pathways. In mammalian brain, only the methylating pathway occurs.

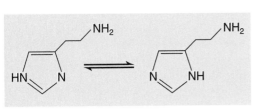

FIG. 3. The two tautomers of histamine.

high K_m for *t*-MH, 3.7 mM [5]. The enzyme is colocalized with histamine in some of the tuberomammillary neurons [6]. The intermediate aldehyde, which has not been isolated, is oxidized to *tele*-methylimidazoleacetic acid (*t*-MIAA). *t*-MH and *t*-MIAA show a simple precursor-product relationship in various types of studies: Both metabolites decrease in brain after treatment of rats with the HMT inhibitor metoprine; *t*-MH accumulates and *t*-MIAA falls in regions of rat brain after treatment of rats with the monoamine oxidase inhibitor pargyline; levels of the two compounds are correlated in samples of cisternal cerebrospinal fluid of monkey; during diurnal cycles measured in monkey cisternal cerebrospinal fluid, changes in levels of *t*-MIAA follow those of *t*-MH [4,5].

Histamine Has a High Turnover Rate in Brain

The concentrations of histamine, *t*-MH, and *t*-MIAA in regions of brain are highly correlated; the highest concentrations are found in the hypothalamus. Turnover rates of histamine vary over 50-fold in different regions of brain. The total amount of turnover is highest in hypothalamus, but rate constants are highest in the caudate nucleus and cortex [4,5,13]. The relatively low rate constant in hypothalamus implies that only a portion of the histamine there is turning over; the presence of histamine-containing cell bodies, as well as nerve terminals, in the hypothalamus can account for the low rate constant. The steady-state levels of histamine in brain are low. The half-lives of histamine in rat cortex and caudate nucleus are about 11 min, much shorter than the half-lives, 71 and 48 min, respectively, of dopamine [13].

Diamine Oxidase

The other major route of histamine metabolism in peripheral tissues is direct oxidative deamination by diamine oxidase to form imidazoleacetaldehyde and then imidazoleacetic acid (IAA) (Fig. 2). That the aldehyde is an intermediate was shown by the formation of imidazole ethanol after inhibition of aldehyde dehydrogenase. This route of metabolism to form IAA, while important in mammalian peripheral tissues, does not occur in mammalian brain. Although IAA (and its riboside and ribotide) is found in rat brain [3,4], it arises from a source other than histamine. Brain IAA probably results from

transamination of histidine to form imidazolepyruvic acid, which is oxidatively decarboxylated to IAA. The nervous systems of some invertebrates have been shown to form imidazoleacetic acid from histamine [4].

Other Pathways

Some invertebrates lack both the methylating and the oxidative pathways [3,4]. In *Aplysia,* the only histamine metabolite is γ-glutamylhistamine [4]. In mast cells, γ-glutamylhistamine is formed and incorporated into proteins.

Tele-methylhistamine has negligible activity on histamine receptors, but other histamine metabolites are active on other receptors

IAA has activity on γ-aminobutyrate (GABA) receptor$_1$ (see Chap. 18), showing potency similar to GABA and similar sensitivity to blockade by bicuculline [3,4]. IAA also blocks uptake of GABA. IAA enters mammalian brain from peripheral tissues [3,4]. IAA acts like GABA on the GABA-benzodiazepine-chloride receptor complex, increasing the affinity of the receptor for benzodiazepines. In contrast, *t*-MIAA *decreases* the affinity of the receptor for benzodiazepines. In this system, *t*-MIAA acts at a distinct site, since bicuculline blocks the effects of both GABA and IAA but not the effect of *t*-MIAA.

RECEPTORS AND SECOND MESSENGERS

The density of H$_1$ receptors in brain regions varies among species

Most information concerning distribution of the H$_1$ receptor in brain [7] has been based on high-affinity binding of the labeled histamine antagonist pyrilamine (i.e., mepyramine) or of labeled doxepin, an antidepressant drug with very high affinity for the H$_1$ receptor. Autoradiography shows that the

CA3 region of the hippocampus has a high density of H_1 receptors in rat brain and a low density in guinea pig brain. In brain of primates, the caudate nucleus, putamen, cortex, and hippocampus are rich in H_1 receptors [7]. There is no similarity between the regional distribution of the H_1 receptor and the regional distribution of histamine, its metabolites, the enzymes that synthesize and metabolize histamine, or histaminergic nerve endings. Other transmitter systems also show lack of concordance among their components.

Binding of H_1 agonists to the H_1 receptor is modulated by Na^+ and GTP, which decrease the affinity of the receptor for histamine [7]. The H_1 receptor cloned from bovine adrenal medulla (GenBank accession number 90430) [17] is a 56-kDa protein, which, like other receptors coupled to G proteins, has seven transmembrane domains (see Chap. 10). Two N-glycosylation sites are present. Transmembrane domain five has threonine and asparagine residues, unlike the catecholamine and H_2 receptors. The sequence identities of H_1 receptor transmembrane domains are 40.7 percent with canine H_2 receptor and 44.3 percent with the m_1 muscarinic receptor (see Chap. 11). The resemblance to the muscarinic receptor explains the high affinity of muscarinic receptors for many H_1 receptor antagonists and some of the side effects of administered H_1 antagonists [3,4].

Stimulation of the H_1 receptor is associated with increased formation of cAMP and cGMP, increased phosphoinositide turnover, and ion shifts

Stimulation of H_1 receptors in conventionally prepared homogenates of brain does not increase cAMP formation, but in slices or a cell-free preparation containing large vesicular sacs or synaptoneurosomes, stimulation of the H_1 receptor increases cAMP formation [7] (see also Chaps. 10 and 21). The increased cAMP formation on stimulation of the H_1 receptor is indirect, dependent on stimulation of H_2 receptors and the presence of adenosine. The effect of adenosine is especially interesting since, as noted above, immunocytochemistry suggests that histamine and adenosine may coexist in the same neurons (see also Chap. 19).

Histamine-stimulated cGMP formation in neural tissues is also linked to the H_1 receptor [7]. This effect of histamine requires Ca^{2+}. Increased glycogenolysis after stimulation of H_1 receptors in brain slices is mediated by increased cytosolic Ca^{2+}, which could depend on H_1 stimulation of the turnover of the phosphoinositides (see Chap. 20). Hydrolysis of the phosphoinositides produces both inositol phosphates and a 1,2-diacylglycerol, mainly 1-stearoyl-2-arachidonyl-sn-glycerol. In many cells, inositol-1,4,5-trisphosphate has been shown to elevate cytosolic Ca^{2+}; Ca^{2+} and diacylglycerol are required for maximal activation of protein kinase C. This is discussed fully in Chap. 20. Electrophysiological effects of H_1 receptor stimulation are mostly excitatory: increase in firing rate, depolarization, facilitation of signal transmission, and reduced K^+ conductance [7].

The association of H_1 receptors with more than one second messenger may be attributed to interaction among second-messenger systems

Products of the phosphoinositides influence other second messengers. In neuroblastoma cells, stimulation of H_1 receptors increases phosphoinositide turnover, thereby releasing arachidonate. Increases in cGMP formation are also observed. Both effects are blocked not only by H_1 antagonists but also by inhibitors of the lipoxygenase pathway of arachidonate metabolism (see Chap. 23). Thus, lipoxygenase product(s) of arachidonate, for example, hydroxyeicosatetraenoic acids and leukotrienes, influence the cGMP response, acting like a *tertiary* messenger(s) [4].

H$_2$ receptors from three species have been cloned and expressed

The H$_2$ receptors of dog (GenBank accession number M32701) [18], human (GenBank accession number M64799) [19], and rat (GenBank accession number S57565) [20] are very similar. The human H$_2$ receptor sequence has 87 percent amino acid identity and that of the rat 82 percent identity to that of the dog. Like other G protein-coupled receptors, the H$_2$ receptors have seven hydrophobic transmembrane domains, and *N*-glycosylation at the N terminus. But in all three species, transmembrane domain 5 differs from that domain of catecholamine receptors and of the H$_1$ receptor in having a threonine and an aspartate residue.

The striatum of guinea pig and basal ganglia of primates have especially dense concentrations of H$_2$ receptors, more so than have hippocampus and cortex [6,7]. The electrophysiological effects of H$_2$ stimulation are inhibitory or excitatory: decrease in firing rate, hyperpolarization, or facilitation of signal transmission (block of K$^+$ conductance [gK$^+$ Ca^{2+}]) [7].

H$_2$ receptors are directly linked to adenylyl cyclase through a G protein [3–7] (see Chap. 21). H$_2$-stimulation is highest in homogenates of the guinea pig hippocampus and cortex. However, homogenates of other regions of guinea pig brain and of the brain of some other species show slight or nondetectable responses of H$_2$-linked adenylyl cyclase activity even when the *slices* respond to H$_2$ agonists with increased cAMP formation and when autoradiography and electrophysiology show the H$_2$ receptor to be present.

On some nonmammalian neurons, histamine produces electrophysiological effects that are blocked by appropriate concentrations of H$_2$ antagonists but are unaffected by guanylyl nucleotides. A similar dissociation is found in the atrium response. The chronotropic effect of histamine on guinea pig atria is mediated by the H$_2$ receptor, and binding studies show K_B values consistent with presence of the H$_2$ receptor, but binding is unaffected by a guanylyl nucleotide and histamine does not stimulate atrial adenylyl cyclase activity. It is possible that a distinct histamine receptor exists with similar affinities for H$_2$ agonist and antagonists but with a different transducing system, one not associated with a G protein.

Postulated mechanism of H$_2$ receptor activation

Application of quantum chemical calculations led to a hypothesis concerning the mechanism of activation of H$_2$ receptors by histamine and other H$_2$ agonists [21], a proposal that has been supported by subsequent work [22]. The proposed proton relay mechanism (Fig. 4) is based on tautomerism of the imidazole ring (Fig. 3). It is known from both experimental and theoretical studies that the tautomeric preference of histamine changes with ionization of the side chain amino group. As the free base, where the side chain amino group is uncharged, i.e., -NH$_2$, the more stable tautomer has the proton in the *pros*-nitrogen of the ring; as the monovalent cation, where the side chain amino group is protonated, i.e., -NH$_3^+$, the more stable tautomer has the proton on the *tele*-nitrogen. In the hypothesized mechanism, the cationic side chain amino group of histamine interacts with an anionic site of the receptor, while the *tele*-NH and *pros*-N interact with additional sites on the receptor. The effect of the interaction of the cationic amino group with an anionic site is to confer on the ring the properties of the free base of histamine: the *pros*-N becomes more nucleophilic and becomes protonated by the receptor; and the *tele*-NH releases its proton to the receptor. This charge relay triggers the response of the H$_2$ receptor molecule to stimulation by histamine. An analogous shift could account for stimulation by the specific H$_2$ agonist dimaprit (Fig. 4). The threonine and aspartate bonds in transmembrane domain 5, which are distinct to H$_2$ receptors [18–20], could form the hydrogen bonds necessary for the charge relay. Binding of the

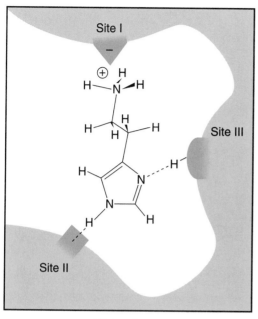

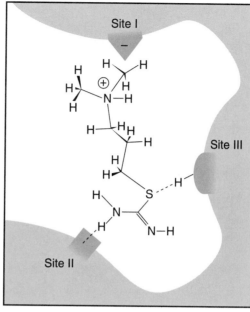

Histamine   Dimaprit

FIG. 4.   Proposed activation of the H_2 receptor. The protonated side chain N of histamine or the analogous protonated N of dimaprit (the specific H_2 agonist), interacts with site I, an anionic site on the receptor, e.g., aspartate, which triggers shifts of the protons at sites II and III.

cationic amino group to aspartate could trigger the postulated tautomeric shift.

Stimulating the H_3 presynaptic receptor reduces release of endogenous histamine

The synaptic release of histamine is influenced by Ca^{2+} and Mg^{2+}, as is the release of other biogenic amines (see Chaps. 9 and 12). Histamine can reduce presynaptic histamine release through reduction of Ca^{2+} influx into axonal terminals. A K^+-induced increase in histamine synthesis is also inhibited presynaptically by histamine. The H_3 presynaptic autoreceptor is linked to both effects [7]. The H_3 autoreceptor, which is coupled to a G protein, is especially prominent in the cortex and basal ganglia [7]. Treatment with an antagonist of the H_3 receptor results in reduced brain levels of histamine by increasing histamine release.

The effects of histamine on neurons are slow in onset and of long duration, like the effects of norepinephrine and 5-hydroxytryptamine, and different from the rapid and brief effects of amino acid transmitters

Like norepinephrine and 5-hydroxytryptamine, histamine potentiates the effects of amino acids on many mammalian neurons. Of special interest are observations showing state dependence [4]. Some osmosensitive neurons in the supraoptic nucleus that fail to respond to iontophoretically applied histamine do respond after injection of hypertonic NaCl [7]. This may be another example of a neuromodulator role of histamine [4]. In *Aplysia* too, there is evidence that histamine functions as a modulator. The C2 cells, rich in histamine, project to cells that potentiate feeding behavior by releasing 5-hydroxytryptamine. C2 cells fire when stimuli are applied to the perioral area of *Aplysia*, and they continue to fire as long as rhythmic mouth movements persist. Since mechanical stimuli to the mouth generate spikes, C2 is probably a primary mechanosensory afferent neuron. The C2 cell requires a high rate of axon input to pass proprioceptive information to the follower cell; in its normal state it does not convey information. Its role in feeding, then, is modulatory rather than obligatory [4].

Among the functions to which histamine may contribute are arousal, locomotor activity, analgesia, regulation of biological rhythms, thermoregulation, feeding, drinking, and release of neuropeptides

The rapid turnover of histamine in the hypothalamus, its high density of histaminergic fibers, and its content of histamine receptors may be consonant with some of these functions. Most observations supporting these and other postulated functions derive from observations on the effects of injected histamine [5–7]. Perhaps the least equivocal attributions to functions of *endogenous* histamine are its roles in secretion of neuropeptides. Histamine in hypothalamus contributes to release of corticotropin-releasing hormone, prolactin, and vasopressin [5–7].

Histaminergic systems are present in peripheral nerves and ganglia, as revealed by immunocytochemistry. Histamine may modulate activities of the gastrointestinal [23] and vascular [24] systems, the latter, at least in part, by modulating adrenergic activity.

ACKNOWLEDGMENTS

The author is grateful to the many investigators whose work forms the basis for this chapter and apologizes to authors whose papers could not be cited because of space limitation. The reader is referred to the selected recent key references and reviews for earlier citations.

REFERENCES

1. Kwiatkowski, H. Histamine in nervous tissue. *J. Physiol.* 102:32–41, 1943.
2. Green, J. P. Histamine and the nervous system. *Fed. Proc.* 23:1095–1102, 1964.
3. Hough, L. B., and Green, J. P. Histamine and its receptors in the nervous system. In A. Lajtha, (ed.), *Handbook of Neurochemistry.* New York: Plenum, 1984, Vol. 6, pp. 145–211.
4. Prell, G. D., and Green, J. P. Histamine as a neuroregulator. *Annu. Rev. Neurosci.* 9: 209–254, 1986.
5. Hough, L. B. Cellular localization and possible functions for brain histamine: Recent progress. *Prog. Neurobiol.* 30:469–505, 1987.
6. Watanabe, T., and Wada, H. *Histaminergic Neurons: Morphology and Function.* Boston: CRC, 1991.
7. Schwartz, J. C., and Haas, H. L. (eds.), *The Histamine Receptor. Receptor Biochemistry and Methodology.* New York: Wiley-Liss, 1992, Vol. 16.
8. Dale, H. H. Foreword. *Handb. Exp. Pharmacol.* 18:XXVI–XXXV, 1966.
9. Green, J. P. Histamine receptors. In H. Y. Meltzer, W. E. Bunny, J. T. Coyle, K. L. Davis, and I. J. Kopin (eds.), *Psychopharmacology, The Third Generation of Progress.* New York: Raven, 1987, pp. 273–279.
10. Joseph, D. R., Sullivan, P. M., Yang, Y.-M., et al. Characterization and expression of the complementary DNA encoding rat histidine decarboxylase. *Proc. Natl. Acad. Sci. U.S.A.* 87: 733–737 and 746, 1990.
11. Yamamoto, J., Yatsunami, K., Ohmori, E., et al. cDNA-derived amino acid sequence of L-histidine decarboxylase from mouse mastocytoma P-815 cells. *FEBS Lett.* 276:214–218, 1990.
12. Bayliss, D. A., Wang, Y.-M., Zahnow, C. A., Joseph, D. R., and Millhorn, D. E. Localization of histidine decarboxylase mRNA in rat brain. *Mol. Cell. Neurosci.* 1:3–9, 1990.
13. Green, J. P., and Khandelwal, J. K. Histamine turnover in regions of rat brain. *Adv. Biosci.* 51:185–194, 1985.
14. Borchardt, R. T., and Matuszewska, B. *S*-Adenosylmethionine-dependent transmethylation of histamine: Purification and partial characterization of guinea pig brain and rat kidney histamine *N*-methyltransferase. *Adv. Biosci.* 51:163–172, 1985.

5. Gitomer, W. L., and Tipton, K. F. Purification and kinetic properties of ox brain histamine *N*-methyltransferase. *Biochem. J.* 233:669–676, 1986.

6. Nishibori, M., Oishi, R., Itoh, Y., and Saeki, K. Purification and partial characterization of histamine *N*-methyltransferase from bovine brain. *Neurochem. Int.* 19:135–141, 1991.

7. Yamashita, M., Fukui, H., Sugama, K., et al. Expression cloning of a cDNA encoding the bovine histamine H_1 receptor. *Proc. Natl. Acad. Sci. U.S.A.* 88:11515–11519, 1991.

8. Gantz, I., Schäffer, M., Del Valle, J., et al. Molecular cloning of a gene encoding the histamine H_2 receptor. *Proc. Natl. Acad. Sci. U.S.A.* 88:429–433, and 5937, 1991.

9. Gantz, I., Munzert, G., Tashiro, T., Schäffer, M., Wang, L., and Yamada, T. Molecular cloning of the human histamine H_2 receptor. *Biochem. Biophys. Res. Commun.* 178:1386–1392, 1991.

20. Trailffort, E., Ruat, M., Arrang, J. M., Leurs, R., Piomelli, D., and Schwartz, J. C. Expression of a cloned rat histamine H_2 receptor mediating inhibition of arachidonate release and activation of cAMP accumulation. *Proc. Natl. Acad. Sci.* 89:2649–2653, 1992.

21. Green, J. P., Johnson, C. L., and Weinstein, H. Histamine as a neurotransmitter. In M. A. Lipton, A. DiMascio, and K. F. Killam (eds.), *Psychopharmacology, a Generation of Progress.* New York: Raven, 1978, pp. 319–332.

22. Pardo, L., Mazurek, A. P., Osman, R., and Weinstein, H. Theoretical studies of the activation mechanism of histamine H_2 receptors: Dimaprit and the receptor model. *Int. J. Quant. Chem. Quant. Biol. Symp.* 16:281–290, 1989.

23. Rangachari, P. K. Histamine: Mercurial messenger in the gut. *Am. J. Physiol. (Gastroint. Liver Physiol.)* 262:G1–G13, 1992.

24. Campos, H. A., and Briceno, E. Two models of peripheral sympathetic autoregulation: Role of neuronal histamine. *J. Pharmacol. Exp. Ther.* 261:943–950, 1992.

CHAPTER 15

Opioid Peptides and Opioid Receptors

Eric J. Simon and Jacob M. Hiller

Basic Neurochemistry: Molecular, Cellular, and Medical Aspects, 5th Ed., edited by G. J. Siegel et al. Published by Raven Press, Ltd., New York, 1994. Correspondence to Eric J. Simon, Departments of Psychiatry and Pharmacology, New York University Medical Center, 550 First Avenue, New York, New York 10016.

Opium is one of the oldest medications known to humans. Its efficacy in relieving pain and diarrhea has been known for thousands of years. During the nineteenth century morphine was recognized to be the principal alkaloid responsible for most of the beneficial effects of opium. It is also responsible for opium's undesirable side effects, the most important of which is the development of addiction upon chronic use.

Developments in the neurochemical and neuropharmacological aspects of opiate research, most of which have occurred during the past two decades, are discussed in this chapter. The field is a very active and rapidly moving one, and the reader will find in the reference list a number of books and reviews that provide detailed information and complete literature citations [1–7].

HISTORICAL SUMMARY

Discovering stereospecificity of opiate action was a critical advance

The hypothesis that specific receptors for opiates exist in the central nervous system of animals and humans arose from pharmacological studies of narcotic analgesics and from the large-scale efforts mounted in many industrial, governmental, and university laboratories to attempt synthesis of a nonaddictive analgesic. Many very useful compounds have been synthesized, and some of these are in clinical use. However, synthesis of the perfect nonaddictive analgesic has not yet been achieved. A large body of important information regarding the structural requirements for pharmacological action resulted from this work. It was recognized that many of the actions of opiates, such as analgesia and addiction liability, are stereospecific, i.e., these activities reside in only one of the enantiomers of a racemic mixture. It was also shown that relatively small alterations in parts of the morphine molecule result in drastic changes in its pharmacology. The most interesting and important such change is the substitu-

tion of the methyl on the tertiary amino group by an allyl or cyclopropylmethyl group that endows the resulting molecule with potent and specific antagonistic activity against many of the pharmacological actions of morphine and related opiates. Some antagonists (e.g., nalorphine, cyclazocine) retain part of their analgesic or "agonist" potency (agonist/antagonist drugs), whereas others (e.g., naloxone and naltrexone) become pure antagonists, devoid of detectable agonist properties.

Stereospecificity was explained by postulating specific receptors for opiates

The remarkable stereospecificity and structural constraints placed on these drugs for many of their actions are most readily explicable by the existence of highly specific binding sites to which these drugs must attach to exert their effects. Binding to these sites or "receptors" is presumed to trigger a series of reactions that result in the observed response. Antagonists are thought to act by binding to the receptors with high affinity, but they seem to lack the ability to trigger the subsequent events (see Chap. 10).

Although the receptor postulate for the actions of opiates has existed for several decades, the biochemical demonstration of its validity did not occur until 1973, when three laboratories simultaneously and independently reported the existence of stereospecific opiate binding, which represented the major portion of total binding to animal brain homogenates [8–10]. Stereospecific binding is represented by that portion of the bound labeled opiate that is displaceable by an unlabeled opiate but not by its inactive enantiomer. There is now good evidence that these binding sites are pharmacological opiate receptors.

Why do animal tissues contain receptors for plant opioid alkaloids?

The existence of opiate receptors is now firmly established for all vertebrates examined, from hagfish to humans, as well as for some invertebrates. This gave rise to the questions as to why so many species should be endowed with highly specific receptors for alkaloids produced by opium poppies and why such receptors have survived the eons of evolution. A physiological function that confers a selective advantage on the organism that carries them seemed probable. Such a function required the existence of endogenous substances, which are the real ligands of the receptors. The possibility that an endogenous analgesic system exists was also supported by the finding, dating back to 1969, that electrical stimulation of the central gray region of the brain produced powerful, long-lasting analgesia [11], but the idea of an endogenous analgesic substance was only conceived later.

Opiate-like activity is found in the brain and pituitary gland

When none of the known neurotransmitters or hormones were found to be bound to opiate receptors with high affinity or to be active in bioassays specific for opiates, the search for novel endogenous substances with opiate-like (opioid) activity began. The first reports of the existence of such substances came simultaneously from John Hughes in Hans Kosterlitz's laboratory and from Terenius and Wahlström. The presence of opioid activity in extracts of the pituitary was first reported by Goldstein and his group.

The identification of the first endogenous opioids was accomplished by Hughes and Kosterlitz and their collaborators [12], who found that the opioid activity present in aqueous extracts of pig brain resided in two pentapeptides, Tyr-Gly-Gly-Phe-Met and Tyr-Gly-Gly-Phe-Leu, which they named methionine (met)-enkephalin and leucine (leu)-enkephalin, respectively (enkephalin is from the Greek for "in the head").

The finding of opioid activity in the pituitary and the observation by Hughes and coworkers that the met-enkephalin sequence is present in the pituitary hormone, β-lipo-

tropin (β-LPH), as residues 61–65, led to the discovery of three longer peptides with opioid activity, all representing sequences present in β-LPH. These peptides were named α-, β-, and τ-endorphin, following a suggestion by E. J. Simon that the term endorphin (a contraction of endogenous and morphine) might be an appropriate and useful term for endogenous substances with opioid activity. More recently, Goldstein and coworkers [13] discovered another potent endogenous opioid peptide, not derived from β-LPH, which they named dynorphin. At least 12 currently known peptides have opioid activity. Since it is now evident that the primary function of opiate receptors is to bind endogenous opioids, they have been renamed opioid receptors and will be so referred to henceforth in this chapter.

OPIOID RECEPTORS

Properties and distribution of opioid receptors provide important leads toward the elucidation of function

Opioid binding sites are found in the central nervous system and in a number of peripheral tissues (isolated guinea pig ileum and vasa deferentia from several species are peripheral tissues extremely useful as *in vitro* bioassay systems for opiates and their receptors). They are tightly attached to cell membranes, and cell fractionation experiments suggest that they exist predominantly in the synaptic region. Stereospecific binding is saturable and of high affinity, ranging from 10^{-11} to 10^{-7} M for substances with strong to moderate opioid activity. The pH optimum for binding is in the physiological range (pH 7 to 8).

Biochemical Properties of Opioid Receptors Were Elucidated

Biochemical studies have indicated that opioid binding is highly sensitive to various proteolytic enzymes and to a large number of reagents capable of reacting with amino acids and functional groups present in proteins. Thus, opioid binding is inhibited by sulfhydryl reagents, such as *N*-ethylmaleimide (NEM) and iodoacetate. Results of these studies suggested that proteins play an essential role in specific opioid binding. Recent studies, using immobilized plant lectins able to bind specific sugars, have shown the existence of sugar moieties in opioid receptors, indicating that these integral membrane proteins are glycoproteins. The role of lipids in opioid binding is less clear. Binding is highly sensitive to some preparations of phospholipase A, but not to phospholipases C and D. Phospholipids may have a role in holding receptors in their proper conformation in the membrane lipid bilayer.

The evidence that opioid receptors can exist in different conformational states is of considerable interest. In brief, results from our laboratory and from S. H. Snyder's laboratory at Johns Hopkins University showed that sodium ions in the incubation medium increase the affinity of antagonist binding while decreasing that of agonist binding. The suggestion that this is due to a conformational change was supported by our finding that sodium decreases the rate of inactivation of receptor sulfhydryl groups by sulfhydryl reagents, such as NEM. Both effects are highly specific for sodium; only lithium has been found to have a similar though weaker effect. The knowledge that opioid binding sites have this kind of plasticity may prove important in our understanding of the steps subsequent to opioid binding that lead to the observed physiological responses.

Distribution of Opioid Receptors

Detailed studies of the distribution of opioid binding sites within the central nervous system have been carried out in a number of species, including humans, monkeys, cows, guinea pigs, and rats. The early experiments were done by dissecting and homogenizing discrete regions of the brain and spinal cord and binding labeled opiates to the homogenates. More recent studies have used autoradiography of brain and spinal cord slices to achieve detailed mapping of receptors even in subnuclei of various regions. Two methods have been used successfully: (a) injection of animals with labeled opioids and examination of tissue slices made at various times and (b) the incubation of tissue slices from various central nervous system regions with labeled opioids *in vitro*. The results from many different laboratories can be summarized by stating that large differences exist in the levels of opioid binding sites between different central nervous system regions. Moreover, the areas rich in opioid receptors tend to be in, or associated with, the limbic system, and in all areas that have been implicated in pain perception and modulation and some of the other actions of opiate drugs. Table 1 summarizes the regions containing high receptor levels and the putative opiate (or opioid) responses mediated by these regions.

The question of presynaptic or postsynaptic localization of opioid receptors has been investigated in numerous ways; there is evidence for both. As will be discussed in the next section, there are multiple types of opioid receptors. It is not yet known whether some types of receptors are presynaptic and some postsynaptic or whether a given type can have either location.

Multiple types of opioid receptors have been found to exist

The existence of multiple opioid peptides and the knowledge that receptors for classical neurotransmitters often exist in multiple forms led scientists to search for multiple classes of opioid receptors. The first evidence for multiple opioid receptors came from experiments of Martin and co-workers [14] in chronic spinal dogs. Striking differences in pharmacological responses to different narcotic analgesics and their inability to substitute for each other in suppressing withdrawal symptoms in addicted dogs led them to postulate the existence of three types of receptors. These were named for the prototype drugs used: μ for morphine, κ for

TABLE 1.   Location of opioid receptors proposed to mediate specific opioid effects

Opioid effect	Location of opioid receptors
ANALGESIA	
Spinal (body)	Laminae I and II of dorsal horn
Trigeminal	Substantia gelatinosa of trigeminal nerve
Supraspinal	Periaqueductal gray matter, medial thalamic nuclei, intralaminar thalamic nuclei, ?striatum
AUTONOMIC REFLEXES	
Suppression of cough Orthostatic hypotension } Inhibition of gastric secretion	Nuclei tractus solitarius, commisuralis, ambiguous and locus coeruleus
Respiratory depression	Nucleus tractus solitarius, parabrachial nuclei
Nausea and vomiting	Area postrema
Meiosis	Superior colliculus, pretectal nuclei
ENDOCRINE EFFECTS	
Inhibition of vasopressin secretion	Posterior pituitary
Hormonal effects	Hypothalamic infundibulum, hypothalamic nuclei, accessory optic system, ? amygdala
BEHAVIORAL AND MOOD EFFECTS	Amygdala, nucleus stria terminalis, hippocampus, cortex, medial thalamic nuclei, nucleus accumbens, ? basal ganglia
MOTOR RIGIDITY	Striatum

From Atweh and Kuhar, *Br. Med. Bull.* 39:47–52, 1983, with permission from Churchill Livingstone, Edinburgh.

ketocyclazocine, and σ for SKF 10047 (*N*-allylnormetazocine).

Following the discovery of the enkephalins, Kosterlitz's group provided evidence for yet another receptor type [15]. They found that the electrically evoked contractions of the isolated guinea pig ileum were much more sensitive to inhibition by morphine and related opiate alkaloids than by enkephalins, whereas the opposite was observed with the mouse vas deferens. They suggested that the two bioassay systems contained different populations of receptors. The major receptors present in the guinea pig myenteric plexus seem to prefer opiates and resemble Martin's μ receptors, whereas the vas deferens seems to contain a preponderance of receptors that exhibit higher affinity for enkephalins and their analogs. These new receptors were named δ (deferens) receptors. *In vitro* binding competition studies in guinea pig brain homogenates supported the existence of these two receptor types.

Opioid-binding sites of the κ type have also been confirmed by results of *in vitro* binding studies, though this proved more difficult because of the low level of such sites present in the rat, the animal used in the early experiments. More importantly, all κ opiates known at that time also exhibited high affinity for μ and δ sites. Only when μ and δ sites were saturated with ligands selective for them could κ sites be demonstrated.

The σ-opioid receptors are also present in the central nervous system. However, the fact that actions mediated by these receptors are not reversed by naloxone and the finding that there appears to be overlap between σ sites and binding sites for the nonopiate drug of abuse phencyclidine (angel dust) have led to the suggestion that σ receptors should not be defined as opioid receptors.

A large amount of evidence from many laboratories supports the existence of μ-, δ-, and κ-opioid receptors. Table 2 describes the agonist and antagonist ligands, both selective and nonselective, most commonly used for research on the three major types of opioid receptors. A number of other receptor types have been postulated (e.g., ϵ, ι, and λ), as well as receptor subtypes (e.g., μ_1, μ_2, κ_1, κ_2). The reader is referred to the review articles listed at the end of this chapter for details on these topics.

The major types of opioid receptors differ in their regional distribution in the central nervous system

The existence of multiple types of opioid receptors appears to be well established and is supported by the finding that the three major types of opioid receptors vary significantly in their distribution within the central nervous system. The techniques developed for the differential labeling of μ, δ, and κ

receptors in crude membrane preparations were found useful in autoradiography, a technique that permits much more detailed mapping. These include the use of highly selective tritiated ligands, when these are available, and, when these are not available, the use of a labeled nonselective ligand together with unlabeled selective ligands to saturate receptor types other than the one under study. Results of these studies carried out in rat and guinea pig brain by a number of laboratories are briefly summarized. Opioid receptors of the μ type are found in cortical layers I and IV and in the caudate putamen, amygdala, thalamus, periaqueductal gray matter, median raphe, hypothalamus, and hippocampus, while δ binding is seen in cortical layers II, III, and V and in the cau-

TABLE 2.　Ligands commonly used in studies of the endogenous opioid system

Compound	Type AG	Type ANT	Structure
Morphine	μ		Alkaloid
Naloxone		μ, δ (κ)	Alkaloid, with *N*-allyl substituent on basic nitrogen atom
Naltrexone		μ, δ (κ)	Alkaloid, with cyclopropylmethyl substituent on basic nitrogen atom
Levorphanol	μ		Morphinan
Cyprodime		μ	Morphinan
DAGO	μ		Tyr-D-Ala-Gly-MePhe-Gly-ol, an enkephalin analog
Dermorphin	μ		Tyr-D-Ala-Phe-Gly-Tyr-Pro-Ser-NH$_2$, a native peptide from frog (genus *Phyllomedusa*) skin
Morphiceptin	μ		Tyr-Pro-Phe-Pro-NH$_2$, a peptide derived from β-casein
CTOP		μ	D-Phe-Cys-Tyr-D-Trp-Orn-Thr-Pen-Thr-NH$_2$, cyclic octapeptide related to somatostatin
Leu-enkephalin	δ, μ		Tyr-Gly-Gly-Phe-Leu
DADLE	δ, μ		Tyr, D-Ala-Gly-Phe-D-Leu
DSLET	δ_2		Tyr-D-Ser-Gly-Gly-Phe-Leu-Thr
DPDPE	δ_1		[D-Pen^2, D-Pen^5]enkephalin, cyclic peptide
Deltorphin	δ_2		Tyr-D-Met-Phe-His-Leu-Met-Asp-NH$_2$, a native peptide from frog skin
Naltrindole		δ_2	6,7-Indole analog of naltrexone
ICI 174864		δ	*N,N*-diallyl-Tyr-Aib-Aib-Phe-Leu
D-Prodyn	κ		Tyr-Gly-Gly-Phe-Leu-Arg-Arg-Ile-Arg-D-Pro-Lys
Ethylketocyclazocine	κ	μ, δ	Benzomorphan
Bremazocine	κ	μ, δ	Benzomorphan
U50,488H	κ		Benzeneacetamide
U69,593	κ_1		Benzeneacetamide
Nor-binaltorphimine		κ	Dimeric naltrexone derivative

(AG) Agonist; (ANT) Antagonist. Parentheses denote very low affinity.

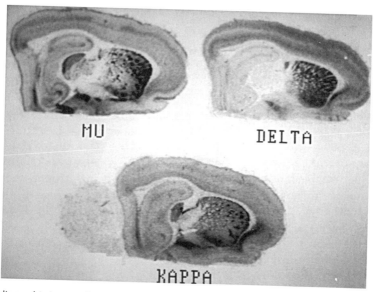

MU

DELTA

KAPPA

FIG. 1. Autoradiographic images showing the localization of μ-, δ-, and κ-opioid-binding sites in rat brain. Sagittal sections were taken 3.9 mm lateral to midline. The labeling of μ-binding sites was carried out with [³H]DAGO, a highly μ-selective enkephalin analog; δ-binding sites were labeled with [³H]DSTLE, an enkephalin analog selective for δ sites. [³H]Bremazocine, a high-affinity universal ligand, was used to label κ sites in the presence of saturating concentrations of selective μ and δ ligands. Differences in the distribution of μ-, δ-, and κ-opioid-binding sites are notable in the cortex, hippocampus, thalamus, and caudate putamen. (From Ofri, D., Fan, L. Q., Simon, E. J., and Hiller, J. M., *Brain Res.* 581:252–260, 1992.)

date putamen, amygdala, pontine and septal nuclei, and olfactory bulb and tubercle. The κ receptors are located in cortical layers V and VI, caudate putamen, amygdala, thalamus, hypothalamus, hippocampus, substantia nigra, nucleus accumbens, n. tractus solitarius, parabrachial n., and zona incerta. While overlap of receptor types clearly exists, their general anatomical localization is relatively distinct. Figure 1 shows examples of autoradiographic images of brain slices, illustrating the differential distribution patterns of μ-, δ-, and κ-opioid receptors.

A question that is more difficult to answer is whether different types of opioid receptors represent different conformations of a single receptor molecule or whether some or all of the different types are separate molecular entities. Though the distribution data favor the latter, they do not prove it. Experiments bearing on this subject will be summarized in the following sections.

What are the functions and endogenous ligands of the different receptor types?

The current notion as to the identity of the endogenous ligands for the three major types of receptors is that δ receptors mediate the effects of enkephalins, while κ receptors seem to bind and mediate the actions of the peptides derived from the precursor prodynorphin (see below). These assignments should be regarded as preliminary, but there is even more uncertainty about the endogenous ligands of the μ receptor. It has been suggested that it is the receptor for β-endorphin or for the recently found endogenous morphine alkaloids. Alternatively, it may be an isoreceptor for the enkephalins.

There is evidence that the major types of opioid receptors use cAMP as their second messenger. Experiments done mainly in NG108-15 cells, but also in brain homogenates, indicate that the activation of opioid receptors results in inhibition of adenylyl cyclase activity. They appear to be coupled to adenylyl cyclase via one of the inhibitory guanine nucleotide regulatory proteins (G_i proteins). A large family of stimulatory and inhibitory G proteins has been found to exist. There is also evidence that opioid receptors may be coupled directly to ion channels via a so-called G_o (G other) protein. Uncoupling of opioid receptors from their G proteins results in a binding site that binds agonists with low affinity, whereas antagonists continue to bind with high affinity.

There has also been progress in delineating the ionic channels involved in the effects mediated by the three major opioid receptor types. Briefly, the evidence suggests that binding to μ and δ receptors leads to the opening of potassium channels, whereas binding to κ sites results in the closing of calcium channels [16].

The functions of the various types of opioid receptors are not yet delineated. With the recent availability of highly selective ligands, the elucidation of physiological function should become easier. It is hoped that sufficient functional specialization will be found to permit the synthesis of drugs with highly specific effects and absence of undesired side effects. Currently, it appears as though all three major receptor types are involved in pain modulation (analgesia); δ receptors have been implicated in cardiovascular effects of opioid peptides, while κ receptors seem to play a role in salt and water balance.

Further knowledge of receptor structure and function requires their isolation and purification. This is also the only way the molecular distinctiveness of different receptor types (or lack thereof) can be definitively established. There are two ways to accomplish this: (a) by linking receptors covalently to a labeled ligand by affinity labeling or crosslinking and then isolating the labeled complex; and (b) by isolating and purifying active receptor molecules. These approaches are discussed in the next two sections.

Isolation and purification of opioid receptors can be monitored by covalent attachment of labeled ligand

The earliest attempt to isolate prelabeled opioid binding sites did not involve covalent binding but the use of a very-high-affinity ligand, etorphine, which dissociates sufficiently slowly to survive extraction and assay. In 1975 a [³H]etorphine-labeled macromolecular complex was solubilized with a nonionic detergent and found to have properties consistent with its being an etorphine-opioid receptor complex [17]. The complex was useful for characterization but was not sufficiently stable to permit extensive purification.

Isolation of δ Receptors

Since that time a large number of potentially useful affinity and photoaffinity ligands for opioid binding sites have been prepared. The only one that has been successfully used to purify the receptor is fentanylisothiocyanate (FIT) and a more potent analog, known as "superFIT." Klee and associates [18] have purified to homogeneity a [³H]superFIT-receptor complex isolated from the neuroblastoma-glioma hybrid cell line NG108-15. Since these cells are known to contain only δ receptors, the isolated glycoprotein must be a binding unit of the δ receptor. It was found to have a molecular weight of 58 kDa on sodium dodecylsulfate polyacrylamide gel electrophoresis (SDS-PAGE).

Separation of μ and δ Receptors

More recently, affinity-crosslinking has been used to isolate binding proteins from both μ and δ receptors [19]. Iodination of the tyrosine in the 1-position of β-endorphin destroys its ability to bind to receptors. However, a second tyrosine is present in human β-endorphin (β-end$_h$), and advantage has been taken of this fact to prepare [¹²⁵I]labeled human β-endorphin with the label in tyrosine-27. This material was found to have high affinity for both μ- and δ-binding sites.

but very low affinity for κ sites. The binding and crosslinking of [^{125}I]β-end$_h$ to tissues containing either μ or δ sites or both was now possible. Membranes crosslinked in this manner were solubilized in SDS, separated on SDS-PAGE, and the gels submitted to autoradiography. A number of labeled bands were seen, all of which were opioid binding site-related, since labeling could be prevented by carrying out binding assays in the presence of excess unlabeled opioids.

For this discussion, two bands revealed by SDS-PAGE are of importance: a band of $M_r = 65,000$, present in all tissues containing μ sites, including rat thalamus with a large preponderance of μ sites, and a 53-kDa band, present in tissues containing δ sites, including NG108-15 cells, which contain only δ sites. Further support for the hypothesis that the 65-kDa protein is the major μ-binding protein was obtained by showing that it fails to be crosslinked when binding of [^{125}I]β-end$_h$ is carried out in the presence of the highly selective μ ligand DAGO. Similarly, the putative major δ-binding protein (53 kDa) is not labeled when binding is carried out in the presence of the highly specific δ ligand DPDPE.

This work represents the first evidence indicating that μ- and δ-binding sites may be distinct molecules. The results do not, however, distinguish between differences in the polypeptides (primary gene products) or in post-translational modifications. This information will only be available when the total amino acid sequences of the various opioid receptor types are known. Very recently, the amino acid sequence of δ receptors has been elucidated (see below).

Active opioid-binding sites can be extracted from membranes and purified

The first step in the isolation of opioid-binding sites is their solubilization from the cell membranes with which they are tightly associated, a step that proved more difficult than anticipated. However, several laboratories have now developed methods to extract solu-

ble active binding sites from membranes derived from a variety of tissues. Digitonin, CHAPS, and Triton X-100 have been the detergents most frequently used.

The first receptor type to be separated in its active form was the κ receptor. In our laboratory [20] this was accomplished by sucrose density gradient centrifugation of a digitonin extract of guinea pig brain. Two peaks of opioid binding were obtained. The first was found to be virtually pure κ sites, while the second peak contained a mixture of μ and δ sites. A similar separation was achieved by Chow and Zukin [21] using molecular exclusion chromatography of CHAPS extracts of rat brain membranes.

The purification to homogeneity of active opioid-binding sites has been accomplished for the μ-opioid receptor in several laboratories. The first such purification was achieved in our laboratory [22]. Digitonin extracts of bovine striatal membranes were purified by two major chromatographic steps, ligand affinity chromatography on immobilized β-naltrexyl-6-ethylenediamine and lectin affinity chromatography on a column of wheat germ agglutinin-agarose. The total purification obtained was 60,000- to 70,000-fold, with a specific activity of opioid binding of ca. 12,000 to 14,000 pmol/mg protein. These values are in excellent agreement with the theoretical values for a protein of 65 kDa containing a single binding site. The purified receptor exhibits a single band of $M_r = 65,000$ on SDS-PAGE.

Active δ sites have not yet been purified, but a κ site from frog brain has been purified. It is not known whether this site is identical to mammalian κ receptors.

The major opioid receptors have been cloned and sequenced

A very significant advance in research on opioid receptors occurred recently with the cloning of the δ-opioid receptor. Two laboratories [23,24], headed by C. Evans of the UCLA Medical School and B. L. Kieffer of the Ecole Supérieure de Biotechnologie,

Strasbourg, France, independently and simultaneously published the δ-opioid receptor sequence from cDNA libraries derived from the RNA of NG108-15 cells. Both laboratories constructed a plasmid that can be transfected either into bacteria or (transiently) into eukaryotic cells. The plasmid used drives expression of the inserted cDNA in the eukaryotic cells. The researchers screened their libraries by assaying for functional receptor expression in the transfected cells. Both groups assayed radiolabeled ligand binding using [^{125}I]DADLE (Evans) or [^{3}H]DTLET (Kieffer). To minimize the number of operations, pools of clones were assayed. Plasmid DNA from a ligand binding pool was isolated and transfected into bacteria to make more DNA for transfected eukaryotic cells. Repeated cycling led to the isolation of a pure clone. The cDNA obtained by both groups encoded a protein having 372 amino acids and considerable homology to G protein-coupled receptors. The ligand-binding profile of the transfected COS cells was that of δ-opioid receptors. Functional coupling to second-messenger systems was demonstrated by the reduction of forskolin-stimulated increase in cAMP by DPDPE. The deduced amino acid structure has considerable homology with receptors for somatostatin (37 percent amino acid identity), angiotensin (31 percent identity), interleukin-8 (22 percent identity), and the receptor for N-formyl peptide (21 percent identity). The second and third domains of the seven transmembrane domains of this molecule contain aspartate residues that may provide a counter ion for the amino groups of δ ligands. The COOH-terminal domain contains a number of cysteine residues that may undergo palmitoylation, and the N terminus contains two potential N-glycosylation sites. In addition, multiple consensus sequences for phosphorylation appear on several cytoplasmic domains, which may mediate the observed regulation of receptor function in response to opioid exposure.

The similarity of the cloned δ-receptor to somatostatin receptors was the basis for the ability of Yasuda et al. [25] to clone the mouse κ-opiate receptor cDNA. While screening a mouse brain cDNA library with probes against conserved regions of the somatostatin receptor family, these investigators identified two unique clones with 35 to 40 percent identity with SSTR1. Following expression of the clones in COS cells, they found that neither bound radiolabeled somatostatin analogs. One of the cloned receptors proved to be identical to the δ receptor cloned from NG108-15 cells. The other clone, however, could be specifically labeled with the κ-selective agonist [^{3}H]U69,543, indicating that the cloned receptor is a κ-opioid receptor. This was confirmed by pharmacological analysis of the receptor, which showed that κ-selective ligands potently bound to the receptor. In contrast, ligands selective at μ, δ, or σ receptors did not bind to this clone. The high affinity of this cloned receptor for U50,488 and U69,543 as well as nor-BNI indicates that it is a κ$_1$-receptor subtype. Binding to this κ receptor was stereospecific, consistent with the opiate nature of the binding site. The cloned κ receptor can associate with pertussis-toxin-sensitive G proteins and mediates agonist inhibition of adenylyl cyclase activity in a naloxone-reversible manner, indicating that it is a functional opiate receptor.

Most recently, low-stringency hybridization of cDNA probes, based on the structure of the cloned mouse δ receptor, resulted in the cloning of cDNA encoding a μ-opioid receptor. When the cDNA was transfected into COS cells, opioid binding with a typical μ pharmacological profile was observed [26; G. Uhl, *private communication*].

OPIOID PEPTIDES

Progress has been rapid in our knowledge of the biosynthesis and molecular genetics of the opioid peptides

The relatively large number of opioid peptides isolated in recent years, the sequence of which begins with either met- or leu-en-kephalin, is a reflection of the complexity of the endogenous opioid system. Investigators have used various approaches to study the biosynthesis of opioid peptides. These include use of the classical technique of incorporation of labeled amino acids into cultures of cells known to synthesize the peptide in question and the use of antibodies to demonstrate the presence of peptides in putative precursor proteins. Recombinant DNA technology has been used to determine the amino acid sequence of polypeptide precursors from the nucleotide sequence of mRNA isolated from cells that produce the precursor and for the study of the structure of the genes that code for the precursor proteins.

The major opioid peptides are cleavage products of three distinct proteins, which are the primary products of three genes

These precursor proteins are proopiomelanocortin (POMC), which contains β-LPH and gives rise to β-, α-, and τ-endorphin; pro-enkephalin, whose cleavage products are met-enkephalin, leu-enkephalin, met-enkephalin-arg[6]-phe[7], met-enkephalin-arg[6]-gly[7]-leu[8], and peptide E; and prodynorphin, the precursor protein of α-neo-eudorphin, β-neo-endorphin, dynorphin A-(1-8), dynorphine A-(1-17), and dynorphin B (rimorphin). The amino acid sequences of these opioid peptides are listed under their respective precursor proteins in Table 3. These proteins are the products of three separate genes. Precursor protein and gene structures are depicted in Figs. 2 and 3.

Proopiomelanocortin

POMC is also the precursor of the nonopioid hormones adrenocorticotropin (ACTH) and α-, β-, and τ-melanocyte-stimulating hormones (MSH) (see Chap. 16). Its discovery [27,28] is of considerable importance since it was the first time a precursor was found to give rise to several different biologically active peptides. It was also the first of the three opioid peptide precursors to be sequenced [29]. The major source of POMC

TABLE 3. Opioid precursors and major active opioid peptide products

Precursor (No. of amino acids)	Peptide	Structure[a]
POMC		
Human (267)	β-Endorphin	YGGFLTSEKSQTPLVTLFKNAIIKKNAYKKGE
	γ-Endorphin	YGGFLTSEKSQTPLVTL
	α-Endorphin	YGGFLTSEKSQTPLVT
Proenkephalin (A)		
Human (269)	Met-enkephalin	YGGFM
	Leu-enkephalin	YGGFL
	Heptapeptide	YGGFMRF
	Octapeptide	YGGFMRGL
	Peptide E	YGGFLRRQFKVVTRSQQDPNAYYEELFDV
Prodynorphin (Proenkephalin B)		
Porcine (256)	α-Neo-endorphin	YGGFLRKYPK
	β-Neo-endorphin	YGGFLRKYP
	Dynorphin A (1-17)	YGGFLRRIRPKLKWDNQ
	Dynorphin A (1-8)	YGGFLRRI
	Leumorphin (dynorphin B [1-29])	YGGFLRRQFKVVTRSQQDPNAYYEELFDV
	Dynorphin B (rimorphin)	YGGFLRRQFKVVT

[a] (A) Ala; (D) Asp; (E) Glu; (F) Phe; (G) Gly; (H) His; (I) Ile; (K) Lys; (L) Leu; (M) Met; (N) Asn; (P) Pro; (Q) Gln; (R) Arg; (T) Thr; (S) Ser; (V) Val; (W) Trp; (Y) Tyr.

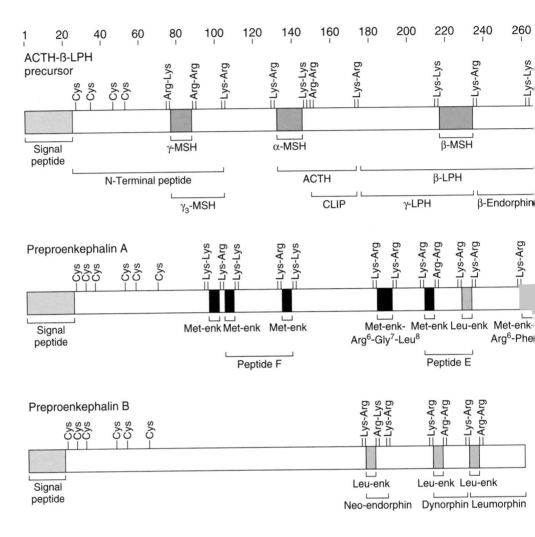

FIG. 2. Diagrammatic representation of structures of opioid peptide precursors. Met-enkephalin (Met-enk), leu-enkephalin (Leu-enk), signal peptides, and MSH units are shown. Cysteine and dibasic acid residues are shown *above* and major peptides derived from each precursor *below* each diagram. (LPH) lipotropin; (CLIP) corticotropin-like intermediate lobe peptide. (From Imura, H., *J. Endocrinol.* 107:147–157, 1985.)

is the pituitary gland; in its intermediate lobe, β-endorphin, the 31-amino acid C-terminal peptide of β-LPH, is the predominant active opioid peptide product. The gene coding for POMC contains two introns (areas within the gene not transcribed into mRNA) and three exons (areas transcribed into mRNA). Post-translational processing of precursor proteins is tissue specific. Pairs of basic amino acid residues border each of the

peptides in the precursor molecule and are the presumed targets of proteolytic cleavage. Processing of POMC in the arcuate nucleus of the brain appears to be similar to that in the intermediate lobe of the pituitary. Post-translational modification may also lead to inactivation of opioid peptides. Thus, *N*-acetylation of the N-terminal tyrosine of β-endorphin produces a peptide devoid of activity at the opioid receptor.

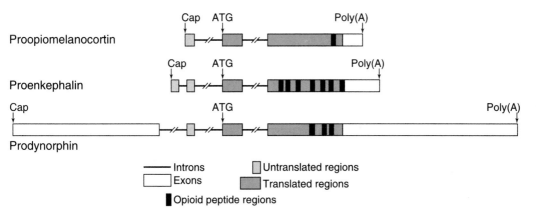

FIG. 3. The opioid peptide gene family. (Cap) start of transcription; (ATG) start of translation; (Poly A) start of polyadenylation; opioid peptide regions refer to met-enkephalin and/or leu-enkephalin. (From Hollt, V. In Almeida, O. F. X., and Shippenberg, T. S., [eds.], *Neurobiology of Opioids.* Heidelberg: Springer-Verlag, 1991, p. 12.)

Proenkephalin

Proenkephalin was first discovered in bovine adrenal cortex, where enkephalin biosynthesis was elucidated [30]. It contains one copy of leu-enkephalin, four copies of met-enkephalin, and one copy each of a met-enkephalin C-terminal-extended heptapeptide and octapeptide, all separated by basic dipeptides, where processing generally takes place (Fig. 2). Human proenkephalin (267 amino acids) is encoded by a gene containing four exons and five introns. An N-terminal signal peptide, 24 amino acids in length, is present in the precursor protein. A body of evidence exists supporting the finding that proenkephalin in the bovine adrenal medulla is identical to that in the brain. The processing of this precursor in the brain appears to be more complete in that free enkephalins are the principal cleavage products, whereas high-molecular-weight enkephalin-containing peptides predominate in the adrenal medulla.

Prodynorphin

Prodynorphin, the most recent of the opioid peptide precursors to be characterized, has been isolated from mammalian tissues, such as brain, anterior pituitary, adrenal gland, spinal cord, and reproductive organs. Sequencing of the human prodynorphin gene revealed four exons and three introns. The amino acid sequence of leu-enkephalin is repeated three times in the precursor. All active opioid peptides processed from prodynorphin are C-terminal extensions of leu-enkephalin. They are α- and β-neo-endorphin, dynorphin A (1-17), dynorphin A (1-8), and dynorphin B (1-29), also called leumorphin, processed at double basic amino acids that serve as processing signals. However, it is likely that enzymes able to cleave at single arginine sites exist, as demonstrated by the formation of dynorphin A (1-8) and rimorphin by the cleavage between isoleucine-8 and arginine-9 of dynorphin A and between threonine-13 and arginine-14 of leumorphin, respectively.

Processing of peptide precursor proteins is dependent on the enzymes present in the tissue

The proteolytic enzymes responsible for processing of precursors to produce the biologically active peptides have been studied in great detail and several have been cloned and sequenced. A detailed discussion of this subject is beyond the scope of this chapter (for review, see Chap. 22 in ref. 1). The distribution of processing enzymes responsible for particular types of cleavage, leading to the production of various opioid peptides, is not uniform. Therefore, the nature of the products derived from a given precursor molecule is dependent on the type of enzyme a neuronal cell body or its proximal dendrites is programmed to manufacture. Thus, for example, dynorphin A (1-8) may be the principal product of prodynorphin in one area of the brain while longer forms of dynorphin are abundant in other brain areas.

Similarities are observed among precursors and genes of opioid peptides

It is of great interest to note that POMC, proenkephalin, and prodynorphin possess many shared characteristics. The three precursor proteins contain almost the same number of amino acids. All possess multiple sequences of opioid peptides contained in the C-terminal half of the molecule, and these peptides are almost always framed by pairs of basic amino acids. In addition, all contain a cysteine-rich N-terminal sequence preceded by very similarly sized signal peptides. Six separate cysteine residues in the N-terminal regions of proenkephalin and prodynorphin have almost equivalent placement. Finally, amino acid sequence homology between proenkephalin and prodynorphin exceeds 50 percent.

The structural organization of the gene encoding the three precursors also exhibits impressive similarities in the placement and sizes of their respective introns and exons. Thus, it has been suggested that these genes have developed by evolution from a common gene.

Distribution and tissue levels of opioid peptides can be measured by several techniques

To study the anatomical distribution and tissue levels of opioid peptides, highly specific and sensitive methods for their identification and quantitation are needed. Assays making use of highly specific polyclonal antibodies,

generated against opioid peptides or opioid peptide-protein conjugates in rabbits and other animals, and monoclonal antibodies, raised by hybridoma technology, have been developed. Radioimmunoassays (RIAs) have been developed for all members of the three opioid peptide families. They measure the amount of peptide present in a tissue or plasma extract by competition with radiolabeled peptide for binding to the specific antibody. RIAs with sensitivities enabling them to detect femtomoles of a given peptide have been developed. Since a number of the antibodies employed in these assays demonstrate some degree of immunological cross-reactivity, a preparatory step using high-pressure liquid chromatography has often been employed to separate the peptide of interest from other cross-reacting peptides.

Immunohistochemical techniques have proven extremely useful in mapping the distribution of opioid peptides. These methods consist of incubating an opioid peptide antibody with freeze-dried sections of tissue. The antigen-antibody complex is then visualized by the use of a second antibody (against the first) conjugated with a fluorescent marker or radioactive label or by the peroxidase-antiperoxidase method of Sternberger.

Peptidergic axons are widely distributed

RIAs and immunohistochemical techniques have been used for the detailed mapping of β-endorphin, enkephalin, and dynorphin in the central nervous system. Results of these studies are summarized below. It was noted early that areas of the brain that contain nerve fibers and terminals and that transport and release opioid peptides occur much more frequently than areas in the brain containing cell bodies that produce opioid peptides.

β-Endorphin

Major concentrations of β-endorphin are found in the arcuate nucleus of the medial basal hypothalamus and the nucleus of the solitary tract, which lies within the medulla oblongata; however, nerve fibers containing β-endorphin have been found to project from these two centers to many areas of the brain. From the arcuate nucleus, β-endorphin-containing tracts project forward through the preoptic area, around the anterior commissure, and into the periaqueductal region of the diencephalon. Midline structures containing β-endorphin include the anterior paraventricular nucleus and the locus coeruleus. Neurons containing β-endorphin project laterally from the nucleus of the solitary tract to many pontine reticular sites and from there continue into the medulla to innervate the nuclei raphe magnus, reticularis gigantocellularis, paragigantocellularis, and reticularis lateralis.

Enkephalins

The most widely distributed opioid peptides are the enkephalins, which are found in many neuronal systems from the telencephalon to the spinal cord. The enkephalins have been shown to form local circuits or to be transported via lengthy neuronal projections to areas distant from the cell bodies in which they were synthesized. The distributions of leu-enkephalin and met-enkephalin have so far been found to be identical. In all areas, the level of leu-enkephalin is lower than that of met-enkephalin. This finding is in accord with the ratio of copies of these two pentapeptides in the proenkephalin precursor molecule. The enkephalins have their highest concentration in the globus pallidus, followed by, in descending order of concentration, the remainder of the telencephalon (except for low concentrations in the hippocampus and cortical areas), the diencephalon, pons, mesencephalon, and cerebellum.

Dynorphins

In general, the anatomical localization of peptides derived from the prodynorphin precursor follows the distribution map established for the enkephalin peptides. Dynorphins have their highest concentrations in the posterior pituitary and the hypothalamus. RIAs have shown high concentrations to be present in the amygdala, septum, spinal cord, midbrain, and striatum. Somewhat lower levels have been detected in the hippocampus, thalamus, and pons, and very low concentrations occur in the cortex and cerebellum.

There is a problem in matching the localization of opioid peptides and their putative receptors

Finally, it should be noted that a poor correlation exists between the anatomical distribution of opioid peptide-containing nerve fibers and terminals and the distribution of the major types of opioid-binding sites. The following are a few examples of these incongruous distribution patterns. The caudate and various cortical areas possess high concentrations of opioid-binding sites but low concentrations of opioid peptides. This is in contrast to the situation seen in the globus pallidus, which has a very high concentration of enkephalin but only low levels of δ-opioid-binding sites. The same is true for the substantia nigra and the hippocampus, which receive dense innervation from the dynorphin system but have sparse populations of κ-type opioid-binding sites. On the other hand, areas of dense κ binding have been autoradiographically identified in the hypothalamus, an area possessing the highest concentration of dynorphin.

The reasons for discrepancies between peptide and receptor localization are at present obscure. They may be due to the use of ligands for receptor labeling that have less than optimal specificity or to conditions employed for *in vitro* labeling studies, either of which could lead to labeling of only high-affinity receptors when it may be the low-affinity receptors that are more closely aligned with the release sites of the peptides.

How is the expression of opioid peptide precursors regulated?

Methods described for the localization of opioid peptides leave open the question of whether genes coding for their precursors are expressed in the same cells. The possibility that the peptides may be synthesized at a distance and transported to their site of storage or action is especially relevant to the central nervous system. Another important question is whether changes in peptide levels resulting from physiological, pharmacological, or pathological alterations are due to changes in gene expression or to other events, such as altered transport, precursor processing, breakdown, or release. Answers are now possible through the use of modern methods of molecular biology. Gene expression, i.e., the level of mRNA, can be measured by hybridization with suitable labeled oligonucleotide probes prepared from the known nucleotide sequence of the cDNA (or mRNA) coding for the peptide precursor. The amount of labeled hybrid can be measured by dot blots on nitrocellulose. The size of the message can be determined by Northern blot analysis. The technique of *in situ* hybridization permits the cellular localization of a specific mRNA (see Chaps. 24 and 25).

These techniques have already been widely applied to opioid peptides, especially to proenkephalin. For example, it has long been known that enkephalin levels are very low in rat adrenals but increase 10- to 15-fold following surgical denervation. This increase was shown by Udenfriend and coworkers to be due to increased gene expression, since a comparable increase in the level of proenkephalin mRNA was observed. This provides evidence for transcriptional and/or translational control of enkephalin biosynthesis. This technique also led to the unexpected finding of high levels of proenkephalin message in rat testis, ovary, and heart. All these tissues have barely measurable levels of enkephalin. The significance of the presence of untranslated mRNA is not understood.

In situ hybridization has been used to define the cellular distribution of proenkephalin mRNA in the caudate putamen and cerebellar cortex of the rat. The subpopulations of cells that express the message were delineated.

Many physiological functions are suggested for endogenous opioids

The putative functions of opioid peptides have been deduced from their observed pharmacological effects, their anatomical distribution in regions known to control various physiological and behavioral functions, as well as from the effects of the administration of the opiate antagonist naloxone. One should be aware that pharmacological activity is only indicative of physiological function. Our understanding of how and under what conditions a given peptide activates a physiological mechanism is still incomplete, and much remains to be learned.

Physiological and behavioral effects

The properties of opioid peptides can best be summarized by stating that their pharmacological effects are remarkably similar to those of the plant-derived and synthetic opiate alkaloids. Physiological areas in which the endogenous opioid system seems to have a role include pain perception, stress mechanisms, respiratory regulation, temperature control, tolerance development, and physical dependence, as well as modulation of diuretic and cardiovascular functions. Behavioral patterns that seem to be under the influence of opioid peptides include sexual behavior, feeding and drinking, grooming, and locomotor and operant behavior. Opioid peptides may also serve a role in memory storage and recall (see Chap. 50). Like opiates, opioid peptides interact with the endocrine system, producing increases in the release of growth hormone, ACTH, prolactin, and antidiuretic hormone and decreases in the circulating levels of thyrotropin, luteinizing hormone, and follicle-stimulating hormone (see Chaps. 16 and 49). A very large, relatively recent area of exploration is the interaction between the central nervous system and the immune system. Here, too, the endogenous opioid peptides appear to have a role.

Inhibitors of the enzymatic degradation of enkephalins produce their pharmacological effects by increasing extracellular levels of endogenous opioid peptides

Transmission signals that are triggered by amine or amino acid neurotransmitters are terminated mainly by their removal from the synaptic cleft by specific re-uptake mechanisms. In contrast, cessation of signals initiated by the binding of neuropeptides, e.g., enkephalins, is accomplished through enzymatic cleavage of the biologically active peptide into inactive fragments by peptidases. These peptidases include, but are not limited to, neutral metalloendopeptidase ("enkephalinase," EC 3.4.24.11) and aminopeptidase-N, which hydrolyzes the Gly^3-Phe^4 bond and the Tyr^1-Gly^2 bond of enkephalin, respectively. The distribution of neutral metalloendopeptidase in the central nervous system was found to overlap the anatomical localization of the enkephalins. A relatively good correspondence was also found with the distribution of μ and δ receptors. Subcellular fractionation studies indicate that this peptidase is a membrane-bound enzyme in which the active site faces the extracellular space.

Evidence that enkephalinase inhibitors prevent, to varying degrees, the hydrolysis of exogenous enkephalin in synaptic membrane preparations containing peptidases was clearly demonstrable. Since confirmation of this finding in the whole animal was difficult, investigators resorted to brain slices, where the topographic relationship between the stores of opioid peptides and concentrations of peptidases are maintained. It was found that following K^+-induced depolarization of the slices, recovery of enkephalins released into the bathing medium was increased by 100 percent in the presence of peptidase inhibitors.

Pharmacological testing by intracere-broventricular or intrathecal administration of bestatin or amastatin (inhibitors of aminopeptidase) or of thiorphan, acetorphan, phosphoramidon, or kelatorphan (inhibitors of neutral metalloendopeptidase) potentiates the antinociceptive activity of exogenous enkephalins and, most importantly, reduces, in a naloxone-reversible manner, responses to various noxious stimuli (for review see Chap. 23 in ref. 1). Peak effects are seen with the combined administration of inhibitors of both peptidases. Many studies have shown that enkephalinase inhibitors provide protection to endogenous opioids and thus mimic the pharmacological effects of opioids. In Table 4 an assortment of opioid-associated effects elicited by enkephalinase inhibitors and their susceptibility to reversal by naloxone are compared with the effects evoked by the administration of exogenous opioids. Besides the obvious clinical application of these selective peptidase inhibitors as analgesics, these substances are being investigated as potential antidepressant, antihypertensive, and antidiarrheal agents.

Endogenous opioids may have a role in disease

The participation of opioid peptides and their receptors in a number of pathological conditions has been investigated. The finding that, in rats, naloxone can rapidly reverse the hypotensive effects of bacterial endotoxin (commonly used as a model of human septic shock) led to the hypothesis that the profound hypotension produced during shock may be mediated via the endogenous opioid peptides. The psychopathological states of schizophrenia and depression have also been investigated. Based on the finding that the major behavioral response after intraventricular injection of β-endorphin in rats was the induction of catatonia, two essentially opposite hypotheses have been developed for a role of opioid peptides in schizophrenia (see also Chap. 47). One holds that catatonic symptoms may be the result of ex-

TABLE 4.   Pharmacological properties of enkephalinase inhibitors compared with those of exogenous opiates

Tests	Effect of enkephalinase inhibitors	Antagonism by naloxone	Effect of exogenous opiates
Analgesia	Weak and selective	Yes	Strong and general
Tolerance to analgesia	±		+++
Inhibition of nociceptive neurons firing	++	Partial	+++
Changes in turnover of cerebral monoamines	++	Yes	++
Changes in seizure susceptibility	++	Yes	+++
Behavioral despair	++	Yes	++
Conditioned reinforcement	+	Yes	++
Inhibition of micturition reflexes	++	Yes	+++
Castor oil diarrhea	++	Yes	+++
Withdrawal symptoms	±		+++
Central cardiovascular effects	−		++
Respiratory depression	−		+++

From Schwartz et al. *Trends Pharmacol. Sci.* 6:472–476, 1985.

cess opioid peptides, and the second argues that a deficiency in opioid peptide content could account for this behavior. The former hypothesis justified the administration of opiate antagonists to schizophrenic patients, and the latter hypothesis was the rationale for administering opioid peptides and their analogs. Variable results have been reported with both regimens. The administration of naloxone to patients with endogenous depression has given promising results in the hands of some investigators.

Possible roles for opioids are suggested in neuromodulation and neurotransmission

The ability of opioid peptides to inhibit the release of various neurotransmitters, such as epinephrine, dopamine, acetylcholine, and substance P, supports their possible function as neuromodulators. In those instances in which opioid receptors are located postsynaptically, the peptides may function as neurotransmitters. Additional evidence supporting their role in synaptic transmission comes from the finding that they are largely located in nerve terminals and that they can be released from nervous tissue in response to depolarization in a calcium-dependent manner.

ACKNOWLEDGMENTS

The research carried out in the authors' laboratory was supported by grant DA-00017 from the National Institute on Drug Abuse.

REFERENCES

1. Herz, A., Akil, H., and Simon, E. J. *Handbook of Experimental Pharmacology, Vol. 104/I, Opioids I.* Heidelberg: Springer-Verlag, 1993.
2. Hollt, V. Opioid peptide processing and receptor selectivity. *Annu. Rev. Pharmacol. Toxicol.* 26:59–77, 1986.
3. Almeida, O. F. X., and Shippenberg, T. S. *Neurobiology of Opioids.* Berlin: Springer-Verlag, 1991.
4. Simonds, W. F. The molecular basis of opioid receptor function. *Endocrine Rev.* 9:200–212, 1988.
5. Simon, E. J., and Hiller, J. M. Solubilization and purification of opioid binding sites. In G. W. Pasternak (ed.), *The Opiate Receptors.* Clifton, NJ: Humana, 1988, pp. 165–194.
6. Illes, P. Modulation of transmitter and hormone release by multiple neuronal opioid receptors. *Rev. Physiol. Biochem. Pharmacol.* 112: 139–233, 1989.
7. Simon, E. J. Opioid receptors and endogenous opioid peptides. *Med. Res. Rev.* 11: 357–374, 1991.

8. Simon, E. J., Hiller, J. M., and Edelman, I. Stereospecific binding of the potent narcotic analgesic ^{3}H-etorphine to rat brain homogenate. *Proc. Natl. Acad. Sci. U.S.A.* 70:1947–1949, 1973.

9. Terenius, L. Stereospecific interaction between narcotic analgesics and a synaptic plasma membrane fraction of rat cerebral cortex. *Acta Pharmacol. Toxicol.* 32:317–320, 1973.

10. Pert, C. B., and Snyder, S. H. Opiate receptor: Demonstration in nervous tissue. *Science* 179:1011–1014, 1973.

11. Liebeskind, J. C., Mayer, D. J., and Akil, H. Central mechanisms of pain inhibition: Studies of analgesia from focal brain stimulation. In J. J. Bonica (ed.), *Advances in Neurology. International Symposium on Pain,* Vol. 4, New York: Raven, 1974, pp. 261–268.

12. Hughes, J., Smith, T. W., Kosterlitz, H. W., Fothergill, L. A., Morgan, B. A., and Morris, H. R. Identification of two related pentapeptides from the brain with potent opiate agonist activity. *Nature* 258:577–579, 1975.

13. Goldstein, A., Tachibana, S., Lowney, L. I., Hunkapiller, M., and Hood, L. Dynorphin (1-13), an extraordinarily potent opioid peptide. *Proc. Natl. Acad. Sci. U.S.A.* 76:6666–6670, 1979.

14. Martin, W. R., Eades, C. G., Thompson, J. A., Huppler, R. E., and Gilbert, P. E. The effects of morphine- and nalorphine-like drugs in the nondependent and morphine-dependent chronic spinal dog. *J. Pharmacol. Exp. Ther.* 197:517–532, 1976.

15. Lord, J. A. H., Waterfield, A. A., Hughes, J., and Kosterlitz, H. W. Endogenous opioid peptides: Multiple agonists and receptors. *Nature* 267:495–499, 1977.

16. North, R. A. Opioid receptor types and membrane ion channels. *Trends Neurosci.* 9:114–117, 1986.

17. Simon, E. J., Hiller, J. M., and Edelman, I. Solubilization of a stereospecific opiate-macromolecular complex from rat brain. *Science* 190:389–390, 1975.

18. Simonds, W. F., Burke, T. R., Jr., Rice, K. C., Jacobson, A. E., and Klee, W. A. Purification of the opiate receptor of NG 108-15 neuroblastoma-glioma hybrid cells. *Proc. Natl. Acad. Sci. U.S.A.* 82:4974–4978, 1985.

19. Howard, A. D., De la Baume, S., Gioannini, T. L., Hiller, J. H., and Simon, E. J. Covalent labeling of opioid receptors with radioiodinated human β-endorphin. *J. Biol. Chem.* 260:10833–10839, 1985.

20. Itzhak, Y., Hiller, J. M., and Simon, E. J. Solubilization and characterization of μ, δ and κ opioid binding sites from guinea pig brain: Physical separation of κ receptors. *Proc. Natl. Acad. Sci. U.S.A.* 81:4217–4221, 1984.

21. Chow, T., and Zukin, R. S. Solubilization and preliminary characterization of mu and kappa opioid receptor subtypes from rat brain. *Mol. Pharmacol.* 24:203–212, 1983.

22. Gioannini, T. L., Howard, A. D., Hiller, J. M., and Simon, E. J. Purification of an active opioid-binding protein from bovine striatum. *J. Biol. Chem.* 260:15117–15121, 1985.

23. Kieffer, B. L., Befort, K., Gaveriaux-Ruff, C., and Hirth, C. G. The δ-opioid receptor: Isolation of a cDNA by expression cloning and pharmacological characterization. *Proc. Natl. Acad. Sci. U.S.A.* 89:12048–12052, 1992.

24. Evans, C. J., Keith, D. E. Jr., Morrison, H., Magendzo, K., and Edwards, R. H. Cloning of a delta opioid receptor by functional expression. *Science* 258:1952–1955, 1992.

25. Yasuda, K., Raynor, K., Kong, H., Breder, C., Takeda, J., Reisine, T., and Bell, G. Cloning and functional comparison of kappa and delta opioid receptors from mouse brain. *Proc. Natl. Acad. Sci. U.S.A.* 90:6736–6740, 1993.

26. Chen, Y., Mestek, A., Liu, J., Hurley, J. A., and Yu, L. Molecular cloning and functional expression of a μ-opioid receptor from rat brain. *Mol. Pharmacol.* 44:8–12, 1993.

27. Mains, R. E., Eipper, B. A., and Ling, N. Common precursor to corticotropins and endorphins. *Proc. Natl. Acad. Sci. U.S.A.* 74:3014–3018, 1977.

28. Roberts, J. L., and Herbert, E. Characterization of a common precursor to corticotropin and β-lipotropin: Cell-free synthesis of the precursor and identification of corticotropin peptides in the molecule. *Proc. Natl. Acad. Sci. U.S.A.* 74:4826–4830, 1977.

29. Nakanishi, S., Inoue, A., Kita, T., et al. Nucleotide sequence of cloned cDNA for bovine corticotropin-β-lipotropin precursor. *Nature* 278:423–427, 1979.

30. Lewis, R. V., Stern, A. S., Kimura, S., Rossier, J., Stein, S., and Udenfriend, S. A 50,000-dalton protein in adrenal medulla that may be a common precursor of [Met]- and [Leu]enkephalin. *Science* 208:1459–1461, 1980.

Neuropeptides

MICHAEL J. BROWNSTEIN

Basic Neurochemistry: Molecular, Cellular, and Medical Aspects, 5th Ed., edited by G. J. Siegel et al. Published by Raven Press, Ltd., New York, 1994. Correspondence to Michael J. Brownstein, Laboratory of Cell Biology, National Institute of Mental Health, National Institutes of Health, Bethesda, Maryland 20892.

PEPTIDERGIC NEURONS

Peptides serve as chemical messengers in the central nervous system and the periphery

The discovery of neurosecretory cells in vertebrates by Ernst Scharrer led to the proposal that there were "peptidergic neurons" and to the subsequent amplification of this concept [1]. Initially, the term peptidergic neurons referred to neurosecretory cells in the hypothalamus that released vasopressin and oxytocin directly into the circulation from nerve terminals in the posterior pituitary. Now we know that peptidergic neurons have a broad distribution and that there are a great many biologically active peptides.

Two lines of work led to the broadening of the definition of the peptidergic neuron. The first of these involved studies of "releasing factors"—hypothalamic hormones the existence of which was suggested by G. W. Harris and his coworkers (for historical development, see Fink [2]). These studies

culminated in the isolation and characterization of a tripeptide-releasing factor, thyrotropin-releasing hormone [3]. The latter effort represented a landmark event in the historical development of the field of neuroendocrinology and provided impetus for the discovery of the peptide-releasing and release-inhibiting hormones. The second major development was the detection of substance P by von Euler and Gaddum in 1931 and its isolation and characterization by Leeman and Mroz. Substance P was concentrated in specific extrahypothalamic areas such as sensory ganglia, and this alerted physiologists to the possibility that peptides might act as neurotransmitters.

Peptidergic neurons occur throughout the animal kingdom. In fact, in lower invertebrates, such as annelids, at least one-half of the cerebral ganglion is thought to consist of such neurons [1]. Amino acid sequences are known for several of the invertebrate neuropeptides: the red chromatotropin and FMRFamide of crustaceans; the adipokinetic hormone and proctolin of insects; and the egg-laying hormone and peptides A and B of *Aplysia*.

Many peptide structures appear to be phylogenetically conserved, since vertebrate peptide homologs have been detected in invertebrates, and vice versa. In addition, there seem to be significant redundancies of peptide structure, i.e., there are families of structurally similar molecules. Members of these families have different functions and distributions and act on different receptors.

PEPTIDES INVOLVED IN HYPOTHALAMIC AND PITUITARY FUNCTION

The pituitary is composed of anterior or distal, intermediate, and posterior or neural lobes

The posterior pituitary is of neuronal origin; it arises from the floor of the hypothalamus and is connected to the median eminence of the hypothalamus by a stalk (Fig. 1). The anterior and intermediate parts of the pituitary originate from epithelial cells that migrate up from the roof of the embryonal mouth cavity (Rathke's pouch). The three parts of the pituitary eventually join one another and take up residence beneath the diencephalon, those derived from Rathke's pouch becoming most rostral.

Axons of large neurons in the supraoptic and paraventricular hypothalamic nuclei travel through the median eminence and stalk to the posterior pituitary, where they terminate near blood vessels. Thus the posterior pituitary is best thought of as a part of the brain from which secretion of hormones into the peripheral circulation occurs. In humans, the hormones in question are vasopressin and oxytocin (Fig. 1). They are members of a large family of peptides. As shown in Table 1, the members of this family are structurally similar, differing from one another by only one or two amino acids. They are all nine residues in length and have a cysteine bridge.

Normally, separate populations of mag-

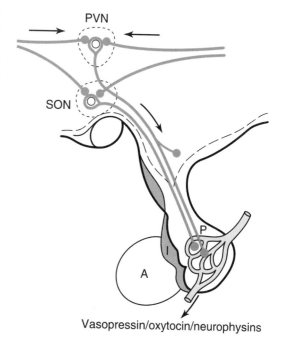

Vasopressin/oxytocin/neurophysins

FIG. 1. The hypothalamoneurohypophysial system. Magnocellular neurons in the supraoptic nucleus (SON) and paraventricular nucleus (PVN) of the hypothalamus project via the median eminence to the posterior pituitary (P). There they release their hormones into capillaries. The magnocellular neurons are influenced by both ascending and descending afferents. Note that the axons of some neurons in the PVN terminate in the zona externa of the median eminence and release their contents into the portal capillary plexus. (A) anterior lobe; (I) intermediate lobe.

nocellular neurons synthesize and secrete vasopressin and oxytocin along with their so-called carrier proteins, the neurophysins. When it is released into the bloodstream, vasopressin, or antidiuretic hormone, stimulates water conservation by the kidney. Without this hormone, animals have to consume large amounts of water each day to replace their fluid losses. If water is not freely available, depletion of body fluids and cardiovascular collapse rapidly ensue. As its name suggests, vasopressin also increases arterial blood pressure. Until recently, this was regarded by many to be a nonphysiological effect of the peptide, but now vasopressin's role in regulating blood pressure is accepted.

TABLE 1.   Neurohypophysial hormones[a]

VASOTOCIN (NONMAMMALIAN VERTEBRATES)

Ile-Tyr-Cys
  | |
Gln-Asn-Cys-Pro-*Arg*-Gly-NH$_2$

OXYTOCIN-LIKE PEPTIDES

Oxytocin (mammals)
  Ile-Tyr-Cys
    | |
  Gln-Asn-Cys-Pro-Leu-Gly-NH$_2$

Mesotocin (Australian marsupials, birds, reptiles, amphibians, lungfish)
  Ile-Tyr-Cys
    | |
  Gln-Asn-Cys-Pro-Ile-Gly-NH$_2$

Isotocin (bony fish)
  Ile-Tyr-Cys
    | |
  Ser-Asn-Cys-Pro-Ile-Gly-NH$_2$

Glumitocin (rays)
  Ile-Tyr-Cys
    | |
  Ser-Asn-Cys-Pro-Gln-Gly-NH$_2$

Valitocin (sharks)
  Ile-Tyr-Cys
    | |
  Gln-Asn-Cys-Pro-Val-Gly-NH$_2$

Aspargtocin (sharks)
  Ile-Tyr-Cys
    | |
  Asn-Asn-Cys-Pro-Leu-Gly-NH$_2$

VASOPRESSIN-LIKE PEPTIDES

Arginine vasopressin (placental, marsupial, and egg-laying mammals)
  Phe-Tyr-Cys
    | |
  Gln-Asn-Cys-Pro-*Arg*-Gly-NH$_2$

Lysine vasopressin (placental and marsupial mammals)
  Phe-Tyr-Cys
    | |
  Gln-Asn-Cys-Pro-*Lys*-Gly-NH$_2$

Phenypressin (marsupials)
  Phe-Phe-Cys
    | |
  Gln-Asn-Cys-Pro-*Arg*-Gly-NH$_2$

Moderate to severe dehydration is associated with an outpouring of vasopressin. Theoretically, this outpouring could be triggered either by the decrease in plasma volume that is associated with dehydration or an increase in plasma osmolality; the latter seems to be the more important factor.

Mechanosensitive cation channels on magnocellular neurons allow them to respond to changes in osmolality that result in their shrinking or swelling. Cells elsewhere in the body that are sensitive to changes in osmolality or blood pressure also influence vasopressin secretion.

A number of neurotransmitters alter the firing patterns of vasopressin-producing neurons and affect the release rate of the hormone

Acetylcholine, histamine, and angiotensin are especially potent in releasing vasopressin; norepinephrine has the opposite action. Many other neurotransmitters present in a variety of ascending and descending pathways probably participate in controlling vasopressin secretion, mediating changes in its release in response to pain, stress, hemorrhage, transfusion, orthostasis, and anoxia.

Oxytocin, the second neurohypophysial hormone to be characterized, plays an important role in reproduction and lactation. The word oxytocin ("quick birth") was coined because the hormone stimulates uterine contractions. There is no doubt that oxytocin is secreted during parturition, but its precise role in promoting the orderly evacuation of the fetus from the uterus is still debated.

The part played by oxytocin in milk ejection is clearer. When suckling commences, afferent stimuli from the teats cause release of oxytocin from the posterior pituitary. Oxytocin activates a contractile mechanism, and alveolar milk is expressed through the lactiferous ducts into the sinuses or cisterns connecting to the teat ducts. In the absence of oxytocin, only the milk stored in the cisterns is available to the suckling infant.

Recently, oxytocin-producing magnocellular neurons have been shown to synthesize vasopressin when female animals are lactating. Consequently, vasopressin and oxytocin are released together in response to nursing. The former helps the mother to compensate for an acute volume loss.

Magnocellular hypothalamic neurons do not have an exclusive franchise for the production of vasopressin and oxytocin

Several additional populations of neurons in the brain seem to make vasopressin and oxytocin, and there are also cells in the periphery that produce these hormones. It should be clear from the above that, like many other biologically active peptides, these function in a number of ways. Released into the bloodstream, they act as neurohormones. Released into the pituitary portal plexus (see below), they function as releasing hormones, stimulating the secretion of adrenocorticotropic hormone (ACTH). Released at synapses in the central and peripheral nervous systems, they act as neurotransmitters or neuromodulators. Finally, released by non-neuronal cells in the periphery, they act on adjacent cells as paracrine mediators or on the same cells that released them as autocrine agents.

Growth hormone and prolactin have similar primary structures and, to an important degree, similar functions

Growth hormone probably affects metabolic processes in all tissues of the body. Its most obvious action is to cause growth of the immature animal by stimulating elongation of long bones and by stimulating protein biosynthesis at the expense of sugar and fat stores. Some of the actions of growth hormone are mediated by another group of peptides, the somatomedins, which are made in the liver. The effects of prolactin, on the other hand, seem to result from the direct influence of this hormone on target cells. Although prolactin can stimulate protein biosynthesis just as growth hormone does, its only certain physiological function is to stimulate lactation in the breast that has been primed with estrogen, progesterone, glucocorticoids, insulin, and thyroxine.

Thyroid-stimulating hormone (TSH), luteinizing hormone (LH), and follicle-stimulating hormone (FSH), as well as human chorionic gonadotropin (CG), are glycoproteins formed from two peptide subunits called α- and β-chains. Fifteen to 30 percent of the total weight of the molecules is contributed by their sugar moieties (polymers of fucose, mannose, galactose, N-acetylglucosamine, N-acetylgalactosamine, and sialic acid) and the rest by the peptide chains. The amino acid sequence of the α-chain, which is not biologically active, seems to be the same in TSH, LH, FSH, and CG. The biologically active β-chains differ in primary structure.

TSH increases the volume and vascularization of the thyroid gland and stimulates the synthesis and release of thyroid hormones. It also promotes lypolysis in adipose tissue, but the physiological importance of this extrathyroid effect is not understood.

In women, FSH causes growth and development of the ovarian follicle. Subsequently, LH acts on the follicle, causing it to mature and secrete estrogens. LH then induces ovulation and participates in transforming the follicle into the progesterone-secreting corpus luteum. In men, FSH promotes spermatogenesis, and LH stimulates androgen production by the testis (Leydig cells).

Adrenocorticotropic hormone (corticotropin or ACTH), α-melanocyte-stimulating hormone (α-MSH), β-MSH, β-lipotropic hormone (β-LPH), and β-endorphin constitute a family of peptides that are synthesized as parts of a common precursor molecule, pro-opiocortin [4], which has a molecular weight of about 31 kDa. This glycoprotein has β-LPH (β-endorphin and β-MSH) on its C-terminal end, ACTH (α-MSH) in the middle, and γ-MSH near the N-terminal end.

In all species studied, ACTH has 39 amino acid residues. Its first 24 amino acids are constant from species to species. The first 13 amino acids of ACTH are required for the only significant physiological action of the hormone, adrenocorticotropic activity. Adding the next seven amino acids one at a time progressively enhances the molecule's potency. The remaining 19 amino acids are not required for optimum biological activity.

Melanotropic and small nonsecretory cells comprise the intermediate lobe of the pituitary gland. α-MSH contains the first 13 amino acids of ACTH. It is *N*-acetylated and C-amidated and, consequently, resistant to most peptidases.

β-MSH, β-LPH, α-MSH, and ACTH secreted from the anterior and/or intermediate lobes of the pituitary have seven amino acids in common (ACTH residues 4 to 10). These residues are the minimum required for melanotropic activity in amphibians and reptiles. The role of MSH in mammals is still unknown. In fact, humans have a vestigial intermediate pituitary and have little or no circulating α-MSH.

The anterior pituitary is an organ that is separate from, but regulated by, the brain

The anterior pituitary is connected to the hypothalamus by a special portal vascular system [5] (Fig. 2). This system consists of two connected capillary beds, one in the external zone of the median eminence and the other in the pituitary. Axons of a variety of neurons terminate adjacent to portal capillaries in the median eminence. Some of the nerve endings in the median eminence release hypothalamic hormones that enter the portal vessels and travel to the anterior pituitary (undiluted by blood from the general circulation). Others release neurotransmitters that probably influence by presynaptic mechanisms the secretion of the hypothalamic hormones.

On reaching the anterior pituitary, hypothalamic hormones stimulate or inhibit the synthesis and secretion of tropic hormones made in the pituitary. A number of releasing hormones and release-inhibiting hormones are present in the hypothalamus. Four releasing hormones—TRH, gonadotropin-releasing hormone (GnRH), corticotropin-releasing hormone (CRH), and growth hormone-releasing hormone (GHRH)—and one release-inhibiting hormone (growth hormone release-inhibiting hormone or somatostatin) have been isolated and characterized (see Table 2). A number of other peptides—vasopressin, oxytocin, vasoactive intestinal polypeptide, enkephalin, substance P, and cholecystokinin, to name a few—may be involved in regulating anterior pituitary function as well.

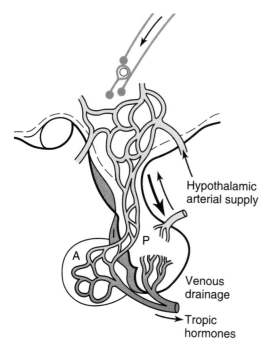

Hypothalamic arterial supply

P

A

Venous drainage

Tropic hormones

FIG. 2. Control of anterior pituitary function. Releasing hormones and release-inhibiting hormones are secreted into portal capillaries in the zona externa of the median eminence. The hormones travel to the anterior pituitary; there they act on tropic hormone-producing cells. These cells secrete into the general circulation; tropic hormones may also travel back to the brain through the portal vessels. Cells that make releasing or release-inhibiting hormones are excited or inhibited by other neurons. Furthermore, release of hypothalamic hormones may be modulated in the median eminence by a presynaptic mechanism. A, anterior lobe; P, posterior pituitary.

The general properties of the hypothalamic hormones are outlined in Table 3. It is noteworthy that the properties of a releasing factor (or release-inhibiting factor) are quite similar to those of a neurotransmitter. Indeed, the releasing factors are best thought of as a special class of chemical messengers that act on a variety of cells, among them cells in the anterior pituitary.

TRH stimulates the secretion of thyrotropin and prolactin; GnRH stimulates the secretion of LH and FSH; CRH stimulates ACTH and β-endorphin release; and GHRH stimulates growth hormone secretion. Somatostatin inhibits the secretion of growth hormone, thyrotropin, and prolactin *in vitro,* but it seems unlikely that somatostatin participates in regulating prolactin *in vivo.* Dopamine, on the other hand, is a potent inhibitor of prolactin secretion and is found in high concentrations in the median eminence. Hence, it has been suggested that dopamine is a prolactin release-inhibiting hormone.

In addition to controlling anterior pituitary function, the hypothalamic hormones may act in the central nervous system and the periphery

GnRH, for example, induces mating behavior in female rats. This orchestration of reproductive phenomena—mating and ovulation—by a single peptide may represent a special case. Peptides may also mediate diverse and unrelated events.

In addition to acting within the central nervous system, hypothalamic hormones function in the periphery. Thus, somatostatin has been shown to play an important role outside the brain in the pancreas and gastrointestinal tract. It inhibits the secretion of insulin, glucagon, and gastrin and decreases gastric acidity. Conversely, a number of peptides first isolated from gut extracts and thought of as gastrointestinal hormones are now known to operate in the brain.

The neuroendocrine system is a hierarchy, with higher centers regulating lower ones

The hierarchical control of secretory activity involves feedback loops (Fig. 3). Thus, changes related to secretory activity are detected by a control center, and the information is used to adjust the output of the control mechanism in an appropriate way. Consequently, Fig. 3 could be redrawn with many extra arrows pointing upward to indicate feedback.

Negative, or inhibitory, feedback is the usual means of maintaining a particular level

TABLE 2. Amino acid sequences of representative mammalian biologically active peptides

Adrenocorticotropic hormone
H-Ser-Tyr-Ser-Met-Glu-His-Phe-Arg-Trp-Gly-Lys-Pro-Val-Gly-Lys-Lys-Arg-Arg-Pro-Val-Lys-Val-Tyr-Pro-Asn-Gly-Ala-Glu-Asp-Glu-Leu-Ala-Glu-Ala-Phe-Pro-Leu-Glu-Phe-OH

Angiotensin II
H-Asp-Arg-Val-Tyr-Ile-His-Pro-Phe-OH

Atrial natriuretic polypeptide (one of three peptides in this family)
Arg-Asp-Met-Arg-Gly-Gly-Phe-Cys-Ser-Ser-Arg-Arg-Leu-Ser
Ile
Gly-Ala-Gln-Ser-Gly-Leu-Gly-Cys-Asn-Ser-Phe-Arg-Tyr

Bradykinin
H-Arg-Pro-Pro-Gly-Phe-Ser-Pro-Phe-Arg-OH

Calcitonin
Asn-Gly-Cys
Leu
Ser-Thr-Cys-Met-Leu-Gly-Thr-Tyr-Thr-Gln-Asp-Phe-Asn-Lys-Phe-His-Thr-Phe-Pro-Gln-Thr-Ala-Ile-Gly-Val-Gly-Ala-Pro-NH$_2$

Calcitonin gene-related peptide
Thr-Asp-Cys-Ala
Ala-Thr-Cys-Val-Thr-His-Arg-Leu-Ala-Gly-Leu-Leu-Ser-Arg-Ser-Gly-Gly-Val-Val-Lys-Asn-Asn-Phe-Val-Pro-Thr-Asn-Val-Gly-Ser-Lys-Ala-Phe-NH$_2$

L-Carnosine
N-β-alanyl-L-histidine

Cholecystokinin octapeptide
Asp-Tyr(SO$_3$)-Met-Gly-Trp-Met-Asp-Phe-NH$_2$

Corticotropin-releasing hormone
Ser-Glu-Glu-Pro-Pro-Ile-Ser-Leu-Asp-Leu-Thr-Phe-His-Leu-Leu-Arg-Glu-Val-Leu-Glu-Met-Ala-Arg-Ala-Glu-Gln-Leu-Ala-Gln-Gln-Ala-His-Ser-Asn-Arg-Lys-Leu-Met-Glu-Ile-Ile-NH$_2$

Dynorphin A
Tyr-Gly-Gly-Phe-Leu-Arg-Arg-Ile-Arg-Pro-Lys-Leu-Lys-Trp-Asp-Asn-Gln

β-Endorphin
H-Tyr-Gly-Gly-Phe-Met-Thr-Ser-Glu-Lys-Ser-Gln-Thr-Pro-Leu-Val-Thr-Leu-Phe-Lys-Asn-Ala-Ile-Ile-Lys-Asn-Ala-Tyr-Lys-Lys-Gly-Glu-OH

Galanin
Gly-Trp-Thr-Leu-Asn-Ser-Ala-Gly-Tyr-Leu-Leu-Gly-Pro-His-Ala-Ile-Asp-Asn-His-Arg-Ser-Phe-His-Asp-Lys-Tyr-Gly-Leu-Ala-NH$_2$

Gastrin-releasing peptide (the mammalian equivalent of bombesin)
Ala-Pro-Val-Ser-Val-Gly-Gly-Gly-Thr-Val-Leu-Ala-Lys-Met-Tyr-Pro-Arg-Gly-Asn-His-Trp-Ala-Val-Gly-His-Leu-Met-NH$_2$

Gonadotropin-releasing hormone (also called luteinizing hormone-releasing hormone [LHRH])
pGlu-His-Trp-Ser-Tyr-Gly-Leu-Arg-Pro-Gly-NH$_2$

Growth hormone-releasing hormone
Tyr-Ala-Asp-Ala-Ile-Phe-Thr-Asn-Ser-Tyr-Arg-Lys-Val-Leu-Gly-Gln-Leu-Ser-Ala-Arg-Lys-Leu-Leu-Gln-Asp-Ile-Met-Ser-Arg-Gln-Gln-Gly-Glu-Ser-Asn-Gln-Glu-Arg-Gly-Ala-Arg-Ala-Arg-Leu-NH$_2$

Leu-enkephalin
H-Tyr-Gly-Gly-Phe-Leu-OH

α-Melanocyte-stimulating hormone
Acetyl-Ser-Tyr-Ser-Met-Glu-His-Phe-Arg-Trp-Gly-Lys-Pro-Val-NH$_2$

Met-enkephalin
H-Tyr-Gly-Gly-Phe-Met-OH

TABLE 2.   *(continued)*

Neurotensin
  pGlu-Leu-Tyr-Glu-Asn-Lys-Pro-Arg-Arg-Pro-Tyr-Ile-Leu-OH
NPY
  Tyr-Pro-Ser-Lys-Pro-Asp-Asp-Pro-Gly-Glu-Asp-Ala-Pro-Ala-Glu-Asp-Met-Ala-Arg-Tyr-Tyr-Ser-Ala-Leu-Arg-His-
  Tyr-Ile-Asn-Leu-Ile-Thr-Arg-Gln-Arg-Tyr-NH$_2$
Somatostatin (the shorter of two active forms is shown)
  Lys-Thr-Phe-Thr-Ser-Cys-Gly-Ala-H
      | |
  Trp-Phe-Phe-Asn-Lys-Cys-OH
Substance P (one member of a peptide family that also includes substance K and neurokinin B)
  H-Arg-Pro-Lys-Pro-Glu-Glu-Phe-Phe-Gly-Leu-Met-NH$_2$
Thyrotropin-releasing hormone
  pGlu-His-Pro-NH$_2$
Vasoactive intestinal peptide (one member of a peptide family that also includes parathyroid hormone, calcitonin,
secretin, gastric inhibitory polypeptide, and growth hormone-releasing hormone)
  H-His-Ser-Asp-Ala-Val-Phe-Thr-Asp-Asn-Tyr-Thr-Arg-Leu-Arg-Lys-Glu-Met-Ala-Val-Lys-Lys-Tyr-Leu-Asn-Ser-Ile-
  Leu-Asn-NH$_2$

of output in the face of uncontrolled or unpredictable disturbances. For example, an increase in the blood level of adrenocorticosteroids causes a decrease in the release of ACTH from the anterior pituitary. This, in turn, results in a decrease in the secretion rate of corticosteroids, and they return toward their original level. Gonadal steroids and thyroxine also exert negative feedback control over their respective tropic hormones.

There is evidence for positive, or stimulatory, feedback as well as negative feedback. Implantation of estrogen in the rat pituitary during a critical period of the estrous cycle causes advancement of ovulation, which is

TABLE 3.   Criteria for assessing the physiological role of any proposed substance as a releasing factor

1. The putative releasing factor must be extractable from hypothalamic or stalk-median eminence tissue
2. It must be present in hypophysial portal blood in greater amounts than in systemic blood (i.e., it is released into the portal capillaries)
3. Varying concentrations of the substance in portal vessel blood should be related to varying secretion rates of one of the anterior pituitary hormones under a number of different experimental and environmental conditions
4. The factor should stimulate (or inhibit) secretion of one or more anterior pituitary hormones when administered *in vivo* or *in vitro*. Inhibitors, if available, should antagonize the actions of the endogenous peptide and block (or stimulate) anterior pituitary hormone secretion
5. Target cells should have receptors for the candidate peptides; e.g., corticotropes should, and indeed do, have CRH binding sites

After Harris [33].

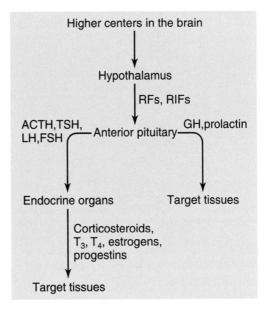

FIG. 3.   Neuronal control of anterior pituitary function. (RF) releasing factor; (RIF) release-inhibiting factor.

probably due to an increase in the plasma level of LH. By acting on the developing ovarian follicle, the LH causes a further increase in estrogen level. Unlike negative feedback systems, positive feedback controls are inherently unstable. Once set in motion, they rapidly produce a high level of activity. For example, estrogen stimulation of LH secretion seems responsible for the peak of LH output that triggers ovulation when the follicle is mature. Inhibitory mechanisms are required for turning off positive feedback control loops. Inhibition by LH of its own

secretion may provide such a mechanism in the example cited above.

In general, the higher a regulatory center is in the neuroendocrine hierarchy, the more opportunities it has to be fed back on, positively or negatively. Theoretically, the feedback control of a center can be mediated by the secretory product of the center itself (this sort of feedback—releasing hormones onto the very cells that make them—is termed ultrashort feedback), by the secretory products of lower centers, or by reflexes triggered by these secretory products. Cells

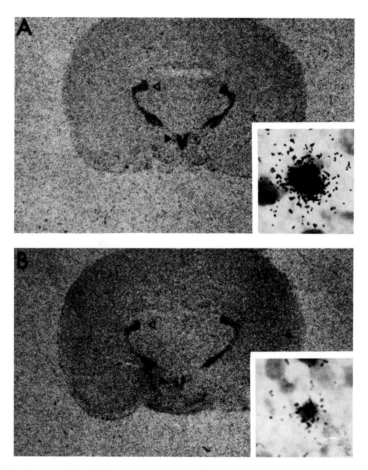

FIG. 4.   *In situ* hybridization histochemistry of TRH mRNA-containing cells in the paraventricular nucleus (PVN) of the hypothalamus and the reticular nucleus of the thalamus. The autoradiographic hybridization signal on X-ray film appears as an area of darkening over the PVN *(solid arrowhead)* and reticular nucleus *(open arrowhead)* of a rat treated with propylthiouracil (PTU) **(A)** and of a PTU-treated rat injected with T_3 **(B).** The hybridization appears as dense clusters of grains over individual cell bodies within the PVN of a PTU-treated rat *(inset **A**)* and of a PTU-treated rat injected with T_3 *(inset **B**).* Each inset shows the most intensely labeled cells within the respective PVN [31].

a the anterior pituitary and in the hypothalamus are sensitive to peripheral hormone levels. These hormone-brain and hormone-pituitary interactions are responsible for so-called long-feedback effects. For example, repeated injection of exogenous thyroxine into an animal with an isolated pituitary will cause atrophy of its thyroid gland, just as in the intact animal. This is taken to indicate that the isolated pituitary gland, in addition to maintaining a low rate of TSH secretion, is sensitive to the level of thyroxine in the general circulation. Increasing the thyroxine level inhibits the TSH release and produces atrophy of the target organ. There is also evidence that thyroxine affects the synthesis and secretion of TRH (Fig. 4).

After stalk section, the thyroid is unresponsive to many of the stimuli that would have increased its secretory activity in the intact animal, such as environmental stress. The input to the pituitary-thyroid axis from these stimuli must be mediated via TRH secretion into the hypophysial portal system. Similar observations have been made for ACTH and the gonadotropic hormones.

Feedback control of brain centers by adenohypophysial tropic hormones is referred to as internal or short feedback. There is evidence that each of the tropic hormones except prolactin may act on the hypothalamus in such an inhibitory short loop. Since the pressure in pituitary portal vessels is low, blood flow in this vascular system is probably bidirectional, although predominantly toward the pituitary (Fig. 2). Therefore, pituitary secretions can return to the median eminence, to the cerebrospinal fluid, and, finally, to the rest of the brain either directly by this route or indirectly (and much diluted) through systemic circulation. Peripheral hormones must be carried to the brain through the general circulation. Once there, these peripheral hormones act, along with pituitary tropic hormones, on a variety of neurons that are involved in neuroendocrine regulation (for more detail, see Lightman and Everitt [6]).

EXPERIMENTAL APPROACHES TO THE STUDY OF NEUROPEPTIDES

There is no single best approach to the detection and isolation of biologically active neuropeptides

One general paradigm that has been used with success [7] is presented in Table 4. In this approach, the biochemist is directed by the biological phenomenon of interest, that is, the bioactivity of the peptide. The biological assay may be either a physiologically relevant one, as was the case for the hypothalamic releasing factors (see above), or a reproducible response to the peptide in a neuronal or non-neuronal tissue that may have no apparent relationship to its actual

TABLE 4. Steps in the analysis of a neuropeptide[a]

1. Development of a quantitative bioassay
2. Evidence that the biologically active material is peptidic in nature
3. Development of extraction and separation procedures for maximum yields of the purified peptide
4. Chemical and physical characterization of the pure peptide (e.g., molecular weight determination and amino acid composition)
5. Obtain amino acid sequence of the peptide
6. Chemical synthesis of the peptide (which is then tested for bioactivity using quantitative bioassay)
7. Produce antibodies to peptide
8. Characterization of antibodies using synthetic analogs of the peptide (purification of antibodies)
9. Development of immunologic assays and procedures for use on neural tissues (e.g., radioimmunoassay and immunocytochemistry)
10. Isolation of cDNA that encodes the peptide's precursor. Characterization and chromosomal localization of the gene that gives rise to the precursor. Development of methods for detecting and measuring the precursor's mRNA (Northern blotting, *in situ* hybridization histochemistry)
11. Development of binding assays for studying peptide receptors. Isolation of cDNAs encoding these receptors

[a] Although it is highly desirable to have at the outset a biological activity of the peptide that can be monitored by a quantitative bioassay, not all studies on peptides begin with this step; however, the value of a bioassay is emphasized by its role in the establishment of purity criteria for the isolated and the synthetic peptides.

physiological role in the nervous system, as was the case for substance P and the sialogogical bioassay [7]. In some cases, if it is feasible, even a complex behavioral response can be used as the basis for a bioassay.

Development of a quantitative bioassay depends on effective extraction of the peptide

The extraction should be done under conditions that protect the peptide from degradative processes (e.g., proteolytic enzymes), and a solvent should be used in which the peptide is highly soluble. Methods for preventing degradation of the peptide during extraction include microwave treatment or freezing of the tissue with liquid nitrogen, adding protease inhibitors to the extraction solvent, and boiling the tissue in dilute acid. In addition to the problems of degradation, one must also attend to the problem of recovery. Peptides tend to bind to glass surfaces, may be associated with binding proteins, and may be destroyed by such processes as oxidation and esterification of sensitive amino acid residues during extraction. Obviously, the initial extraction step is critical and often must be tailored to the specific peptide being extracted and to the specific tissue from which it is to be extracted [7].

Even with a good extraction procedure, one may find that the biological activity in the extract is altered or masked by other substances that are coextracted. Only by sequential separation steps and bioassay at each step can one determine if this is indeed the case. Herein lies the major value of the quantitative bioassay. The bioassay provides a major criterion for purity of the peptide as it is being fractionated. The aim is to subject the extract to a variety of sequential separation procedures until the isolated peptide is at maximum and constant specific activity (i.e., where the units of biological activity per amount of peptide are maximal and constant). In addition, the bioassay can be used early to determine whether the bioactive sub-

stance is a peptide. Preliminary evidence of its peptidic nature can be obtained by evaluating its size by molecular filtration chromatography, by determining whether it maintains activity after boiling at neutral pH (most, but not all, peptides do), and by determining whether the bioactivity is destroyed by incubation of the material with proteolytic enzymes (e.g., pronase, trypsin) or by acid hydrolysis.

A variety of separation procedures can be used to isolate a purified peptide

Procedures include molecular filtration chromatography (which also provides information about the size of the peptide), selective extractions in diverse solvents, ion-exchange chromatography, thin-layer chromatography, high-voltage electrophoresis, and, where possible, specific affinity chromatography. The latter procedure is particularly efficacious, as it provides a large purification in a single step because of a specific property of the peptide (i.e., it may bind specifically to a protein and be eluted from a column on which this protein is attached only in the presence of an excess of a competing ligand). High-performance liquid chromatography (HPLC) has proven especially useful for peptide separation. The point of using these separation procedures is to generate a pure peptide. One criterion of purity has already been discussed; that is, the peptide is at maximum and constant specific biological activity. Several other criteria should also be fulfilled: N-terminal and C-terminal analyses of the peptide show that there is only one N-terminal and one C-terminal amino acid, and analysis of the amino acid composition of the peptide demonstrates that the molar ratios of its constituent amino acids remain constant integrals throughout sequential fractionation procedures.

After a peptide has been isolated in sufficient quantity (50 pmol to 1 nmol, depending on whether it is N-terminally derivatized), its amino acid sequence can be determined by automated Edman degradation and/or fast atom bombardment mass spectroscopy [8]. Alternatively, a partial sequence for the peptide can be used to generate oligonucleotide probes for screening a cDNA library. The amino acid sequence of the peptide can be inferred from the sequence of its precursor protein. Ultimately, the peptide can be synthesized chemically in large quantities, and the purified molecule can be compared with the natural product and bioassayed.

Tatemoto and Mutt [9] have devised another strategy for identifying and purifying biologically active peptides. They recognized the fact that many such peptides are C-terminally amidated and developed a method for detecting amidated amino acids liberated when peptides are hydrolyzed. Using this method they have found a number of novel species that subsequently proved to be quite active *in vivo* and *in vitro*, e.g., peptide histidine-isoleucine (PHI) related to vasoactive intestinal peptide (VIP), neuropeptide Y (NPY), and galanin. Care must be taken not to jump too quickly to the conclusion that a new "biologically active" peptide is a chemical messenger [10].

Characterization of peptide precursors by molecular biological techniques has also led to the discovery of novel peptides. It is not uncommon for a precursor to contain more than one active agent. In addition, differential splicing of peptide genes can give rise to mRNAs encoding different products; witness the case of calcitonin and the calcitonin gene-related peptide [11].

Immunological techniques can be used to study neuropeptide distribution and cellular compartmentation

Radioimmunoassay (RIA) techniques can detect extremely low (femtomole) levels of peptides. Immunological reactions are relatively specific, and RIAs require little technical investment [12]. Similarly, the techniques of immunocytochemistry provide a unique morphological approach to the cellular and subcellular localization of peptides even in a tissue as heterogeneous as the brain.

The production of antibodies to a peptide involves the immunization of rabbits, goats, mice, or guinea pigs with a peptide that has been emulsified in Freund's adjuvant. Relatively impure peptides can be used for immunization, and slight denaturation of the antigens may actually improve their immunogenicity. Small peptides that may not be antigenic can be made so by coupling them to larger proteins, such as bovine serum albumin or thyroglobulin. Antibody concentration tends to increase with repeated immunization, reaching a maximum after about three to five immunizations. The presence and characteristics of the antibody are usually tested, using RIA methods [12], after each reimmunization.

Despite the obvious power of RIA for the analysis of peptides, there are many potential pitfalls and sources of artifacts that may confront the naive user. It must be remembered that, even in the best of cases, the unique value of RIA is its extraordinary sensitivity and simplicity. Its specificity, however, is based on immunological reactions with antigenic determinants that may be shared by diverse molecules (e.g., prohormones versus peptide hormones). Hence, in a strict sense, peptides cannot be shown to exist in a tissue by means of immunological procedures. What is measured is specific peptide-like immunoreactivity, and definitive proof of a specific peptide's presence in the tissue still requires a biochemical approach.

The principle of immunocytochemistry is to detect the antigen in tissue by light and electron microscopy using a labeled antibody

The various markers for antibodies include covalently bound fluorescent molecules, ferritin, enzymes (peroxidase), and radioactive substances. The recent uses of enzymatic and radioactive markers in antigen-antibody complexes have greatly enhanced the sensitivity of this method and have reduced some of the problems inherent in covalent labeling of the antibodies. Although immunocytochemical techniques are extremely useful and provide a unique approach to the cellular localization of peptides, proof of specificity of the immunoreaction is very difficult to obtain. It is generally agreed that the specificity manifested by antiserum in an RIA does not guarantee specificity in an immunocytochemical procedure that uses the same antiserum, partly because of the much higher antisera dilutions used in RIA [7]. One approach used to deal with this problem is to purify the antibodies by means of affinity chromatography, that is, to produce so-called monospecific antibodies. In this approach, purified antigen is covalently coupled to Sepharose beads. Specific antibody will attach to the beads, and, after removing nonspecific antibodies by washing, the specific antibodies can be selectively eluted and used. Another approach is to adsorb out the specific antibody in the immunocytochemical procedure by the addition of excess antigen as a control for nonspecific labeling [13]. In any case, evidence for the detection of a "specific" peptide by immunocytochemistry is usually regarded as less compelling than evidence obtained by RIA methods. As with RIA, the peptide visualized immunocytochemically is referred to as "specific-peptide-like immunoreactivity."

In situ hybridization histochemistry has been employed extensively to study the distribution of peptidergic cells

In situ hybridization histochemistry is based on the use of labeled oligonucleotide or RNA probes complementary to mRNAs of interest. By adjusting hybridization and wash conditions carefully, it is possible to minimize "noise" (nonspecific binding of the probe to tissue elements) and to maximize signal (binding of the probe to the specific mRNA that is to be visualized). The sensitivity of the method has improved with time; currently, 10 or fewer copies of transcript per cell can be detected. In addition, by including standards on the slides, the techniques can be made roughly quantitative.

As with immunocytochemistry, control experiments performed to validate the results of *in situ* hybridization histochemistry are not perfect. Accepted controls include (i) developing a Northern blot made with mRNA from the tissue that is being studied and showing that the probe used detects a single band of the correct size; (ii) using two or more probes directed at different parts of the mRNA of interest and showing that the resulting signals have the same distributions; and (iii) using a sense-strand probe corresponding to one's antisense probe and showing that there is no signal.

As discussed below, immunocytochemistry and *in situ* hybridization histochemistry provide somewhat different information. The former allows the investigator to visualize peptides in axons and, following colchicine treatment, in cell bodies. The latter allows cell bodies to be visualized because the highest levels of mRNAs are found in neuronal perikarya, though it should be noted that mRNAs have been detected in both dendrites and axons of neurons.

The application of molecular biological methods to study neuropeptides has had an important impact on research relating to identification of neuropeptides. A molecular biological approach has been used to isolate cDNAs encoding neuropeptide precursors, precursor-processing enzymes, and peptide receptors. Many genes corresponding to the peptide precursor cDNAs have been isolated, and the structures of these genes have been examined. In the case of a few of these genes, the regulatory domains responsible for tissue-specific expression or the level of transcription have been characterized.

PEPTIDE DISTRIBUTION IN THE NERVOUS SYSTEM

One reason for studying the distribution of peptides in the central nervous system is to determine whether they are present in neurons

The peptide's presence in neurons must be shown first if it is to be considered a neurotransmitter candidate. By examining the neuroanatomy of peptidergic systems, one does much more than satisfy this criterion, however. If one function of a peptide is known, its distribution can hint at the role of brain areas where it is found. For example, the presence of LHRH in the septum and preoptic areas suggested (but certainly did not guarantee) that these regions might be involved somehow in reproduction. Indeed, these regions may provide the anatomical substrate for LHRH-induced lordotic behavior (see Chap. 49).

If the central role of a peptide is a mystery, as was the case with substance P, looking at its distribution may provide clues about its actions. The presence of large amounts of substance P in the dorsal part of the spinal cord hinted that it might mediate pain sensation. In addition to providing a starting point for physiological and behavioral studies, neuroanatomical studies are necessary as first steps for biochemical and cell biological investigations. Conversely, the demonstration that specific cells in which a peptide has been visualized are capable of manufacturing the peptide provides a final vindication of the anatomical data.

Many peptides have unique distributions reflecting the location of neuronal perikarya that produce them and the processes that store and release them

Peptides that are produced as parts of the same precursor typically have very similar distributions, but need not be identically distributed; variations in post-translational processing of a precursor in the different cells that make it can give rise to variations in the products formed.

Axons and nerve endings are especially rich in peptides

The cell bodies seem to manufacture peptide precursors and send them down the axons rather rapidly, so that peptide levels in perikarya are normally not very high. For this reason, peptidergic cell bodies have proven difficult to visualize immunocytochemically. Agents such as colchicine that block axonal transport have been used by immunohistochemists to promote the build-up of peptides in cell bodies. After colchicine treatment, peptide-containing perikarya that are impossible to see otherwise can sometimes be visualized.

Anatomists interested in neuropeptides have introduced a nonimmunological technique, *in situ* hybridization histochemistry

In situ hybridization histochemistry is based on the ability of radiolabeled DNA that is complementary to a specific mRNA to bind to mRNA in tissue sections. The technique is relatively sensitive, and, because mRNA is confined mainly to the cell body, it is useful for mapping peptidergic perikarya. In addition, it can be used to detect changes in mRNA levels that follow pharmacological, physiological, or surgical manipulations (see Siegel [14] and Fig. 3).

There is nothing about the anatomy of central peptidergic neurons that distinguishes them from other classes of neurons: some are large, some small; some are local-circuit neurons, and others project to distant regions. Consequently, in the absence of immunological staining techniques, peptide-producing neurons cannot be separated from their nonpeptide-producing neighbors. Indeed, peptides coexist with one another or with non-peptide transmitters in many neurons. There is growing evidence that, at different times or under different circumstances, neurons may actually release different transmitters.

Many peptides were found in unexpected places

Pituitary tropic hormones, such as prolactin and growth hormone, have been shown to be present in the brain and seem to be in specific populations of neurons. Insulin has also been detected in brain extracts. Hormones present in the blood or in structures that are in close proximity to the brain, such as the pituitary or pineal gland, may not be made by central neurons; they may be taken up and stored by them. Alternatively, part of the hormone in the brain may be made endogenously, and part may be provided by an outside source.

In addition to demonstrating that numerous gut and pituitary hormones are widely distributed in the central nervous system, workers in this field have shown that hypothalamic hormones are not as narrowly distributed as they were at first thought to be. Somatostatin, for example, is found both inside the hypothalamus and outside it. In fact, only about one-quarter of the somatostatin in the brain is in the hypothalamus. Therefore, it has been suggested that somatostatin may act as a neurotransmitter at sites other than the median eminence. Similarly, based on their widespread distributions, it has been suggested that TRH and CRH may be central neurotransmitters. (For specific information on neuroanatomical studies of peptidergic pathways, the reader should consult detailed reviews of this topic, e.g., Björklund and Hökfelt [15].)

BIOSYNTHESIS OF NEUROPEPTIDES

Much of our understanding of peptide biosynthesis comes from studies on tissues other than brain

To date, the mechanisms for the biosynthesis of neuronal peptides appear to be similar to those mechanisms found in other eukaryotic tissues. Two major alternatives exist: (a) the synthesis of oligopeptides by enzymatic mechanisms, that is, synthetases; and (b) synthesis by conventional ribosomal protein synthesis mechanisms, usually as a prohormone that is degraded by limited proteolysis to specific peptide products in the cell before release. Mechanism (a) is used for small peptides, such as carnosine (β-alanyl-L-histidine) and glutathione (γ-L-glutamyl-L-cysteinyl-glycine), which are found in various eukaryotic tissues (including brain) and are synthesized by such enzymes as carnosine synthetase and γ-glutamyl-L-cysteine (plus tripeptide) synthetase, respectively. Larger peptides, such as insulin, nerve growth factor, ACTH, endorphin, vasopressin, and oxytocin, appear to be synthesized as prohormones.

If protein synthesis inhibitors block peptide synthesis, there is presumptive evidence for the prohormone mode of synthesis

If protein synthesis inhibitors like cycloheximide or puromycin do not block the synthesis of a peptide, a search for a specific enzymatic mechanism is in order. Another approach is to employ RIAs for the peptide to see whether on biochemical separation (e.g., gel filtration) higher molecular weight, heterogeneous immunoreactive forms of the peptide can be detected. This also represents presumptive evidence, but not proof, of a prohormone ("big" forms of insulin, ACTH, growth hormone, calcitonin, and other peptides have been detected by this method).

Biosynthesis of a peptide from a prohormone can be studied by means of pulse-chase labeling

A tissue known to contain substantial quantities of the peptide of interest is exposed to radioactive amino acids for a short time (pulse). Immediately after this pulse, a larger form of the peptide should be detected. The tissue, having been pulsed in this manner, is then exposed to a large excess of nonradioactive amino acids to dilute out the radioactive amino acids (chase) or, alternatively tissue is exposed to protein synthesis inhibitors to block *de novo* protein synthesis. The minimum requirement in these experiments is to show that radioactivity associated with the higher molecular weight precursor (or prohormone) decreases with time after the chase or addition of inhibitor. Concurrently, there is an increase in the radioactivity of the peptide product. To demonstrate this, it is necessary in many cases (particularly with heterogeneous tissue such as brain) to use an antibody to the peptide that also reacts with the precursor in a quantitative immunoprecipitation procedure to detect all of the relevant labeled molecules. Labeled presumptive precursors can be purified from the immunoprecipitates and evaluated for the presence of the peptide sequence by limited proteolysis mapping *in vitro* and by analysis of amino acid sequences.

The use of cell-free protein-synthesizing systems (e.g., wheat germ and reticulocyte *in vitro* systems) and polyribosomes from the tissue of interest can lead to the synthesis of the prohormone

Cell-free protein-synthesizing systems have the advantage of also identifying the preprohormone, that is, the prohormone with a characteristic peptide still attached to its N terminus that is used as a signal to direct the prohormone into the cisternae of the endoplasmic reticulum.

Isolation of DNA complementary to mRNAs that encode peptide precursors is used to characterize propeptides

The various methods described above have in large measure been superseded by paradigms involving the use of recombinant DNA. The sequences of almost all of the neu-

ropeptide precursors are now known [16–18].

The cDNAs that encode precursors can be put to many uses:

1. They can be used to probe genomic libraries for their respective genes. Regulatory domains of these genes can be studied.
2. cDNA probes can be used for Northern blotting to measure mRNA levels.
3. cRNA and cDNA probes can be generated for *in situ* hybridization histochemistry.
4. cDNAs can be expressed, intact or mutated, to examine intracellular sorting or to make substrates for studies of processing enzymes.

Development of the prohormone concept

The discovery in 1967 by Steiner and Dyer [19] that insulin is synthesized in a large precursor form as proinsulin provided the impetus for further studies, which have shown that this is a common mode of biosynthesis of eukaryotic peptides destined for secretion. The studies on proinsulin offer a useful intellectual and experimental paradigm. Proinsulin is a single polypeptide chain ordered as follows: NH_2-(B-chain)-Arg-Arg-(C-peptide)-Lys-Arg-(A-chain)-COOH. The presumed function of the C peptide is to ensure the correct folding and sulfhydryl oxidation between the A and B chains in proinsulin. The higher rate (15 times) of mutation in the C peptide than in the insulin moiety suggests that the C peptide may not have a physiological function; however, immunoassay of C peptide may be a useful differential diagnostic procedure for hypoglycemia.

The transformation of proinsulin to insulin in the β-cells appears to take place in the secretory granule and involves proteolytic cleavage by an endopeptidase followed by removal of C-terminal basic amino acid residues by an exopeptidase. The half-time of conversion is about 1 hr. The insulin is maintained in the granule in a crystalline form (in combination with zinc). This system leads to several important generalizations: (a) peptide hormones can be synthesized in larger precursor forms (i.e., as prohormones); (b) post-translational processing of the prohormone occurs in the secretory granule; and (c) peptides other than the known biologically active one(s) will emerge from this biosynthetic mechanism, and, if processing occurs intragranularly, all will be released simultaneously by the cell.

The intracellular compartmentation [20] following synthesis of the protein on the rough endoplasmic reticulum (RER) is determined, in part, by the translocational process itself. The initial N-terminal amino acid sequence of the protein serves as a signal for the protein to traverse the RER membrane and enter the cisternae, where the signal sequence is immediately cleaved off. Similar signal sequences exist for secreted proteins and some intrinsic membrane proteins (see Chap. 24). The prohormone, plus its transient N-terminal sequence, which usually contains 20 to 30 amino acids, is referred to as a preprohormone.

Peptide biosynthesis in neurons also involves propeptide precursors

The first hypothesis for the existence of a prohormone came from studies on the nervous system. In 1964, Sacks and Takabatake hypothesized that vasopressin, a nonapeptide, and neurophysin, a protein of about 10,000 M_r, were formed by post-translational processing of a common precursor protein. Two precursors of neurophysin (~20,000 M_r each), one associated with vasopressin synthesis and the other with oxytocin synthesis, were identified in pulse-chase and immunoprecipitation experiments on the rat hypothalamoneurohypophysial system [21], and, subsequently, DNAs complementary to the RNAs that encode the precursors were isolated [22].

Neuropeptide precursors appear to be processed in much the same way as insulin. Sulfhydryl oxidation and proximal glycosyla-

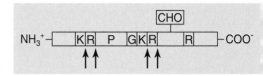

FIG. 5.   A general peptide precursor.

tion take place in the RER cisternum. In the Golgi apparatus, they are further glycosylated and sorted into secretory granules. In the granule, the precursors come in contact with a variety of peptidases and with enzymes that add functional groups to specific amino acids.

A general peptide precursor is depicted in Fig. 5. This propeptide has already had its signal sequence removed. It has two pairs of basic residues: lysine (K) and arginine (R). As is true for insulin, the first step in processing such a protein is cleavage at the paired basic amino acids by an endopeptidase. The cleavage can occur between the two amino acids or on the C-terminal side of the pair (arrows). In the former case, basic residues are left attached to both the N terminus and the C terminus of the peptide P. Trimming enzymes are required to remove these appendages—a basic-residue-specific aminopeptidase and a basic-residue-specific carboxypeptidase, called carboxypeptidase H, and referred to above.

Note that the precursor in Fig. 5 has a single arginine (R) residue. Some precursors (e.g., that of vasopressin) are cleaved at single basic residues. The enzyme(s) responsible for this are thought to be different from the paired-base-specific endopeptidases. The converting endopeptidases have proven to be difficult to isolate and characterize. A large number of candidate proteases were partially purified, but it was difficult to demonstrate that any one of them played an important role *in vivo*. This is no longer the case, however. Following the discovery of KEX2, a paired-base-specific endoprotease involved in peptide precursor processing in yeast, similar proteases were found in mammalian cells. KEX2 and its mammalian coun-

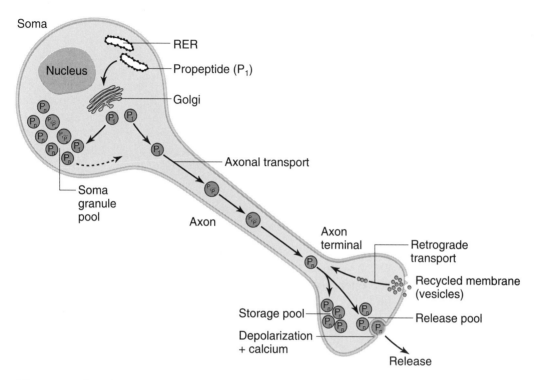

FIG. 6. Hypothetical model of biosynthesis, translocation, processing, and release of peptides in a peptidergic neuron. (RER) rough endoplasmic reticulum; (P_1) propeptide or precursor molecule; ($P_1 \cdots P_n$) intermediates between P_1 and P_n; (P_n) final peptide product of processing. (From Gainer et al. [32].)

terparts, PC2 and PC3, have been shown to cleave a number of peptide precursors *in vitro*. In addition, PC2 and PC3 are found in a number of peptide-producing cells. These proteins are unlikely to be the only processing proteases, however. Additional enzymes should be isolated in the future. It is also worth noting that peptide precursors are not the only substrates for these enzymes. For example, it is evident from its primary structure that the carboxypeptidase H translation product can undergo proteolytic processing.

The glycine (G) just N-terminal to the second KR pair in the precursor is required for peptide P to be amidated. The amidating enzyme, propeptide amidating monooxygenase, requires molecular oxygen, ascorbic acid, and Cu^{2+}. The glycine will donate its amino group to the amino acid that precedes it.

A number of other enzymes may act to modify peptides. α-MSH and β-endorphin both undergo *N*-acetylation; cholecystokinin and gastrin are tyrosine sulfated. In theory, peptides can also be carboxymethylated or phosphorylated.

Since precursor processing appears to take place in the secretory granules during axonal transport, one would expect all of the products generated from a precursor protein to be released during stimulus-induced exocytosis. A hypothetical model of the peptidergic neuron is illustrated in Fig. 6.

SECRETION OF NEUROPEPTIDES

The neuropeptide secretion mechanism appears to be similar to that of conventional neurotransmitter secretion [23]. The principal events in the release of neuropeptides occur as follows: The propagated action potential depolarizes the nerve terminal and induces an influx of Ca^{2+}, which produces exocytosis and extrusion of secretory granule (or vesicle) contents into the extracellular space. The dependence of the stimulus-secretion coupling on extracellular Ca^{2+} is well established [24], and various morphological features of the exocytotic process have been visualized in freeze-fracture studies. Retrieval of the granule membranes after exocytosis is in large vacuoles [25], but, in contrast to cholinergic terminals, where recycling of vesicle membrane occurs (Chap. 11), little is known at present about the fates of the retrieved peptidergic granule membranes.

Peptide secretion from nerve terminals depends on Ca^{2+} entry during depolarization

This feature of the basic mechanism has been used as a criterion for the physiological relevance of stimulation-induced release of peptides from a variety of experimental preparations. The release experiments are usually performed on either thin tissue slices, or blocks, or on synaptosomes, isolated nerve endings, prepared from a specific brain area incubated in a well-oxygenated physiological medium. After an initial washing of the tissue by repeated changes of medium, a stimulus is applied. The stimulus may be field electrical stimulation, depolarization by an excess of K^+, or the addition of veratridine (Na^+ channel activation) to the medium. In all cases, removal of Ca^{2+} from the medium should prevent secretion of the peptides. In some cases, the membrane depolarization step is bypassed by direct application of a Ca^{2+} ionophore (e.g., A23187), which causes an increase in intracellular Ca^{2+} and thus induces exocytosis. Release experiments can also be done in the intact animal either by using push-pull cannulas in specific brain regions [26] or by monitoring the cerebrospinal fluid for peptide release after specific brain areas have been stimulated.

Recently, another method has been developed to detect peptide release *in vivo*. It involves implanting antibody-coated "microprobes" into specific areas of the brain for short periods of time. The probes are then removed and placed in a solution of radiolabeled peptide. The latter will only bind to regions of the probe to which peptide has not already bound *in vivo*. Binding of labeled peptide is detected autoradiographically. The method is invasive, but it does little damage to the tissue studied.

Peptidergic neurosecretory cells tend to fire in bursts, with each burst followed by inactivity

This temporal pattern of release *in vivo*, although poorly understood, is significant; it suggests that periodicity is important for sustained secretory activity in these cells. Periodicity may also be important to the target organ; this has been elegantly demonstrated in a study in which monkeys with hypothalamic lesions that abolish LH and FSH release by the pituitary were infused with GnRH. Infusion of GnRH failed to restore LH and FSH secretion, whereas once-hourly infusion of GnRH re-established normal hormone release. Thus, the cyclic pattern of GnRH delivery to the target organ was more important than the amount delivered. The intermittent delivery may avoid down-regulation or desensitization of the GnRH receptors in the target tissue.

INACTIVATION MECHANISMS

The time course and extent of neurotransmitter action are determined, in part, by the mechanisms involved in the reduction of the neurotransmitter concentration around the receptor. This can occur by diffusion of the substance away from the receptor; by reuptake by the presynaptic terminals or surrounding glia, or both; or by enzymatic degradation of the substance (see Chap. 9). So far there have been no convincing data to indicate that reuptake of neuropeptides akes place, and enzymatic degradation appears to be the principal mechanism for inactivation of neuropeptides.

In general, proteolytic enzymes are described as either exopeptidases or endopeptidases (proteinases). Exopeptidases hydrolyze peptides from either their C- or N-terminal regions by removal of single amino acids (or dipeptides). Endopeptidases cleave internal bonds of proteins and peptides. They often show specificity with regard to the nature of the peptide bond (e.g., trypsin hydrolyzes exclusively at basic amino acid [lysine and arginine] residues) but rarely are specific to only one substrate. The probable reason is that the specificity of limited proteolysis is determined by the three-dimensional structure (conformation) of the peptide substrate and of the protease [27]. The substrate region containing the susceptible peptide bond must match the active site of the enzyme for hydrolysis to occur. Thus, proteases may degrade diverse substrates with conformational homologies.

Keeping the above caveats about protease specificity in mind, it is worth noting that enzymes that show selective degradation of biologically active peptides have been found in various tissues, including brain. Many neuropeptides have groups blocked by N-terminal acetylation, C-terminal amidation, or addition of N-terminal pyroglutamate. These prevent the action of exopeptidases. Therefore, relatively specific endopeptidases are involved in their degradation.

PEPTIDE RECEPTORS

Biological effects are correlated with binding measurements

A great deal can be learned about the affinity and specificity of a biological receptor for its natural ligand by means of dose-response measurements either in the whole animal or in isolated organs *in vitro*. Alternatively, binding of radiolabeled agonists or antagonists

TABLE 5. Characteristics of ligand-receptor interactions

BIOLOGICAL ACTIVITY

The labeled ligand should have the same biological potency as its unlabeled parent compound

HIGH AFFINITY

Concentrations of ligand as low as those that are biologically effective should specifically bind to receptors

REVERSIBILITY

Agonists with rapidly reversible biological actions should dissociate rapidly from their binding sites

STRUCTURAL OR STERIC SPECIFICITY

Binding of a labeled ligand and displacement of this ligand by other agonists or antagonists should quantitatively reflect the biological potencies of the agonists and antagonists treated

SATURABILITY

A biologically relevant concentration of ligand should saturate specific binding sites

to whole cells, suspension of plasma membranes, or solubilized membrane components can be studied. The latter is fast, relatively simple to perform, and serves as a first step in receptor purification. It must be undertaken cautiously, however, because not all binding is to biologically relevant sites (i.e., receptors). Several criteria must be satisfied to establish that the interaction of a ligand with any given preparation represents binding to a receptor (Table 5) (see also Chap. 10 for detailed discussions of receptor quantification).

Whenever possible, quantitative comparisons between binding and biological effects should be made. The activation of a ligand-dependent, membrane-localized enzyme, such as adenyl cyclase, might be measured at the same time that binding is determined. Similar sets of parallel measurements can sometimes be made on isolated membrane preparations, but there is no guarantee that ligand-induced modulation of enzyme activity will be the same in the intact cell as in an isolated membrane.

Intact homogeneous populations of cells cannot easily be obtained from the brain for direct comparisons of binding and biological activity. Nevertheless, it is possible to compare binding of a variety of agonists and antagonists and, in this way, to determine the structural specificity of binding sites in the central nervous system. Thus, most of the criteria listed in Table 5 can be met. To the extent that cells or membranes harvested from the central nervous system are heterogeneous, though, little can be learned by comparing the properties of receptors of various brain regions. Meaningful comparisons of this sort can be made only by isolating purified populations of plasma membranes from cells and measuring the number of receptors per milligram of membrane (see Chap. 10).

Biologically active peptides can be labeled and used in binding studies

Common problems encountered in studies of peptide receptors have included (a) difficulties in labeling the peptide: iodinated peptides may be inactive and tritiation may prove difficult or may yield a product with too low a specific activity; and (b) enzymatic degradation of the labeled peptide.

Insulin, for example, can be iodinated without losing its biological activity, and its degradation by peptidases in membrane preparations can be inhibited by bacitracin [28]. Although the density of insulin receptors on cells is low, specific binding of insulin to cells and membranes can be detected by using radioiodinated insulin (1,000 Ci/mmol). It would be difficult, if not impossible, to study insulin binding by using a tritiated ligand; but tritiated ligands have been used successfully to study other classes of receptors, among them the receptors for the opioid peptides (Chap. 15). The latter are unique in that they can be occupied by members of a large group of well-characterized nonpeptide agonists and antagonists. Labeled antagonists with high affinities for the opiate receptor and with conveniently long receptor-antagonist half-lives have been used in lieu of the peptides to study binding sites in the brain and elsewhere.

Agonists and antagonists have been synthesized that are resistant to peptidase action. These should prove to be useful ligands for binding studies of the receptors and receptor purification by affinity chromatography.

RECEPTOR CLONING

Complementary DNAs encoding several neuropeptide receptors have now been isolated (Table 6, and see ref. 29). With the exception of the receptors for ANP and the VIP-related peptides, all of these have been members of a single G protein-coupled receptor superfamily. They have seven hydrophobic membrane-spanning domains, sites

TABLE 6.   Cloned G protein-coupled peptide receptors

Adrenocorticotropic hormone
Angiotensin II
Bradykinin
Bombesin
Calcitonin
Endothelin
Follicle-stimulating hormone
Gastrin
Growth hormone-releasing hormone
Interleukin 8
Leuteinzing hormone/chorionic gonadotropin
Melanocyte-stimulating hormone
Neuromedin K
Neuropeptide Y
Opiate
Oxytocin
Peptide YY
Parathyroid hormone
Somatostatin
Substance K
Substance P
Thrombin
Thyrotropin-releasing hormone
Thyroid-stimulating hormone
Vasopressin
Vasoactive intestinal peptide

for glycosylation on their extracellular N termini, and sites for phosphorylation by regulatory kinases. To date, no peptide except *N*-acetylAspGlu has been found to act through a ligand-gated ion channel type receptor, but there is reason to believe that such peptide receptors exist.

Many neuropeptide receptor cDNAs have been isolated by expression cloning. The first such cDNA encoded the substance K receptor. *Xenopus* oocytes were used for these experiments. When RNA is injected into this cell, it is translated efficiently. RNA encoding a receptor that mediates an increase in intracellular Ca^{2+} can be detected electrophysiologically after applying ligand to oocytes two to three days after injecting RNA. Alternatively, efflux of radiolabeled calcium or Ca^{2+}-induced light production by aequorin can be used to detect the presence of receptors.

Initially, a library is prepared in a vector that has a phage promoter (T7, T3, or SP6) upstream of the cDNA. This allows mRNA to be produced *in vitro* using the cDNA as a template. Progressively smaller sublibraries are screened; ultimately, a single clone is obtained.

Other expression cloning techniques have been used successfully in the last few years. DNA prepared from sublibraries has been transfected into mammalian cell lines, and the expressed receptors have been detected by means of autoradiography or binding assays. This usually requires the use of an iodinated ligand.

After one member of a receptor family has been cloned, additional members can sometimes be cloned by screening cDNA or genomic libraries with probes based on the structure of the first cDNA. This was true of the vasopressin receptors. The first of these, the V1a subtype, was cloned by means of expression in *Xenopus* oocytes. Subsequently, the V1b and V2 subtypes were cloned based on their similarities to the V1a receptor. The V1a and V1b receptors mediate an increase in intracellular Ca^{2+}; stimulation of the V2 receptor results in increases in cAMP. The V1a receptor is found in very high levels in the rat liver where it stimulates glycogenolysis and regeneration following injury. It is also found in specific populations of cells in the central nervous system. The V1b receptor is present on the membranes of ACTH-producing cells in the anterior pituitary, and the V2 receptor is present in the kidney where it mediates the antidiuretic actions of vasopressin. The vasopressin receptors are much more similar to one another than they are to any of the other members of the G protein-coupled receptor superfamily, except for the oxytocin receptor. This is not surprising, because vasopressin and oxytocin are very similar in structure.

The above description of vasopressin receptors shows that, just as there are multiple muscarinic, noradrenergic, and dopaminergic receptor subtypes, there are multiple receptors for some of the biologically active peptides. These should react with specific agonists and antagonists, and they stimulate different second-messenger responses—presumably by interacting with different G proteins—in different tissues. They provide a new opportunity to develop useful pharmaceutical agents. This is not the only clinically important outcome of receptor cloning, however. The V2 receptor has been shown to be defective in a rare inherited disorder, X-linked nephrogenic diabetes insipidus. The urine of people with this problem does not concentrate in response to vasopressin. Therefore, they have to drink more water than others or face rapid dehydration, fever, and even coma. The disorder can now be diagnosed prenatally or perinatally.

PEPTIDES AND NEURONAL FUNCTION

Hypothalamic peptides are physiologically important messages in the regulation of the anterior pituitary by brain, but the situation for the rest of the brain is less clear. Extensive pharmacological evidence suggests that there are a variety of peptide receptors in extrahypothalamic areas. In addition, expo-

TABLE 7.   Potential sites and mechanisms of neuropeptide action

---

Acts as a conventional neurotransmitter in a synaptic pathway

Influences a synaptic pathway by its presynaptic action
    Affects amount and time course of transmitter release
    Affects transmitter reuptake at synapse
    Alters "releasable" and "nonreleasable" transmitter pools
    Affects transmitter biosynthesis

Influences a synaptic pathway by its postsynaptic action on receptor
    Alters receptor sensitivity
    Affects receptor-ionophore coupling
        Kinetics
        Specific ionic conductances

Influences a synaptic pathway by its effects on electrogenesis
    Change in electrically excitable membrane properties
        Resting conductance
        Spike threshold
        Intracellular electrical resistance (length constant)
        Current-voltage relations of membrane
        Coupling resistance at electrotonic junctions
        Alters electrogenic pump activity
    Excitation-coupled phenomena
        Muscle contraction
        Metabolic processes

---

sure of the nervous system to specific peptides often produces profound changes in the biochemistry and physiology of the nervous system as well as specific modifications of behavior (Table 7). Immunocytochemical procedures can demonstrate that neurons containing biologically active peptides are distributed throughout the brain. Nevertheless, it is still not possible to state whether peptides play a unique role in neuronal function.

Can neuropeptides act as neurotransmitters?

The work on invertebrate peptides proves that they can. Although the criteria for the identification of a neurotransmitter are well established (Chap. 9), it is often difficult to satisfy them in any specific case. Thus, although substance P fulfilled many of the desiderata of a candidate for primary afferent

transmitter, its time course of action was too slow in comparison with natural afferent activity, and hence its candidacy as the primary afferent transmitter was not credible. However, substance P might be associated specifically with slow-conducting fibers in pain pathways [30]. The point is that, unless the neuronal circuit in which the peptide may be involved is understood and amenable to experimental analysis, it is extremely difficult to evaluate the status of any putative transmitter. Peptides often seem to serve as neuromodulators, i.e., they affect the responses elicited by other agents. It should be apparent that the criteria for identification of neuromodulators are identical to those of neurotransmitters and that the use of the term does not obviate the necessity for rigorous analysis of the mechanisms of action of the substance in question.

Neurochemists are as excited about neuropeptides as they were about monoamines in the early 1960s. This is in part because the peptides are so potent biologically and in part because they are present in discrete systems of neurons. Undoubtedly many peptides remain to be discovered and characterized. In fact, the number of peptides two to ten amino acids long that might theoretically exist is astronomical ($>10^{13}$). There are 10^{10} neurons in the human brain, so it is possible, although unlikely, that each neuron makes its own unique peptide.

REFERENCES

1. Scharrer, B. Peptidergic neurons: Facts and trends. *Gen. Comp. Endocrinol.* 34:50–62, 1978.
2. Fink, G. The development of the releasing factor concept. *Clin. Endocrinol.* 5(Suppl.): 245s–260s, 1976.
3. Guillemin, R. Peptides in the brain: The new endocrinology of the neuron. *Science* 202: 390–402, 1978.
4. Mains, R. E., Eipper, B. A., and Ling, N. Common precursor to corticotropins and endorphins. *Proc. Natl. Acad. Sci. U. S. A.* 74: 3014–3018, 1977.

5. Green, J. D., and Harris, G. W. The neurovascular link between the neurohypophysis and adenohypophysis. *J. Endocrinol.* 5:136–146, 1947.

6. Lightman, S. L., and Everitt, B. J. (eds.), *Neuroendocrinology.* Boston: Blackwell, 1986.

7. Leeman, S. E., Mroz, E. A., and Carraway, R. Substance P and neurotensin. In H. Gainer (ed.), *Peptides in Neurobiology.* New York: Plenum, 1977, pp. 99–144.

8. Marshak, D. R., and Fraser, B. A. Structural analysis of brain peptides. In J. B. Martin, M. J. Brownstein, and D. T. Krieger (eds.), *Brain Peptides Update.* New York: Wiley, 1987, pp. 9–36.

9. Tatemoto, K., and Mutt, V. Isolation of two novel candidate hormones using a chemical method for finding naturally occurring polypeptides. *Nature* 285:417–418, 1980.

10. Koller, K. J., and Brownstein, M. J. Use of a cDNA clone to identify a supposed precursor protein containing valocin. *Nature* 325:542–545, 1987.

11. Rosenfeld, M. G., Mermod, J.-J., Amara, S. G., Swanson, L. W., Sawchenko, P. E., et al. Production of a novel neuropeptide encoded by the calcitonin gene via tissue-specific RNA processing. *Nature* 304:129–135, 1983.

12. Yalow, R. S. Radioimmunoassay: A probe for the fine structure of biological systems. *Science* 200:1236–1242, 1978.

13. Swaab, D. F., Pool, C. W., and Van Leeuwen, F. W. Can specificity ever be proved in immunocytochemical staining? *J. Histochem. Cytochem.* 25:388–389, 1977.

14. Siegel, R. E. *In situ* hybridization histochemistry. In J. B. Martin, M. J. Brownstein, and D. T. Krieger (eds.), *Brain Peptides Update.* New York: Wiley, 1987, pp. 81–100.

15. Björklund, A., and Hökfelt, T. (eds.), *Handbook of Chemical Neuroanatomy.* New York: Elsevier, Vol. 4, 1985.

16. Martin, J. B., Brownstein, M. J., and Krieger, D. T. (eds.), *Brain Peptides Update.* New York: Wiley, 1987.

17. Iverson, L. L., Iverson, S. D., and Snyder, S. H. (eds.), *Handbook of Psychopharmacology. Neuropeptides.* New York: Plenum, Vol. 16, 1983.

18. Hökfelt, T., Fuxe, K., and Pernow, B. *Coexistence of Neuronal Messengers: A New Principle in Chemical Transmission.* (Progress in Brain Research, Vol. 68.) New York: Elsevier, 1986.

19. Steiner, D. F., and Dyer, P. E. The biosynthesis of insulin and a probable precursor of insulin by a human islet cell adenoma. *Proc. Natl. Acad. Sci. U. S. A.* 57:473–480, 1967.

20. Palade, G. Intracellular aspects of the process of protein synthesis. *Science* 189:347–358, 1975.

21. Russell, J. T., Brownstein, M. J., and Gainer, H. Biosynthesis of vasopressin, oxytocin, and neurophysins: Isolation and characterization of two common precursors (propressophysin and prooxyphysin). *Endocrinology* 107:1880–1891, 1980.

22. Richter, D., and Ivell, R. Gene organization, biosynthesis, and chemistry of neurohypophysial hormones. In H. Imura (ed.), *The Pituitary Gland. Comprehensive Endocrinology.* New York: Raven, 1985, pp. 127–148.

23. Douglas, W. W. How do neurones secrete peptides? Exocytosis and its consequences, including "synaptic" vesicle formation, in the hypothalamo-neurohypophysial system. *Prog. Brain Res.* 39:21–39, 1973.

24. Thorn, N. A., Russell, J. T., Torp-Pedersen, C., and Treiman, M. Calcium and neurosecretion. *Ann. N.Y. Acad. Sci.* 307:618–639, 1978.

25. Nordman, J. J., and Morris, J. F. Membrane retrieval at neurosecretory axon endings. *Nature* 261:723–725, 1976.

26. Gaddum, J. H. Push-pull cannulae. *J. Physiol. (Lond)* 155:1–2, 1961.

27. Neurath, H., and Walsh, K. A. Role of proteolytic enzymes in biological regulation (a review). *Proc. Natl. Acad. Sci. U. S. A.* 73:3825–3832, 1976.

28. Cuatrecasas, P. Insulin receptor of liver and fat cell membranes. *Fed. Proc.* 32:1838–1846, 1973.

29. Seeman, P. *Receptor Tables. Vol. 1: Receptor Amino Acid Sequences of G-Linked Receptors.* Toronto: University of Toronto, 1992.

30. Collu, R., et al. (eds.), *Central Nervous System Effects of Hypothalamic Hormones and Other Peptides.* New York: Raven, 1979.

31. Koller, K. J., Wolff, R. S., Warden, M. K., and Zoeller, R. T. Thyroid hormones regulate levels of thyrotropin-releasing-hormone mRNA in the paraventricular nucleus. *Proc. Natl. Acad. Sci. U. S. A.* 84:7329–7333, 1987.

32. Gainer, H., Sarne, Y., and Brownstein, M. J. *J. Cell Biol.* 73:366–381, 1977.

33. Harris, G. W. Humours and hormones. The Sir Henry Dale Lecture of 1971. *J. Endocrinol.* 53:ii–xii, 1972.

CHAPTER 17

Excitatory Amino Acid Transmitters

RAYMOND DINGLEDINE AND CHRIS J. MCBAIN

Basic Neurochemistry: Molecular, Cellular, and Medical Aspects, 5th Ed., edited by G. J. Siegel et al. Published by Raven Press, Ltd., New York, 1994. Correspondence to Raymond Dingledine, Department of Pharmacology, University of North Carolina, CB 7365, Faculty Laboratory Office Building, Room 1106, Chapel Hill, North Carolina 27599.

The amino acids glutamate and aspartate, and perhaps certain of their analogs, mediate most of the excitatory synaptic transmission in the brain. The realization that glutamatergic pathways are involved in such diverse processes as epilepsy, ischemic brain damage, and learning, and that they influence the development of normal synaptic connections in the brain, is of great practical interest. Studies of the functions of excitatory amino acid receptors were dominated by electrophysiological approaches until molecular cloning revealed the sequences of an increasingly heterogeneous family of receptors. Thus, the neurochemistry and protein chemistry of these receptors and their transmitters are resurfacing as major research thrusts.

In the rest of this chapter we follow the practice of naming this family of receptors after one of their prominent neurotransmitter agonists and so use the term "glutamate receptor" to refer to all excitatory amino acid receptors. A series of reviews covering the pharmacology, physiology, molecular biology, and neuropathological involvement of glutamate receptors [1–3] provides a worthwhile supplement to the material presented in this chapter.

THREE FUNCTIONAL CLASSES OF IONOTROPIC GLUTAMATE RECEPTOR

Most glutamate receptors are ionotropic; i.e., the agonist binding sites and associated ion channel are incorporated into the same macromolecular complex. Agonists act to increase the probability that the channel will open. The N-methyl-D-aspartate (NMDA), α-amino-3-hydroxy-5-methyl-4-isoxazole-propionic acid (AMPA), and kainate (KA) classes of glutamate receptor are members of the superfamily of *ligand-gated ion channels*, which include the nicotinic acetylcholine receptors, γ-aminobutyric acid$_A$ (GABA$_A$) receptors, inhibitory glycine receptors, and 5-hydroxytryptamine$_3$ (5-HT$_3$) receptors, among others. The aminocyclopentyl dicarboxylic acid (ACPD) and L-2-amino-4-phosphonopropionic acid (L-AP4) subtypes of glutamate receptor, in contrast, are coupled through G proteins to intracellular effectors, similar to the muscarinic acetylcholine, GABA$_B$, and β-adrenergic receptors.

NMDA receptors have multiple regulatory sites

The NMDA receptor is one of the most tightly regulated neurotransmitter receptors. There are no fewer than five distinct binding sites for endogenous ligands that influence the probability of ion channel opening (Fig. 1). These consist of two different agonist recognition sites (for glutamate and glycine) and a polyamine regulatory site that promote receptor activation, and separate recognition sites for Mg^{2+} and Zn^{2+} that act to inhibit ion flux through agonist-bound receptors.

NMDA receptor agonists are typically short-chain dicarboxylic amino acids such as glutamate, aspartate, and NMDA. Acting at the conventional agonist binding site, glutamate is the most potent agonist endogenous to the mammalian brain, followed (in order

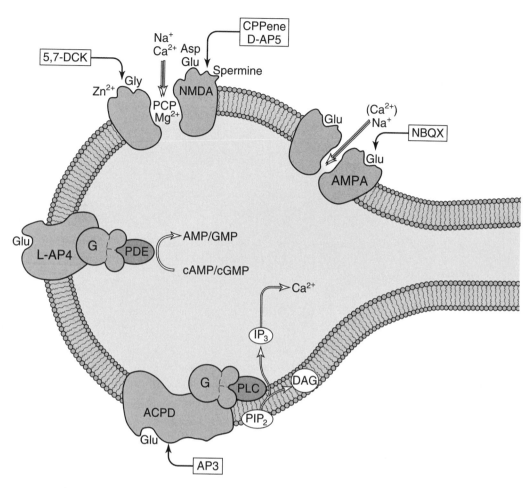

FIG. 1. Molecular views of four types of glutamate receptors. Two heteromeric ionotropic receptors are shown, the NMDA and AMPA receptors, and two metabotropic receptors, the L-AP4 and ACPD receptors. Competitive antagonists of each receptor are boxed. The NMDA receptor channel is additionally blocked by Mg^{2+} and phencyclidine (PCP). Zn^{2+} is a negative modulator, and polyamines such as spermine are positive modulators, of NMDA channel activation. Both L-AP4 and ACPD receptors are metabotropic in that they are coupled via G proteins (G) to intracellular enzymes, phospholipase C (PLC) for the ACPD receptor, and phosphodiesterase (PDE) for the L-AP4 receptor. Phospholipase C catalyzes the production of inositol 1,4,5-trisphosphate (IP_3) and diacylglycerol (DAG) from phosphatidylinositol 4,5-bisphosphate (PIP_2). The resulting increase in cytoplasmic IP_3 triggers release of Ca^{2+} from intracellular stores.

of potency) by L-homocysteate, aspartate, cysteinesulfinate, and quinolinate [4]. NMDA itself, although a very selective agonist at these receptors, is 30-fold less potent than glutamate in electrophysiological assays.

Competitive antagonists of NMDA receptors can be formed from the corresponding agonists by extending the carbon chain, sometimes in a ring structure. The following structural features often increase the potency of these compounds as antagonists: selection of the D-enantiomer, replacement of the ω-carboxyl group with a phosphonic acid group, and incorporation of an unsaturated bond in the carbon chain. Numerous competitive antagonists of this recognition site are available, and include D-2-amino-5-phosphonopentanoic acid (D-AP5) and 3-(2-carboxypiperazin-4-yl)1-propenyl-1-phosphonic acid (2R-CPPene), the latter having a K_d of approximately 40 nM in binding and functional studies. These compounds are polar and penetrate the blood-brain barrier only poorly, although recently several NMDA receptor blockers have been developed that have good access to the brain from the blood.

The NMDA receptor is unique among all known neurotransmitter receptors in its requirement for the simultaneous binding of two different agonists for activation. In addition to the conventional agonist binding site typically occupied by glutamate, the binding of glycine appears to be required for receptor activation [5]. This finding went unnoticed for many years because glycine is a contaminant of most laboratory solutions in a concentration high enough (>50 nM) to occupy a substantial fraction of its binding sites on the NMDA receptor. Because neither glycine nor glutamate acting alone can open this ion channel, they are referred to as "co-agonists" of the NMDA receptor [5]. The glycine site on the NMDA receptor is pharmacologically distinct from the classical inhibitory glycine receptor (see Chap. 18) in that it is not blocked by strychnine and is not activated by β-alanine. Several small analogs of glycine, including serine and alanine, can act as agonists at this site. In both cases the D-isomer is 20- to 30-fold more potent than the L-isomer. Bicyclic compounds and derivatives of either kynurenic acid or quinoxalinedicarboxylic acid are competitive antagonists of the glycine site. Interestingly, most glycine site antagonists in these two series also block competitively the agonist recognition site of AMPA receptors (see below), suggesting possible structural similarities in the two ligand recognition sites. Halogenation of both ring structures typically induces a large increase in potency, with 5,7-dichlorokynurenic acid (5,7-DCK) being a very potent (K_d = 60 nM) and highly selective glycine-site antagonist.

One or more modulatory sites that bind polyamines such as spermine and spermi-dine are also found on NMDA receptors. Occupancy of the polyamine site does not appear to be required for receptor activation, but in low micromolar concentrations these polyamines increase the ability of glutamate and glycine to open ion channels [6]. The positive modulatory action is achieved by increasing the frequency of opening of individual receptor channels [7]. At higher concentrations, however, polyamines produce a voltage-dependent block of the ion channel and thus inhibit receptor activation [7]. Interestingly, although polyamines such as spermine and spermidine are synthesized intracellularly, the rapid time course of polyamine action suggests that their binding site faces the extracellular fluid. Whereas some naturally occurring polyamines such as spermine and spermidine are "agonists" at the positive modulatory polyamine site, certain triamines such as diethylenetriamine can block the action of the agonists without themselves exerting any effect on glutamate or glycine; such compounds are antagonists of the polyamine site.

Thus, glutamate, glycine, and certain polyamines act in concert to open NMDA ion channels. In contrast, a very important brake on NMDA receptor activation is provided by extracellular Mg^{2+}, which exerts a voltage-dependent block of the open ion channel [8]. Other voltage-dependent blockers of NMDA receptor channels include MK-801, the anesthetic ketamine, and the recreational drug of abuse phencyclidine (PCP). These blockers (and Mg^{2+}) exhibit varying degrees of voltage dependence and therefore probably recognize somewhat different domains in the channel of the NMDA receptor.

Another endogenous blocker of the NMDA receptor is Zn^{2+}, but in contrast to Mg^{2+} the block by extracellular Zn^{2+} is nearly independent of voltage. Therefore, Zn^{2+} and Mg^{2+} must also bind to separate sites on NMDA receptors. Several glutamatergic pathways in the brain concentrate Zn^{2+} and release it upon stimulation, but the precise role of Zn^{2+} in excitatory synaptic transmission mediated by NMDA receptors is unknown.

In addition to the regulatory mechanisms discussed above, the ability of glutamate and glycine to activate NMDA receptors is greatly influenced by extracellular pH and the state of phosphorylation of the receptor. The more alkaline the pH, in the range of 6.8 to 8.4, the higher the channel opening frequency in the presence of given concentrations of agonists [9]. This suggests that an ionizable histidine in the NMDA receptor may play a role in receptor activation. In another modulatory process, a slow loss of the ability of even high concentrations of agonists to activate NMDA receptors in excised membrane patches from central neurons could be countered by the inclusion of an ATP-regenerating system in the solution bathing the cytoplasmic face of the membrane [10]. Phosphorylation of one or more key amino acid residues on the NMDA receptor may be necessary for sustained activation.

AMPA receptors are selectively blocked by quinoxalinediones

This second functional class of ionotropic glutamate receptor was historically termed the "quisqualate receptor" but has undergone a name change in recognition of the discovery of metabotropic receptors, which are activated by low concentrations of quisqualate but not AMPA. AMPA receptors are widespread throughout the central nervous system (CNS) and appear to serve as the synaptic receptor for fast excitatory synaptic transmission mediated by glutamate. AMPA receptors can be distinguished from NMDA receptors by selective agonists (AMPA for AMPA receptors and aspartate and NMDA for NMDA receptors). Aspartate apears to be inactive at AMPA receptors. Selective antagonists for AMPA receptors also exist. Certain quinoxalinediones, notably 6-nitro-7-sulphamobenzo[f] quinoxaline-2,3-dione (NBQX), are potent and selective competitive antagonists of AMPA receptors but have a weak or no effect on other receptors. With the probable exception of NBQX, however, most quinoxalinediones have some affinity for the glycine site of NMDA receptors.

Kainate receptors are defined by agonist selectivity

An AMPA- and NMDA-insensitive component of [³H]glutamate binding to brain membranes exists and is potently competed for by the algal toxins kainic and domoic acids. The pharmacological profile of kainate receptors, which can also be specifically labeled by 1 to 10 nM [³H]kainate, differs from that of AMPA receptors in agonist rank order. For kainate receptors studied by radioligand binding, the order of agonist potency is kainate > glutamate > AMPA, whereas for AMPA receptors it is AMPA > glutamate > kainate. Autoradiographic studies reveal a high density of [³H]kainate binding sites at some synapses (see below), making it likely that these receptors have a synaptic function. Unfortunately, selective antagonists of kainate receptors are not yet available, making it difficult to study their physiological role in synaptic transmission.

METABOTROPIC RECEPTORS ARE COUPLED THROUGH G PROTEINS

Metabotropic glutamate receptors are so named because they are linked by G proteins to cytoplasmic enzymes. Metabotropic receptor activation produces, in different cell types, increases in intracellular Ca^{2+} concentration mediated by phosphoinositide hydrolysis, release of arachidonic acid mediated by phospholipase D activation, and increases or decreases in cyclic AMP (cAMP) levels. Excellent recent reviews of the molecular and pharmacological aspects of metabotropic receptors are available [2,3].

L-AP4 receptors are found on retinal bipolar cells

The existence of a metabotropic glutamate receptor can be inferred from the actions of

L-AP4, a γ-phosphonyl derivative of gluta-mate. Although L-AP4 has been shown to prevent glutamate release from presynaptic nerve terminals, the strongest evidence for a distinct L-AP4 receptor is provided by results of studies in the retina, where both L-AP4 and glutamate hyperpolarize a class of reti-nal bipolar neurons. This is unusual since other neurons in the vertebrate CNS are de-polarized by glutamate. The hyperpolariza-tion is brought about by activation of a G protein that appears in turn to activate a phosphodiesterase (see Fig. 1), which hydro-lyzes a cyclic nucleotide that maintains the cation channels in an open state [11]. No selective blockers of L-AP4 receptors are known, nor have the binding sites been con-vincingly radiolabeled.

ACPD activates another class of metabotropic receptor

The L-AP4 receptor described above can be considered a type of metabotropic receptor. Occupancy of another metabotropic recep-tor by an aminocyclopentyl dicarboxylic acid derivative, *trans*-ACPD, or by quisqualate, ibotenate, or glutamate, activates phospholi-pase C to cause the hydrolysis of phosphoino-sitides to inositol 1,4,5-trisphosphate (IP_3), which in turn quickly releases Ca^{2+} from in-tracellular stores (see Fig. 1). Of the above agonists, the most selective by far is *trans*-ACPD, the effects of which are insensitive to blockers of the conventional ionotropic re-ceptors, D-AP5 and NBQX. 2-Amino-3-phos-phonopropionic acid (L-AP3) is a weak an-tagonist of phospholipase C-linked meta-botropic gutamate receptors at some sites.

Metabotropic receptors modulate synaptic ion channels

Metabotropic receptors have now been shown to exert a wide variety of modulating effects on both excitatory and inhibitory syn-aptic transmission, as expected if receptor activation is coupled to multiple effector en-zymes. The closure of Na-selective ion chan-nels in retinal bipolar neurons by glutamate and L-AP4 acting on metabotropic receptors has already been discussed. Many other ef-fects of metabotropic receptors on neuronal excitability have been demonstrated [3]. For example, metabotropic receptor activation closes voltage-dependent K^+ M-channels and Ca^{2+}-dependent K^+ channels in hippocampal neurons, which produces a slow excitation. In cerebellar granule cells, however, metabo-tropic receptors increase the activity of Ca^{2+}-dependent K^+ channels, leading to a reduc-tion in excitability. The second messengers and enzymes responsible for the various ef-fects of metabotropic receptors have not been elucidated. Perhaps the most interest-ing example from an integrative point of view is the finding that in hippocampal pyra-midal cells, metabotropic receptor activation by ACPD potentiates currents through NMDA receptors. This effect is reduced by protein kinase C inhibitors and may there-fore [12] be caused by a reduction in the affinity of the NMDA channel for its blocking ion, Mg^{2+}.

GLUTAMATE AND ASPARTATE ARE THE MAJOR EXCITATORY TRANSMITTERS

Glutamate and aspartate meet many of the criteria of a neurotransmitter

Of the amino acids in the adult CNS, L-gluta-mate and L-aspartate are the most likely can-didates for neurotransmitter action at excita-tory amino acid receptors and are used by some of the most widely distributed neu-ronal types. Glutamate and aspartate are present in high concentrations in the CNS and are released in a Ca^{2+}-dependent man-ner on electrical stimulation *in vitro*. Both have powerful excitatory effects on neurons when iontophoresed *in vivo*. High-affinity uptake systems are located in nerve terminals of many neuronal pathways. Selective binding sites can be demonstrated by both autoradiographic and pharmacological techniques *in vitro.*

The unequivocal identification of glutamate and aspartate as neurotransmitter candidates has been hampered by their involvement in many other functions. For example, glutamate is incorporated into proteins, is involved in fatty acid synthesis, contributes to the regulation of ammonia levels and the control of osmotic and anion balance, and serves as a precursor for GABA (see Chap. 18) and for various Krebs cycle intermediates. It is therefore not surprising that glutamate should be the most abundant amino acid in the CNS. Its concentration is almost six times that of the principal inhibitory neurotransmitter GABA. The transmitter pool of glutamate may constitute approximately 30 percent of the total glutamate concentration in the CNS.

Metabolism of glutamate and aspartate

Glutamate and aspartate are nonessential amino acids that do not cross the blood-brain barrier; therefore, they are not supplied to the brain by the circulation. Instead, they are synthesized from glucose and a variety of other precursors. Synthetic and metabolic enzymes for glutamate and aspartate have been localized to the two main compartments of the brain, neurons and glial cells. The synthesis and metabolism of glutamate and aspartate are more dependent on the interaction between nerve terminals and glial cells than are the synthesis and metabolism of most other groups of neurotransmitters (Fig. 2). Glutamic acid is in a metabolic pool with α-oxoglutaric acid and glutamine. Glutamate is released from nerve terminals and, to a large extent, is taken up into glial cells where it is converted to glutamine. Glutamine is believed to be cycled back to the nerve terminal where it participates in the replenishment of the transmitter pool of glutamate and GABA.

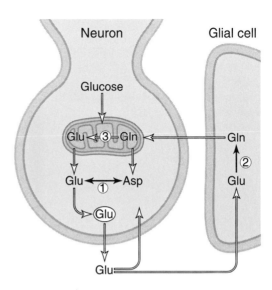

FIG. 2.   Metabolism of glutamate in synaptic structures. Glutamate is synthesized and stored within synaptic endings of the nerve terminal. Synthesis of transmitter pools of glutamate is likely to involve two major synthetic pathways. The conversion of glutamine to glutamate involves the enzymatic action of glutaminase (3) within the mitochondrial compartment. Glutamate formation also occurs by a process of transamination (1). Newly synthesized glutamate is then packaged and stored in high concentration within synaptic vesicles. After release of glutamate from the nerve terminal into the synaptic cleft, it is taken up into glial cells and converted into glutamine (2). Glutamine is then cycled back to the nerve terminal where it participates in the replenishment of transmitter stores of glutamate.

The transmitter pool of glutamate is stored in synaptic vesicles

Synaptic vesicles actively accumulate glutamate through a Mg^{2+}-ATP-dependent process. This uptake mechanism is inhibited by substances that destroy the electrochemical gradient. The concentration of glutamate within synaptic vesicles is thought to be in excess of 20 mM. It has been shown that synaptic vesicles can be stained with a highly specific glutamate antibody, supporting the idea that glutamate acts as a neurotransmitter [13]. Vesicular uptake distinguishes the transmitter pool of glutamate from other pools. Aspartate is neither an inhibitor nor a substrate for this uptake mechanism. A vesicular uptake mechanism for aspartate has not yet been demonstrated, somewhat weakening the case for considering aspartate to be a neurotransmitter.

Glutamate and aspartate are potent neuroexcitants

Historically, the most compelling evidence that glutamate and aspartate function as neurotransmitters has come from the observation that at low concentrations, they excite most cells in the CNS. Under physiological conditions the major role of synaptically released glutamate is to interact with receptors on adjacent cells. Receptor activation opens postsynaptic cation channels, which depolarizes the postsynaptic membrane and increases the likelihood that a postsynaptic cell will fire an action potential. Studies of glutamate and aspartate physiology have revealed that their interactions with receptors is complex and, as stated above, several subtypes of glutamate receptor are known to exist throughout the CNS. Molecular biological approaches (described below) have revealed another level of complexity of these receptors, and it is likely that a multitude of receptor subtypes exist. In functional terms, it is convenient to classify ionotropic glutamate receptors as AMPA- or NMDA-preferring. Both classes of receptors are present on most neurons of the CNS, although there are a few notable exceptions. There is evidence to suggest that on many cell types, AMPA and NMDA receptors are clustered together within the same postsynaptic densities. This close apposition results in the simultaneous activation of these receptors. The integration of current flow through the two receptor systems endows the cell with a powerful means of regulating neuronal excitation.

Activation of AMPA receptors

The interaction of glutamate with AMPA receptors increases the probability that an associated ion channel will open and permit ions to flow through the membrane. Activation of AMPA receptors is thought to underlie the

vast majority of "fast" synaptic transmission in the CNS. The concentration of glutamate required to half-maximally activate these receptors is approximately 15 μM, about three orders of magnitude less than the concentration thought to be contained within synaptic vesicles. Therefore, synaptically released glutamate has a high probability of interacting with its receptor on the adjacent cell. It has already been noted that aspartate has little or no affinity for AMPA receptors.

Current flow through AMPA-activated channels has been shown to occur in discrete conductance states of the channel (see Chap. 4). Glutamate-activated, single-channel currents through AMPA receptors in outside-out patches of cerebellar granule cells have at least four conductance states, ranging in amplitude from 1 to 30 pS [14]. Openings of channels to conductance states greater than 30 pS are infrequent. It remains to be determined, however, which conductance states actually underlie postsynaptic potentials. Activation of AMPA receptors by glutamate (or AMPA) is followed rapidly by desensitization of the receptor; i.e., following exposure to agonist, channels open for only several milliseconds, then abruptly close despite the continued presence of the ligand. The mechanism of desensitization is poorly understood, but this process may control the time course of excitatory postsynaptic potentials (EPSPs) at certain synapses and/or prevent prolonged activation of the receptor.

Ion flow through AMPA receptors

Current flow through AMPA receptors is largely carried by the movement of Na^+ from the extracellular face to the intracellular compartment. Measurement of reversal potential (i.e., the membrane potential at which the driving force for current flow is equal on both membrane faces so the net current flow is zero) indicates a nonspecific increase in permeability to monovalent cations. Since the reversal potential of current flow through this channel is close to 0 mV,

A. AMPA receptors

B. NR1-NMDA receptor

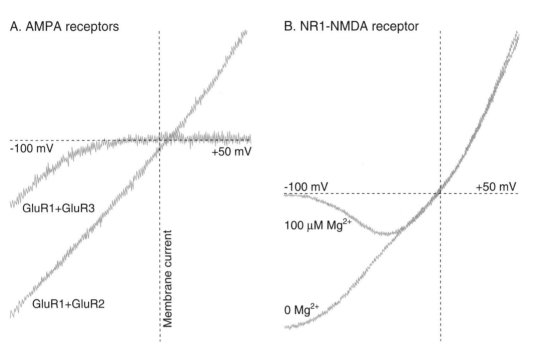

FIG. 3. Current-voltage relationships for AMPA and NMDA receptors. Receptors can be expressed in *Xenopus* oocytes by microinjection of *in vitro*-transcribed RNA encoding various glutamate receptor subunits. Oocytes were voltage-clamped to permit measurement of ionic currents flowing across the plasma membrane following exposure to agonists. In the presence of an agonist, the membrane potential was slowly ramped from −100 mV to +50 mV and the membrane current recorded. The *horizontal dashed line* shows zero membrane current. Although these current-voltage relationships were obtained from recombinant receptors, each of these patterns is found in studies of native glutamate receptors. **A:** Coexpression of GluR1 and GluR3 produces a receptor that exhibits striking inward rectification in that virtually no outward ionic flux is present. Coexpression of GluR1 and GluR2, however, produces a receptor with a nearly linear current-voltage relationship. **B:** Receptors formed from homomeric NR1A subunits exhibit a roughly linear current-voltage relationship in the absence of Mg^{2+}, but in the presence of Mg^{2+}, current flux through NMDA receptor channels becomes progressively smaller as the membrane potential is made more negative. At −100 mV the NMDA-induced current is virtually abolished by Mg^{2+}.

an outward current carried by K^+ must counterbalance the inward flow of Na^+ ions. The current-voltage relationship for these AMPA receptors is roughly linear (GluR1 + GluR2; Fig. 3A, see below). Since Cs^+ can substitute for K^+ in maintaining the reversal potential close to zero, it is likely that these channels do not discriminate well among Na^+, K^+, and Cs^+ [15]. The contribution of anionic currents appears to be negligible at these receptors. It was recently reported that some AMPA receptors on neurons and astrocytes in diverse structures such as the striatum, hippocampus, and cerebellum are permeable to Ca^{2+}. The translocation of Ca^{2+} from

the extracellular space to the intracellular compartment plays a key role in the regulation of a variety of second-messenger systems (see Chap. 20). Therefore, this Ca^{2+} permeability is likely to be of great significance in neuronal excitation by glutamate receptors, particularly in instances where NMDA receptors do not appear to operate. Some AMPA receptor channels that are permeable to Ca^{2+} exhibit a rectifying type of current-voltage relationship (Fig. 3A).

Activation and block of NMDA receptors

NMDA receptors have properties that set them apart from other conventional ligand-gated receptors. At resting membrane potentials (-70 to -50 mV), activation of NMDA receptors results in little current flow. At membrane potentials more negative (hyperpolarized) than about -50 mV, the concentration of Mg^{2+} in the extracellular fluid of the brain is sufficient to virtually abolish ion flux through NMDA receptor channels even in the presence of the coagonists glutamate and glycine. Thus, although glutamate (or aspartate) is bound to the receptive site and the channel "activated," the entry of Mg^{2+} into the channel pore blocks the movement of monovalent ions across the channel. In the presence of Mg^{2+} ions the current-voltage relationship of this receptor has a region of slope negativity, illustrated by a characteristic J-shaped current-voltage relationship (Fig. 3B). As the membrane potential is made less negative or even positive, the affinity of Mg^{2+} for its binding site decreases, and the block becomes ineffective. Depolarization-induced relief from voltage-dependent channel block by Mg^{2+} is at the root of several of the most interesting aspects of NMDA receptor function (see below). The relief of this block causes the resulting current-voltage relationship, like that of most AMPA receptors, to be linear (Fig. 3B).

Patch-clamp and fluctuation analyses have demonstrated that activation of the NMDA receptor channel complex, in a Mg^{2+}-free solution, results in current flow through channels with a predominant conductance of about 50 pS [8,15]. Openings to lower conductance states of 35 and 18 pS have also been found in central neurons. In the presence of low concentrations of extracellular Mg^{2+}, channel behavior is very different at negative holding potentials. The dehydration of Mg^{2+} as it enters the ion channel is apparently so slow that it substantially impedes permeation of Mg^{2+} through the channel. Rather, Mg^{2+} moves in and out of the open channel on a time scale of tens to hundreds of microseconds, giving rise to a "flickery" channel block in single-channel recordings. This blocking action is mimicked by a variety of divalent cations, e.g., Co^{2+},

Mn^{2+}, and Ni^{2+}, but not Zn^{2+}. The potency of block by these divalent cations is correlated with their substitution rate constant for water molecules in the inner hydration shell, suggesting that the slow replacement of water around divalent cations may be a major factor in controlling the permeability of these ions through NMDA receptor channels.

Ion flow through NMDA receptors

Like AMPA receptors, activation of NMDA receptors results in a nonspecific increase in permeability to the monovalent cations Na^+ and K^+. Although activation of NMDA receptors results in appreciable current flow and tends to depolarize the cell membrane toward threshold for action potential firing, this is unlikely to be the primary role of this receptor when activated at typical resting membrane potentials because NMDA receptors are highly permeable to divalent cations. Calcium is about 10-fold more permeable than Na^+. Several other divalent cations are also permeant through the NMDA receptor channel. The permeability sequence of these ions is $Ca^{2+} > Ba^{2+} > Sr^{2+} \gg Mn^{2+}$ [16]. Thus, an important role of NMDA receptors may be to inject Ca^{2+} into the postsynaptic membrane.

Synaptic activation of glutamate receptors

Synaptic release of glutamate results in a two-component excitatory postsynaptic current (EPSC) at most central synapses. There is considerable evidence to suggest that AMPA and NMDA receptors are colocalized at most excitatory synapses. Activation of AMPA receptors mediates a component that has a rapid onset and decay whereas the component mediated by NMDA receptor activation has a slower rise time and a decay component lasting up to several hundred milliseconds (Fig. 4). The decay time of the NMDA receptor component is approximately 100 times longer than the mean open time of the channel. The prolonged activation of NMDA receptors is thought to be due to the high affinity of glutamate, which dissociates slowly

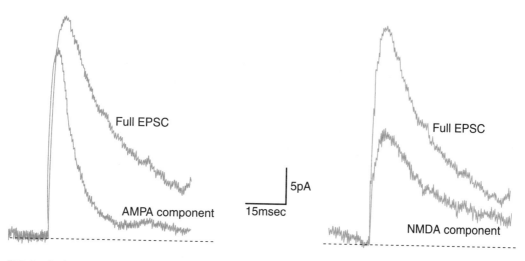

FIG. 4. Excitatory postsynaptic currents (EPSCs) of hippocampal neurons, which are comprised of both AMPA and NMDA receptor components. EPSCs recorded from a neuron in the rat hippocampal slice preparation were voltage-clamped by a patch pipette at a membrane potential of +50 mV. In the *left panel* the EPSC is shown before and after treatment with D-AP5, an NMDA receptor blocker that reveals the component of the EPSC mediated solely by AMPA receptors. Likewise, in the *right panel,* the EPSC is shown in the absence and presence of CNQX, which blocks the AMPA component to isolate the NMDA component. The AMPA component of the full EPSC rises rapidly and is of brief duration. In contrast, NMDA receptor-mediated components rise slowly and contribute to the prolongation of the synaptic event.

from its receptor. In contrast, AMPA receptors have a lower affinity for glutamate, which dissociates rapidly from AMPA receptors. Thus, both AMPA and NMDA components of the EPSC could be produced by a nearly instantaneous rise and fast decay of free transmitter in the synaptic cleft, not unlike that of acetylcholine at the neuromuscular junction. The slower time course of NMDA receptor activation may provide a mechanism by which temporal or spatial summation can occur after a conditioning input. The resulting summed depolarization may allow other synaptic inputs or nonsynaptic membrane channels to initiate action potential firing.

Physiological implications of calcium ion flow through NMDA receptors: synaptic plasticity

The high permeability of NMDA receptor channels for divalent cations has many implications for cell function. Calcium concentration within the cell interior is heavily buff-

ered to about 100 nM. The elevation of cytoplasmic Ca^{2+} by Ca^{2+} entry through NMDA receptor channels may lead to the transient activation of a variety of Ca^{2+}-activated enzymes, including protein kinase C, phospholipase A_2, phospholipase C, Ca^{2+}/calmodulin-dependent protein kinase II, nitric oxide synthase, and a number of endonucleases. Activation of each of these enzymes has been shown to occur as a result of Ca^{2+} entry following amino acid receptor activation.

Long-term potentiation (LTP) is a robust form of synaptic enhancement that can last up to several weeks *in vivo* and is perhaps the best-studied form of synaptic plasticity (see Chap. 50). It is an activity-dependent increase in synaptic efficacy that may underlie some forms of learning and memory in the mammalian brain. At synapses between hippocampal cornu ammonis (CA) 3 and CA1 pyramidal cells, LTP has an absolute requirement for postsynaptic NMDA receptor activation. Only the AMPA receptor component of the EPSP is enhanced, however, since the resulting enhanced EPSC can be blocked by AMPA receptor antagonists but is unaffected by NMDA receptor antagonists. Thus, the NMDA receptor-mediated component is necessary for LTP formation, yet its properties appear to be unchanged by LTP. The precise mechanisms of LTP formation have not been identified, and both pre- and post-synaptic mechanisms have been implicated. The postsynaptic contribution to LTP is reasonably well understood. An NMDA receptor-mediated rise in postsynaptic Ca^{2+} concentration is necessary for LTP. Either NMDA receptor antagonists or injection of a Ca^{2+} chelator into the postsynaptic neuron can block LTP. Secondary activation of several Ca^{2+}-dependent postsynaptic enzymes, including nitric oxide synthase and Ca^{2+}/calmodulin–dependent protein kinase II, has been postulated. A presynaptic component of LTP expression would require retrograde signaling from postsynaptic spines back to presynaptic terminals. One of the short-lasting diffusible gases, nitric oxide or carbon monoxide, may have a role in this process. Postsynaptic Ca^{2+} entry is known to result in the formation of nitric oxide from L-arginine by nitric oxide synthase, a Ca^{2+}/calmodulin-dependent enzyme. Nitric oxide is thought to diffuse out of postsynaptic cells and cross the synaptic cleft, where neurotransmitter release is increased by an unknown mechanism. The extremely short lifetime of nitric oxide and therefore its limited diffusion capabilities make it a good candidate for a synapse-specific retrograde messenger.

MOLECULAR CLONING OF GLUTAMATE RECEPTOR SUBUNITS

Nine families can be defined by structural homologies

The cloning by expression of the first glutamate receptor complementary DNA (cDNA) (GluR1) in late 1989 [17] triggered a predictable frenzy of activity that has already led to the identification of more than 16 genes that encode structurally related proteins. An excellent review of this field is available [2].

All of the subunits of the ionotropic glutamate receptors appear to be similar in topology to those of other ligand-gated ion channels in having four presumptive membrane-spanning domains, although this conclusion currently relies completely on interpretation of hydropathy plots. GluR1 is predicted to be 889 amino acids long, compared to about 480 amino acids for nicotinic, $GABA_A$, or glycine receptor subunits. The extra length in GluR1 is due to an unusually large N-terminal extracellular domain. Currently, seven families of ionotropic glutamate receptor subunits and two metabotropic receptor families have been identified. The structural homologies among the ionotropic subunits are shown in Fig. 5. Within a given family, members show about 80 percent identity at the amino acid level over the ~400 amino acid stretch of membrane-spanning regions. Between families, however, a lower degree of identity exists (50–55 percent or less).

Metabotropic receptor genes

In addition to the ionotropic receptors discussed above, six genes in two structural families of metabotropic receptors (mGluR1–mGluR6) have been identified [2,18], with mGluR1 existing as three splice variants. These genes appear to encode typical seven-membrane-spanning proteins, and like the ionotropic receptors, they possess an unusually large extracellular domain preceding the membrane-spanning segments. Studies with recombinant receptors expressed in *Xenopus* oocytes or mammalian cell lines suggest that mGluR1 and mGluR5 are linked through a G protein to activation of phospholipase C, whereas mGluR2, mGluR3, and mGluR4 inhibit the adenylyl cyclase cascade. mGluR1 and mGluR5 may encode the IP_3-generating metabotropic receptor defined in functional studies (see Fig. 1), but whether mGluR2, mGluR3, and mGluR4 genes encode L-AP4 receptors (see Fig. 1) is a subject for future study. However, functional studies of recombinant metabotropic receptors have necessarily involved expression in non-neuronal cells, and the degree of prom-

Ionotropic gutamate receptors

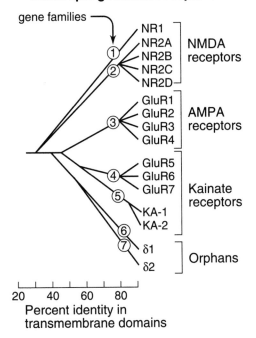

FIG. 5.   Structural relationships among cloned glutamate receptor subunits. The protein sequences were compared within the presumed transmembrane domains and their flanking regions. Each subunit shown is coded by a different gene, and gene families (enumerated for clarity) are formed by subunits that are highly related. For example, the GluR1 through GluR4 subunits form a family since they are about 83 percent identical in amino acid sequence with each other over this region, but only about 50 percent identical with the GluR5 through GluR7 family and even less (about 30 percent) with the NMDA receptor subunits. Functional roles for the two orphan subunits have not yet been defined.

iscuity in G protein coupling between receptor and effector is unknown. One should therefore approach the issue of receptor-effector coupling with some caution. The identity of the G proteins and effectors associated with any of the metabotropic receptor gene products in *neurons* is currently unknown.

Ionotropic glutamate receptors are heteromeric subunit assemblies

Based on analogy with nicotinic acetylcholine receptors, the ligand-gated ion channel receptors are likely to be multimeric assem-blies of individual subunits. Of great significance was the realization that the structural grouping of glutamate receptor subunits also delineated them functionally (see Fig. 5). Advantage has been taken of techniques for expressing functional receptors in *Xenopus* oocytes and in mammalian cells lacking native glutamate receptors. A significant feature of the glutamate receptors is that different subunit combinations produce functionally different receptors; this predicts that a very large family of glutamate receptors may exist in the brain.

GluR1 through GluR4 subunits (also named GluR-A through GluR-D, or in mouse $\alpha1-\alpha4$) coassemble with one another to form proteins with the functional profile of AMPA receptors. Thus, when *Xenopus* oocytes are injected with mixtures of GluR1 through GluR4 RNAs, receptors are formed and exhibit the potency sequence AMPA > domoate > kainate. The median effective concentration (EC_{50}) of kainate is greater than 30 μM, the response to AMPA desensitizes rapidly, and 6-cyano-7-nitroquinoxaline-2,3-dione (CNQX) has a K_d of less than 1 μM, all features predicted from studies of AMPA receptors in the brain.

Subunits of the GluR5 through GluR7 and KA-1 or KA-2 families, on the other hand, appear to coassemble into functional *kainate* receptors when studied in heterologous expression systems. Results of experiments with radioligands demonstrate that homomeric GluR5, GluR6, and GluR7 receptors expressed in mammalian cell lines bind [^{3}H]kainate with an affinity of approximately 80 to 100 nM. Such homomeric receptors may correspond to the ''low-affinity'' kainate binding sites identified earlier in studies of plasma membranes from brain. Homomeric KA-1 receptors, on the other hand, bind kainate with an affinity of 4 nM and may correspond to the ''high-affinity'' kainate binding site in brain. None of these homomeric receptors is insensitive to AMPA, giving credence to the old notion of distinct kainate and AMPA receptors.

GluR6 encodes functional homomeric receptors in *Xenopus* oocytes having a kainate receptor profile in that the order of agonist potency is kainate > glutamate ≫ AMPA. Kainate is more potent ($K_D = 1$ μM) and CNQX is less potent ($K_D = 4$ μM) in homomeric GluR6 receptors than in receptors formed from the AMPA receptor subunits GluR1 through GluR4. Although GluR7, KA-1, KA-2, and GluR5 are virtually inactive when expressed alone, GluR5 and KA-2 coassemble to form a functional receptor in *Xenopus* oocytes. Likewise, KA-1 imparts weak AMPA sensitivity to GluR6 receptors [19].

To date, two NMDA receptor (NR) subunit families have been identified [20], one apparently represented by a single gene and the other by four genes (see Fig. 5) encoding proteins of about 900 and 1,450 amino acids. Homomeric NR1 receptors possess the full complement of pharmacological features of bona fide NMDA receptors, including dependence on glycine, voltage-dependent block by Mg^{2+} (see Fig. 3B) and PCP, and competitive block by D-APV. All agonist and regulatory binding sites are thus encoded by a single gene. Agonist-induced cation currents are very small in homomeric NR1 receptors, however, but are increased more than 100-fold by coexpression with one of the NR2 subunits. This suggests that most NMDA receptors in the brain are probably heteromeric receptors, as is likely to be the case with AMPA and kainate receptors.

Splice variants and RNA editing increase receptor heterogeneity

Splice variants that impart functional differences and/or different cellular expression patterns have been found for most of the subunits shown in Fig. 5. The first splice variants to be described are the so-called "flip" and "flop" versions of the AMPA receptor subunits GluR1 through GluR4 [21]. The messenger RNA (mRNA) encoding each of these subunits exists in two versions differing by a 115-bp segment. Within this encoded cassette of 38 amino acids that lie in the putative third cytoplasmic loop, the two alternative versions differ by only 9 to 11 amino acids, which are mostly conservative substitu-

tions. Nonetheless, the flip and flop splice variants give rise to receptors that differ in the relative amplitudes of their responses to glutamate and kainate and differ in their regional distribution in the brain. Additional C-terminal splice isoforms of GluR4 exist and are differentially expressed in the cerebellum, one predominantly in granule cells and the other in Bergman glial cells. Alternative splicing of GluR5 near the C terminus has also been demonstrated. Alternative exon selection within the large N-terminal extracellular domain influences agonist dose-response curves in the NR1 NMDA receptor subunit gene. These results suggest that all or most of the primary RNA transcripts of the AMPA, kainate, and NMDA receptor subunits undergo alternative splicing.

An important form of regulation appears to be achieved by editing of the primary RNA transcripts for the AMPA and kainate receptor subunits. GluR1 and GluR3, when expressed individually or in combination, form receptor channels that exhibit substantial Ca^{2+} permeability and an inwardly rectifying current-voltage relationship (see Fig. 3A), but the incorporation of GluR2 into these receptors reduces Ca^{2+} permeability and linearizes the current-voltage relationship. To investigate the structural determinants of ion permeability in AMPA and kainate receptors, conventional protein engineering techniques including site-directed mutagenesis were used to construct mutant receptor subunits for both receptor families. A single amino acid within a putative transmembrane domain was found to determine divalent ion permeability of the AMPA receptor [22]. A glutamine (Q) resides in this position in GluR1 and GluR3, but an arginine (R) is present in GluR2; this site has thus been named the "Q/R site." Interestingly, the genomic DNA sequence has a glutamine codon in this position, even for subunits such as GluR2 in which the mature mRNA has an arginine codon in this site. Evidently, RNA editing is employed to control the amino acid encoded by this critical codon [23]. RNA editing and associated changes in ionic permeability have also been demonstrated for some kainate receptor subunits. The conditions under which neurons utilize RNA editing to regulate the permeability properties of their glutamate receptors remain to be demonstrated.

Given this combination of internal and C-terminus splice variants and Q/R editing, it is likely that four to eight or more mature RNAs can be made from each of the 16 known genes encoding ionotropic receptor subunits. Thus, neurons have a very large degree of flexibility in constructing a potentially huge number of receptors. The actual degree of glutamate receptor heterogeneity utilized by neurons is a major unanswered question today.

CELLULAR DISTRIBUTION OF GLUTAMATE AND ITS RECEPTORS

Glutamate-like immunoreactivity at asymmetrical cortical synapses

Electron microscopic analysis of glutamate immunoreactive puncta within the cortex has shown that many of these structures are axon terminals [24]. Most glutamate-positive axon terminals form asymmetrical synaptic contacts on small- and medium-caliber dendritic shafts and spines. Glutamate-positive axon terminals on cell bodies are extremely rare. Likewise, axon terminals making symmetrical synapses (presumably inhibitory) do not contain glutamate immunoreactivity.

Autoradiography reveals the distribution of glutamate receptors

The existence of multiple genes encoding NMDA, AMPA, and kainate receptor subunits suggests a myriad of receptor subtypes. Autoradiographic approaches have determined that the three broad classes of glutamate receptor are differentially distributed throughout the CNS. The regional distributions of these receptors are in reasonable agreement with known target areas of excitatory amino acid pathways and with their pathophysiological function. Radioligand binding studies using [³H]AMPA (or [³H]

glutamate together with kainate and NMDA to prevent binding to other receptors) have shown that AMPA receptors are distributed throughout the entire CNS. The highest concentrations of these receptors are found in the hippocampus, cortex, lateral septum, striatum, and the molecular layer of the cerebellum.

On the basis of NMDA-displaceable [³H]glutamate binding, the highest levels of NMDA receptors in the CNS are within the strata oriens and radiatum of the hippocampal formation and the inner portion of the dentate gyrus molecular layer (Fig. 6). Results of studies with radioligand have shown that NMDA receptors are localized at postsynaptic densities and are present in high density in the cerebral cortex, hippocampus, striatum, septum, and amygdala. The distributions of AMPA and NMDA receptors are similar, as expected if these receptors act in concert to excite the postsynaptic membrane (see above).

Although the vast majority of excitatory synapses are thought to use AMPA receptors, an intriguing subtype of glutamate receptor that exhibits high affinity for [³H]kainate exists. These receptors are largely expressed in the CA3 region of the hippocampus (Fig. 6), cortex, and lateral septum. The function of these receptors is at present unclear but their distribution corresponds to those areas especially vulnerable to the neurotoxic actions of kainate. In sensory neurons of rat dorsal root ganglion, there is a population of amino acid receptors that is activated by kainate and domoate but not AMPA or quisqualate. The properties of these receptors are thus different from those of conventional AMPA receptors found in higher centers. The glutamate receptors present on dorsal root ganglia are likely to be of the kainate subtype.

In situ hybridization and the use of subunit-specific antibodies complement results of autoradiographic studies

In situ hybridization studies of AMPA, kainate, and NMDA subunit mRNAs reveal

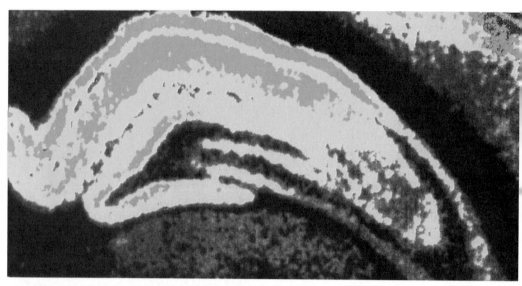

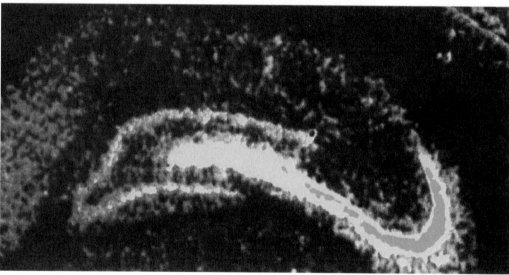

FIG. 6. Autoradiography of NMDA and kainate receptor distribution within the hippocampus. In the hippocampus, high concentrations of NMDA-sensitive [³H]ʟ-glutamate-binding sites **(A)** are found in the termination zone of the Schaffer-collateral/commissural pathway in the CA1 region and also in the granule cell layers. High concentrations of kainate-sensitive [³H]ʟ-glutamate binding sites, on the other hand, are found in the termination zone of the mossy fiber pathway **(B)** in the CA3 region. (From Cotman, C. W., Monaghan, D. T., Ottersen, O. P., and Storm-Mathisen, J. *Trends Neurosci.* 10:273–280, 1987.)

prominent expression throughout the CNS. Regional variations exist in expression of mRNAs encoding GluR1 through GluR4. For example, in the hippocampus, GluR1, GluR2, and GluR3 are expressed uniformly throughout the granule and pyramidal cell layers. In contrast, GluR4 mRNA levels are relatively high in CA1 and dentate gyrus but are low in CA3 and CA4 pyramidal cell layers. In the cerebral cortex, GluR2 is found throughout all layers; in layers III and IV, GluR1 and GluR3 occur in low levels whereas GluR4 mRNA is prominent in this area.

Antibodies raised to the GluR1 subunit can be used as high-affinity probes for receptors containing this subunit. The distribution of antibodies to the GluR1 subunit parallels that of GluR1 mRNA as determined by *in situ* hybridization. Moreover, immunocytochemistry at the electron microscopic level demonstrates that GluR1 subunits are concentrated in postsynaptic densities, as expected for a neurotransmitter receptor.

The distribution of GluR5 is distinct from the distribution of the AMPA receptor subunits GluR1 through GluR4. The most intense signals for GluR5 mRNA are in the cingulate gyrus, piriform cortex, amygdala, and lateral septum. Similarly, mRNAs encoding

the subunits KA-1 and KA-2 show patterns of expression different from those of RNAs encoding AMPA receptor subunits. The selectively high expression of KA-1 and GluR6 mRNAs in the CA3 region of the hippocampus closely corresponds to autoradiographically determined high-affinity kainate binding sites. In contrast, mRNAs for KA-2 are found throughout the entire CNS and dorsal root ganglia.

The mRNAs encoding NMDA receptor subunits are also differentially distributed. Expression of NR1 mRNA is nearly ubiquitous in the CNS. In contrast, the four NR2 genes show differential patterns of expression (Fig. 7). NR2A, like NR1, is present throughout the forebrain and the cerebellum. NR2B and NR2C, however, have a more

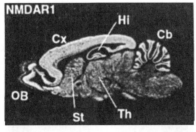

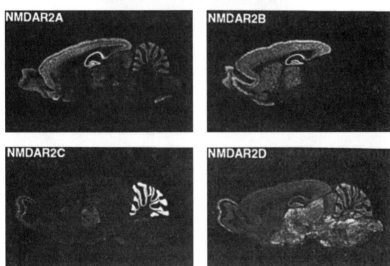

FIG. 7. Regional distribution of mRNAs encoding the five NMDA receptor genes in adult rat brain, by *in situ* hybridization. (OB) olfactory bulb; (Cx) cortex; (Hi) hippocampus; (Cb) cerebellum; (Th) thalamus; (St) striatum. (From Nakanishi [2].)

limited distribution. NR2B is expressed in highest levels in the forebrain and NR2C in the cerebellum where NR2B mRNA is not detected. NR2D expression seems virtually complementary to that of NR2A in being high in the midbrain and hindbrain but low in the forebrain.

In conclusion, *in situ* hybridization has highlighted regional differences in mRNA expression of subunits encoding glutamate receptors. These differences illustrate the likely heterogeneity of glutamate receptors throughout the CNS. Together with differences in electrophysiological properties of different subunit combinations expressed in cell lines or oocytes, the patterns of subunit expression throughout the CNS predict the existence of multiple subtypes of AMPA, kainate, and NMDA receptors.

GLUTAMATE MAY MEDIATE CERTAIN NEUROLOGICAL DISORDERS

Glutamate and aspartate as excitotoxins

Glutamate and structurally related ligands, in addition to their powerful excitatory effects at glutamate receptors, are potent neurotoxins. That glutamate and other amino acids act as neurotoxins was first realized in the 1970s when these agents were given orally to immature animals. Acute neurodegeneration was observed in those areas not well protected by the blood-brain barrier, notably the arcuate nucleus of the hypothalamus. The mechanisms of neurodegeneration are divergent and activation of all classes of ionotropic glutamate receptor has been implicated. Neurodegeneration, e.g., following an ischemic insult, may involve mechanisms resembling a pathological exaggeration of LTP-like phenomena, i.e., the neuronal insult results partially from AMPA receptor activation with concomitant NMDA receptor involvement and Ca^{2+} influx. Indeed, a close correlation exists between neurotoxic potency and affinity of glutamate receptors for a range of agonists. That is, the more able a compound is to depolarize neurons, the greater the likelihood of that agent causing neuronal toxicity.

When administered in high doses, glutamate produces adverse effects such as nausea, abdominal pain, flushing, and warming of the upper part of the body, along with a burning feeling in the chest. Higher doses may precipitate asthmatic reactions. These adverse reactions of glutamate, which are attenuated by atropine and exaggerated by physostigmine, have been referred to as *"Chinese restaurant syndrome."* This syndrome probably has little to do with an action of glutamate at central excitatory amino acid receptors.

Intracerebroventricular injection of kainate causes selective lesions

Intracerebroventricular injection of kainic acid has been shown to result in a well-characterized pattern of neuronal cell damage. In the hippocampus, kainic acid causes an axon-sparing selective lesion of the CA3 pyramidal neurons, an area rich in KA-1 and GluR6 mRNA expression (see above). The consequences of kainic acid lesioning are cell death and epileptiform discharges in cells normally innervated by the damaged pyramidal neurons. Other cell types in the hippocampus are relatively unharmed. This suggests that activation of kainate receptors may be responsible for this toxic effect of kainic acid.

Ischemic cell damage

Prolonged periods of anoxic insult to neuronal tissue, e.g., during cardiac arrest or thrombotic stroke, often result in ischemic cell damage and neurotoxicity. Oxygen deprivation precipitates a depletion of energy stores within neuronal and glial cell compartments with a concomitant acidosis and release of free radicals (Fig. 8). The depletion of energy stores affects cellular metabolism, energy-dependent ionic pumps, and the ability of cells to maintain resting mem-

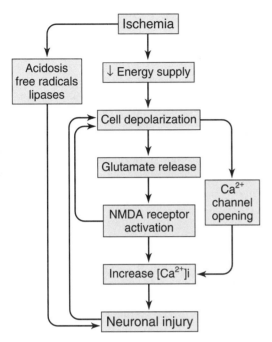

FIG. 8. Potential paths leading to neuronal injury resulting from an episode of ischemic insult. An ischemic episode initiates a complex pathway involving the depletion of cellular energy stores and the release of free radicals. The energy depletion permits sustained activation of glutamate receptors and the consequent entry of Ca^{2+} via NMDA receptors and voltage-gated Ca^{2+} channels. The elevation of intracellular Ca^{2+} levels causes excessive activation of a variety of Ca^{2+}-dependent enzymes. Excessive neuronal depolarization results in neuronal injury and often cell death.

brane potential. Consequently, depolarization of cells results in action potentials and the release of glutamate from presynaptic terminals. The released glutamate activates postsynaptic AMPA and NMDA receptors. The entry of Ca^{2+} through the NMDA receptor complex and voltage-sensitive Ca^{2+} channels increases the intracellular concentration of Ca^{2+}. As described above, an elevation of intracellular Ca^{2+} will trigger a cascade of second-messenger systems, many of which remain activated long after the initial stimulus is removed. The inability of a population of cells to maintain a resting potential precipitates a positive feedback loop that leads to neuronal cell injury or death. Animal models of ischemic cell injury have highlighted the

potential benefits of suitable "neuroprotectants" targeted to the glutamate receptor family. In some stroke models, for example, administration of an NMDA receptor blocker even several hours after the initial insult results in substantial protection of the hippocampus and striatum, two of the regions most heavily damaged by interruption in blood supply.

Epileptiform activity involves glutamate receptor activation

Involvement of excitatory amino acids in epilepsy and ischemic neuronal damage is well documented. A large number of animal models of epilepsy and neurodegeneration have clearly implicated a causal role for the glutamate receptor family (see Chap. 43). Excessive stimulation of glutamatergic pathways or pharmacological manipulation resulting in glutamate receptor activation can precipitate seizures. Epileptiform activity usually results from AMPA receptor activation; as seizure activity intensifies, an increased involvement of NMDA receptors is observed. Results of studies with a variety of animal models have shown that NMDA receptor antagonists can reduce the intensity and duration of seizure activity. Antagonism of AMPA receptor activation usually prevents *initiation* of the seizure-like event. This suggests that epileptiform activity depends on the interplay between synaptic AMPA and NMDA receptors. Evidence from human tissue supports the role of amino acids in epilepsy. For example, in patients with refractory complex partial seizures with an associated structural focus, surgically removed hippocampal tissue shows an up-regulation of AMPA and NMDA receptors.

Neurodegenerative disorders

Disorders of excitatory amino acid transmission have also been implicated in amyotrophic lateral sclerosis (ALS) and the chronic neurodegenerative diseases olivopontocerebellar atrophy and Huntington's chorea.

Neurolathyrism is a spastic disorder occurring in East Africa and India. It is associated with the dietary consumption of the chick pea *Lathyrus sativus*. The glutamate-like excitant β-*N*-oxalylamino-L-alanine has been identified as the toxin in this plant. Its action at AMPA receptors in the spinal cord may be responsible for the observed degeneration of lower and upper motor neurons.

The high incidence of ALS observed in residents of the Pacific island of Guam was determined to be due to the dietary ingestion of the cycad *Cyas circinalis*. This seed contains an amino acid, β-*N*-methylamino-L-alanine (BMAA). In the presence of bicarbonate, BMAA becomes excitotoxic through a mechanism involving the activation of AMPA and NMDA receptors. Its action can be blocked by the NMDA receptor antagonist D-AP5. An important topic for future research will be to identify the roles, if any, that overactivation of glutamate receptors plays in such neurological disorders.

SUMMARY

Research directed toward understanding the functions of glutamate receptors has progressed in parallel with the expansion of neuroscience research in the past decade. Indeed, demonstrations that glutamate receptors are involved in numerous physiological and pathophysiological phenomena continue to fuel a substantial fraction of neuroscience research. With the cloning and now mutagenesis of the glutamate receptors, the application of the patch voltage clamp, and the refinement of neuroanatomical techniques, new opportunities have arisen to address the basic functions of these nearly ubiquitous neurotransmitter receptors. The application of molecular biological approaches has been particularly instructive. For example, we now know that at least some native glutamate receptors are heterooligomeric proteins like nicotinic acetylcholine receptors. Some of the structural domains

responsible for ion permeation have been identified, and we know that different combinations of subunits assemble into receptors with different functional properties. The latter realization is quite important since it suggests that new therapeutic strategies might be devised that take advantage of the molecular diversity of these receptors.

Current and future research will seek to determine which subunit combinations are permissible *in situ*, the genetic regulation of glutamate receptor functions, and the precise roles of glutamatergic pathways and receptor subtypes in neurological disorders, development, and learning. Realization of these goals will require a coordinated effort from multiple disciplines.

REFERENCES

1. The pharmacology of excitatory amino acids. A TIPS special report. *Trends Pharmacol. Sci.* 1990.
2. Nakanishi, S. Molecular diversity of glutamate receptors and implications for brain function. *Science* 258:597–603, 1992.
3. Schoepp, D. D., and Conn, P. J. Metabotropic glutamate receptors in brain function and pathology. *Trends Pharmacol. Sci.* 14:13–20, 1993.
4. Patneau, D., and Mayer, M. L. Structure activity relationships for amino acid transmitter candidates acting at *N*-methyl-D-aspartate and quisqualate receptors. *J. Neurosci.* 10: 2385–2399, 1990.
5. Kleckner, N. W., and Dingledine, R. Requirement for glycine in activation of NMDA receptors expressed in *Xenopus* oocytes. *Science* 241:835–837, 1988.
6. Williams, K., Romano, C., Dichter, M. A., and Molinoff, P. B. Modulation of the NMDA receptor by polyamines. *Life Sci.* 48:469–498, 1991.
7. Rock, D. M., and Macdonald, R. L. The polyamine spermine has multiple actions on *N*-methyl-D-aspartate receptor single-channel currents in cultured cortical neurons. *Mol. Pharmacol.* 41:83–88, 1991.
8. Nowak, L., Bregestovski, P., Ascher, P., Herbet, A., and Prochiantz, A. Magnesium gates glutamate-activated channels in mouse central neurones. *Nature* 307:462–465, 1984.

9. Traynelis, S. F., and Cull-Candy, S. G. Pharmacological properties and H$^+$ sensitivity of excitatory amino acid receptor channels in rat cerebellar granule neurones. *J. Physiol. (Lond.)* 443:727–763, 1991.

10. MacDonald, J. F., Mody, I., and Salter, M. W. Regulation of *N*-methyl-D-aspartate receptors revealed by intracellular dialysis of murine neurones in culture. *J. Physiol. (Lond.)* 414:17–34, 1989.

11. Nawy, S., and Jahr, C. E. Suppression by glutamate of cGMP-activated conductance in retinal bipolar cells. *Nature* 346:269–271, 1990.

12. Chen, L., and Mae Huang, L.-Y. Protein kinase C reduces Mg^{2+} block of NMDA-receptor channels as a mechanism of modulation. *Nature* 356:521–523, 1992.

13. Storm-Mathisen, J., Leknes, A. K., Bore, A. T., et al. First visualization of glutamate and GABA in neurones by immunocytochemistry. *Nature* 301:517–520, 1983.

14. Cull-Candy, S. G., and Usowicz, M. M. On the multiple-conductance single channels activated by excitatory amino acids in large cerebellar neurones of the rat. *J. Physiol. (Lond.)* 415:555–582, 1989.

15. Mayer, M. L., and Westbrook, G. L. The physiology of excitatory amino acids in the vertebrate central nervous system. *Prog. Neurobiol.* 28:197–291, 1987.

16. Mayer, M. L., and Westbrook, G. L. Permeation and block of *N*-methyl-D-aspartic acid receptor channels by divalent cations in mouse cultured central neurones. *J. Physiol. (Lond.)* 394:501–527, 1987.

17. Hollmann, M., O'Shea-Greenfield, A., Rogers, S. W., and Heinemann, S. F. Cloning by functional expression of a member of the glutamate receptor family. *Nature* 342:643–648, 1989.

18. Tanabe, Y., Masu, M., Ishii, T., et al. A family of metabotropic glutamate receptors. *Neuron* 8:169–179, 1992.

19. Herb, A., Burnashev, N., Werner, P., et al. The KA-2 subunit of excitatory amino acid receptors shows widespread expression in brain and forms ion channels with distantly related subunits. *Neuron* 8:775–785, 1992.

20. Meguro, H., Mori, H., Araki, K., et al. Functional characterization of a heteromeric NMDA receptor channel expressed from cloned cDNAs. *Nature* 357:70–74, 1992.

21. Sommer, B., Keinanen, K., Verdoorn, T. A., et al. Flip and flop: A cell specific functional switch in glutamate-operated channels of the CNS. *Science* 249:1580–1585, 1990.

22. Hume, R. I., Dingledine, R., and Heinemann, S. F. Identification of a site in glutamate receptor subunits that controls calcium permeability. *Science* 253:1028–1032, 1991.

23. Sommer, B., Kohler, M., Sprengel, R., and Seeburg, P. H. RNA editing in brain controls a determinant of ion flow in glutamate-gated channels. *Cell* 67:11–19, 1991.

24. DeFelipe, J., Conti, F., VanEyck, S., and Manzoni, T. Demonstration of glutamate-positive axon terminals forming asymmetric synapses in cat neocortex. *Brain Res.* 455:162–165, 1988.

CHAPTER 18

GABA and Glycine

TIMOTHY M. DeLOREY AND RICHARD W. OLSEN

Basic Neurochemistry: Molecular, Cellular, and Medical Aspects, 5th Ed., edited by G. J. Siegel et al. Published by Raven Press, Ltd., New York, 1994. Correspondence to Richard W. Olsen, Department of Pharmacology, UCLA School of Medicine, Center for Health Sciences, 10833 LeConte Avenue, Los Angeles, California 90024-1735.

γ-Aminobutyric acid (GABA) is the major inhibitory neurotransmitter in the mammalian central nervous system (CNS). It was discovered in 1950 by Roberts and Awapara. Electrophysiological studies between 1950 and 1965 suggested a role for GABA as a neurotransmitter in the mammalian CNS. Since then, GABA has met the five classical criteria for assignment as a neurotransmitter: It is present in the nerve terminal, it is released from electrically stimulated neurons, there is a mechanism for reuptake of the released neurotransmitter, its application to target neurons mimics the action of inhibitory nerve stimulation, and specific receptors exist.

In view of the ubiquitous nature of GABA in the CNS, it is perhaps not too surprising that its functional significance should be far-reaching. A growing body of evidence suggests a role for altered GABAergic function in neurological and psychiatric disorders of humans, including Huntington's chorea, epilepsy, tardive dyskinesia, alcoholism, schizophrenia, sleep disorders, and Parkinson's disease. Pharmacological manipulation of GABAergic transmission is an effective approach for the treatment of anxiety [1]. In addition, it has been suggested that the depressant anesthetic actions of barbiturates result from an enhancement of inhibitory synaptic transmission mediated by $GABA_A$ receptors [2].

GABA SYNTHESIS, UPTAKE, AND RELEASE

GABA is formed *in vivo* by a metabolic pathway referred to as the GABA shunt

The GABA shunt is a closed loop process with the dual purpose of producing and conserving the supply of GABA. GABA is present in high concentrations ($\mu M/g$) in many brain regions. These concentrations are about 1,000 times higher than concentrations of the classical monoamine neurotransmitters in the same regions. This is in accord with the powerful and specific actions of GABAergic neurons in these regions. Glucose is the principal precursor for GABA production *in vivo,* although pyruvate and other amino acids can also act as precursors. The first step in the GABA shunt is the transamination of α-ketoglutarate, formed from glucose metabolism in the Krebs cycle, by GABA α-oxoglutarate transaminase (GABA-T) into glutamic acid (Fig. 1). Glutamic acid decarboxylase (GAD) catalyzes the decarboxylation of glutamic acid to form GABA. GAD appears to be expressed only in cells that use GABA as a neurotransmitter. GAD, localized with antibodies or messenger RNA (mRNA) hybridization probes, serves as an excellent marker for GABAergic neurons in the CNS. GABA is metabolized by GABA-T to form succinic semialdehyde. To conserve the available supply of GABA, this transamination generally occurs when the initial parent compound, α-ketoglutarate, is present to accept the amino group removed from GABA, reforming glutamic acid. Therefore, a molecule of GABA can only be metabolized if a molecule of precursor is formed. Succinic semialdehyde can be oxidized by succinic semialdehyde dehydrogenase (SSADH) into succinic acid and can then reenter the Krebs cycle, completing the loop.

GABA release into the synaptic cleft is stimulated by depolarization of presynaptic neurons. GABA diffuses across the cleft to the target receptors on the postsynaptic surface. The action of GABA at the synapse is terminated by reuptake into both presynaptic nerve terminals and surrounding glial cells. The membrane transport systems mediating reuptake of GABA are both temperature- and ion-dependent processes. These transporters are capable of bidirectional neurotransmitter transport. They have an absolute requirement for extracellular Na^+ ions with an additional dependence on Cl^- ions. The GABA transporter is a 70- to 80-kDa glycoprotein with multiple transmembrane regions; it has no sequence homology with GABA receptors. Pharmacological and kinetic studies suggest the possibility of a vari-

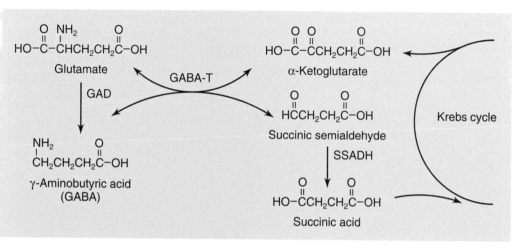

FIG. 1.   Reactions of the GABA shunt that are responsible for the synthesis, conservation, and metabolism of GABA.

ety of subtypes of GABA transporter [3]. GABA taken back up into nerve terminals is available for reutilization, but GABA in glia is metabolized to succinic semialdehyde by GABA-T and cannot be resynthesized in this compartment since glia lack GAD. GABA can ultimately be recovered from this source by a circuitous route involving the Krebs cycle (see [4]). GABA is converted to glutamine and transferred back to the neuron, where glutaminase can convert it to glutamate and allow it to reenter the GABA shunt (see Chap. 17). The ability of the reuptake system to transport GABA against a concentration gradient has been demonstrated using synaptosomes. Under normal physiological conditions, the ratio of internal to external GABA is about 200. The driving force for this reuptake process is supplied by the movement of Na^+ down its concentration gradient.

GABA RECEPTOR PHYSIOLOGY AND PHARMACOLOGY

GABA receptors have been identified electrophysiologically and pharmacologically in all regions and levels of the brain

Because GABA is widely distributed and utilized throughout the CNS, early GABAergic drugs have had very generalized effects on CNS function. The development of more selective agents has led to the identification of at least two distinct classes of GABA receptors, termed $GABA_A$ and $GABA_B$. They differ in their pharmacological, electrophysiological, and biochemical properties. Less is known about the $GABA_B$ receptor, primarily due to the limited number of pharmacological agents selective for this site. Originally, $GABA_B$ receptors were identified by their insensitivity to the $GABA_A$ antagonist bicuculline and the $GABA_A$ agonists isoguvacine, 4,5,6,7-tetrahydroisoxazolo[5,4-c]pyridin-3-ol (THIP), and 3-aminopropane sulfonic acid (APS). The GABA analog $(-)$baclofen [β-(4-chlorophenyl)-γ-aminobutyric acid] was found to be a potent and selective $GABA_B$ agonist. Recent findings suggest that the $GABA_B$ receptors are indirectly coupled to K^+ channels, can decrease Ca^{2+} conductance, and can inhibit cyclic AMP production via intracellular mechanisms mediated by guanine nucleotide-binding proteins (G proteins). $GABA_B$ receptors can cause both postsynaptic and presynaptic inhibition. Presynaptic inhibition may occur as a result of $GABA_B$ receptors on nerve terminals causing a decrease in the influx of Ca^{2+}, thereby reducing the release of neurotransmitters.

$GABA_A$ receptor pharmacology and

function are vastly different from those of the GABA$_B$ receptor. Electrophysiological studies of the GABA$_A$ receptor complex indicate that it mediates an increase in membrane conductance with an equilibrium potential near the resting level of -70 mV. This conductance increase is often accompanied by a membrane hyperpolarization, resulting in an increase in the firing threshold and, consequently, a reduction in the probability of action potential initiation (i.e., neuronal inhibition). This reduction in membrane resistance is accomplished by the GABA-dependent facilitation of Cl$^-$ ion permeation through a receptor-associated channel. Electrophysiological data [5] suggest that there are two GABA recognition sites per receptor complex. An increase in the concentration of GABA results in an increase in the mean channel open time due to opening of doubly-liganded receptor forms which exhibit open states of long duration. It has been demonstrated using a membrane preparation from rat brain that the increase in the ionic permeability of the GABA$_A$ receptor complex is transitory in the continuing pres-

ence of agonist [6]. This phenomenon is known as desensitization and is rapidly reversible. The molecular mechanism of desensitization is not understood and various hypotheses remain under investigation. Protein phosphorylation has been suggested as playing an important role in the desensitization process. In addition, Cash and Subbarao [6] have proposed the existence of GABA binding sites specific for the initiation of desensitization that are distinct from sites mediating opening of the Cl$^-$ channel.

The GABA$_A$ receptor is part of a larger GABA/benzodiazepine chloride ion channel macromolecular complex

The complex includes five major binding domains (Fig. 2). These include binding sites for GABA, benzodiazepines, barbiturates, picrotoxin (localized in or near the Cl$^-$ channel), and the anesthetic steroids. These binding domains serve to modulate the receptor's response to GABA stimulation. In addition, other drugs, including ethanol and penicillin, have been reported to have an ef-

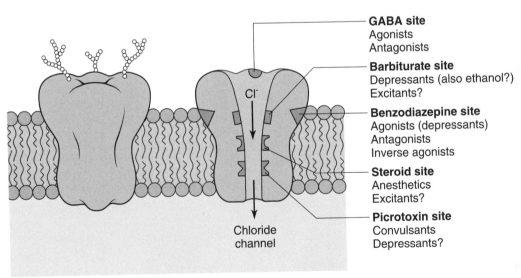

FIG. 2.   Structural model of the GABA$_A$/benzodiazepine receptor-chloride (Cl$^-$) ionophore complex. The *cut-away view* demonstrates targets for a variety of compounds that influence the receptor complex. No specific drug receptor location is implied.

fect on this receptor [7]. An integral part of this complex is the Cl$^-$ channel. The GABA binding site is the site directly responsible for opening the Cl$^-$ channel. A variety of agonists bind to this site and elicit GABA-like responses. One of the most useful agonists is the compound muscimol, a naturally occurring GABA analog isolated from the hallucinogenic mushroom *Amanita muscaria*. It is a potent and specific agonist at GABA$_A$ receptors and has been a valuable tool for pharmacological and radioligand binding studies [8]. Other GABA agonists include THIP, APS, imidazoleacetic acid, and β-hydroxy-γ-amino-*n*-butyric acid. The classical GABA$_A$ receptor antagonist is the convulsant bicuculline, which reduces current by decreasing the opening frequency and mean open time of the channel [7]. Detailed kinetic studies of the effect of bicuculline have not been reported, but it is likely that bicuculline produces its antagonistic effects on GABA$_A$ receptor currents by competing with GABA for binding to the GABA$_A$ receptor. Whether bicuculline binds to one or both of the GABA binding sites remains unclear.

The benzodiazepine binding site was first discovered in 1977 [9,10]

Benzodiazepine receptor binding sites were found to copurify with the GABA binding sites [11]. In addition, benzodiazepine receptors are immunoprecipitated with monoclonal antibodies that were developed to recognize the protein containing the GABA binding site. This indicates that the benzodiazepine receptor is an integral part of the GABA$_A$ receptor-Cl$^-$ channel complex.

Benzodiazepine agonists represent the newest group of agents in the general class of depressant drugs, which also includes barbiturates, that show anticonvulsant, anxiolytic, and sedative-hypnotic activity. Well-known examples include diazepam (Valium) and chlordiazepoxide (Librium), which are often prescribed for their anxiolytic effects. The mechanism of action of benzodiazepine agonists is to enhance GABAergic transmission. From electrophysiological studies, it is known that these benzodiazepines increase the probability of channel opening in response to GABA, thus accounting for their pharmacological and therapeutic actions [12]. In addition, the benzodiazepine site has been shown to be allosterically coupled to the barbiturate and picrotoxin sites [2]. Benzodiazepine receptors are heterogeneous with respect to affinity for certain ligands. A wide variety of nonbenzodiazepines, such as β-carbolines, cyclopyrrolones, and imidazopyridines, also bind to the benzodiazepine site.

Measurements of mean channel open times show that barbiturates act by increasing the proportion of channels opening to the longest open state (9 msec) while reducing the proportion opening to the shorter open state (1 and 3 msec), resulting in an overall increase in mean channel open time and Cl$^-$ flux [7]. Phenobarbital and pentobarbital are two of the most commonly used barbiturates. Phenobarbital has been used to treat patients with epilepsy since 1912. Pentobarbital is also an anticonvulsant, but it has sedative side effects.

Channel blockers, such as the convulsant compound picrotoxin, cause a decrease in mean channel open time. Picrotoxin works by preferentially shifting opening channels to the briefest open state (1 msec). Thus, both picrotoxin and barbiturates appear to act on the gating process of the GABA$_A$ receptor channel, but their effects on the open states are opposite each other. Experimental convulsants like pentylenetetrazol and the cage convulsant *t*-butyl bicyclophosphorothionate (TBPS) also act to block the Cl$^-$ channel. The antibiotic penicillin is a channel blocker with a net negative charge. It has been shown to block the channel by interacting with the positively charged amino acid residues within the channel pore, consequently occluding Cl$^-$ passage through the channel [7].

Neuroactive steroids, such as the synthetic steroid alphaxalone, have been found to enhance GABA$_A$ receptor current by increasing mean channel open time

It is not clear how this enhancement occurs. These steroids act directly on the membrane receptor protein rather than through the classical genomic mechanism mediated by soluble high-affinity cytoplasmic steroid hormone receptors. Alphaxalone has been used to induce anesthesia, a phenomenon thought to be closely associated with the GABA$_A$ receptor. Recent work has shown that reduced progesterone and corticosterone derivatives exert sedative and hypnotic effects *in vivo* [13] and are found to be potent modulators of GABA$_A$ receptor function *in vitro*. Thus, endogenous steroids may influence CNS function under certain physiological or pathological conditions. Neuroactive steroids have been shown to enhance agonist binding to the GABA site and to allosterically modulate benzodiazepine and TBPS binding. These effects are similar to the effects of barbiturates and led to the hypothesis that the neurosteroid binding site may be closely associated with but not identical to the barbiturate site. Like barbiturates, high concentrations of neurosteroids directly activate the GABA$_A$ receptor.

The neurochemical actions of ethanol in the central nervous system remain obscure

Recently, direct evidence of ethanol augmentation of GABA-mediated Cl$^-$ flux was reported [14]. The similarity between the actions of ethanol and sedative drugs such as benzodiazepines and barbiturates that enhance GABA action suggests that ethanol may exert some of its effects by enhancing the function of the GABA receptor.

There have been numerous studies on the role of GABA$_A$ receptors in anesthesia. A considerable amount of evidence has been compiled to suggest that general anesthetics, including barbiturates, volatile gases, steroids, and alcohols, enhance GABA-me-

diated Cl$^-$ conductance. For example, a strong positive correlation exists between anesthetic potencies and the stimulation of GABA-mediated Cl$^-$ uptake. This is seen with barbiturates and anesthetics in other chemical classes [2,15]. Barbiturates at pharmacological concentrations are known to allosterically increase binding of benzodiazepines and GABA to their respective binding sites. A proper assessment of this phenomenon requires not only a behavioral model of anesthesia but also *in vitro* models for the study of receptor function (e.g., Cl$^-$ flux) and binding.

While electrophysiological techniques have been useful for the identification and study of GABA receptors, this approach has limitations. The experiments are often difficult and time-consuming to perform. In addition, a quantitative estimate of GABA receptor density and identification of receptor subtypes are not usually possible. Problems such as these, along with the need to make the GABA receptor more available for general study, gave rise to the development and acceptance of radioligand binding assays for the study of the GABA receptor [16]. Binding methodologies were adopted to avoid problems with the GABA reuptake system, which could result from the presence of free endogenous GABA released by homogenization. These methodologies included tissue lysis; thorough washing, sometimes with low levels of detergent; removal of sodium; and ice-cold incubation steps to remove endogenous GABA; disabling of the transport system; and denuding of the complex of endogenous compounds. Using these procedures, the mammalian GABA$_A$ receptor has been well characterized.

CLONING GABA RECEPTORS

The GABA$_A$ receptor was first cloned [17] using partial protein sequences for two polypeptides in the purified protein [11]

Verification of these complementary DNAs (cDNAs) as GABA receptor subunits was made by expression in *Xenopus* oocytes of GABA-activated channels [17,18]. Sequencing revealed that the $GABA_A$ receptor is a member of a superfamily of ligand-gated ion channels. This family includes the nicotinic acetylcholine receptor, strychnine-sensitive glycine receptor, and some of the excitatory amino acid receptors. Our current understanding of the molecular structure of the $GABA_A$ receptor-ionophore complex is that it is a heteropentameric glycoprotein of about 275 kDa composed of combinations of α, β, γ, δ, and ρ polypeptide subunits [17,19,20]. The subunits are 50 to 60 kDa and have about 20 to 30 percent sequence identity between classes (α, β, γ, δ, ρ). A variety of subunit isoforms have been reported (α_{1-6}, β_{1-4}, γ_{1-3}). About 70 percent sequence identity is shared between the isoforms of each subunit class (Fig. 3). This suggests that the genes probably evolved from a common ancestral sequence. About 10 to 20 percent homology exists between $GABA_A$ subunit polypeptides and those of other members of the ligand-gated ion channel gene superfamily. Differential distribution of $GABA_A$ receptor subtype mRNAs in brain is consistent with data indicating variation in physiological function, pharmacology, and biochemistry of different brain regions. It is likely that different combinations with differing pharmacologies and conductances are expressed in different neuronal populations. *In situ* hybridization has revealed that mRNAs encoding subunits of $GABA_A$ receptors unit subtype mRNAs are distributed differentially in both rat and cow brain [19,20]. For example, the distributions of the three major α-subunit subtypes α_1, α_2, and α_5 are very different [21] (Fig. 4); i.e., multiple protein isoforms occur in brain depending on a tissue-dependent subunit composition. The subunit composition is currently unknown but will be deduced by a combination of determining which polypeptides are present in a given cell, which ones can be isolated together as an oligomer, and what pharmacological properties can be reconstituted from recombinant subunits of known combinations.

Each $GABA_A$ subunit contains four putative α-helical membrane-spanning domains (M_1–M_4) with a predominantly hydrophobic character. One or more membrane-spanning regions from each subunit form the walls of the channel pore. The sequences of these transmembrane segments are highly conserved between the subunits of the $GABA_A$ receptor as well as between members of the gene superfamily. The region between M_3 and M_4 contains a long, variable putative intracellular domain. This and other intracellular domains may contribute to the subtype specificity and may participate in intracellular regulatory mechanisms.

Photoaffinity-labeling of the $GABA_A$ receptors suggests that the binding sites for benzodiazepines are localized on the α-subunit, and binding sites for GABA ligands are primarily on β-subunits, although it appears that all of the subunits are capable of binding GABA and activating Cl^- channels [19].

Reconstitution of $GABA_A$ receptors from recombinant polypeptides expressed in heterologous cells reveals that the nature of the α- and β-subunit subtypes determines the pharmacological specificity at the GABA and benzodiazepine sites, and that the γ-subunits are necessary for sensitivity to benzodiazepines [22]. Some $GABA_A$ receptors apparently lack benzodiazepine binding sites altogether or have a novel pharmacological profile at this site; these receptors may be

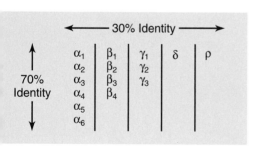

FIG. 3. Homology between peptide sequences making up the subunits of the $GABA_A$ receptor. Percent sequence identity between polypeptide isoforms of a single subunit class (e.g., α_1) and those comparing sequence identity between different subunit classes (e.g., α vs. β) are approximate values.

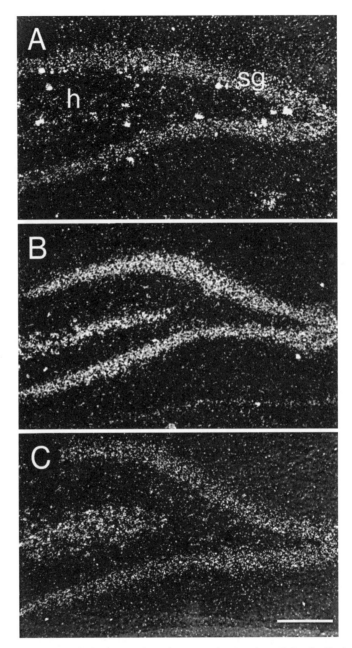

FIG. 4.   Autoradiograph of *in situ* hybridization histochemistry, showing the cellular distribution of the mRNA fo the α_1, α_2, and α_5-subunits in the dentate gyrus. **A:** α_1 mRNA is present in granule cells within the hilus (h) and stratum granulosum (sg). **B:** α_2 mRNA is abundant in CA4 pyramidal cells and granule cells. **C:** α_5 mRNA is present in lower levels than α_1 or α_2 mRNA. Scale bar, 200 μm. (Photograph courtesy of Dr. Nicholas Brecha; from MacLennar et al. [21] with permission.)

associated with the δ-subunit, may lack the γ-subunits, or may contain a unique low abundance α-subunit such as α_6.

Successful cloning of the $GABA_A$ receptor subunits and deduction of the corresponding amino acid sequences have led to the finding that phosphorylation sites are present on all of the subunits. However, phosphorylation of the β- and γ-subtypes appears to hold more promise of physiological significance than phosphorylation of the α-subunits. The β-subunits contain a consensus sequence for phosphorylation by cyclic AMP-dependent protein kinase [17]. As noted above, phosphorylation of this subunit has been suggested to control desensitization of the $GABA_A$ receptor, which occurs on exposure to GABA. The catalytic subunit of protein kinase A, when applied intracellularly to mouse spinal cord neurons, reduces $GABA_A$ receptor current [23]. In addition, there is a protein kinase C consensus phosphorylation site on some α-subunits and a splice variant of the γ_2-subunit [24]. The physiological significance of these observations remains unknown.

GLYCINE RECEPTOR

Glycine was first proposed to act as a neurotransmitter in mammalian spinal cord in 1965

Glycine is widely recognized as a major inhibitory neurotransmitter in the vertebrate CNS, especially the spinal cord (see [4] for review). Like GABA, it inhibits neuronal firing by gating Cl^- channels but with a characteristically different pharmacology. Glycine has met the physiological criteria to be designated a neurotransmitter.

Glycine is synthesized from glucose and other substrates in the brain

The immediate precursor of glycine is serine, which is converted to glycine by the activity of the enzyme serine hydroxymethyltrans-ferase (SHMT). As for GABA, Ca^{2+}-dependent release of glycine and specific postsynaptic receptors have been demonstrated. Glycine's action is terminated by its reuptake by a high-affinity transporter system. Synaptosomal uptake of radioactive glycine has been demonstrated in spinal cord and lower brainstem. In supraspinal regions, glycine can be taken up by transport systems that have lower affinity and specificity for glycine. The metabolic disposal of glycine is unclear, but it has been shown that glycine can be converted to a variety of other substances. However, none of these mechanisms has been shown to be associated with glycine neurons.

GLYCINE RECEPTOR PHYSIOLOGY AND PHARMACOLOGY

A number of amino acids can activate, to varying degrees, the glycine receptor

The amino acids that can activate the glycine receptor include β-alanine, taurine, L-alanine, L-serine, and proline. GABA is inactive at this receptor. There are only a few known antagonists of glycine receptors. They include the plant alkaloid strychnine, which is highly selective for the glycine receptor, and the amidine steroid RU 5135, which is somewhat less selective. Both compounds bind the glycine receptor with nanomolar affinities. The binding site for glycine is believed to be closely related to the site for antagonist binding but it may not be identical [25]. Current findings suggest that at least three molecules of glycine are required to activate the glycine receptor [26]. The physiological significance of multiple binding sites for glycine is unclear.

CLONING GLYCINE RECEPTORS

Glycine receptors belong to the same gene superfamily as the $GABA_A$ receptor

The native receptor is a macromolecular complex of about 250 kDa composed of a combination of two homologous polypeptides identified as α (48 kDa) and β (58 kDa). It has been proposed that the glycine receptor, like the other members of the family, consists of a quasisymmetrical pentameric arrangement forming a central ion pore [26]. There is approximately 50 percent amino acid sequence identity between the α- and β-subunits. In addition, a 93-kDa polypeptide is believed to be associated with the glycine receptor. Photoaffinity-labeling of the glycine receptor suggests that the binding sites for glycine and strychnine are found on the 48-kDa polypeptide (α-subunit). The α- and β-subunits span the postsynaptic membrane and are believed to be glycosylated. Like the GABA$_A$ receptor subunits, the glycine receptor subunits (α and β) each have four hydrophobic segments (M$_1$–M$_4$) which probably span the lipid bilayer as α helices. Unlike the α- and β-subunits, the 93-kDa polypeptide is a highly hydrophilic protein, cytoplasmically localized at postsynaptic membranes. It appears that the 93-kDa polypeptide is a peripheral component of the glycine receptor serving to anchor the glycine receptor in the postsynaptic membrane by attaching it to cytoskeletal elements [26].

Currently, four isoforms of the α-subunit but only one form of β have been cloned. The α$_2$ polypeptide represents a subunit primarily expressed neonatally, whereas the α$_3$ is found primarily postnatally. The developmental stage at which the α$_4$ mRNA accumulates is currently unknown, but α$_4$ transcripts are only found in very low levels in adult rodent brain.

Functional expression of the α$_1$, α$_2$, and α$_3$ transcripts in frog oocytes generates glycine-gated Cl$^-$ channels that are blocked by nanomolar levels of strychnine. A variant of the α$_2$ assembles a channel with a much lower affinity for strychnine and is thought to correspond with the strychnine-insensitive glycine receptor found neonatally in rat spinal cord.

Immunocytochemical mapping with monoclonal antibodies raised against α-subunit antigen gives results similar to those obtained in autoradiographic studies of [³H]strychnine binding sites. Although the majority of sites are found in spinal cord and brainstem, a small but significant population is found in higher brain regions. Interestingly, the β-subunit mRNA is abundant in many brain regions where neither [³H]strychnine binding nor known α-subunit mRNAs are found. The implication of this finding is presently unclear.

There is now little doubt that GABA and glycine are the major rapid-acting inhibitory neurotransmitters in the mammalian brain

The roles of these two neurotransmitters are clearly distinct, both chemically and physiologically. Diversity of subunit isoforms has been exhibited in both GABA$_A$ and glycine receptors. Recent studies suggest a varied pharmacology and physiology associated with differing isoform combinations. An understanding of the nature of these combinations should assist in the development of a new series of therapeutic agents which interact with GABA$_A$ or glycine receptors in a more specific manner than currently available drugs.

REFERENCES

1. Enna, S. J., and Möhler, H. Gamma-aminobutyric acid (GABA) receptors and their association with benzodiazepine recognition sites. In H. Y. Meltzer (ed.), *Psychopharmacology: The Third Generation of Progress.* New York: Raven Press, 1987, pp. 265–272.
2. Olsen, R. W., Sapp, D. M., Bureau, M. H., Turner, D. M., and Kokka, N. Allosteric actions of central nervous system depressants including anesthetic on subtypes of the inhibitory γ-aminobutyric acid$_A$ receptor-chloride channel complex. *Ann. N. Y. Acad. Sci.* 625: 145–154, 1991.
3. Guastella, J., Nelson, N., Nelson, H., et al. Cloning and expression of a rat brain GABA transporter. *Science* 24:1303–1306, 1990.
4. McGeer, P. L., and McGeer, E. G. Amino acid

neurotransmitters. In G. Siegel, B. Agranoff, R. W. Albers, and P. Molinoff (eds.), *Basic Neurochemistry*, 4th ed. New York: Raven Press, 1989, pp. 311–332.

5. Sakmann, B. Elementary steps in synaptic transmission revealed by currents through single ion channels. *Neuron* 8:613–629, 1992.

6. Cash, D. J., and Subbarao, K. Channel opening of γ-aminobutyric acid receptor from rat brain: Molecular mechanisms of the receptor response. *Biochemistry* 26:7562–7570, 1987.

7. Macdonald, R. L., and Twyman, R. E. Biophysical properties and regulation of $GABA_A$ receptor channels. *Semin. Neurosci.* 3:219–230, 1991.

8. Krogsgaard-Larsen, P., Brehm, L., and Schaumburg, K. Muscimol, a psychoactive constituent of *Amanita muscaria,* as a medicinal chemical model structure. *Acta Chem. Scand. Ser. B* 35:311–324, 1981.

9. Möhler, H., and Okada, T. Benzodiazepine receptor: Demonstration in the central nervous system. *Science* 198:849–851, 1977.

10. Squires, R. F., and Braestrup, C. Benzodiazepine receptors in rat brain. *Nature* 266:732–734, 1977.

11. Sigel, E., Stephenson, F. A., Mamalaki, C., and Barnard, E. A. A γ-aminobutyric acid/benzodiazepine receptor complex of bovine cerebral cortex: Purification and partial characterization. *J. Biol. Chem.* 258:6965–6971, 1983.

12. Study, R. E., and Barker, J. L. Diazepam and (−)-pentobarbital: Fluctuation analysis reveals different mechanisms for potentiation of γ-aminobutyric acid responses in cultured central neurons. *Proc. Natl. Acad. Sci. U. S. A.* 78:7180–7184, 1981.

13. Majewska, M. D., Harrison, N. L., Schwartz, R. D., Barker, J. L., and Paul, S. M. Steroid hormone metabolites are barbiturate-like modulators of the GABA receptor. *Science* 232:1004–1007, 1986.

14. Suzdak, P. D., Schwartz, R. D., Skolnick, P., and Paul, S. M. Ethanol stimulates gamma-aminobutyric acid receptor-mediated chloride transport in rat brain synaptoneurosomes. *Proc. Natl. Acad. Sci. U. S. A.* 83:4071–4075, 1986.

15. Allan, A. M., and Harris, R. A. Anesthetic and convulsant barbiturates alter gamma-aminobutyric acid-stimulated chloride flux across brain membranes. *J. Pharmacol. Exp. Ther.* 238:763–768, 1986.

16. Zukin, S. R., Young, A. B., and Snyder, S. H. γ-Aminobutyric acid binding to receptor sites in the rat central nervous system. *Proc. Natl. Acad. Sci. U. S. A.* 71:4802–4807, 1974.

17. Schofield, P R., Darlison, M. G., Fujita, N., et al. Sequence and functional expression of the $GABA_A$ receptor shows a ligand-gated receptor super-family. *Nature* 328:221–227, 1987.

18. Miledi, R., Parker, I., and Sumikawa, K. Synthesis of chick brain GABA receptors by frog oocytes. *Proc. R. Soc. Lond. [Biol.]* 216:509–515, 1982.

19. Olsen, R. W., and Tobin, A. J. Molecular biology of GABA-A receptors. *FASEB J.* 4:1469–1480, 1990.

20. Lüddens, H., and Wisden, W. Function and pharmacology of multiple $GABA_A$ receptor subunits. *Trends Pharmacol. Sci.* 12:49–51, 1991.

21. MacLennan, A. J., Brecha, N., Khrestchatisky, M., et al. Independent cellular and ontogenetic expression of mRNAs encoding three α-polypeptides of the rat $GABA_A$ receptor. *Neuroscience* 43:369–380, 1991.

22. Pritchett, D. B., Lüddens, H., and Seeburg, P. H. Type I and type II $GABA_A$-benzodiazepine receptors produced in transfected cells. *Science* 245:1389–1392, 1989.

23. Porter, N. M., Twyman, R. E., Uhler, M. D., and Macdonald, R. L. Cyclic AMP-dependent protein kinase decreases $GABA_A$ receptor current in mouse spinal neurons. *Neuron* 5:789–796, 1990.

24. Whiting, P., McKernan, R. M., and Iversen, L. L. Another mechanism for creating diversity in γ-aminobutyrate type A receptors: RNA splicing directs expression of two forms of $γ_2$ subunit, one of which contains a protein kinase C phosphorylation site. *Proc. Natl. Acad. Sci. U. S. A.* 87:9966–9970, 1990.

25. Young, A. B., and Snyder, S. H. The glycine synaptic receptor: Evidence that strychnine binding is associated with the ionic conductance mechanism. *Proc. Natl. Acad. Sci. U. S. A.* 71:4002–4005, 1974.

26. Langosch, D., Becker, C.-M., and Betz, H. The inhibitory glycine receptor: A ligand-gated chloride channel of the central nervous system. *Eur. J. Biochem.* 194:1–8, 1990.

Purinergic Systems

JOEL LINDEN

Purines such as ATP and adenosine play a central role in the energy metabolism of all life forms. This fact probably delayed recognition of other roles for purines as autocrine and paracrine substances and neurotransmitters. Today it is recognized that purines are released from neurons and other cells and produce widespread effects on multiple organ systems by binding to cell-surface purinergic receptors. ATP is a classical neurotransmitter that is packaged into neuronal secretory granules and released in quanta in response to action potentials. In addition, ATP is released from non-neuronal sources including platelets, mast cells, and possibly endothelial cells, and large amounts escape from damaged cells. A number of ectoenzymes are involved in the rapid metabolism of ATP to adenosine in the extracellular space. Adenosine is not a classical neurotransmitter because it is not stored in neuronal synaptic granules or released in quanta. It is generally thought of as a neuromodulator that gains access to the extracellular space in part from the breakdown of extracellular ATP, and in part by translocation from the cytoplasm of cells by nucleoside transport proteins. Adenosine thus acts as a metabolic messenger that imparts information about the intracellular metabolism of a

Basic Neurochemistry: Molecular, Cellular, and Medical Aspects, 5th Ed., edited by G. J. Siegel et al. Published by Raven Press, Ltd., New York, 1994. Correspondence to Joel Linden, Departments of Internal Medicine and Physiology, University of Virginia, 1010 Cobb Hall, Hospital Drive, Box 158, Health Sciences Center, Charlottesville, Virginia 22908.

TABLE 1.   Purinergic receptor classes

	Adenosine receptors			
	A_1	A_{2a}	A_{2b}	A_3
Agonists	CCPA ≥ R-PIA > NECA	WRC 0090 = CGS 21680 ≥ NECA	NECA ≫ CGS 21680	NECA ≥ R-PIA ≫ CGS 21680
Radioligands	[³H]CCPA, [³H]CHA, [¹²⁵I]ABA, [¹²⁵I]APNEA	[³H]CGS 21680, [¹²⁵I]APE	None	[¹²⁵I]ABA, [¹²⁵I]APNEA
Antagonists	CPXª = XAC > BW-A1433 > KF-17837 > N-0861	KF-17837 > BW-A1433 = XAC > CPX	XAC > BW-A1433 > CPX	ABOPX > BW-A1433 > XAC
Radioligands	[³H]CPX, [¹²⁵I]BW-A844, [³H]XAC	None	None	[¹²⁵I]ABOPX
Brain distribution	Hippocampus, cerebellum, cortex, striatum, thalamus	Striatum, nucleus accumbens, olfactory bulb	Pars tuberalis	(Low levels) cortex, striatum, olfactory bulb
Effectors	↓ Adenylyl cyclase ↓ Ca²⁺ channels ↑ K⁺ channels ↑↓ Phospholipase C	↑ Adenylyl cyclase	↑ Adenylyl cyclase	↓ Adenylyl cyclase

ª CPX is sometimes abbreviated as DPCPX.
ᵇ Desensitizing agonist.
(CCPA) 2-chloro-N^6-cyclopentyladenosine; (R-PIA) R-N^6-phenylisopropyladenosine; (NECA) 5'-N-ethylcarboxami-doadenosine; (WRC 0090) 2-[2-(4-methylphenyl)ethoxy]adenosine; (CGS 21680) 2-(p-2-carboxyethyl)phenethyl-amino)-5'-N-ethylcarboxamidoadenosine; (ABA) N^6-aminobenzyladenosine; (APE) 2-[2-(4-aminophenyl)ethylami-no]adenosine; (CHA) N^6-cyclohexyladenosine; (APNEA) N^6-2-(4-amino-3-iodo-phenyl)ethyladenosine; (CPX) 8-cyclopentyl-1,3-dipropylxanthine. (Continued on next page.)

particular cell to extracellular-facing receptors on the same and adjacent cells. Extracellular adenosine is rapidly removed, in part by reuptake into cells and in part by degradation to inosine. Receptors for both ATP and adenosine are very widely distributed in the nervous system as well as in other tissues.

Drury and Szent-Gyorgyi [1] first noted effects of adenyl purines on cardiac and vascular contractility in 1929, but it was not until 34 years later that Berne identified a physiological role for adenosine as a mediator of coronary vasodilation in response to myocardial hypoxia. In 1970 Sattin and Rall [2] and Shimizu and coworkers [3] reported that adenosine stimulates cyclic AMP formation in the brain and proposed that these effects are mediated by cell-surface receptors. Subsequently, Burnstock proposed that purines can act as neurotransmitters.

PURINERGIC RECEPTORS

Based on physiological responses of various tissues to purines, Burnstock deduced that there are distinct receptors that bind adenosine or ATP, designated P_1 and P_2 purinergic receptors, respectively [4]. It is now known that there are *families* of both adenosine and ATP receptors. In addition to adenosine, some adenosine analogs activate adenosine receptors but not ATP receptors, and some ATP analogs activate ATP receptors but not adenosine receptors (Fig. 1). However, not all purines activate purinergic receptors. For example, adenine, guanosine, inosine, and uric acid do not activate adenosine or ATP receptors. The development of synthetic compounds that activate purinergic receptors has been important for elucidating how purinergic receptors function because some

TABLE 1   *(continued)*

		ATP receptors		
P_{2x}	P_{2y}	P_{2z}	P_{2t}	P_{2u}
APCPP $\gg$ 2-MeS-ATP	2-MeS-ATP > APCPP	ATP-α-S > 2-MeS-ATP	ADP > 2-MeS-ADP	UTP = ATP
[^{3}H]APCPP	[^{35}S]ADPβS	[^{3}H]2-MeS-L-ATP	[^{32}P]2-MeS-ADP	[^{35}S]ADPβS
ANAPP$_3$,[b] suramin	RB2, suramin	2-MeS-L-ATP	2-Cl-ATP	Suramin

(XAC) xanthineamino congener; (BW-A844) 3-aminophenethyl-8-cyclopentyl-1-propylxanthine; (KF-17837) 1,3,7-tripropyl-8-(3,4-dimethoxystyryl)xanthine; (N-0861) N^6-endonorbornan-2-yl-9-methyladenine; (ABOPX) 3-amino-benzyl-8-(4-oxyacetate)-1-propylxanthine; (BW-A1433) 1,3-dipropyl-8-(4-acrylate)xanthine; (APCPP) α,β-methylene ATP; (MeS) methylthio; (ADPβS) adenosine-5'-β-thiodiphosphate; (RB2) reactive blue 2; (ANAPP$_3$) 3-O-(3[N-(4-azido-2-nitrophenyl)amino]propionyl) adenosine 5'-triphosphate.

of these compounds are more potent than the parent purines, and most are more stable than adenosine and ATP, which have short biological half-lives.

Purinergic receptors are located on the surface of cells and hence bind purines in the extracellular space. There is also an adenosine binding site located intracellularly on the enzyme adenylyl cyclase. This is referred to as the "P-site" of adenylyl cyclase, and binding of adenosine and other purines, notably 3'-AMP, 2'-deoxy-3'-AMP, and 2',5'-dideoxyadenosine, to this site inhibits enzyme activity [5]. The P-site was named on the basis of the fact that adenosine analogs with unmodified purine substituents can bind to it. Molecules modified in the ribose portion can bind to the P-site. There are a number of other intracellular binding sites for adenosine and ATP, both of which are substrates and allosteric modulators of nu-merous enzymes. Because of their intracellular location and distinct pharmacology, these intracellular binding sites are not usually considered to be purinergic receptors.

There are distinct classes of cell-surface purinergic receptors that bind adenosine or ATP

Multiple types of purinergic receptors were proposed on the basis of observations that adenosine and ATP analogs produce physiological responses in various organ systems with distinct structure-activity profiles. In some instances these differences in physiological responses have been confirmed by results of radioligand binding assays. The nomenclature of purinergic receptor subtypes and the identity of selective agonists and antagonists are listed in Table 1.

Adenosine receptors are activated by

A

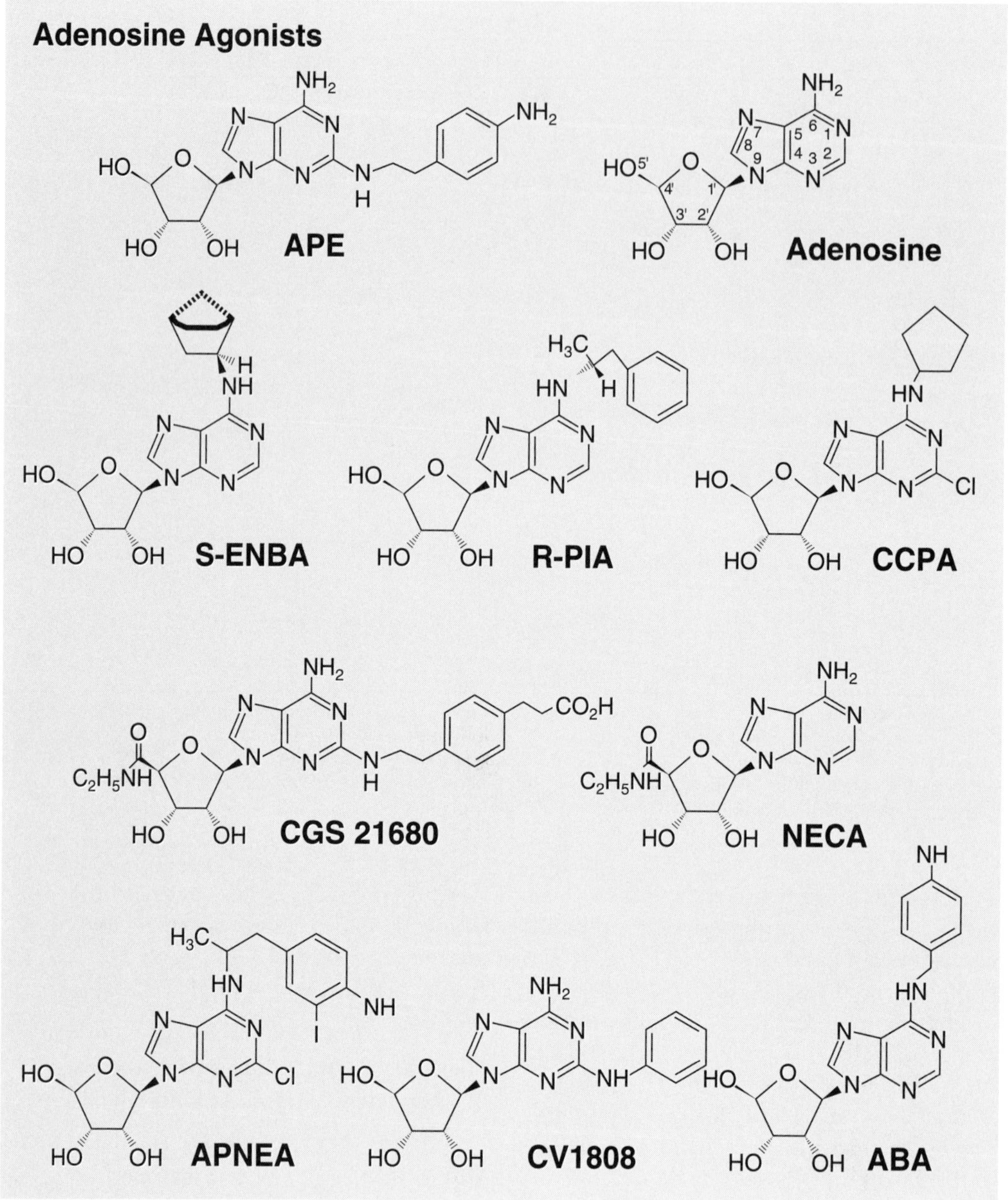

Adenosine Agonists

FIG. 1. Structures of purinergic drugs. Refer to the legend of Table 1 for abbreviations. (S-ENBA) *S*-endonorboronyla-denosine; (CV1808) 2-phenylaminoadenosine; (NBTI) nitrobenzylthioinosine.

adenosine, but not by guanosine, cytosine, or uridine. A number of high-affinity, selective antagonists have been synthesized, and some of these are listed in Table 1. Generally, P_2 receptors are activated by ATP, but an excep-tion is the P_{2t} receptor that is found exclu-sively on platelets and megakaryocytes. The P_{2t} receptor is activated by ADP and blocked by ATP. It is notable that ADP is a major con-stituent of platelet secretory granules. P_2 pu-

B

Adenosine Antagonists

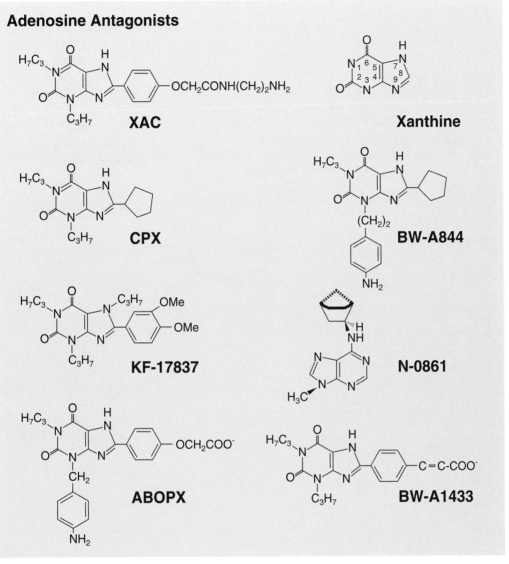

XAC

Xanthine

CPX

BW-A844

KF-17837

N-0861

ABOPX

BW-A1433

C

Adenosine Transport Inhibitors

NBTI

Dipyridamole

FIG. 1.   *(continued)*

rinergic receptors generally are not activated by pyrimidine triphosphates (uridine triphosphate [UTP] or cytosine triphosphate [CTP]) with the exception of the P_{2u} receptor, which is so named because it is activated equally well by ATP and UTP. A problem that continues to hamper the study of ATP receptors is the absence of selective antagonists, and the compounds that are listed as ATP receptor antagonists in Table 1 are nonselective, low-affinity compounds.

Xanthines block adenosine, but not ATP receptors

One of the criteria initially used to distinguish adenosine and ATP receptors was selective blockade of the former by xanthines (see Fig. 1) such as caffeine (1,3,7-trimethylxanthine) and theophylline (1,3-dimethylxanthine). These xanthines occur naturally in coffee, tea, and chocolate, and their well-known stimulant action has been attributed to blockade of adenosine receptors in the

A

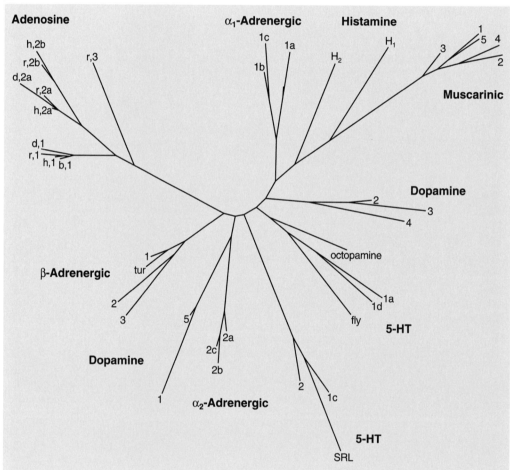

FIG. 2. **A:** Homologies between adenosine and cationic amine receptors. A *tree* constructed using distance criteria was generated by comparing the nucleotide sequences on only the highly conserved transmembrane regions of the receptors. (r) rat; (d) dog; (h) human; (tur) turkey; (SRL) a putative serotonin receptor; (5-HT) 5-hydroxytryptamine. (Tree construction by William Pearson and Kevin Lynch of the University of Virginia.)

B

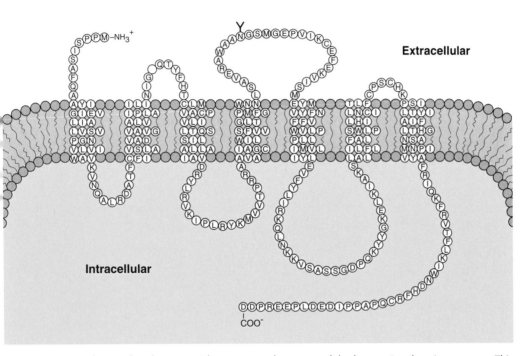

FIG. 2. *(continued)* **B:** Deduced amino acid sequence and structure of the human A_1 adenosine receptor. This typical adenosine receptor is a member of the large family of guanine nucleotide-binding protein-coupled receptors that span the plasma membrane seven times. Unusual features of adenosine receptors are short amino termini lacking N-linked glycosylation sites. These are found instead on extracellular loop 2 (as pictured). The ligand binding pocket is thought to be formed by amino acids in transmembrane segments 2, 3, and 7. GTP-binding proteins are thought to interact with juxtamembranous regions of intracellular loops 2 and 3 and the carboxyl terminus.

central nervous system. Recently, 8-phenyl-xanthines and 8-cycloalkylxanthines were synthesized and characterized as adenosine receptor antagonists that are thousands of times more potent and, in some cases, more selective for individual adenosine receptor subtypes than are caffeine and theophylline.

Purinergic receptor subtypes have been cloned using a homology-screening protocol

Oligonucleotides were designed on the basis of similarities among genes encoding the superfamily of receptors that interact with guanosine triphosphate (GTP)-binding proteins (G proteins), all of which contain seven hydrophobic membrane-spanning segments [6,7]. The superfamily includes receptors for biogenic amines and a variety of other hor-

mones and neurotransmitters. Once the first adenosine receptors were identified, several adenosine receptor subtypes were cloned in quick succession (Table 2). All of the adenosine receptors consist of a single subunit 35 to 46 kDa in molecular mass. The similarity of adenosine receptors to the cationic amine receptors is illustrated in Fig. 2A. Figure 2B shows the structure of the human A_1 adenosine receptor which has features shared by the other members of this family. The receptors have one or two consensus sequences for N-linked glycosylation (NXS/T) in their second extracellular loop. It is thought that these glycosylation sites may be involved in targeting receptors for expression on the cell surface. Adenosine receptors also contain multiple serine and threonine residues on the third intracellular loop or near the car-

TABLE 2.   Properties of cloned adenosine receptor subtypes[a]

Receptor subtype	Predominant locations	Clone/accession no.	Mass (Da)	mRNA size (kb)	No. of amino acids
A_1	Brain, spinal cord, testis, fat, heart	Canine/X14051 Rat/M69045, M64299 Bovine/X63592, M86261 Human	36,511–36,699	3.5, 5.5	326
A_{2a}	Striatum	Canine/X14052 Rat Human/M97370	44,707–45,060	2.6	410–412
A_{2b}	Large intestine, cecum, bladder	Rat/M91466 Human/M97759	36,333–36,367	1.8, 2.2	332
TGPCR1 A_3	Testis	Rat/X59249, M94152	36,512	1.5	319

[a] Accession numbers refer to the Genbank or EMBL databases.

boxyl terminus. These may become phosphorylated and lead to receptor desensitization during prolonged exposure to adenosine. The greatest similarities in the structure of the adenosine receptor subtypes are found in the transmembrane segments, particularly in segments 2, 3, and 7. This suggests that these segments may be aligned next to each other in the plane of the membrane bilayer to form a ligand binding pocket. ATP receptors have also begun to be cloned. These are distinct from adenosine receptors and as yet are poorly characterized.

METABOLISM OF ATP AND ADENOSINE

The concentration of adenosine in the interstitial fluid of brain and other tissues is increased when oxygen supply exceeds oxygen demand. The effect of adenosine is to increase oxygen delivery by dilating most vascular beds and to decrease oxygen demand by reducing cellular energy utilization. In the brain this is usually manifested as a decrease in neuronal firing and in the release of excitatory neurotransmitters.

As described above, ATP is released as a neurotransmitter or cotransmitter. In addition, it is abundant in granules released from mast cells and basophils and is released from damaged tissues and possibly from endothelial cells. Large amounts of ADP are released from activated platelets. Another possible source of extracellular purine nucleotide is cyclic AMP, which is actively secreted from some types of cells. Adenine nucleotides are rapidly degraded by a series of ectonucleotidases (Fig. 3). 5'-Nucleotidase, which converts AMP to adenosine, exists both in the cytosol and as a membrane-associated ectoenzyme. Ecto-5'-nucleotidase is a homodimer that is linked to the plasma membrane through a glycosyl-phosphatidylinositol lipid anchor. This enzyme is competitively inhibited by α,β-methylene ADP (AOPCP). In cytochemical studies, ecto-5'-nucleotidase has been found to be associated with plasma membranes of glial cells and astrocytes, particularly near synaptic terminals. Cytosolic 5'-nucleotidases are involved in the formation of adenosine during increased metabolic activity. Even a small decrease in ATP can lead to a large increase in the substrate for this enzyme, AMP, because under normal conditions the concentration of ATP is about 50 times higher than that of AMP.

Adenosine and homocysteine are

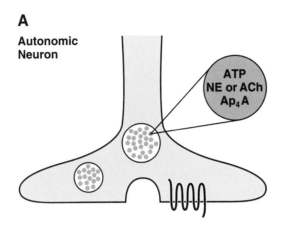

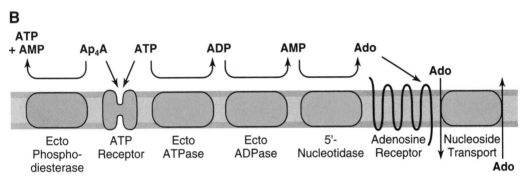

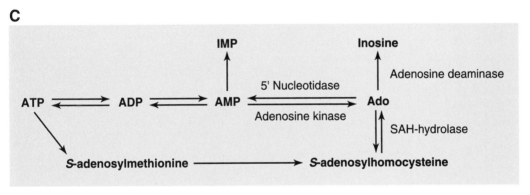

FIG. 3. Purine release and metabolism. **A:** Adenine nucleotides are schematically depicted as being stored as cotransmitters in synaptic granules (see *enlargement*) of a typical autonomic neuron. (NE) norepinephrine; (ACh) acetylcholine; (Ap₄A) diadenosine tetraphosphate. **B:** ATP and diadenosine tetraphosphate (Ap₄A) are degraded to adenosine by a series of ectoenzymes. Adenosine (Ado) accumulates in hypoxic, ischemic, or metabolically active cells and can be transported to the interstitial space by a membrane-associated nucleoside transport protein. Both pre- **(A)** and post- **(B)** junctional adenosine receptors are depicted as traversing the plasma membrane seven times as is typical of receptors that interact with GTP-binding proteins. A different structure is depicted for a postjunctional ATP receptor since some (e.g., P₂ₓ), but not all (e.g., P₂ᵧ) of these are receptor-operated channels. Refer to the text for additional discussion. **C:** The major pathways of intracellular adenosine metabolism are also shown. (IMP) inosine monophosphate; (SAH) *S*-adenosylhomocysteine.

formed from the hydrolysis of *S*-adenosylho-mocysteine (SAH) by the enzyme SAH hydrolase. Attempts to measure intracellular adenosine are complicated by the fact that over 90 percent of intracellular adenosine may be weakly bound to this enzyme. SAH is formed from *S*-adenosylmethionine (SAM), which is a cofactor in transmethylation reactions. Although SAH is the precursor of a sizable fraction of adenosine under resting conditions, most adenosine is derived from the 5-nucleotidase pathway during conditions of hypoxia, ischemia, or metabolic stress.

Adenosine can be transported across cell membranes in either direction by a membrane-associated facilitated nucleoside transport protein. A second Na^+-dependent nucleoside transport process is found in some tissues, including renal epithelia and choroid plexus [8]. Most degradation of adenosine is intracellular, as evidenced by the fact that inhibitors of adenosine transport such as dipyridamole (see Fig. 1) increase interstitial levels of adenosine. Dipyridamole is used clinically to elevate adenosine in coronary arteries and produce coronary vasodilation. In high doses, dipyridamole can accentuate adenosine receptor-mediated actions in the central nervous system, resulting in sedation, anticonvulsant effects, decreased locomotor activity, and decreased neuronal activity. Other inhibitors of facilitated adenosine transport include nitro-benzylthioinosine and mioflazine.

After extracellular adenosine is taken up into cells, it can be reincorporated into the nucleotide pool upon phosphorylation by the cytosolic enzyme adenosine kinase. In normoxic resting tissues, most adenosine is rephosphorylated since the K_m of adenosine kinase is 10 to 100 times lower than the K_m of adenosine deaminase. Deamination, leading to a large accumulation of inosine, becomes the major pathway of adenosine metabolism when adenosine levels are elevated, because the kinase becomes saturated with substrate. Most adenosine deaminase activity is cytosolic, but there is some ectoadenosine deam-inase activity that can deaminate adenosine in the extracellular space. Investigation of these metabolic pathways has been fostered by the availability of specific inhibitors of some of these enzymes. Adenosine kinase is competitively inhibited by iodotubercidin and 5'-deoxy-5'-amino-adenosine. Adenosine deaminase is competitively inhibited by deoxycoformycin and by erythro-9-[2-hydroxy-3-nonyl]adenine (EHNA). These drugs, by elevating adenosine, have been found to produce adenosine-like actions in laboratory animals.

ADENOSINE RECEPTORS

A_1 adenosine receptors

A_1 receptors were originally characterized on the basis of their ability to inhibit adenylyl cyclase in adipose tissue. A number of other G protein-mediated effectors of A_1 receptors have subsequently been discovered; these include activation of K^+ channels, extensively characterized in striatal neurons [9], and inhibition of Ca^{2+} channels, extensively characterized in dorsal root ganglion cells [10]. The effectors of A_1 adenosine receptors and other purinergic receptor subtypes are summarized in Table 3.

The binding of ligands to rat A_1 receptors is greatly enhanced by the addition of aryl or cycloalkyl substituents to the N^6 position of adenosine or to the 8-position of xanthines. Conformationally constrained bicyclic compounds have even greater affinities (see Fig. 1). Thus, for rat A_1 receptors it is widely accepted that R-N^6-phenylisopropyladenosine (R-PIA) binds more tightly than 5'-N-ethylcarboxamidoadenosine (NECA). A complicating factor in this structure-activity profile stems from the observation that there are marked species differences in ligand binding. Thus, N^6-substituted adenosine analogs are potent agonists and 8-aryl-substituted xanthines are potent antagonists in rat, but these compounds have lower affinity for canine and guinea pig receptors, and the

TABLE 3. Effectors of purinergic receptors

Receptor	Effector
A_1	Inhibit adenylyl cyclase
	Increase K^+ channel conductance
	Decrease Ca^{2+} channel conductance
	Increase or decrease phospholipase C activity
A_{2a}	Activate adenylyl cyclase
A_{2b}	Activate adenylyl cyclase
	Activate phospholipase C (*Xenopus* oocytes)
A_3	Inhibit adenylyl cyclase
P_{2u}	Activate phospholipase C
P_{2x}	Increase Ca^{2+} channel conductance (receptor-gated channel)
P_{2y}	Activate phospholipase C
	Activate phospholipase D
	Activate phospholipid base exchange activity
P_{2t}	Inhibit adenylyl cyclase
P_{2z}	Increase ionic conductance (receptor-gated channel?)

pharmacology of other species, including that of humans, has not yet been studied in great detail.

A_1 adenosine receptors are widely distributed in the central nervous system (Fig. 4). These receptors have been extensively characterized in brain because they are expressed in high density (0.5–1.0 pmol/mg membrane protein), and because of the development of several high-affinity radioligands (see Table 1). In the periphery, adenosine A_1 receptors are found in the heart where they produce negative inotropic, chronotropic, and dromotropic responses [11]; in adipose tissue where they inhibit lipolysis and enhance insulin-stimulated glucose transport; and in kidney where they reduce glomerular filtration pressure and produce an antidiuresis.

Many of the central actions of adenosine can be attributed to inhibition of Ca^{2+}-dependent excitatory neurotransmitter release. Most of these effects appear to be presynaptic and are mediated by G proteins coupled to inhibition of N-type Ca^{2+} channels and stimulation of K^+ channels. However, in

some instances, adenosine produces excitatory effects in the central nervous system. For example, in the nucleus tractus solitarius (NTS), adenosine increases glutamate release and elicits excitatory cardiovascular effects [12]. Both excitatory and inhibitory effects of adenosine have been noted in hippocampal slices [13]. Activation of A_1 receptors has been shown to produce a species-dependent activation or inhibition of the phosphatidylinositol pathway in cerebral cortex. In other tissues, activation of A_1 receptors results in synergistic activation of the phosphatidylinositol pathway in concert with Ca^{2+}-mobilizing hormones or neurotransmitters [14]. Effects of adenosine that have been attributed to activation of central A_1 receptors include sedation, anticonvulsant activity, analgesia, and neuroprotection. In spinal cord, adenosine can be derived from capsaicin-sensitive, small-diameter primary afferent neurons and potentiates the antinociceptive action of norepinephrine [15]. Opiates have been shown to induce release of adenosine from brain slices and synaptosomes and the spinal cord [16], and some of the effects of opiates are blocked by adenosine receptor antagonists. It has also been suggested that some of the behavioral effects of alcoholic beverages may be mediated by adenosine because intoxicating concentrations of ethanol can block adenosine transport.

A_2 adenosine receptors

A_2 receptors were originally characterized on the basis of their ability to stimulate cyclic AMP accumulation in neuronal tissues. Based on substantial differences in binding affinity for adenosine, these were divided into A_{2a} and A_{2b} subtypes, a subdivision that has subsequently been confirmed by results of molecular cloning (see Table 2). CGS 21680 binds with much higher affinity to A_{2a} than to A_{2b} receptors. Adenosine analogs with alkoxy- or alkamino substitutions on the 2-position also are selective A_{2a} agonists. 8-Styrylxanthines such as KF-17837 have been

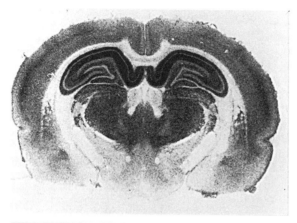

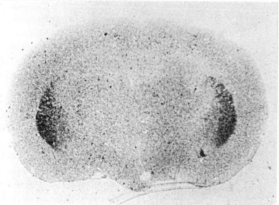

FIG. 4.   Distribution of A_1 and A_{2a} receptors in rat brain. *Top:* Autoradiograph of the binding of the A_1-selective radioligand [^{3}H]cyclohexyladenosine to a slice of rat brain. Note the widespread distribution of A_1 receptors and the particularly high density of receptors in the hippocampus. *Bottom:* Autoradiograph of the binding of the A_{2a}-selective radioligand [^{125}I]APE. Note the restricted striatal distribution. (Photograph courtesy of Dr. Kevin Lee of the University of Virginia.)

reported to be selective antagonists of the A_{2a} receptor.

In the central nervous system, A_{2a} receptors are restricted to the striatum, nucleus accumbens, and olfactory tubercle (see Fig. 4). A_{2a} adenosine receptors are coexpressed with D_2 dopamine receptors in a subset of striatal neurons [17]. Activation of A_{2a} adenosine receptors enhances cyclic AMP formation, whereas activation of D_2 dopamine receptors inhibits cyclic AMP formation. The administration of drugs that stimulate dopamine receptors, such as apomorphine and L-DOPA, to rodents with a unilateral lesion of the nigrostriatal pathway induces a turning behavior contralateral to the lesioned side due to the development of supersensitivity of dopamine receptors in the denervated striatum. Methylxanthines, which block adenosine receptors, also produce such turn-ing behavior and potentiate the effects of dopamine agonists. On the other hand, adenosine agonists inhibit D_2-mediated behaviors. These findings suggest that modulation by adenosine of striatal dopaminergic systems contributes to the psychomotor depressant effects of adenosine agonists and to the psychomotor stimulatory effects of methylxanthines. Since rodent turning behavior is an experimental model of Parkinson's disease, A_{2a}-selective adenosine receptor antagonists may have potential as antiparkinsonian drugs [18].

A_2 receptors present on sensory nerves in the carotid body, aortic body, pulmonary circulation, and elsewhere produce excitatory sensory input. These receptors have been implicated in the production of dyspnea and pain of angina pectoris, ulcer, and the human blister base preparation.

A_3 adenosine receptors

Prior to their cloning, the existence of A_1 and A_2 receptors had been postulated based on results of binding assays with radioligands and the study of physiological and biochemical responses to various ligands. After these receptors were cloned, a search for related genes revealed an unexpected receptor in the adenosine family, designated A_3. The term "A_3" was also used to designate a putative A_1-like receptor in heart and autonomic neurons, but such a receptor has not been proven to exist, and this old, pharmacologically postulated A_3 receptor is distinct from the A_3 receptor that has been cloned. In current usage, A_3 refers to the cloned receptor. In the rat, the A_3 transcript is found almost exclusively in testes. However, the transcript for similar sheep and human receptors is modestly expressed throughout the brain and heavily expressed in pineal, lung, and spleen. It is not yet known which, if any, of the central effects of adenosine are mediated by A_3 receptors.

Uncloned adenosine receptors

Subtle differences in the pharmacological properties of A_1 receptor-mediated responses in brain, autonomic ganglia, neuromuscular synapses, heart, and fat have led to as yet unsubstantiated suggestions that subtypes of A_1 receptors may exist. Since A_1 adenosine receptors have been shown to be capable of coupling to GTP-binding proteins in both the G_i and G_o families, it is possible that some of these pharmacological differences are produced because receptors couple to different G proteins in different tissues.

2-Phenylaminoadenosine (CV 1808, see Fig. 1) and several related compounds have been shown to activate a K^+ conductance in striatal neurons and coronary artery smooth muscle cells [19]. It is notable in this regard that blockade of ATP-sensitive K^+ channels with hypoglycemic sulfonylureas such as glybenclamide greatly attenuate hypoxia- and adenosine-mediated coronary vasodilation. This suggests a possible linkage between ATP-sensitive K^+ channels that are highly expressed in the central nervous system and an as yet unspecified adenosine receptor. Pharmacological characterization of ligands that activate K^+ currents in striatal neurons and smooth muscle cells and that compete with [^{3}H]CV 1808 for binding to striatal membranes suggests a novel receptor tentatively designated the A_4 receptor. This putative receptor can be distinguished from other adenosine receptors because it is weakly blocked by xanthines. Xanthine-resistant relaxant effects of adenosine noted in tracheal and vascular tissues also suggest that xanthine-resistant adenosine receptors that have not yet been cloned may exist or that adenosine may produce some of its actions by nonreceptor-mediated intracellular actions.

ATP RECEPTORS

Like P_1 (adenosine) receptors, it is clear that P_2 (ATP) receptors have a very wide tissue distribution. Although ATP and adenine nucleotides play a central role in intracellular energy metabolism and do not readily traverse the plasma membrane, there are several sources of extracellular ATP which permit it to gain access to cell-surface receptors and hence play an important role in cellular signaling [20]. In the autonomic nervous system ATP is released as a cotransmitter from both sympathetic and parasympathetic neurons. ATP can also be released from synaptosomal preparations of cortex, hypothalamus, and medulla. In cortical synaptosomes a portion of ATP that is released is coreleased with acetylcholine or norepinephrine, but the majority is released from neurons that are neither adrenergic nor cholinergic. In affinity-purified cholinergic nerve terminals, ATP and acetylcholine are coreleased in a ratio of $1:10$. The ATP that is released is rapidly broken down by widely distributed 5'-nucleotidases, resulting in the formation of adenosine (see Fig. 3). Excitatory effects of ATP on neurons in the central nervous system have been noted in cuneate nucleus, cerebellar Purkinje cells, cells in the sensory vestibular and trigeminal nuclei, and cortex. In many instances ATP has been noted to have biphasic or inhibitory effects, attributed in part to its breakdown to adenosine.

P_{2t} receptors

P_{2t} receptors are found exclusively on platelets, their precursor megakaryocyte cells, and certain cultured hematopoietic cells such as K562 leukemia cells. They can be distinguished from other P_2 receptors in that ADP is the most potent natural agonist, and ATP is a competitive antagonist. ADP acts via a G protein to inhibit cyclic AMP accumulation, mobilize intracellular Ca^{2+}, and stimulate granule secretion. The responses of platelets to ADP are prevented by activators of protein kinase C such as phorbol 12-myristate 13-acetate.

P_{2y} and P_{2u} receptors

P_{2y} receptors have been extensively characterized in turkey erythrocytes as well as in liver and endothelial cells. They couple via a G protein, G_q, to activate phospholipase C and produce an inositol 1,4,5-trisphosphate-dependent mobilization of intracellular Ca^{2+}. A possibly distinct P_{2u} receptor has been proposed on the basis of the fact that in some tissues the pyrimidine nucleotide UTP has a similar effect [21]. Although the putative P_{2u} receptor is also activated by purine nucleotides, its activation by UTP represents an exception to the classification of these receptors as "purinergic" since UTP is a pyrimidine.

P_{2y} receptors found on endothelial cells elicit a Ca^{2+}-dependent release of endothelium-dependent relaxing factor (EDRF) and vasodilation. A secondary activation of a Ca^{2+}-sensitive phospholipase A_2 increases the synthesis of endothelial prostacyclin, which limits the extent of intravascular platelet aggre-gation following vascular damage and platelet stimulation. The P_{2y}-mediated vasodilation opposes a vasoconstriction elicited by P_{2x} receptors found on vascular smooth muscle cells that elicit an endothelial-independent excitation (i.e., constriction). P_{2y} receptors are also found on adrenal chromaffin cells and platelets, where they modulate catecholamine release and aggregation, respectively. P_{2y} receptors on chromaffin cells have been found to bind diadenosine polyphosphates such as diadenosine tetraphosphate (Ap_4A, see Fig. 3) and diadenosine pentaphosphate (see Fig. 1) with high affinity. Diadenosine polyphosphates are costored with ATP and catecholamines in chromaffin cells and possibly in neuronal secretory granules, and trigger P_{2y} receptor-mediated Ca^{2+} mobilization [22]. Although the ratio of dinucleotides to ATP is low (approximately 1:10), the metabolism of dinucleotide polyphosphates by ectophosphodiesterases is much slower than the metabolism of nucleotides by ectonucleotidases; thus, receptor-mediated effects of dinucleotide polyphosphates may become accentuated with time and distance from release sites.

In addition to activating phospholipase C, the P_{2y} receptor of rat liver has been shown to be coupled via G proteins to phospholipase D and to distinct phospholipid base exchange enzymes that stimulate the incorporation of choline into phospholipids [23]. Base exchange activity may serve to replenish the phosphatidylcholine depleted from the plasma membranes as a result of prolonged activation of phospholipase C.

P_{2x} receptors

P_{2x} receptors have in many instances been shown to activate a receptor-operated channel that triggers rapid (<1 msec) Ca^{2+} entry into cells. These receptors are found in the gastrointestinal tract, veins and arteries, the genitourinary tract, urinary bladder, vas deferens, nictitating membrane and cardiac muscle, and pheochromocytoma (PC-12) cells. Receptor-operated fast channels are also found in the central nervous system, where they respond to ATP as well as to serotonin, acetylcholine, and glutamate, each of which binds to distinct receptor-operated channels. Pharmacological characterization of the P_2 receptor in the rat medial habenula suggests that the neuronal receptor is similar to the P_{2x} receptor found in the periphery [24]. The ATP-gated channels show inward rectification, unlike N-methyl-D-aspartate (NMDA)-gated channels, which become blocked by Mg^{2+} at negative potentials. Thus, Ca^{2+} can enter ATP-gated channels in neurons that have not been depolarized.

P_{2z} receptors

ATP^{4-}, a minor form of purine nucleotide that is not complexed with divalent cations, has been proposed to activate putative P_{2z} receptors found on various blood cells (erythrocytes, lymphocytes, macrophages, and neutrophils) and mast cells. It has been suggested that ATP is a mediator of cell-to-cell spread of Ca^{2+} in mast cells and may contribute to inflammatory responses [25].

REFERENCES

1. Drury, A. N., and Szent-Gyorgyi, A. The physiological activity of adenine compounds with especial reference to their action upon the mammalian heart. *J. Physiol.* (*Lond.*) 68: 213–237, 1929.
2. Sattin, A., and Rall, T. W. The effect of adenosine and adenine nucleotides on the cyclic adenosine 3′,5′-phosphate content of guinea pig cerebral cortex slices. *Mol. Pharmacol.* 6: 12–23, 1970.
3. Shimizu, H., Creveling, C. R., and Daly, J. Stimulated formation of adenosine 3′,5′-cyclic phosphate in cerebral cortex: Synergism between electrical activity and biogenic amines. *Proc. Natl. Acad. Sci. U.S.A.* 65: 1033–1040, 1970.
4. Burnstock, G. A basis for distinguishing two types of purinergic receptor. In L. Bolis and R. W. Straub (eds.), *Cell Membrane Receptors for Drugs and Hormones: A Multidisciplinary Approach*. New York: Raven Press, 1978, pp. 107–118.
5. Johnson, R. A., Yeung, S-M. H., Bushfield, M., Stubner, D., and Shoshani, I. 'P'-site-mediated inhibition of adenylyl cyclase and its physiological implications. In S. Imai and M. Nakazawa (eds.), *Role of Adenosine and Adenine Nucleotides in the Biological System*. Amsterdam: Elsevier, 1991, pp. 43–55.
6. Liebert, F., Parmentier, M., Lefort, A., Dinsart, C., Van Sande, J., Maenhaut, C., Simons, M.-J., Dumont, J. E., and Vassart, G. Selective amplification and cloning of four new members of the G protein-coupled receptor family. *Science* 244:569–572, 1989.
7. Linden, J., Tucker, A. L., and Lynch, K. R. Molecular cloning of adenosine A_1 and A_2 receptors. *Trends Pharmacol. Sci.* 12:326–328, 1991.
8. Spector, T., and Huntoon, S. Specificity and sodium-dependence of the active nucleoside transport system in choroid plexus. *J. Neurochem.* 42:1048–1052, 1984.
9. Trussel, L. O., and Jackson, M. B. Adenosine-activated potassium conductance in cultured striatal neurons. *Proc. Natl. Acad. Sci. U.S.A.* 82:4857–4861, 1985.
10. Dolphin, A. C., Forda, S. R., and Scott, R. H. Calcium-dependent currents in cultured rat dorsal root ganglion neurons are inhibited by an adenosine analogue. *J. Physiol.* (*Lond.*) 373:47–61, 1986.
11. Belardinelli, L., Linden, J., and Berne, R. M. The cardiac effects of adenosine. *Prog. Cardiovasc. Dis.* 32:73–97, 1989.
12. Mosqueda-Garcia, R., Tseng, C.-J., Appalsamy, M., Beck, C., and Robertson, D. Cardiovascular excitatory effects of adenosine in the nucleus of the solitary tract. *Hypertension* 18:494–502, 1991.
13. Okada, Y., Sakurai, T., and Mori, M. Excitatory effect of adenosine on neurotransmission is due to increase of transmitter release in the hippocampal slices. *Neurosci. Lett.* 142: 233–236, 1992.
14. Linden, J. Structure and function of the A_1 adenosine receptor. *FASEB J.* 5:2668–2676, 1991.
15. Sawynok, J., Reid, A., and Isbrucker, R. Adenosine mediates calcium-induced antinociception and potentiation of noradrenergic antinociception in the spinal cord. *Brain Res.* 524: 187–195, 1990.

16. Sawynok, J., Sweeney, M. I., and White, T. D. Adenosine release may mediate spinal analgesia by morphine. *Trends Pharmacol. Sci.* 10:186–189, 1989.

17. Fink, J. S., Weaver, D. R., Rivkees, S. A., Peterfreund, R. A., Pollack, A. E., Adler, E. M., and Reppert, S. M. Molecular cloning of the rat A_2 adenosine receptor: Selective co-expression with D_2 dopamine receptors in rat striatum. *Mol. Brain Res.* 14:186–195, 1992.

18. Ferre, S., Von Euler, G., Johansson, B., Fredholm, B. B., and Fuxe, K. Stimulation of high-affinity adenosine A_2 receptors decreases the affinity of dopamine D_2 receptors in rat striatal membranes. *Proc. Natl. Acad. Sci. U.S.A.* 88:7238–7241, 1991.

19. Cornfield, L. J., Hu, S., Hurt, S. D., and Sills, M. A. [^{3}H]2-Phenylaminoadenosine ([^{3}H]CV 1808) labels a novel adenosine receptor in rat brain. *J. Pharmacol. Exp. Ther.* 263:552–561, 1992.

20. Hoyle, C. H. V., and Burnstock, G. ATP receptors and their physiological roles. In T. Stone (ed.), *Adenosine in the Nervous System.* London: Academic Press, 1991, pp. 43–76.

21. O'Connor, S. E., Dainty, I. A., and Leff, P. Further subclassification of ATP receptors based on agonist studies. *Trends Pharmacol. Sci.* 12:137–141, 1991.

22. Castro, E., Pintor, J., and Miras-Portugal, M. T. Ca^{2+}-stores mobilization by diadenosine tetraphosphate, Ap_4A, through a putative P_{2y} purinoceptor in adrenal chromaffin cells. *Br. J. Pharmacol.* 106:833–837, 1992.

23. Siddiqui, R. A., and Exton, J. H. Phospholipid base exchange activity in rat liver plasma membranes. Evidence for regulation by G-protein and P_{2y}-purinergic receptor. *J. Biol. Chem.* 267:5755–5761, 1992.

24. Edwards, F. A., Gibb A. J., and Colquhoun, D. ATP receptor-mediated synaptic currents in the central nervous system. *Nature* 359:144–147, 1992.

25. Osipchuk, Y., and Cahalan, M. Cell-to-cell spread of calcium signals mediated by ATP receptors in mast cells. *Nature* 359:241–244, 1992.

CHAPTER 20

Phosphoinositides

BERNARD W. AGRANOFF AND STEPHEN K. FISHER

BACKGROUND / 418

CHEMISTRY OF THE INOSITOL LIPIDS AND PHOSPHATES / 419

THE INOSITOL PHOSPHATES / 422

DIACYLGLYCEROL / 424

FUNCTIONAL CORRELATES OF PHOSPHOINOSITIDE-LINKED RECEPTORS IN THE NERVOUS SYSTEM / 425

REFERENCES / 428
ADDITIONAL REFERENCES / 428

Basic Neurochemistry: Molecular, Cellular, and Medical Aspects, 5th Ed., edited by G. J. Siegel et al. Published by Raven Press, Ltd., New York, 1994. Correspondence to Bernard W. Agranoff, Mental Health Research Institute, Departments of Biological Chemistry and Psychiatry, University of Michigan, 1103 E. Huron, Ann Arbor, Michigan 48104-1687.

BACKGROUND

A growing number of ligands, including neurotransmitters, neuromodulators, and hormones, have been shown to exert their physiological action via an intracellular second-messenger system in which the activated receptor-ligand complex stimulates the turnover of inositol-containing phospholipids. In this chapter, the biochemical and cellular basis of this ubiquitous pathway, as well as its pharmacological significance, is examined in the context of the nervous system. A brief review of the sequence of the discoveries that have led to our current view provides an understanding of the technological and conceptual obstacles that were overcome in the process.

Stimulation of secretion is accompanied by incorporation of inorganic phosphate into phospholipids

In 1953, Hokin and Hokin [1] reported that slices of pancreas incubated with labeled inorganic phosphate ($^{32}P_i$) exhibited increased phospholipid labeling under conditions of stimulation by muscarinic agents, such as carbamoylcholine (carbachol). Although unphysiologically high concentrations of carbachol were required to produce maximal stimulation, both the lipid labeling and the secretion of amylase into the medium were blocked when the alkaloid atropine, a known muscarinic receptor antagonist, was also present. They had thus discovered a biochemical "handle" with which to investigate receptor action. The observed labeling was confined to two quantitatively minor phospholipid components: phosphatidate (PA) and phosphatidylinositol (PI). This demonstration of receptor-stimulated lipid labeling was quickly extended and generalized to a number of other ligands, each in the presence of an appropriate tissue (e.g., thyrotropin in the presence of thyroid tissue). The avian salt gland, which secretes sodium chloride (NaCl) nonexocy-

totically in the presence of carbachol, also supported a muscarinic stimulation of PA and PI labeling. In each tissue, it was necessary to use whole cells, in the form of slices, minces, or dissociated cells, to elicit the effect. An apparent exception was found in studies with brain homogenates, which support muscarinic stimulation of lipid labeling even though they are broken-cell preparations. It was eventually found that the stimulated lipid labeling in brain homogenates is mediated by a nerve-ending fraction. These pinched-off organelles may be regarded as resealed anucleate neurons in which the vectorial inside-outside relationship has been preserved. Hence, the generalization that whole cells are required for demonstration of ligand-stimulated lipid labeling was upheld. More recently, however, there have been successful demonstrations of ligand-stimulated breakdown of phosphoinositides in membrane preparations supplemented with guanine nucleotides.

Inorganic phosphate incorporation into lipids has been shown to involve a cycle of glycerolipid breakdown and reutilization

A few years after the initial reports of receptor-mediated labeling of lipids, a unique metabolic relationship between PA and PI was elucidated via the liponucleotide intermediate cytidine diphosphate diacylglycerol (CDP·DAG). CDP·DAG is formed from cytidine triphosphate (CTP) and PA, and it serves as the biosynthetic precursor of PI (see Chap. 5); however, under conditions of ligand-stimulated labeling of PA and PI, there is no enhancement of incorporation of labeled glycerol into either of these lipids. This result indicates that the observed stimulated incorporation of $^{32}P_i$ into PA and PI must involve a cycle in which there is degradation and reutilization of the glycerolipid backbone. It was initially proposed that PI breakdown is stimulated as a result of receptor activation, with the release and reutilization of diacylglycerol (DAG). It is now known that in most, if not all, instances of stimulated inositol lipid turnover, the initiating step is the breakdown of a phosphorylated derivative of PI (phosphatidylinositol 4,5-bisphosphate [PI(4,5)P_2;PIP$_2$]) rather than of PI itself, as discussed below. Although it was known that highly phosphorylated inositol lipids are present in tissues, particularly in brain, there were few techniques for their convenient extraction from tissue incubations or for their separation using thin-layer chromatographic (TLC) systems. It was partly for this reason that their role in transmembrane signaling was not recognized earlier. Acidified lipid extraction solvents such as chloroform-methanol-HCl ensure complete extraction of all of the inositol lipids, and TLC systems incorporating oxalate salts in the silica gel matrix have facilitated their separation [2].

Following the initial demonstration of stimulated PI and PA labeling, the broad distribution of this effect became evident. A review of the field in 1975 [3] identified over 60 examples. A common pattern appeared: Elevation of intracellular Ca^{2+} in the activated cells either was demonstrated or could be reasonably inferred. It was less clear at the time whether the elevated intracellular Ca^{2+} was the cause or the result of the stimulated labeling of lipids. This matter was clarified in 1983 by the demonstration by Streb et al. that inositol trisphosphate [I(1,4,5)P_3], a cleavage product of PI(4,5)P_2, serves as a mediator of intracellular Ca^{2+} release [4]. Thus, lipid breakdown precedes Ca^{2+} release. To better understand the events leading to PIP$_2$ breakdown and its resynthesis, it is useful to review the underlying structural chemistry.

CHEMISTRY OF THE INOSITOL LIPIDS AND PHOSPHATES

The three quantitatively major phosphoinositides are structurally and metabolically re-lated. These phosphoinositides consist of PI and the two polyphosphoinositides, phosphatidylinositol 4-phosphate (PIP) and PIP$_2$ (Fig. 1).

PI consists of a DAG moiety, which is phosphodiesterified to *myo*-inositol, a 6-carbon polycyclic alcohol. PI is phosphorylated to PIP in a reaction requiring ATP and catalyzed by PI 4-kinase, an integral membrane enzyme that is activated by detergents. PI(4)P is further phosphorylated via PIP kinase to PIP$_2$ (Fig. 2). This enzyme is found in both brain membranes and cytosol and does not phosphorylate PI.

Recently a new family of inositol lipids, the 3-phosphoinositides, was described. The enzyme PI 3-kinase is cytosolic and in contrast to PI 4-kinase, is strongly inhibited by detergents. This enzyme will also phosphorylate PI(4)P to PI(3,4)P_2 and PI(4,5)P_2 to PI(3,4,5)P_3. Although brain is enriched in PI 3-kinase, the significance of the 3-phosphoinositides in the nervous system is unknown (see 3-phosphoinositides, below).

There exists an unusual uniformity in the fatty acid composition of the inositol lipids. All three of the major phosphoinositides are enriched in the 1-stearoyl, 2-arachidonoyl (ST/AR) *sn*-glycerol species (~80 percent in brain). The polyphosphoinositides [PI(4)P and PI(4,5)P_2] are present in much lower amounts than PI and are believed to be localized predominantly, if not exclusively, to the inner leaflet of plasma membranes. The brain is the best-known source of the polyphosphoinositides. The total amount of the three phosphoinositides in brains that had been extracted following focused microwave treatment to minimize postmortem degradation was estimated to be 78, 4, and 14 nmol/mg of neostriatal protein for PI, PIP, and PIP$_2$, respectively (Van Dongen et al., cited in ref. 2). Although postmortem breakdown is rapid, a considerable fraction of brain phosphoinositide appears to be in a slowly degraded pool.

The phosphoinositides differ from other phospholipids, such as phosphatidylethanolamine, phosphatidylcholine, and phosphatidylserine, in that they contain no nitrogen. They share this property with the phosphatidylglycerol series, which are also formed from the precursor CDP·DAG (see Chap. 5). *myo*-Inositol is one of nine possible isomers of hexahydroxycyclohexane. It has one axial and five equatorial hydroxyls and is by far the most prevalent isomer in nature. Its distinctive configuration can be easily understood by regarding its cyclohexane chair configuration as a turtle in which the axial hydroxyl is the head, while the four limbs and tail serve as the five equatorial po-

sitions (see Fig. 1). In all of the phosphoinositides, DAG is affixed to the D-1 hydroxyl, the turtle's right front leg, via a phosphodiester linkage with the *sn*-3 position of glycerol. Using the D (for dextro isomer) numbering convention, looking down at the turtle from above and proceeding counterclockwise, the head is then at position D-2, while the left front leg is D-3, etc. At present, there are no known brain phosphoinositides containing cyclitols other than *myo*-inositol, nor are there as yet examples in which the inositol is diesterified to DAG at a position other than D-1.

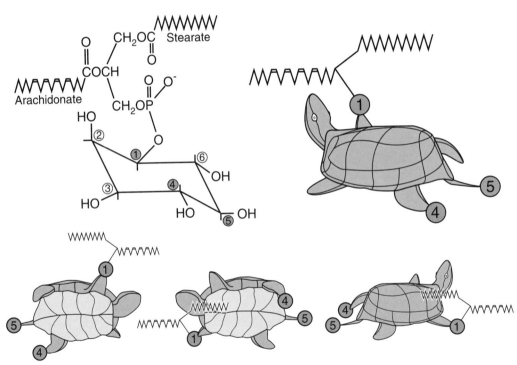

FIG. 1.   Stereochemistry of the inositol lipids. Inositol lipids characteristically contain stearic acid (18:0) and arachidonic acid (20:4 ω6) esterified to the 1 and 2 position of *sn*-glycerolphosphate, respectively. The phosphate *(dark circles)* is diesterified to the 1 position of D-*myo*-inositol. *myo*-Inositol in its favored chair conformation has five equatorial hydroxyls and one axial hydroxyl. Looking at the chair from above and counting counterclockwise, the axial hydroxyl is then in position 2. As indicated by the *drawing on the right,* the inositol molecule can be conveniently viewed as a turtle in which the diacylglycerol phosphate moiety is attached to the right front leg (position 1), next to the raised head (the axial hydroxyl in position 2). The other equatorial hydroxyls are represented by the remaining limbs and the tail. Phosphatidylinositol (PI) can be phosphorylated at position 4 (the rear left leg), or the rear left leg as well as the tail (positions 4 and 5 as shown), to yield phosphatidylinositol 4-phosphate [PI(4)P] and phosphatidylinositol 4,5-bisphosphate [PI(4,5)P₂], respectively. Once these relationships are understood, inositol phosphates can be seen from many vantage points without losing sight of their steric configurations, as indicated by three views of PI(4,5)P₂ in the lower portion of the drawing.

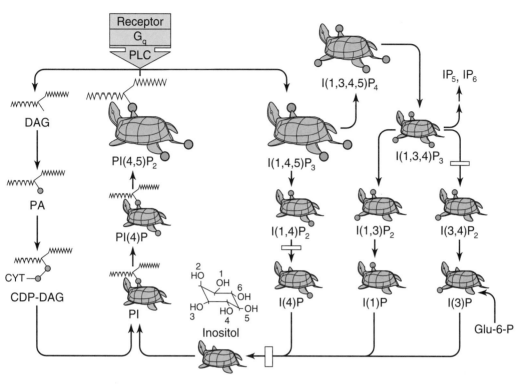

FIG. 2. Pathways of phosphoinositide degradation and resynthesis. Receptor-mediated breakdown of PIP_2 via PI-PLC (PLC) leads to the formation of DAG and $I(1,4,5)P_3$. The latter is metabolized via either 5-phosphatase or 3-kinase pathways to yield $I(1,4)P_2$ and $I(1,3,4,5)P_4$, respectively. Successive dephosphorylations of these two inositol phosphates result in the formation of $I(4)P$, $I(1)P$, and $I(3)P$. $I(3)P$ may also be synthesized from glucose 6-phosphate (Glu-6-P). Inositol monophosphates are then cleaved by monophosphatase to regenerate inositol. Li^+ blocks the dephosphorylation reactions indicated by *open bars*. DAG, when released, is metabolized in the plasma membrane to form phosphatidic acid (PA) via the action of DAG kinase. PA is subsequently converted to CDP·DAG, and in the presence of inositol, to PI. $PI(4,5)P_2$ is then regenerated by the action of specific kinases on PI and $PI(4)P$.

The 3-phosphoinositides

Recent studies indicated the presence of small amounts of additional inositol lipids that are characterized by the presence of a phosphate group at the D-3 position of the inositol ring, i.e., the 3-phosphoinositides. These lipids [$PI(3)P$, $PI(3,4)P_2$, and $PI(3,4,5)P_3$] are present in both neural and nonneural tissues at concentrations well below those found for either $PI(4)P$ or $PI(4,5)P_2$. At present, the physiological role of the 3-phosphoinositides is unknown, but unlike their more highly expressed counterparts, these lipids do not serve as substrates for phosphoinositidase C (PI-PLC), the enzyme known to be activated in stimulated phosphoinositide turnover (see below).

Phosphoinositides are cleaved by a family of phosphoinositidase C isozymes

At least three isozymes (β, γ, and δ) of PI-PLC exist in tissues including brain; each is a product of a separate gene and is an immunologically distinct entity [5]. They have been extensively purified, the complementary DNA (cDNA) sequences elucidated, and antibodies raised to all three enzymes. Despite the similarity of function, only two regions of amino acid homology exist, one of 150 and a second of 120 amino acid residues which are 54 and 42 percent identical among the isozymes. In addition, PI-PLC-γ exhibits some amino acid sequences that are found in nonreceptor tyrosine kinases (*src*, GTPase-activating protein, and α-spectrin). Differences in the regional and cellular distribution of PI-PLC isozymes are observed. For example, whereas PI-PLC-γ is distributed uniformly within neurons in all brain regions, PI-PLC-β is most concentrated within specific brain regions, such as cerebral cortex, hippocampus, and globus pallidus. In contrast, PI-PLC-δ is preferentially localized to glial cells.

PI-PLC activity is present in both membranes and cytosol. Although PI-PLC will catalyze the breakdown of all three major lipids, when assayed under conditions that mimic those present in the intracellular ionic environment (pH 7, high K^+, $[Ca^{2+}] \leq 1$ μM), $PI(4,5)P_2$ and $PI(4)P$, rather than PI, are the preferred substrates. Nanomolar concentrations of Ca^{2+} are required for PI-PLC activity, and increases in cytosolic Ca^{2+} concentrations that occur following receptor activation may serve to further increase enzyme activity, particularly for PI.

Cleavage of PIP_2 initiates two cycles: one in which the DAG backbone is conserved and recycled, and one in which inositol is reutilized

As indicated above, it can be inferred that a cycle operates in which DAG is conserved. To this end, the enzyme DAG kinase was sought and found. It converts the DAG released on phosphoinositide cleavage to PA, which can then be converted to PI via CDP·DAG (see Fig. 2; also see Chap. 5). Although the latter steps are those seen in the *de novo* biosynthesis of inositol lipids, it is likely that net synthesis and stimulated lipid turnover occur in separate and distinct metabolic compartments: The receptor-stimulated cycle is likely to be confined to the plasma membrane, whereas the various steps in the *de novo* pathway occur in the mitochondrial and/or endoplasmic reticular fractions. The coreleased inositol mono-, di-, and trisphosphates are eventually cleaved by phosphatases to regenerate free inositol, which may then combine with CDP·DAG to form PI via PI synthase. Sequential phos-

phorylation of PI to PIP_2 via PIP closes both loops of this double cycle, as depicted in Fig. 2.

THE INOSITOL PHOSPHATES

D-myo-inositol 1,4,5-trisphosphate $[I(1,4,5)P_3]$ is a second messenger that liberates Ca^{2+} from the endoplasmic reticulum via intracellular receptors

Of the three inositol phosphates formed upon PI-PLC-activated cleavage of the phosphoinositides, $I(1,4,5)P_3$ is unique in its ability to mobilize Ca^{2+} (Fig. 3). This observation is one of the key arguments that PIP_2 breakdown, rather than that of PIP or PI, initiates the cellular responses to receptor activation. When directly injected into cells, or added to permeabilized cells or membrane fractions, $I(1,4,5)P_3$ elicits an increased release of Ca^{2+} from a store that has been associated with the endoplasmic reticulum. That specific receptor sites mediate the action of $I(1,4,5)P_3$ was first indicated by the presence of binding sites in membrane fractions obtained from distinct brain regions, notably the cerebellum, the brain region most enriched in these receptors [6]. The purified receptor is a glycoprotein, has a molecular weight of 260 kDa on sodium dodecyl sulfate-polyacrylamide gel electrophoresis (SDS-PAGE), and is highly selective for $I(1,4,5)P_3$. In brain, the binding of $I(1,4,5)P_3$ to its receptor is rendered sensitive to Ca^{2+} at physiologically relevant concentrations of the ion by the presence of a 300-kDa protein, calmedin, thought to play a regulatory role in Ca^{2+} homeostasis. *In vivo*, the IP_3 receptor is comprised of four noncovalently bound identical subunits that collectively form a single transmembrane pore. Each subunit possesses an IP_3 binding site, and when three to four of these sites are occupied by IP_3, a conformation change in the receptor complex occurs such that an open ion channel is formed and Ca^{2+} is released. Activation of phosphoinositide-linked receptors frequently results in os-

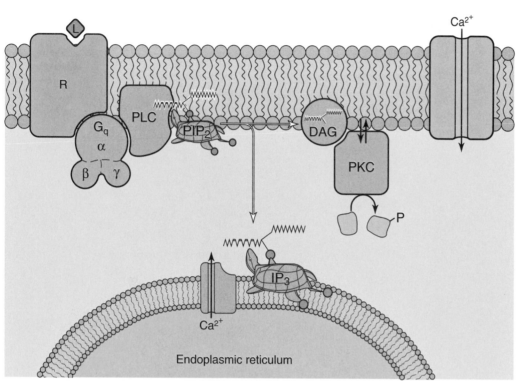

FIG. 3. Linkage between receptor activation, phosphoinositide hydrolysis, and Ca^{2+} signaling. Occupancy of a cell-surface receptor by ligand results in the activation of phosphoinositide-specific phospholipase C (PLC), which is mediated through an intervening guanine nucleotide-binding protein (G_q). Phosphatidylinositol 4,5-bisphosphate (PIP_2) is phosphodiesteratically cleaved by PLC to yield DAG and inositol 1,4,5-trisphosphate (IP_3). DAG activates protein kinase C (PKC), following its translocation (⬆⬇) from cytosol to plasma membrane, and results in the phosphory-lation of specific proteins. When released, three to four molecules of IP_3 interact with a specific IP_3 receptor present in the endoplasmic reticulum and Ca^{2+} is liberated, raising its concentration in the cytosol. In addition, the activation of PLC results in the influx of Ca^{2+}, which continues for as long as the ligand occupies the receptor. The molecular mechanism whereby PLC activation results in the opening of this Ca^{2+} channel is yet to be determined.

cillations of the intracellular Ca^{2+} signal. Whether IP_3 directs such oscillations is not presently known. Neural and nonneural forms of the IP_3 receptor may exist and be formed by alternative gene splicing [7,8].

The metabolism of inositol phosphates leads to regeneration of free inositol

$I(1,4,5)P_3$ can be metabolized either by a 5'-phosphatase (a membrane-bound enzyme) to yield inositol 1,4-bisphosphate $[I(1,4)P_2]$ or by a cytosolic inositol phosphate 3-kinase to form inositol 1,3,4,5-tetrakisphosphate $[I(1,3,4,5)P_4]$ (see Fig. 2). Both of these ac-tivities may be regarded as "off signals," ter-minating the action of $I(1,4,5)P_3$. The $I(1,4)P_2$ that results from 5-phosphatase ac-tion is dephosphorylated further to inositol 4-monophosphate $[I(4)P]$ and then to free inositol. $I(1,3,4,5)P_4$, which itself has been suggested to possess a second-messenger function in facilitating the entry of Ca^{2+} into cells, also serves as a substrate for the same 5-phosphatase that acts on $I(1,4,5)P_3$, with the resultant formation in this instance of inositol 1,3,4-trisphosphate $[I(1,3,4)P_3]$. Un-like its 1,4,5-trisphosphate isomer, $I(1,3,4)P_3$ is ineffective at mobilizing intracellular Ca^{2+}. $I(1,3,4)P_3$ can be further metabolized to inositol 1,3-bisphosphate [I(1,3)P$_2$] or inositol 3,4-bisphosphate [I(3,4)P$_2$] (see Fig. 2). These compounds are then dephosphorylated by 4- or 3-phosphatases to yield inositol 3- or 1-monophosphates, respectively.

A single enzyme, inositol monophosphatase, leads to the regeneration of free inositol. This enzyme exhibits similar affinities for all five of the equatorial inositol monophosphate hydroxyls. Inositol 2-phosphate, not produced in this degradative pathway, is a poor substrate, attributable to the axial configuration of the phosphate. The enzyme is inhibited by Li$^+$ in an uncompetitive manner; i.e., the degree of inhibition is a function of substrate concentration. It should be noted that unlike most other tissues, brain can synthesize inositol *de novo* by the action of inositol monophosphate synthase, which cyclizes glucose 6-phosphate to form I(3)P. The enzyme has been localized immunohistochemically to the brain vasculature [9].

The action of Li$^+$ on inositol monophosphatase has greatly facilitated the use of [^{3}H]inositol in the study of stimulated phosphoinositide turnover [10]. In the presence of both Li$^+$ and a phosphoinositide-linked ligand, the amount of labeled intracellular inositol phosphates that accumulates following a preincubation with [^{3}H]inositol can be stimulated as much as 50-fold, whereas the presence of either Li$^+$ or ligand alone has very little effect on [^{3}H]inositol monophosphate accumulation. Although ligand-activated turnover is initiated by PIP$_2$ breakdown and the generation of I(1,4,5)IP$_3$, this product is quickly degraded. It is thus far more convenient to use an indirect measurement of the accumulation of labeled inositol monophosphates in the presence of Li$^+$ than to attempt to measure the transient appearance of labeled I(1,4,5)IP$_3$ a few seconds after ligand addition.

Higher inositol phosphates

In contrast to the intracellular roles proposed for I(1,4,5)P$_3$ and I(1,3,4,5)P$_4$, extra-cellular roles for IP$_5$ and IP$_6$ have been entertained, based on the ability of these inositol phosphates to regulate heart rate and blood pressure when injected into the nucleus tractus solitarius [11]. The involvement of inositol 1,3,4,5,6-pentakisphosphate in the allosteric regulation of hemoglobin has been known for many years. IP$_6$ (phytate) is a well-known component of plant seeds. More recently, demonstration of specific IP$_6$ binding sites in brain and anterior pituitary gland supports the possibility of a role for these inositol polyphosphates in mammalian brain [12].

Cyclic inositol phosphates

When PI is cleaved by PI-PLC, two inositol monophosphates are released in relatively equal amounts: D-*myo*-inositol 1-phosphate [I(1)P] and D-*myo*-inositol 1:2 cyclic phosphate [I(c1,2)P]. Similarly, there is evidence that PI(4,5)P$_2$ breakdown results in the production of I(c1:2,4,5)P$_3$, the cyclic analog of I(1,4,5)P$_3$. A cyclase which cleaves I(c1:2)P$_1$ to I(1)P is inactive against the higher analogs, a result suggesting that the latter are degraded by phosphatases to the cyclic monophosphate prior to cleavage of the cyclic phosphate ring. A specific function for the cyclic inositol phosphates is not yet known. Although I(c1:2,4,5)P$_3$ is able to mobilize intracellular Ca^{2+}, it is less effective than I(1,4,5)P$_3$. It is also less well cleaved by the 5′-phosphatase, potentially extending its lifetime as a second messenger.

DIACYLGLYCEROL

Protein kinase C, a widely distributed protein kinase requiring the presence of phosphatidylserine and Ca^{2+}, is activated by DAG

Protein kinase C (PKC) consists of a catalytic and a regulatory subunit. The latter appears to be the site of DAG, phosphatidylserine, and Ca^{2+} binding, as well as providing an attachment site of the enzyme to membranes.

PKC is particularly enriched in brain. It is possible that PKC-mediated phosphorylation of receptors, G proteins, or the PI-PLC affects the receptor-mediated breakdown of PIP_2 and thus exerts feedback control on signal transduction. It was recently shown that four subtypes of PKC exist and are coded by separate but interrelated genes. One form of PKC, designated βII, is brain-specific (see also Chap. 22).

Since $I(1,4,5)IP_3$ production leads to increased intracellular Ca^{2+} which in turn stimulates PKC action, the two messengers DAG and $I(1,4,5)IP_3$ generally act in concert. DAG can, however, arise in cells from sources other than the phosphoinositides. For example, it can be generated from the action of a phosphatidylcholine (PC)-specific phospholipase C or from the transfer of phosphorylcholine from PC to ceramide in the synthesis of sphingomyelin (see Chap. 5). If the DAG released from stimulated phosphoinositide turnover specifically activates cellular PKC, one might expect ST/AR DAG to be a particularly effective activator of the enzyme. It turns out to be only marginally better than other long-chain fatty acyl DAGs; however, chemical analysis indicates that brain DAG is enriched in the ST/AR species. It would therefore seem that ST/AR DAG is *de facto* the principal activator of PKC *in vivo,* even though the enzyme shows little specificity for it. Superior synthetic DAG analogs for experimental purposes include the relatively soluble species, 1-oleoyl, 2-acetyl *sn*-glycerol (OAG).

Of particular value in studying the function of PKC are the phorbol esters. These tumor-promoting plant products and their synthetic derivatives are able to penetrate whole cells and can thus be added to tissue incubations. Many inferences regarding the intracellular actions of PKC are based on results of studies with the phorbol esters in whole cells. Since these substances, like DAG, may produce feedback inhibition of signal transduction at a number of metabolic levels, results of experiments using phorbol esters in whole cells are often complex and must be interpreted cautiously.

Protein kinase C regulates the activity of a large number of proteins, the phosphorylation of which can result in increases or decreases in their catalytic activity

Of particular interest are the actions of PKC on ion channels, since in this way phosphorylation may directly affect signal transduction. In platelets, PKC activity is associated with the phosphorylation of a 40-kDa protein. PKC itself has homology with DNA-binding proteins, and it has been postulated that it may also play a direct role in the regulation of macromolecular synthesis.

If DAG is an intracellular messenger that activates PKC, what then is the "off signal" that terminates its action? Phosphorylation of DAG to PA in the lipid-labeling cycle could serve this purpose. Additional possibilities include the action of DAG lipase, which can cleave DAG to fatty acid and monoacylglyceride (MAG). Although this hydrolytic activity can be demonstrated, it should be noted that for the labeling cycle to remain truly regenerative, it would be necessary to then reacylate MAG to DAG. Such deacylation-reacylation reactions could be of importance in the generation of arachidonate for prostanoid synthesis from inositide intermediates (see Chap. 23).

FUNCTIONAL CORRELATES OF PHOSPHOINOSITIDE-LINKED RECEPTORS IN THE NERVOUS SYSTEM

The complexity of the brain is reflected by a wide array of diverse receptors coupled to stimulation of phosphoinositide turnover

A large number of pharmacologically distinct receptors are linked to the activation of PI-PLC. Table 1 summarizes the presently known extent of this diversity [13]. Phosphoinositide hydrolysis elicited by the activation of muscarinic, adrenergic, histaminergic, serotonergic, glutamatergic, and endothelin

TABLE 1.   Pharmacological profile of receptor-activated phosphoinositide hydrolysis in neural tissues

Receptor	Subtype(s)
Muscarinic	m_1 and m_3
Adrenergic	α_{1A} and α_{1B}
Histaminergic	H_1
Serotonergic	5-HT$_2$ and 5-HT$_{1c}$
Glutamatergic	Metabotropic
Endothelin	
Purinergic	P_2
Thromboxane	A_2
Prostaglandin	E_2
Bradykinin	B_2
Vasopressin	V_1
Nerve growth factor	
Cholecystokinin	
Neuropeptide Y	
Neurotensin	
Gastrin-releasing peptide	
Bombesin	
Substance P	
Oxytocin	
Eledoisin	
Neurokinin	
Vasointestinal peptide	
Angiotensin	
Gonadotropin-releasing hormone	
Platelet-activating factor	
Thyrotropin-releasing hormone	

receptors is reliably observed in brain slices, primary cultures of neurons and glia, and cultured neurotumor cells. For the other receptors listed, much of the evidence linking them to phosphoinositide hydrolysis is limited to studies performed with either neurotumor cells or other neural-derived tissues. In some instances the same transmitter may be linked to multiple mechanisms of signal transduction. For example, acetylcholine interacts with two subtypes of muscarinic receptors to increase phosphoinositide hydrolysis. Other subtypes of muscarinic receptor are linked to inhibition of adenylyl cyclase activity while nicotinic cholinergic receptors are ligand-gated ion channels.

What is the physiological significance of stimulated phosphoinositide turnover in the nervous system?

Because the nervous system is so enriched in the components of the phosphoinositide signaling system, it is not ideal for examining the signal transduction of a single ligand in detail. There is, in addition, likely to be convergence of several receptors on any given brain cell type. Hence, the best-understood models of signal transduction via stimulated phosphoinositide turnover are extraneural, for example, secretion by the salivary or pancreatic glands, and activation of platelets by thrombin or leukocytes by chemotactic peptides. It is likely that there are diverse roles for the phosphoinositide-associated messengers in the nervous system, ranging from mediating the primary signal of neurotransmission to modulating neuronal signals, secretion, and perhaps even contraction.

Does the sharing of a single system by multiple cell-surface receptors lead to degeneracy of the signal?

Given the brain's necessity for a wide variety of extracellular messengers, such as neurotransmitters and hormones, it would seem that sharing intracellular messengers would lead to degradation of signal and loss of information. In the case of the nervous system, it may be that there are anatomically discrete second-messenger domains within a single cell. Video-enhanced microscopic methods for studying Ca^{2+} signaling [14] may offer an experimental approach to address this possibility. It is also possible that the sharing of second-messenger systems has useful physiological value, for example, in heterologous desensitization. Thus, if the loss of response to a given receptor can lead to loss of response to another receptor, this suggests the sharing of one or more steps in the transduction process. Such sharing could be part of a physiological process whereby various neuronal inputs are integrated intracellularly.

Receptor activation of PI-PLC occurs through a guanine nucleotide-binding (G) protein

As is well documented for adenylyl cyclase-linked receptors, activation of a G protein intervenes between agonist occupancy of cell-surface receptors and resultant enhanced intracellular PI-PLC activity. Nonhydrolyzable analogs of GTP increase PI-PLC activity when added to brain membranes that have been prelabeled with [³H]inositol, and furthermore, they promote the action of agonists added to the same tissue preparation. The activation of PI-PLC is usually insensitive to either pertussis or cholera toxins, thus excluding the involvement of G_i, G_o, or G_s (see Chap. 10). Recently, the α-subunit of a novel pertussis toxin-insensitive G protein (G_q: molecular weight = 42 kDa) was purified from brain and shown in reconstitution experiments to specifically activate the β isozyme of PI-PLC [15]. Other G proteins that positively regulate the activity of PI-PLC may also exist. In addition, brain may possess an inhibitory G protein that represses the activity of PI-PLC in a pertussis toxin-sensitive manner [16].

Does the action of Li⁺ on the phosphoinositide labeling cycle explain the therapeutic action of Li⁺ in manic depressive psychosis?

It has been suggested that the uncompetitive inhibition of inositol monophosphatase by Li⁺ serves as the basis of its therapeutic action in affective disorders. The inositol depletion hypothesis proposes that monophosphatase inhibition *in vivo* lowers inositol levels in cells that are most actively producing inositol monophosphate, i.e., have maximally activated their phosphoinositide-linked receptors. This selectivity is the result of the uncompetitive nature of the Li⁺ inhibition, since the degree of inhibition is proportional to the amount of substrate, i.e., inositol monophosphate. PI synthase is slowed by lack of inositol. Thus, overactive cells are thought to be differentially inhibited. Although clinically therapeutic doses of Li⁺ do achieve sufficiently high levels of Li⁺ in the brain (about 1 mM) to inhibit the monophosphatase, experiments in rats with even higher doses produce only a 25 percent lowering of brain inositol. This degree of lowering of brain inositol would not appear to be sufficiently near the K_m of PI synthase to slow PI synthesis. It has also been observed that Li⁺ must be administered for many days before a therapeutic effect is seen. This suggests that delayed effects of Li⁺, such as regulation of enzymes, might better correlate with the clinical effect. While the inositol depletion hypothesis appears attractive in many respects, its validity remains to be demonstrated.

What is the role of PI-anchored proteins?

In both neural and nonneural tissues, a growing number of proteins have been shown to be linked to the outer membrane leaflet via a glycosidic linkage. The common structural features of this attachment are an ethanolamine residue with an amide linked to the terminal carboxyl group of the protein, a mannose-containing glycan, and a nonacetylated glucosamine residue linked to the D-6 position (the turtle's right hind leg) of *myo*-inositol via a glycosidic linkage. Although as noted above, the phosphoinositides contain predominantly stearate and arachidonate, these substituents are no longer dominant in PI anchors, being replaced by myristate, octadecanoate, or docosanoate. In rat pheochromocytoma cells, the addition of nerve growth factor stimulates the production of myristate-labeled DAG and an inositol glycan. The latter has been proposed to serve as a second messenger. D-Chiroinositol may in some instances replace *myo*-inositol. Not only does the fatty acid composition of PI anchors differ from that associated with signal transduction, but degradation requires forms of PI-PLC that are specific for the glycosylated form of PI. While unique roles in the nervous system have not been demonstrated, it is interesting that various brain-specific proteins, including myelin basic protein, acetylcholinesterase, and Thy-1, are PI-anchored.

ACKNOWLEDGMENTS

The auspices of the Fogarty scholar-in-residence award program are acknowledged with thanks (B. W. A.).

REFERENCES

1. Hokin, L. E., and Hokin, M. R. Effects of acetylcholine on the turnover of phosphoryl units in individual phospholipids of pancreas slices and brain cortex slices. *Biochim. Biophys. Acta* 18:102–110, 1955.
2. Hajra, A. K., Fisher, S. K., and Agranoff, B. W. Isolation, separation and analysis of phosphoinositides from biological sources. In A. A. Boulton, G. B. Baker, and L. A. Horrocks (eds.), *Neuromethods (Neurochemistry) (Vol. 8: Lipids and Related Compounds)*. Clifton, N.J.: Humana Press, 1988, pp. 211–255.
3. Michell, R. H. Inositol phospholipids and cell surface receptor function. *Biochim. Biophys. Acta* 415:81–147, 1975.
4. Streb, H., Irvine, R. F., Berridge, M. J., and Schulz, I. Release of Ca^{2+} from a nonmitochondrial intracellular store in pancreatic acinar cells by inositol-1,4,5-trisphosphate. *Nature* 306:67–69, 1983.
5. Rhee, S. G., Suh, P.-G., Ryu, S.-H., and Lee, S. Y. Studies of inositol phospholipid-specific phospholipase C. *Science* 244:546–550, 1989.
6. Worley, P. F., Baraban, J. M., and Snyder, S. H. Inositol 1,4,5-trisphosphate receptor binding: Autoradiographic localization in rat brain. *J. Neurosci.* 9:339–346, 1989.
7. Danoff, S. K., Ferris, C. D., Donath, C., Fischer, G. A., Munemitsu, S., Ullrich, A., Snyder, S. H., and Ross, C. A. Inositol 1,4,5-trisphosphate receptors: Distinct neuronal and nonneuronal forms derived by alternative splicing differ in phosphorylation. *Proc. Natl. Acad. Sci. U.S.A.* 88:2951–2955, 1991.
8. Nakagawa, T., Okano, H., Furiuchi, T., Aruga, J., and Mikoshiba, K. The subtypes of the mouse inositol 1,4,5-trisphosphate receptor are expressed in a tissue-specific and developmentally specific manner. *Proc. Natl. Acad. Sci. U.S.A.* 88:6244–6248, 1991.
9. Wong, Y.-H. H., Kalmbach, S. J., Hartman, B. K., and Sherman, W. R. Immunohistochemical staining and enzyme activity measurements show *myo*-inositol-1-phosphate synthase to be localized in the vasculature of brain. *J. Neurochem.* 48:1434–1442, 1987.
10. Berridge, M. J., Downes, C. P., and Hanley, M. R. Lithium amplifies agonist-dependent phosphatidylinositol resposnes in brain and salivary glands. *Biochem. J.* 206:587–595, 1982.
11. Vallejo, M., Jackson, T., Lightman, S., and Hanley, M. R. Occurrence and extracellular actions of inositol pentakis- and hexakisphosphate in mammalian brain. *Nature* 330: 656–658, 1987.
12. Nicoletti, F., Buno, V., Cavallaro, S., Copani, A., Sortino, M. A., and Canonico, P. L. Specific binding sites for inositolhexakisphosphate in brain and anterior pituitary. *Mol. Pharmacol.* 37:689–693, 1990.
13. Fisher, S. K., Heacock, A. M., and Agranoff, B. W. Inositol lipids and signal transduction in the nervous system: An update. *J. Neurochem.* 58:18–38, 1992.
14. Tsien, R. Y., and Poenie, M. Fluorescence ratio imaging: A new window into intracellular ionic signaling. *Trends Biochem. Sci.* 11: 450–455, 1986.
15. Smrcka, A. V., Hepler, J. R., Brown, K. O., and Sternweis, P. C. Regulation of polyphosphoinositide-specific phospholipase C activity by purified G_q. *Science* 251:804–807, 1991.
16. Litosch, I. Guanine nucleotides mediate stimulatory and inhibitory effects on cerebral-cortical membrane phospholipase C activity. *Biochem. J.* 261:245–251, 1989.

ADDITIONAL REFERENCES

Downes, C. P., and MacPhee, C. H. *myo*-Inositol metabolites as cellular signals. *Eur. J. Biochem.* 193:1–18, 1990.

Irvine, R. F. Inositol phosphates and Ca^{2+} entry: Towards a proliferation or a simplification? *FASEB J.* 6:3085–3091, 1992.

Majerus, P. W. Inositol phosphate biochemistry. *Annu. Rev. Biochem.* 61:225–250, 1992.

Reitz, A. B. (ed.), *Inositol Phosphates and Derivatives. Synthesis, Biochemistry, and Therapeutic Potential.* ACS Symposium Series 463. Washington, D.C.: American Chemical Society, 1991.

Shinomura, T., Mishima, S., Asaoka, Y., Yoshida, K., Oka, M., and Nishizuka, Y. Degradation of phospholipids and protein kinase C activation for the control of neuronal functions. *Adv. Exp. Med. Biol.* 318:361–373, 1992.

CHAPTER 21

G Proteins and Cyclic Nucleotides in the Nervous System

ERIC J. NESTLER AND RONALD S. DUMAN

Basic Neurochemistry: Molecular, Cellular, and Medical Aspects, 5th Ed., edited by G. J. Siegel et al. Published by Raven Press, Ltd., New York, 1994. Correspondence to Eric J. Nestler, Division of Molecular Psychiatry, Departments of Psychiatry and Pharmacology, Yale University School of Medicine and Connecticut Mental Health Center, 34 Park Street, New Haven, Connecticut 06508.

THE SECOND-MESSENGER HYPOTHESIS

The mechanisms by which extracellular agents, such as neurotransmitters and circulating hormones, act on plasma membrane receptors to produce alterations in intracellular processes have been one of the most intensely investigated areas in the biomedical sciences for several decades. One of the seminal advances in this field came in the late 1950s when Earl Sutherland and his colleagues demonstrated that epinephrine induces glycogenolysis in the liver by stimulating the synthesis of an intracellular second messenger, adenosine 3′,5′-cyclic monophosphate (cyclic AMP or cAMP). Since that time, cAMP and other small molecules (e.g., guanosine 3′,5′-cyclic monophosphate [cGMP], Ca^{2+}, nitric oxide [NO], and the metabolites of phosphatidylinositol and of arachidonic acid) have been shown to serve a myriad of second-messenger roles in the nervous system. These messengers mediate many of the actions of hormones and neurotransmitters on diverse aspects of neuronal function (Fig. 1). In recent years, attention has also been given to a class of guanine nucleotide-binding proteins, termed "G proteins," as the factors that typically "couple" plasma membrane receptors to the generation of intracellular second messengers (see Fig. 1). This chapter reviews the roles of G proteins and the proteins involved in the synthesis and metabolism of the cyclic nucleotides, cAMP and cGMP, in the nervous system.

G PROTEINS

With the exception of synaptic transmission mediated via receptors that contain intrinsic enzymatic activity or that form ion channels, the family of membrane proteins known as G proteins appears to be involved in all other transmembrane signaling in the nervous system. G proteins, first identified and characterized by Rodbell, Gilman, and others, are named because of their ability to bind the

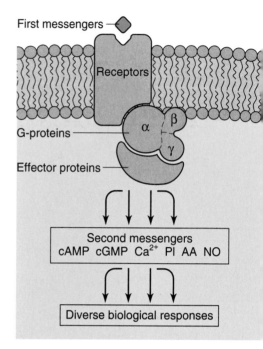

FIG. 1. Schematic illustration of the second-messenger hypothesis. This hypothesis states that many types of first messengers in the brain, through the activation of specific plasma membrane receptors and G proteins, stimulate the formation of intracellular second messengers, which mediate many of the biological responses of the first messengers in target neurons. Prominent second messengers in the brain include cAMP, cGMP, Ca^{2+}, the metabolites of phosphatidylinositol (PI) (e.g., inositol trisphosphate and diacylglycerol) and of arachidonic acid (AA) (e.g., prostaglandins, prostacyclins, thromboxanes, leukotrienes), and nitric oxide (NO).

guanine nucleotides, guanosine triphosphate (GTP) and guanosine diphosphate (GDP). The proteins also possess an intrinsic GTPase activity. Many types of effector proteins are known to be influenced by G proteins; these include ion channels, adenylyl cyclase, phospholipase C (which catalyzes the hydrolysis of phosphatidylinositol), phospholipase A_2 (which catalyzes the hydrolysis of arachidonic acid), and phosphodiesterase (PDE) (in rod outer segments).

Multiple forms of G proteins exist in the nervous system

Three types of G protein were identified in early studies. G_t, termed "transducin," was identified as the G protein that couples rhodopsin to regulation of photoreceptor cell function, and G_s and G_i were identified as the G proteins that couple plasma membrane receptors to the stimulation and inhibition, respectively, of adenylyl cyclase, the enzyme that catalyzes the synthesis of cAMP.

Since that time, a multitude of G protein subunits have been identified by a combination of biochemical and molecular cloning techniques. In addition to G_t, G_s, and G_i, the other major types of G protein in brain are designated G_o, G_{olf}, G_{gust}, G_z, G_q, and G_{11-16}. Moreover, for each of these types of G protein, multiple subtypes that show unique distributions in the brain and periphery are known.

Each G protein is a heterotrimer composed of single α-, β-, and γ-subunits

The different types of G protein contain distinct α-subunits, which are responsible for their specific functional activity. The types of G protein α-subunit known to exist, categorized on the basis of their structural homologies, are listed in Table 1. As a first approximation, the different types of α-subunit share common β- and γ-subunits, although there are an increasing number of known subtypes for these subunits as well, which may possess different physiological activities [1]. The apparent mass of β-subunits is 35 to 36 kDa; that for the γ-subunits is 5 to 10 kDa.

TABLE 1.   Heterotrimeric G protein α-subunits in brain

Class	kDa[a]	Toxin-mediated ADP-ribosylation	Effector protein(s)
G_s family			
$G_{\alpha S1}$	52	Cholera	Adenylyl cyclase (activation)
$G_{\alpha S2}$	45	↓	↓
$G_{\alpha olf}$	45		
G_i family			
$G_{\alpha i1}$	41	Pertussis	⎰ Adenylyl cyclase (inhibition)
$G_{\alpha i2}$	40	↓	Ion channels (inhibition or activation)
$G_{\alpha i3}$	41		Phospholipase C (activation)
			⎱ ?Phospholipase A_2
$G_{\alpha o1}$	39	Pertussis	⎰ Ion channels (inhibition or activation)
$G_{\alpha o2}$	39	↓	?Phospholipase C (activation)
			⎱ ?Phospholipase A_2
$G_{\alpha t1}$	39	⎰ Cholera and	⎰ Phosphodiesterase (activation) in rods
$G_{\alpha t2}$	39	⎱ pertussis	⎱ and cones
$G_{\alpha gust}$	40	Unknown	?Phosphodiesterase (activation) in taste epithelium
$G_{\alpha z}$	40	None	Adenylyl cyclase (inhibition)
G_q family[b]	42–44		
$G_{\alpha q}$		None	Phospholipase C (activation)
$G_{\alpha 11}$			Unknown
$G_{\alpha 12}$			
$G_{\alpha 13}$			
$G_{\alpha 14}$			
$G_{\alpha 15}$			
$G_{\alpha 16}$		↓	↓

[a] Values shown reflect apparent M_r obtained by gel electrophoresis in most cases. The values shown for $G_{\alpha gust}$, G_z, and $G_{\alpha 11}$ through $G_{\alpha 16}$ reflect calculated mass based on their amino acid sequence.
[b] $G_{\alpha 12}$ and $G_{\alpha 13}$ are sometimes categorized as a separate family.
(?) indicates that the association between the particular G proteins and effector proteins shown in the table remains tentative.

The functional activity of G proteins involves their dissociation and reassociation in response to extracellular signals

This is shown schematically in Fig. 2. In the resting state, G proteins exist as heterotrimers that are bound to GDP and are not associated with extracellular receptors or intracellular effector proteins (Fig. 2A). When a ligand binds to (and activates) a receptor, it produces a conformational change in the receptor, which causes it to associate with the α-subunit of the G protein (Fig. 2B). This,

in turn, alters the conformation of the α-subunit and leads to (1) the exchange of GTP for GDP on the α-subunit, (2) the dissociation of a βγ-subunit complex from the α-subunit, and (3) the release of the receptor from the G protein (Fig. 2B and C). This process generates a free α-subunit bound to GTP, which is biologically active and can regulate the functional activity of effector proteins within the cell. In addition, there is increasing evidence that complexes of free βγ-subunits may also have biological activity [1–6]. The system returns to its resting state when

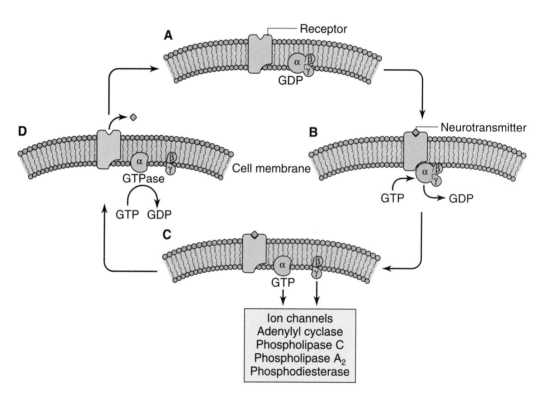

FIG. 2.   Schematic illustration of G protein function in the brain. **A:** Under basal conditions, G proteins exist in cell membranes as heterotrimers composed of single α-, β-, and γ-subunits and are not associated physically with neurotransmitter receptors. In this situation, the α-subunits are bound to GDP. **B:** Upon activation of the receptor by its ligand (e.g., neurotransmitter), the receptor physically associates with the α-subunit, which leads to the binding of GTP to the α-subunit and the displacement of GDP. **C:** GTP binding induces the generation of free α-subunit by causing the dissociation of the α-subunit from its β- and γ-subunits and from the receptor. Free α-subunit, bound to GTP, is functionally active and directly regulates a number of effector proteins, which, depending on the type of α-subunit and cell involved, can include ion channels, adenylyl cyclase, phospholipase C, phospholipase A₂, and phosphodiesterase. It is also possible that free βγ-subunit complexes directly regulate some of these effector proteins. **D:** GTPase activity intrinsic to the α-subunit degrades GTP to form GDP. This leads to the reassociation of the α- and βγ-subunits, which, along with the dissociation of ligand from the receptor, leads to restoration of the basal state. (From Hyman and Nestler [35].)

the ligand is released from the receptor and the GTPase activity that resides in the α-subunit hydrolyzes GTP to GDP (Fig. 2D). The latter action leads to reassociation of the free α-subunit with the $\beta\gamma$-subunit complex to restore the original heterotrimer.

G proteins have also been reported to undergo phosphorylation by cAMP-dependent and Ca^{2+}-dependent protein kinases and by protein tyrosine kinases. However, the effect of phosphorylation on G protein function and its role in the regulation of physiological processes have not yet been defined.

G proteins couple some neurotransmitter receptors directly to ion channels

In most such cases, it appears that the α-subunit released from the G protein-receptor interaction directly gates (i.e., opens or closes) a specific ion channel [7]. One of the best-established examples of this type of mechanism in brain is the coupling of opiate, α_2-adrenergic, D_2 dopaminergic, muscarinic cholinergic, $5\text{-}HT_{1A}$ serotonergic, and $GABA_B$ receptors to the activation of an inward rectifying K^+ channel via pertussis toxin-sensitive G proteins (i.e., subtypes of G_o and/or G_i). Some of these same neurotransmitter receptors have been shown to be similarly coupled to voltage-dependent Ca^{2+} channels via the same types of G proteins, although the channels are inhibited by this interaction. It is likely that other types of ion channels are also coupled to neurotransmitter receptors via G proteins. In addition, a direct action of $\beta\gamma$-complexes on ion channels has been proposed [4].

G proteins regulate intracellular levels of second messengers

G proteins control intracellular cAMP levels by mediating the ability of neurotransmitters to activate or inhibit adenylyl cyclase. Examples of neurotransmitters that regulate cAMP levels in the nervous system are given in Table 2.

TABLE 2.   Examples of neurotransmitter regulation of adenylyl cyclase

Neurotransmitter	Neurotransmitter receptor	
	Inhibition	Stimulation
Norepinephrine, epinephrine	α_2-Adrenergic	β-Adrenergic (β_1 and β_2) α_1-Adrenergic[a]
Dopamine	D_2	D_1, D_5
Serotonin	$5\text{-}HT_{1A}$, $5\text{-}HT_{1B}$, $5\text{-}HT_{1D}$	$5\text{-}HT_4$
Histamine		H_2
Acetylcholine	m_2, m_4, m_5	
GABA	$GABA_B$	$GABA_B$[a]
Adenosine	A_1	A_2
Somatostatin	S-R[b]	
Opioids	μ, δ, and κ	κ
Vasoactive intestinal peptide (VIP)		VIP-R[b]
Neuropeptide Y	Y_1, Y_2, Y_3	
Neurotensin	NT-R[b]	
Corticotropin-releasing factor		CRF-R[b]
Cannabinoids	R[c]	
Glutamate	$mGLU$[d]	Most subtypes[e]

[a] Activation of these receptors leads to conditional stimulation of adenylyl cyclase, in that such stimulation is observed in brain slices in the presence of agents (e.g., β-adrenergic receptor agonists) which directly stimulate the enzyme via G_s.
[b] Many of the neuropeptide receptors that regulate adenylyl cyclase have not yet been cloned. As a result, subtypes of the receptors have not been definitively established.
[c] The endogenous ligand(s) for this cannabinoid binding receptor remain(s) unknown.
[d] Metabotropic glutamate receptors (mGLU), which belong to the family of G protein-coupled receptors, are reported to inhibit adenylyl cyclase in addition to stimulating phospholipase C.
[e] Glutamate can stimulate adenylyl cyclase activity indirectly by increasing cellular levels of Ca^{2+} (secondary to membrane depolarization), which in conjunction with calmodulin can then activate Ca^{2+}/calmodulin-sensitive forms of the enzyme.

The mechanism by which neurotransmitters stimulate adenylyl cyclase is well established. Activation of those neurotransmitter receptors that couple to G_s results in the generation of free $G_{\alpha s}$ subunits which bind to and directly activate adenylyl cyclase. In addition, free $\beta\gamma$-subunit complexes have been shown to influence certain subtypes of adenylyl cyclase (see below). A similar mechanism appears to be the case for $G_{\alpha olf}$, a type of G protein (structurally related to $G_{\alpha s}$) that is enriched in olfactory epithelium and mediates the ability of odorant and odorant receptors to stimulate adenylyl cyclase [36].

The mechanism by which neurotransmitters inhibit adenylyl cyclase and decrease neuronal levels of cAMP has eluded definitive identification. By analogy with the action of G_s, it was proposed originally that activation of neurotransmitter receptors that couple to G_i results in the generation of free $G_{\alpha i}$ subunits, which could bind to, and thereby directly inhibit, adenylyl cyclase. However, the inhibition of adenylyl cyclase by $G_{\alpha i}$ has been difficult to demonstrate in cell-free reconstitution experiments. Alternative possibilities are that free $\beta\gamma$-subunit complexes, generated by the release of $G_{\alpha i}$, might directly inhibit certain forms of adenylyl cyclase or might bind free $G_{\alpha s}$ subunits in the membrane [3]. Sequestration of $G_{\alpha s}$ would then decrease basal stimulation of adenylyl cyclase. In addition to G_i, there is evidence that $G_{\alpha z}$ (which can be considered a subtype of the G_i family based on sequence homologies) can also mediate inhibition of adenylyl cyclase [8].

The transducin family of G proteins mediates signal transduction in the visual system (see Chap. 7) by regulating specific forms of PDE, an enzyme that catalyzes the metabolism of cyclic nucleotides. $G_{\alpha t}$ activates PDE via direct binding to the enzyme. $G_{\alpha gust}$ (also referred to as gustducin) shares a high degree of homology with $G_{\alpha t}$ [39]. It is enriched in taste epithelium, and it has been suggested that it mediates signal transduction in this tissue via the activation of a distinct form of PDE.

The ability of neurotransmitter receptors to stimulate the phosphatidylinositol second-messenger pathway is mediated by the activation of phospholipase C, which catalyzes the hydrolysis of phosphatidylinositol into the second messengers inositol trisphosphate and diacylglycerol. It now appears that neurotransmitter-induced activation of phospholipase C is mediated via G proteins [37,38]. In most cases, G_q is involved, and it is thought that $G_{\alpha q}$ binds to and directly activates certain forms of phospholipase C. In other cases, subtypes of G_i and/or G_o may be involved. The mechanism by which G proteins mediate neurotransmitter regulation of arachidonic acid metabolism, via the activation or inhibition of phospholipase A_2, is less well understood, but may also involve subtypes of G_i or G_o. In each of these cases, possible roles for $\beta\gamma$-complexes in the regulation of enzyme activity have been proposed and in some cases demonstrated [6,40].

In addition to the heterotrimeric G proteins, other forms of G proteins play important roles in cell function

These proteins, like the heterotrimeric G proteins, bind guanine nucleotides, possess intrinsic GTPase activity, and cycle through GTP- and GDP-bound forms (see Fig. 2). One unifying feature of the various classes of G proteins is that the binding of GTP increases the proteins' affinity for some target molecule, whereas the binding of GDP decreases that affinity.

One major class of G protein, termed the "small G proteins," has mass of 20 to 35 kDa [9,37]. Examples of small M_r G proteins and their possible functional roles are given in Table 3. The best-characterized small M_r G protein is the ras family, a series of related proteins of ~21 kDa. These proteins were identified originally as the oncogene products of *rat* sarcoma viruses. Subsequently, normal cellular homologs of viral ras were identified. Normal cellular homologs of oncogenes are often referred to as proto-oncogenes. The physiological functions of ras remain unknown. The proteins have been implicated in mediating signal transduction pathways in diverse tissues, including brain. For example, ras can influence intracellular cAMP levels and the activities of several protein kinases through as yet unknown mechanisms (see Chap. 22). In addition, a role for

TABLE 3.   Examples of small M_r G proteins

Class	Possible cellular function
Ras	Signal transduction (regulation of cAMP and Ca^{2+} pathways and of several protein kinases)
	Assembly of macromolecular complexes
Rab3	Localized to synaptic vesicles where it may regulate vesicle traffic and/or exocytosis
Rho	Assembly of cytoskeletal structures (e.g., actin microfilaments)
ARF	ADP-ribosylation of $G_{\alpha s}$[a]
	Assembly and function of Golgi complex

[a] ARF is required for cholera toxin-mediated ADP-ribosylation of $G_{\alpha s}$; it may also play a role in endogenous ADP-ribosylation.
(ARF) ADP-ribosylation factor.

ras in the macromolecular assembly of protein complexes in cell membranes has been proposed.

Other types of G proteins are the eukaryotic initiation and elongation factors. These proteins play a critical role in ribosomal assembly and protein translation. Dynamin, a member of the kinesin family which appears to mediate sliding between microtubules, is also a G protein.

Some G proteins can be modified by ADP-ribosylation

Among the tools that facilitated the discovery and characterization of G proteins were the bacterial toxins, cholera and pertussis toxins, which were known to influence adenylyl cyclase activity. It was subsequently shown that these actions of the toxins are achieved by their ability to catalyze the addition of an ADP-ribose group (donated from nicotinamide-adenine dinucleotide [NAD]) to specific amino acid residues in certain G protein α-subunits.

Cholera toxin catalyzes the ADP-ribosylation of a specific arginine residue in $G_{\alpha s}$ and $G_{\alpha t}$. This covalent modification inhibits the intrinsic GTPase activity of these α-subunits and thereby "freezes" them in their activated (free) state (see Fig. 2C). Through

this mechanism, cholera toxin stimulates adenylyl cyclase activity and photoreceptor transduction mechanisms (see Chap. 7). The ability of cholera toxin to ADP-ribosylate G_s may require the presence of a distinct protein, termed "ADP-ribosylation factor," or ARF. ARF, which is itself a small M_r G protein (see Table 3), is also ADP-ribosylated by cholera toxin [9].

In contrast, pertussis toxin catalyzes the ADP-ribosylation of a specific cysteine residue in $G_{\alpha i}$, $G_{\alpha o}$, and $G_{\alpha t}$. This covalent modification inactivates these α-subunits such that they cannot exchange GDP for GTP in response to receptor activation (see Fig. 2B). Pertussis toxin thus blocks the ability of neurotransmitters to inhibit adenylyl cyclase, or to influence the gating of K^+ and Ca^{2+} channels, in target neurons. However, since $G_{\alpha z}$ is not a substrate for pertussis toxin, the toxin may not be able to block neurotransmitter-mediated inhibition of adenylyl cyclase in all cases. The G_q and G_{11} through G_{16} types of G protein α-subunit are not known to undergo ADP-ribosylation.

A third type of bacterial toxin, diphtheria toxin, is known to catalyze the ADP-ribosylation of eukaryotic elongation factor, the functional activity of which is inhibited by this reaction. Moreover, a botulinum toxin ADP-ribosylates, and disrupts the function of, the small M_r G protein rho (see Table 3).

In the absence of bacterial toxins, brain and peripheral tissues are known to contain endogenous ADP-ribosyltransferases, which catalyze the ADP-ribosylation of numerous cellular proteins [10,29]. Although most of the substrates for endogenous ADP-ribosylation in brain remain unknown, recent evidence indicates that $G_{\alpha s}$ and ARF are among them. This has led to the suggestion that ADP-ribosylation may represent a mechanism by which G protein function is regulated *in vivo*. In addition, there is evidence that endogenous ADP-ribosylation of cellular proteins may be regulated by second messengers (see below). Recent evidence supports an important role for endogenous ADP-ribosylation in the regulation of neuronal function: Levels of ADP-ribosylation are dramatically altered in the CA1 region of the hippocampus in association with long-term potentiation, considered to be a cellular model of learning and memory [11].

G proteins in the pathophysiology of disease

G proteins have been shown to be involved in the etiology of several disease states. Some pituitary adenomas are caused by mutations in $G_{\alpha s}$, which alter its functional activity [12]. Different types of mutations in $G_{\alpha s}$ are responsible for pseudohypoparathyroidism, a rare hereditary disease in which target tissues are resistant to the physiological actions of parathyroid hormone despite the existence of a normal number of functionally active hormone receptors [13].

Recently, neurofibromatosis type 1, a familial disorder characterized by multiple benign tumors of certain glial cells, was shown to be due to a mutation in the gene that codes for GTPase activation protein, or GAP (see [14]). GAP functions in the cell by stimulating the intrinsic GTPase activity in the ras family of small M_r G proteins. This distinguishes ras from the α-subunits of the heterotrimeric G proteins whose GTPase activity is not dependent on an activator protein. The mutation in GAP that leads to neurofibromatosis renders GAP unable to activate the GTPase activity of ras. This means that the GTP-bound form of ras remains active for abnormal periods of time and leads, through an as yet unknown mechanism, to abnormal cell growth. The critical importance of the small M_r G proteins in cell growth and differentiation is highlighted by the consideration, as noted above, that several forms of these proteins are proto-oncogenes. This means that mutations in these proteins that result in alterations in their regulatory properties can lead to oncogenesis. Ras in particular has been implicated in several human cancers including colorectal adenocarcinoma.

In addition to their involvement in specific disease states, levels of heterotrimeric G protein subunits have been shown to be altered in specific regions of the central nervous system in response to chronic exposure to many types of psychoactive drugs. This has been shown for antidepressant drugs, lithium (used in the treatment of mania and depression), opiates, cocaine, and alcohol (see [15,16]). Evidence has been presented to suggest that drug-induced alterations in levels of G proteins contribute to the therapeutic or addictive actions of these drugs on the brain.

ADENYLYL CYCLASE

Regulation of cAMP formation by neurotransmitter receptors as well as by intracellular messenger pathways is determined by the activity of the enzyme adenylyl cyclase (also referred to as adenylate cyclase). Adenylyl cyclase can also be activated by forskolin, a plant diterpene that has been useful in studies of enzyme regulation and purification. The substrate for adenylyl cyclase is a complex of Mg^{2+} and ATP. In addition, free divalent cation (e.g., free Mg^{2+}), in excess of ATP, is a requisite cofactor for enzyme activity. As shown in Fig. 3, adenylyl cyclase forms cAMP by creating a cyclic phosphodiester bond with the α-phosphate group of ATP, with the concomitant release of pyrophosphate, which provides energy for the reaction.

There are multiple forms of adenylyl cyclase

Results of biochemical and molecular cloning studies indicate the existence of several forms of adenylyl cyclase that comprise a distinct enzyme family [17–20]. To date, four distinct forms of the enzyme have been definitively identified; these are referred to as types I through IV. There is also more preliminary evidence for at least two additional enzymes, types V and VI. Each of these enzymes is membrane-bound. These various forms of adenylyl cyclase are differentially

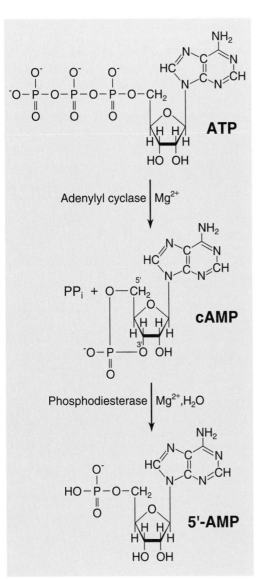

FIG. 3.   The chemical pathways of the synthesis and degradation of cAMP. cAMP is synthesized from ATP by the enzyme adenylyl cyclase with the release of pyrophosphate (PP$_i$) and is hydrolyzed into 5'-AMP by the enzyme phosphodiesterase. Both reactions require Mg^{2+}.

regulated and display distinct distributions in nervous and nonnervous tissues. Type I adenylyl cyclase is found predominantly in brain. Type II is expressed at highest levels in brain but is also found at lower levels in lung and olfactory tissue. Type III is highly enriched in olfactory epithelium. Type IV ap-

pears to be widely distributed and is present at high levels in brain. In addition, a soluble form of adenylyl cyclase has been identified in sperm, but has not yet been cloned.

Adenylyl cyclase types I through IV, the best-characterized forms of the enzyme, display some amino acid homology within specific (conserved) segments of the molecule, but have limited overall sequence homology. However, the four enzymes appear to be similar in their overall topographical structure [17,20], which is illustrated in Fig. 4. Hydropathicity profiles of their amino acid sequences indicate that adenylyl cyclase proteins contain two large hydrophobic regions, each of which consists of six putative membrane-spanning domains. There are two large cytoplasmic domains, one between the two hydrophobic regions and the other at the carboxy terminus of the protein. The cytoplasmic domains are the most highly conserved portions of the four different adenylyl cyclase proteins, and they are similar to each other within a given enzyme molecule. Moreover, there is some homology between these domains and the catalytic domains of certain

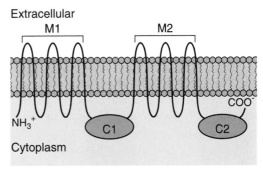

FIG. 4.   Schematic illustration of the proposed topographical structure of the four membrane forms of adenylyl cyclase. Hydropathicity profiles predict that adenylyl cyclase contains two hydrophobic regions (M1 and M2), each of which contains six membrane-spanning regions, and two relatively less hydrophobic regions (C1 and C2), which are thought to be located in the cytoplasm. The catalytic domains may be located within C1 and C2, and both are necessary for functional activity of the enzyme. The carboxy (COO$^-$) half of the protein determines whether βγ-subunit complexes inhibit (type I) or stimulate (types II and IV) adenylyl cyclase.

guanylyl cyclases (the enzyme that catalyzes the synthesis of cGMP—see below). These domains are thought to contain nucleotide binding sites, and both appear to be necessary for catalytic activity; there is no enzymatic activity when only one of the domains is expressed, but activity is reinstated when the two halves of the molecule are coexpressed [20]. The adenylyl cyclases are glycosylated and contain several potential sites for phosphorylation (see below).

The topographical structure of the adenylyl cyclase proteins resembles that of membrane transporters and ion channels. However, there is currently no convincing evidence of a transporter or channel function for mammalian adenylyl cyclases. The structural similarity may indicate that these functionally divergent protein families are derived in an evolutionary sense from related proteins.

The different forms of adenylyl cyclase are regulated by distinct mechanisms

The type I through IV enzymes differ in their ability to be regulated by Ca^{2+} and calmodulin [20]. Types I and III are stimulated by Ca^{2+}/calmodulin complexes, whereas types II and IV are insensitive.

Although adenylyl cyclase types I through IV are each stimulated by activated $G_{\alpha s}$ (i.e., $G_{\alpha s}$ bound to GTP), they differ in their regulation by $\beta\gamma$-subunit complexes [4,7]. In the presence of $G_{\alpha s}$, addition of $\beta\gamma$-complexes inhibits type I, does not affect type III, and stimulates types II and IV adenylyl cyclases. Studies with chimeras of the different enzyme types indicate that the stimulatory effect of $\beta\gamma$ resides in the carboxy half of the molecule [20]. These studies utilized "noncovalent" chimeras, where the amino half of the type I enzyme (containing the first membrane-spanning and cytoplasmic domains) is coexpressed in cultured cells with the carboxy half of either the type I or the type II enzyme (containing the second membrane-spanning and cytoplasmic domains). Depending on whether the carboxy portion is from type I or II, the coexpressed chimera is either inhibited or stimulated, respectively, by $\beta\gamma$-complexes. In addition to the different forms of adenylyl cyclase showing differential responses to $\beta\gamma$-subunits, it is likely that different forms of β- and γ-subunits influence the various forms of adenylyl cyclase in different ways [1]. The soluble form of adenylyl cyclase from sperm is stimulated by Ca^{2+}/calmodulin, but does not appear to be influenced by G proteins.

The differential sensitivity of adenylyl cyclase types I through IV to $\beta\gamma$- and Ca^{2+}/calmodulin complexes suggests that complex pathways exist for the regulation of cAMP formation [2,20]. Examples of these pathways, most of which remain hypothetical, are illustrated schematically in Fig. 5. In cells which contain type I adenylyl cyclase (Fig. 5A), cAMP formation is stimulated by extracellular signals that increase Ca^{2+} entry into the cells, as well as by those signals that activate receptors coupled to G_s. Cells expressing type I adenylyl cyclase may have inherently high levels of cAMP formation due to basal stimulation by Ca^{2+}/calmodulin. In fact, the high levels of adenylyl cyclase enzymatic activity in brain relative to other tissues may be explained in this way. This high level of enzyme activity could also underlie the requirement for additional mechanisms by which this type of adenylyl cyclase is inhibited: cAMP formation may be inhibited in these cells not only by signals that activate receptors coupled to G_i, but also by additional signals that activate receptors coupled to other G proteins (e.g., G_o and G_q) leading to release of $\beta\gamma$-subunits. This could provide a mechanism for keeping "in check" the high cAMP synthetic capacity present in brain, as well as provide multiple mechanisms for the regulation of cAMP formation by a variety of extracellular signals.

A very different situation may exist in cells that express type II adenylyl cyclase (Fig. 5B). In these cells, enzyme activity is not stimulated by Ca^{2+}/calmodulin, but is increased by signals that activate receptors coupled to G_s, as well as by additional signals that acti-

A

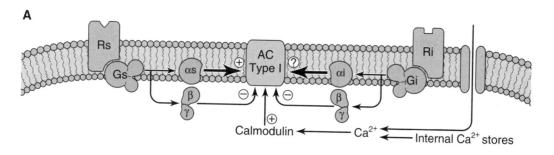

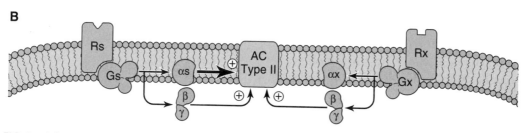

B

FIG. 5.   Schematic illustration of the mechanisms by which the activity of adenylyl cyclase types I and II may be regulated. Adenylyl cyclase types I and II can be distinguished by their sensitivity to Ca^{2+}/calmodulin and regulation by G proteins. **A:** Since adenylyl cyclase type I is stimuluated by Ca^{2+}/calmodulin, it is hypothesized that an increase in cellular Ca^{2+} levels, which can result from either increased entry of Ca^{2+} into the cell or increased release of Ca^{2+} from internal stores, will activate the enzyme. Adenylyl cyclase type I, like types II through IV, is activated by $G_{\alpha s}$ (αs). In addition, in the presence of activated $G_{\alpha s}$, the type I enzyme is inhibited by $\beta\gamma$-subunits. The potency of $G_{\alpha s}$ to activate the enzyme is some 10- to 20-fold higher than that of $\beta\gamma$-complexes to inhibit it, so that activation of enzyme activity is the predominant effect when only stimulatory receptors and G_s are activated. G_i (αi) is generally thought to mediate inhibition of adenylyl cyclase. Although the mechanism of G_i action remains unknown, the release of $\beta\gamma$-subunits from G_i could be involved. Not shown in the figure is the additional possibility that the source of the inhibitory $\beta\gamma$-complexes is a G protein other than G_s or G_i. Adenylyl cyclase type III, like the type I enzyme, is stimulated by Ca^{2+}/calmodulin, but is not affected by $\beta\gamma$-complexes. **B:** Adenylyl cyclase type II is not sensitive to Ca^{2+}/calmodulin and, in the presence of activated $G_{\alpha s}$, is stimulated by $\beta\gamma$-complexes. The receptors (Rx) and G protein α-subunits (Gx, αx) that provide the $\beta\gamma$-subunits for this type of regulation are unknown, but could conceivably involve receptors coupled to various types of G protein systems (e.g., G_o, G_q, etc.). Type IV adenylyl cyclase exhibits regulatory properties similar to those shown for the type II enzyme. Note: While the same $\beta\gamma$-complexes are shown for all the G proteins listed, there are several known subtypes of β- and γ-subunits that may influence the various types of adenylyl cyclase in different ways. (Rs) stimulatory receptor; (Ri) inhibitory receptor.

vate receptors coupled to other G proteins through the generation of free $\beta\gamma$-subunit complexes. This may provide a mechanism by which cAMP formation is regulated in an integrated manner by multiple extracellular stimuli. In fact, there are several examples in brain of interactions between receptors coupled to G_s and those coupled to other G proteins. For example, stimulation of adenylyl cyclase activity in cerebral cortex by activation of β-adrenergic receptors (which are coupled to G_s) is potentiated by activation of α_1-adrenergic or $GABA_B$ receptors, which are not coupled to G_s and which alone have little or no effect on cAMP formation [21]. This potentiation could result from release of free $\beta\gamma$-complexes from the G proteins coupled to α_1-adrenergic or $GABA_B$ receptors (e.g., G_o and/or G_q). However, these potentiating effects are dependent on extracellular Ca^{2+} and may also, therefore, be mediated by activation of Ca^{2+}-dependent intracellular pathways.

Still additional mechanisms for the regulation of adenylyl cyclase activity are provided by reports that the enzyme can be regulated through phosphorylation by cAMP-dependent protein kinase or by protein kinase C (see [22]). Effects of protein kinase C provide a mechanism by which activation of the Ca^{2+} and phosphatidylinositol pathways stimulates adenylyl cyclase. This provides a connection between receptors linked to stimulation of adenylyl cyclase and those linked to the turnover of membrane phosphoinositides.

Adenylyl cyclase is subject to long-term regulation in the nervous system

Prolonged exposure of cells to agonists at particular receptors typically leads to desensitization of receptor function, whereas prolonged exposure to antagonists may lead to sensitization of receptor function. Increasing evidence suggests that desensitization and sensitization can be achieved, depending on the receptor and cell type involved, through alterations in the receptors themselves as well as through alterations in the proteins distal to the receptor that mediate receptor function.

Processes of receptor desensitization and sensitization are best established for receptors coupled (positively or negatively) to the cAMP system. Agonist- and antagonist-dependent changes in these receptors themselves are discussed elsewhere (see Chap. 12). Postreceptor changes that contribute to receptor desensitization and sensitization can include alterations in G proteins (see above), adenylyl cyclase, cAMP-dependent protein kinase, and substrates for protein kinase. As one example, coordinate modification in each of these steps has been associated with processes of opioid tolerance and dependence [16]. Agonist- and antagonist-induced alterations in adenylyl cyclase appear to involve its phosphorylation by various protein kinases and could conceivably also involve regulation of its genetic expression.

In addition to regulation of adenylyl cyclase mediated through effects of agonists or antagonists on receptors, some drugs have direct effects on the adenylyl cyclase protein. For example, lithium, widely used in the treatment of bipolar depressive disorders, inhibits adenylyl cyclase activity by interfering with the enzyme's Mg^{2+} binding sites, but leads to increases in adenylyl cyclase expression after chronic administration [15].

The importance of adenylyl cyclase in neuronal function is further emphasized by the demonstration that the rutabaga mutation in the fruit fly *Drosophila*, which shows memory and learning deficits, involves the loss of Ca^{2+}/calmodulin-sensitive adenylyl cyclase [23].

GUANYLYL CYCLASE

Guanylyl cyclase (also referred to as guanylate cyclase) catalyzes the synthesis of cGMP from GTP in a reaction analogous to that shown in Fig. 3 for adenylyl cyclase. Two major classes of guanylyl cyclase are known to exist, identified originally on the basis of their subcellular distribution: membrane-bound or soluble [24,25]. Figure 6 illustrates possible mechanisms by which these types of guanylyl cyclases are regulated by extracellular signals.

Membrane-bound forms of guanylyl cyclase are plasma membrane receptors

These transmembrane proteins possess cell-surface domains that function as neuropeptide receptors and intracellular domains that contain guanylyl cyclase catalytic activity. The binding of ligand to, and consequent activation of, the receptor domain leads to the activation of the catalytic domain.

These enzymes also contain a third domain, which is referred to as the "protein kinase domain" based on its structural homology to protein kinases. It is thought that this domain contains an ATP binding site, which is required for guanylyl cyclase activity. Indeed, the binding of ATP to this site may

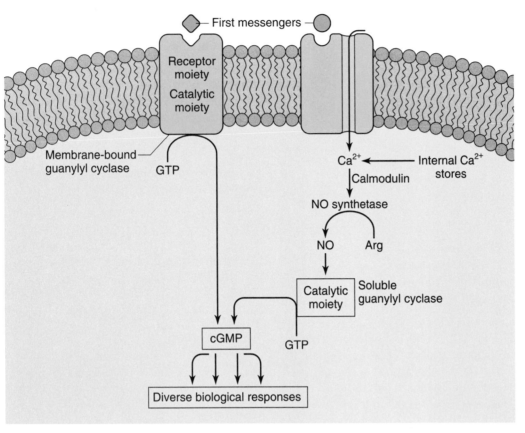

FIG. 6.   Schematic illustration of the mechanisms by which first messengers stimulate guanylyl cyclase. Two major classes of guanylyl cyclase are known: membrane-bound and soluble. The membrane-bound forms contain extracellular receptor moieties that recognize specific first messengers (e.g., atrial natriuretic peptide) and a catalytic moiety that synthesizes cGMP from GTP. The soluble forms contain the catalytic moieties only and are activated by nitric oxide (NO). First messengers stimulate NO synthesis by increasing cellular levels of Ca^{2+}, which in conjunction with calmodulin activates NO synthetase. First messengers increase cellular Ca^{2+} levels in most cases by depolarizing neuronal membranes and thereby activating voltage-dependent Ca^{2+} channels and increasing the flux of Ca^{2+} into the cell (e.g., nerve impulses, glutamate, acetylcholine, substance P). In some cases, Ca^{2+} can enter the cell directly via activated ligand-gated ion channels as shown in the figure (e.g., as with N-methyl-D-aspartate glutamate receptors). In still other cases, first messengers can increase intracellular Ca^{2+} levels by stimulating the release of Ca^{2+} from internal stores.

play a role in transducing the effect of a ligand binding to the receptor domain to the activation of enzyme activity in the catalytic domain.

Three forms of membrane-bound guanylyl cyclase, with mass of ~120 kDa, have been identified in mammalian tissues by molecular cloning [24,25]. Two of these are plasma membrane receptors for atrial natriuretic peptide (ANP) and related peptides. Atrial natriuretic peptide is a 28 amino acid

peptide isolated originally from cardiac atria and involved in the regulation of sodium excretion and blood pressure. Several variant forms of ANP have been identified, including a so-called brain natriuretic peptide (BNP). Increasing evidence suggests that these peptides play important roles as extracellular signals in diverse tissues including brain. It appears that activation of guanylyl cyclase, and the subsequent increase in cellular cGMP levels, mediate some of the cellular actions of these peptides on target tissues.

The third known form of guanylyl cyclase is activated by a bacterial enterotoxin, although the natural ligand for the receptor moiety of the protein is not yet known. The membrane-bound forms of guanylyl cyclase, which can be considered "signal-transducing enzymes," are structurally homologous to other signal-transducing enzymes, such as certain protein tyrosine kinases and phosphatases, which also possess receptor moieties in their extracellular (amino terminus) domain and enzyme catalytic activity in their intracellular domain (see Chap. 22).

Soluble forms of guanylyl cyclase are activated by nitric oxide

These enzymes are homologous to the catalytic domains of the membrane-bound forms of guanylyl cyclase. They are thought to be heterodimers, because they appear to exist, under physiological conditions, as complexes of α- and β-subunits, each with mass of 70 to 80 kDa [24]. Both types of subunit contain catalytic domains, but the enzyme is only functionally active in a heterodimeric state. This can be seen as similar to the situation for adenylyl cyclase, which contains two catalytic entities within a single polypeptide chain (see Fig. 4). Multiple isoforms of α- and β-subunits of guanylyl cyclase have been cloned, and they exhibit distinct tissue and cellular distributions. It is possible that brain contains numerous species of guanylyl cyclase, with distinct functional and regulatory properties, formed by the heterodimerization of the α- and β-subunits.

A major advance in our understanding of guanylyl cyclase regulation was the demonstration that NO serves as an intracellular signal that controls the activity of soluble forms of guanylyl cyclase. It is thought that NO activates these enzymes via interactions with their heme prosthetic groups. It is through the generation of NO that numerous neurotransmitters, including glutamate, acetylcholine, substance P, histamine, and bradykinin, are thought to activate guanylyl cyclase and increase cellular levels of cGMP in brain and elsewhere. Similarly, all organic nitrates (e.g., nitroglycerin, nitroprusside) used in the treatment of ischemic heart disease induce vasodilation through activation of soluble guanylyl cyclase and increased levels of cGMP.

Nitric oxide functions as an intracellular second messenger

The synthesis of NO is catalyzed by an enzyme termed "NO synthetase" [26,27]. This enzyme converts arginine into free NO and citrulline in a reaction that requires a tetrahydrobiopterin cofactor and the reduced form of nicotinamide-adenine dinucleotide phosphate (NADPH). Only certain types of neurons contain NO synthetase, such that the enzyme exhibits a highly specific localization in the brain. NO synthetase is a Ca^{2+}/calmodulin-sensitive enzyme; the binding of Ca^{2+}/calmodulin complexes to the enzyme results in the activation of catalytic activity (see Fig. 6). Thus, neurotransmitters that increase cellular Ca^{2+} levels would be expected to stimulate guanylyl cyclase activity in those neurons that contain NO synthetase.

It has been hypothesized that NO serves as an *intercellular* messenger. According to this scheme, NO, generated in response to an increase in intracellular Ca^{2+} levels in one neuronal cell, might diffuse out of the cell and into a second neuron, where it would stimulate guanylyl cyclase activity and produce various physiological effects. It has been suggested that NO plays a role in long-term potentiation [28], a cellular model of learning in the nervous system (see Chap. 50).

It is important to note that in addition to guanylyl cyclase, certain ADP-ribosyltransferases may also be NO-stimulated enzymes [29]. This means that some of the physiological actions of NO may be mediated through the ADP-ribosylation of specific G proteins or other cellular proteins (see above).

PHOSPHODIESTERASES

Given the role of cyclic nucleotides in signal transduction pathways, it is not surprising that the metabolism, as well as the synthesis, of these second messengers is highly regulated. Such metabolism is achieved by a large number of enzymes, the PDEs, which catalyze the conversion of cAMP and cGMP into 5′-AMP and 5′-GMP via hydrolysis of 3′-phosphoester bonds (see Fig. 3).

There are multiple forms of PDE in brain

Five major families of PDE, shown in Table 4, have been delineated based primarily on two criteria: (1) the mechanisms for regulation of enzyme activity, and (2) the kinetic properties of the enzymes for hydrolyzing cyclic nucleotides [30–33]. This latter property is denoted as the K_m of the enzyme for

TABLE 4.   Classification and selected properties of cyclic nucleotide phosphodiesterases (PDEs)

Family	Some regulatory and kinetic characteristics	Selective inhibitors[a]
I	"Ca^{2+}/calmodulin-stimulated PDE" Regulated by Ca^{2+}/calmodulin High K_m (low affinity)	Trifluoperazine Vinpocetine
II	"cGMP-stimulated PDE" Regulated by cGMP High K_m (low affinity)	
III	"cGMP-inhibited PDE" Regulated by cGMP Low K_m (high affinity)	Milrinone Enoximone Amrinome[b]
IV	"cAMP-specific PDE" Physiological regulators unknown Low K_m (high affinity)	Rolipram Ro 20-1724
V	"cGMP-specific PDE" Regulated by transducin Low K_m (high affinity)	Dipyridamole

[a] In addition to the relatively specific inhibitors listed in this table, there are a number of compounds, particularly the methylxanthines (e.g., theophylline, isobutylmethylxanthine, caffeine), which inhibit most major forms of PDE.

[b] The compounds listed here are among a large number that have been developed as specific inhibitors of PDE III.

cAMP or cGMP. A low K_m value signifies high affinity for substrate; for example, a low-K_m PDE typically has a K_m of less than 1 μM.

The PDE I family is stimulated by Ca^{2+}/calmodulin and consists of several subtypes in brain and peripheral tissues [30–33]. Two isozymes of PDE I, with molecular weights of 61 and 63 kDa, account for more than 90 percent of total brain PDE activity. Immunocytochemical studies have revealed that high levels of these enzymes are localized in synaptic densities, in the dendritic fields of cerebellar Purkinje cells, and in cerebral cortical pyramidal cells. An additional isozyme with a mass of 75 kDa has been identified in brain. Each of these enzymes exhibits relatively high K_m values for cGMP and cAMP.

The activity of PDE I isozymes can be regulated under physiological conditions by extracellular signals that influence intracellular Ca^{2+} levels. There is also evidence that these enzymes are regulated by protein phosphorylation [30]. The 61- and 63-kDa isozymes are good substrates for cAMP-dependent and Ca^{2+}/calmodulin-dependent protein kinase, respectively; phosphorylation decreases the functional capacity of the enzymes by decreasing their affinity for Ca^{2+}/calmodulin.

Two PDE families are regulated by cGMP, one that is stimulated (PDE II) and one that is inhibited (PDE III). cGMP-stimulated PDE II has a high K_m for cAMP and cGMP. There are at least two cyclic nucleotide binding sites on PDE II isozymes: One is presumably the catalytic site, the other may be a high-affinity site that allosterically regulates the catalytic activity of the enzyme. PDE II can be activated 10- to 50-fold by concentrations of cGMP that are found in cells. However, stimulation is transient since cGMP is also a substrate for the enzyme and is therefore rapidly metabolized. Results of immunohistochemical studies demonstrate that PDE II is found throughout the brain. In contrast, there is currently no evidence for the presence of cGMP-inhibited PDE III in brain. Instead, PDE III, which has a low K_m for cAMP, is enriched in heart and in vascular tissues, where it regulates cardiac and smooth muscle contraction.

PDE IV, which is also known as the cAMP-specific, low-K_m PDE, is found in many tissues and is abundantly expressed in the central nervous system. Multiple isozymes have been identified. However, little is known about their regulation under physiological conditions. In liver, PDE IV isozymes are regulated by insulin, presumably through phosphorylation. There are also reports that guanine nucleotides stimulate the activity of PDE IV, which would suggest regulation by as yet unidentified G proteins.

The best-known members of the PDE V family are the light-activated photoreceptor isozymes [34]. In addition, members of this family exist in lung and platelet, but to date there is no evidence for their presence in brain. The PDE V family is also referred to as the cGMP-specific PDEs. They show 50-fold selectivity for cGMP relative to cAMP. Activation of photoreceptor PDE in rod and cone outer segments is mediated by transducin, a G protein specific to retina (see above). These PDEs are multimeric enzymes, composed of α-, β-, and γ-subunits. They are inactive in the dark; light results in their activation via a complex biochemical cascade (see Chap. 7 for more detail).

The PDE enzymes show a distinctive molecular structure

Members of each of the five PDE families have been characterized by molecular cloning [31,32]. All of the enzymes thus far identified in mammalian tissues include a highly conserved region of approximately 270 amino acids within the carboxy end of the enzyme, which corresponds to their catalytic domain. Within this region, all of the cAMP-specific PDE enzymes (e.g., PDE IV) contain an identical sequence that represents the cAMP binding domain. A similar sequence is found in the regulatory subunit of cAMP-dependent protein kinase (see Chap. 22). Those PDEs that have high-affinity cGMP binding sites that apparently serve an alloste-

ric function (e.g., PDE II) share a distinct conserved region within their amino acid sequence. Some PDEs are membrane-associated, although the molecular basis of this association has not been clearly established. Hydropathicity profiles are predictive of transmembrane domains, but models of the topographical structure of these enzymes have not yet been developed.

PDE inhibitors offer promise for pharmacological therapeutics

This may not be surprising given the widespread role of cyclic nucleotides in the regulation of cell function [30,32]. The best examples of drugs that influence PDEs are the methylxanthines; these drugs are used therapeutically in the treatment of obstructive pulmonary disease, and are responsible for the stimulant properties of coffee, tea, and related substances. Inhibition of PDE contributes to some of the clinical effects of these drugs.

Other examples of PDE inhibitors with possible clinical usefulness are inhibitors of PDE III or IV (see Table 4). Based on the localization of PDE III to heart and vascular tissue and the effect of cAMP on muscle contraction and relaxation in these tissues, a large number of PDE III inhibitors have been developed for possible clinical application to the treatment of cardiovascular disease. Inhibitors of PDE IV are being developed as possible antidepressants; the rationale for this application comes from the observation that many antidepressant treatments appear to increase cAMP function in brain acutely. It is speculated that persistent increases in cAMP levels may lead to the long-term adaptive changes in the brain thought to underlie the antidepressant effects of these agents. There is also indirect evidence for the importance of PDE IV isozymes in neuronal function [23]. For example, the dunce mutation in *Drosophila*, which results in learning and memory deficits, involves loss of function of a cAMP-specific PDE.

FUNCTIONAL ROLES FOR cAMP AND cGMP

Over the last three decades, cAMP has been shown to serve as an intracellular second messenger for numerous extracellular signals in the nervous system. In fact, the number of functional processes regulated by cAMP is too large to enumerate in detail. It is important, however, to review the general types of effects that cAMP exerts in neurons.

cAMP can be viewed as subserving two major functions in the nervous system

First, cAMP mediates some short-term aspects of synaptic transmission: Some rapid actions of certain neurotransmitters on ion channels that do not involve activation of ligand-gated channels are mediated through cAMP. Second, cAMP, along with other intracellular messengers, plays a central role in mediating various aspects of synaptic transmission: Numerous effects of neurotransmitters on target neuron functioning, both short term and long term, are achieved through intracellular messengers. This includes regulation of the general metabolic state of target neurons, as well as modulatory effects on neurotransmitter synthesis, storage, and release; neurotransmitter receptor sensitivity; cytoskeletal organization and structure; and neuronal growth and differentiation. This also includes those long-term actions of neurotransmitters that are mediated through alterations in neuronal gene expression (see Chap. 24).

It is important to emphasize that a role for cAMP and other intracellular messengers is not limited to actions of neurotransmitters mediated through G protein-linked receptors. Thus, although activation of ligand-gated ion channels may lead to changes in membrane potential that are independent of intracellular messengers, activation of these channels also leads to numerous additional (albeit slower) effects that are mediated through intracellular messengers. For example, activation of certain glutamate receptor ion channels leads rapidly to membrane depolarization and more slowly to increases in celular levels of cAMP (e.g., by activation of Ca^{2+}/calmodulin-sensitive forms of adenylyl cyclase). cAMP then mediates several other effects of glutamate on the neurons. By virtue of numerous interactions between cAMP and other intracellular messenger pathways, these pathways play the central role in coordinating a myriad of neuronal processes and adjusting neuronal function to environmental cues [35].

Most of the effects of cAMP on cell function are mediated through protein phosphorylation

By far the most important mechanism through which cAMP exerts its myriad physiological effects is through the specific activation of cAMP-dependent protein kinases. This was first demonstrated by Krebs and his coworkers for cAMP regulation of glycogenolysis, and shortly thereafter shown to be a widespread mechanism by Greengard and his colleagues. Indeed, cAMP-dependent protein kinase is now known to phosphorylate virtually every type of neural protein; this accounts for the ability of cAMP to influence so many diverse aspects of neuronal function. The ability of cAMP to activate protein kinases, and the role of protein phosphorylation in the regulation of neuronal function, is covered in greater detail in Chap. 22.

How do a wide variety of neurotransmitters and hormones produce tissue- and cell-specific biological responses, if many such responses are mediated by the same intracellular messengers, cAMP and cAMP-dependent protein kinase? Specificity is achieved at several levels: at the level of tissue-specific receptors for the neurotransmitter or hormone, at the level of different subtypes of GTP-binding protein, and at the level of tissue-specific substrate proteins for protein kinase. Only tissues that express specific receptors will respond to a given neurotransmitter or hormone. Moreover, since all cells contain similar catalytic subunits of cAMP-dependent protein kinase (see Chap. 22), the nature of the proteins phosphorylated in a given tissue depends on the types and amounts of proteins expressed in that tissue and on their accessibility to protein kinase.

There are a small number of exceptions to the rule that the physiological effects of cAMP in mammals are achieved through activation of cAMP-dependent protein kinases. The best-established exception is cation channels in olfactory epithelium, which directly bind, and are thereby gated by, cAMP. However, even in the case of ion channels, cAMP regulation of ion channels appears to be most commonly achieved through protein phosphorylation.

The mechanism by which cGMP produces its physiological effects is less well established

It has been more difficult to identify second-messenger actions of cGMP compared to those of cAMP. This probably reflects the lower concentrations of cGMP in most tissues, and the likelihood that cGMP plays a less widespread role in cell function. Nevertheless, physiological actions of cGMP are being identified. The best-studied action is in the retina, where cGMP mediates the effects of light on cation channels in rod outer segments by directly binding to the channels or to closely associated proteins. In addition, cGMP has been shown to activate and inhibit different forms of PDE, as discussed earlier in this chapter, also through direct binding to the enzymes.

In addition to such direct actions of cGMP on effector proteins, many physiological effects of cGMP are probably mediated through the activation of cGMP-dependent protein kinase and the subsequent phosphorylation of specific substrate proteins (see Chap. 22). For example, the ability of neurotransmitters to influence ion channels in target neurons is mediated through increased cellular levels of cGMP, the activation of cGMP-dependent protein kinase, and the subsequent phosphorylation of the chan-

nels (or some associated proteins). As another example, in certain neuronal cell types, neurotransmitters that increase cGMP levels, through the activation of cGMP-dependent protein kinase and the phosphorylation and activation of DARPP-32 (dopamine- and cAMP-regulated phosphoprotein of 32 kDa, an inhibitor of protein phosphatase 1), would alter the phosphorylation state of the numerous proteins dephosphorylated by this protein phosphatase (see Chap. 22).

FUTURE PERSPECTIVES

Over the past several decades, great progress has been made in our understanding of signal transduction pathways in the brain. The identification and characterization of G proteins and the enzymes that control the synthesis and metabolism of cyclic nucleotides in the nervous system represent an important advancement. However, our knowledge of these systems is far from complete. Undoubtedly, new subtypes of G proteins, adenylyl and guanylyl cyclases, and PDEs will be identified in the future, each with distinct functional and regulatory properties. In addition, the numerous neuronal proteins that are regulated by cyclic nucleotides and protein kinases must be more fully explored. The nature and functional consequences of interactions between cyclic nucleotide pathways and other intracellular signal transduction pathways also need to be better characterized.

Studies aimed at obtaining a more complete understanding of signal transduction in the brain will require an integrated approach, combining the expertise of molecular and cell biology, electrophysiology, pharmacology, neuroanatomy, and behavior. This work, which may well occupy the next several decades, will lead ultimately to the delineation of the actions of cyclic nucleotides and other second messengers in the nervous system, under normal and pathophysiological conditions.

REFERENCES

1. Kleuss, C., Scherubl, H., Hescheler, J., Schultz, G., and Wittig, B. Different β-subunits determine G-protein interaction with transmembrane receptors. *Nature* 358: 424–426, 1992.
2. Federman, A. D., Conklin, B. R., Schrader, K. A., Reed, R. R., and Bourne, R. Hormonal stimulation of adenylyl cyclase through Gi-protein βγ subunits. *Nature* 356:159–161, 1992.
3. Tang, W., and Gilman, A. G. Type-specific regulation of adenylyl cyclase by G protein βγ subunits. *Science* 254:1500–1503, 1991.
4. Okabe, K., Yatani, A., Evans, T., Ho, Y., Codina, J., Birnbaumer, L., and Brown, A. βγ dimers of G proteins inhibit atrial muscarinic K⁺ channels. *J. Biol. Chem.* 265:12854–12858, 1990.
5. Pitcher, J. A., Inglese, J., Higgins, J. B., Arriza, J. L., Casey, P. J., Kim, C., Benovic, J. L., Kwatra, M. M., Caron, M. G., and Lefkowitz, R. J. Role of βγ subunits of G-proteins in targeting the β-adrenergic receptor kinase to membrane-bound receptors. *Science* 257: 1264–1267, 1992.
6. Katz, A., Wu, D., and Simon, M. I. Subunits βγ of heterotrimeric G protein activate β2 isoform of phospholipase C. *Nature* 360: 686–689, 1992.
7. Birnbaumer, L. G proteins in signal transduction. *Annu. Rev. Pharmacol. Toxicol.* 30: 675–705, 1990.
8. Wong, Y. H., Conklin, B., and Bourne, H. Gz-mediated hormonal inhibition of cyclic AMP accumulation. *Science* 255:339–342, 1992.
9. Hall, A. The cellular functions of small GTP-binding proteins. *Science* 249:635–640, 1990.
10. Williams, M. B., Li, X., Gu, X., and Jope, R. S. Modulation of endogenous ADP-ribosylation in rat brain. *Brain Res.* 592:549–556, 1992.
11. Duman, R. S., Terwilliger, R. Z., and Nestler, E. J. Alterations in nitric oxide-stimulated endogenous ADP-ribosylation associated with long-term potentiation in rat hippocampus.
12. Landis, C. A., Masters, S. B., Spada, A., Pace, A., Bourne, H., and Vallar, L. GTPase inhibiting mutations activate the alpha chain of Gs and stimulate adenylyl cyclase in human pituitary tumours. *Nature* 340:692–696, 1989.
13. Farfel, Z., Brickman, A., Kaslow, H., Brothers, V., and Bourne, H. Defect of receptor-cyclase coupling protein in pseudohypoparathyroidism. *N. Engl. J. Med.* 303:237–242, 1980.
14. Daston, M., Scrable, H., Nordlund, M., Sturbaum, A., Nissen, L., and Ratner, N. The protein product of the neurofibromatosis type 1 gene is expressed at highest abundance in neurons, Schwann cells, and oligodendrocytes. *Neuron* 8:415–428, 1992.
15. Colin, S., Chang, H., Mollner, S., et al. Chronic lithium regulates the expression of adenylate cyclase and Gi-protein α subunit in rat cerebral cortex. *Proc. Natl. Acad. Sci. U.S.A.* 88:10634–10637, 1991.
16. Nestler, E. J. Molecular mechanisms of drug addiction. *J. Neurosci.* 12:2439–2450, 1992.
17. Krupinski, J., Coussen, F., Bakalyar, H., et al. Adenylyl cyclase amino acid sequence: Possible channel- or transporter-like structure. *Science* 244:1558–1564, 1989.
18. Bakalyar, H. A., and Reed, R. R. Identification of a specialized adenylyl cyclase that may mediate odorant detection. *Science* 250: 1403–1406, 1990.
19. Feinstein, P., Schrader, K., Bakalyar, H., et al. Molecular cloning and characterization of a Ca²⁺/calmodulin-insensitive adenylyl cyclase from rat brain. *Proc. Natl. Acad. Sci. U.S.A.* 88: 10173–10177, 1991.
20. Gao, B., and Gilman, A. G. Cloning and expression of a widely distributed (type IV) adenylyl cyclase. *Proc. Natl. Acad. Sci. U.S.A.* 88:10178–10182, 1991.
21. Duman, R. S., and Enna, S. J. Modulation of receptor-mediated cyclic AMP production in brain. *Neuropharmacology* 26:981–986, 1987.
22. Bookbinder, L. H., Moy, G. W., and Vacquier, V. D. In vitro phosphorylation of sea urchin sperm adenylate cyclase by cyclic adenosine monophosphate-dependent protein kinase. *Mol. Reprod. Dev.* 28:150–157, 1991.
23. Dudai, Y. Neurogenetic dissection of learning and short-term memory in *Drosophila. Annu. Rev. Neurosci.* 11:537–563, 1988.
24. Koesling, D., Bohme, E., and Schultz, G. Guanylyl cyclases, a growing family of signal-transducing enzymes. *FASEB J.* 5:2785–2792, 1991.
25. Yuen, P. S. T., and Garbers, D. L. Guanylyl cyclase-linked receptors. *Annu. Rev. Neurosci.* 15:193–225, 1992.
26. Hope, B. T., Michael, G. J., Knigge, K. M., and Vincent, S. R. Neuronal NADPH diaphorase is a nitric oxide synthase. *Proc. Natl. Acad. Sci. U.S.A.* 88:2811–2814, 1991.

27. Bredt, D. S., and Snyder, S. H. Nitric oxide, a novel neuronal messenger. *Neuron* 8:3–11, 1992.

28. Haley, J. E., Wilcox, G. L., and Chapman, P. F. The role of nitric oxide in hippocampal long-term potentiation. *Neuron* 8:211–216, 1992.

29. Duman, R. S., Terwilliger, R. Z., and Nestler, E. J. Endogenous ADP-ribosylation in brain: Initial characterization of substrate proteins. *J. Neurochem.* 57:2124–2132, 1991.

30. Beavo, J. A. Multiple isozymes of cyclic nucleotide phosphodiesterase. *Adv. Second Messenger Phosphoprotein Res.* 22:1–37, 1988.

31. Beavo, J. A., and Reifsnyder, D. H. Primary sequence of cyclic nucleotide phosphodiesterase isozymes and the design of selective inhibitors. *Trends Pharmacol. Sci.* 11:150–155, 1990.

32. Nicholson, C. D., Challiss, J., and Shahid, M. Differential modulation of tissue function and therapeutic potential of selective inhibitors of cyclic nucleotide phosphodiesterase isoenzymes. *Trends Pharmacol. Sci.* 12:19–27, 1991.

33. Strada, S. J., and Thompson, W. J. (eds.), *Adv. Cyclic Nucleotide Protein Phosphorylation Res. Cyclic Nucleotide Phosphodiesterases*, Vol. 16, New York: Raven, 1984.

34. Stryer, L. Cyclic GMP cascade of vision. *Annu. Rev. Neurosci.* 9:87–119, 1986.

35. Hyman, S. E., and Nestler, E. J. *The Molecular Foundation of Psychiatry.* Washington, D.C.: American Psychiatric Press, 1993.

36. Jones, D. T., and Reed, R. R. Golf: An olfactory neuron specific-G protein involved in odorant signal transduction. *Science* 1989;244:790–795.

37. Bourne, H. R., Sanders, D. A., and McCormick, F. The GTPase superfamily: a conserved switch for diverse cell functions. *Nature* 1990;348:125–132.

38. Simon, M. I., Strathmann P., and Gautam, N. Diversity of G proteins in signal transduction. *Science* 1991;252:802–808.

39. McLaughlin, S. K., McKinnon, P. J., and Margolskee, R. F. Gustducin is a taste-cell-specific G protein closely related to the transducins. *Nature* 1992;357:563–569.

40. Camps, M., Carozzi, A., Schnabel, P., Scheer, A., Parker, P. J., and Gierschik, P. Isozyme-selective stimulation of phospholipase C-β2 by G protein βγ-subunits. *Nature* 1992;360:684–686.

CHAPTER 22

Protein Phosphorylation and the Regulation of Neuronal Function

ERIC J. NESTLER AND PAUL GREENGARD

Basic Neurochemistry: Molecular, Cellular, and Medical Aspects, 5th Ed., edited by G. J. Siegel et al. Published by Raven Press, Ltd., New York, 1994. Correspondence to Eric J. Nestler, Division of Molecular Psychiatry, Departments of Psychiatry and Pharmacology, Yale University School of Medicine and Connecticut Mental Health Center, 34 Park Street, New Haven, Connecticut 06508.

PROTEIN PHOSPHORYLATION IS A FINAL COMMON PATHWAY

Protein phosphorylation is a final common pathway of fundamental importance in biological regulation. Virtually all types of extracellular signals, both inside and outside the nervous system, are known to produce many of their diverse physiological effects by regulating the state of phosphorylation of specific phosphoproteins in their target cells. Examples of the large number of molecular pathways involving protein phosphorylation that have been revealed over the past 20 years are shown schematically in Fig. 1. The view that protein phosphorylation is the major molecular currency through which protein function is regulated in response to extracellular stimuli is supported by over a generation of research [1]. Thus, although proteins are known to be covalently modified in many other ways, e.g., by ADP-ribosylation, acylation (acetylation, myristoylation), carboxymethylation, tyrosine sulfation, and glycosylation, none of these mechanisms is as widespread and readily subject to regulation by physiological stimuli as is phosphorylation. This chapter presents an overview of the vital role played by protein phosphorylation in the regulation of neuronal function.

Protein phosphorylation systems consist of a protein kinase, a protein phosphatase, and a substrate protein

These components interact according to the scheme shown in Fig. 1. A substrate protein is converted from the dephospho form to the phospho form by a protein kinase, and the phospho form is converted back to the dephospho form by a protein phosphatase.

Protein kinases are classified as protein serine/threonine kinases, which phosphorylate substrate proteins on serine or threonine residues, or as protein tyrosine kinases, which phosphorylate substrate proteins on tyrosine residues. Most phosphorylation (>95 percent) of proteins occurs on serine residues; a small amount (~3–4 percent), on threonine residues; and very little (<1 percent), on tyrosine residues. In all cases, the kinases catalyze the transfer of the terminal (γ) phosphate group of ATP to the hydroxyl moiety in the respective amino acid residue; Mg^{2+} is required for this reaction. Protein phosphatases catalyze the cleavage of this phosphoester bond through hydrolysis.

Phosphorylation of a protein alters that protein's charge since phosphate groups are highly negatively charged, which can then alter the protein's conformation or shape

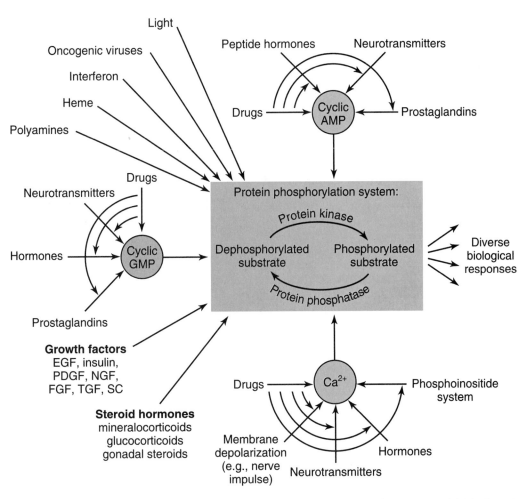

FIG. 1. Schematic diagram of the role played by protein phosphorylation in mediating some of the biological effects of a variety of regulatory agents. Many of these agents regulate protein phosphorylation through altering intracellular levels of a second messenger, cyclic AMP, cyclic GMP, or Ca^{2+}. Other agents appear to regulate protein phosphorylation through mechanisms that do not involve these second messengers. Most drugs regulate protein phosphorylation by affecting the ability of first messengers to alter second-messenger levels *(curved arrows)*. A small number of drugs (e.g., phosphodiesterase inhibitors, Ca^{2+} channel blockers, lithium) regulate protein phosphorylation by directly altering second-messenger levels *(straight arrows)*. (EGF) epidermal growth factor; (PDGF) platelet-derived growth factor; (NGF) nerve growth factor; (FGF) fibroblast growth factor; (TGF) transforming growth factor; (SC) somatomedin C. (From Nestler and Greengard [1].)

and ultimately its functional activity. A change in the state of phosphorylation of a protein can be achieved physiologically through increases or decreases in the activity of either a protein kinase or a protein phosphatase. Examples of each of these mechanisms are known to occur in the nervous system; however, activation of specific protein kinases is the best-studied mechanism

through which extracellular signals regulate protein phosphorylation in neural tissue.

Some individual steps in the molecular pathways through which extracellular signals regulate neuronal function through protein phosphorylation are shown in Fig. 2. Extracellular signals, or first messengers, in the nervous system include a variety of neurotransmitters, hormones, and trophic factors,

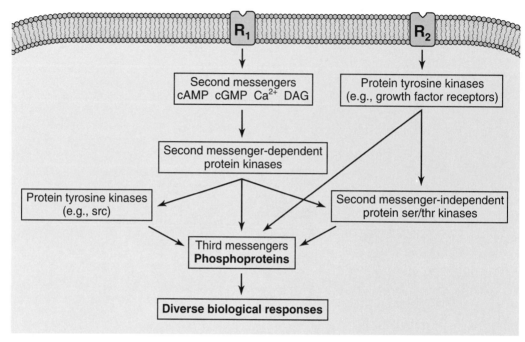

FIG. 2. Signals in the brain. Extracellular signals (first messengers) produce specific biological responses in target neurons via a series of intracellular signals (second, third messengers, etc.). Second messengers in the brain include cyclic AMP (cAMP), cyclic GMP (cGMP), Ca^{2+}, and diacylglycerol (DAG). cAMP and cGMP produce most of their effects through the activation of cAMP-dependent and cGMP-dependent protein kinases, respectively. The former enzyme exhibits a broad substrate specificity and the latter a more restricted specificity. Ca^{2+} exerts many of its effects through the activation of Ca^{2+}-dependent protein kinases, as well as through a variety of physiological effectors other than protein kinases. Ca^{2+} activates protein kinases in conjunction with calmodulin (enzymes termed Ca^{2+}/calmodulin-dependent protein kinases) or diacylglycerol (enzymes termed protein kinase C). There are at least five types of Ca^{2+}/calmodulin-dependent protein kinase and multiple isoforms of protein kinase C in brain. Ca^{2+}/calmodulin-dependent protein kinase II and protein kinase C exhibit broad substrate specificities and are likely to mediate many of the second-messenger actions of Ca^{2+}. Not illustrated in the figure is the point that some protein phosphatases can also be regulated directly by second messengers, for example, calcineurin, which is activated by Ca^{2+} and calmodulin. Brain also contains a large number of other protein serine/threonine kinases (some of which are listed in Table 2) that are not activated directly by second messengers, but seem to be regulated indirectly by second messengers and second-messenger-dependent protein kinases and by protein tyrosine kinases. The brain and other tissues contain two major classes of protein tyrosine kinases. Some of these enzymes are physically associated with plasma membrane receptors (e.g., most growth factor receptors) and become activated upon ligand binding to the receptors. Others are not physically associated with receptors (e.g., src) and are activated by as yet unknown mechanisms.

as well as light and nerve impulses themselves. In most established cases, these first messengers activate protein kinases indirectly by increasing the intracellular level of a second messenger in target neurons. Prominent second messengers in the nervous system that directly activate protein kinases include cyclic AMP (cAMP), cyclic GMP (cGMP), Ca^{2+}, and diacylglycerol (a major metabolite of phosphatidylinositol). The next steps in these pathways involve activa-

tion of specific classes of protein kinase and the subsequent phosphorylation of specific substrate proteins, leading, through one or more steps, to specific biological responses.

The brain has extraordinarily active systems for protein phosphorylation compared with non-neuronal tissue

cAMP-dependent and Ca^{2+}-dependent protein phosphorylation is much more prominent in extracts of cerebral cortex and cerebellum than in various non-neuronal tissues including liver, kidney, heart, and lung (Fig. 3). The more prominent protein phosphorylation observed in neuronal tissue probably reflects higher concentrations of various protein kinases as well as higher concentrations and larger numbers of substrate proteins. Neuronal tissue, because it contains a myriad of distinct cell types, might be expected to contain a larger variety of substrate proteins than non-neuronal tissue.

PROTEIN KINASES

Protein kinases differ in their cellular and subcellular distribution, substrate specificity, and regulation by cellular messengers

Among the most prominent protein kinases in the brain are those activated by (and named for) the second messengers cAMP, cGMP, Ca^{2+}, and diacylglycerol [1,2].

cAMP-dependent protein kinase is composed of catalytic and regulatory subunits

The holoenzyme of the protein kinase, which consists of a tetramer of two catalytic (C) and two regulatory (R) subunits, is inactive; cAMP activates the holoenzyme by binding to the R subunits, thereby causing dissociation of the holoenzyme into free R and free (active) C subunits. Three C subunits (of about 40 kDa) and four R subunits (of 50–55 kDa) have been cloned from mammalian tissues [2,3]. The three C subunits, designated $C\alpha$, $C\beta$, and $C\gamma$, exhibit a very similar and broad substrate specificity (i.e., they phosphorylate a large number of physiological substrate proteins) and can probably be considered isoforms of the enzyme. The four R subunits consist of two forms each of type I and type II proteins. $RII\alpha$ and $RII\beta$, but not $RI\alpha$ and $RI\beta$, undergo autophosphorylation, as described below. Most of the R and C sub-

units of protein kinase show a wide cellular and subcellular distribution in the brain.

cGMP-dependent protein kinase is a dimer of two identical subunits

Each subunit, with a molecular mass of ~75 kDa, contains a regulatory (cGMP binding) domain and a catalytic domain. As with the cAMP-dependent enzyme, cGMP activates the inactive holoenzyme by binding to the regulatory domain of the molecule; however, unlike the cAMP-dependent enzyme, activation of the cGMP-dependent holoenzyme is not accompanied by dissociation of the subunits. cGMP-dependent protein kinase shows a much more limited cellular distribution and substrate specificity than cAMP-dependent protein kinase. This reflects the smaller number of second-messenger actions of cGMP in the regulation of cell function.

Multiple forms of Ca^{2+}-dependent protein kinase exist in the nervous system

The Ca^{2+}-dependent protein kinases are divided into two subclasses. One is activated by Ca^{2+} in conjunction with the Ca^{2+}-binding protein calmodulin and is referred to as Ca^{2+}/calmodulin-dependent protein kinase. The brain contains at least five types of Ca^{2+}/calmodulin-dependent protein kinase, each with very different properties. Ca^{2+}/calmodulin-dependent protein kinase II, like the cAMP-dependent enzyme, exhibits a broad cellular distribution and substrate specificity, and can be considered a "multifunctional protein kinase" in that it probably mediates many of the second-messenger actions of Ca^{2+} in many types of neurons. By analogy to cGMP-dependent protein kinase, Ca^{2+}/calmodulin-dependent protein kinase II contains a regulatory domain which, in the resting state, binds to and inhibits a catalytic domain; this inhibition is relieved when Ca^{2+}/calmodulin binds to the regulatory domain. Several isoforms of this enzyme with mass of 50 to 60 kDa have been cloned. The

A

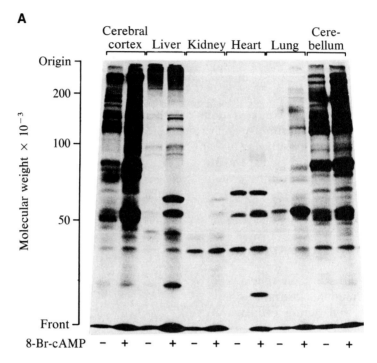

B

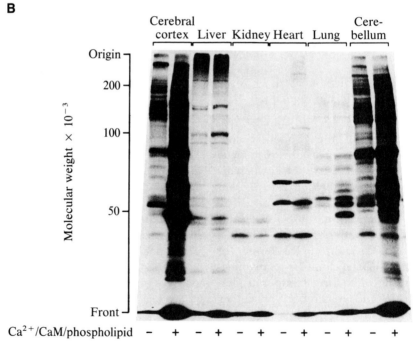

enzyme exists under physiological conditions as multimeric complexes of the same or distinct isoforms [4].

The other four types of Ca^{2+}/calmodulin-dependent protein kinase are phosphorylase kinase, myosin light-chain kinase, and Ca^{2+}/calmodulin-dependent protein kinases I and III [1,2,5]. These enzymes appear to phosphorylate only a limited number of substrate proteins under physiological conditions, and each may therefore mediate relatively few second-messenger actions of Ca^{2+} in the nervous system.

The other subclass of calcium-dependent protein kinase is activated by Ca^{2+} in conjunction with diacylglycerol and phosphatidylserine or other phospholipids and is referred to as Ca^{2+}/diacylglycerol-dependent protein kinase or protein kinase C [6]. Multiple forms of protein kinase C have been cloned, with the brain known to contain at least seven species of the enzyme. The variant forms of protein kinase C exhibit different cellular distributions in brain and different regulatory properties. For example, they differ in the relative ability of Ca^{2+} and diacylglycerol to activate them. However, these enzymes show similar substrate specificities and can, as a result, be considered isoforms. Protein kinase C exists under physiological conditions as single polypeptide chains of about 80 kDa. Each polypeptide contains a regulatory domain which, in the resting state, binds to and inhibits a catalytic domain; this inhibition is relieved when Ca^{2+} and/or diacylglyc-

erol bind to the regulatory domain. Protein kinase C exhibits a broad substrate specificity and mediates numerous second-messenger functions of Ca^{2+} in target neurons.

There is direct evidence that second-messenger-dependent protein kinases mediate numerous physiological actions of extracellular signals

The intracellular injection of cAMP-dependent protein kinase, cGMP-dependent protein kinase, Ca^{2+}/calmodulin-dependent protein kinase II, or protein kinase C into particular types of neurons has been shown to mimic specific physiological responses (e.g., regulation of ion channels, neurotransmitter release, gene transcription) to known neurotransmitters in those neurons [1,7,8]. Where specific inhibitors of the kinases are available, their injection has been shown to block the ability of the neurotransmitters to elicit those responses. Taken together, these findings demonstrate that activation of these second-messenger-dependent protein kinases is both a necessary and sufficient step in the sequence of events by which certain first messengers produce some of their physiological effects. Most of the earlier injection studies were performed with invertebrate neurons because of their relatively large size and the ease with which they can be identified. In more recent years, as electrophysiological techniques have become increasingly sophisticated, it has been possible to obtain

---

FIG. 3.   Autoradiographs showing **(A)** cAMP-dependent and **(B)** Ca^{2+}-dependent endogenous protein phosphorylation in extracts of rat tissues. Various tissues were removed from rats shortly after decapitation and were homogenized and then centrifuged at low speed ($700 \times g$) for 10 min to remove nuclei and large cellular debris. Aliquots (each containing 150 μg of protein) were incubated with $[\gamma^{-32}P]ATP$ for 1 min at 30°C in the presence (+) or absence (−) of 10 μM 8-bromo (8-Br)-cAMP **(A)** or 0.5 mM free Ca^{2+} plus 10 μg/ml calmodulin (CaM) plus 50 μg/ml phosphatidylserine **(B)**. The reaction was terminated by the addition of sodium dodecyl sulfate (SDS), and the samples were analyzed by SDS-polyacrylamide gel electrophoresis and autoradiography. Cerebral cortex and cerebellum exhibit much more prominent cAMP-dependent and Ca^{2+}-dependent protein phosphorylation than do the non-neuronal tissues liver, kidney, heart, and lung. (S. I. Walaas and P. Greengard, *unpublished observations.*) (From Nestler and Greengard [1].)

similar results in vertebrate nervous systems, including mammalian neurons.

The brain contains several types of protein serine/threonine kinases that are not directly regulated by the second messengers cAMP, cGMP, Ca^{2+}, and diacylglycerol

Examples of such enzymes are listed in Table 1. They include enzymes that were identified originally in association with a particular substrate protein, but have been shown recently to play a more widespread role in signal transduction in the brain [9,10]. An example is a family of protein kinases referred to alternatively as MAP kinase (*m*icrotubule-*a*ssociated *p*rotein kinase or *m*itogen-*a*ctivated *p*rotein kinase) or ERK (*e*xtracellular by *r*egulated protein *k*inase). Known substrate proteins for the MAP kinases include, in addition to MAPs, tyrosine hydroxylase and the Jun family of transcription factors. Although MAP kinases are not activated directly by second messengers, second messengers and the extracellular signals that generate them are known to regulate MAP kinase activity indirectly. For example, cAMP (through the acti-

vation of cAMP-dependent protein kinase) and Ca^{2+} (through the activation of protein kinase C) activate MAP kinases in a variety of cell types. The precise mechanisms remain unknown, but appear to involve activation of the small M_r GTP-binding protein ras (see Chap. 21), and the subsequent activation (through several steps) of a kinase which phosphorylates and activates MAP kinase. Some of the physiological effects of MAP kinase are achieved, at least in some cell types, through phosphorylation and activation of another protein kinase, termed rsk (named originally as *r*ibosomal *S6 k*inase) [11].

The view is emerging that intracellular processes are controlled by complex webs of a large number of interregulated protein kinases, which have only recently begun to be identified. These protein kinases are subject to regulation by extracellular signals via second messengers and second-messenger-dependent protein kinases, as well as by receptor-regulated protein tyrosine kinases (Fig. 2).

The brain contains many types of protein tyrosine kinases

Two major classes of enzyme are involved, as illustrated in Fig. 2. In one, the kinase is physically part of a plasma membrane receptor, such that binding of a ligand to the receptor results in activation of the intrinsic tyrosine kinase activity. This is the case for many types of trophic factor receptors, including those for insulin, insulin-like growth factor, and epidermal growth factor, all present in the nervous system.

The other class of protein tyrosine kinase lacks an extracellular receptor moiety. Src kinase (M_r ~60,000) is the prototypical example of this type of enzyme. Extracellular signals appear to regulate the activity of this type of protein tyrosine kinase through two general types of mechanisms. In one, the protein kinase becomes physically associated with a specific plasma membrane receptor when the receptor itself is activated by its ligand. Transient association with the recep-

TABLE 1.   Examples of protein serine/threonine kinases not regulated directly by second messengers[a]

Casein kinases I and II

MAP (*m*icotubule-*a*ssociated protein) kinases I, II, and III

Rhodopsin kinase

βARK (β-adrenergic receptor kinase)

βARK-related enzymes

Rsk (ribosomal S6 kinases)

Cdc kinases

Mos/raf kinases

Double-stranded RNA–dependent protein kinase

Neurofilament kinase

[a] This list is not intended to be comprehensive. The protein kinases listed are present in many cell types in addition to neurons and are included here because among their multiple functions in the nervous system is apparently the regulation of neuron-specific phenomena. Not included are other protein kinases present in diverse tissues (including brain) that play a role in generalized cellular processes, such as intermediary metabolism, and that may not play a role in neuron-specific phenomena.

or then results in activation of the protein kinase. This may be the case for the nerve growth factor receptor, which activates a protein tyrosine kinase termed trk. In the other mechanism, the protein tyrosine kinase does not associate with receptors, but is activated indirectly by second messengers (see Fig. 2). Although there is growing evidence for this mechanism in the brain (e.g., membrane depolarization, which causes an increase in cellular Ca^{2+} levels, increases protein tyrosine kinase activity in nervous tissue), the detailed steps involved remain unknown.

The transforming agents of several oncogenic viruses are protein tyrosine kinases. In fact, this class of enzyme was first identified through the study of oncogenes, and two of the enzymes mentioned above (i.e., src, trk) are the normal cellular homologs of oncogene products. The association of protein tyrosine kinases with transformation, and later with growth factor receptors, led to the early view that these enzymes play an important role in cell division and growth. However, several lines of evidence suggest that protein tyrosine kinases play an important role in the regulation of adult neuronal function, including signal transduction, in addition to a role in the regulation of growth and differentiation. The adult brain contains very high levels of protein tyrosine kinase activity, compared to most other tissues. In addition, protein tyrosine kinase activity is enriched, along with some of its substrate proteins, in synaptic fractions of brain where it can be regulated by numerous extracellular signals in specific brain regions (e.g., see [12]).

The brain contains numerous proteins that are phosphorylated on tyrosine residues. Notable examples are synaptophysin (a synaptic vesicle-associated phosphoprotein), the nicotinic acetylcholine receptor, phospholipase C (the enzyme that catalyzes the breakdown of phosphatidylinositol into inositol trisphosphate and diacylglycerol), and numerous cytoskeletal proteins. However, it has not yet been established in most cases which type of enzyme phosphorylates which substrate protein under physiological conditions.

Many types of protein kinases undergo autophosphorylation

The autophosphorylation of most protein kinases is associated with an increase in kinase activity. In some instances, such as with the insulin receptor-associated protein tyrosine kinase, autophosphorylation is an obligatory step in the sequence of molecular events through which those kinases are activated. In other instances, such as with type II cAMP-dependent protein kinase, autophosphorylation may represent a positive feedback mechanism through which the kinases are activated to a greater extent, in this case by enhancing the rate of dissociation of the R and C subunits. In the case of Ca^{2+}/calmodulin-dependent protein kinase II, autophosphorylation causes the catalytic activity of the enzyme to become independent of Ca^{2+} and calmodulin. This means that the enzyme, activated originally in response to elevated levels of cellular Ca^{2+}, remains active after Ca^{2+} levels have returned to baseline. By this mechanism, neurotransmitters that activate Ca^{2+}/calmodulin-dependent protein kinase II can produce relatively long-lived alterations in neuronal function.

PROTEIN PHOSPHATASES

Much less is known about protein phosphatases than about protein kinases. This reflects the general inclination in biological research to concentrate on "turn-on" processes as opposed to "turn-off" processes. It also reflects the greater technical difficulties associated with the study of protein phosphatases. However, despite these difficulties, a systematic characterization of protein phosphatases in the nervous system has been initiated in recent years. This work has indicated that many first messengers elicit physiological responses in the brain through the regulation of protein phosphatases as well as protein kinases. Protein phosphatases, like protein kinases, are classified as protein serine/threonine phosphatases or protein tyrosine phosphatases, based on the amino acid residues they dephosphorylate.

The brain contains at least four types of protein serine/threonine phosphatases that differ in their physicochemical properties, substrate specificity, and regulation by cellular messengers

The enzymes, each of which has been cloned, are designated protein phosphatase 1, 2A, 2B, and 2C [13–15]. Several additional species of enzyme have been isolated by molecular cloning, although their biochemical and physiological properties are as yet unknown. Two mechanisms for the physiological regulation of protein serine/threonine phosphatases have been described. A phosphatase may be activated directly on binding a second messenger. This is analogous to the regulation of second-messenger-dependent protein kinases. Protein phosphatase 2B (calcineurin), which is activated upon binding Ca^{2+} and calmodulin, displays this type of regulation. Alternatively, a phosphatase may be regulated indirectly by second messengers through a class of proteins referred to as "protein phosphatase inhibitors." In this case, second messengers activate protein kinases, which then phosphorylate phosphatase inhibitors. Phosphorylation of the inhibitor proteins then regulates their phosphatase inhibitory activity, leading to changes in the state of phosphorylation of other cellular proteins. Protein phosphatase 1, which is inhibited by three known types of inhibitor proteins (see below), displays this type of regulation. Finally, recent evidence suggests that protein phosphatases may also be regulated by direct phosphorylation catalyzed by protein kinases; protein phosphatase 2A has been reported to be phosphorylated and inactivated by several protein tyrosine kinases [16].

The brain contains high levels of protein tyrosine phosphatase activity

The precise number and detailed characteristics of such enzymes, and the mechanisms through which extracellular or intracellular signals regulate their activity, remain to be determined [14–17]. In non-neural tissues, certain types of protein tyrosine phosphatase (e.g., an enzyme termed CD45) contain moieties that are structurally related to plasma membrane receptors. It is presumed that these enzymes are regulated directly by binding as yet unidentified ligands. This would be analogous to the regulation of receptor-associated protein tyrosine kinases by binding growth factors.

There are four known species of protein phosphatase inhibitor proteins

Inhibitor 1, inhibitor 2, and DARPP-32 (*dopamine-* and *cAMP-regulated phosphoprotein of 32 kDa*) all inhibit protein phosphatase 1, while G substrate inhibits protein phosphatase activity in cerebellar extracts [1,7]. Inhibitor 1 is a substrate for cAMP-dependent protein kinase; DARPP-32, a substrate for cAMP-dependent and cGMP-dependent protein kinases (as well as other protein kinases—see below); G substrate, for cGMP-dependent protein kinase; and inhibitor 2, for glycogen synthase kinase 3. The phosphorylation of inhibitor 1, DARPP-32, and G substrate leads to activation of their phosphatase inhibitory activity, whereas the phosphorylation of inhibitor 2 leads to inactivation of its phosphatase inhibitory activity. All four inhibitors are low-molecular-weight, acid-soluble, heat-stable proteins with an elongated tertiary structure; are phosphorylated on threonine residues; and exhibit some homology in their amino acid composition. These considerable similarities suggest that the proteins were derived, in the course of evolution, from some common precursor.

Inhibitors 1 and 2 appear to be widely distributed in various tissues, including brain, whereas DARPP-32 and G substrate how a much more restricted distribution. DARPP-32 (discussed below) is enriched in neurons that express D_1 dopamine receptors, and G substrate is localized to cerebellar Purkinje cells. Some neuronal cell types thus appear to contain unique species of phosphatase inhibitor proteins.

NEURONAL PHOSPHOPROTEINS

Many types of neuronal proteins are regulated by phosphorylation

As shown in Table 2, these include enzymes involved in neurotransmitter biosynthesis, proteins that regulate cellular levels of second messengers, autophosphorylated protein kinases, protein phosphatase inhibitors, proteins involved in the regulation of transcription and translation, cytoskeletal proteins, synaptic vesicle-associated proteins, neurotransmitter receptors, and ion channels. Regulation of these proteins by phosphorylation has been reviewed in detail [1,2,8,18,19].

Through phosphorylation of these many types of proteins, protein phosphorylation is involved in carrying out or regulating diverse processes in the nervous system. Protein phosphorylation affects neurotransmitter biosynthesis, axoplasmic transport, neurotransmitter release, generation of postsynaptic potentials, ion channel conductance, neuronal shape and motility, elaboration of dendritic and axonal processes, development and maintenance of differentiated properties of neurons, and gene expression.

Protein phosphorylation is an important mechanism of memory

The phosphorylation of any of the aforementioned types of proteins can be viewed as "molecular memory," a change in the structure and function of a protein that reflects perturbation of a specific signal transduction pathway in a specific neuronal cell type. Behavioral learning and memory may be established through the accumulation of many types of such phosphorylation events. Short-term memory may involve the phosphorylation of presynaptic or postsynaptic proteins in response to synaptic activity, which would result in transient facilitation or inhibition of synaptic transmission. Long-term memory may involve phosphorylation of proteins that play a part in the regulation of gene expression, which would result in more permanent modifications of synaptic transmission. For example, long-term potentiation (LTP), one of the most extensively studied electrophysiological models of memory, now seems to be initiated through short-term changes in Ca^{2+}-dependent protein phosphorylation and maintained by longer-term changes in gene expression. However, the specific pre- and postsynaptic proteins regulated in this manner are still unknown (see [8,20], Chap. 50).

Neuronal phosphoproteins exhibit great diversity in the number and types of amino acid residues phosphorylated

The complexity of intracellular regulation is underscored by the now well-established observation that many, perhaps even most, proteins are phosphorylated on more than one amino acid residue by more than one type of protein kinase. This is referred to as "multisite" phosphorylation. Depending on the protein, phosphorylation of different residues can lead to similar or opposite changes in that protein's function. In some cases, phosphorylation of one residue can influence the ability of other residues to undergo phosphorylation. The phosphorylation of neuronal proteins by more than one protein kinase can serve to integrate the activities of multiple intracellular pathways to achieve coordinated regulation of cell function.

Brain phosphoproteins reflect regional and subcellular diversity

Some neuronal phosphoproteins are present ubiquitously in all types of nerve cells,

TABLE 2. Classes of neuronal proteins regulated by phosphorylation[a]

Enzymes involved in neurotransmitter biosynthesis and degradation
    Tyrosine hydroxylase
    Tryptophan hydroxylase

Neurotransmitter receptors
    Nicotinic acetylcholine receptor
    β-Adrenergic receptor
    α_2-Adrenergic receptor
    $GABA_A$ receptor
    Muscarinic cholinergic receptor
    Glutamate receptor

Ion channels
    Voltage-dependent Na^+, K^+, Ca^{2+} channels
    Ligand-gated channels
    Ca^{2+}-dependent K^+ channels
    Nonspecific cation channel

Enzymes and other proteins involved in the regulation of second-messenger levels
    G proteins
    Phospholipases
    Adenylyl cyclase
    Guanylyl cyclase
    Phosphodiesterases
    IP_3 (inositol 1,4,5-trisphosphate) receptor

Protein kinases
    Autophosphorylated protein kinases (whereby most protein kinases phosphorylate themselves)
    Protein kinases phosphorylated by other protein kinases (many examples)

Protein phosphatase inhibitors
    DARPP-32
    Inhibitors 1 and 2

Cytoskeletal proteins involved in neuronal growth, shape, and motility
    Actin
    Tubulin
    Neurofilaments (and other intermediate filament proteins)
    Myosin
    Microtubule-associated proteins
    Actin-binding proteins

Synaptic vesicle proteins involved in neurotransmitter release
    Synapsins I and II
    Clathrin
    Synaptophysin
    Synaptobrevin

Transcription factors
    Cyclic AMP response element-binding proteins (CREB)
    Immediate-early gene products (such as Fos, Jun, and Zif)
    Steroid and thyroid hormone receptors

Other proteins involved in transcription or mRNA translation
    RNA polymerase
    Topoisomerase
    Histones and nonhistone nuclear proteins
    Ribosomal protein S6
    eIF (eukaryotic initiation factor)
    eEF (eukaryotic elongation factor)
    Other ribosomal proteins

Miscellaneous
    Myelin basic protein
    Rhodopsin
    Neural cell adhesion molecules
    Myristoylated, alanine-rich C kinase substrate of 87 kDa (MARKS)
    Growth-associated protein of 43 kDa (GAP, aka B-50)

[a] This list is not intended to be comprehensive, but is intended instead to indicate the wide variety of neuronal proteins regulated by phosphorylation. Some of the proteins are specific to neurons, but most are present in cell types in addition to neurons and are included because among their multiple functions in the nervous system is the regulation of neuron-specific phenomena. Not included are the many phosphoproteins present in diverse tissues (including brain) that play a role in generalized cellular processes, such as intermediary metabolism, and that do not appear to play a role in neuron-specific phenomena.

whereas others are expressed in specific subsets of neurons. The specific localization of phosphoproteins to certain neuronal cell types has made it possible to use antisera or nucleotide probes against these proteins or their messenger RNAs (mRNAs) to study anatomical, developmental, and pathophysiological aspects of the neurons in which the proteins occur. An example of this is discussed in more detail below (see DARPP-32).

The phosphorylation of a protein can influence its functional activity in several ways

For many proteins, a change in charge and conformation, due to the addition of phosphate groups, results in alterations in their intrinsic functional activity. For example, the catalytic activity of an enzyme can be switched on or off, or an ion channel can be opened or closed. For many other proteins, phosphorylation-induced changes in charge and conformation result in alterations in the affinity of the proteins for other molecules. For example, phosphorylation alters the affinity of numerous enzymes for their cofactors and end-product inhibitors, phosphorylation of receptors can alter their affinity for G proteins, and phosphorylation of some nuclear transcription factors alters their DNA binding properties.

Phosphorylation can represent the primary mechanism through which a protein is regulated physiologically or it can exert a modulatory influence on the function of a protein. This point is illustrated by consideration of ion channels. Phosphorylation of some ion channels represents the primary mechanism through which the channels are gated, i.e., opened or closed. This is the case, e.g., for a nonspecific cation channel in noradrenergic neurons of the locus coeruleus, which is activated by phosphorylation of the channel (or a closely associated protein) by cAMP-dependent protein kinase. In contrast, phosphorylation of most other channels, e.g., voltage-gated Na^+, K^+, and Ca^{2+} channels, plays a modulatory role by altering

the sensitivity of the channels to open or close in response to a change in membrane potential.

To illustrate some of the roles played by protein phosphorylation in the regulation of nervous system function, six well-characterized neuronal phosphoproteins are discussed in detail.

Tyrosine hydroxylase is the rate-limiting enzyme in the biosynthesis of the catecholamine neurotransmitters dopamine, norepinephrine, and epinephrine

A number of extracellular signals have been shown to stimulate catecholamine biosynthesis *in vivo*, and this effect appears to be mediated through increases in the catalytic activity of tyrosine hydroxylase (see also Chap. 12). It now appears that such changes in the catalytic activity of tyrosine hydroxylase are achieved through cAMP-dependent and Ca^{2+}-dependent phosphorylation of the enzyme [1,21].

Tyrosine hydroxylase is a tetramer of identical 60-kDa subunits. The enzyme is a substrate for several protein kinases: cAMP-dependent protein kinase, Ca^{2+}/calmodulin-dependent protein kinase II, and protein kinase C. One site (serine 40) of tyrosine hydroxylase is phosphorylated by all three kinases, whereas a second site (serine 19) is phosphorylated only by Ca^{2+}/calmodulin-dependent protein kinase II. Phosphorylation of either site by Ca^{2+}/calmodulin-dependent protein kinase II requires the presence of an "activator" protein, which has been cloned. Phosphorylation appears to increase the catalytic activity of tyrosine hydroxylase by increasing the V_{max} of the enzyme and the affinity of the enzyme for its pterin cofactor and by decreasing the affinity of the enzyme for its end-product inhibitor. Tyrosine hydroxylase also contains additional serine residues that are phosphorylated by other protein kinases. For example, the enzyme is phosphorylated on serine 31 by MAP kinase, which is also thought to increase the catalytic activity of the enzyme [9].

Regulation of Phosphorylation

The state of phosphorylation of tyrosine hydroxylase is regulated by stimuli that increase Ca^{2+} or cAMP levels in neurons, including nerve impulses and certain neurotransmitters in well-defined regions of the nervous system, in the adrenal medulla, and in cultured pheochromocytoma cells. In addition, tyrosine hydroxylase phosphorylation is stimulated by nerve growth factor in certain cell types, possibly through activation of MAP kinase. These changes in the phosphorylation of tyrosine hydroxylase have been shown to correlate with changes in the catalytic activity of the enzyme and in the rate of catecholamine biosynthesis.

Several key questions remain with regard to the regulation of tyrosine hydroxylase by phosphorylation. What is the precise effect of the phosphorylation of each specific serine residue on the catalytic activity of the enzyme? How does the phosphorylation of multiple residues affect enzyme activity? Does the phosphorylation of one residue affect the ability of the others to be phosphorylated? Tyrosine hydroxylase provides a striking example of how multiple intracellular messengers and protein kinases converge functionally through the phosphorylation of a single substrate protein. Phosphorylation of tyrosine hydroxylase by cAMP-dependent and Ca^{2+}-dependent protein kinases and by MAP kinase enables a catecholaminergic cell to adjust its rate of neurotransmitter biosynthesis to a host of external stimuli and to changing physiological needs.

Rhodopsin mediates the effects of light on retinal rod cells

Rhodopsin represents 90 percent of the integral protein of rod outer segment membranes. It has a molecular mass of approximately 40 kDa and is composed of the protein opsin and the prosthetic group 11-*cis*-retinal. Light induces the isomerization of 11-*cis*-retinal to all-*trans*-retinal, which in turn leads to a conformational change in rhodopsin. This change then initiates a biochemical cascade that leads to a transient hyperpolarization of rod outer segments (see Chapter 7). Rhodopsin is phosphorylated by rhodopsin kinase, which plays an integral role in the process by which rod outer segments become adapted, or desensitized, to light [22].

Rhodopsin kinase is a predominantly cytosolic second-messenger-independent protein kinase of 68 kDa. It phosphorylates light-adapted, but not dark-adapted, rhodopsin; the conformational change induced in rhodopsin by light renders it an effective substrate for rhodopsin kinase. Neither form of rhodopsin is phosphorylated by any known second-messenger-dependent protein kinase. Rhodopsin kinase phosphorylates rhodopsin on multiple serine and threonine residues, which are localized in a small region of the C-terminal portion of the protein, the part of the rhodopsin molecule that is exposed to the cytosol of rod outer segments. The state of phosphorylation of rhodopsin is regulated *in vivo* by changes in environmental lighting.

To understand the role of rhodopsin phosphorylation in the regulation of rod outer segment function, it is necessary to review the role of rhodopsin itself. Light leads to hyperpolarization of rod outer segment membranes via a molecular cascade (see also Chap. 7). Light induces a conformational change in rhodopsin such that light-adapted rhodopsin, referred to as R*, binds to a complex consisting of transducin (a GTP-binding membrane protein) and GDP. This leads to an exchange of GTP for GDP, which in turn causes dissociation of R* and the β- and γ-subunits of transducin from the complex. The resulting complex of GTP and the α-subunit of transducin then activates the enzyme cGMP-phosphodiesterase, which leads to decreases in cGMP levels and consequently to hyperpolarization of rod outer segments. R* acts catalytically in this cascade;

once released from the R*:transducin:GTP complex, it is able to activate many additional transducin:GDP complexes. However, it is known that rod outer segments become adapted to light after very brief periods of time. This means that mechanisms exist to reverse rapidly the ability of R* to activate transducin:GDP complexes. The phosphorylation of rhodopsin represents such a mechanism [22].

Phospho-R*, like dephospho-R*, is able to activate the transducin/phosphodiesterase cascade. An additional protein, referred to as arrestin, a 48-kDa protein present at high levels in rod outer segment cytosol, plays a necessary role in quenching phospho-R*. Arrestin binds with high affinity to phospho-R* but not to dephospho-R* or to dark-adapted rhodopsin, and the formation of arrestin:phospho-R* complexes makes phospho-R* unavailable for any further activation of the transducin/phosphodiesterase system. The kinetics of the various steps in this pathway are such that R* activates numerous molecules of transducin before undergoing phosphorylation by rhodopsin kinase and sequestration by arrestin.

Desensitization of the β-Adrenergic Receptor

Activation and desensitization of β-adrenergic receptor-stimulated adenylyl cyclase are analogous to the regulation of rod outer segment phosphodiesterase by rhodopsin [23,24] (Fig. 4). Thus, the binding of a β-

A

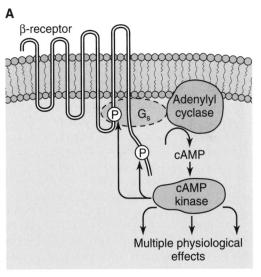

B

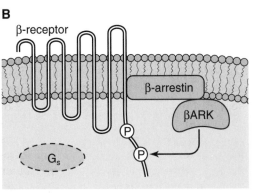

FIG. 4.   Scheme illustrating desensitization of the β-adrenergic receptor mediated by receptor phosphorylation. **A:** Activation of the β-adrenergic receptor by its ligand results, via coupling with G_s, in stimulation of adenylyl cyclase, increased cellular levels of cAMP, and stimulation of cAMP-dependent protein kinase, which mediates the physiological effects of β-receptor activation through the phosphorylation of numerous cellular proteins. The protein kinase also phosphorylates several serine residues in the third cytoplasmic and C-terminus domains of the receptor. As a mechanism of negative feedback, such phosphorylation decreases the ability of the ligand to stimulate adenylyl cyclase, although the molecular mechanism for this desensitization in receptor function remains unknown. **B:** Activation of the β-adrenergic receptor by its ligand results in a conformational change in the receptor, which renders it an effective substrate for β-adrenergic receptor kinase (βARK). βARK phosphorylates the receptor at several serine/threonine residues in its C-terminal domain. Such phosphorylation leads to the functional "uncoupling" of the receptor from G_s, thereby resulting in desensitization. This uncoupling does not occur as a result of receptor phosphorylation per se, but rather requires the action of an additional protein, termed β-arrestin, which appears to interact preferentially with the phosphorylated receptor to prevent its activation of G_s.

adrenergic agonist (analogous to light) to its receptor (analogous to rhodopsin) leads, through an interaction with a GTP-binding protein designated G_s (analogous to transducin), to the activation of adenylyl cyclase (analogous to phosphodiesterase). Occupation of the β-adrenergic receptor by agonist also leads to desensitization of the receptor; binding of the agonist to the receptor induces a conformational change in the receptor that renders it an effective substrate for β-adrenergic receptor kinase (or βARK), a second-messenger-independent protein kinase (analogous to rhodopsin kinase). Phosphorylation of the receptor prevents its association with G_s and consequently leads to decreased activation of adenylyl cyclase. An additional protein, β-arrestin (analogous to arrestin in rod outer segments), is involved in this uncoupling process.

In addition to the functional similarities between the rhodopsin and β-adrenergic receptor systems, there are also structural homologies. Rhodopsin and the β-adrenergic receptor show considerable similarities in their primary and tertiary structures, and they belong to the family of G protein-coupled receptors that contain seven transmembrane domains (see Chap. 10). Transducin and G_s, which belong to a family of heterotrimeric GTP-binding proteins, consist of virtually identical β- and γ-subunits and similar α-subunits, which can substitute for each other in the activation of phosphodiesterase and adenylyl cyclase (see Chap. 21). Finally, rhodopsin kinase and βARK are homologous proteins, as are arrestin and β-arrestin. The structural and functional similarities of these two systems are consistent with the possibility that analogous systems may be widespread in the nervous system. Increasing evidence now suggests that many members of the G protein-coupled receptor family are phosphorylated by receptor-associated protein kinases and that such phosphorylation mediates desensitization of these receptors (see [25]).

The nicotinic acetylcholine receptor mediates synaptic transmission at nicotinic cholinergic synapses

It has been known for many years that prolonged exposure of the nicotinic receptor to acetylcholine leads to a decrease in the sensitivity of the receptor to acetylcholine, a process referred to as desensitization (see Chap. 11). Phosphorylation of the receptor by cAMP-dependent protein kinase, protein kinase C, or protein tyrosine kinase enhances the rate at which desensitization of the receptor develops in response to acetylcholine [19].

The nicotinic acetylcholine receptor is a 250-kDa protein complex that consists of four types of subunits (α, β, γ, and δ) with a stoichiometry of $\alpha_2\beta\gamma\delta$ (see Chap. 11). The various subunits of the receptor are effective substrates for three distinct protein kinases: (a) cAMP-dependent protein kinase phosphorylates single serine residues in the γ- and δ-subunits; (b) protein kinase C phosphorylates single serine residues in the α- and δ-subunits; and (c) protein tyrosine kinase phosphorylates single tyrosine residues in the β-, γ-, and δ-subunits. The serine residues phosphorylated by the cAMP-dependent and Ca^{2+}-dependent enzymes on the δ-subunit appear to represent distinct sites.

Receptor Desensitization Mediated by Protein Phosphorylation

Results of studies involving reconstitution of purified acetylcholine receptor into phospholipid vesicles have provided direct evidence for a functional role of receptor phosphorylation. Purified receptor phosphorylated by cAMP-dependent protein kinase prior to reconstitution was shown to desensitize in the presence of acetylcholine at a rate seven to eight times faster than that of dephosphorylated receptor, as measured by quench-flow kinetic techniques. Other properties of the receptor, namely, the affinity of the receptor for acetylcholine, the rate of ion transport through activated receptor channels, and the mean time that activated receptor channels remain open, were found to be unaffected by receptor phosphorylation. Consistent with these observations *in vitro* was the demonstration that forskolin, which increases cellular cAMP levels by activating the enzyme adenylyl cyclase, dramatically increased the rate of desensitization of the nicotinic receptor in intact muscle preparations. It now appears that cAMP-dependent phosphorylation of the receptor in skeletal muscle is stimulated by calcitonin gene-related peptide (CGRP), which is colocalized with acetylcholine in motor nerve terminals (Fig. 5). Since greater frequency of stimulation is required to release CGRP than acetylcholine from motor nerve endings, CGRP-mediated desensitization of the receptor may serve a negative feedback role on the function of the synapse during periods of intense stimulation.

Phorbol esters, agents that specifically activate protein kinase C, also increase the rate of desensitization of the nicotinic receptor in cultured myotubes. This suggests that phosphorylation of the receptor by protein kinase C has an effect on receptor function similar to that of phosphorylation by cAMP-dependent protein kinase. This is interesting in light of the fact that the serine residues in the δ-subunit that are phosphorylated by the two kinases appear to be located 16 amino acid residues from each other. Furthermore, the tyrosine residue that appears to be phosphorylated in this subunit is located between these two sites, consistent with the fact that phosphorylation of the receptor by protein tyrosine kinase also accelerates receptor desensitization.

Further work is needed to elucidate the precise molecular mechanisms through which phosphorylation of the receptor by each protein kinase results in alterations in the kinetics of receptor desensitization. It will also be important to ascertain whether phosphorylation of the receptor by one kinase alters the ability of the other kinases to phosphorylate and regulate its properties. Moreover, the first messengers that regulate receptor desensitization, in muscle as well as

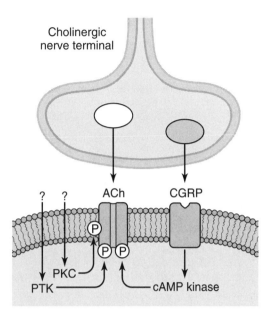

FIG. 5. Scheme illustrating desensitization of the nicotinic cholinergic receptor mediated by receptor phosphorylation. Acetylcholine released from cholinergic nerve terminals activates the nicotinic cholinergic receptor. Calcitonin gene-related peptide (CGRP), which is colocalized with acetylcholine in some cholinergic nerve terminals, is also released under conditions of intense nerve stimulation. CGRP activates its receptor, which is coupled via Gₛ to the activation of adenylyl cyclase and of cAMP-dependent protein kinase. The protein kinase then phosphorylates single serine residues in the γ- and δ-subunits of the nicotinic receptor, which results in desensitization of receptor function. The receptor is also known to be phosphorylated at distinct residues by protein kinase C and by a protein tyrosine kinase, which also results in receptor desensitization. The first messengers that stimulate these pathways of desensitization have not been established. There is some evidence that acetylcholine, via depolarization-induced Ca²⁺ entry, activates the protein kinase C pathway.

in brain, via the activation of cAMP-dependent protein kinase, protein kinase C, or protein tyrosine kinase need to be identified.

The synapsins, originally discovered as phosphoproteins in particulate synaptic fractions of brain, regulate the release of neurotransmitter from nerve endings

The synapsins represent a family of four synaptic vesicle-associated phosphoproteins

[1,26,27]. They are expressed primarily in neurons, where they are associated with small synaptic vesicles in virtually all nerve terminals throughout the central and peripheral nervous systems. Synapsins Ia and Ib (referred to collectively as synapsin I) are derived from a single gene by alternative splicing and exhibit M_r values of 86,000 and 80,000, respectively. Synapsins IIa and IIb, also derived from a single gene, exhibit M_r values of 74,000 and 55,000, respectively.

Regulation of Neurotransmitter Release by Synapsin I Phosphorylation

Synapsin I possesses a head or globular domain that is phosphorylated on one serine residue (site 1) by cAMP-dependent protein kinase and by Ca^{2+}/calmodulin-dependent protein kinase I. It also possesses a tail or filamentous domain that is phosphorylated on two other serine residues (sites 2 and 3) by Ca^{2+}/calmodulin-dependent protein kinase II. Phosphorylation of synapsin I occurs in the intact nervous system in response to nerve impulses and to a variety of neurotransmitters acting at presynaptic receptors (Fig. 6). It appears that dephosphosynapsin I binds to both vesicles and actin. Synapsin I thereby "cages" the vesicles; i.e., it inhibits their availability for release.

Phosphorylation of synapsin I on its tail domain by Ca^{2+}/calmodulin-dependent protein kinase II decreases its affinity for synaptic vesicles, and the subsequent dissociation of the protein from the vesicles "decages" them and readies them for neurotransmitter release without affecting the release mechanism per se. This scheme is supported by a series of experiments with the squid giant synapse and the goldfish Mauthner cell, in which the injection of dephosphosynapsin I, but not phosphosynapsin I, into nerve terminals inhibits spontaneous and impulse-evoked neurotransmitter release, whereas injection of Ca^{2+}/calmodulin-dependent protein kinase II facilitates neurotransmitter release. Similar effects of synapsin I and of the protein kinase are seen in studies with

permeabilized rat brain synaptosomes, indicating that analogous mechanisms operate in mammalian neurons. Phosphorylation of synapsin I on its tail domain also decreases its affinity for actin; this may contribute further to the phosphorylation-induced decaging of vesicles within the nerve terminal and to the subsequent facilitation of neurotransmitter release [28].

The Synapsins May Also Play a Role in the Regulation of Synaptogenesis

The introduction of synapsin I into embryonic spinal neurons in cultured *Xenopus* embryos has been shown to promote the maturation of synapses [29]. A similar effect has been demonstrated for synapsin II when transfected into cultured neuroblastoma cells. This action of the synapsins is associated with the appearance of a number of other synaptic vesicle-associated proteins. The mechanisms by which the synapsins influence the expression of other proteins and promote the differentiation of synaptic nerve terminals have not yet been established. Nevertheless, these results indicate that in addition to regulating neurotransmitter release at fully functional synapses, the synapsins may also participate in the functional maturation of synapses during development and possibly even synaptogenesis in the adult nervous system.

DARPP-32, originally discovered as a phosphoprotein in soluble fractions of brain, is a protein phosphatase inhibitor enriched in dopaminoceptive neurons

DARPP-32 was discovered during a study of the regional distribution of neuronal phosphoproteins in rat brain. It is one of several substrates for cAMP-dependent protein kinase that are highly concentrated in the basal ganglia [7]. DARPP-32 has an apparent mass of 32 kDa by sodium dodecyl sulfate polyacrylamide gel electrophoresis (SDS-PAGE), but its actual molecular mass based on sequencing data is ~23 kDa. It is phos-

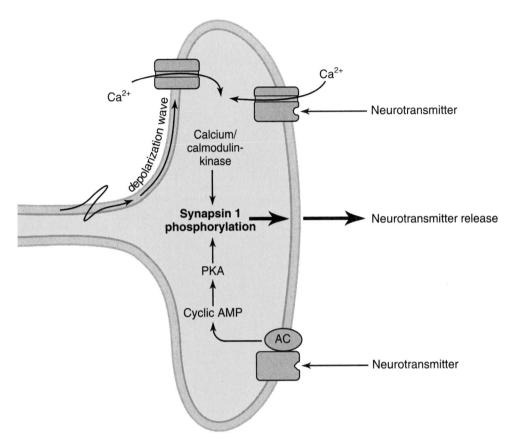

FIG. 6. Schematic diagram of the regulation of synapsin I phosphorylation in nerve terminals. Nerve impulses stimulate synapsin I phosphorylation through depolarization of the nerve terminal plasma membrane, an increase in free Ca^{2+} levels, and the activation of Ca^{2+}/calmodulin-dependent protein kinases. Phosphorylation of synapsin I then modulates neurotransmitter release. Phosphorylation of synapsin I appears to be involved in various Ca^{2+}-dependent mechanisms of regulation of neurotransmitter release, including the phenomenon of posttetanic potentiation. Some neurotransmitters stimulate (or inhibit) synapsin I phosphorylation by binding to presynaptic receptors and thereby altering Ca^{2+} levels and Ca^{2+}/calmodulin-dependent protein kinase activity. Such phosphorylation (or dephosphorylation) of synapsin I may be involved in Ca^{2+}-dependent mechanisms through which certain neurotransmitters acting on presynaptic receptors of axon terminals regulate neurotransmitter release. Other neurotransmitters stimulate (or inhibit) synapsin I phosphorylation by binding to other presynaptic receptors and thereby altering adenylyl cyclase (AC) activity, leading to changes in cAMP levels and cAMP-dependent protein kinase (PKA) activity. Such phosphorylation (or dephosphorylation) of synapsin I may be involved in cAMP-dependent mechanisms through which neurotransmitters acting on receptors of axon terminals regulate neurotransmitter release. Nerve impulse conduction would be expected to stimulate synapsin I phosphorylation in all nerve terminals throughout the nervous system. In contrast, most neurotransmitters would be expected to stimulate synapsin I phosphorylation only in certain nerve terminals. (Modified from Nestler, E. J., and Greengard, P. *Prog. Brain Res.* 60:323–340, 1986.)

phorylated *in vitro* on a single threonine residue by cAMP-dependent or by cGMP-dependent protein kinase. Phospho-DARPP-32, but not the dephospho form of the protein, inhibits protein phosphatase 1 with a K_i of about 1 nM. In contrast, it is not an effective inhibitor of protein phosphatases 2A, 2B, or 2C. DARPP-32 is also phosphorylated on serine residues by casein kinases I and II; such phosphorylation influences the ability of the threonine residue to be phosphorylated by cAMP-dependent protein kinase.

DARPP-32 is highly enriched in neurons in the brain that possess D_1 dopamine receptors, and it appears to be present in all such neurons. It is also present in renal tubular epithelial cells, parathyroid hormone-producing cells in the parathyroid gland, and tanocytes, all of which are known to express the D_1 receptor. However, DARPP-32 has been found in one cell type that does not express D_1 dopamine receptors, namely, choroid epithelial cells.

Regulation of DARPP-32 Phosphorylation and Its Functional Role

The state of phosphorylation of DARPP-32 is regulated in D_1 dopaminoceptive neurons by the neurotransmitter dopamine, which acts through increases in cAMP levels and activation of cAMP-dependent protein kinase (see Chap. 21). DARPP-32 phosphorylation can also be stimulated in these and other cell types by other types of hormones and neurotransmitters that activate pathways in which levels of cAMP or cGMP are changed. Changes in the phosphorylation state of DARPP-32, through the activation of its phosphatase inhibitory activity, indirectly influence the phosphorylation state of other proteins, and thereby mediate some of the effects of dopamine and other first messengers on cell function.

The full spectrum of proteins regulated in this way by DARPP-32 phosphorylation has not yet been identified, although the electrogenic ion pump Na,K-ATPase represents one target protein [30]. Regulation of this protein by DARPP-32 provides a mechanism through which alteration in DARPP-32 phosphorylation can lead to changes in the electrical excitability of neurons and in ion transport properties of nonexcitable peripheral tissues.

Several types of physiological actions for DARPP-32 can be envisioned. First, DARPP-32, phosphorylated and activated in response to dopamine (or another first messenger) and cAMP (or cGMP), can act as a positive feedback signal for these messengers by reducing the dephosphorylation of other substrates for the same protein kinase. Second, DARPP-32 can reduce dephosphoryla-

tion of substrate proteins for other protein kinases and, in so doing, can mediate the effects of first- and second-messenger systems on one another. Third, DARPP-32, through its phosphorylation by cAMP (or cGMP)-dependent protein kinase and its dephosphorylation by Ca^{2+}/calmodulin-dependent protein phosphatase (calcineurin), can integrate certain physiological effects of first messengers that influence the cAMP and Ca^{2+} systems.

An example of this latter mechanism is illustrated in Fig. 7. In this scheme, extra-

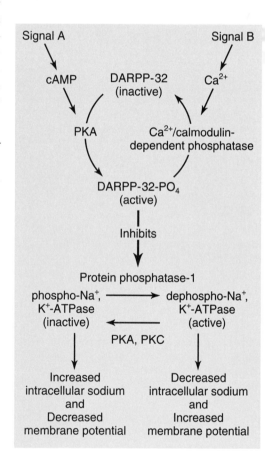

FIG. 7. Scheme illustrating hypothetical role of DARPP-32 in mediating effects of first messengers with opposing physiological actions in regulation of Na,K-ATPase activity. This scheme, involving bidirectional control of Na,K-ATPase activity, may be applicable to various tissues, including brain and kidney. (PKA) cAMP-dependent protein kinase; (PKC) protein kinase C. (From Pessin et al. [30].)

cellular signals that activate the cAMP pathway would phosphorylate and activate DARPP-32, whereas extracellular signals that activate the Ca^{2+} pathway would dephosphorylate and inactivate DARPP-32. Changes in DARPP-32 activity would then lead to altered activity of protein phosphatase 1 and, as a result, to altered dephosphorylation of Na,K-ATPase, a prominent substrate for this enzyme. Changes in the phosphorylation state of the Na,K-ATPase would result in altered sodium transport across the cell membrane and, in excitable cells, to an altered membrane potential. Considerable evidence has been obtained to support this scheme in several cell types [30]. Moreover, the scheme can account for some of the antagonist actions of dopamine (acting through cAMP) and glutamate (acting through Ca^{2+}) on neuronal excitability in striatal neurons.

Anatomical Uses of DARPP-32

DARPP-32 is one of several phosphoproteins that are enriched in the basal ganglia; two of the others are designated ARPP-21 and ARPP-19. The restricted distribution of these proteins makes them useful tools for the identification and ultrastructural study of specific subclasses of neurons in the nervous system and for the morphological analysis of the dendritic and axonal projections of these cells. For example, these proteins have been used to identify the specific cellular targets of psychotropic drugs (including antipsychotic drugs and cocaine) on the basal ganglia and to study the pathophysiology of neuropsychiatric disorders that involve the basal ganglia, such as Huntington's disease, Tourette's syndrome, and tardive dyskinesia (see also Chap. 44).

CREB is a prototypical example of a transcription factor whose physiological activity is regulated by phosphorylation

CREB (*c*yclic AMP *r*esponse *e*lement-*b*inding protein) is one of a family of proteins that mediate effects of cAMP on gene expression [8,31]. CREB binds to a specific sequence of DNA (called a cAMP response element, or CRE) in the promoter (regulatory) regions of genes and thereby increases or decreases the rate at which those genes are transcribed.

The details of the mechanism by which CREB influences gene expression have not been established, but the prevailing view is that in the basal (or unstimulated) state, CREB is bound to its CRE but does not alter transcriptional rates. Stimulation of a cell by a first messenger that increases cAMP levels leads to activation of cAMP-dependent protein kinase and to the translocation of free catalytic subunit of the protein kinase into the nucleus where it phosphorylates CREB on a single residue (serine 133). Such phosphorylation then activates transcriptional activity, presumably by enabling CREB to interact with and facilitate the activity of the RNA polymerase II complex, which mediates the initiation of transcription. Stimulation of a cell by first messengers that increase cellular Ca^{2+} levels similarly activates CREB, possibly through the activation of Ca^{2+}/calmodulin-dependent protein kinases I and/or II and the phosphorylation of serine 133 or a nearby residue. The regulation of CREB by phosphorylation is illustrated in Fig. 8.

The number of neural genes known to contain CREs is growing as more and more genes are cloned. Prominent examples are tyrosine hydroxylase, β_2-adrenergic receptors, c-*fos*, proenkephalin, somatostatin, and vasoactive intestinal polypeptide (VIP). The expression of these genes is thought to be regulated in part at their CREs by the phosphorylation of CREB or a CREB-like protein.

Consideration of CREB highlights the view that among the many cellular processes regulated by protein phosphorylation is gene transcription. This view is further underscored by the knowledge that virtually all classes of transcription factors undergo phosphorylation by cAMP-dependent, Ca^{2+}-dependent, and/or other protein kinases. Even transcription factors, the effects of which are regulated primarily through alterations in their own transcription (e.g., fos and jun and

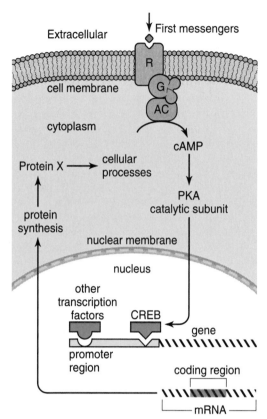

FIG. 8. Schematic illustration of the role played by CREB phosphorylation in mediating some of the actions of cAMP, and those first messengers that act through cAMP, on gene transcription. Some first messengers increase or decrease cellular levels of cAMP through receptor (R) interactions with specific G proteins (G) and the activation or inhibition of adenylyl cyclase (AC). Increased or decreased levels of cAMP lead to corresponding changes in cAMP-dependent protein kinase (PKA) activity by increasing or decreasing, respectively, levels of free catalytic subunit of the enzyme. Some free catalytic subunit translocates to the nucleus where it phosphorylates CREB already bound to CREs in specific genes. The phosphorylation of CREB activates its transcriptional activity and leads to changes in the rate at which those genes are transcribed.

other immediate early gene transcription factors), are influenced by phosphorylation. For example, c-*fos* is heavily phosphorylated on a series of serine residues in the C-terminal region of the protein by several types of protein kinase. The likely functional importance of these phosphorylation sites is indicated by the fact that the difference between c-fos (the normal cellular form of the protein) and v-fos (the viral oncogene product) is a frame-shift mutation in the v-Fos protein, which obliterates the phosphorylated serine residues. It is possible that the loss of these phosphorylation sites removes a mechanism by which the cell can regulate the protein, thereby leading to cellular transformation.

CELLULAR MESSENGER SYSTEMS INTERACT AT VARIOUS LEVELS OF PROTEIN PHOSPHORYLATION PATHWAYS

cAMP, cGMP, Ca^{2+}, and the numerous extracellular signals that act through these second messengers are known to regulate many of the same physiological processes

The effects of these signals may be synergistic or antagonistic. Furthermore, many other cellular messengers, e.g., second-messenger-independent protein serine/threonine kinases and protein tyrosine kinases and phosphatases, also influence the same processes. Thus, rather than being generated through a single molecular pathway, most physiological responses represent the complex product of the coordinated actions of multiple cellular messengers involving multiple molecular pathways.

It is now apparent that such pathways frequently converge at various levels of protein phosphorylation systems. The cAMP, cGMP, and Ca^{2+} second-messenger systems are known to interact with each other and with other prominent cellular messenger systems. These interactions have been shown to occur at multiple levels of protein phosphorylation pathways: at the level of the intracellular concentration of second messengers, at the level of protein kinases, at the level of protein phosphatases, at the level of the same substrate protein, and at the level of different substrate proteins. These interactions, too numerous to elaborate here, have been reviewed elsewhere; some illustrative examples are presented below [1,8].

Cellular Messengers

As examples of interactions at the level of the concentration of cellular messengers, adenylyl cyclase and guanylyl cyclase are each regulated by Ca^{2+}. cAMP and cGMP appear to alter cellular Ca^{2+} levels by regulating the flux of Ca^{2+} into neurons and the sequestration of Ca^{2+} by intracellular organelles. G proteins, which play a role in generating each of these second messengers (see Chap. 21), are also phosphorylated and regulated by cAMP-dependent and Ca^{2+}-dependent protein kinases. In addition, prostaglandins regulate cellular levels of cAMP and cGMP and influence the activity of Ca^{2+}/calmodulin-dependent protein kinase II. Diacylglycerol, derived from the breakdown of phosphatidylinositol, allows the activation of certain forms of protein kinase C to occur at lower Ca^{2+} concentrations. In addition, cyclic nucleotides and Ca^{2+} have been reported to regulate the generation of these lipid messengers, in part through the phosphorylation of phospholipases, which are also substrates for protein tyrosine kinases.

Protein Kinases

As examples of interactions at the level of protein kinases, cAMP-dependent protein kinase phosphorylates certain Ca^{2+}/calmodulin-dependent protein kinases and thereby alters their catalytic activity, and protein tyrosine kinases are regulated by both cAMP-dependent protein kinase and protein kinase C. Other examples of protein kinases phosphorylating each other are given earlier in this chapter under the discussion of MAP kinases.

Protein Phosphatases

As an example of interactions at the level of protein phosphatases, calcineurin, a Ca^{2+}/calmodulin-dependent protein phosphatase, dephosphorylates and inactivates DARPP-32, an inhibitor of protein phosphatase 1.

Substrate Proteins

As examples of interactions at the level of the same substrate protein, many phosphoproteins are phosphorylated at the same or at distinct residues by more than one protein kinase, as discussed above for tyrosine hydroxylase, the nicotinic acetylcholine receptor, synapsin I, DARPP-32, and CREB. Indeed, multisite phosphorylation of proteins appears to be the rule rather than the exception. This type of interaction includes numerous substrates, such as the nicotinic acetylcholine receptor, that are phosphorylated on serine residues by second-messenger-dependent protein kinases and on tyrosine residues by protein tyrosine kinases. Finally, interactions can occur at the level of different substrate proteins, with distinct substrates for cAMP-dependent, Ca^{2+}-dependent, and protein tyrosine kinases each regulating the same physiological process.

The extraordinary complexity in biological systems underscores the difficulty in determining the precise molecular basis of a given physiological process. The central role of protein phosphorylation as a regulatory mechanism that mediates the actions of many individual cellular messengers and of interactions among them imbues the study of protein phosphorylation with a unique potential: to provide an experimental framework within which to unravel the layers of molecular steps that underlie and regulate cell function.

PROTEIN PHOSPHORYLATION MECHANISMS IN DISEASE

The study of protein phosphorylation has helped clarify the mechanisms involved in the causes and manifestation of disorders of the nervous system. Two illustrative examples are given here: Alzheimer's disease and opiate addiction.

Abnormal phosphorylation of specific neural proteins may contribute to the development of Alzheimer's disease

Alzheimer's disease is a serious, dementing illness of enormous medical and societal importance. It involves the degeneration of specific types of neurons in the brain. An invariable feature of Alzheimer's disease is the appearance of amyloid plaques. These plaques contain the β/A4 amyloid protein and there is evidence suggesting that the accumulation of β/A4 contributes to neuronal degeneration and that mutations in the gene that codes for this protein are involved in a small number of cases of familial Alzheimer's disease.

β/A4 is derived from amyloid precursor protein (APP) through proteolytic processing. In normal cells, APP is processed predominantly into fragments that are not associated with disease states. It is not yet known why APP is cleaved anomalously to yield β/A4 to a greater extent in Alzheimer's disease. However, increasing evidence indicates that signal transduction pathways involving protein phosphorylation are potent regulators of APP cleavage, and can alter the rates of cleavage both at normal sites and at sites yielding putative amyloidogenic fragments [32].

The role of protein kinase C in this process has received the most attention. Activators of protein kinase C, or inhibitors of protein phosphatase 1 (e.g., okakaic acid), dramatically stimulate APP proteolysis, whereas protein kinase C inhibitors diminish cleavage of the protein. The finding that protein kinase C regulates APP processing raises the possibility that agents that regulate this protein kinase (or specific protein phosphatases) might prove to be useful in the clinical management of Alzheimer's disease. Further support for the potential clinical utility of drugs that influence protein kinases or protein phosphatases in Alzheimer's disease is the evidence that aberrant phosphorylation mechanisms (i.e., excessive phosphorylation of neurofilament and MAPs) may contribute

to the formation of neurofibrillary tangles, another component of Alzheimer structural pathology.

Up-regulation of the cAMP pathway is one mechanism underlying opiate addiction

The mechanisms by which opiates induce tolerance, dependence, and withdrawal in specific target neurons have been a major focus of research for many years. The inability to account for prominent aspects of opiate addiction on the basis of alterations to endogenous opioid peptides, or in opiate receptors, has shifted attention to postreceptor mechanisms [33].

The noradrenergic neurons of the locus coeruleus have provided a useful model system for the study of opiate addiction. Acutely, opiates inhibit these neurons, in part by inhibiting the synthesis of cAMP through inhibition of adenylyl cyclase. These neurons become tolerant to opiates (their firing rates return to normal levels with continued exposure to the drug), and they become dependent on opiates (their firing rates increase far above control levels upon removal of the drug). These changes in the electrical excitability of locus coeruleus neurons mediate many of the physical signs and symptoms associated with opiate withdrawal syndromes.

Increasing evidence indicates that a chronic opiate-induced up-regulation of the cAMP pathway (manifested by increased levels of adenylyl cyclase, cAMP-dependent protein kinase, and several phosphoprotein substrates for the protein kinase) contributes to opiate tolerance, dependence, and withdrawal exhibited by locus coeruleus neurons [33]. This up-regulated cAMP pathway can be viewed as a homeostatic response of the neurons to persistent inhibition of the cells by opiates. In the chronic opiate-treated state, the up-regulated cAMP pathway helps return neuronal firing rates to control levels (i.e., tolerance). Upon abrupt removal of the opiate, e.g., following the administration of an opiate receptor antagonist, the up-regulated cAMP system, now unopposed, accounts for part of the withdrawal activation of the cells.

Results of other studies have indicated that up-regulation of the cAMP pathway may be a common mechanism by which a number of neuronal cell types respond to chronic opiates and develop tolerance and dependence. There is also evidence that similar mechanisms involving alterations in the cAMP second-messenger and protein phosphorylation pathway may mediate aspects of addiction to other types of drugs of abuse, for example, cocaine and alcohol.

CONCLUSIONS

Twenty-five years ago, little information was available concerning the molecular machinery by which chemical and electrical stimuli produce diverse physiological responses in various types of neurons. In fact, there was not even a conceptual framework available through which one could approach this subject. As a result of work since that time, it has become apparent that the study of protein phosphorylation provides such an approach. The injection of protein kinases and protein kinase inhibitors into neurons has demonstrated a direct causal relationship between the activation of specific protein kinases and the generation of specific physiological responses to extracellular signals in the nervous system. Virtually every type of neuronal protein, and therefore every type of neural process, is now known to be regulated by protein phosphorylation. The protein kinase/protein phosphatase system, by controlling the phosphorylation state of substrate proteins of every conceivable category, provides the flexibility required for regulating a variety of neuronal processes having widely different temporal characteristics. By studying protein phosphorylation mechanisms, it should be possible to develop a progressively more complete understanding of the molecular basis of innumerable types of neuro-

physiological phenomena, from the shortest lived to the longest lived, and from the most simple to the most complex.

REFERENCES

1. Nestler, E. J., and Greengard, P. *Protein Phosphorylation in the Nervous System.* New York: Wiley, 1984.
2. Hunter, T., and Sefton, B. M. (eds.). Protein phosphorylation. Part A. *Methods Enzymol.* 200: 1991.
3. Cadd, G., and McKnight, G. S. Distinct patterns of cAMP-dependent protein kinase gene expression in mouse brain. *Neuron* 3: 71–79, 1989.
4. Hanson, P. I., and Schulman, H. Neuronal Ca^{2+}/calmodulin-dependent protein kinases. *Annu. Rev. Biochem.* 61:559–601, 1992.
5. Picciotto, M. R., Czernik, A. J., and Nairn, A. C. Characterization of calcium/calmodulin-dependent protein kinase I: cDNA cloning and identification of autophosphorylation site. *J. Biol. Chem.* [in press] 1993.
6. Kikkawa, U., Kishimoto, A., and Nishizuka, Y. The protein kinase C family: Heterogeneity and its implications. *Annu. Rev. Biochem.* 58: 31–44, 1989.
7. Hemmings, H. C., Jr., Nairn, A. C., McGuinness, T. L., Huganir, R. L., and Greengard, P. Role of protein phosphorylation in neuronal signal transduction. *FASEB J.* 3:1583–1592, 1989.
8. Hyman, S. E., and Nestler, E. J. *The Molecular Foundation of Psychiatry.* Washington, D.C.: American Psychiatric, 1993.
9. Haycock, J. W., Ahn, N. G., Cobb, M. H., and Krebs, E. G. ERK1 and ERK2, two microtubule-associated protein 2 kinases, mediate the phosphorylation of tyrosine hydroxylase at serine-31 in situ. *Proc. Natl. Acad. Sci. U.S.A.* 89:2365–2369, 1992.
10. Tuazon, P. T., and Traugh, J. A. Casein kinase I and II—multipotential serine protein kinases: Structure, function, and regulation. *Adv. Second Messenger Phosphoprotein Res.* 23: 123–164, 1991.
11. Wood, K. W., Sarneck, C., Roberts, T. M., and Blenis, J. *ras* mediates nerve growth factor receptor modulation of three signal-transducing protein kinases: MAP kinase, Raf-1, and RSK. *Cell* 68:1041–1050, 1992.

12. Bading, H., and Greenberg, M. E. Stimulation of protein tyrosine phosphorylation by NMDA receptor activation. *Science* 253: 912–914, 1991.

13. Cohen, P. The structure and regulation of protein phosphatases. *Annu. Rev. Biochem.* 58: 453–508, 1989.

14. Hunter, T., and Sefton, B. M. (eds.). Protein phosphorylation. Part B. *Methods Enzymol.* 201: 1991.

15. Shenolikar, S., and Nairn, A. C. Protein phosphatases: Recent progress. *Adv. Second Messenger Phosphoprotein Res.* 23:1–121, 1991.

16. Chen, J., Martin, B. L., and Brautigan, D. L. Regulation of protein serine-threonine phosphatase type-2A by tyrosine phosphorylation. *Science* 257:1261–1264, 1992.

17. Fischer, E. H., Charbonneau, H., and Tonks, N. K. Protein tyrosine phosphatases: A diverse family of intracellular and transmembrane enzymes. *Science* 253:401–406, 1991.

18. Hershey, J. W. B. Protein phosphorylation controls translation rates. *J. Biol. Chem.* 264: 20823–20826, 1989.

19. Huganir, R. L., and Greengard, P. Regulation of neurotransmitter receptor desensitization by protein phosphorylation. *Neuron* 5: 555–567, 1990.

20. Madison, D. V., Malenka, R. C., and Nicoll, R. A. Mechanisms underlying long-term potentiation of synaptic transmission. *Annu. Rev. Neurosci.* 14:379–397, 1991.

21. Zigmond, R. E., Schwarzschild, M. A., and Rittenhouse, A. R. Acute regulation of tyrosine hydroxylase by nerve activity and by neurotransmitters via phosphorylation. *Annu. Rev. Neurosci.* 12:415–461, 1989.

22. Lolley, R. N., and Lee, R. H. Cyclic GMP and photoreceptor function. *FASEB J.* 4: 3001–3008, 1990.

23. Lefkowitz, R. J., Hausdorff, W. P., and Caron, M. G. Role of phosphorylation in desensitization of the β-adrenoceptor. *Trends Pharmacol. Sci.* 11:190–194, 1990.

24. Kobilka, B. Adrenergic receptors as models for G protein-coupled receptors. *Annu. Rev. Neurosci.* 15:87–114, 1992.

25. Liggett, S. B., Ostrowski, J., Chesnut, L. C., Kurose, H., Raymond, J. R., Caron, M. G., and Lefkowitz, R. J. Sites in the third intracellular loop of the α_{2A}-adrenergic receptor confer short term agonist-promoted desensitization. *J. Biol. Chem.* 267:4740–4746, 1992.

26. De Camilli, P., Benfenati, F., Valtorta, F., and Greengard, P. The synapsins. *Annu. Rev. Cell Biol.* 6:433–460, 1990.

27. Valtorta, F., Benfenati, F., and Greengard, P. Structure and function of the synapsins. *J. Biol. Chem.* 267:7195–7198, 1992.

28. Benfenati, F., Valtorta, F., Chieregati, E., and Greengard, P. Interaction of free and synaptic vesicle-bound synapsin I with F-actin. *Neuron* 8:377–386, 1992.

29. Lu, B., Greengard, P., and Poo, M-M. Exogenous synapsin I promotes functional maturation of developing neuromuscular synapses. *Neuron* 8:521–529, 1992.

30. Pessin, M. S., Snyder, G. L., Halpain, S., Girault, J-A., Aperia, A., and Greengard, P. DARPP-32/protein phosphatase-1/Na^+/K^+ ATPase system: A mechanism for bidirectional control of cell function. In *Proceedings of the 1992 Wenner Gren International Symposium.* Stockholm [in press] 1993.

31. Montminy, M. R., Gonzalez, G. A., and Yamamoto, K. K. Regulation of cAMP-inducible genes by CREB. *Trends Neurosci.* 13:184–188, 1990.

32. Gandy, S., and Greengard, P. Amyloidogenesis in Alzheimer's disease: Some possible therapeutic opportunities. *Trends Pharmacol. Sci.* 13:108–113, 1992.

33. Nestler, E. J. Molecular mechanisms of drug addiction. *J. Neurosci.* 12:2439–2450, 1992.

CHAPTER 23

Eicosanoids

LEONHARD S. WOLFE AND LLOYD A. HORROCKS

ESSENTIAL FATTY ACIDS

The dietary essentiality in mammals of certain polyunsaturated fatty acids of the n-6 family, particularly linoleic acid (Z,Z or all-*cis*-9,12-octadecadienoic acid) and arachidonic acid (Z,Z,Z,Z or all-*cis*-5,8,11,14-eicosatetraenoic acid), has been known since the pioneering studies of George and Mildred Burr in 1929 on feeding young rats for several months on a fat-free diet. The symptoms included growth retardation, scaly derma-titis, increased transepidermal water loss, and reproductive failure. The essentiality of fatty acids of the n-3 family, particularly α-linoleic acid (Z,Z,Z-9,12,15-octadecatrienoic acid), initially was uncertain but is now firmly established (see also Chap. 5). Deficiency of 18:3 n-3 does not influence reproductive function or growth, but is associated with altered central nervous system (CNS) and visual functions. Diets with minimal 18:3 n-3 and no or very low amounts of n-3 long chain polyenoic acids cause neurological prob-

Basic Neurochemistry: Molecular, Cellular, and Medical Aspects, 5th Ed., edited by G. J. Siegel et al. Published by Raven Press, Ltd., New York, 1994. Correspondence to Leonhard S. Wolfe, Montreal Neurological Institute, 3801 University Street, Montreal, Quebec H3A 2B4, Canada.

lems, altered learning behavior, lower visual acuity thresholds, and abnormal electroretinograms in rodents, monkeys, and human infants. Young adults on total parenteral nutrition, with only safflower oil as a source of lipid, also have neurological and visual problems. These functional changes are associated with a reduction of the normally high levels (45–60 percent) of 22:6 n-3 or docosahexaenoic acid in ethanolamine and serine glycerophospholipids of the rod outer segments of photoreceptors in the retina. Synaptic membranes are also particularly rich in 22:6 n-3. There is now much evidence that polyenoic acids of both the n-6 and n-3 families are crucial to the normal functioning of excitable membranes in the CNS and retina [1]. This chapter deals with a family of physiologically active derivatives of the n-6 series, most notably arachidonate.

EICOSANOIDS: GENERAL PROPERTIES AND BIOSYNTHETIC REACTIONS

The generic name "eicosanoids" was introduced by Corey in 1980 to denote a group of oxygenated products derived enzymatically from 20 carbon polyunsaturated fatty acids. The major precursor of these compounds is arachidonic acid, and the pathways that lead to the eicosanoids are known collectively as the "arachidonate cascade" [2]. Docosahexaenoic acid can also be enzymatically oxygenated to generate products termed "docosanoids." Fatty acids of the n-3 series, such as eicosapentaenoic acid (EPA) and docosahexaenoic acid (DHA), important constituents of some fish oils, are now coming into prominence as dietary agents that can modify the production of eicosanoids in human tissues. These substances may affect pathophysiological responses in a number of human diseases, such as myocardial infarction and rheumatoid arthritis.

The general field of eicosanoids is now very complex, but there are a number of general features that can help us to understand the importance of these varied and potent biologically active substances. Eicosanoids are formed by virtually every tissue in the body and are widely distributed in the animal kingdom, being found in invertebrates, such as coral, sea urchins, and arthropods, and even in plants. The biological activities of individual prostaglandins vary from organ to organ in a given species and may differ markedly from species to species. Even in different stages of development or in different phases of organ function (as occurs, for example, in the uterus), an individual prostaglandin may have different biological effects. It is only in the past 10 years that the important involvement of eicosanoids in synaptic signal transduction pathways, ion channel activities, and modulation of neurotransmitter release has been discovered [3].

There are three major pathways in the arachidonate cascade in mammalian organisms that initiate stereospecific oxygenations of arachidonic acid released from membrane phospholipids: (1) the cyclooxygenase pathway or prostaglandin G/H synthase, which forms prostaglandins and thromboxanes; (2) the lipoxygenase pathways, which form leukotrienes, lipoxins, and other specific hydroperoxy- and hydroxyeicosatetraenoic acids; and (3) the epoxygenase pathways, which transform arachidonic acid, through the monooxygenase activity of cytochrome P_{450}, to epoxyeicosatetraenoic acids.

In lower organisms and plants, prostanoids can be synthesized by the allene oxide synthase pathway, which is also a P_{450} enzyme. Figure 1 illustrates these various pathways. Release of arachidonic acid from membrane phospholipids occurs after a wide variety of stimuli to receptors on cells—hormones, neurotransmitters, antibodies, growth factors, proteins, peptides, toxins—as well as pathological conditions including inflammation, vascular shock, burns, brain trauma, hypoxia, ischemia, seizures, and immune reactions. Eicosanoids themselves can stimulate arachidonic acid release in specific organs. The release of arachidonic acid and its transformation into metabolites are local, and the

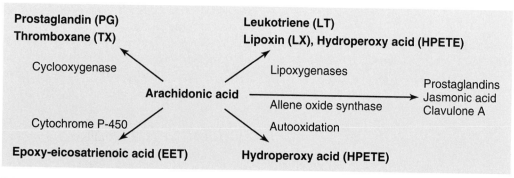

FIG. 1.   Scheme of various ways in which arachidonic acid may be oxygenated. Arachidonic acid is converted enzymatically to prostaglandins and thromboxanes by cyclooxygenase; to leukotrienes, lipoxins, and hydroperoxy acids by lipoxygenases; and to epoxy derivatives by cytochrome P_{450}. In plants and lower organisms, an allene oxide synthase can form prostaglandins, as well as other compounds. Various isomers of hydroperoxy acids can be formed by nonenzymic autooxidation.

effects of the eicosanoids occur in the immediate vicinity of their formation. At these sites the compounds rarely act in isolation, but reinforce, sensitize, or antagonize many ongoing cellular processes, particularly stimulus-secretion-coupled events. Enzyme reactions in tissues such as liver, lung, and kidney (dehydrogenases, desaturases, β- and ω-oxidases, reductases, acetylases) convert the parent eicosanoids into multiple biologically inactive metabolites that are then excreted in the urine [3]. The naturally active compounds thus are not found in significant concentrations in the systemic circulation. Once formed, the compounds act as bioregulators of responses to second messengers, such as cyclic adenosine monophosphate (cAMP), inositol trisphosphate and inositol tetrakisphosphate (and their cyclic derivatives), and diacylglycerol (DAG), which affects calcium mobilization, specific protein binding, and the activity of protein kinases. Many of the genes coding for the eicosanoid-specific enzymes have now been cloned. Their evolutionary origin is ancient and involves both the animal and plant kingdoms.

MECHANISMS OF ARACHIDONATE RELEASE FROM NEURAL MEMBRANES

Under normal conditions, the level of eicosanoid precursor arachidonate in the cytosol is extremely low because the re-esterification of this fatty acid through acyltransferases into membrane phospholipids prevails over its release. During cell stimulation the release of arachidonate is catalyzed by several direct and indirect enzymic pathways. The direct pathway involves the stimulation of phospholipase A_2 (PLA_2). One indirect pathway requires the activation of phospholipase C, followed by DAG and monoacylglycerol lipases (Fig. 2). A second indirect pathway releases arachidonate via a lysophospholipase preceded by PLA_2. The hydrolysis of phospholipids by phospholipase D (PLD) produces phosphatidic acid, which can then be hydrolyzed by a phosphatidic acid–specific PLA_2. The action of a phosphatase on phosphatidic acid generates DAG, which can be hydrolyzed by DAG and monoacylglycerol lipases. Arachidonate can also be transferred from one phospholipid class to another, via acyl group transfer under the action of coenzyme A (CoA)-dependent and CoA-independent transacylases [4]. This trafficking of arachidonate among different phospholipids, termed the "remodeling pathway," is still poorly understood, but is the key factor in delivering arachidonate to the appropriate phospholipid acceptor prior to PLA_2-catalyzed hydrolysis. This is generally regarded as the rate-limiting step in the formation of oxygenated metabolites of arachidonic acid

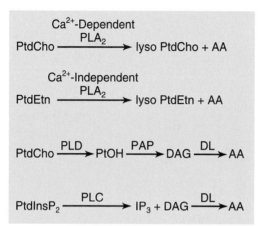

FIG. 2.   Phospholipases involved in the release of arachidonic acid (AA). (PLA$_2$) phospholipase A$_2$; (PLD) phospholipase D; (PLC) phospholipase C; (DAG) 1,2-diacylglycerol; (DL) diacylglycerol lipase; (IP$_3$) inositol 1,4,5-trisphosphate; (PtdCho) phosphatidylcholine; (lyso PtdCho) lysophosphatidylcholine; (PtdEtn) phosphatidylethanolamine; (lyso PtdEtn) lysophosphatidylethanolamine; (PtdInsP$_2$) phosphatidylinositol bisphosphate; (PAP) phosphatidic acid phosphohydrolase.

as well as in the formation of platelet-activating factor (PAF). When arachidonic acid is hydrolyzed from 1-*O*-alkyl-linked species of phospholipids, lysoplatelet-activating factor is formed, which can then be acetylated to form PAF (Fig. 3). A second mechanism of PAF synthesis (not shown) involves the transfer of phosphocholine from CDP-choline to alkylacetylglycerol. PAF is a potent autacoid

mediator that interacts with specific membrane binding sites, causing an increase in intracellular Ca^{2+} levels, activation of PLA$_2$ and phospholipase C, and stimulation of other second-messenger producing systems.

Although the relative contributions of these pathways to the release of arachidonate are still obscure, the importance of the direct deacylation of phospholipids by PLA$_2$ and the action of di- and monoacylglycerol lipases preceded by phospholipase C has been clearly established.

Regulation of phospholipases A$_2$

Phospholipases may be classified as Ca^{2+}-dependent PLA$_2$ and Ca^{2+}-independent PLA$_2$ [5,6]. The Ca^{2+}-dependent phospholipases require Ca^{2+} at the active site [7]. The level of Ca^{2+} concentration necessary to stimulate PLA$_2$ in many assay systems is much higher than that achieved with any physiological stimuli. Thus, factor(s) other than Ca^{2+} may be involved in agonist-induced stimulation of PLA$_2$.

In the case of the macrophage cell line RAW 264.7, PLA$_2$ activity is almost entirely cytosolic when cells are homogenized in the presence of Ca^{2+} chelators. In the presence of a high concentration of Ca^{2+} (>1 mM), there is a loss of cytosolic activity and a concomitant increase in membrane-associated

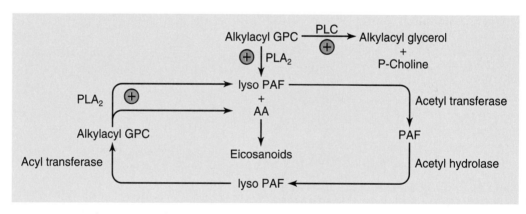

FIG. 3.   Diagram showing PAF cycle and its relationship to phospholipases and eicosanoids. (PAF) platelet-activating factor; (GPC) glycerophosphocholine; (Lyso PAF) lysoplatelet-activating factor; (AA) arachidonic acid; (PLA$_2$) phospholipase A$_2$; (PLC) phospholipase C. Stimulation of PLA$_2$ and PLC activities by PAF is indicated by plus signs.

activity, reflecting a regulatory role for Ca^{2+} in the activation of PLA_2 by promoting its association with membrane. In fact, it was recently reported that a 140 amino acid fragment from the N-terminal end of PLA_2 is involved in its binding to the plasma membrane in response to Ca^{2+}. PLA_2 activity of the synaptosomal membrane is regulated by the phosphorylation/dephosphorylation process. Ca^{2+}/calmodulin-dependent protein kinase II phosphorylates PLA_2 and inhibits its activity [5–7].

PLA_2 activity is regulated by PLA_2 inhibitory and PLA_2 stimulatory proteins. In mammalian tissues, antiinflammatory steroids induce the synthesis of PLA_2 inhibitory proteins called lipocortins, members of the annexin superfamily of Ca^{2+}-dependent lipid-binding proteins. The concentration of these proteins is rather low in brain. During cell stimulation, annexins are phosphorylated by protein kinase C (PKC), resulting in loss of their inhibitory activity. The mechanism of regulation of PLA_2's by annexins is not fully understood, although it has been proposed that annexins bind to phospholipids and block access of the enzyme to its substrate [8].

PLA_2 stimulatory protein has also been partially purified from rat cerebral cortex. It is phosphorylated by PKC. It has been suggested that phosphorylation of stimulatory protein regulates PLA_2 activity in neurons. PLA_2 stimulatory protein may play a pivotal role in the propagation of inflammatory diseases.

Peroxidation of membrane phospholipids is accompanied by an increased activity of PLA_2. Vitamin E, a well-known antioxidant, inhibits PLA_2 activity by associating with the membrane [9]. This process may be involved in remodeling of membranes.

PLA_2 activity is also regulated by G proteins. The dissociation of the α-subunit from the $\beta\gamma$-subunits of G protein activates PLA_2, whereas the recombination of free α and $\beta\gamma$ to form $\alpha\beta\gamma$ heterotrimer turns off PLA_2 activation. (G proteins are discussed in Chap. 10.) Free fatty acids may also play an important role in the regulation of PLA_2 activity [10].

PAF stimulates the release of arachidonic acid in human and rabbit polymorphonuclear leukocytes, guinea pig peritoneal macrophages, 3T3 fibroblasts, and human endothelial cells. This release is brought about by PLA_2. The involvement of the Ca^{2+} influx and a G protein has been proposed during the PLA_2 activation process.

A Ca^{2+}-independent PLA_2 was recently purified from brain. This enzyme is active against ethanolamine plasmalogen and phosphatidylethanolamine, but nothing is known about its regulation. The corresponding enzyme from heart is active toward choline and ethanolamine plasmalogen and is stimulated and stabilized by ATP.

Regulation of phospholipase C

Multiple forms of phospholipase C have been purified from mammalian brain, and phospholipase C-γ has been sequenced. It contains regions of homology with tyrosine kinase. Epidermal growth factor (EGF) or platelet-derived growth factor (PDGF) stimulation of 3T3 fibroblasts results in phosphorylation of phospholipase C-γ by tyrosine kinase. EGF or PDGF also induces a translocation of phospholipase C-γ from cytosol to membranes, suggesting that regulation of phospholipase C involves a phosphorylation/dephosphorylation process that is accompanied by translocation of this enzyme from cytosol to membrane [10].

Phospholipase C activity is also regulated by G proteins. The stable analogs of GTP induce the stimulation of phospholipase C in cerebral cortex preparations. Phospholipase C-linked G protein is pertussis toxin-insensitive, whereas PLA_2-linked G protein is pertussis toxin-sensitive. PAF stimulates polyphosphoinositide turnover in platelets and neutrophils as a result of the activation of phosphoinositide-specific phospholipase C by PAF. While the mechanism of stimulation of phospholipase C is poorly defined, the involvement of G protein(s) and tyrosine kinase(s) has been proposed.

Regulation of diacylglycerol and monoacylglycerol lipases

Regulation of DAG and monoacylglycerol lipases is also a complex process. The enzymic activities may be regulated by free fatty acids that are end products of their catalytic action. *In vitro* this inhibition can be reversed by fatty acid-free bovine serum albumin. A treatment of neuron-enriched primary cultures with bradykinin results in a three- to fourfold increase in the specific activity of DAG and monoacyglycerol lipases, and this stimulation can be blocked by a bradykinin antagonist. DAG requires no metal ion, and homogeneous preparations of microsomal and plasma membrane DAG lipases are not affected by Ca^{2+}. However, in the membrane-bound state, the microsomal DAG lipase activity is stimulated by a high concentration of Ca^{2+}, whereas the enzyme activity in plasma membrane is not affected by Ca^{2+}. The differential response of DAG lipases in the membrane-bound state may result from differences in the membrane lipid composition of the two membranes.

Regulation of phospholipase D

PLD is regulated by two distinct mechanisms. One mechanism, activated by receptor-linked agonists, involves a G protein. In cell-free preparations from cerebral cortex, the stable GTP analog, guanosine 5'-(γ-thio) triphosphate, produces a dose-dependent stimulation of PLD activity [10]. The identity of the G protein involved in PLD regulation remains to be established.

The other mechanism involves PKC. Tumor-promoting phorbol esters stimulate PLD activity in brain preparations and several types of neuronal and glial cultures. In most preparations, PLD is activated by both phorbol esters and GTP (γS), suggesting that the two regulatory mechanisms coexist in a cell. However, PKC inhibitors and PKC down-regulation do not attenuate PLD activity in receptor-stimulated cell cultures.

In some brain preparations, PLD activity is stimulated by Ca^{2+}. PLD activation by sphingoid bases and membrane-permeant synthetic DAGs may be a consequence of membrane perturbation, favoring substrate availability to the enzyme. PLD activity is also regulated by G proteins, but the identity of this G protein remains to be established. Phorbol ester stimulates PLD activity, indicating the involvement of PKC in the regulation of PLD.

CYCLOOXYGENASE PATHWAYS: PROSTAGLANDINS AND THROMBOXANES

A brief history of the discovery of the various prostaglandins and the technical advantages that made their identification possible may be found in the fourth edition of *Basic Neurochemistry*. The structures and biosynthetic relationships of the prostaglandins and thromboxanes are shown in Fig. 4. Naturally occurring prostaglandins contain a cyclopentane ring and a *trans* (E) double bond between C-13 and C-14 and a *(S)*hydroxyl group at C-15. Thromboxane A_2 (TXA_2) is highly unstable and contains a six-membered ring with a bicyclic oxitane-oxane structure. Prostaglandin H synthase (PGHS-1) is a constitutive bifunctional enzyme with two different catalytic activities: (a) a cyclooxygenase that catalyzes the formation of prostaglandin G_2 (PGG_2) from arachidonate and (b) a hydroperoxidase activity that reduces PGG_2 to prostaglandin H_2 (PGH_2). The enzyme is a 72-kDa membrane-associated protein existing as a homodimer. Molecular cloning indicates that the protein initially contains a signal peptide that is cleaved when it traverses the endoplasmic reticulum during synthesis. The native enzyme is a hemoprotein containing one protoporphyrin IX per subunit and is glycosylated at three asparagine residues. Aspirin competes with

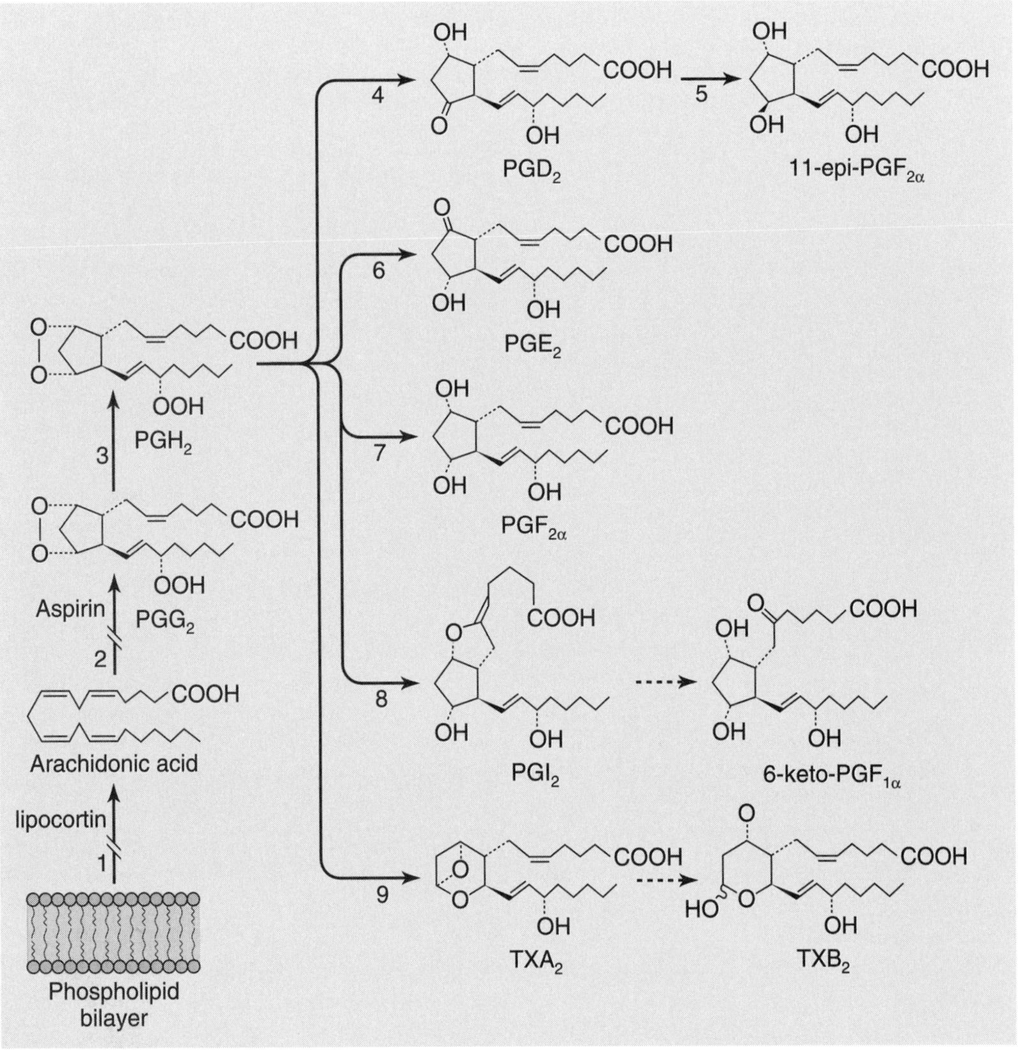

FIG. 4.   The arachidonic acid cascade: cyclooxygenase pathways. The nomenclature of enzymes is as follows: (1) phospholipase A_2; (2) prostaglandin (PG) endoperoxide synthase (cyclooxygenase); (3) prostaglandin endoperoxide synthase (hydroperoxidase); (4) PGD synthase (PGH-D isomerase); (5) PGF synthase (PGD_2 11-ketoreductase); (6) PGE synthase (PGH-E isomerase); (7) PGF synthase (PGH-F isomerase); (8) PGI synthase; (9) thromboxane (TX) synthase. The *broken lines* indicate nonenzymic processes.

arachidonate for binding and acetylates serine 530, which leads to irreversible cyclooxygenase inactivation. Other nonsteroidal antiinflammatory drugs cause reversible inhibition by competing with arachidonate binding, e.g., ibuprofen (Advil). Antiinflammatory steroids act by inhibition of transcription of the PGH synthase gene or promotion of the synthesis of lipocortin, a member of the annexin family of phospholipid-binding proteins. Very recently a second prostaglandin H synthase (PGHS-2) that is inducible by growth factors and cytokines was discovered. The induction of the transcription of the PGHS-2 gene is inhibited by glucocorticoids [2,3,11,12].

The formation of prostaglandins E_2 (PGE_2), D_2 (PGD_2), $F_{2\alpha}$ ($PGF_{2\alpha}$), I_2 (PGI_2), and 11-epi-PGF$_{2\alpha}$ and TXA$_2$ from PGH$_2$ is catalyzed by their respective synthases. The synthesis of these prostanoids appears to be cell-specific. For example, cultured rat astroglial cells synthesize 10 times more prostaglandins than neural cells in primary culture.

PGD$_2$ synthase or PGH$_2$ D-isomerase is a glycosylated membrane-bound enzyme, as determined by molecular cloning. From the deduced amino acid sequence from the complementary DNA (cDNA), the enzyme becomes a member of the lipocalin superfamily, which comprises secretory molecule transporters. In brain this enzyme shows unique developmental changes in activity and cellular location. The highest enzyme activity occurs during neural differentiation and synaptogenesis. However, in mature rats the enzyme activity shifts to the oligodendrocytes. PGE$_2$ synthase is unique in requiring glutathione (GSH) as cofactor. The anionic form of glutathione *S*-transferase catalyzes the isomerization of PGH$_2$ to PGE$_2$. PGF$_{2\alpha}$ synthase, from molecular cloning, is a member of the aldehyde reductase family of proteins. It also catalyzes the formation of 11-epi-PGF$_{2\alpha}$ from PGD$_2$ [3]. PGI$_2$ synthase and TXA$_2$ synthase are both hemoproteins and probably members of the cytochrome P$_{450}$ protein family. Like PGH synthase, both enzymes undergo "suicide" inactivation during catalysis.

Prostaglandins and thromboxanes probably exit cells by a specific transporter, act on specific receptors in the local environment, and then become catabolized to inactive products in the circulation after passage through the lung, liver, and kidney. The initial steps are catalyzed by oxidation to the 15-keto compounds by NADH-dependent 15-hxdroxyprostaglandin dehydrogenases, then reduction of the Δ13 double bond, followed by β- and ω-oxidations. PGI$_2$ and TXA$_2$ are nonenzymatically hydrolyzed to the 6-keto-PGF$_{1\alpha}$ and thromboxane B$_2$ (TXB$_2$) before subsequent modifications by oxidation reactions. Measurement of blood and urine metabolites by gas chromatography-mass spectrometry (GC-MS) methods has become an important means to determine total body eicosanoid formation under normal physiological and pathological conditions.

LIPOXYGENASE PATHWAYS

Distinct mammalian lipoxygenases that exist catalyze the insertion of oxygen into the *(S)* configuration at positions 5, 12, and 15 of arachidonic acid and also produce hydroperoxy and hydroxy analogs of certain other polyenoic fatty acids (Fig. 5). The 5-lipoxygenase that forms leukotrienes is particularly important in inflammatory cells [2,13]. Leukotriene A$_4$ (LTA$_4$) is enzymatically converted to leukotriene B$_4$ (LTB$_4$). Cloning studies have shown that this is a bifunctional enzyme with LTA$_4$ hydrolase activity and also contains a zinc binding site and aminopeptidase activity. The efficient conversion of LTA$_4$ to leukotriene C$_4$ (LTC$_4$) is catalyzed by the GST-Yn$_1$Yn$_1$ isozyme of glutathione *S*-transferase. Leukotrienes D$_4$ (LTD$_4$) and E$_4$ (LTE$_4$), the principal peptidoleukotrienes in the slow-reacting substance of anaphylaxis, are formed from LTC$_4$ by γ-glutamyltranspeptidase and a dipeptidase. Human platelets and brain contain a 12-lipoxygenase. The unstable intermediate 12*(S)*-hydroperoxy-5,8,14-*cis*-10-*trans*-eicosatetraenoic acid (12-HPETE) can be metabolized to epoxy derivatives termed "hepoxilins" by a cytochrome P$_{450}$ enzyme. These compounds are of particular interest in the nervous system and in CNS ischemia (see Chap. 42). The 15-lipoxygenase has been characterized in human reticulocytes, eosinophils, and pulmonary epithelial cells. Its biological significance remains to be determined.

BRAIN EICOSANOIDS

Release of prostaglandins into superfusates of cerebral cortex, cerebellum, and spinal cord and into the cerebral ventricles *in vivo*, and increased synthesis and release after stimulation of neural pathways, have been

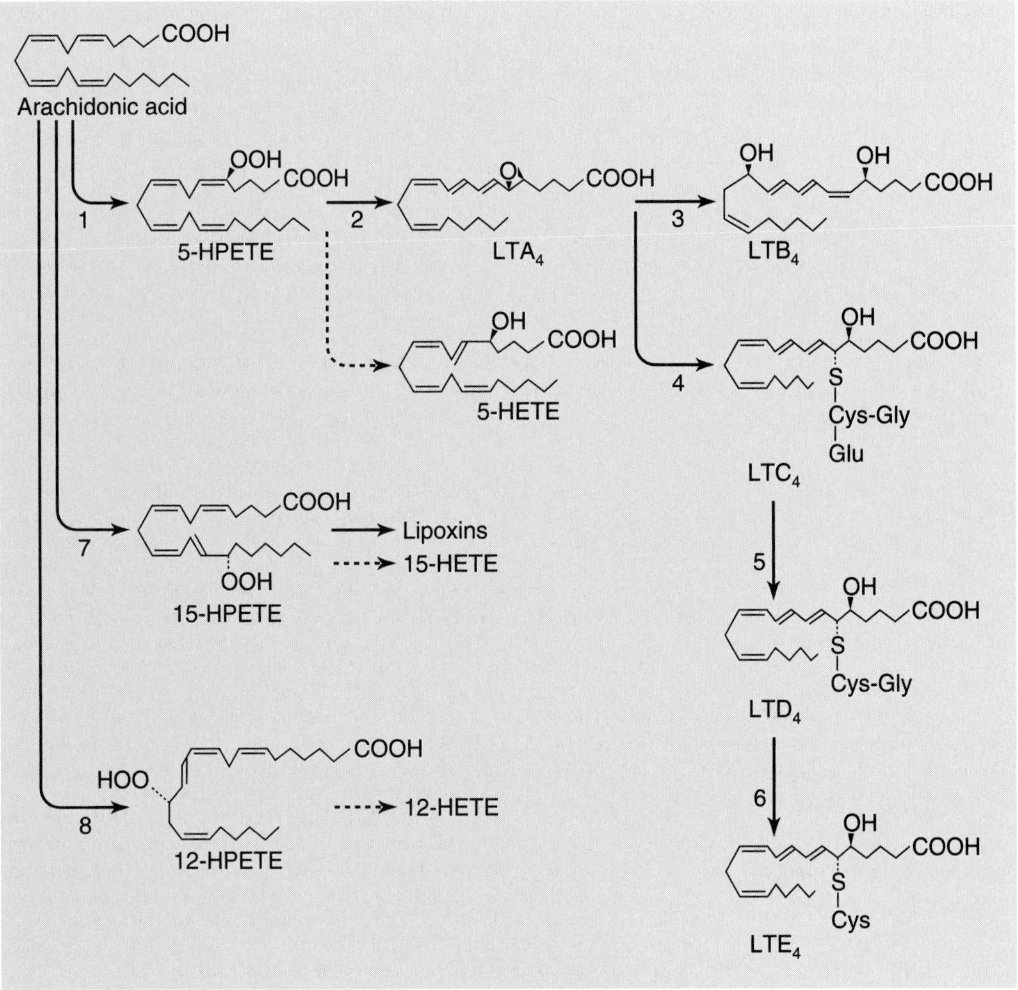

FIG. 5.   The arachidonic acid cascade: lipoxygenase pathways. The nomenclature is as follows: (1) 5-(S)-li-poxygenase (activated by 5-lipoxygenase-activating protein [FLAP]; (2) leukotriene (LT) A_4 synthase; (3) LTA_4 hydrolase; (4) LTC_4 synthase; (5) γ-glutamyltranspeptidase; (6) dipeptidase; (7) 15-(S)-lipoxygenase; (8) 12-(S)-lipoxygenase. 5-HETE, 15-HETE, and 12-HETE are the corresponding reduction products of the hydroperoxyeicosatetraenoic acids. Abbreviations used are defined in the text and in Fig. 1.

clearly demonstrated. The basal content of prostaglandins in quick-frozen cerebral neocortex (rat, gerbil, human) is at the limit of detection, measured by specific GC-MS analyses or even by radioimmunoassay. However, Hayaishi found the highest basal levels in the olfactory bulb and pineal gland, followed by the hypothalamus (see [3]).

Interpretation of the meaning of basal levels of prostaglandins is controversial. Endogenous synthesis of prostaglandins can occur in dissected brain regions, even in the cold. The brain regions most difficult to dissect have the highest content, and this raises the question of whether this reflects actual basal levels or biosynthesis from endogenously released arachidonic acid post mortem [3]. There is good documentation that incubated intact brain tissue can synthesize prostaglandins (PGE_2, $PGF_{2\alpha}$, PGI_2, PGD_2) and TXB_2 during short incubation periods. In rodent brain, PGD_2 is quantitatively the most important cyclooxygenase product. Cat brain differs in that $PGF_{2\alpha}$ and TXB_2 are the principal products and PGD_2 formation is exceedingly small. In human cortex and hypothalamus, PGD_2 is formed and rapidly metabolized. Basal levels of eicosanoids in brain tissue may not represent the real concentrations of the compounds at the neuronal or glial cell level or in synaptic regions, where the concentrations may be considerably higher. Furthermore, in human brain, PGD_2 may be rapidly converted enzymatically into 11-epi-$PGF_{2\alpha}$ (9-α,11-β-PGF_2). This reaction has been found to take place in human neocortex and may account in part for the low levels of PGD_2 found in human brain. Other human tissues can form PGD_2 in very significant amounts.

In the brain, regional differences of PGD_2, PGE_2, and PGF_2 synthetic enzyme activity do occur. Induction of seizures in convulsion-prone gerbils or in rats by electroshock or convulsant drugs (metrazole, bicuculline) markedly increases arachidonic acid release and formation of PGE_2 and $PGF_{2\alpha}$. The cerebral cortex and hippocampus show by far the largest increases, with considerably less effect observed at the level of the hypothalamus.

The leukotrienes (LTB_4, LTC_4, LTD_4) and monohydroxyeicosatetraenoic acids (HETEs) are synthesized by lipoxygenase pathways in brain, and these products are not derived from contamination with leukocytes or other blood elements. The concentrations of LTC_4 in brain are in the picomolar range, with the highest levels in the hypothalamus, median eminence, nucleus accumbens, and olfactory bulb. LTC_4 is reported to mediate luteinizing hormone release specifically from rat anterior pituitary cells at concentrations of 10^{-14} to 10^{-11} M. There is no effect on release of growth hormone. The effect of LTC_4 appears to differ from the action of hypothalamic luteinizing hormone-releasing hormone (LHRH). LTC_4 action is rapid, whereas LHRH action is much slower. Indeed, LTC_4 acts in leukocytes as a secretagogue. Furthermore, by im-

munocytochemical methods, a specific group of LTC_4-reacting neurons has been found in the median eminence. LTC_4 action may be related to the immediate release of preformed stored hormone, whereas LHRH peptide action is directed toward synthesis of new hormone at the nuclear level. There is no doubt that these studies are uncovering unexpected new roles for leukotrienes in brain in modulation of neurohormone and, possibly, neurotransmitter release. An efficient transport system for LTC_4 has been found in the choroid plexus. A further development in the leukotriene story in brain is the finding of increased LTB_4-, LTC_4-, and LTD_4-like immunoreactivity in gerbil brain after ischemia and reperfusion and after brain injury and subarachnoid hemorrhage. Since LTC_4 is a potent vasoconstrictor and increases vascular permeability, particularly in the lung, it is possible that it may be an important initiator of the formation of cerebral ischemic edema and may constrict small cerebral blood vessels. Although some workers have reported that LTC_4 or arachidonic acid injected directly into the brain parenchyma induces breakdown of the blood-brain barrier (BBB), and that inhibition of arachidonic acid conversion to leukotrienes prevents vasogenic edema, other investigators, employing open cranial window techniques, could find no effect on the BBB, even at pharmacological concentrations. Nevertheless, leukotrienes do cause venous and arterial vasoconstriction, and it is clear that 5-lipoxygenase activity is present in brain and can lead to the synthesis of 5-HPETE and 5-HETE, as well as the biologically active leukotrienes.

Tissue slices of cerebral cortex and homogenates from mouse and rat brain synthesize a number of HETEs. After addition of the calcium ionophore A 23187 and arachidonic acid (75 μM), microgram amounts of 12-HETE are formed far in excess of the formation of prostaglandins and thromboxanes. The formation of 12-HETE is particularly high in rat cerebral cortex and hippocampal slices and in rat pineal gland,

and it is formed in bovine retina. 12-HETE is synthesized by mouse neuroblastoma cells in culture, suggestive of a neuronal origin. Also of interest is that 12-HETE is formed in human skin and increases in hyperproliferative diseases, such as psoriasis.

EICOSANOIDS AS SECOND MESSENGERS AND MODULATORS OF SYNAPTIC TRANSMISSION

Prostaglandins

The interaction of prostaglandins in the autonomic nervous system has been given much attention. Stimulation of sympathetic or parasympathetic nerves is associated with release of prostaglandins, principally PGE_2 and $PGF_{2\alpha}$. The release rate is, in general, related to the stimulus frequency, and it returns to basal levels when stimulation ceases. The postsynaptic effector cell membrane is judged the most likely site of synthesis because receptor blockade by drugs (hyoscine, atropine, phenoxybenzamine, dibenzyline) inhibits prostaglandin release. Addition of neurotransmitter also stimulates prostaglandin release. Investigations by Hedqvist and co-workers (see [3]) on stimulation of sympathetic nerves to various organs (heart, oviduct, spleen, vas deferens) revealed that effector responses are inhibited by PGE_1 and PGE_2, but not by the PGF series of prostaglandins. Such inhibition can be produced by picogram to nanogram amounts well within the range seen physiologically. Hedqvist proposed that endogenous PGE_2, formed and released from the postsynaptic effector membrane during stimulation, inhibits the release of norepinephrine from presynaptic terminals; however, there is evidence both for and against the role of prostaglandins in inhibiting the exocytotic release of norepinephrine from sympathetic nerve endings [3,12].

Release of PGE_2 in the CNS may also be involved in the regulation of neurotransmitter release. The stimulated release of norepinephrine and dopamine from rat cerebral cortex and neostriatum *in vitro* is reduced by PGE_2. The disappearance of dopamine histofluorescence in the neostriatum of rats pretreated with a tyrosine hydroxylase inhibitor is prolonged when PGE_2 is infused into the carotid artery. The physiological significance of prostaglandins at peripheral and central noradrenergic synapses is still far from clear. PGE prostaglandins can reduce calcium conductance, and this may underlie an inhibitory action on transmitter release. Subtypes of PGE_2 receptors have been identified in brain and adrenal medulla and found to be coupled to a G protein, but so far they have not been purified and cloned.

A large body of evidence, principally from Hayaishi's group, indicates that PGD_2 in the brain functions as a sleep-inducing agent in the preoptic area of the hypothalamus [14]. In rat brain, PGD_2, administered by intracerebral or intraventricular injection, induces sedation, catalepsy, sleep, and hypothermia in a dose-related manner. It also potentiates hexobarbitone hypnosis and has an anticonvulsant action. Selenium compounds ($SeCl_4$, Na_2SeO_3, and ebselen, an antiinflammatory organic selenium compound) inhibit selectively PGD_2 synthase. In rats, introduction of these compounds into the third ventricle by microdialysis inhibits sleep and activates behavior, with a moderate elevation of temperature and an increase in food and water intake. Intraventricular administration of PGD_2 also has a suppressive effect on the pulsatile release of luteinizing hormone; however, *in vitro* studies in which the medial basal hypothalamus of the rat was superfused showed that PGD_2 has no effect on the release of LHRH but does induce release of luteinizing hormone from the pituitary gland. Of much interest is that PGD_2 also increases serotonin content and turnover in brain. In the rodent brain at least, a neuromodulatory action of PGD_2 appears to exist, particularly on serotoninergic neurons that are known to have widespread projections to the cerebral cortex. Various prostaglandins have modulatory effects on hormone release from the hypothalamic-pituitary axis by modulation of neurotransmitter release, particularly dopamine. On the other hand, PGE_2 is an endogenous compound that induces wakefulness and hyperthermia, particularly in response to systemic pyrogens and the cytokine interleukin-1. Thus, in the hypothalamus these prostaglandins are involved in the regulation of the sleep-wake cycle, temperature, hypothalamopituitary functions, and food and water intake. While the function of $PGF_{2\alpha}$ in brain is still uncertain, its function in other tissues is well characterized. For example, in corpus luteal cells, it stimulates hydrolysis of inositol phospholipids and induces luteolysis. Recently it was shown that astrocytes possess a $PGF_{2\alpha}$ receptor coupled to phospholipase C and mediated by a GTP-binding protein, G_p.

PGE prostaglandins stimulate cAMP formation in many tissues, including cerebral cortex slices *in vitro*. Synergism of action on adenylate cyclase occurs with combinations of hormones and prostaglandins in intact brain tissue, but the meaning of these complex interactions is far from clear. Homogenization destroys this hormonal responsiveness. There is growing appreciation, however, that high concentrations of intracellular cAMP are associated with inhibition of cell growth in various cell lines in culture. Mouse neuroblastoma cells in culture respond to dibutyryl cAMP, PGE_1, and PGE_2 with a striking morphological differentiation, including the development of neuritic processes, a result that suggests that PGE prostaglandins play a role in cellular differentiation. Another aspect of the relationship between cAMP and PGE prostaglandins that is of particular relevance to the CNS is that morphine and related drugs inhibit the stimulation of cAMP formation by PGE prostaglandins . These studies raise the possibility that some of the pharmacological effects of opiates are related to inhibition of the action of endogenously produced prostaglandins on cAMP levels in the brain.

Lipoxygenase metabolites

The invertebrate and mammalian nervous systems have an active 12-(S)-lipoxygenase that catalyzes the conversion of arachidonic acid into 12-HPETE [15]. This intermediate can be metabolized to 12-HETE, the 12-keto compound, hepoxilin β_3 (10-hydroxy-11,12 epoxyeicosatrienoic acid), and hepoxilin A (8-hydroxy-11,12 epoxyeicosatrienoic acid) or oxidatively cleaved at carbon 12 to form 12-ketododecatrienoic acid. This would have been of little interest to the neuroscientist were it not for the discovery of some remarkable properties of these compounds in the mechanosensory neurons of the marine mollusk *Aplysia californica*. In these neurons, 12 lipoxygenase metabolites of arachidonic acid act as second messengers and may also participate in the communication of local groups of cells. In the sensory neurons of *Aplysia*, serotonin and the molluscan tetrapeptide, FMRFamide, close and open, respectively, a specialized subclass of potassium ion channels termed "K^+S," named because serotonin inactivates the channel (see also Chap. 50). Patch-clamp studies have shown that opening of the K^+S channel can be mimicked by 12-HPETE. Furthermore, this metabolite exerts a dual action, causing firstly a fast depolarization, followed by a slow hyperpolarization. The fast depolarization appears to be mediated by the 12-keto metabolite of 12-HPETE, whereas the slow hyperpolarization results from the activity of the cytochrome P_{450} monooxygenase, which forms the 11,12 epoxy metabolite, hepoxilin A_3 [3]. All of these metabolites are actively produced by neural tissue of *Aplysia*. Of further interest is the finding that 12-HPETE is a potent inhibitor of Ca^{2+}/calmodulin-dependent protein kinase, which catalyzes the phosphorylation of synapsin I in mammalian synaptic endings [16]. Thus, 12-lipoxygenase metabolites may also regulate neurotransmitter release and modulate synaptic strength. There are other examples of the modulation of potassium currents by arachidonic acid and its lipoxygenase metabolites, e.g., the G protein-gated muscarinic K^+ channel in atrial cardiac myocytes and similar channels in smooth muscle.

Long-term potentiation (LTP) of synaptic transmission [17] (see also Chap. 50) has been loosely implicated in learning and memory and has been the subject of intense investigation and controversy, particularly on whether its maintenance is determined by presynaptic or postsynaptic events. It seems clear that induction of LTP involves activation of glutamate receptors, which cause sufficient depolarization of the postsynaptic cell membrane to relieve the Mg^{2+} blockade of the *N*-methyl-D-aspartate (NMDA) type of receptors. Calcium enters the cell via the NMDA receptor ion channel and initiates the cascade of events that results in persistent enhancement of synaptic transmission. Recently it was shown that arachidonic acid and lipoxygenase metabolites are likely involved in the induction and expression of LTP. Glutamate and NMDA release arachidonic acid from hippocampal slices through activation of membrane-bound brain PLA_2 and markedly stimulate the formation of 12-HETE [18]. It has also been shown that following the induction of LTP, there is a small but rapid release of arachidonic acid and the synthesis of 12-HETE. The noncompetitive NMDA receptor antagonist MK-801 prevents this release. Lipoxygenase inhibitors and MK-801 also block the induction of LTP. It is uncertain what the individual roles of arachidonic acid and/or 12-lipoxygenase metabolites are. A current hypothesis is that arachidonic acid, released from postsynaptic membranes during induction of LTP, reaches the presynaptic terminals by free diffusion and facilitates the release of glutamate; i.e., it acts as a retrograde messenger. Caution is needed in this interpretation since another candidate molecule is nitric oxide synthesized from L-arginine by the constitutive calmodulin-dependent nitric oxide synthase. Analogs, such as N^G-nitro-L-arginine, block the induction of LTP in an arginine-reversible manner and so does bathing the hippocampal slices with hemoglobin, which binds nitric oxide but does not penetrate cells. Both nitric oxide and arachidonic acid may act as retrograde messengers in LTP but as yet this is far from proven.

In summary, arachidonic acid and eicosanoids exert both intracellular and intercellular actions in the nervous system. Their roles as second messengers or lipid mediators in neurotransmitter signal transduction and their paracrine influences on neighboring neurons and glia have been, and undoubtedly will continue to be, clarified.

EICOSANOIDS IN CNS PATHOLOGY

Seizures

Levels of eicosanoids are markedly increased as early as 30 sec after the onset of seizures. The highest levels of eicosanoids are reached between 2 and 6 min after the onset of seizure activity. The major metabolites are PGD_2, followed by $PGF_{2\alpha}$, PGE_2, TXB_2, and 6-keto-$PGF_{1\alpha}$. After about 30 min, eicosanoid levels nearly approach the basal value. Cyclooxygenase inhibitors, such as indomethacin, flurbiprofen, and diclofenac, block convulsion-induced eicosanoid synthesis without affecting the latency time or appearance of the clonic seizures. This clearly shows that the rise of cerebral eicosanoid concentration is secondary to the convulsive state [19].

The levels of sulfidopeptide leukotrienes are also increased following tonic-clonic seizures in the brain of spontaneously convulsing gerbils. Once again, the highest levels of the above leukotrienes are produced 6 min after seizure onset. The molecular mechanism of eicosanoid release after the onset of seizure activity is not fully understood. However, based on the release of arachidonic acid, one can speculate that stimulation of phospholipases and lipases may be involved. The fact that pretreatment of animals with dexamethasone decreases seizure-induced arachidonic acid release indicates the activation of PLA_2. Induction of seizures is also accompanied by increased levels of 1-stearoyl-2-arachidonoyl-*sn*-glycerol and inositol 1,4,5-trisphosphate, suggesting the involvement of phosphoinositide-specific phospholipase C. 1-Stearoyl-2-arachidonoyl-*sn*-glycerol can be hydrolyzed to fatty acids and glycerol by diacyl- and monoacylglycerol lipases. Increased availability of arachidonic acid in bicuculline-induced convulsing animals is accompanied by increased activity of eicosanoid-forming enzymes (see also Chap. 20).

Brain inflammation

Inflammation is defined as a complicated response of tissue involving several cell types (e.g., polymorphonuclear leukocytes, macrophages, lymphocytes, and mast cells) and many putative mediators and modulators (histamine, kinins, interferons, prostaglandins, thromboxanes, and leukotrienes). These mediators act in concert to amplify the inflammatory response, which is characterized by edema, hyperthermia, and loss of function [3,13]. The evidence that cyclooxygenase products are important mediators of signs of inflammation is conclusive; prostaglandins have been detected in inflammatory exudate at biologically active concentrations, and the cyclooxygenase is selectively inhibited by nonsteroidal antiinflammatory drugs (e.g., aspirin and indomethacin). LTB_4 has potent chemotactic and degranulating effects on polymorphonuclear leukocytes and produces polymorphonuclear leukocyte accumulation in the brain tissue *in vivo*. Synovial fluid from patients with rheumatoid arthritis and gout contains elevated levels of LTB_4.

The HPETE and HETE compounds formed from arachidonic acid via different lipoxygenase pathways are pharmacologically less active than LTB_4. However, they may also induce cell influx into the area of inflammation. Cysteinyl-leukotrienes (LTC_4, LTD_4, and LTE_4) may be involved in enhancement of vascular permeability, with extravascular plasma leakage and edema formation [20]. These leukotrienes are biosynthesized in inflammatory cells (e.g., macrophages, eosinophils) and there is good

evidence that they are formed in increased amount at inflammatory sites.

Brain injury and ischemia

Stimulation of phospholipases and lipases during ischemia results in the generation of free fatty acids, including arachidonic acid, which, during reperfusion, is either metabolized by cyclooxygenase to eicosanoids and lipid peroxides or converted to leukotrienes and hydroxy fatty acid by lipoxygenase. Among the vasoactive eicosanoids, thromboxane and prostacyclin are the most potent. They affect hemostasis and vascular integrity in an opposing manner. Thromboxane induces platelet aggregation and vasoconstriction, whereas prostacyclin inhibits platelet aggregation and produces vasodilation. Thus, the generation of eicosanoids during ischemia and reperfusion contributes to the onset of the alterations in the microcirculation [21–24].

The conversion of PGG_2 to PGH_2 by hydroperoxidase produces free radicals. The generation of free radicals in the hydrocarbon core of the cell membrane may induce a cross-linking reaction with membrane phospholipids and proteins, thereby changing the microenvironment and structure of the proteins and irreversibly affecting the plasma membrane and mitochondrial functions. This may be responsible for brain damage during ischemic injury and reperfusion. Fatty acid hydroperoxides that are produced in high concentration during ischemic insult inhibit the reacylation of phospholipids, and this inhibition may constitute another important mechanism of irreversible brain damage (see also Chap. 42).

Because leukotrienes enhance vascular permeability and are potent vasoconstrictors, they are known to exacerbate cellular damage caused by cerebral ischemia. Their concentration is increased significantly during ischemia and reperfusion, and abnormal effects on brain function can be antagonized by inhibitors of leukotriene synthesis. Leukotrienes also induce the reduction of Na,K

ATPase activity by which brain edema is produced during ischemic injury and reperfusion.

Cerebral vasospasm

Cerebral vasospasm is caused by subarachnoid hemorrhage or trauma and may lead to cerebral ischemia. The mechanism for this vasospasm is not known. It is proposed that constriction of the arteries is caused by endogenous substances whose synthesis and/or release is stimulated as a result of hemorrhage or mechanical stimuli. Prostaglandins are key mediators in the above process. Both PGE_2 and $PGF_{2\alpha}$ are potent constrictors of cerebral vessels and produce prolonged vasospasm when given intracisternally. The formation of prostaglandins within the arterial wall may be more important in the pathogenesis of vasospasm than the level of prostaglandins in cerebrospinal fluid [25,26].

PGI_2, because of its vasodilating activity and ability to inhibit platelet aggregation, is most important under physiological conditions. It is suggested that cerebral vasospasm may be a result of the decreased synthesis of this prostaglandin. The fact that cerebral vessels synthesize both vasodilator and vasoconstrictor prostaglandins indicates that an imbalance in the synthesis of either may result in vasospasm and migraine. Like PGE_1, PGI_2 also prevents release of degradative enzymes such as lysosomal proteases and phospholipases, acts as an antiinflammatory agent in these tissues, directly promotes epidermal growth, and relaxes vascular smooth muscle. Abnormal PGI_2 production is reported to occur in human and experimental models of atherosclerosis [27].

TXA_2 has a potent spasmogenic activity when applied topically to cerebral vessels. The constrictor activity of thromboxane on cerebral vessels is similar to that of $PGF_{2\alpha}$ and approximately twice that produced by serotonin.

Leukotrienes are also potent vasoconstrictors, and their biosynthesis is significantly increased in cerebral vasospasm.

REFERENCES

1. Innis, S. M. Essential fatty acids in growth and development. *Prog. Lipid Res.* 30:39–103, 1991.
2. Smith, W. L., Borgeat, P., and Fitzpatrick, F. A. The eicosanoids: Cyclooxygenase, lipoxygenase, and epoxygenase pathways. In D. E. Vance and J. Vance (eds.), *Biochemistry, Lipoproteins and Membranes.* New York: Elsevier Science Publishers B.V., 1991, Chap. 10, pp. 297–325.
3. Shimizu, T., and Wolfe, L. S. Arachidonic acid cascade and signal transduction. *J. Neurochem.* 55:1–15, 1990.
4. Snyder, F., Lee, T-C., and Blank, M. L. The role of transacylases in the metabolism of arachidonate and platelet activating factor. *Prog. Lipid Res.* 31:65–86, 1991.
5. Clark, J. D., Lin, L-L., Kriz, R. W., et al. A novel arachidonic acid-selective cytosolic PLA_2 contains a Ca^{2+}-dependent translocation domain with homology to PKC and GAP. *Cell* 65:1043–1051, 1991.
6. Hirashima, Y., Farooqui, A., Mills, J. S., and Horrocks, L. A. Identification and purification of calcium-independent phospholipase A_2 from bovine brain cytosol. *J. Neurochem.* 59:708–714, 1992.
7. Clark, M. A., Özgür, L. E., Conway, T. M., Dispoto, J., Crooke, S. T., and Bomalaski, J. S. Cloning of a phospholipase A_2-activating protein. *Proc. Natl. Acad. Sci. U.S.A.* 88:5418–5422, 1991.
8. Flower, R. J. Lipocortin and the mechanism of action of the glucocorticoids. *Br. J. Pharmacol.* 94:987–1015, 1988.
9. van Kuijk, F. J. G. M., Sevanian, A., Handelman, G. J., and Dratz, E. A. A new role for phospholipase A_2: Protection of membranes from lipid peroxidation damage. *Trends Biochem. Sci.* 12:31–34, 1987.
10. Farooqui, A. A., Hirashima, Y., and Horrocks, L. A. Brain phospholipases and their role in signal transduction. In N. G. Bazan, G. Toffano, and M. Murphy (eds.), *Neurobiology of Essential Fatty Acids.* New York: Plenum Press, 1992, pp. 11–25.
11. Sigal, E. The molecular biology of mammalian arachidonic acid metabolism. *Am. J. Physiol.* 260:L13–L28, 1991.
12. Galli, C., and Petroni, A. Eicosanoids and the central nervous system. *Ups. J. Med. Sci. Suppl.* 48:133–144, 1990.

13. Samuelsson, B., Dahlén, S. E., Lindren, J. Å., Rouzer, C. A., and Serhan, C. N. Leukotrienes and lipoxins: Structures, biosynthesis, and biological effects. *Science* 237:1171–1176, 1987.

14. Hayaishi, O. Molecular mechanisms of sleep-wake regulation: Roles of prostaglandins D_2 and E_2. *FASEB J.* 5:2575–2581, 1991.

15. Piomelli, D., and Greengard, P. Lipoxygenase metabolites of arachidonic acid in neuronal transmembrane signalling. *Trends Pharmacol. Sci.* 11:367–373, 1990.

16. Piomelli, D., and Greengard, P. Bidirectional control of phospholipase A_2 activity by Ca^{2+}/calmodulin-dependent protein kinase II, cAMP-dependent protein kinase, and casein kinase II. *Proc. Natl. Acad. Sci. U.S.A.* 88: 6770–6774, 1991.

17. Bliss, T. V. P., Errington, M. L., Lynch, M. A., and Williams, J. H. Presynaptic mechanisms in hippocampal long-term potentiation. In *Symposia on Quantitative Biology, The Brain.* New York: Cold Spring Harbor Laboratory Press, 1990, Vol. LV, pp. 119–129.

18. Pellerin, L., and Wolfe, L. S. Release of arachidonic acid by NMDA-receptor activation in the rat hippocampus. *Neurochem. Res.* 16: 983–989, 1991.

19. Hertting, G., and Seregi, A. Synthesis, origin and involvement of eicosanoids in the convulsing brain. In N. G. Bazan (ed.), *Lipid Mediators in Ischemic Brain Damage and Experimental Epilepsy.* Basel: Karger, 1990, Vol. 4, pp. 162–189.

20. Unterberg, A., Schmidt, W., Wahl, M., Ellis, E .F., Marmarou, A., and Baethmann, A. Evidence against leukotrienes as mediators of brain edema. *J. Neurosurg.* 74:773–780, 1991.

21. Galli, C., Petroni, A., Bertazzo, A., and Sarti, S. Arachidonic acid and its metabolites during cerebral ischemia and recirculation. In A. I. Barkai and N. G. Bazan (eds.), *Arachidonic Acid Metabolism in the Nervous System: Physiological and Pathological Significance.* New York: The New York Academy of Sciences, 1989, Vol. 559, pp. 352–364.

22. Hsu, C. Y., Liu, T. H., Xu, J., et al. Arachidonic acid and its metabolites in cerebral ischemia. In A. I. Barkai and N. G. Bazan (eds.), *Arachidonic Acid Metabolism in the Nervous System: Physiological and Pathological Significance.* New York: The New York Academy of Sciences, 1989, Vol. 559, pp. 282–295.

23. Chen, S. T., Hsu, C. Y., Hogan, E. L., Halushka, P. V., Linet, O. I., and Yatsu, F. M. Thromboxane, prostacyclin, and leukotrienes in cerebral ischemia. *Neurology* 36: 466–470, 1986.

24. Braquet, P., Spinnewyn, B., Demerle, C., et al. The role of platelet-activating factor in cerebral ischemia and related disorders. In A. I. Barkai and N. G. Bazan (eds.), *Arachidonic Acid Metabolism in the Nervous System: Physiological and Pathological Significance.* New York: The New York Academy of Sciences, 1989, Vol. 559, pp. 296–312.

25. Macdonald, R. L., and Weir, B. K. A. A review of hemoglobin and the pathogenesis of cerebral vasospasm. *Stroke* 22:971–982, 1991.

26. Yokota, M., Tani, E., and Maeda, Y. Biosynthesis of leukotrienes in canine cerebral vasospasm. *Stroke* 20:527–533, 1989.

27. Moncada, S. Biology and therapeutic potential of prostacyclin. *Stroke* 14:157–172, 1983.

PART THREE

Molecular Neurobiology

CHAPTER 24

Gene Expression in the Mammalian Nervous System

ALLAN J. TOBIN

Basic Neurochemistry: Molecular, Cellular, and Medical Aspects, 5th Ed., edited by G. J. Siegel et al. Published by Raven Press, Ltd., New York, 1994. Correspondence to Allan J. Tobin, Department of Biology, University of California, Los Angeles, California 90024-1606.

In confronting the mammalian brain, molecular biologists face a seemingly impossible challenge: How do cells with the same genetic information come to have such diverse cellular phenotypes, each with the capacity to respond characteristically to changes in local environment and in the experience of the organism as a whole? The answers to this question must be based on an understanding of gene expression and its regulation, the subject of this chapter. The material and the viewpoint here are similar to those of several recent chapters and reviews [1–3].

during development and in response to environmental cues has undoubtedly provided unparalleled opportunities for rapid physiological adaptation to varying environments and (in the case of our own species) efficient cultural adaptation through learning and language. More than any other organ, the brain illustrates the tight interaction between heredity and environment in the determination of phenotype, both of cells and of organisms. Moreover, the human brain, whose regulatory complexity is greater than any other organ, has become the major agent for modifying our common environment.

THE CELLULAR COMPLEXITY OF THE BRAIN REQUIRES COMBINATORIAL CODING OF GENE EXPRESSION

The human brain contains more than 10^{12} neurons. Each neuron is arguably unique, with a distinct size, shape, position, and pattern of connections, transmitters, and responses to chemical and electrical cues. But the human genome contains at most only enough information for about 10^6 genes. Even if all these genes were expressed in the brain, there would not be enough information to specify each neuron separately.

As in the case of the immune system, the key to understanding the complexity of the brain lies in combinations. Just as nine-digit zip codes specify each block in the United States, so could a relatively small number of genes specify the unique properties of every cell in the brain. In this chapter I discuss the general principles of gene expression in eukaryotes and show how variations in the processing of genetic information lead to the fantastic diversity of cells in the brain.

With its huge number of potential combinations of expressed genes, the brain has an extraordinarily high informational content. Flexibility in gene regulation in brain cells may explain the rapid spread of mammals into a wide variety of ecological niches. The evolved ability to express distinctive gene combinations in individual cell types

GENE EXPRESSION IN EUKARYOTES

The familiar central dogma of molecular biology states that information flows from DNA to RNA to proteins. Cells copy the information contained in the nucleotide sequence of DNA into corresponding nucleotide sequences of RNA. For structural genes—stretches of DNA that code for proteins—the carrier is *messenger RNA*, or *mRNA*. In eukaryotes, mRNAs are produced in the nucleus and travel to the cytoplasm. There, in association with the ribosomes and other synthetic machinery, each mRNA directs the synthesis of a single type of polypeptide chain, which directly or indirectly assembles into a mature protein.

DNA and RNA each consist of linear chains of four nucleotide building blocks. Information in DNA and RNA is thus contained in dialects of a single language, and the conversion of information from DNA into RNA is called *transcription*.

Each polypeptide consists of linear chains of 20 amino acid building blocks. The information in proteins is thus written in a different language, and the conversion of information from RNA to protein is called *translation*.

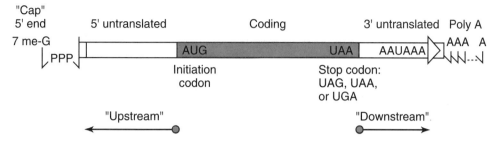

FIG. 1. Structure of a eukaryotic mRNA. A typical eukaryotic mRNA, reading from the 5' end ("upstream") on the left, to the 3' end ("downstream") on the right. The 5' untranslated region is usually 10 to 200 bases long, and the 3'-untranslated region is 50 to 2,000 bases long. The average size of the coding region in abundant mRNAs is about 1,500 bases.

All eukaryotic mRNAs share common features

Each mRNA contains coding information that specifies the sequence of amino acid residues in a type of polypeptide chain. In addition, each mRNA contains noncoding information that includes control signals for translation: (a) an initiation site for translation, a sequence that dictates both the starting site of the polypeptide and the *frame* (phase) in which the triplet code is read; (b) a termination sequence that signals the end of the polypeptide chain; (c) a binding site slightly "upstream" from the initiation site that facilitates binding to ribosomes; and (d) other "upstream" and "downstream" sequences that contribute to the transport and stability of the mRNA. Most eukaryotic mRNAs also contain two additional structures that are added after transcription and are not copied from DNA: (a) an inverted "cap" at the 5' end; and (b) a "tail" for 50 to 150 residues of adenylic acid (poly A) at the 3' end of the mRNA. The sequence AAUAAA in the primary transcript is the usual signal for the addition of poly A some 20 bases downstream (Fig. 1).

Eukaryotic genes contain more information than their corresponding mRNAs

Most eukaryotic genes also contain long stretches of DNA that are transcribed into RNA but are excised before the primary transcript matures into functional mRNA. These interruptions in the structural information for polypeptide synthesis are called *intervening sequences,* or *introns.* In contrast, the coding sequences are called *exons* (Fig. 2).

Mature mRNA usually results from an elaborate process that removes introns and splices together the remaining exons, like so many pieces of film or magnetic tape. DNA and the primary RNA transcript also contain sequences that specify where the splices are to occur. The pattern of splicing of a single transcript can vary from tissue to tissue, as discussed below.

Genes contain still more noncoding sequences. Many of these contribute to the reg-

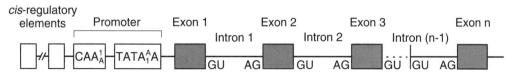

FIG. 2. Structure of a eukaryotic gene.

ulation of gene expression. In particular, some regulatory sequences serve to specify the cells in which a given gene is expressed.

Molecular biologists are now able to create specific alterations in DNA sequences of suspected function. They then can examine the effect of these changes on gene expression in a test system, e.g., in cell-free systems able to transcribe DNA into RNA, in cultured cells programmed to express recombinant DNAs with which they have been transformed (or "transfected"), or even in *transgenic* animals, in which altered genes are transferred to fertilized eggs and become part of the genome (see Chap. 26). Among the sequences identified in this way are (a) *promoters*, which specify the starting point and direction of transcription; (b) cis-*regulatory elements* (also called *response elements* or *enhancers*), which facilitate the transcription of neighboring DNA, independent of the element's orientation, and relatively independent of its position; and (c) termination signals.

DNA regulatory sequences specify the start point and the end point of transcription, as well as the temporal and spatial patterns of expression

Promoters, regulatory elements, and termination signals usually consist of 6–20 base pairs (bp) of DNA, which bind specific proteins. Most eukaryotic promoters, for example, contain the sequence "TATA," embedded in a longer consensus sequence, about 25 bp upstream from the start site of transcription. This "TATA box" specifically binds a transcription factor, TFIID, which interacts with other transcription factors and RNA polymerase II [4]. Similarly, regulatory elements can bind to specific regulatory proteins, called *transcription factors*. The binding of a transcription factor to a regulatory element can either affect the immediate rate of transcription, for example, by increasing or decreasing the probability of initiation by the RNA polymerase complex, or it could produce a stable changes in *chromatin structure*

(the manner in which DNA and nuclear proteins assemble into a compact structure within the nucleus). Changes in chromatin structure can produce a long-term change in the rate of transcription by altering the accessibility of a particular gene to the transcriptional apparatus. In the case of such structural alterations, the continuous presence of the *trans*-acting factor might not be required.

Some stable changes in chromatin structure do occur during *cytodifferentiation,* the process during which a cell acquires its specialized properties. Such changes are often revealed experimentally by changes in the susceptibility of a particular gene (in isolated nuclei) to digestion by added nucleases, suggesting that nuclease susceptibility may be a good index of accessibility to RNA polymerase. Nuclease digestion experiments (especially with DNAse I) have shown that genes actively transcribed (by RNA polymerase) in a particular cell are often more susceptible to digestion; for example, globin genes are preferentially susceptible to digestion by added DNAse I in red cell precursors but not in oviduct [5].

In addition, DNA sequences that bind effector proteins, such as polymerase or an enhancer-binding protein, may have distorted structures that render them hypersensitive to DNAse I digestion. Probes of chromatin structure thus suggest that the pattern of active genes within a given cell type depends on developmental history as well as on the expression of specific effectors at a given moment.

Post-translational events provide additional opportunities for regulation

After mRNAs are translated into polypeptides, still more information processing occurs, with attendant opportunities for developmental regulation. Polypeptides fold into specific conformations and assemble into complexes with other polypeptides. The creation of three-dimensional structures from linear polypeptides depends not only on the amino acid sequence of each polypeptide, but also on the ionic conditions and pH of the surrounding cytosol, as well as on the concentrations of specific *allosteric effectors* (small molecules that alter a protein's conformation and activity). In addition, the covalent structure of each polypeptide may be altered by disulfide bond formation, protease cleavage, glycosylation, phosphorylation, methylation, fatty acid acylation, and covalent linkage to peptides or to membrane lipids. These covalent changes often affect the conformation of individual polypeptides, their association with other polypeptides, and their biological function. The activity of many proteins depends upon their regulated phosphorylation by protein kinases and dephosphorylation by phosphatases.

The flow of information from DNA to functional protein is the same in the brain as in other organs. For many years, however, researchers avoided the brain for mechanistic studies, because of its multiplicity of cell types and the complexity of gene expression. With the advent of recombinant DNA techniques and the polymerase chain reaction (PCR) for studying the expression of specific genes, many molecular biologists have undertaken detailed studies of the structure and expression of genes important to brain function. (See below and Chap. 25 for a discussion of these methods.)

Molecular hybridization techniques allow the detection and measurement of specific DNA and RNA sequences

The identification and quantification of specific sequences in DNA and RNA depend on duplex formation by polynucleotide strands with complementary sequences. The stability of such duplexes depends on the length of the complementary sequences, the degree of matching between the two strands, the temperature, the salt concentration, and the presence of compounds (such as formamide) that interfere with the interactions of the two strands. Researchers can distinguish among exact and inexact matches by

noting the temperature at which duplexes dissociate or "melt." Perfect or near-perfect matches maintain their double-strandedness under stringent conditions, that is, at high temperature and low salt concentration.

Formation of duplexes between previously associated DNA strands is called *reannealing*, or *reassociation*. Formation of duplexes between DNA and RNA, RNA and RNA, or between DNA sequences not originally associated, for example, between genomic and recombinant DNAs is called *hybridization*.

Hybridization techniques are at the center of the technical repertoire of molecular biologists, as discussed in Chapter 25. Hybridization experiments allow researchers to identify DNA fragments, recombinant DNA molecules, and RNAs with specified base sequences. Such identification depends on the use of molecular "probes" of known sequence, usually recombinant DNAs or synthetic oligonucleotides.

Hybridization may be performed (a) in solution; (b) with blots of DNA or RNA onto various supports, most frequently nitrocellulose or nylon membranes; or (c) on tissue sections. Solution hybridization is the best understood and follows the kinetic course of simple bimolecular or pseudomonomolecular reactions. Hybridization to blots of DNA (Southern blots) or to blots of RNA ("Northern" blots, a now accepted jargon that contrasts RNA blots with the DNA blots developed by E. Southern), dot blots, and slot blots—are technically much simpler, however. Hybridization to extracted RNA allows researchers both to identify the sizes of specific mRNAs and their precursors and to estimate the amount of each RNA species in a given extract.

Molecular neurobiologists now use a variant of the polymerase chain reaction—starting with a DNA copy of extracted mRNA (cDNA)—to detect the presence of individual mRNAs and even to determine quantitative changes in their expression. To detect a specific sequence, one does not need a recombinant DNA, but only a pair of specific oligonucleotides that span a known sequence. These oligonucleotides are used as primers for the repetitive replication of the specific DNA sequence that they flank (as discussed in Chap. 25). In addition, a recently described method can copy the mRNA of a single cell into cDNA, which can then be analyzed later by PCR [6]. In this method, oligonucleotide primers, reverse transcriptase (an enzyme that copies RNA into DNA), and appropriate precursors are injected directly into a cell, which serves as a reaction container. The virtue of this approach is that the chosen cell may first be characterized by electrophysiological techniques. This micromethod may thus provide a way of understanding the relationship between the electrophysiological experience of a cell and its pattern of gene expression.

Hybridization of probes for specific mRNAs to tissue sections is called *in situ hybridization* or *hybridization histochemistry*. *In situ* hybridization is especially useful for detecting the cellular distribution of mRNAs in heterogenous tissues such as the brain. Most investigators now use RNA probes labeled with ^{35}S or with a nonradioactive probe (such as digoxigenin) that can be detected by immunohistochemistry. The RNA probes are transcribed *in vitro* from recombinant DNAs containing a sequence of interest attached to sequences that are recognized by specific bacteriophage RNA polymerases.

MORE THAN ONE POLYPEPTIDE CAN ARISE FROM A SINGLE GENE

Most eukaryotic genes are mosaics of exons and introns. In the now established picture of mRNA production, transcription begins at a single promoter and yields a single primary transcript containing all the introns and exons. All primary transcripts are immediately modified by the addition of a "cap" consisting of a 7-methylguanosine residue at the 5' end. Almost all transcripts that will eventually exit to the cytoplasm are further

modified at their 3' ends by the addition of 200 to 250 adenylic residues (poly A). Polyadenylation occurs in the nucleus soon after the termination of transcription. Cytoplasmic nucleases subsequently nibble the poly A tail down to about 50 to 150 residues. Molecular machinery within the nucleus, including ribonucleoprotein particles containing small nuclear RNAs, then cut and splice the primary transcripts to produce mature mRNAs that lack introns.

Although many genes appear to produce only one primary transcript and a unique mature mRNA, other genes produce many alternative forms of primary transcripts and mature mRNAs. Primary transcripts may start or end at different sites and may have more than one site for the addition of poly A, and different splicing events may string together different subsets of exons from a single primary transcript. (In such a case, one mRNA's exon becomes another mRNA's intron, thus fogging definitions. Most investigators now use "exon" to refer to any segment of DNA or RNA that codes for a polypeptide sequence segment in *any* cell.) A single stretch of DNA may thus encode a variety of polypeptides. Sometimes, a single cell may simultaneously express these different polypeptides; in other cases, the pattern of transcription and splicing is subject to developmental regulation. After geneticists spent decades arriving at the textbook definition, "one gene—one polypeptide chain," subsequent studies of gene expression conclusively showed that one gene can encode many different polypeptide chains, often with divergent functions.

Alternative splicing, polyadenylation, and editing of primary transcripts yield alternative RNAs from the same gene

The nervous system provides many examples of the same segment of DNA encoding several polypeptide chains. Two contrasting examples are especially instructive: (a) the multiple mRNAs for myelin basic protein, and (b) the alternative polyadenylation and splicing of a gene that encodes the Ca^{2+}-regulating peptide calcitonin in thyroid and a putative neurotransmitter called calcitonin gene-related peptide (CGRP) in brain.

Transcription of the gene for myelin basic protein appears to begin and end at single sites to yield a single primary transcript containing seven exons and six introns [7]. Alternative patterns of splicing yield at least five species of mRNA that encode five polypeptide chains of slightly different sizes. These polypeptides have common sequences at each end and slightly different sequences in the middle.

No one knows whether these five polypeptides have different functions in myelin, but similar alternative splicing of the neural cell adhesion molecule (N-CAM) results in alternative proteins that either contain or do not contain a transmembrane domain, and the two products differ in their manner of association with the cell membrane (Fig. 3A). An even greater range of functional differences results from alternative splicing of the RNA encoding the potassium channel from the *Shaker* gene of *Drosophila* (see Chap. 4).

In contrast, as illustrated in Fig. 3B, the precursor of the mRNAs for calcitonin and CGRP contains six exons, five introns, and two sites for polyadenylation. In the thyroid, the transcript is polyadenylated at the end of the fourth exon, whereas in neurons, poly A lies at the end of the sixth exon. Splicing in the thyroid yields calcitonin mRNA, which consist of exons 1, 2, 3, and 4; in neurons, however, exon 4 is removed, and exons 5 and 6 are attached to the mRNA. The two mRNAs each encode polypeptides that are precursors of the biologically active peptides. Exons 1 and 6 do not encode translated polypeptide sequence. Post-translational proteolytic processing in both thyroid and brain removes the amino acid sequences encoded by exons 2 and 3, so the final calcitonin peptide in thyroid derives entirely from exon 4, and CGRP in brain from exon 5. Similar alternative patterns of polyadenylation and splicing occur for the common primary transcript for two tachykinin peptides, substance P and

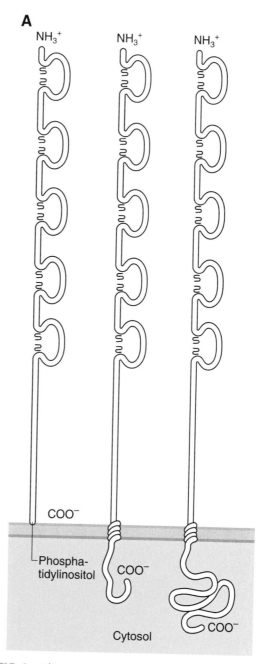

FIG. 3.   Alternative splicing. **A:** Different forms of N-CAM with different membrane-association domains are the products of alternative splicing (redrawn with permission from Alberts, et al. *The Molecular Biology of the Cell, 2nd ed.* Garland Publishing, 1989).

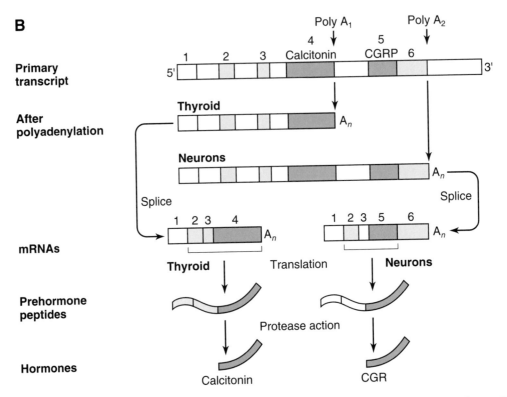

FIG. 3. *(continued).* **B:** Differential processing of the primary transcripts from the calcitonin gene. (Redrawn with permission from Darnell, J., Lodish, H., and Baltimore, D. *Molecular Cell Biology.* New York: Scientific American Books, 1990.)

substance K, and for amyloid precursor protein [8].

Finally, recent work with kinetoplastid protozoa has demonstrated the occurrence of *RNA editing,* a process that changes the sequence of an RNA molecule in a manner not dependent on template DNA [9]. Such a single sequence alteration occurs in the RNA of a glutamate receptor subunit and leads to a functional change in the encoded receptor [10].

mRNA translation and degradation are also subject to modulation

Once mature mRNAs arrive in the cytoplasm, they become subject to further regulation through alterations in the efficiencies of translation and in the rapidity of their degradation [11]. The classic example of transla-

tional control of gene expression is the mRNA contained in the sea urchin egg prior to fertilization: The unfertilized sea urchin egg contains many apparently mature maternal mRNAs, but translation is extremely slow until after fertilization.

The egg yolk protein vitellogenin provides an excellent example of the regulation of mRNA stability: Estrogen increases the half-life of vitellogenin mRNA by about 30-fold. No such changes have been shown in the development of neurons or glia, but studies of the processing and stability of brain RNAs are still in their infancy.

Post-translational processing of single polypeptides can vary among cell types

Even after the production of mature mRNA and its translation into a polypeptide, cells can still regulate the character and amount of biologically active gene products. The 134 amino acid residue polypeptide pro-opio-melanocortin (POMC), for example, is a precursor of at least seven biologically active peptides, including adrenocorticotropic hormone; β-endorphin; β- and γ-lipotropic hormones; and α-, β-, and γ-melanocyte-stimulating hormones (see Chaps. 15 and 16). The pattern of post-translational processing of POMC in turn is likely to depend on the activity of cell-type specific proteases, the products of other developmentally regulated genes.

Other regulatable post-translational processes include covalent modification and the association of a polypeptide with itself or with other proteins to form homo- or hetero-oligomers. Among the most important and best studied covalent modifications are phosphorylations by a variety of kinases (see Chaps. 10, 21, and 22). Here we observe that specific post-translational modifications result from the action of extracellular signals, such as growth factors and neurotransmitters, acting through second messengers, such as cyclic AMP (cAMP), Ca^{2+}, or diacylglycerol. Furthermore, the proteins whose activity is modified by regulated phosphorylations may themselves regulate the expression of other genes. The well-characterized transcription factor CREB (*c*yclic AMP *r*esponse *e*lement-*b*inding protein), for example, is subject to phosphorylation both by cyclic AMP-dependent kinase and calcium/calmodulin-dependent protein kinase (CaM kinase); phosphorylation by either kinase activates the protein and thereby stimulates transcription.

THE SEQUENCE ORGANIZATION OF GENES AND REGULATORY ELEMENTS SUGGEST THEIR EVOLUTIONARY HISTORY

The many steps required for the production of a biologically active protein almost certainly result from the opportunism of evolution. The first genes were probably RNA rather than DNA, and present genes probably resulted from the combination of small coding regions. Like contemporary eukaryotic genes, the earliest genes, we now think, were mosaics of exons and introns. Because genomes continually rearranged in evolutionary time, the duplication and shuffling of exons allowed the sharing of useful structural domains by several or many genes.

Searches of protein sequence databases demonstrate the presence of similar sequence segments in many proteins, and analyses of the three-dimensional structures of proteins reveal nearly identical three-dimensional motifs. This similarity of sequence and structure attests to the common origin (that is, the *homology*) of proteins such as myoglobin and hemoglobin. Similarly, proteins that act as transcription factors share common sequence motifs and appear to have derived from common ancestral motifs.

In speaking about sequence matches at either the amino acid or nucleotide level, one should reserve the word "homology" for its proper evolutionary context—meaning derivation from a common ancestor. Thus myoglobin and hemoglobin are homologous in the same sense as are a bat's wing and a human arm. The commonly used jargon "percent homology" (which thus resembles the expression "percent pregnant") should be replaced by "percent identity" or "percent similarity" to encompass conservative amino acid substitutions.

Sequence matches, however, do not only result from homology and divergent evolution. Sequence similarity can also result from convergent evolution. The common short DNA sequences of transcriptional regulatory elements may result from the selective advantage that these sequences would give for the appropriate cell-specific or temporal expression of the adjacent structural genes. The variable distance between such elements and the regulated genes would greatly increase the chances of a particular sequence arising by chance mutation rather than by divergence from a duplicated ancestral sequence.

Gene rearrangements

Apart from the evolutionary significance of gene rearrangements, we would like to know whether they may contribute to gene regulation in the brain. In the immune systems of vertebrates, DNA rearrangements occur during the development of an individual organism, in the cytodifferentiation of both B and T lymphocytes. In addition, loss and rearrangement of DNA occur during oogenesis in *Drosophila* and amphibia. A recent report proposed that such rearrangement may occur in the brain, but this conclusion has been challenged on technical grounds [12,13]. It seems fair to say that no compelling evidence of gene rearrangement in mammals presently exists outside the immune system.

Multigene families

Duplications and rearrangements of entire ancestral genes (in contrast to the rearrangement of exons alone) were instrumental in the evolution of the many *multigene families* of the contemporary mammalian genome. The characteristics of multigene families include (a) multiple copies; (b) related sequences; (c) parallel (but not necessarily identical) functions of the gene products; and (d) usually distinctive patterns of developmental regulation for individual family members.

Multigene families almost certainly arose by gene duplication, unequal crossing over, and sequence divergence. In many cases (such as the α and β globin families) family members lie next to each other on a single chromosome. In other cases, however, the individual genes of a family have dispersed to different chromosomes.

The nervous system provides many examples of such families whose members differ in their function or their regulation. For example, a two-member multigene family encodes two forms of the GABA-synthesizing enzyme glutamate decarboxylase (GAD_{65} and GAD_{67}). The two GADs fulfill the definitions of a multigene family: (a) they derive from two genes on two different chromosomes, (b) they share about 65% sequence identity, at both the nucleotide and amino acid levels; (c) they both catalyze the decarboxylation of glutamate to form GABA, but with differing enzymatic properties; and (d) they are independently regulated during development and in response to experimental manipulations [14].

The GAD family also illustrates another common characteristic of multigene families—independent selective pressures on individual family members. While the two forms of GAD, GAD_{65} and GAD_{67}, differ at 35% of their amino acid residues in both rats and humans, human and rat GAD_{65} are 96% identical, while human and rat GAD_{67} are 97% identical. This suggests (a) that the two GADs diverged before the evolutionary divergence of rats and humans (and probably before the mammalian radiation); and (b) that natural selection maintained the divergent sequences, presumably because evolutionary success required the functions of both proteins.

Larger multigene families are also important in the determining characteristics of different types of neurons. Examples include

1. The G-protein superfamily that includes genes for the muscarinic acetylcholine receptor (see Chaps. 10, 11, and 21), the β-adrenergic receptor (see Chap. 12), rhodopsin (see Chap. 7), and odorant receptors (see Chap. 8);

2. The ligand-gated channel superfamily that includes the four subunits of the nicotinic acetylcholine receptor (see Chap. 11), the γ-aminobutyric acid ($GABA_A$) receptor, the glycine receptor (see Chap. 18), and some receptors for excitatory amino acids (see Chap. 17);

3. A conductance channel family that includes the voltage-dependent K^+- and Na^+-channel polypeptides (see Chap. 4);

4. A family of neurotrophic factors (the neurotrophins) that includes nerve growth factor, brain-derived growth factor; and also a family of receptors for these neurotrophins; and

5. Families of transporters: one for amine and amino acid neurotransmitters, including GABA, and another for glutamate (see Chap. 3).

Besides the families responsible for the functional properties of neurons, several other gene families encode proteins that regulate transcription (see below).

HYBRIDIZATION TECHNIQUES HAVE ALLOWED ESTIMATES OF THE COMPLEXITY OF GENE EXPRESSION IN THE MAMMALIAN BRAIN

Even before they could study the expression of specific genes in the brain, molecular biologists could address questions regarding the sizes of the brain's transcriptional and translational repertoires. The approach was to use hybridization of appropriate DNAs and RNAs to determine the fraction of an organism's DNA that could form complementary duplexes. Hybridization with mRNA gives an index of how many genes are likely to be translated into protein, while hybridization with nuclear RNA (nRNA) gave an index of how many genes are transcribed. As might be expected, not all DNA is transcribed into RNA, and much more of the informational capacity of the genome is expressed in the brain than in any other tissue.

The haploid genome of a mammal consists of about 3×10^9 nucleotide pairs. If all this DNA specified the amino acid sequences of polypeptides, it could encode 1 million polypeptides, each 1,000 amino acid residues long.

How many genes are expressed in the brain?

A typical eukaryotic gene contains much DNA that does not code for polypeptides, with as much as 95 percent of an organism's DNA specifying introns, known regulatory sequences, and sequences of unknown function, both within and between genes. Some of the unexplained noncoding DNA may have a regulatory role; much of it, however, may represent DNA that makes no contribution to phenotype—such sequences have been called "selfish DNA."

Molecular hybridization experiments permit one to determine the fraction of the genome that is expressed as mRNA. Such experiments show the complexity of gene expression in the brain: The brain contains about two to three times more information in mRNA than other tissues. Similar experiments with nRNA show that the brain as a whole transcribes at least 30 percent of genomic DNA sequences.

Knowing the amount of DNA expressed in mRNA and the average size of mRNA, we can estimate the average number of genes expressed in the brain. The average size of brain-specific mRNAs is almost 5 kilobases (kb), two to three times the average size of the abundant mRNAs expressed in other tissues. Present estimates range from about 30,000 to 200,000 different genes expressed in brain [15]. We do not yet understand why brain-specific mRNAs should be longer, on average, than those of other tissues.

More complex brains do not depend on more genes

Cows, mice, and humans all have about the same amount of DNA per cell, but their brains differ dramatically in both cellular and intellectual complexity. A mouse brain, for example, contains 10–100 fold fewer cells than the human brain, but about the same number of total genes and expressed genes. The greater complexity of the human brain, then, apparently results from factors other than the overall number of expressed genes. It seems likely that the complexity of the brain depends on combinations and interactions at the cellular level.

Does gene expression in the brain differ from that in other organs?

More mRNAs are expressed in the brain than in other organs, and brain-specific mRNAs appear to be larger than those expressed elsewhere. Gene expression in the brain also appears to differ from that in other tissues in the extent of polyadenylation of isolated mRNA. In mammalian tissues other than the brain, more than 90 percent of isolated mRNA molecules contain poly A tails. Almost all mRNA isolated from fetal rat and mouse brains also contains such poly A tails. In adult rodent brains, however, less than 50 percent of isolated mRNA (defined as polysomal RNA that is neither ribosomal RNA nor transfer RNA) contains poly A. RNA lacking poly A is termed (poly A)$^-$ RNA. In other tissues, (poly A)$^-$ RNA makes up less than 10 percent of the total mRNA. Several groups suggested the existence of a large class of brain-specific (poly A)$^-$ mRNA that appears late in development.

An alternative, now generally accepted, explanation for the high level of (poly A)$^-$ RNA in the brain is that the late-appearing, brain-specific mRNAs are substantially larger than the mRNAs expressed in fetal brain [15]. The larger mRNAs are more sensitive to breakage during isolation. If a 5-kb mRNA is cut in two, only the 3' portion will contain a poly A sequence. The 5' portion will appear to be a (poly A)$^-$ mRNA whose size is comparable to that of abundant mRNAs. Although a few mRNAs in higher organisms, notably those encoding the histones, are known not to contain poly A tails, there are at present no defined examples of brain-specific mRNAs that lack poly A.

Although gene expression in the brain is more complicated than in other tissues, it may not be fundamentally different. Rather, the complexity of the brain may result from the utilization of many mechanisms used more sparingly in other tissues.

Patterns of gene expression vary among brain regions and among individual cells

Anatomical boundaries within the brain define regions of the brain that differ in organization, connections, and use of neurotransmitters. Ligand binding studies and immunocytochemistry have shown that specific neurotransmitter-related proteins are differentially distributed; for example, D_2 dopamine receptors are found in highest concentrations in the striatum (see Chap. 12), and the NMDA-type of glutamate receptors are found in highest concentrations in the hippocampus and dentate gyrus (see Chap. 17). Many neurodegenerative diseases preferentially affect specific regions of the brain, for example, the substantia nigra in Parkinson's disease, the striatum in Huntington's disease (see Chap. 44), and the basal forebrain in Alzheimer's disease (see Chap. 45).

In general, individual brain regions are similar in the total number of genes expressed, and molecular hybridization experiments have failed to identify distinctive, regionally confined classes of mRNA. Several groups, however, have identified mRNAs that are preferentially expressed in specific cell populations by taking advantage of subtractive hybridization techniques, which identify mRNAs that are present in one tissue at much higher levels than in another tissue. One mRNA specifically expressed in photoreceptor cells of the mouse retina, for example, is the site of the mutation responsible for a type of retinal degeneration, *rds* (retinal degeneration slow) [16]. (See Chap. 7.)

Immunocytochemistry, ligand binding studies, and *in situ* hybridization to mRNA within individual cells all indicate that various classes of cells differ in their expression of individual mRNAs. For example, GAD_{65} and GAD_{67}, and their corresponding mRNAs, are present in specific cell types in the cerebellum, hippocampus, cortex, thalamus, as well as in other regions of the brain. While virtually all classes of neurons that contain one GAD also contain the other, individual neuron types differ in the relative amounts of the two mRNAs. As illustrated in Fig. 4, for example, Purkinje cells and Golgi cells of the cerebellar cortex both produce GABA, and each cell type contains both GAD_{65} and GAD_{67}. The two cell types contain approximately equal concentrations of GAD_{67} mRNA, but Golgi cells have much greater concentrations of GAD_{65} mRNA. Individual cell types, rather than anatomically

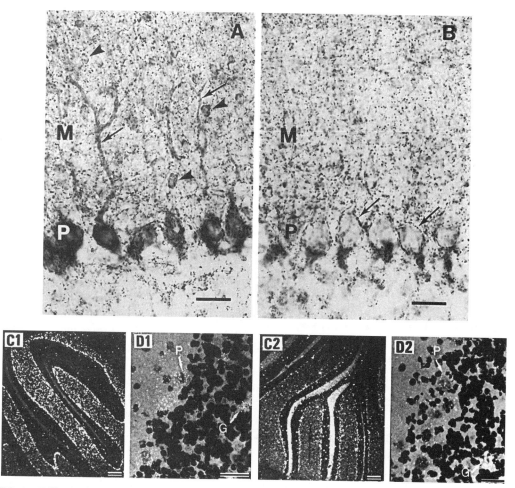

FIG. 4. Differential expression of the two glutamic decarboxylases in the cerebellar cortex. Immunohistochemical localization of **A:** GAD_{67} mostly in Purkinje cell bodies (P) and dendrites *(arrows);* also in probable basket cell neurons *(arrowheads);* (M) molecular layer. **B:** GAD_{65} mostly in axon terminals on Purkinje soma *(arrows)* and in dark-staining clumps at base of Purkinje soma which are probable basket cell terminals. **C1–D2:** Autoradiography following *in situ* hybridization with probes for the two GAD mRNAs. **C1,D1:** GAD_{67} mRNA is expressed at similar levels in Golgi (G) and Purkinje (P) neuronal cell bodies. **C2,D2:** GAD_{65} mRNA is expressed at higher levels in Golgi than in Purkinje neuronal cell bodies. Bar, 1 mm in C1 and C2; bar, 50 μm in D1 and D2.

defined regions, seem to be the units of developmental regulation of gene expression in the brain.

CIS-REGULATORY ELEMENTS AND *TRANS*-ACTING FACTORS CONTRIBUTE TO CELL-SPECIFIC REGULATION

Among the most striking advances since the 4th edition of this book has been the acceler-

ating increase in knowledge of transcriptional regulation. Most of this information has come from three kinds of experiments—the molecular characterization of genes that disrupt the normal development of fruit flies (*Drosophila melanogaster*) and roundworms (*Caenorhabditis elegans*), *in vitro* reconstruction of RNA synthesis from purified proteins and DNAs, and transfection of cells with recombinant DNA molecules. These studies have identified scores of cis-

regulatory DNA elements, DNA sequences whose presence is necessary for the regulated expression of the adjacent structural gene, as well dozens of *trans-acting proteins* (or *transcription factors*), which bind to *cis*-regulatory sequences and either activate or inhibit transcription. An amazingly convergent view has emerged: Not only do invertebrates and vertebrates (and in some cases even yeast) employ the same regulatory strategies, but in many cases they also use very closely related regulatory molecules.

How complex is gene regulation?

Researchers have estimated that 10% of genes in *E. coli* encode regulatory proteins, and 1% of genes in *C. elegans* encode members of the homeobox family, one of 12 identified families in transcription factors. Gene regulation in the mammalian nervous system is likely to be at least as complex as that in bacteria or worms, so we might expect to find at least 10^3–10^4 transcription factors and a corresponding number of *cis*-regulatory sites. While these estimates are daunting from an experimental viewpoint, even 10^4 transcription factors could not individually specify the sets of 10^4–10^5 kinds of protein molecules in each of 10^{12} neurons, much less specify their regulation in response to developmental or experiential cues. The diverse patterns of gene expression in neurons (and in other cells) must therefore result from *combinations* of transcription factors, at least some of which must be responsive to environmental factors.

In vitro studies of eukaryotic transcription underscore the need for cooperation among transcription factors. For most genes, transcription rates are extremely low in the presence of only RNA polymerase II, TFIID, and other members of the TFII-polymerase II complex. Addition of transcription factors greatly increases the rates of transcription.

Cell lines and transgenic mice are commonly used test systems for regulatory sequences

A commonly used strategy for identifying the elements that control gene expression is to use recombinant DNA techniques to construct hybrid genes that contain a suspected regulatory region of one gene and the coding region of another gene (see Chap. 25). The product of the second gene serves as a reporter of the ability of a given test sequence to regulate expression in a particular type of cell. The bacterial enzyme chloramphenicol acetyltransferase is a valuable reporter, since it catalyzes an easily assayed reaction that is not found in eukaryotic cells. The enzymatic activity of the reporter in cells containing a hybrid gene indicates the effectiveness of different test sequences in regulating gene expression. Other useful reporters include bacterial β-galactosidase and firefly luciferase.

Two principal test systems are employed for the expression of hybrid genes: (a) cell lines, and (b) transgenic mice. In the first case, hybrid genes are put into a continuous cell line, and the expression of the reporter gene is monitored. Some experiments measure the transient expression of hybrid genes in the hours or days that they have access to the host cells' machinery for gene expression. Other experiments examine the expression of hybrid genes that have become integrated into host DNA.

Researchers examine the effects, on reporter protein production, of different DNA segments, usually starting with the DNA sequences flanking the 5′ end of the coding sequence. Once they identify putative regulatory segments, researchers identify the nucleotide residues responsible for regulation by testing the effects of site-directed mutations.

One goal of such experiments is to compare the ability of different DNA sequences to regulate gene expression in cell lines with different properties. A particularly interesting set of questions centers on gene regulation in different types of neurons. By what mechanism, for example, are tyrosine hydroxylase and dopamine-β-hydroxylase both expressed in the noradrenergic neurons of the locus coeruleus, but not in the dopaminergic neurons of the substantia nigra?

Recent work with transfected cell lines illustrates the combinatorial and synergistic nature of gene regulation. For example, the tissue-specific transcription of tyrosine hydroxylase in a rat pheochromocytoma cell line depends on two regulatory elements [17]. One of these elements is the AP-1 motif, which binds to the well-characterized transcription factors fos and jun (see below). The other element is related to enhancer elements in the genes encoding immunoglobulin light chain, insulin, and a set of proteins made in the exocrine pancreas. Mutations in either element reduced transcription as did increasing the separation of the two elements. Still more remarkably, combining the two elements activated the otherwise inappropriate expression of a β-globin gene in pheochromocytoma cells.

Cell lines that maintain specific cellular phenotypes are useful for studying gene regulation

Expression of transient or stable hybrid genes in continuous cell lines has allowed the identification of general and specific regulatory sequences for many genes. The paucity of cell lines with well-defined neuronal phenotypes, however, has limited studies of neuronal gene expression.

Most of the cell lines used have derived from naturally occurring or chemically induced tumors. Recently, however, a number of laboratories have begun to generate neuronal cell lines by immortalizing neuronal precursors with oncogenes carried in engineered retroviruses. Potentially, the most valuable of these lines may contain a stably integrated oncogene (the early viral protein large T antigen, Tag, encoded by the oncogenic DNA virus SV40) whose activity is temperature sensitive: At a permissive tempera-

ture, e.g., 33°C, Tag is active, and the cells proliferate as a neoplasm; at a restrictive temperature, e.g., 42°C, Tag is inactive, and the cells revert to a specific neuronal phenotype [18].

Inserting DNA in cells presents another problem for studies of hybrid gene expression. Some cell lines readily take up DNA from coprecipitates with calcium phosphate. Other cell lines do not, and researchers need to use other methods, including the transient opening of the membrane with an electric pulse, known as eletroporation; injection; or infection with engineered viruses, especially retroviruses.

Transgenic mice allow investigations of the pattern of gene expression dictated by *cis*-regulatory elements

The other general approach to the study of regulatory sequences takes advantage of the fact that it is possible to inject exogenous genes into mouse zygotes to produce transgenic mice. After a successful injection, an engineered transgene becomes part of the DNA in all cells, including the germ line. By examining the pattern of gene expression of the reporter gene by immunocytochemistry, for example, researchers can identify the elements that regulate cell-specific gene expression [19]. As more laboratories gain the ability to produce transgenic mice, this approach will undoubtedly contribute much to our understanding of neuronal cytodifferentiation. It seems likely, however, that the cost and complexity of experiments with transgenic mice will make work with cell lines the more common approach.

Families of regulatory factors

Trans-acting regulatory factors interact with the *cis*-regulatory sequences to establish the pattern of gene expression within individual cells. Several methods can detect the specific binding of *trans*-acting factors to specific DNA sequences. These include experiments that measure the ability of bound proteins to prevent the chemical or enzymatic cleavage of specific DNA sequences ("foot-printing") and determination of lowered electrophoretic mobility of a specific DNA fragment when it is bound to a protein (gel retardation) (see Chap. 25). These methods have led to the isolation and characterization of a number of transcription factors. DNAs encoding other transcription factors have been isolated by direct screening of expression libraries for sequences that bind to identified *cis*-regulatory sequences. Still other transcription factors have been identified by the ability of their DNAs to hybridize to related *Drosophila* or *C. elegans* regulatory sequences that were originally identified by genetics.

The transcription factors thus far identified have one of three distinctive structural designs (as illustrated in Fig. 5)—called *helix-turn-helix* (containing three α-helices separated by short turns), *zinc finger* (which contain zinc atoms bound either to the side chains of four cysteine residues or of two cysteine and two histidine residues), and *amphipathic helix* (which contain α-helices with nonpolar side chains extending from one side, allowing the formation of dimers). A finer classification scheme subdivides the known transcription factors into a total of 12 distinctive sets, five of which are listed in Table 1. Each of these 12 families has been the subject of much ongoing research and of periodic review articles. This chapter will discuss three examples of transcription factors that are responsive to signaling molecules.

Each transcription factor usually has several structural domains—(a) a *DNA-binding domain* that recognizes a specific DNA regulatory sequence; (b) an *effector domain* (or *transactivating domain*) that interacts either with another transcription factor (often forming a homo- or hetero-dimer) or with a protein of the transcriptional apparatus, thereby increasing or decreasing the rate of transcription; and, in some cases, (c) a *ligand-binding domain* that binds to a small molecule, thereby changing the activity of the factor.

Many, perhaps most, transcription factors appear to act as dimers—either homodimers or heterodimers with another member of the same family The *cis*-regulatory elements recognized by such dimeric factors are often symmetrical with respect to rotation, so that the sequence (reading from 5′ to 3′) of each strand of DNA is the same within the element (as illustrated in Fig. 5). Though the nomenclature is not strictly correct, these *rotationally* symmetrical sequences are called *palindromes* (which are actually defined to have *mirror* symmetry, as in "Madam, I'm Adam"). The rotational symmetry of *cis*-regulatory elements may explain why transcriptional regulation does not depend on the orientation of enhancer elements, as mentioned above.

Signaling molecules can activate transcription

The best examples of transcriptional regulation by effector molecules involve the actions of (a) second messengers such as cyclic AMP, calcium ions, and diacylglycerol; (b) growth factors; and (c) steroid hormones, thyroid hormone, and retinoic acid. The transcription factors (CREB, fos, and jun) that respond to cyclic AMP and to growth factors are members of the amphipathic helix family: Each contains a characteristic *leucine zipper*, which mediates dimerization. The factors responsible for the response to steroids, thyroid hormone, and retinoic acid are closely related members of the zinc-finger family.

CREB

Cyclic AMP, a "second messenger" whose intracellular concentration changes in response to a variety of hormones and transmitters, stimulates the phosphorylation (by protein kinase A) of many cellular proteins. One such phosphorylated protein is a ubiquitous transcription factor, with a leucine zipper called CREB (cyclic AMP response element-binding protein) [20,21]. In its

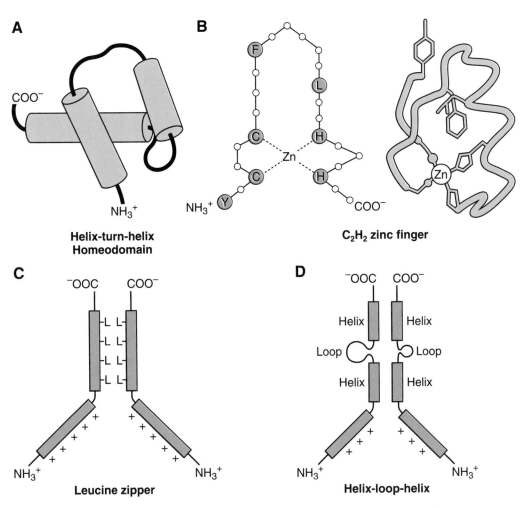

A

**Helix-turn-helix
Homeodomain**

B

C₂H₂ zinc finger

C

Leucine zipper

D

Helix-loop-helix

FIG. 5.   Structure of transcription factors from different families. (From Watson, Gilman, Witkowski, and Zoller, *Recombinant DNA, 2nd ed.,* New York: Scientific American Books, 1991, with permission.)

phosphorylated form, CREB binds to an 8-base *cis*-regulatory sequence called CRE (cyclic AMP response element), which is present in several genes whose transcription is increased by cyclic AMP. So increases in cyclic AMP stimulate protein kinase A, which activates CREB, which stimulates transcription.

fos and jun

Increased intracellular calcium activates protein kinase C, which can in turn activate tran-scription. At least part of the transcriptional effect of calcium is mediated by *fos* and *jun*, two other transcription factors with leucine zippers. (Unlike CREB, which was isolated by virtue of its ability to bind to a previously identified *cis*-regulatory element, fos and jun were first identified as the cellular counter-parts of viral oncogenes, and fos and jun are also called c-fos and c-jun.) A variety of stim-uli, including growth factors and electrical stimulation, lead to a rapid increase (within minutes) in the mRNAs for fos and jun, and they are taken as examples of *immediate early*

TABLE 1. Five families of transcription factors

Class of factor	Examples	Distinguishing characteristics	Interactions
Helix-turn-helix Homeobox	Antennapedia, bithorax, and other *Drosophila* genes; corrsponding genes in mammals, Hox 1, etc.	Highly basic domain of about 60 amino acid residues, highly conserved among family members; distantly related to helix-turn-helix regulators of bacterial transcription	Cascade of interactions among members of this family
POU	Pit-1 (responsible for cell-specific activation of prolactin and growth hormone); Oct-2 (binds to octamer motif in immunoglobulin heavy chain enhancer; Unc-86 (mutations which lead to uncoordinated *C. elegans*); many other family members since discovered	Each contains a homeobox but with about 20/60 amino acid residues matching those of the homeobox factors; additional common segment of about 80 amino acid residues	Can act on DNA as monomer; but some interact with other regulatory proteins; individual members have distinctive temporal and spatial patterns of expression
Zinc finger Nuclear receptors	Receptors for steroid hormones, thyroid hormone, and retinoic acid	Zinc finger formed by four cysteine residues; act as dimers	Steroids, thyroid hormone, retinoic acid
Amphipathic helix Leucine zipper	CREB, fos, jun, and other factors closely related to each of these (CREB relatives, E1A and ATF subfamily; fos relatives, fra-1 and fosB; the jun relatives, junA, junB, and junD)	α-Helix with leucine in every 7th position; forms heterodimer through leucine zipper	Transmitters and hormones that stimulate production of cyclic AMP, acting through protein kinase A; phorbol esters acting via protein kinase C
Helix-loop-helix	MyoD (a transcription factor that can stimulate the differentiation of a fibroblast line into muscle cells); c-myc; E12 and E47 (immunoglobulin enhancer binding proteins); *Drosophila achaete/scute* and *daughterless*	Each contains two conserved α-helical regions of 12–15 amino acid residues, connected by a nonconserved "loop"; helices are amphipathic with hydrophobic side chains extending from one side	Form dimers via amphipathic helices (similar to leucine zipper factors); interactions with other family members (e.g., MyoD and E12/47)

genes, a term borrowed from studies of viral life cycles. The transcription of fos and jun depends at least in part upon the activation of CREB by cyclic AMP-dependent protein kinase A or by calcium/calmodulin kinase [22,23].

Fos and jun form heterodimers via their leucine zippers. The fos-jun heterodimer binds to a previously recognized 7-base pair *cis*-regulatory element called AP-1 or TRE (TPA response element, since it mediates the response to tetradecanoyl-phorbol-acetate, or TPA, which stimulates protein kinase C). Other members of the fos and jun subfamilies can form a large number of different heterodimers, each of which might recognize different *cis*-acting elements or might activate transcription to a different extent.

AP-1 sites, which are similar to CREs, are found in a number of genes, including the prodynorphin gene, which encodes opiate precursors. Fos and jun are therefore candidate regulators of dynorphin expression. Consistent with this hypothesis, painful stimuli trigger the somatotopic expression of fos and jun in the dorsal horn of the spinal cord, allowing the mapping of pain pathways, even in the absence of full knowledge of their actual target genes.

Nuclear Receptors

Steroids, thyroid hormone, and retinoic acid all diffuse across the plasma membrane and bind to specific intracellular receptors (see Chap. 9). The steroid-receptor complex then diffuses into the nucleus, where it interacts with DNA and stimulates the expression of specific genes. Each receptor consists of at least three domains, one of which binds to the hormone, another that consequently binds to a specific *cis*-regulatory element, and another responsible for transactivation. These domains may be switched, experimentally, among the receptor molecules, allowing, for example, the artificial induction by estrogen of a set of genes normally stimulated by glucocorticoids.

Hormones that act on nuclear receptors affect gene expression in many cells, including the nervous system. The action of steroids, however, differs among cell types. Glucocorticoids thus induce the synthesis of tyrosine aminotransferase in the liver and growth hormone in the pituitary, but decrease the synthesis of pro-opiomelanocortin in the pituitary and lead to the death of lymphocytes in the thymus. It seems likely that in each cell type, glucocorticoids act to alter gene expression through the same receptor.

The differentiated state of each cell (its cell type and stage in cytodifferentiation) thus affects its responsiveness to regulation by any given effector.

Families of transcription factors generate complex patterns of gene regulation

Transcription factors interact with ligands, with the transcriptional apparatus, and with each other. They are also subject to covalent modifications (such as phosphorylation) that affect their activity and their localization. A 1991 review [2] enumerated six dimensions of transcriptional regulation: (1) the existence of a large number (perhaps 5,000) of mammalian transcription factors, of which 1,500–2,500 are expected to be brain specific; (2) the combinations of several types of *cis*-regulatory elements in individual genes, providing targets for several transcription factors, as in the case of tyrosine hydroxylase; (3) interactions between members of the same family, such as fos and jun, or different members of the nuclear receptor family; (4) interactions between members of different families, such as the prevention of jun-fos binding to specific AP-1 elements by the glucocorticoid receptor; (5) covalent modifications, such as phosphorylation of CREB; and (6) the regulated partitioning of transcription factors, such as the sequestering of the glucocorticoid receptor by a heat shock protein or of the widely distributed NF-κB transcription factor by a cytoplasmic protein, phosphorylation of which allows the release of NF-κB and its movement into the nucleus.

The explosion of information about gene expression shows no signs of slowing. No one should be surprised by the daunting complexity of gene regulation in general, and in the brain in particular. On the one hand, this continuing and even accelerating progress is dispiriting, since we must constantly assimilate new facts. On the other hand, new data allow us to see repeating patterns (such as the importance of dimers and the still relatively small number of families of transcription factors). However complex these patterns, they must still serve as the basis for understanding both the development of the brain and its plastic changes in response to experience.

ACKNOWLEDGMENTS

This chapter was written in honor of the 90th birthday of Professor John T. Edsall.

I thank Michel Khrestchatisky, who developed many of the basic themes of this chapter for the previous edition of *Basic Neurochemistry*. I am also grateful to the following people for their helpful comments on the present version: Robert Brackenbury, Anthony Campagnoni, Dona Chikaraishi, Luis Covarrubias, Cheryl Craft, Nathaniel Heintz, George Lawless, Gregor Sutcliffe, David Tobin, Rachel Tyndale, and Robert Weatherwax.

REFERENCES

1. Lemke, G. Gene regulation in the nervous system. In Z. Hall (ed.), *An Introduction to Molecular Neurobiology*. Sunderland, MA: Sinauer, 1992, pp. 313–354.
2. He, X., and Rosenfeld, M. G. Mechanisms of complex transcriptional regulation: implications for brain development. *Neuron* 7: 183–196, 1991.
3. Struhl, K. Mechanisms for diversity in gene expression patterns. *Neuron* 7:177–181, 1991.
4. Gill, G., and Tjian, R. Eukaryotic coactivators associated with the TATA box binding protein. *Curr. Opin. Genet. Dev.* 2:236–242, 1992.
5. Evans, T., Felsenfeld, G., and Reitman, M. Control of globin gene transcription. *Annu. Rev. Cell Biol.* 6:95–124, 1990.
6. Eberwine, J., Yeh, H., Miyashiro, K., Cao, Y., Nair, S., Finnell, R., Zettel, M., and Coleman, P. Analysis of gene expression in single live neurons. *Proc. Natl. Acad. Sci. U.S.A.* 89(7): 3010–3014, 1992.
7. Mikoshiba, K., Okano, H., Tamura, T., and Ikenaka, K. Structure and function of myelin

protein genes. *Annu. Rev. Neurosci.* 14: 201–217, 1991.
8. Martins, R. N., Robinson, P. J., Chleboun, J. O., Beyreuther, K., and Masters, C. L. The molecular pathology of amyloid deposition in Alzheimer's disease. *Mol. Neurobiol.* 5: 389–398, 1992.
9. Simpson, L., and Shaw, J. RNA editing and the mitochondrial cryptogenes of kinetoplastid protozoa. *Cell* 57:355–366, 1989.
10. Sommer, B., Köhler, M., Sprengel, R., and Seeburg, P. H. RNA editing in brain controls a determinant of ion flow in glutamate-gated channels. *Cell* 67:11–19, 1991.
11. Atwater, J. A., Wisdom, R., and Verma, I. M. Regulated mRNA stability. *Annu. Rev. Genet.* 24:519–541, 1990.
12. Matsuoka, M., Nagawa, F., Okazaki, K., Kingsbury, L., Yoshida, K., Müller, U., Larue, D. T., Winer, J. A., and Sakano, H. Detection of somatic DNA recombination in the transgenic mouse brain. *Science* 254:81–86, 1991.
13. Abeliovich, A., Gerber, D., Tanaka, O., Katsuki, M., Graybiel, A. M., and Tonegawa, S. On somatic recombination in the central nervous system of transgenic mice. *Science* 257: 404–407, 1992.
14. Erlander, M. G., Tillakaratne, N. J. K., Feldblum, S., Patel, N., and Tobin, A. J. Two genes encode distinct glutamate decarboxylases. *Neuron* 7:91–100, 1991.
15. Sutcliffe, J. G. mRNA in the mammalian central nervous system. *Annu. Rev. Neurosci.* 11: 157–198, 1988.
16. Travis, G. H., Brennan, M. B., Danielson, P. E., Kozak, C. A., and Sutcliffe, J. G. Identification of a photoreceptor-specific mRNA encoded by the gene responsible for retinal degeneration slow (rds). *Nature* 338:70–73, 1989.
17. Yoon, S. O., and Chikaraishi, D. M. Tissue-specific transcription of the rat tyrosine hydroxylase gene requires synergy between an AP-1 motif and an overlapping E box-containing dyad. *Neuron* 9:55–67, 1992.
18. Renfranz, P. J., Cunningham, M. G., and McKay, R. D. G. Region-specific differentiation of the hippocampal stem cell line HiB5 upon implantation into the developing mammalian brain. *Cell* 66:713–729, 1991.
19. Smeyn, R. J., Oberdick, J., Schilling, K., Berrebi, A. S., Mugnaini, E., and Morgan, J. I. Dynamic organization of developing Purkinje

cells revealed by transgene expression. *Science* 254:719–721, 1991.

20. Brindle, P. K., and Montminy, M. R. The CREB family of transcription activators. *Curr. Opin. Genet. Dev.* 2:199–204, 1992.

21. Goodman, R. H. Regulation of neuropeptide gene expression. *Annu. Rev. Neurosci.* 13: 111–127, 1990.

22. Sheng, M., McFadden, G., and Greenberg, M.

E. Membrane depolarization and calcium induce c-*fos* transcription via phosphorylation of transcription factor CREB. *Neuron* 4: 571–582, 1990.

23. Morgan, J. I., and Curran, T. Stimulus-transcription coupling in the nervous system: involvement of the inducible proto-oncogenes *fos* and *jun*. *Annu. Rev. Neurosci.* 14:421–451, 1991.

CHAPTER 25

Molecular Probes for Gene Expression

RICHARD H. GOODMAN AND MALCOLM J. LOW

Basic Neurochemistry: Molecular, Cellular, and Medical Aspects, 5th Ed., edited by G. J. Siegel et al. Published by Raven Press, Ltd., New York, 1994. Correspondence to Richard H. Goodman, Vollum Institute for Advanced Biomedical Research, Oregon Health Sciences University L-474, Portland, Oregon 97201-3098.

Advances in the understanding of ion channel, receptor, and transmitter physiology have become increasingly dependent on recombinant DNA technology. This chapter addresses two issues related to this technology—how molecular probes for neuronal gene expression are obtained and how they are utilized experimentally to analyze neuronal function. The generation of molecular probes usually requires the construction of gene libraries and the screening of such libraries for specific DNA sequences. In this chapter, we address the general approaches for constructing gene libraries and outline some of the techniques that have been used successfully to isolate neural-specific genes. We also describe approaches for quantitating gene expression and characterizing the DNA elements and transcription factors that control gene regulation.

STRUCTURE AND USES OF COMPLEMENTARY DNA

Complementary DNA is a double-stranded copy of messenger RNA and contains the same sequence information as RNA

A *complementary* DNA (cDNA) *library* contains a representation of all of the messenger RNA (mRNA) molecules from a given cell or tissue source. In general, therefore, nonabundant mRNAs are infrequently represented. The differential representation of cDNAs in such a library contrasts with a *genomic library*, which theoretically contains an equal representation of all genes. Another important difference between cDNA and genomic libraries is that the former contains only transcribed sequences. Genomic libraries contain a large amount of nonstructural DNA, including intervening sequences (introns) and flanking DNA, that is never translated into protein (see Chap. 24). This nonstructural DNA can nonetheless be very important in controlling gene expression and can be the locus of pathological mutations associated with neurological disease (see Chap.

26). Thus, the issue of whether to screen a cDNA or genomic library to isolate a neural-specific gene depends on the particular question being asked. In general, it is easier to isolate and characterize a cDNA clone, especially if the cDNA library can be constructed from a source that is rich in the desired mRNA. If an enriched source cannot be identified, it may be desirable to screen a genomic library directly. Regulatory elements that control gene transcription can only be isolated from a genomic library. In practice, genomic clones are generally isolated by using cDNA clones as hybridization probes.

The sequence of cDNA molecules can provide information about proteins that is not available from biochemical analyses

Studies of neuropeptide biosynthesis provide one example of the utility of cDNA cloning. Neuropeptides are generally produced from larger, biologically inactive precursors. The N-termini of these precursors contain signal sequences, 15 to 30 amino acids in length, that are removed during the process of translation. Additionally, many neuropeptides are synthesized as polyproteins, sometimes containing multiple bioactive peptides. Although the precursor *(prohormone)* forms of some neuropeptides have been identified immunochemically, the amounts isolated are often insufficient for structural analysis. Consequently, the only way to predict the primary structure of a precursor protein and to determine whether it contains multiple peptides is by determining the sequence of its cDNA. Examples of novel neuroendocrine peptides predicted entirely through the analysis of cDNA clones include peptide histidine methionine (PHM-27) [1] and the calcitonin gene-related peptide (CGRP) [2]. Complementary DNA sequences have also provided the structures of many ion channels and receptors, which typically are expressed at levels far below those required for biochemical analysis. Finally, it is only through the characterization of cDNA sequences that several novel mechanisms for generating peptide and channel diversity, such as exon-shuffling and RNA editing, have been discovered [3].

Cloned cDNAs are invaluable for studying the regulation of gene expression in the nervous system

The Northern blot technique, which allows the precise characterization and quantitation of specific mRNAs, utilizes radiolabeled cDNA molecules for hybridization to nucleic acids immobilized on nitrocellulose or nylon membranes. *In situ* hybridization histochemistry allows qualitative analysis of specific mRNA species in individual cells. The combination of these two methods provides a powerful technology for examining the molecular biology of gene expression in complex tissues such as the brain.

Cloned cDNAs are used in expression vectors to produce recombinant neurobiological proteins

Cloned cDNAs can be expressed in either bacterial or animal cells, and the choice of a particular expression system generally depends upon the requirement for specific types of post-translational modifications. In some instances, bacterial cells can accomplish all of the biosynthetic steps required for generating biologically active products. Other products require a complex series of processing events that can be performed only by animal cells. The frog oocyte system has been particularly useful for expressing biologically active ion channels and receptors [4]. Other expression systems, particularly those utilizing insect cells, are useful for obtaining large amounts of recombinant proteins [5]. Products can be purified from such expression systems by traditional biochemical approaches, or by creating fusion proteins that contain an easily removable affinity tag [6]. It should be remembered that post-translational modifications may vary in different cell types, so it is important to compare the recombinant gene products to those found in native cells.

Isolating a cDNA clone is frequently the first step toward isolating a gene

A cDNA clone provides an ideal probe for screening a genomic library because it contains long stretches of nucleic acids that are identical with the gene. Low-stringency hybridizations can be used to probe for related members of a multigene family or to screen for homologous sequences in other species. Eukaryotic genes can be highly complex, with multiple intervening sequences separating the individual protein-coding regions. Because a cDNA represents only the exonic sequences, the structure of the cDNA allows an accurate assignment of the splice donor and acceptor sites. Indeed, determining the structure of a gene without knowledge of the cDNA sequence can be exceedingly difficult. The polymerase chain reaction provides an alternative approach for amplifying sequences of genomic DNA that does not require a cDNA probe (see below).

CONSTRUCTION OF cDNA LIBRARIES

cDNA clones of neurobiological interest may be identified by hybridization, immunological, or functional approaches

Hybridization approaches depend on the availability of a cDNA or oligonucleotide probe. Immunological approaches rely on specific antibodies to identify recombinant proteins produced by an expression vector. Functional approaches depend on assays specific for particular biological features of the protein of interest. All of these methods require the construction of a cDNA library, although optimal libraries for use in each method have slightly different features.

The first step in preparing a cDNA library is to isolate intact RNA

The most commonly used methods for isolation of RNA utilize chaotropic agents, such as guanidine isothiocyanate, to denature proteins that cause RNA degradation [7]. RNA is typically separated from DNA and protein by differential precipitation in lithium chloride or by centrifugation through cesium chloride. The polyadenylated fraction of RNA, which represents most of the mRNA pool but only approximately 1 percent of the total cellular RNA, can be purified by affinity chromatography to oligodeoxythymidine (dT) linked cellulose or magnetic beads. The polyadenylate tail at the 3′ end of the RNA binds to the chain of deoxythymidine residues under high-salt conditions and can be eluted in low-salt buffer. A significant fraction of brain mRNA appears to be nonpolyadenylated and cannot be purified on oligo(dT) columns, however (see Chap. 24). Further enrichment for a particular species of mRNA can be achieved by sucrose gradient centrifugation or by denaturing agarose gel electrophoresis. In general, sucrose gradient centrifugation results in a lower degree of purification than gel electrophoresis but is technically easier and allows a greater yield of nondegraded RNA.

Production of cDNA libraries utilizes the enzyme reverse transcriptase to synthesize single-stranded DNA copies of mRNA molecules

Reverse transcriptase is an RNA-dependent DNA polymerase which requires a primer to initiate its activity. Typically, the primer consists of a short chain of oligo(dT) residues, which hybridizes to the 3′ polyadenylate tail of the mRNA. Reverse transcriptase is a 5′- to 3′-directed polymerase. Therefore, the copy produced by the action of reverse transcriptase is complementary to the mRNA template (antisense). If the mRNA sequence is partially known, synthetic oligonucleotide primers can be used instead of oligo(dT) to enrich the library for the desired cDNA. Similarly, either specific or random oligonucleotide primers can be used to increase the likelihood of generating cDNA clones that

represent the 5′ end of the mRNAs, corresponding to the 5′ untranslated and amino-terminal portions of the encoded proteins.

The most commonly used procedure for generating double-stranded cDNA is based on the method of Gubler and Hoffman [8]. This method utilizes reverse transcriptase to synthesize the first cDNA strand, and the RNA is replaced with DNA by using RNAse H and DNA polymerase I. The Gubler and Hoffman technique has proven to be highly efficient, producing as many as 10^6 recombinants from each microgram of starting mRNA. Additionally, cDNA clones generated by this technique are often full-length.

Complementary DNA molecules introduced into bacteria would be rapidly degraded if not inserted into a suitable vector

Many cDNA libraries utilize plasmid vectors, small circular molecules of DNA that contain multiple unique restriction endonuclease sites and one or more antibiotic resistance markers. Plasmids exist within the bacterial cell as episomes which can be separated easily from the chromosomal DNA. Plasmids with relaxed replication characteristics can be amplified many times, increasing the relative amount of foreign DNA in the cell. Most libraries are constructed in bacteriophage vectors which have a much higher cloning efficiency than plasmid vectors and offer several technical advantages.

The insertion of cDNA molecules into a vector is generally accomplished by using synthetic DNA linkers. These linkers, typically small double-stranded fragments of DNA which contain one or two restriction sites, can be added to the flush ends of cDNA molecules by using the enzyme DNA ligase. The blunt-ended linkers tend to add onto the ends of the cDNA as concatamers. By cleaving the "linkered" DNA with the appropriate restriction enzyme, a sticky-ended fragment of cDNA can be generated. This sticky-ended cDNA fragment can be inserted into a plasmid or bacteriophage vector at a site containing complementary sticky ends, sealed using DNA ligase, and passaged in bacteria as a recombinant DNA molecule. To prevent the vector molecule from religating to itself without inserting a cDNA molecule, it is frequently necessary to dephosphorylate the ends of the vector. Linkers have been developed that can insert cDNAs into cloning vectors in specified orientations.

As mentioned above, bacteriophage libraries can be screened far more efficiently than plasmid libraries. While assaying 50,000 to 100,000 bacterial colonies is extremely labor-intensive, screening 10^6 bacteriophage plaques is relatively easy. Furthermore, genetic characteristics have been introduced into bacteriophage vectors to increase the ease of selecting recombinants. For example, the cloning site in λgt10 interrupts the phage repressor gene *(cI)* such that only those that contain a cDNA insert form clear lytic plaques when grown on the appropriate bacterial strain. The cloning site in λgt11, a bacteriophage vector designed primarily for immunological screening, interrupts the *lacZ* gene. Consequently, recombinant λgt11 phage cannot metabolize the indicator X-gal (5-bromo-4-chloro-3-indolyl-β-D-galactoside) and form white plaques, whereas nonrecombinant phages form blue plaques.

SCREENING cDNA LIBRARIES

The procedures required for identifying a particular cDNA clone within a cDNA library depend on the abundance of the specific mRNA. To detect a rare cDNA, it may be necessary to screen as many as 10^6 independent clones. Abundant cDNAs can be identified by screening only a few hundred clones.

Very abundant clones can be identified by screening a cDNA library with a radiolabeled probe generated from total polyadenylated RNA

In practice, this screening would be performed by using the colony hybridization procedure of Grunstein and Hogness [9]. Recombinant bacterial colonies are grown on a nitrocellulose filter, replicated, and then lysed with alkali. The alkali also denatures the plasmid DNA and allows the DNA to become permanently attached to the filter. The filters are washed to remove the bacterial debris, baked to fix the DNA, and then incubated with a radiolabeled probe generated from total polyadenylated RNA. Colonies that contain sequences complementary to the probe can be detected by autoradiography. If, for example, 10 percent of the mRNA molecules encode a single protein and the remainder of the mRNAs encode less abundant species, a cDNA probe generated from the total population of mRNAs would be enriched for the abundant molecule. Colonies detected with this probe are likely to encode the most abundant mRNA species.

Synthetic oligonucleotide probes can be used to detect rare cDNA clones

Frequently, the amino acid sequence of a protein or peptide fragment can be determined through biochemical techniques. Although the precise DNA sequence encoding a peptide might be unknown, it is nonetheless often possible to synthesize a family of oligonucleotides representing all of the combinations of codons that correspond to any peptide sequence. Because of the degeneracy of the genetic code, the number of oligonucleotides required to represent every possible DNA sequence can be quite large. To decrease this number of possibilities, oligonucleotide probes are usually generated from peptide sequences rich in the amino acids methionine, tryptophan, phenylalanine, tyrosine, histidine, glutamine, asparagine, lysine, aspartic acid, glutamic acid, and cysteine, which are encoded by only one or two different codons. To reduce the number of ambiguous codons still further, several additional approaches for generating probes have been utilized. First, deoxyguanosine can be substituted for deoxyadenosine, and deoxythymidine can be used in place of deoxycytosine. These substitutions, which substantially decrease the complexity of an oligonucleotide mixture, can be made because guanosine and thymidine weakly base-pair in a double-stranded DNA molecule. By this simple maneuver, Touchot et al. [10] reduced the complexity of a mixed 20-*mer* from 512 to 61. Another approach to decreasing the complexity of a mixed oligonucleotide is to substitute deoxyinosine, which base-pairs with any of the four deoxynucleotides, at all ambiguous positions. The resultant probe has a low complexity but is not as specific as an oligonucleotide containing the normal nucleotide bases. Additionally, educated guesses can be made about the likelihood of a specific codon being correct by using codon-usage tables that have been developed for different eukaryotic species.

Oligonucleotides synthesized for screening cDNA libraries are usually between 15 and 25 nucleotides long. By adjusting the stringency of hybridization through alteration of the temperature and salt concentration, one can distinguish among sequences that differ by as little as a single nucleotide. The specificity of oligonucleotide probes can be increased further by performing hybridizations in the presence of tetramethylammonium chloride, which eliminates the preferential melting of adenine-thymine (A-T) base-pairs. Using two independent oligonucleotide probes representing discrete portions of the cDNA also increases the specificity of hybridization.

Because hybridization between two nucleic acid sequences is a function of several independent parameters, including the degree of complementarity, the amount of guanine-cytosine (G-C) pairing, and the length of the hybridizing strands, it is often possible to overcome a single probe deficiency by altering some other characteristics. Therefore, an alternative approach for oligonucleotide screening is to use long probes (30–100 nucleotides long) containing a limited number of mismatches. Long probes only 80 percent homologous to the optimal sequence can produce highly specific hybridization signals under conditions of low-stringency hybridization and washing. In general, the hybridization conditions for long-probe screening need to be determined empirically to reduce background binding.

The polymerase chain reaction can be used to isolate cDNA clones that are new members of known gene families

The polymerase chain reaction (PCR) has revolutionized many aspects of molecular biology, including the isolation of cDNA clones encoding neural-specific molecules. PCR selectively amplifies stretches of double-stranded DNA up to 2–3 kb in length and relies on the use of appropriate pairs of oligonucleotide primers, a thermostable form of DNA polymerase, and a repetitive thermal cycling reaction consisting of denaturation, annealing, and polymerization steps. The nucleotide sequence of PCR-amplified DNA can be obtained directly or after subcloning the fragment into a plasmid vector.

PCR cloning has been used widely for identifying novel members of large gene families. A particularly good example is the superfamily of seven transmembrane-containing neurotransmitter and neuropeptide receptors [11]. Although the cytosolic and extracellular domains of receptors in this class are quite divergent, many amino acid residues within the hydrophobic transmembrane segments are conserved. These transmembrane segments have been used to design degenerate oligonucleotide primers for use in PCR. The degenerate PCR approach has also allowed characterization of multiple members of the POU-homeodomain family of neural-specific transcription factors [12] and various ligand and voltage-gated ion channels [13]. A refinement of this strategy is the "nested" PCR approach that uses two separate sets of oligonucleotide primer pairs, one internal to the other, to increase the specificity of the reactions [14]. Because of the ability of PCR to amplify extremely rare sequences, a major problem has been the identification of large numbers of "orphan" receptors, that is, receptors without identified natural ligands or functions. It will take many years for physiologists to "catch up" with the complexity generated by molecular biologists armed with their PCR machines.

IMMUNOLOGICAL AND RECOGNITION SITE SCREENING IN BACTERIAL EXPRESSION SYSTEMS

Hybridization and PCR approaches to isolating cDNA clones require a substantial amount of prior information about the protein of interest. Often, especially for nonabundant proteins, it is difficult or impossible to determine the amino acid sequence of even a small peptide fragment. Immunological screening approaches, particularly those based on bacterial systems, can obviate the need to obtain prior protein sequence information but depend on several assumptions. First, antibody recognition must not depend on post-translational modifications that are only accomplished by eukaryotic cells. This means that glycosylation, phosphorylation, sulfation, and particular patterns of proteolytic cleavage cannot be required for antibody binding. Second, because immunological screening approaches typically demand that the antibody recognize denatured proteins fused to a large bacterial product, the antibody recognition site cannot depend on the protein conformation. Finally, the eukaryotic proteins expressed in bacteria must be protected from bacterial degradation and must not be toxic to the host bacterial cells.

An additional problem in any sort of expression-cloning, whether the screening procedure is immunological or functional, is insuring that the cDNAs are translated in the proper reading frame and orientation. Because a DNA sequence theoretically can be translated in either orientation and in any of three reading frames, the random insertion of a cDNA into an expression vector has only one chance in six of encoding an authentic protein. Although there are methods for directing the orientation of a cDNA into a vector, it is often easier in bacterial systems to scale-up the number of colonies screened. This scaling-up requires a very efficient cloning strategy, however. In bacteriophage expression systems, such as the λgt11 vector, cDNA molecules are inserted into a unique restriction site near the end of the gene encoding the enzyme β-galactosidase. The foreign cDNAs are expressed as fusion proteins in this system, linked to β-galactosidase, and are less likely to be viewed as "foreign" by bacterial degradation systems. Finally, expression of the fusion proteins can be controlled by the inducer isopropyl-β-D-thiogalactopyranoside (IPTG). Thus, it is possible to limit the expression of the potentially toxic fusion proteins until just prior to screening. Immunological screening involves inducing the bacteriophage with IPTG, transferring the fusion proteins to a nitrocellulose filter, and then probing with specific antibody. In general, polyclonal antibodies have been preferable to monoclonals for library screening. Affinity-purified antisera, immunoabsorbed to remove antibodies to bacterial proteins, have been most useful. Binding of the specific antibody is detected by using iodinated staphylococcal protein A or by an alkaline phosphatase-based secondantibody technique.

Unfortunately, because immunological screening often depends on incompletely characterized antibodies and the sequence of the desired protein is typically unknown, it can be difficult to confirm that an immunopositive bacteriophage encodes the appropriate cDNA. It is essential, therefore, to devise a secondary screening procedure to eliminate false-positive cDNA clones. One approach that has been particularly useful for identifying neuropeptide cDNAs has been to combine immunological screening with *in situ* hybridization histochemistry [15]. This combination of methodologies was used to clone the cDNA encoding the precursor to thyrotropin-releasing hormone (TRH), one of the hypothalamic releasing factors. Because the mature TRH molecule is only a tripeptide, oligonucleotide probes are of little use for recognizing the precursor. Furthermore, antisera directed against mature TRH, which is modified at the N-terminal by cyclization of the glutamic acid residue and at the C-terminal by amidation of the proline residue, do not recognize the precursor form of the peptide. Lechan et al. [16] utilized an antiserum directed against a synthetic decapeptide, designed to represent an N- and C-terminal extended form of TRH, to screen a rat hypothalamic λgt11 expression library. Immunopositive clones detected using the antibody were then used in *in situ* hybridization assays of rat brain slices. Only the cDNAs that identified TRH-immunopositive neurons were considered to represent potential TRH precursors. The complexity of neuropeptide anatomy in the central nervous system, as assayed by *in situ* hybridization, in this instance provided a useful adjunct to the relatively nonspecific immunochemical expression cloning approach.

Recognition site screening is a form of expression-cloning designed to identify cDNA clones encoding DNA-binding proteins [17] such as transcription factors. The theoretical basis of this screening strategy is analogous to that described above for immunological screening, but depends on the selective high-affinity binding of transcription factors to short (8–12) nucleotide DNA motifs contained in *cis*-acting genetic regulatory elements. In practice, nitrocellulose filters containing proteins produced by a λ phage expression library are screened with concatamers of a radioactively labeled oligonucleotide representing a proposed genetic regulatory element. Use of a mutated oligonucleotide that no longer binds the transcription factor and is nonfunctional as a transcriptional regulator provides an important negative control. The success of this procedure depends on many variables including the ability of a monomeric factor to bind the oligonucleotide with high affinity, the ability of the factor to bind to DNA in the absence

of post-translational modifications, and the lack of significant nonspecific DNA binding. Rigorous characterization of the DNA-binding specificity of the encoded protein should be confirmed by a combination of DNAse I footprinting and gel shift assays using native and mutated binding site probes (described in a later section). The general utility of this type of screening method has been extended to include screening with protein subunit probes and other types of ligands [18].

EXPRESSION CLONING IN EUKARYOTIC SYSTEMS

As discussed above, bacterial expression systems do not accomplish the post-translational modifications that occasionally are essential for immunological recognition or biological function. It is often necessary, therefore, to rely on eukaryotic expression systems for identifying cDNAs of neurobiological interest. These eukaryotic systems are particularly valuable for cloning cDNAs encoding large membrane proteins such as ion channels or receptors. Because sequences at the amino-termini of many proteins are essential for correct targeting, processing, and folding in eukaryotic cells, a prerequisite for expression cloning in animal cells is to construct a full-length cDNA library. Fortunately, several of the available cloning strategies satisfy this requirement.

Fibroblast cells were used in many early DNA transfection studies

Expression cloning has a long history, beginning with the early studies that resulted in the first identification of oncogenes. DNA-mediated gene transfer techniques were used to introduce high molecular weight DNA from human tumors into mouse fibroblast cell lines. Some specific DNA fragments altered the growth properties of recipient cells, an effect that could be recognized by focus formation or growth in soft agar. Characterization of the sequences of these fragments revealed that they were related to the oncogenic portions of tumor-causing viruses.

Neurobiologists have used similar approaches to identify genes encoding cell-surface receptors. One of the first examples of this approach was the cloning of the low-affinity nerve growth factor (NGF) receptor by Chao et al. [19]. These workers introduced high-molecular-weight human genomic DNA into receptor-deficient mouse fibroblast L-cells. Co-transfection of a gene encoding herpes virus thymidine kinase (TK) into the TK deficient L-cell line allowed selection for cells that had integrated the foreign DNA into their genome. TK^+ cells were then screened for the expression of NGF receptors by an immunological erythrocyte rosette assay. Human DNA encoding the NGF receptor was identified by screening DNA from transfected NGF receptor-positive L-cells with human repetitive sequence DNA. Similar techniques have been used by other investigators to clone cDNAs for neurotransmitter and other growth factor receptors [20].

Frog oocytes provide another highly efficient expression system for cDNA cloning

Another relatively old technique, the frog oocyte translation system, has proven to be particularly useful for cloning cDNAs encoding membrane proteins such as channels and receptors. This procedure, originally developed by Gurdon et al. [21], provides a means of translating mRNAs from most types of eukaryotic cells. Importantly, frog oocytes can perform most of the post-translational modifications required for biological function of membrane proteins. Additionally, the oocyte provides a relatively simple system for performing electrophysiological or biochemical analyses of channels or transport proteins. Receptors that transduce signals through inositol trisphosphate (IP_3) are particularly easy to detect in oocytes. IP_3 liberates Ca^{2+} from intracellular storage pools in these cells, which open Ca^{2+}-activated chloride channels. The opening of these channels can be detected by measuring the voltage gradient or current across the oocyte membrane. Receptors coupled to the cyclic AMP-dependent signal transduction pathway are more difficult to assay in the frog oocyte system.

The RNA used in oocyte injection experiments can be isolated from cells or transcribed from cDNA expression libraries. By microinjecting expressed mRNAs into frog oocytes, one can test the activity of individual pools of cDNA clones. This functional method of cDNA screening generally requires that the cDNA inserts encode the entire protein. Depending on the length of the particular mRNA, this requirement can present an extremely difficult problem. If the membrane protein contains multiple subunits, cloning strategies based on oocyte expression become even more problematic. One approach to overcoming these problems is to use a procedure based on hybridization arrest. In this approach, RNA from a tissue or cell line is allowed to hybridize to a pool of cDNAs in solution. Hybridized and nonhybridized RNA are separated by density gradient centrifugation and are tested in frog oocytes. By assaying sequentially smaller pools of clones, a single cDNA that encodes the receptor or transporter of interest can be identified. Once isolated, the individual cDNA can be used to screen a cDNA or genomic library by hybridization techniques. Proof that the isolated DNA sequences encode an authentic receptor or channel requires that transcribed RNA produce a functional protein.

HYBRIDIZATION ASSAYS USING cDNA PROBES

Complementary DNA probes can be used in at least four types of assays to quantitate gene expression in the nervous system. Three of these assays—the Northern blot, RNAse protection, and *in situ* hybridization assay—utilize radiolabeled probes generated from cDNA molecules. Radiolabeled probes can be prepared by incubating the denatured cDNA with synthetic oligomers and the large fragment of DNA polymerase, or by transcribing the cDNA from the sense strand to produce an antisense RNA. In general, both methods of producing radiolabeled probes are effective, but antisense RNAs have several particular advantages over DNA probes. First, it is easy to control the length of the labeled probe. Probes generated by random-primer labeling of DNA are usually variable in length. Second, antisense RNA is single-stranded. Consequently, back-hybridization to the sense strand does not compete for binding to the target RNA. Third, the binding of RNA-RNA hybrids is stronger than RNA-DNA hybrids. Thus, it is possible to perform hybridization under more stringent conditions. Finally, nonhybridized antisense RNA can be digested with RNAse, decreasing the background caused by free radiolabeled probe. Antisense RNAs are particularly useful for nuclease protection and *in situ* hybridization assays. The interested reader is referred to a recent monograph that discusses these reactions and this methodology in detail [22].

Northern blot assays allow quantitation of specific species of mRNA. These assays are typically performed by electrophoresing RNA on agarose gels containing formamide, glyoxal, or methylmercury, transferring the RNA to an inert support by capillary or electroblotting, and then hybridizing with a radiolabeled probe. In general, the rules governing hybridization of nucleic acids in solution apply fairly well to RNAs immobilized on nitrocellulose filters. Hybridization is therefore dependent on the length of the probe, G-C content, temperature, and salt concentration of the hybridization solution. Hybridizations using antisense RNA probes are usually performed under more stringent conditions than those using cDNA probes.

Occasionally, Northern blot assays cannot distinguish among mRNAs that are closely related in size and sequence. In these instances, RNAse protection assays can be particularly useful. In this procedure, radiolabeled antisense RNA is hybridized to RNA in solution, and the mixture is treated with a combination of ribonucleases and then electrophoresed on a denaturing polyacrylamide gel. Ribonucleases A and T1 preferentially digest single-stranded RNA. Therefore, when the probe is completely hybridized to a complementary sequence of RNA, it is protected from digestion with RNAse. Any divergence between the probe and target RNA allows the probe to be digested at the point of mismatch, resulting in a smaller fragment of radiolabeled RNA. Because the nonhybridized probe is completely degraded by RNAse, the RNAse protection assay is also an extremely sensitive and specific assay for the detection of low-abundance mRNAs. In addition to quantitating low-abundance mRNAs, the RNAse protection assay is used widely to distinguish alternatively spliced forms of the same mRNA and to identify transcriptional initiation sites.

Because neural tissues are so heterogeneous, Northern blot or RNAse protection assays are often inadequate to detect differences in gene expression among individual neuronal nuclei. *In situ* hybridization assays coupled with densitometric analyses of grain counts allow quantitation of specific mRNAs in individual cells within the central nervous system. Probes for these assays include antisense RNA, oligonucleotides, or nick-translated cDNA. *In situ* hybridization assays have been used very effectively to evaluate the changes in neuropeptide mRNA levels after specific physiological events, to detect the expression of genes during development, and to distinguish receptor subtypes in different brain regions [23].

Northern blot, RNAse protection, and *in situ* hybridization assays assess steady-state mRNA levels and do not provide a direct measure of gene expression. These steady-state levels are determined by both synthetic and degradative processes. Therefore, an alteration in specific mRNA content within a cell or tissue can reflect either a change in RNA stability or a change in gene expression. To measure alterations in gene expression directly, the transcriptional run-off assay can be utilized. In this assay, isolated nuclei are incubated with radioactive ribonucleotides and allowed to transcribe *in vitro*. Radiolabeled transcripts are bound to specific cDNAs immobilized on a nitrocellulose or nylon filter. Because the elongation rate is constant, the amount of specific transcript produced is proportional to the transcriptional rate. Although run-off studies cannot be applied to neuronal cells *in situ*, recent attempts to detect mRNA precursors by *in situ* hybridization assays with intron-specific probes have provided encouraging results [24].

PCR has provided an additional method to quantify gene expression in localized areas of the brain. The technique known as coupled reverse transcription PCR (RT-PCR) [25] uses total RNA isolated from small regions of tissue. The RNA is first reverse transcribed to produce single-stranded cDNA. A pair of oligonucleotide primers is then used to amplify the single-stranded cDNA and the amount of the resulting PCR product is, in theory, proportional to the starting quantity of mRNA in the tissue samples. This technique requires a rigorous set of controls to assure its validity, including the empirical optimization of cycle number and input amount of total RNA. Each reaction must also include internal controls. A cloned template of slightly different size to the mRNA but containing the identical oligonucleotide sequences at its two termini is used to control for inter- and intra-assay variability. Additionally, primers are chosen that span an intron so that the inadvertent amplification of genomic, rather than cDNA, sequences can be monitored. Finally, a similarly sized segment of a ubiquitous, unregulated mRNA is co-amplified using a second set of unrelated primers in each reaction. RT-PCR should be particularly useful for quantifying mRNA responses in discrete

small brain regions to physiological or pharmacological stimuli.

CHARACTERIZATION OF GENETIC ELEMENTS INVOLVED IN TRANSCRIPTION

Although a detailed discussion of promoter analysis is beyond the scope of this review, it is clear that many of the recent advances in the understanding of neuronal gene expression have resulted from the identification of regulatory sequences in neural-specific genes and the characterization of proteins that bind to these sequences. Several of the methods that have been used to elucidate these protein-DNA interactions are considered below.

Protein-DNA interactions can be visualized through the use of gel-mobility shift or DNAse I protection assays

The gel-mobility shift assay takes advantage of the fact that the migration of DNA fragments through low ionic strength polyacrylamide gels is retarded when the fragments are bound to protein molecules. In general, these assays are performed by using DNA fragments labeled at the ends with ^{32}P. Because many proteins bind nonspecifically to DNA, it is usually necessary to perform these assays in the presence of a nonspecific competitor such as poly dI:dC. Specificity of binding must be confirmed by additional competition experiments utilizing wild-type or mutated DNA sequences. An advantage of the gel-mobility shift assay is that it is extremely sensitive. Therefore, this technique is typically used to monitor the biochemical purification of transcription factors.

To visualize the region of protein-DNA interaction more precisely, the DNAse I footprint assay has been utilized. This technique is based on the observation that proteins bound to a region of DNA protect the underlying sequences from cleavage by the endonuclease DNAse I. When the DNA fragment is labeled at one end bound to a mixture of proteins, and subjected to cleavage with DNAse I, the protection becomes apparent on a sequencing gel as a blank region in the pattern of labeled DNA fragments. This blank region is also known as a footprint. A modification of this approach is *in vivo* footprinting, in which protein binding to DNA in intact fragments of chromatin can be discerned. The polymerase chain reaction has greatly increased the sensitivity of the *in vivo* footprinting technique.

Functional assays make use of fusion genes containing heterologous reporters

The binding assays described above can identify which sequences of DNA are competent to interact with protein molecules, but do not address the functional implications of these interactions. To determine how a DNA element contributes to transcriptional regulation, a variety of promoter assays have been used. The most common of these assays utilizes the bacterial reporter enzyme chloramphenicol acetyl transferase, which is fused downstream from a functional eukaryotic promoter and putative regulatory region.

The chimeric gene can be introduced into cultured cells, either transiently or stably, and assayed for reporter gene activity. Putative regulatory elements containing specific mutations can also be examined and correlated with their ability to bind *trans*-acting factors. It is essential in these assays to confirm that the fusion gene utilizes the appropriate promoter sequence. This confirmation can be obtained through the use of RNAse protection assays. It is also important to remember that the promoter assay provides an *indirect* measure of transcription. Run-off assays (described above) continue to represent the gold standard for measurements of transcriptional rate.

CONCLUSIONS

New approaches for isolating neural-specific cDNAs and the development of sensitive as- says for measuring gene expression have greatly increased the understanding of neuronal regulation. It is now possible to measure changes in mRNA accumulation at the single-cell level. A major task for the next few years is to develop approaches for measuring gene regulation in real-time. Advances in this area will continue to push the frontiers of our knowledge of the genetic control of neuronal function.

REFERENCES

1. Itoh, N., Obata, K., Yanihara, N., and Okamoto, H. Human preprovasoactive intestinal polypeptide contains a novel PHI-27-like peptide, PHM-27. *Nature* 304:547–549, 1983.
2 Amara, S. G., Jones, V., Rosenfeld, M. G., Ong, E. S., and Evans, R. M. Alternative RNA processing in calcitonin gene expression generates mRNAs encoding different polypeptide products. *Nature* 298:240–244, 1982.
3. Sommer, B., Kohler, M., Sprengel, R., and Seeburg, P. H. RNA editing in brain controls a determinant of ion flow in glutamate-gated channels. *Cell* 67:11–19, 1991.
4. White, M. M. Designer channels: site-directed mutagenesis as a probe for structural features of channels and receptors. *Trends Neurosci.* 8: 364–368, 1985.
5. Summers, M. D., and Smith, G. E. A manual of methods for baculovirus vectors and insect cell culture procedures. *Tex. Agric. Exp. Stn. Bull.* 1555:56, 1987.
6. Hopp, T. P., Prickett, K. S., Price, V. L., Libby, R. T., March, C. J., Cerretti, D. P., Urdal, D. L., and Conlon, P. J. A short polypeptide marker sequence useful for recombinant protein identification and purification. *Biotechnology* 6:1204–1210, 1988.
7. Chirgwin, J. M., Przybyla, A. E., MacDonald, R. J., and Rutter, W. J. Isolation of biologically active ribonucleic acid from sources enriched in ribonuclease. *Biochemistry* 18:5294–5299, 1979.
8. Gubler, U., and Hoffman, B. J. A simple and very efficient method for generating cDNA libraries. *Gene* 25:263–269, 1983.
9. Grunstein, M., and Hogness, D. S. Colony hybridization: a method for the isolation of

cloned DNAs that contain a specific gene. *Proc. Natl. Acad. Sci. USA* 72:3962–3965, 1975.

10. Touchot, N., Chardin, P., and Tavitian, A. Four additional members of the ras gene superfamily isolated by an oligonucleotide strategy: molecular cloning of ypt-related cDNAs from a rat brain library. *Proc. Natl. Acad. Sci. USA* 84:8210–8214, 1987.

11. Dohlman, H. G., Thorner, J., Caron, M. G., and Lefkowitz, R. J. Model systems for the study of seven-transmembrane segment receptors. *Annu. Rev. Biochem.* 60:653–688, 1991.

12. He, X., Treary, M. N., Simmers, D. M., Ingraham, H. A., Swanon, L. W., and Rosenfeld, M. G. Expression of a large family of POU-domain regulatory genes in mammalian brain development. *Nature* 340:35–42, 1989.

13. Vega-Saenz de Miera, E. C., and Lin, J.-W. Cloning of ion channel gene families using the polymerase chain reaction. *Methods Enzymol.* 207:613–619, 1992.

14. Innis, M. A., Gelfand, D. H., Sninky, J. J., and White, T. J. (eds.) *PCR Protocols: A Guide to Methods and Applications.* San Diego: Academic Press, Inc., 1990.

15. Mandel, G., and Goodman, R. H. Using the brain to screen cloned genes. *Trends Neurosci.* 10:101–104, 1987.

16. Lechan, R. M., Wu, P., Jackson, I. M. D., Wolfe, H., Cooperman, S., Mandel, G., and Goodman, R. H. Thyrotropin-releasing hormone precursor: characterization in rat brain. *Science* 231:159–161, 1986.

17. Singh, H., Clere, R. G., and LeBowitz, S. H. Molecular cloning of sequence-specific DNA binding proteins using recognition site probes. *Biotechniques* 7:252–261, 1989.

18. Carr, D., and Scott, J. Blotting and band-shifting: techniques for studying protein-protein interactions. *TIBS* 17:246–249, 1992.

19. Chao, M. V., Bothwell, M. A., Ross, A. H., Koprowski, H., Lanahan, A. A., et al. Gene transfer and molecular cloning of the human NGF receptor. *Science* 232:518–521, 1986.

20. Aruffo, A., and Seed, B. Molecular cloning of a CD28 cDNA by a high-efficient COS cell expression system. *Proc. Natl. Acad. Sci. USA* 84:8573–8577, 1987.

21. Gurdon, J. B., Lane, D. C., Woodland, H. R., and Marbaix, G. Use of frog eggs and oocytes for the study of messenger RNA and its translation in living cells. *Nature* 233:177–182, 1971.

22. Valentino, K. I., Eberwine, J. H., and Barchas, J. D. (eds.). *In Situ Hybridization Applications to Neurobiology.* New York: Oxford University Press, 1987, pp. 1–24, 126–145.

23. Mansour, A., Meador-Woodruff, J. H., Bunzow, J. R., Civelli, O., Alcil, H., and Watson, S. J. Localization of dopamine D_2 receptor mRNA and D_1 and D_2 receptor binding in the rat brain and pituitary: an *in situ* hybridization receptor autoradiographic analysis. *J. Neurosci.* 10:2587–2600, 1990.

24. Herman, J. P., Schafer, M. K.-H., Watson, S. J., and Sherman, T. G. *In situ* hybridization analysis of arginine vasopressin gene transcription using intron-specific probes. *Mol. Endocrinol.* 5:1447–1456, 1991.

25. Camp, T. A., Rahal, J. O., and Mayo, K. E. Cellular localization and hormonal regulation of follicle-stimulating hormone and luteinizing hormone receptor messenger RNAs in the rat ovary. *Mol. Endocrinol.* 5:1405–1417, 1991.

CHAPTER 26

Molecular Genetic Approaches to Inherited Neurological Degenerative Disorders

Kunihiko Suzuki

Traditional molecular biological approaches to genetic neurological disorders, in which the defective gene products responsible for the phenotypes are known, have been well developed and are providing a powerful tool for our understanding of and eventual therapeutic attempts with these disorders. The traditional approach starts with the knowledge of the defective gene products, such as an enzyme deficiency, and reaches the gene and

Basic Neurochemistry: Molecular, Cellular, and Medical Aspects, 5th Ed., edited by G. J. Siegel et al. Published by Raven Press, Ltd., New York, 1994. Correspondence to Kunihiko Suzuki, Brain & Development Research Center, University of North Carolina School of Medicine, Chapel Hill, North Carolina 27599.

its characterization through purification of the gene products and cloning of the gene. Examples of the approaches and recent advances in such genetic disorders are illustrated elsewhere in this book (e.g., Chap. 38). However, the genetic disorders in this category constitute a relatively small proportion of the over 3,000 known human genetic disorders of Mendelian inheritance [1,2]. Recent methodological advances now allow us to approach the genetic causes of the remaining disorders without prior knowledge as to which genes are responsible for the disease. Since the flow of logic in this approach is in the reverse direction of the traditional approach, it is often termed "reverse genetics," i.e., one first tries to obtain the gene responsible for the disorder without knowing its function, and then tries to understand its function and the pathophysiology. The cloning strategy is also termed "positional cloning" since the genes are cloned on the basis of their positions in the genome only [3]. The ongoing project of mapping and sequencing the entire human genome is expected to contribute synergistically to the search for the genes responsible for all types of genetic disorders [4]. A recent review is available covering this subject [5].

If the present revolutionary advances in our molecular genetic understanding of hereditary neurodegenerative disorders are to be of pragmatic value in the future, strategies to achieve the ultimate gene therapy must be devised. Technological progress in this direction has also been noteworthy. Many prokaryotic and eukaryotic systems that allow expression of cloned genes have been developed. The gene transfer technology is progressing rapidly, either as *in vitro* systems with or without being vector-mediated, or as transgenes in the whole animal. Furthermore, the technique of homologous recombination is being used to generate mouse mutant strains in which specific genes are artificially and intentionally rendered inactive ("gene targeting"). This approach allows production of authentic mouse models of human genetic disorders when naturally occurring mutants do not exist among the easily manipulated small laboratory animals. Mutant lines of mice with Gaucher disease (glucosylceramidase deficiency, see Chap. 38), cystic fibrosis, apoprotein E deficiency, and others have been generated, taking advantage of this technology.

REVERSE GENETICS

Linkage analysis is the application of strategies to identify a genetic characteristic with its chromosome and its locus within a chromosome

When the abnormal gene product responsible for a given genetic disease is not known, one would like to first know the location of the responsible gene within the genome. The traditional approach for this analysis is based on two principles. (A) The primary sequence of the human genome is not fixed but varies in different individuals (polymorphisms). Such polymorphisms are statistically more common within introns and other noncoding regions of the genome which constitute most of the genomic sequences. In addition, there are regions of the human genome which are particularly polymorphic. Since such polymorphisms often either generate a new restriction site or abolish an existing site, they can be identified by digestion with appropriate restriction enzymes and observing the size of the generated fragments with a probe spanning the region (*r*estriction *f*ragment *l*ength *p*olymorphism; RFLP). (B) During meiosis, two corresponding pairs of chromosomes line up together and then are separated into two daughter cells that eventually generate the germ cells. Thus, two regions of the genome that are on the same chromosome tend to stay together while those on different chromosomes distribute to the germ cells totally independently from each other. However, the two corresponding chromosomes do not always separate cleanly from each other after coming together during meiosis. A crossover can occur in which the two chromosomes exchange an equivalent portion and generate a new pair of chromosomes. Therefore, even two regions on the same chromosome can become separated on two chromosomes if a crossover occurs between the two regions. It then follows that the closer the two regions are on the chromosome, the more likely they are to stay together. In the extreme case in which the polymorphic marker site is within the gene responsible for the disease, the marker will always be together with the gene. The strategy is, therefore, to find a polymorphic marker that is closely "linked" to affected individuals, and thus to the disease-causing gene, in the family. The physical map of the human genome is being developed rapidly where locations of known DNA sequences are marked [6]. Many of those sequences are known to be polymorphic, i.e., give different RFLP in different individuals, and can thus be used as markers for linkage analyses.

A successful linkage analysis requires DNA materials from family members of affected patients, preferably from as many generations as possible. A set of known polymorphic markers are chosen as probes, genomic DNA prepared from individuals, digested by appropriate restriction enzymes and the RFLP patterns examined for each of the markers. Any markers that do not segregate with or against the disease state are discarded. In clearly X-linked diseases, the chromosomal localization is known and only the markers on the X-chromosome need to be selected for the study. As should be clear from the description, linkage analysis is essentially a statistical procedure that can be facilitated by a computer. Programs have been developed specifically for analyses of the results of complex linkage studies. The results are expressed as the *lod* score [7,8], which gives a statistical estimate, in decimal logarithm, of the relative closeness of the given polymorphic marker to the disease-causing gene. A *lod* score of at least 3, preferably greater, is considered to be an indica-

tion that the gene being searched is "linked" to the marker.

The genes responsible for a number of genetic neurological disorders have been mapped to specific chromosomes and their regions by means of linkage analysis. The first spectacular success of the linkage analysis in the field was the localization of the gene responsible for Huntington's disease [9]. The study was successful partly because of the availability of an enormous pedigree in the Lake Maracaibo region of Venezuela. Since then, chromosomal localizations of many genes responsible for genetic neurodegenerative disorders have been identified, e.g., for familial retinoblastoma, neurofibromatosis I, Charcot-Marie-Tooth disease, myotonic dystrophy, three different forms of "Batten disease" (infantile, late infantile, and the juvenile forms), and ataxia telangiectasia. The catalogue of such diseases continues to expand (Table 1).

TABLE 1. Examples of the genes responsible for genetic neurodegenerative disorders mapped by linkage analysis

Disorder	Chromosome
Infantile "neuronal ceroid-lipofuscinosis"	1
Charcot-Marie-Tooth	1
Huntington	4
Spinal muscular atrophy	5
Spinocerebellar degeneration	6
Friedreich ataxia	9
Torsion dystonia	9
Ataxia telangiectasia	11
Familial retinoblastoma	13
Juvenile neuronal ceroid-lipofuscinosis	16
Neurofibromatosis I	17
Niemann-Pick type C	18
Myotonic dystrophy	19
Late-onset familial Alzheimer's disease	19
Early-onset familial Alzheimer's disease	21
Late-infantile neuronal ceroid-lipofuscinosis	not 1 nor 16

For a more detailed map of known genes relevant to the nervous system and/or causing neurological diseases, see [30].

A few caveats must be kept in mind. For the most part, linkage analyses are effective for Mendelian disorders where single genes are responsible for the disease states. It is not that the principle of linkage analysis is not applicable for multigenic disorders. It is simply a matter of complexity. Analysis of a single-gene Mendelian disorder is already complex enough and any increase in the number of genes that must be taken into the analysis increases the complexity logarithmically. Another potentially complicating factor is that genetically different diseases can manifest themselves with similar clinical phenotypes. For example, what had been classified as Sanfilippo disease has turned out to consist of four distinct genetic diseases caused by genetic defects in four different genes (see Chap. 38). If families gathered for a linkage analysis of "one genetic disease" in fact include more than one genetically distinct disorder, the results of the linkage analysis would confuse, if not totally obscure, any conclusion. It is essential, therefore, to ascertain that all individuals being included in a linkage analysis be within a single genetic complementation group. Despite these theoretical constraints, linkage analysis is being applied to potentially highly complex "disorders" with genetic underlining, such as manic-depressive disorders or schizophrenia.

In some instances, cytologically identifiable deletions or other chromosomal abnormalities associated with the disease can provide the crucial clue as to the location of the responsible gene, a situation fully exploited in the positional cloning of the dystrophin gene, abnormalities of which are responsible for Duchenne and Becker muscular dystrophies [10]. More recently, the chromosomal localization of the gene responsible for Niemann-Pick type C disease has been determined by taking advantage of the fact that an equivalent disease exists both in humans and mice [11]. In this approach, artificially constructed mouse microcells, each containing a single copy of a human chromosome, were used as the human chromosome donor. When fused with cells from affected mice,

the biochemical phenotype of the disease could be corrected only when human chromosome 18 was introduced. The gene localization could further be narrowed down because those cells that lost a portion of chromosome 18 in subsequent subcloning reverted back to the Niemann-Pick type C phenotype.

Localizing the gene to a chromosome and to a specific region of a chromosome is facilitated by obtaining more than one linked marker, particularly two markers that flank the target gene

While varieties of ways to reach the target gene have been devised, the basic principle is to extend the DNA sequence information from the identified linked marker region toward the gene, either contiguously or discontinuously. These procedures are often referred to as "chromosomal walking" and "jumping," respectively. Genomic DNA libraries in the λ phage, cosmids, and more recently in the form of the yeast artificial chromosome (YAC) are commonly used to track down the target gene. Human chromosome-specific YAC clones that collectively give the complete contiguous chromosomal DNA sequence have been constructed. In the primitive "walking," a segment of genomic DNA containing the identified marker is sequenced from the marker region, a new primer is made from the newly sequenced region and used for further sequencing, slowly extending along the stretch of DNA toward the target. In order for this strategy to be effective, the marker must be reasonably close to the target gene, because the number of nucleotides that can be sequenced in one step is still limited. A variation of the "walking" is "jumping." The genomic DNA containing the marker sequence is circularized with the marker region on one end, sequenced across the ligated region, thus obtaining the sequence information some distance away from the marker for the next "jumping."

These procedures are slow and tedious, as attested to by the search for the Huntington's disease gene, which has only recently been cloned [12] although it was first localized to chromosome 4 nearly a decade ago. In some other disorders, however, the positional cloning approach has been successful when no other approaches were feasible. Some of the notable examples of genes responsible for genetic neurological disorders that have been cloned by this strategy include neurofibromatosis-I (von Recklinghausen), familial retinoblastoma, myotonic dystrophy, fragile X syndrome, and Duchenne/Becker muscular dystrophies. Although not a neurological disorder, the cloning of the gene responsible for cystic fibrosis provides an excellent overview of how the positional cloning strategy was successfully employed [13].

The final step of the positional cloning strategy for genetic diseases is elucidation of the function of the cloned gene and mutational analysis of patients. It is *a priori* evident that, if the correct gene has been obtained, the gene structure and the function of its product should be abnormal in affected patients.

When the marker is sufficiently close to the target gene, the polymorphism of the marker sequence itself can be used for diagnosis of affected individuals, even though the gene responsible for the disease has not been identified, because essentially no crossover occurs on the chromosome between the disease-causing gene and the marker

As in the DNA diagnosis based on the disease-causing mutation within the responsible gene, knowledge of the nature of the polymorphism in the family is prerequisite. Conceptually, the disease-causing mutation is merely a polymorphism within the gene and thus is no different from a polymorphism in the marker sequence which is so close to the gene that no crossover occurs.

GENE TRANSFER AND EXPRESSION

When "reverse genetics" (positional cloning) is successful and the gene involved in a particular gene disorder is identified, the next major step is elucidation of its function

Once segments of the gene are available, isolation of its transcript in the form of cDNA is a relatively straightforward procedure in principle with the standard recombinant DNA technology. Thus, we assume that both the genomic and cDNA sequences are characterized and available. This also means that the primary amino acid sequence of the gene product is known. Not infrequently, the sequence information itself may suggest the function of the product by its similarity to other proteins of known function. It may be homologous (i.e., evolutionarily related) to other proteins or may be merely similar due to similar functions. Subscription to up-to-date data of recorded nucleotide sequences (NCBI-GenBank) and protein sequences (SWISS-PROT) are available inexpensively on CD-ROMs together with the information on Medlar references and the retrieval software from the National Center for Biotechnology Information ("Entrez"). Commercial molecular biology softwares can then be used to evaluate possible similarity of the gene and its product with those in the database. Many methodologies are available to transfer and express genes on different levels of organization.

Cell-free expression (*in vitro* translation)

cDNA including the entire protein coding sequence can be subcloned into a suitable plasmid vector with flanking RNA polymerase promoters and then transcribed with a capping analogue to a translatable mRNA. The protein coded by the cDNA can then be generated in any of the commercially available *in vitro* translation systems, such as rabbit reticulocyte or wheat germ lysate. The *in vitro* translation product is useful to test immunological reactivity but is often functionally inactive since no post-translational processing takes place. Proteolytic trimming, glycosylation, phosphorylation, and other modifications are often essential for functional activity. The quantity of the gene product that can be generated by *in vitro* translation is very limited.

Expression in living cells

A large number of expression systems are available that use living cells, either in culture or in the form of frog oocyte. Isolated genes, cDNAs, or mRNAs generated from cDNAs can be expressed. They may be prokaryotic or eukaryotic, for transient or stable expression, or integrated and regulated expression or overexpression systems. Each type has its own characteristic advantages and disadvantages and is used in accordance with the purpose of experiments.

The frog oocyte system is a cellular equivalent of the *in vitro* translation system in that mRNA appropriately generated from cloned cDNA is directly injected into fertilized frog eggs. The frog produces unusually large eggs, which permits direct manual injection of a relatively large quantity of mRNA. The injected mRNA is translated by the intrinsic metabolic machinery within the egg and processed to form functional proteins. Thus, the function of the produced protein can be tested, if known or suspected. This system allows only a brief, transient expression of the exogenously injected mRNA and again the quantity that can be generated is very small. Nevertheless, the system has been used widely in neurobiology because many expressed membrane proteins, such as receptors, are integrated into the oocyte membrane and their functions can be studied by sophisticated tools, such as patch clamping.

Perhaps one of the most commonly used mammalian cells for transient expression is the COS-1 cells, which are transformed African green monkey kidney cells. When transfected by cDNAs subcloned into appropriate plasmid vector, such as pSVL, which includes the SV40 late promoter in the

upstream of the cloned cDNA, a minor proportion of COS-1 cells generate the gene product, which can then be tested for its known or suspected function. The expression is transient with the peak activity occurring between 1 and 4 days after transfection. Unless some mechanism is used to select the transfected cells, no more than 10–20% of the cells in the culture express the exogenous gene. Even for these limitations, this system is widely used for its simplicity and technical ease. For more stable expression of cloned genes, many hosts and suitable vectors have been devised, which allow stable integration of the exogenous genes.

When a large quantity of the gene product is required, several overexpression systems can be utilized, some prokaryotic and other eukaryotic. A prokaryotic system has been used successfully to produce milligram quantities of human GM2 activator protein [14]. In this example, the gene product was generated by a recombinant plasmid, pHX17, in *E. coli*, strain M15/pREP4, as a fusion protein attached to six histidine residues bridged to the mature activator protein sequence by a three-amino acid sequence specific for the coagulation factor Xa. Characteristically for proteins generated by prokaryotes, the GM2 activator was not processed. However, the unprocessed fusion protein was fully functional in activating hydrolysis of GM2 ganglioside by β-hexosaminidase A. The fusion protein could be purified to near homogeneity by a single step of nickel affinity chromatography. After renaturation, and digestion with Factor Xa, GM2 activator protein was identical in primary amino acid sequence with the native mature, processed protein in the tissue.

While the prokaryotic over-expression system can produce preparative quantities of cloned gene products, the lack of post-translational processing limits its usefulness when the protein requires such modifications for functional activity. A mammalian system utilizing BHK cells is widely used to overcome such limitations. Another extensively used system utilizes a unique property of an insect virus, baculovirus [15]. This virus is pathogenic only to certain types of insects (butterflies and moths) and thus does not pose a hazard to human workers. It contains a gene coding for the polyhedrin protein, which is generated in an enormous quantity within infected insect tissues. When the cloned cDNA is inserted into the virus just downstream of the polyhedrin gene promoter, the infected insect cells produce large quantities of the protein coded by the cloned gene, driven by the strong polyhedrin gene promoter. The protein is secreted into the culture medium. The human GM2 activator and human sphingolipid activator (SAP) genes have been expressed in the baculovirus system, generating milligram quantities of processed activator proteins. The quantity of the protein that can be produced by the baculovirus system varies widely from less than 1 mg to over 100 mg per liter of culture medium. Estimated by its activating capacity to hydrolyze GM2 ganglioside, approximately 5 mg of the GM2 activator protein per liter of the culture medium was produced by the above recombinant baculovirus. More recently, recombinant baculovirus constructs including the hexa-histidine tail and either the Factor Xa or enterokinase cleavage sequence have become commercially available, thus permitting the same one-step purification of the generated protein by nickel affinity chromatography. Generally, proteins produced by the baculovirus system undergo post-translational processing similar to that for the native protein in mammalian tissues and are functionally active [16], although subtle differences, for example, in the glycosylation pattern, have been described. However, the large quantity of the generated protein tends to overload the intracellular processing machinery and only a small proportion actually undergoes the normal processing. Most are excreted without any processing or with only incomplete processing. One drawback of the baculovirus overexpression system is that the virus eventually kills the host insect cells. Thus, a large amount of the desired protein can be obtained only for up to several days. New infection needs to be started with new cultured insect cells every time.

In vivo transfer and expression

Various attempts have been made to introduce and express foreign genes directly in a living organism. A somewhat naive approach of direct injection of dystrophin cDNA into muscles proved to be effective in establishing reasonably stable local expression in the tissue [17]. More usual are procedures that utilize various vectors, most commonly, viral vectors. Viruses have evolved an efficient machinery to introduce and replicate themselves into the host and express their genetic materials. In principle, therefore, genes that are foreign to a virus can be inserted into the viral genome and be expressed within infected hosts. More of virus-mediated gene transfer and expression will be discussed below under the section "Gene Therapy." Similarly, introduction and expression of foreign genes by transplantation of tissues/organs have been attempted extensively as means of treatment of genetic disorders and will be covered later.

Transgenic mouse

The term "transgenic mouse" refers to mice genetically manipulated by a technology that permits stable integration and expression of exogenous DNA fragments into the genome of the entire organism [18,19]. The technology combines recombinant DNA and mouse biology.

Conventional Transgenic Mice

The principle of the traditional transgenic experiment involves construction of a suitable exogenous gene preparation with an appropriate promoter, its injection into fertilized mouse embryo at the stage of the zygote with a glass pipette, and implantation of the injected egg back into the oviduct of a pseudopregnant host female mouse prepared by

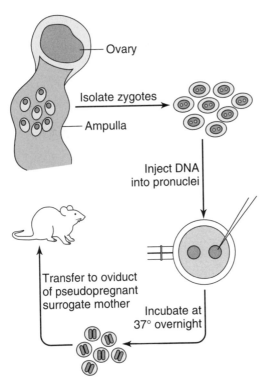

FIG. 1.   Procedure for the conventional transgenic experiment. (Reproduced from [18] by permission.)

mating a virgin female mouse with a vasectomized male (Fig. 1). The injected DNA randomly integrates itself into the embryo genome with a certain statistical probability. The pseudopregnant mouse serves as the host to carry the embryo to the term. Those mice with the stably integrated exogenous gene will carry it in all the cells of the body and should express its product. The efficiency of integration of the exogenous DNA into the mouse genome ranges from a few percent to over 10% of injected eggs. The transgene can be driven by its own native promoter or by an artificially introduced promoter according to the experimental design. When unregulated overexpression of the exogenous gene is desired, an unregulated strong promoter can be placed upstream of the injected gene. On the other hand, attempts have been made to regulate the gene expression in the transgenic animals by using developmentally regulated promoter

(e.g., the native promoter for myelin protein genes, which should be turned on at the time of myelination) or a manipulatable promoter, such as the metalothionein gene promoter, which can be regulated by exogenously provided heavy metals. The traditional transgenic mice can thus express the introduced foreign gene, as if it were a native gene in its genome. The source of the exogenous gene is not a factor in the conventional transgenic expression. In principle, genes from any eukaryotic sources can be expressed in mice. A major limitation of this technology is the randomness of the site of integration of the injected DNA. There is always a statistical probability that the exogenous DNA sequence is integrated in such a way that a native gene sequence is disrupted and thus rendered inactive. Such a transgene may be incompatible with life or may produce varying degrees of abnormality, depending on the function of the disrupted native gene. In fact, a whole group of transgenic mice with unintended insertional mutations of endogenous genes are known [20]. This unpredictable disruption of native genes must be kept in mind when the clinical and biochemical phenotypes of conventional transgenic mice are evaluated.

TARGETED GENE DISRUPTION: MOUSE MODEL OF GENETIC DISEASE

A recent development of the homologous recombination technology and further manipulation of the mouse reproductive biology have made it possible to target specific endogenous genes for disruption [21]

This technology allows one in principle to duplicate in mice specific genetic defects found in humans. The aim of this manipulation is not to express exogenous genes but to specifically inactivate or otherwise manipulate endogenous genes. The underlying mechanistic principle of this technology is that of homologous recombination. When an exogenous DNA sequence is integrated into the mouse genome, there is an extremely small but nonrandom, finite probability that it inserts itself at the site where the native sequence is similar to that of the exogenous sequence. For homologous recombination to occur, the two sequences must be as nearly identical as possible. Homologous genes even from closely related mammalian species are not similar enough, particularly with respect to introns. Recent studies indicate that the probability of homologous recombination can be dramatically greater when the gene to be used to disrupt the endogenous gene is derived from the same strain of mice as that of the recipient cells.

The principle of generating a mouse model of a genetic disease involves the steps illustrated in Fig. 2. Since the efficiency of true homologous recombination is far below

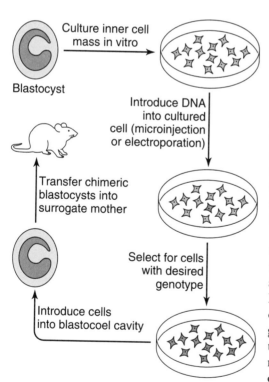

Culture inner cell mass in vitro

Blastocyst

Introduce DNA into cultured cell (microinjection or electroporation)

Transfer chimeric blastocysts into surrogate mother

Select for cells with desired genotype

Introduce cells into blastocoel cavity

FIG. 2.   Procedure for the gene targeting experiment. (Reproduced from [18] by permission.)

that of random integration, direct injection into individual zygotes is impractical. The critical additional component for this technology is a culture of embryonic stem cells (ES cells). These are undifferentiated multipotential cells from mouse blastocysts which can develop into any type of cells and organs in the body. Under certain specific culture conditions, they can be maintained with their multipotential characteristics intact. In order to increase the probability of obtaining recombinant ES cells to pragmatic feasibility, a mechanism for selection, either positive (such as resistance to antibiotics) and/or negative (thymidine kinase), is usually constructed into the exogenously introduced DNA sequence. The exogenous DNA sequence is introduced into ES cells, commonly now by electroporation. Those cells in which the introduced sequence integrates itself into the homologous sequence in the host genome are selected and injected into the cavity of a mouse embryo at the stage of the blastocyst. The injected blastocyst is implanted in a pseudopregnant host female mouse. Thus, the embryo consists of two types of cells each with different genetic make-up: the native cells of the blastocyst and the injected ES cells. Since both are multipotential, the embryo develops into a whole animal that is chimeric with varying proportions of both cells. If, for example, strains of different fur colors are used for the host and the ES cells, the chimera will exhibit stripes and patches of two different fur colors, a procedure often used for easy identification of the resultant chimeras.

Since these transgenic mice are genetically chimeric, an additional step is required to obtain a genetically homogeneous mouse strain in which a specific gene is inactivated. It is necessary to select chimeras that produce recombinant germ cells. Unless the germ cells have the genotype of the ES cells, the resultant offspring will be of the host genotype. When the disrupted gene is located on the X chromosome, only male chimeras producing sperm of the recombinant genotype are needed. For autosomal genes, suitable males and females must be obtained. Since the statistical probability of both alleles being disrupted is infinitesimally small, these chimeras will be "carriers" of the disrupted gene. Crosses between them should produce homozygous mice with both genes inactivated. The strain then can be maintained as for any other autosomal recessive mutant strains of mice.

The number of artificially generated insertional mutations is increasing at an accelerating pace. Notable among them are an equivalent of Gaucher disease, in which the glucosylceramidase gene is inactivated [22], cystic fibrosis [23], and a recently described mutant with inactivated myelin P0 protein [24]. On the other hand, one of the early "successes" turned out to be a disappointment. The hypoxanthine phosphoribosyltransferase (HPRT) gene was inactivated in the mouse for the purpose of producing a mouse model of human Lesch-Nyhan disease. Despite the complete inactivation, "affected" mice were clinically normal. The most likely explanation is that the mouse has active uricase and thus can bypass the defective HPRT. Undoubtedly we will see more mouse models of genetic neurological disorders generated with this technology in the near future, since they provide invaluable tools for studies of pathogenesis and eventual gene therapy of these disorders.

GENE THERAPY

In a broad sense, the term "gene therapy" should encompass any attempts at treating genetic diseases caused by defective genes by introduction and expression of normally functional genes [25,26]. Such attempts were made before the advent of molecular biological technologies in the form of organ/tissue transplantations and are, to a limited extent, still made. Earlier, organ transplantations were employed to provide the body with normal gene products missing in patients. In some instances, the transplan-

tation was indicated for other medical reasons, such as the kidney transplantation in Fabry disease in which kidney failure is one of the prominent clinical manifestations. Cultured fibroblasts were transplanted for their ready availability. The amniotic membrane was used because of its immunological inactivity. Generally, somatic organ implantations have been of limited effectiveness, particularly in those genetic disorders in which clinical and pathological involvement of the central nervous system is prominent, because the normal gene products produced by the implanted organs did not effectively reach the brain. However, promising results have been reported with normal bone marrow transplantation into patients with some genetic neurological disorders, most notably in mucopolysaccharidoses [27]. In the twitcher mouse mutant, which is a naturally occurring mouse model of human globoid cell leukodystrophy (Krabbe disease, galactosylceramidase deficiency) (see Chap. 38), allogeneic bone marrow transplantation effectively alleviated the disease process and prolonged the life span of affected mice by a factor of 3 [28]. Bone marrow transplantation has also been attempted in other animal models.

The narrow definition of "gene therapy" is treatment of genetic diseases on the gene level *utilizing recombinant DNA technologies*. Organ/tissue transplantation is, therefore, not within this narrow definition of gene therapy. Direct injection of exogenous genes such as the one described above for expression of dystrophin in muscle appears limited in future potential. Virus-mediated transfer and expression of normal genes are currently actively pursued by many laboratories. Highly promising results have been obtained in tissue culture systems and also in some animal models of human genetic diseases. The most commonly employed viral vectors are retroviruses because of their well-characterized properties and the efficient and relatively nondiscriminatory capacity to infect various cellular types. If a retrovirus is appropriately modified with an inserted exogenous gene, it can infect the target cells and produce the gene product lacking in the host cell. For stable expression of the virus genome, the retrovirus must be integrated into the host genome, and the integration requires mitosis of the host cells. This property seriously limits the usefulness of retroviruses as the vector for gene therapy of genetic diseases of the central nervous system, because most neurons and glia in the mature brain are postmitotic and do not replicate easily. Use of replication defective herpes simplex 1 overcomes this disadvantage of the retrovirus, since it does not need to be integrated into the host cell genome for its expression. Thus, the exogenous gene engineered into herpes simplex 1 virus can be expressed in postmitotic cells and actively replicating cells with similar efficiency. This ability to replicate and express its own genome independent of the host cell replication further provides an advantage in that there is much less risk of inadvertently disrupting important host genes by random integration.

Transfer and expression of normal genes as the means of treating genetic diseases, as described above, are applicable only to those diseases in which the normal functions of the genes are lacking ("deficiency disease"). While some genetic diseases of autosomal dominant inheritance may well be caused by lack of sufficient quantity of the normal gene products, e.g., essential structural components, and thus are "deficiency diseases," some others may well be due to detrimental effects of mutant gene products. In these disorders, providing normal genes and their products will not be an effective treatment. Similarly, gene therapy will not be effective in conditions in which a gene overdose might be the underlying mechanism, such as in Down's syndrome.

For obvious reasons, gene therapy utilizing the experimental design of the transgenic mouse cannot be readily applied to human patients. However, transgenic technology has been shown to effectively "cure" the clinical, pathological, and bio-

chemical abnormalities in the mouse model of β-glucuronidase deficiency (mucopolysaccharidosis type VII; see Chap. 38) [29].

UNIQUE NATURE OF GENETIC DISORDERS AFFECTING THE BRAIN

We have considered molecular genetic approaches to genetic neurological disorders. While the principle is no different between neurological and non-neurological disorders, biological uniqueness of the nervous system must always be taken into consideration. The essentially postmitotic nature of most neurons and glial cells in the mature central nervous system and the consequent consideration for selection of suitable vectors for gene transfer have been already commented on. It will be useful to consider here some other properties of the nervous system that differentiate it from other organs and tissues. First, the anatomical and cellular structure of the brain is much more complex than other organs, consisting of specialized regions and cell types with unique functional roles: neurons, astrocytes, oligodendroglia, microglia, etc. Expressions of intrinsic genes are highly complex with respect to regions and cellular types, as well as during development. In fact, expressions of certain genes are taken as determinants or markers of the cell types, such as glial fibrillary acid protein (GFAP) in astrocytes, or many myelin-specific proteins and UDP-gal:ceramide galactosyltransferase, which catalyzes the last step of galactosylceramide biosynthesis, in the myelin-forming cells, Schwann cells, and oligodendrocytes. Some receptors may be specific for certain neurons in certain regions and perhaps only during a certain period in brain development. These factors surely render different regions and cellular components of the brain differently susceptible to any genetic abnormalities in different developmental stages. One can only consider, for example, the intrigue of Huntington's disease, a dominantly expressed genetic disorder. An abnormality in only one of the yet-to-be-identified pair of genes on chromosome 4, present in every single cell, causes a disease in which the nervous system develops and functions perfectly well until middle age when a specific small group of neurons start degenerating while other brain constituents apparently continue to function normally. Thus, more than for any other organs, variables such as the anatomical regions, cell types, and developmental stages are critical.

Equally critical is the question of plasticity of developing brain, particularly when treatment of degenerative genetic disorders is contemplated. The brain repairs itself poorly compared to other organs. Even if effective means to treat the disease is found, it would be of only academic interest if the treatment cannot be initiated before the brain sustains irreparable damage. Most genetic lysosomal disorders (Chap. 38) affect the brain early and severely. Affected fetuses diagnosed and aborted at 20 weeks of gestation always show obvious neuropathology. Affected newborns therefore must have advanced damage to their brain. Even if a perfect "cure" is available, it may have to start *in utero* to be pragmatically meaningful. These considerations emphasize the necessity to learn much more about normal developmental processes of the brain and its plasticity or lack thereof than we know now.

REFERENCES

1. McKusick, V. A. *Mendelian Inheritance in Man. Catalogs of Autosomal Dominant, Autosomal Recessive, and X-Linked Phenotypes.* 8th Ed. Baltimore, MD: The Johns Hopkins University Press, 1988.
2. Beaudet, A. L., Scriber, C. R., Sly, W. S., Valle, D., Cooper, D. N., McKusick, V. A., and Schmidke, J. Genetics and biochemistry of variant human phenotypes. In C. R. Scriver, A. L. Beaudet, W. S. Sly, and D. Valle (eds.), *The Metabolic Basis of Inherited Disease.* 6th edition. New York: McGraw-Hill, 1989, pp. 3–163.
3. Lehrach, H., and Bates, G. Approaches to identifying disease gene. In J. Brosius, R. T. Fremeau (eds.), *Molecular Genetic Approaches to Neuropsychiatric Diseases.* New York: Academic Press, 1991, pp. 3–17.
4. Cantor, C. R., and Smith, C. L. Mapping and sequencing the human genome. In J. Brosius, R. T. Fremeau (eds.), *Molecular Genetic Approaches to Neuropsychiatric Diseases.* New York: Academic Press, 1991, pp. 19–34.
5. Davis, M. B., Rosenberg, R. N., and Harding, A. E. Molecular genetics and neurological disease: an introduction. In R. N. Rosenberg, S. B. Prusiner, S. DiMauro, R. L. Barchi, and L. M. Kunkel (eds.), *The Molecular and Genetic Basis of Neurological Disease.* Boston: Butterworth-Heinemann, 1993, pp. 3–20.
6. NIH/CEPH Collaborative Mapping Group. A comprehensive genetic linkage map of the human genome. *Science* 258:67–86, 1992. (Available in an expanded version as one of the reprint series of *Science.*)
7. Ott, J. Principle of human genetic linkage analysis. In J. Brosius and R. T. Fremeau (eds.), *Molecular Genetic Approaches to Neuropsychiatric Diseases.* New York: Academic Press, 1991, pp. 35–53.
8. Buckler, A., and Housman, D. *Methods of Genome Analysis: A Gene Hunter's Guide.* New York: WH Freeman, 1992.
9. Gusella, J. F., Wexler, N., Conneally, P. M., Naylor, S. L., Anderson, M. A., Tanzi, R. E., Watkins, P. C., Ottina, K., Wallace, M. R., Sakaguchi, A. Y., Young, A. B., Shoulson, I., Bonila, E., and Martin, J. B. A polymorphic DNA marker genetically linked to Huntington's disease. *Nature* 306:234–238, 1983.
10. Koening, M., Hoffman, E., Bertelson, C., Monaco, A., Feener, C., and Kunkel, L. Complete cloning of the Duchenne muscular dystrophy (DMD) cDNA and preliminary genomic organization of the DMD gene in normal and affected individuals. *Cell* 50:509–517, 1987.
11. Kurimasa, A., Ohno, K., and Oshimura, M. Restoration of the cholesterol metabolism in 3T3 cell lines derived from the sphingomyelinosis mouse (spm/spm) by transfer of a human chromosome 18. *Hum. Genet.* [in press], 1993.
12. Huntington's Disease Collaborative Group. A novel gene containing a trinucleotide repeat that is expanded and unstable on Hunting-

ton's disease chromosomes. *Cell* 72:971–983, 1993.

13. Tsui, L.-C., and Buchwald, M. Biochemical and molecular genetics of cystic fibrosis. *Adv. Hum. Genet.* 20:153–266, 1991.

14. Klima, H., Klein, A., Schwarzmann, G., Suzuki, K., and Sandhoff, K. Over-expression of a functionally active human GM2-activator protein in E. coli. *Biochem. J.* 292:571–576, 1993.

15. O'Reilly, D. R., Miller, L. K., and Luckow, V. A. *Baculovirus Expression Vectors: A Laboratory Manual.* New York: WH Freeman, 1992.

16. Luchow, V. A., and Summers, M. D. Trends in the development of baculovirus expression vectors. *Biotechnology* 6:47–55, 1988.

17. Wolff, J. A., Malone, R. W., Williams, P., Chong, W., Acsadi, G., Jani, A., and Felgner, P. L. Direct gene transfer into mouse muscle in vivo. *Science* 247:1465–1468, 1990.

18. Popko, B., Germ-line manipulation of the mouse in neuroscience. In J. Brosius and R. T. Fremeau (eds.), *Molecular Genetic Approaches to Neuropsychiatric Diseases.* New York: Academic Press, 1991, pp. 429–447.

19. Sedivy, J. M., and Joyner, A. L. *Gene Targeting.* New York: WH Freeman, 1992.

20. Meisler, M. H. Insertional mutation of "classical" and novel genes in transgenic mice. *Trends Genet.* 8:341–344, 1992.

21. Magin, T. M., and Melton, D. W. Gene targeting. In R. N. Rosenberg, S. B. Prusiner, S. DiMauro, R. L. Barchi, and L. M. Kunkel (eds.), *The Molecular and Genetic Basis of Neurological Disease.* Boston: Butterworth-Heinemann, 1993, pp. 29–39.

22. Tybulewicz, V. L. J., Tremblay, M. L., LaMarca, M. E., Willemsen, R., Stubblefield, B. K., Winfield, S., Zablocka, B., Sidransky, E., Martin, B. M., Huang, S. P., Mintzer, K. A., Westphal, H., Mulligan, R. C., and Ginns, E. I. Animal model of Gaucher's disease from targeted disruption of the mouse glucocerebrosidase gene. *Nature* 357:407–410, 1992.

23. Snouwaert, J. N., Brigman, K. K., Latour, A. M., Malouf, N. N., Boucher, R. C., Smithies, O., and Koller, B. H. An animal model for cystic fibrosis made by gene targeting. *Science* 257:1083–1088, 1992.

24. Giese, K. P., Martini, R., Lemke, G., Soriano, P., and Schachner, M. Mouse P0 gene disruption leads to hypomyelination, abnormal expression of recognition molecules, and degeneration of myelin and axons. *Cell* 71: 565–576, 1992.

25. Jinnah, H., Gage, F., and Friedmann, T. Gene therapy and neurologic disease. A neurologic gene map. In R. N. Rosenberg, S. B. Prusiner, S. DiMauro, R. L. Barchi, and L. M. Kunkel (eds.), *The Molecular and Genetic Basis of Neurological Disease.* Boston: Butterworth-Heinemann, 1993, pp. 969–976.

26. Verma, I. M. Gene therapy. *Sci. Am.* 262: 68–84, 1990.

27. Krivit, W., Whitley, C. B., Chang, P.-N., Shapiro, E., Belani, K. G., Snover, D., Summers, C. G., and Blazer, B. Lysosomal storage diseases treated by bone marrow transplantation: Review of 21 patients. In F. L. Johnson and C. Pochedly (eds.), *Bone Marrow Transplantation in Children.* New York: Raven Press, 1990, pp. 261–287.

28. Suzuki, K., and Suzuki, K. The twitcher mouse: A model of human globoid cell leukodystrophy (Krabbe disease). In R. E. Martensson (ed.), *Myelin, Biology and Chemistry.* Boca Raton, FL: CRC Press, 1992, pp. 745–759.

29. Kyle, J. W., Birkenmeier, E. H., Gwynn, B., Vogler, C., Hoppe, P. C., Hoffmann, J. W., and Sly, W. S. Correction of murine mucopolysaccharidosis VII by a human β-glucuronidase transgene. *Proc. Natl. Acad. Sci. USA* 87: 3914–3918, 1990.

30. Harding, A. E., and Rosenberg, R. N. A neurologic gene map. In R. N. Rosenberg, S. B. Prusiner, S. DiMauro, R. L. Barchi, and L. M. Kunkel (eds.), *The Molecular and Genetic Basis of Neurological Disease.* Boston: Butterworth-Heinemann, 1993, pp. 21–24.

PART FOUR

Cellular Neurochemistry

CHAPTER 27

Axonal Transport and the Neuronal Cytoskeleton

RICHARD HAMMERSCHLAG, JANET L. CYR, AND SCOTT T. BRADY

Basic Neurochemistry: Molecular, Cellular, and Medical Aspects, 5th Ed., edited by G. J. Siegel et al. Published by Raven Press, Ltd., New York, 1994. Correspondence to Richard Hammerschlag, Division of Neurosciences, Beckman Research Institute of the City of Hope, Duarte, California 91010.

NEURONAL ORGANELLES IN MOTION

The axon comprises a major portion of the total volume and surface area in most neurons and may extend several thousand cell body diameters. Since the genetic material and effectively all of the protein synthesis machinery are localized to the cell body, a supply line is maintained to provide structural and functional materials to sites all along the length of the axon. Insights as to how neurons accomplish this task can be obtained by viewing living axons with video-enhanced light microscopy [1,1a] (Fig. 1).

Such video images reveal an array of organelles moving down the axon toward the nerve terminal (anterograde direction) as well as returning to the cell body (retrograde direction). The movements create patterns as engrossing as the ant farms of our childhood and initially appear as chaotic. Some organelles glide smoothly, while others move in fits and starts. On closer examination, an underlying order emerges: The organelles moving in the anterograde direction are typically fainter and smaller but more numerous than those moving retrograde, and all organelles appear to travel along gently curving fibrils. Occasionally, two organelles are seen to travel in opposite directions along the same fibril, appearing destined for a head-on collision but seeming to pass through each other; other organelles hop from one fibril to another. The images imply, and other studies confirm, that the organelles represent membrane-bound packets of materials en route to a variety of intraneuronal destinations. The fibrils, for their part, have been identified by electron microscopy and immunocytochemistry as microtubules, a critically important component of the axonal cytoskeleton. Unseen in the video images, because they occur orders of magnitude more slowly, are the dynamic movements of the fibrils and other structural elements of the axoplasm.

The life cycle of these organelles, their kinetics and molecular cargo, the molecular motors driving their transport, and the substrates along which these movements track constitute interrelated aspects of what is broadly termed axonal transport. A primary aim of this chapter is to provide an understanding of intraneuronal traffic. As a basis for achieving this goal, we begin by reviewing the current picture of the neuronal cytoskeleton which provides the structural support and vectorial tracks that allow axonal transport to occur.

ULTRASTRUCTURE AND MOLECULAR ORGANIZATION OF THE AXON

The three major elements of the axonal cytoskeleton—microtubules, neurofilaments and microfilaments—have long been identifiable in electron micrographs, but considerable debate has occurred regarding the detailed organization of these components. Issues under contention included identification of axoplasmic domains in which particular cytoskeletal components predominate, the nature of cross-bridges between components, and interaction of organelles with cytoskeletal structures. A variety of models

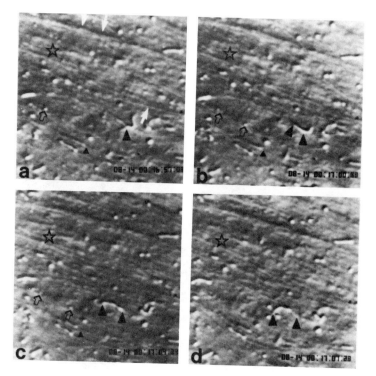

FIG. 1. Sequential video images of fast axonal transport in isolated axoplasm from the squid giant axon. In this preparation, anterograde axonal transport proceeds in the direction from *upper left* to *lower right* (from 10 o'clock toward 4 o'clock). The field of view in these stills is approximately 20 µm, and the images were recorded in real time on videotape. The large, sausage-shaped structures (▲) are mitochondria. Medium-sized particles *(open arrows)* most often move in the retrograde (right to left) direction. Most structures of this size are lysosomal or prelysosomal organelles. The majority of moving particles in these images are faint and moving rapidly (~2 µm/sec), so they are difficult to catch in still images; however, in the region above the *star,* a number of these organelles can be visualized in each panel. The entire field contains faint parallel striations (like those indicated by the *white arrows* in panel **a**) that correspond to the cytoskeleton of the axoplasm, primarily microtubules. The movement of membranous organelles is along these structures, although organelles can occasionally be seen to switch tracks as they move (see the mitochondrion indicated by *large triangles*). (From Brady et al., *Science* 218:1129–1131, 1982.)

were put forth, but each was subject to concerns about possible artifacts of chemical fixation or dehydration-induced shrinkage. The development of protocols that minimize these potential sources of tissue distortion has greatly clarified our view of the cytoskeleton. For example, unfixed tissues may be frozen extremely rapidly to minimize ice crystal damage, then etched and rotary-shadowed or freeze-substituted under vacuum to reveal aspects of internal structure [2]. Further, many of the constituents of structures visualized by video and electron microscopy have been identified by electron immunocyto-chemistry. The images produced by these various methods have provided a foundation for our currently accepted picture of the axon's cytoarchitecture.

In a cross-sectional view, most of the axon is filled with 8–12 nm structures (neurofilaments) separated from each other by side-arm spacers (Fig. 2). Within this field are two types of specialized regions: areas containing larger tubular elements 24 nm in diameter (microtubules), and areas of fuzzy material associated with the microtubules and with the internal side of the axon surface which contain 4–6 nm fibers (microfilaments). Membrane-bound organelles, including mitochondria, appear preferentially associated with the regions containing microtubules and microfilaments. Longitudinal views of axons reveal arrays of neurofilaments and microtubules, as well as sidearms that appear to connect cytoskeletal elements to each other and to membrane-bounded organelles (Fig. 3). However, these images are static, and other approaches are needed to provide information about the dynamics of the neuronal cytoskeleton.

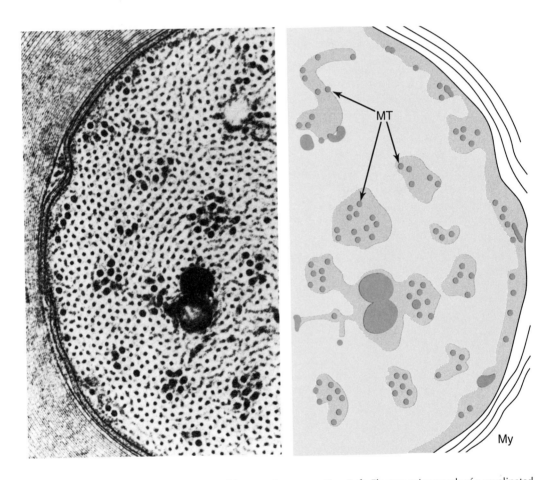

FIG. 2.   The cytoskeleton and organization of the axon in cross section. **Left:** Electron micrograph of a myelinated toad axon in cross section taken near a Schmidt-Lanterman cleft; axon diameter is slightly reduced and the different domains within the axoplasm emphasized. **Right:** Diagram to highlight key features of the axoplasm. Portions of the myelin sheath surrounding the axon can be seen *(My)*. Most of the axonal diameter is taken up by the neurofilaments *(clear area)*. There is a minimum distance between neurofilaments and other cytoskeletal structures that is determined by the sidearms of the neurofilaments. (These sidearms are visible between some of the neurofilaments in the electron micrograph, **left.**) The microtubules *(MT)* (●) tend to be found in bundles and are more irregularly spaced. They are surrounded by a fuzzy material that is also visible in the region just below the plasma membrane *(stippled areas,* **right**). These areas are thought to be enriched in actin microfilaments and presumably contain other SCb proteins as well. The *stippled regions* with embedded microtubules are also the location of membranous organelles in fast axonal transport *(larger, filled irregular shapes,* **right**). Both microtubule and microfilament networks need to be intact for the efficient movement of organelles in fast transport. (Electron micrograph provided by Dr. Alan Hodge; adapted from Hodge and Adelman. In *Structure and Function in Excitable Cells.* New York: Plenum, 1983, pp. 75–111.)

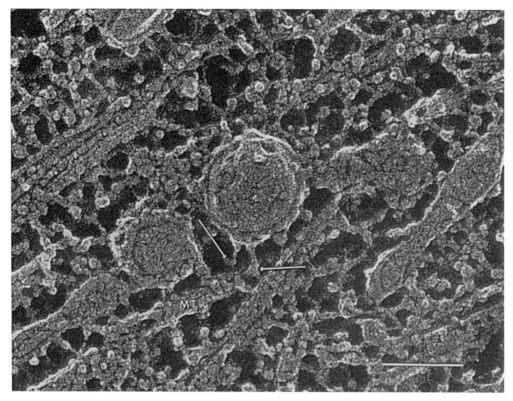

FIG. 3. The axonal cytoskeleton in longitudinal section. Quick-freeze, deep etch electron micrograph of a region of rat spinal cord neurite rich in membrane-bounded organelles and microtubules. *Arrows* point to rod-shaped structures that appear as cross bridges between organelles and microtubules. The bar at the *lower right* indicates 100 nm. (From Hirokawa et al., *Cell* 56:867–878, 1989.)

COMPONENTS OF THE NEURONAL CYTOSKELETON

The importance of neurofilaments (NFs), microtubules (MTs), and microfilaments (MFs) for the development, maintenance, and regeneration of nerve fibers is well documented, although many details of their activities are still being delineated [3]. A prime example is the considerable range of research underway on the phosphorylation states of various cytoskeletal elements. Such studies include findings that phosphate groups may be a determinant in the regulation of axonal caliber by NFs, while hyperphosphorylation of a specific microtubule-associated protein may be a causal factor in the formation of neurofibrillary tangles, a hallmark of Alzheimer's disease.

Neurofilaments make up the bulk of axonal volume in large myelinated fibers

Intermediate filaments of the nervous system appear as solid, rope-like fibrils 8–12 nm in diameter and may be tens or even hundreds of micrometers long. In neurons, they have sidearms that limit packing density, while glial intermediate filaments lack sidearms and may be very tightly packed. While most neurons, astrocytes, Schwann cells, and many associated cell types contain large numbers of intermediate filaments, oligodendrocytes and some neurons have none. Thus, these structures are not essential for cell survival. Intermediate filaments nevertheless serve important functional roles and may represent a substantial fraction of total protein synthesis in neurons and other cell types [4]. Neuronal intermediate filaments exhibit an unusual degree of metabolic stability, which makes them well suited for a role in stabilizing and maintaining neuronal morphology [3,5]. The existence of NFs was established for many years before much was known about their biochemistry or properties. NFs could be seen in early electron micrographs, and many traditional histological procedures visualize neurons as a result of a specific interaction of metals with NFs.

The primary type of intermediate filament in neurons is formed from three subunit polypeptides, the NF triplet, that were initially identified from axonal transport studies. The apparent molecular weights for the NF subunits vary widely across species, but mammalian forms typically range from 180 to 200 kDa for the high molecular weight subunit (NFH), 130 to 170 kDa for the middle subunit (NFM), and 60 to 70 kDa for the low molecular weight subunit (NFL). Molecular genetic analyses have shown that the three NF subunits are distinct polypeptides, each coded by a separate gene [4].

NFs play a critical role in determining axonal caliber [3,5]. They have characteristic sidearms, unique among intermediate filaments, which are formed by the NFM and NFH carboxyl terminal regions [4]. Although all three NF subunits contribute to the NF central core, only the NFM and NFH subunits contribute to sidearms. The NFM and NFH have unusually high levels of phosphorylation [3]. In some species, NFH has 50 or more repeats of a consensus phosphorylation site at its carboxyl terminus and levels of NFH phosphorylation indicate that most of these sites are phosphorylated *in vivo*. Phosphorylation of NFH and NFM sidearms alters charge density on the NF surface, repelling adjacent NFs with similar charge. The high density of surface charge from phosphate groups on NF sidearms make it difficult to imagine a stable interaction between NFs and other structures of like charge. Although many reports refer to crossbridges between NFs, direct studies of interactions between NFs provide little evidence of crosslinks between NFs or between NFs and other cytoskeletal structures [3].

Other intermediate filaments are found in the nervous system as well. Intermediate filament proteins constitute a superfamily which contains five classes, including the nuclear lamins [4]. The NF triplets are class IV intermediate filament proteins, which are expressed only in neurons and have a characteristic domain structure that can be recognized from both primary sequence and gene structure. Class III intermediate filaments are a diverse family that includes vimentin (characteristic of fibroblasts, embryonic neurons, and some endothelial cells) and glial filament acidic protein (a marker for astrocytes and some Schwann cells). Recently, two additional class III intermediate filament proteins, peripherin and α-internexin [3,4], have been described that are unique to neurons and may be coexpressed with the NF triplet. Each has a characteristic pattern of expression during development and regeneration in specific neuronal populations. Intermediate filaments made from class III subunits disassemble more readily under physiological conditions than class IV intermediate filaments [4], so the presence of class III intermediate filament subunit proteins may produce more dynamic structures.

Neuronal populations vary in their number of NFs, the polypeptide composition of those NFs, and the NF phosphorylation levels [3,5]. Both expression and phosphorylation of the NF triplet are regulated during development, maintenance, and regeneration [3]. The pattern of expression for NFs suggest that they contribute to the plasticity of the neuronal cytoskeleton and help determine the stability of neuronal morphologies. NFs represent an efficient and successful mechanism for creating and maintaining neuronal architecture.

Microtubules provide both dynamic structural elements and tracks for organelle traffic

Neuronal MTs are small tubules 24 nm in diameter with walls made up of 12–14 protofilaments which can be visualized in high-resolution electron micrographs [6,6a]. In many cases, sidearms can be visualized projecting from the surface of the MT [2]. These may appear to interact with other MTs or with other structures, but such interactions are likely to be transient in nature. Axonal MTs may be very long, with lengths in excess of 100 μm, but they are not continuous with the cell body. Axonal MTs contain segments that are unusually stable to treatments that depolymerize MTs in other cells, but they constitute a relatively dynamic component of the axonal cytoskeleton [3,7].

MTs serve multiple roles in neurons. They provide a structural framework for many axons and dendrites [5], representing a major determinant of neuronal size and morphology. Many neurons and neuronal regions including small unmyelinated fibers, many dendrites, some neuronal cell bodies, and all arthropod neurons contain few or no NFs, leaving MTs to serve as primary structural elements. A second critical role for MTs is in intracellular transport. Two families of molecular motors found in the nervous system mediate MT-based motility: kinesins and dyneins [8]. The properties of these motors and their role in axonal transport will be considered later. Finally, MTs play essential roles during neuronal growth and development.

Neuronal MTs are biochemically and physiologically diverse, with compositions that vary according to their location, such as axons or dendrites. Even within a single MT, distinct domains exist that vary in composition and degrees of stability. Stable domains are preserved as short MT segments when labile domains depolymerize and may serve to nucleate or organize MTs in axons, particularly during regeneration [3,7].

The primary polypeptides of MTs are alpha and beta tubulins [6,6a]. Multiple genes exist for both alpha and beta tubulins, including brain-specific isoforms [3,6,6a]. Expression of these genes is regulated in development, during regeneration, and in different classes of neurons. Tubulins are highly conserved throughout nature and are subject to a variety of post-translational modifications including acetylation and detyrosination, but the physiological significance of these modifications is not well understood. While some of the best-defined post-translational modifications correlate with increased MT stability *in vivo*, the *in vitro* properties of MTs containing modified tubulins are largely unaffected [3,6,6a]. In most cases, the tubulins are altered during assembly into MTs, but modifications are rapidly reversed following disassembly. Other post-translational modifications of tubulins exist that may affect MT stability [3,6,6a,7].

MTs *in vivo* invariably include members of a heterogeneous set of polypeptides known as microtubule-associated proteins (MAPs) [6,6a]. MAPs interact with MTs rather than with free tubulin and maintain a constant stoichiometry with the tubulin in MTs through cycles of assembly and disassembly. Some MAPs are widely distributed in both neuronal and non-neuronal tissues. Other MAPs are neuron specific and have differential distributions within neurons. For example, MAP2, a high molecular weight MAP, is restricted to dendrites. MAP2 mRNA is transported into dendrites where MAP2 may be locally synthesized [9], but the protein is also thought to be transported. Another class of neuronal MAPs, tau proteins, have a characteristic pattern of phosphorylation in which axonal tau is phosphorylated at sites different from those phosphorylated on tau located in cell bodies and dendrites.

MAPs are differentially expressed during development and regeneration [6,6a], but their specific functions are still being defined. MAPs are thought to stimulate MT formation and stabilize existing MTs *in vivo*. MAPs may contribute to the formation of stable MTs or may preferentially associate with stable MTs. Although MAPs are often described as forming MT crossbridges, there is no evidence that they stably crosslink MTs to other MTs or to nonmicrotubule structures. While transient interactions between MTs certainly occur, MTs are not connected as a crosslinked network. Instead, MTs can slide relative to one another, a property that is likely to be important for their axonal transport [3,10,10a].

Microfilaments play critical roles in neuronal growth and secretion

The third major class of cytoskeletal elements is perhaps the oldest and most diverse. MFs comprise actin subunits arranged like two strings of pearls intertwined to form fibrils 4–6 nm in diameter. A remarkable variety of proteins have been found to interact with actin MFs, ranging from myosin motors to crosslinkers to bundling proteins to anchoring proteins [3,11–13].

Actin MFs are found throughout neurons and glia, but are particularly concentrated in presynaptic terminals, dendritic spines, growth cones, and the subplasmalemmal cortex. Under most circumstances, neuronal MFs are short and organized into a meshwork. In the axonal cytoplasm, MFs are most apparent in the vicinity of MTs and near the plasma membrane. While the existence of many MF-associated proteins in the nervous system is well documented, less is known about their distribution and normal function. The prominent actin bundles seen in fibroblasts or other non-neuronal cells in culture are not characteristic of neurons and most neuronal actin MFs are less than 1 μm in length [3,5,7]. One location containing longer MFs and more elaborate organization is the growth cone, which contains bundles of MFs in the filopodia as well as a more dispersed actin network [13].

MFs and associated proteins such as spectrin form the membrane cytoskeleton, which is thought to be important for cell shape, cell to cell interactions, and distribution of membrane proteins. One key role for MFs is to mediate the interaction of the neuron with the surrounding extracellular matrix and neighboring cells. All adhesion sites including tight junctions and adhesion plaques have interactions with the MF cytoskeleton either directly or indirectly. The existence of the cortical MF meshwork also tends to restrict access to the plasma membrane and is likely to modulate both regulated and constitutive secretion. Similarly, the interior MF matrix appears to be critical for keeping membrane-bounded organelles in the vicinity of the MTs and may be important in targeting of organelles to specific functional domains such as the presynaptic terminal.

Cytoskeletal structures in the neuron overlap in distribution and functions

Although the three major classes of cytoskeletal elements have been considered separately, they interact extensively *in vivo*. Situations where this interplay is apparent include regenerating nerve fibers and maintenance of neuronal morphologies. For example, MTs and MFs play complementary roles in both growth cone and neurite, while NFs are more important in the neurite [3,13,14]. MFs are critical in sprouting and attachment, but are less critical for elongation of the neurite over short distances. Disrupting MTs in the growth cone and distal neurite does not affect sprouting, but inhibits neurite elongation. While NFs are excluded from the growth cone proper, stopping at the neck of the growth cone, the NFs help stabilize the shaft of the growing neurite.

MTs and MFs play a variety of roles in growth cones. MTs display a large repertoire of different behaviors, consistent with roles in both elongation and consolidation of neurite growth. One particularly important function is the delivery of material to the growth cone via axonal transport (see below). MTs also play a role in steering of the growth cone [10,10a], which is a critical element in choosing the correct path during development or regeneration. The experimental evidence indicates that interactions between MFs and MTs appear responsible for most directed growth cone motility, which is homologous with other types of cell migrations. Studies of MF function in growth cones, using fluorescent probes and video microscopy, suggest that they represent critical components of filopodia and lamellopodia [13]. MFs may also be involved in targeting material to specific domains in the growth cone and neurite [3]. Finally, the neuronal cytoskeleton provides an essential framework for intra-axonal transport processes that maintain form and function of the neuron.

DISCOVERY AND DEVELOPMENT OF THE CONCEPT OF FAST AND SLOW COMPONENTS OF AXONAL TRANSPORT

A special set of challenges is presented by the large size and extent of many neurons

Since virtually all neuronal protein synthesis takes place in the cell body, which may represent only 0.1% of the total cell volume, growth and maintenance of neuronal processes require the timely, efficient delivery of material to axonal and dendritic domains. The concept that materials must be transferred from cell body to axon was suggested by Ramón y Cajal and other pioneers of neuroscience during the early part of this century. For many years, the existence of such transport processes could only be inferred.

The first experimental evidence for axonal transport resulted from studies on peripheral nerve regeneration that were stimulated by the desire to improve treatment of limb injuries sustained during World War II. In the classic work of Weiss and Hiscoe (see [15] for review), surgical constriction of a sciatic nerve branch led to morphological changes in the nerve that directly implicated the cell body as the source of materials for axon regrowth. After several weeks, the axon appeared swollen proximal to the constriction, but shriveled on the distal side. Following removal of the constriction, a bolus of accumulated axoplasm slowly moved down the nerve at 1–2 mm/day, very nearly the rate observed for outgrowth of a regenerating nerve. Weiss and Hiscoe concluded that the cell body supplies a bulk flow of material to the axon. This view dominated the field for two decades, but the characteristics of

this slow flow of material did not seem adequate to explain some aspects of nerve growth and function.

Cell biologists subsequently provided convincing arguments for the necessity of this intracellular transport. Neuronal protein synthesis was almost completely restricted to the cytoplasm surrounding the nucleus (translational cytoplasm, which includes polysomes, rough endoplasmic reticulum, and the Golgi complex [16]), and ribosomes were undetectable in the axon. If proteins cannot be synthesized in the axon, then materials necessary for axonal function have to be supplied by transport from the cell body. Axonal transport must be a normal, ongoing process in neurons. By the mid-1960s, the use of radioactive tracers confirmed the existence of a slow "bulk flow" component of transport. Using autoradiography, Droz and colleagues [14] elegantly showed that systemically injected [^{3}H]-amino acids were incorporated into nerve cell proteins and transported along the sciatic nerve as a wavefront of radioactivity. These methods demonstrated that newly synthesized proteins were transported, but some responses of the neuron occurred too rapidly to be readily explained solely by a slow "flow."

Shortly thereafter, radiolabeling studies detected a small proportion of protein traveling down the axon at a considerably faster rate. Such fast rates of transport were confirmed by histochemical labeling of endogenous materials but, unlike slow transport, movement of faster components was observed both toward and away from the cell body. These findings expanded the concept of axonal transport: materials move in both anterograde and retrograde directions at rates that vary by as much as three orders of magnitude [15].

At first, emphasis was placed on characterizing the fast and slow rates of transport. The kinetics of axonal transport have been analyzed by injection of radioactive amino acids into the vitreous of the eye, into dorsal root ganglia, and into ventral spinal cord—procedures that label retinal gan-

A

B

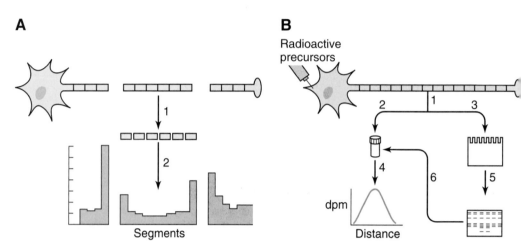

FIG. 4. Schematic diagram of two common methods for analyzing the component rates of axonal transport. **A:** Accumulation of transported material can be studied at a focal block of axonal transport caused by a cut, a crush, a cold block, or a ligature. This approach is a variation of that employed by Weiss and Hiscoe [6] and has been used most often in studies of fast axonal transport [2,8]. In this example, two cuts have been made in order to detect both anterograde and retrograde transport. After time for accumulation at the ends, the nerve segments are cut into uniform segments for analysis *(step 1)*. Each segment is analyzed either for radioactivity in labeled nerves or for enzyme activity, and the rate of accumulation is estimated *(step 2)*. **B:** With segmental analysis, the nerve must be pulse-labeled, usually with radioactive precursors. After an appropriate injection-sacrifice interval to label the rate component of interest, the nerve is also cut into segments *(step 1)*. In some cases, only a single segment is used as a "window" onto the transport process. Each segment is analyzed both by counting the radioactivity in an aliquot *(step 2)* and by gel electrophoresis *(step 3)*, where each lane corresponds to a different segment. The amount of radioactivity in different polypeptides can be visualized with fluorography *(step 5)* and individual bands cut out of the gel *(step 6)* for analysis by liquid scintillation counting. The distribution of either total radioactivity or radioactivity associated with a specific polypeptide can then be plotted *(step 4)*; dpm, disintegrations per minute. (Adapted from Brady. In *Neuromethods, Vol. 1: General Neurochemical Techniques.* Clifton, NJ: Humana Press, 1986, pp. 419–476.)

glion, sensory and motor neurons, respectively. In the case of fast transport, a wavefront of labeled protein was detected traveling away from the cell body at 250–400 mm/day in mammals. Using this approach, slow transport rates of approximately 1 mm/day were observed. Rates for fast transport could also be determined by measuring the amount of a transported substance such as acetylcholinesterase and norepinephrine accumulating at a nerve constriction over a few hours, well before bulk accumulation of axoplasm was detectable. These two approaches for studying axonal transport—locating a radiolabeled wavefront by analysis of successive nerve segments and monitoring the accumulation of materials at a constriction with time (Fig. 4)—generated considerable informa-

tion on the kinetics and on the metabolic and ionic requirements of axonal transport [15]. Such findings formed the basis for more detailed characterization of materials moving in axonal transport and for studies that have begun to reveal the underlying molecular mechanisms.

Fast and slow components of axonal transport differ in both their constituents and their rates

Fast transport is bidirectional and many proteins moved in fast anterograde transport return in the retrograde direction. In contrast, proteins transported at slow rates are degraded when they reach their destination and are not detected in the retrograde component. Subcellular fractionation studies showed that proteins in fast anterograde and retrograde transport were predominantly membrane-associated, while most slowly transported materials were recovered in the soluble fraction.

When labeled polypeptides traveling down the axon are analyzed by SDS poly-acrylamide gel electrophoresis, materials traveling away from the cell body can be grouped into five distinct rate components [3,5]. Each component is characterized by a unique set of polypeptides moving coherently down the axon (Fig. 5) [3,5]. As polypeptides associated with each rate class were identified, most were seen to move only with a single rate and proteins that had common functions or interacted with each other moved together. These observations led to a new view of axonal transport, the Structural Hypothesis [3,5]. This model can be stated simply: Proteins and other molecules move down the axon as components of discrete subcellular structures rather than as individual molecules (Table 1).

The Structural Hypothesis was formulated in response to the observation that rate components of axonal transport move as discrete waves, each with a characteristic rate and a distinctive composition. Advantages of this model include the ability to explain coherent transport of functionally related proteins and the relatively small numbers of motor molecules in neurons. The only assumption made is that the number of elements that can interact with transport motor complexes is limited, so transported material must be packaged appropriately to be moved. The different rate components result from packaging of transported material into different cytologically identifiable structures. In other words, the faster rates reflect transport of proteins preassembled into membranous organelles, including vesicles and mitochondria, or contained in the lumen of these organelles (Fig. 6). The slower rates comprise proteins that are cytoskeletal components, so tubulin and MAPs move as microtubules, and neurofilament proteins move as assembled neurofilaments. Cytoplasmic proteins that are not integral components of a cytoskeletal element may be associated with and transported with these structures (Fig. 7).

Although five distinct major rate components have been identified, the original broad categories of fast and slow transport remain useful. All membrane-associated proteins move in one of the fast rate components, while cytoplasmic and cytoskeletal proteins move as part of the slow components. Current studies indicate that the various types of anterogradely transported organelles move down the axon by a common motor molecule (see below). The differing rates of fast anterograde transport appear to result from the different sizes of organelles, with the increased drag on larger structures resulting in a slower net movement. Less is known about the molecular mechanisms of slow transport, but key insights have been gained in recent years.

Features of fast axonal transport demonstrated by biochemical and pharmacological approaches are apparent from video images

Video microscopy of axoplasm, as described briefly at the beginning of this chapter, has

TABLE 1.   Major rate components of axonal transports

Component	Rate (mm/day)	Structure and composition
Fast transport		
Anterograde	200–400	Small vesiculotubular structures, neurotransmitters, membrane proteins and lipids
Mitochondria	50–100	Mitochondria
Retrograde	200–300	Lysosomal vesicles and enzymes
Slow transport		
SCb	2–8	Microfilaments, metabolic enzymes, clathrin complex
SCa	0.2–1	Neurofilaments and microtubules

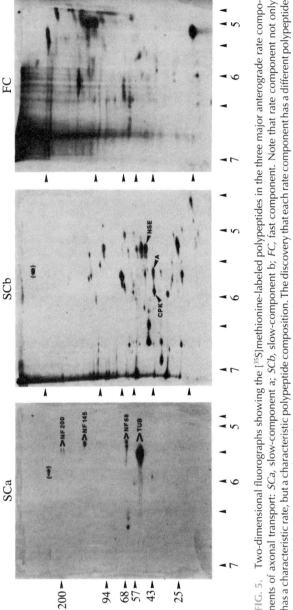

FIG. 5. Two-dimensional fluorographs showing the [^{35}S]methionine-labeled polypeptides in the three major anterograde rate components of axonal transport: *SCa*, slow-component a; *SCb*, slow-component b; *FC*, fast component. Note that rate component not only has a characteristic rate, but a characteristic polypeptide composition. The discovery that each rate component has a different polypeptide composition led to the Structural Hypothesis [10]. (From Tytell et al. *Science* 214:179–181, 1981; illustration provided by Dr. Michael Tytell.)

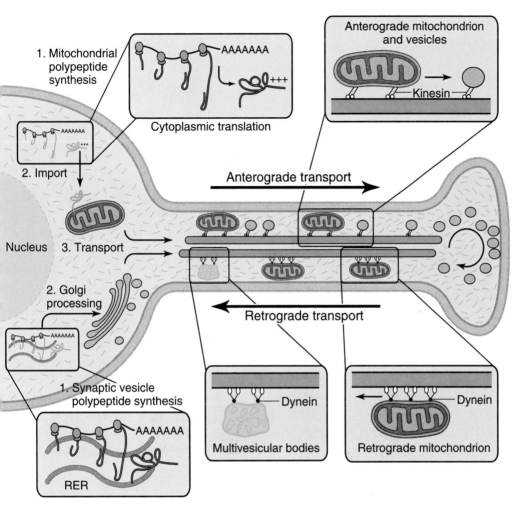

FIG. 6. Schematic illustration of the movement of membrane-associated material in fast axonal transport. Fast axonal transport represents the movement of membrane-bounded organelles along axonal microtubules in both the anterograde and retrograde directions. Two major classes of membrane-bounded organelles that are synthesized and packaged by different pathways are depicted. Synaptic vesicle polypeptides are translated on endoplasmic reticulum-bound ribosomes at which time membrane proteins become properly oriented within the lipid bilayer and secretory polypeptides enter into the lumen of the endoplasmic reticulum. These polypeptides are further processed within the Golgi apparatus where the appropriate post-translational modifications and sorting of polypeptides destined for the axon occur. Once these polypeptides are packaged into vesicular organelles and the appropriate motor molecules are present, the organelles are transported down the axon utilizing axonal microtubules as "tracks" at rates of 200–400 mm/day. Movement in the anterograde direction is believed to be mediated by the molecular motor kinesin while the force necessary to move retrograde organelles is thought to be generated by cytoplasmic dynein. Unlike the synthesis of vesicular polypeptides, mitochondrial polypeptides that are supplied by the host cell are synthesized on cytoplasmic ribosomes and contain a targeting sequence that directs the polypeptides to the mitochondria. Following assembly and the association of motor molecules, the mitochondria move down the axon at rates of 50–100 mm/day. Mitochondria can also be detected moving back toward the cell body in the retrograde direction. The morphology of retrogradely transported mitochondria is distinctly different from that of mitochondria moving in the anterograde direction and is believed to represent degenerating organelles that are not metabolically active.

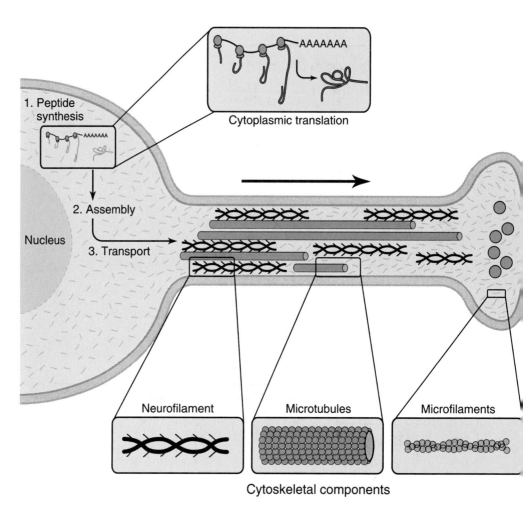

FIG. 7. Schematic illustration of the movement of cytoskeletal elements in slow axonal transport. Slow axonal transport represents the movement of cytoplasmic constituents including cytoskeletal elements and soluble enzymes of intermediary metabolism at rates of 0.2–2 mm/day which are at least two orders of magnitude slower than those observed in fast axonal transport. As proposed in the Structural Hypothesis and supported by experimental evidence, cytoskeletal components are believed to be transported down the axon in their polymeric forms, not as individual subunit polypeptides. Cytoskeletal polypeptides are translated on cytoplasmic polysomes and then are assembled into polymers prior to transport down the axon in the anterograde direction. In contrast to fast axonal transport, no constituents of slow transport appear to be transported in the retrograde direction. Although the polypeptide composition of slow axonal transport has been extensively characterized, the motor molecule(s) responsible for the movement of these cytoplasmic constituents have not yet been identified.

provided key insights into molecular mechanisms of fast axonal transport. The video images of moving organelles directly confirm the bidirectionality of fast transport inferred from accumulation of radiolabeled materials on both sides of a nerve crush and demonstrate that different populations of organelles move in each direction. Anterograde and retrograde rates of organelle movement are comparable to those detected for radiolabeled membrane-associated proteins. Early observations that transport is inhibited by agents that disrupt MTs are consistent with the movement of organelles along fibrils identified as MTs by correlated video and electron microscopy. Video microscopy reveals that organelle movement continues in apparently normal fashion in axons isolated from their cell bodies and even in axoplasm extruded from its plasma membrane. The implication is that transport must be driven by local energy-generating mechanisms, as predicted from observations that application of a cold block or metabolic poison (dinitrophenol or cyanide) to a discrete region of nerve inhibits transport locally [15].

Axonal transport is an adaptation of intracellular transport phenomena common to all cell types

Until recently, axonal transport was understood mainly at a descriptive level, in terms of the components, rates, and pharmacological sensitivities of transport processes. Current research is beginning to probe the molecular mechanisms that underlie movements detected both by direct video visualization and by radioactive tracer methods. Such studies have benefited from considering axonal transport in the broader cell biological context of intracellular transport and contractile phenomena. For example, the well-characterized intracellular pathways for secretion of digestive enzymes in pancreas, hormones in the neurohypophysis, and immunoglobulins in plasma cells as well as for membrane proteins such as acetylcholine receptor in muscle have served as valuable models for examining fast transport pathways in neurons (Fig. 8) [17,18]. The basic structures required for transport and secretion are similar in these non-neuronal cells and the same motor molecules have a wide cellular distribution. While neurons do exhibit molecular specializations, much can be learned by comparing neuronal and non-neuronal processes.

FAST AXONAL TRANSPORT

Although fast axonal transport represents the movement of membrane-bounded or-

ganelles, not all membrane components are destined for the axon. As a result, the first stage of transport must be the synthesis, sorting, and packaging of materials into subpopulations of organelles. Once assembled, organelles destined for the axon must be committed to the transport machinery and moved down the axon. Finally, organelles must be targeted and delivered to specific domains in the axon including axolemma, nodes of Ranvier, and presynaptic terminals.

Newly synthesized membrane and secretory proteins destined for the axon travel by fast anterograde transport

The constituents of a membrane-bounded organelle include integral membrane proteins, secretory products, membrane phospholipids, cholesterol, and gangliosides. The neuron expends a significant fraction of the total energy utilized by axonal transport to move these materials at rates 2–3 orders of magnitude faster than rates for slow transport. As predicted by the Structural Hypothesis and as is apparent in video microscopy, these rapid translocations are achieved by packaging materials into organelles rather than by conveying each as a separate molecule (see also Fig. 6). Clearly, an understanding of how organelles are formed in the cell body and routed to the fast-transport system in the axon is essential [17,18].

In all cell types, secretory and integral membrane proteins are synthesized on polysomes bound to the endoplasmic reticulum. Secretory proteins enter the lumen of the reticulum, whereas membrane proteins become oriented within the bilayer of the membranes (Figs. 6, 8). In contrast, components of the cytoskeleton and enzymes of intermediary metabolism are synthesized on so-called free polysomes, which are actually associated with the cytoskeleton. Newly formed membrane-associated proteins must then be transferred to the Golgi apparatus for processing and post-translational modification, including glycosylation, sulfation, and proteolytic cleavage, as well as for sorting. The

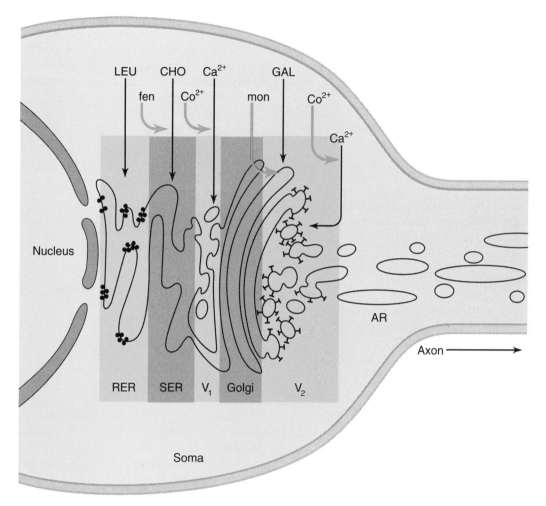

FIG. 8. Summary of pharmacological evidence indicating that newly synthesized membrane and secretory proteins in neurons reach the axons by a pathway similar to that utilized for intracellular transport in non-neuronal cells [4]. Incorporation sites are indicated for several precursors of materials in fast axonal transport: leucine *(LEU)* for proteins, choline *(CHO)* for phospholipids, and galactose *(GAL)* for glycoproteins and glycolipids. Sites of action for several inhibitors are also indicated, including fenfluramine *(fen)*, monensin *(mon)*, and Co^{2+}. One possible site for Ca^{2+}-mediated vesicle fusion is at the transition from rough endoplasmic reticulum *(RER)* and smooth endoplasmic reticulum *(SER)* to the Golgi apparatus *(GA)* via one type of transition vesicle *(V₁)*. The subsequent budding of vesicles *(V₂)* off the GA, presumably mediated by clathrin-coated vesicles, is a second site for Ca^{2+} involvement. The microtubule guides for the axonal vesiculotubular structures in transport and the axoplasmic reticulum *(AR)* are not shown.

pathways for transfer between endoplasmic reticulum and Golgi are being elucidated and involve both a microtubule-dependent step and sorting events mediated by G proteins [19]. After progressing through the different elements of the Golgi, vesicles bud off from the trans-Golgi membrane, and are routed to their target sites via microtubules

and motor molecules. A key point is that membrane and secretory proteins become associated with membranes either during or immediately following their synthesis and maintain this association throughout their lifetime in the cell.

Evidence that a similar sequence of events occurs in neurons was first obtained by electron microscope autoradiography: radiolabeled protein appeared to pass from the rough endoplasmic reticulum to the Golgi apparatus before entering the axon [17]. This pathway has been confirmed and expanded by radiolabeling proteins in the presence of pharmacological agents that inhibit particular events or disrupt selected structures on the intracellular pathway (Fig. 8) [17]. For example, inhibiting synthesis of either protein or phospholipid leads to a proportional decrease in the amount of both protein and phospholipid in fast-transport, whereas application of these inhibitors to the axon has no effect on transport. This suggests that fast axonal transport depends on *de novo* synthesis and assembly of membrane components.

Passage through the Golgi apparatus is obligatory for most proteins destined for fast transport

Fast-transported proteins appear to leave the endoplasmic reticulum in association with transfer vesicles that bud off and undergo Ca^{2+}-dependent fusion with the Golgi apparatus. The requirement that all proteins destined for fast axonal transport (except those associated with the mitochondria) traverse the Golgi stacks, where some are post-translationally modified and all are presumably sorted and packaged, was demonstrated by pharmacological studies with the Na+ ionophore, monensin [17]. This drug selectively disrupts the Golgi stacks and concomitantly depresses the amount of all fast-transport proteins entering the axon.

Transfer from the Golgi apparatus to the fast transport system appears to be mediated by clathrin-coated vesicles. When such vesicles were isolated from [³H]leucine-labeled dorsal root ganglia and the resulting [³H]proteins co-electrophoresed on two-dimensional gels with [³⁵S]methionine-labeled fast-transport proteins from a separate preparation of sciatic nerve, most of the [³⁵S]proteins were found to comigrate with coated-vesicle [³H]proteins [20]. Coated ves-

icles, however, are rarely observed in axons, and clathrin, the major coat protein, is primarily a slow-transport protein [3,7,29]. Thus, it is likely that the Golgi-derived coated vesicles shed their coats prior to undergoing fast transport, and travel down the axon either as individual uncoated vesicles or as so-called vesiculotubular structures (Fig. 8).

Anterograde transport moves synaptic vesicles, axolemmal precursors, and mitochondria down the axon

Fast anterograde transport represents the movement of membrane-bounded organelles along MTs away from the cell body at rates ranging in mammals from 250 to 400 mm/day or 3 to 5 µm/sec [3,8]. Anterograde transport provides newly synthesized components essential for neuronal function and maintenance.

Ultrastructural studies have demonstrated that the material moving in fast anterograde transport includes many small vesicles and tubulovesicular structures as well as mitochondria and dense core vesicles [21,21a]. Material in fast anterograde transport is needed for supply and turnover of both intracellular membrane compartments (i.e., mitochondria and endoplasmic reticulum) as well as the plasma membrane and secretory vesicles. The actual rate of transport appears to be largely determined by size with the smallest organelles in almost constant motion, while mitochondria and larger structures frequently pause for a slower average rate.

A variety of materials move in fast anterograde transport. Materials being transported include membrane-associated enzymes, neurotransmitters, neuropeptides, and membrane lipids. Most are synthesized in the cell body and are transported intact, but some processing events occur in transit. For example, neuropeptides may be generated by proteolytic degradation of propeptides. This biochemical heterogeneity extends to the organelles themselves. The population of small organelles are particularly varied in function and composition. Some correspond to synaptic vesicle precursors and contain neurotransmitters and associated proteins, while others may contain channel proteins or other materials destined for the axolemma [3]. Biochemical and morphological studies have provided a description of the materials transported in fast transport, but were not as well suited for identifying underlying molecular mechanisms involved in translocation.

Video microscopy has provided key insights into mechanism through direct observation of organelle movements while precise control of experimental conditions is maintained. As indicated above, fast axonal transport continues unabated in isolated axoplasm from giant axons of the squid for several hours [1,22]. Isolated axoplasm has no plasma membrane or other permeability barriers, and can be maintained in an active state. The use of video microscopy to study transport in isolated axoplasm led to rigorous dissection of the mechanisms for fast axonal transport using biochemical and pharmacological approaches. These observations confirmed and extended earlier studies in demonstrating many properties of fast anterograde transport.

Retrograde transport carries exogenous material, including trophic factors, and endogenous material, including used membrane constituents, to the cell body

The organelles moving in retrograde transport are heterogeneous in structure and larger on average than the small vesiculotubular structures common in anterograde transport [21,21a]. Multivesicular or multilamellar bodies are common and these are thought to represent carriers of materials to be delivered to lysosomal compartments in the cell body. The larger size of these retrograde organelles affects the rate of transport by increasing drag caused by interactions with cytoplasmic structures [8].

Both morphological and biochemical studies indicate that organelles returning in retrograde transport differ from those in anterograde transport [21]. The turnaround or conversion from anterograde to retrograde transport appears to require repackaging of membrane components. The mechanisms of repackaging are incompletely understood, but certain protease inhibitors will inhibit turnaround without affecting either anterograde or retrograde movement [23,23a]. The specificities of effective protease inhibitors implicate a thiol protease, but the identity of the responsible enzyme is unknown. Consistent with this proposal, protease treatment of purified synaptic vesicles affects the directionality of their movements in axoplasm and presynaptic terminal. Fluorescent synaptic vesicles normally move predominantly in the anterograde direction, but protease treatment of these vesicles blocks movement altogether or results in retrograde transport [23,23a].

The uptake of exogenous materials by endocytosis in distal regions of the axon can result in the return of trophic substances and growth factors to the cell body [24,24a]. These factors assure the survival of the neuron and may modulate neuronal gene expression. Changes in the return of trophic substances play critical roles during development and regeneration of fibers. Retrograde transport of exogenous substances also provides a pathway for viral agents to enter the central nervous system [24,24a]. Once retrograde transported material reaches the cell body, the cargo may be delivered to the lysosomal system for degradation, to nuclear compartments for regulation of gene expression, or to the Golgi complex for repackaging.

Molecular sorting mechanisms ensure delivery of proteins to discrete membrane compartments

While the pathways by which selected membrane-associated proteins are guided through the cell body to the fast transport system have been established in general terms, many intriguing questions regarding the selection process itself are beginning to be addressed [25,25a]. How is it that certain membrane proteins remain in the cell body (for example, the glycosyltransferases of the Golgi membranes) while others are packaged for delivery to the axon? Among transported proteins, how do some reach the axolemma (sodium and potassium channels) while others travel the length of the axon to reside in the nerve terminal (a presynaptic receptor or synaptic vesicle) or enter the synaptic cleft (a secreted neuropeptide)? Finally, how are organelles such as the synaptic vesicle directed toward the axon and a presynaptic terminal, but not to dendritic arbors? This question becomes even more compelling for the dorsal root ganglion cell where the central branch of a single axonal process has presynaptic terminals, while the peripheral branch of the same axon has none.

The answers to these questions remain incomplete, but some mechanisms have begun to emerge. The most detailed information comes from studies on polarized epithelial cells in which the identity of molecular destination signals that deliver newly synthesized proteins selectively to either their basolateral or apical membranes have been sought. These mechanisms are relevant to the neuron, because viral proteins that normally go to basolateral membranes end up in dendritic compartments, while those targeted to apical compartments are moved into the axon [26]. However, the underlying mechanisms appear to be complex. Signals may be "added on," in the form of posttranslational modifications including glycosylation and phosphorylation or "built in," in the form of discrete amino acid sequences [25,25a]. Both mechanisms appear to operate in cells depending on the destination. For example, addition of mannose-6-phosphate residues directs lysosomal enzymes from the Golgi to the lysosomes, while amino acid sequences have been identified that direct proteins into the nucleus or into mitochondria. In general, targeting signals are likely used in directing proteins to specific organelles, while other mechanisms serve to direct the organelles to appropriate final destinations.

Specific membrane components need to be delivered to their sites of utilization and not left at inappropriate sites [3]. A synaptic vesicle must be delivered to presynaptic terminals along with other materials needed for neurotransmitter release, but serves no function in an axon or cell body. The problem is compounded because many presynaptic terminals are not at the end of an axon. Often, numerous terminals occur sequentially along a single axon making *en passant* contacts with multiple targets. Thus, synaptic vesicles cannot merely move to the end of axonal microtubules. Targeting of synaptic vesicles then becomes a more complex problem. Similar complexities arise with membrane proteins destined for the axolemma or a nodal membrane.

One proposed mechanism for targeting of organelles in the axon may have general implications. The synapsin family of phosphoproteins [27], which are concentrated in presynaptic terminals, may be involved in targeting synaptic vesicles to the terminal. Dephosphorylated synapsin binds tightly to both synaptic vesicles and actin MFs, while phosphorylation releases them [27]. Dephosphorylated synapsin inhibits axonal transport of membrane organelles in isolated axoplasm, while phosphorylated synapsin at similar concentrations has no effect [28]. Cycles of phosphorylation and dephosphorylation may target synaptic vesicles to presynaptic terminals by changing the affinity of synapsin for MFs and vesicles. When a synaptic vesicle passes through a region rich in dephosphorylated synapsin, the vesicle will be crosslinked to the available MF matrix by synapsin. Such crosslinked vesicles would be removed from fast axonal transport and are effectively targeted to a synapsin- and MF-rich domain, the presynaptic terminal. Calcium-activated kinases subsequently mobilize the targeted vesicles for transfer to active zones and neurotransmitter release [27,28]. Variations on this mechanism may be a general mechanism for targeting membrane-bounded organelles to specific domains [3].

Finally, virtually all the attention in this chapter has focused on axonal transport, but dendritic transport is also an established phenomenon [9]. Since dendrites usually include a post-synaptic region while axons terminate in presynaptic elements, the dendritic and axonal transport systems each receive a number of unique proteins. Evidence for such sorting mechanisms comes from studies in cultured hippocampal neurons using two different viruses, one of which buds from the basolateral surface of epithelial cells while the other buds from the opposing, apical surface. Basolateral-targeted viral glycoproteins were transported exclusively to the dendritic processes of cultured neurons, whereas glycoproteins of the apical-budding virus were found preferentially in axons [26]. An added level of complexity for intraneuronal transport phenomena is the intriguing evidence that mRNA is routed into dendritic but not axonal domains where it is implicated in local protein synthesis at the base of dendritic spines, such spines serving as post-synaptic sites [9].

SLOW AXONAL TRANSPORT

Cytoplasmic and cytoskeletal elements move coherently at slow transport rates

Two major and one or more minor rate components have been described for slow axonal transport. All represent movement of cytoplasmic constituents including cytoskeletal elements and soluble enzymes of intermediary metabolism [29]. Cytoplasmic and cytoskeletal elements in axonal transport move with rates at least two orders of magnitude slower than fast transport. In favorable systems, the coherent movement of neurofilaments and microtubule proteins [3,5,30] provides strong evidence for the Structural Hypothesis. Particularly striking evidence was provided by pulse-labeling experiments in which NF proteins moved over periods of

weeks as a bell-shaped wave with little or no trailing of NF protein [3,5,39]. Similarly, co-ordinated transport of tubulin and MAPs makes sense only if MTs are being moved, since MAPs do not interact with unpolymerized tubulin [6,7].

Slow Component a (SCa) comprises largely cytoskeletal proteins, NFs, and MT protein. Rates of transport for SCa proteins in mammalian nerve range from 0.2–0.5 mm/day in optic axons to 1 mm/day in motor neurons of the sciatic nerve, and can be even slower in poikilotherms such as goldfish. Although the polypeptide composition of SCa is relatively simple, the relative contribution of SCa to slow transport varies considerably [5,30]. For large axons (i.e., alpha motor neurons in the sciatic nerve), the amount of SCa is a large fraction of the total protein in slow transport, while the amount of material in SCa is relatively reduced for smaller axons (i.e., optic axons). The amount and phosphorylation state of SCa protein in the nerve is the major determinant of axonal diameter.

Slow Component b (SCb) represents a complex and heterogeneous rate component, including hundreds of distinct polypeptides ranging from cytoskeletal proteins like actin [29] and tubulin in some nerves (see [30]) to soluble enzymes of intermediary metabolism [29] such as the glycolytic enzymes. The structural correlate of SCb is not as easily identified as the MTs and NFs of SCa. The actin is presumed to be in the form of MFs, but actin represents only 5–10% of the protein in SCb. Most proteins in SCb may be associated into labile aggregates that interact transiently with the cytoskeleton. Polypeptides such as HSP70, a constitutively expressed member of the heat shock family, may serve to organize these complexes during transport [3,7].

While these two rate components can be identified in all nerves examined to date, the rates and the precise compositions may vary between nerve populations [30]. For example, SCa and SCb are readily resolved as discrete waves moving down optic axons, but the differences in rate are smaller in the axons of sciatic nerve motor neurons so the two peaks overlap. Moreover, virtually all tubulin moves with SCa in the optic axons, while a significant fraction of the axonal tubulin moves at SCb rates in sciatic nerve axons. In each nerve, certain polypeptides may be used to define the kinetics for a given slow component of axonal transport. For SCa, those signature polypeptides are the NF triplet proteins, while actin, clathrin, and calmodulin serve a similar role for SCb.

Axonal growth and regeneration are mediated by slow axonal transport

The rate of axonal growth during development and regeneration of a nerve is roughly equivalent to the rate of SCb in that neuron. This reflects the critical roles played by the slow components of axonal transport in growth and regeneration. During development, SCb proteins are prominant and relatively little NF protein is detectable. Tubulin can be detected moving at both SCb and SCa rates. Once an appropriate target is reached and synaptogenesis begins, there is an upregulation of NF protein synthesis and a gradual slowing of slow transport.

Axonal regeneration involves a complex set of cell body and axonal responses to a lesion. Downregulation of NF triplet and upregulation of specific tubulin isotypes are hallmarks of cell body responses to a lesion [7,14]. In CNS neurons that fail to regenerate, changes in NF and tubulin expression are reduced or absent. Since changes in protein expression do not alter axonal cytoskeletal composition until after a growth cone has formed and extended for some distance, such changes in expression do not affect neurite growth, but may reflect activation of a cellular program for neurite growth [3,5,7,14].

MT stability plays a critical role in regeneration. Axonal MTs must be disassembled as part of reorganizing the cytoskeleton for growth, then reassembled for neurite extension. Specific tubulin genes are upregulated during axonal growth or regeneration, and there are characteristic changes in axonal transport of tubulin with an increase in the fraction of tubulin moving at SCb rates [13]. MAPs are differentially expressed during development, but less is known about changes during regeneration.

Differences in CNS and PNS regeneration are apparent even when comparing branches of single axons. Since CNS and PNS glia differ in many respects, attempts to explain lack of CNS regeneration have focused on variations in glial environments. CNS regeneration in PNS environments provides compelling evidence that functional CNS regeneration is possible [31,31a]. Elements in the glial environment affecting regeneration are being identified [31,31a], but molecular differences between axons in a PNS environment and comparable axons in a CNS environment remain poorly understood.

Cytoskeletal proteins are maintained in distinct domains

Progress has been made toward identification of targeting mechanisms of cytoskeletal and cytoplasmic proteins and some general principles have begun to emerge. Since cytoplasmic constituents move only in the anterograde direction, differential metabolism appears to be the key to targeting of cytoplasmic and cytoskeletal proteins. Concentration of actin and other proteins in the presynaptic terminal can be explained by the slower turnover of such proteins in the presynaptic terminal relative to neurofilament proteins and tubulin [32,32a]. Proteins with slow degradative rates in the terminal accumulate and reach a higher steady-state concentration. Alteration of the rate of degradation for a protein will cause a change in the rate of accumulation for that protein. For example, inhibition of calpains will cause the appearance of neurofilament rings in the presynaptic terminal [32,32a].

Differential turnover of polypeptides may be accomplished in at least two ways.

Proteases may have specificities that allow them to act on some proteins, but not others. Alternatively, post-translational modifications such as ubiquitination or phosphorylation may affect susceptibility of a protein to degradation. This latter mechanism has been proposed to explain the differential distribution of MAPs in the axon and dendrites. For example, axonal tau has a phosphorylation pattern that is different from tau in cell bodies and dendrites, although there is no direct evidence that this differential phosphorylation affects tau stability *in vivo*. Similarly, MAP2 is absent from axons [3,6], and exogenous MAP2 appears to be preferentially degraded in axonal compartments. However, MAP2 is also synthesized locally on mRNA transported into dendrites [9], so multiple mechanisms may be involved.

Properties of slow transport suggest its molecular mechanisms

The information available about the mechanisms of slow axonal transport is relatively limited. These processes are energy dependent and require an intact axonal cytoskeleton. Indirect evidence suggests that MTs play a critical role, because the transport of NFs can be pharmacologically uncoupled from MT transport without eliminating slow transport. In contrast, all agents that disrupt MTs appear to block slow transport of all components. This does not rule out a role for the MF cytoskeleton in slow transport movements, if the MTs are needed to couple motive force with other elements of the cytoskeleton.

The macroscopic rates measured by radiolabel experiments should not be taken to reflect maximum rates for the motors involved. As with the fast transport of mitochondria, the net rate of slow component proteins reflects both the rate of actual movement and the fraction of a given time interval that a given structure is moving. The elongate shape of cytoskeletal structures and their potential for multiple interactions

mean that net displacements are discontinuous. If a structure is moving at a speed of 2 μm/sec, but on average only moves at that rate for 1 second out of every 100 seconds, then the average rate for the structure will translate to only 0.02 μm/sec.

MT movements in growing neurites have been visualized directly in an elegant series of studies [10,10a]. Tubulin may be tagged with a caged fluorescein group, which can be visualized when uncaged by the correct illumination. Labeled tubulins may be injected into a *Xenopus* oocyte where they remain as the oocyte develops into an embryo. In the early embryo, much of the tubulin remains tagged because protein synthesis is initially limited. When the caged fluorescent tubulin is locally photoactivated in a neurite, patches of fluorescent tubulin can be seen to move down the axon. Fluorescent patches remained discrete during movements in the anterograde direction at slow transport rates as predicted by the Structural Hypothesis.

Observations of MTs containing fluorescent tubulin could also be made using rhodamine tubulin [10]. Under favorable conditions, individual fluorescent MTs can be detected moving in neurites and growth cones. These MTs translocate as intact structures. In the growth cone, they appeared to be pulled and even bent in conjunction with growth cone movements. When combined with studies of axonal transport using radiolabels and direct observations of individual MTs with video microscopy, there is little doubt that MTs and NFs can and do move in the axon as intact cytoskeletal structures [3,5,10].

MOLECULAR MOTORS: KINESIN, DYNEIN, AND MYOSIN

Prior to 1985, the only molecular motors identified in vertebrate cells were myosins and flagellar dyneins. Myosins were purified from nervous tissue, but no clear functions were established. Given the evidence that fast axonal transport was microtubule-based, many investigators looked for dynein in cell cytoplasm, but met with little success. Moreover, the characteristic biochemical properties of fast transport were not consistent with either myosin or dynein [8]. Extensive characterization of fast axonal transport pharmacology and biochemistry created a picture of organelle transport distinct from muscle contraction or flagellar beating.

A striking difference between fast axonal transport and myosin- or dynein-based motility was discovered during studies on ATP analogues and axonal transport. Adenylyl-imidodiphosphate (AMP-PNP), a non-hydrolyzable analogue of ATP, is a weak competitive inhibitor of both myosin and dynein. When AMP-PNP is perfused into axoplasm, bidirectional transport stops within minutes [1,22]. Both anterograde and retrograde moving organelles freeze in place on the microtubules. Inhibition of fast axonal transport by AMP-PNP strongly suggested that fast axonal transport involved a new class of motor, unrelated to either myosin or dynein [22]. The polypeptides making up this new type of motor molecule were soon identified and the new motor was named kinesin [33,33a]. Directly or indirectly, this discovery has led to the identification of many new molecular motors in vertebrate cells and has transformed our understanding of cellular motility. All three classes of molecular motor proteins, kinesins, dyneins, and myosins, are now known to represent families of proteins with a variety of different functions [8].

Kinesins mediate anterograde transport in a variety of organisms and tissues

Since their discovery, the kinesins have been extensively characterized with regard to biochemical, pharmacological, immunochemical, and molecular properties [8]. Kinesin is a long, rod-shaped protein, approximately 80 nm in length with two heads, a shaft, and a tail domain. The holoenzyme comprises two heavy chains (molecular weight 115–130 kDa) and two light chains (62–70 kDa) for a total molecular weight of 380 kDa. High-resolution electron microscopic immunolocalization of kinesin subunits and molecular genetic studies indicate that the heavy chains are arranged in parallel, forming the heads and much of the shaft, while light chains are localized to the fan-shaped tail region [8]. Binding of kinesin to MTs is stabilized by AMP-PNP and this property is the basis for many purification schemes. Kinesin is an MT-activated ATPase with minimal basal activity [8,33,33a]. MTs will glide across glass surfaces coated with kinesin with a polarity consistent with a role in anterograde transport (movement is toward the MT-plus end) [8,33,33a].

In neurons and other cell types, kinesin is associated with a variety of membrane-bounded organelles, ranging from synaptic vesicles to mitochondria to coated vesicles to lysosomes. The molecular basis of kinesin and other molecular motor interactions with membrane is not well understood. In the case of kinesin, the interaction is thought to involve the light chains of kinesin along with the carboxyl terminals of the heavy chains.

Kinesin has been purified from many different sources including squid, bovine, chicken, *Drosophila*, and sea urchins. The kinesins are now recognized to represent the first member identified in a family of related proteins with highly conserved motor domains [8,34]. Many kinesin-related proteins are involved with cell division, but precise functions are still being defined. Only a few of these related proteins have been examined biochemically. One of these kinesin-related proteins from *Drosophila*, ncd, is even an MT-minus-end-directed motor. The significance of these kinesin-related proteins for the nervous system remains to be determined. Experiments indicate that the kinesins are involved in the movement of membrane-bounded organelles by fast axonal transport. Strong evidence exists for a kinesin role in anterograde transport. However, a variety of kinesin isoforms exist, and the complexities of kinesin function in the nervous system are only beginning to be understood.

Cytoplasmic dyneins are motors for retrograde axonal transport

One indirect result of the discovery of kinesin was identification of the cytoplasmic form of dynein in nervous tissue, which had been sought for so long [8,35]. Cytoplasmic dynein and kinesin are both associated with MTs by incubation of nucleotide-depleted brain extracts and released by addition of ATP. Dyneins move MTs *in vitro* with a polarity opposite of kinesin, consistent with minus end transport.

Cytoplasmic dyneins are 40-nm-long complexes of high molecular weight (1.6×10^6 daltons). The polypeptide composition is complex and includes two heavy chains and a number of light chains [8,35]. Less is known about the distribution and properties of cytoplasmic dyneins in the nervous system than for kinesin. Immunocytochemistry in nonneuronal cells showed reactivity on mitotic spindles and a punctate pattern in interphase cells presumed to represent dynein bound to membranous organelles. The functions of cytoplasmic dyneins are not as well defined as those for kinesin. They are widely thought to serve as the motor for retrograde axonal transport [35] and have been found to accumulate on both sides of a ligation. An additional possibility for cytoplasmic dynein function is as a candidate for the motor moving MTs in slow axonal transport [8].

Myosins and microfilaments contribute to growth cone motility

Myosins were the first class of molecular motors identified in vertebrate cells, first in muscle and then in nonmuscle cells. In recent years, the number of myosins has increased and now includes three distinct classes [11,11a,12,12a], each of which may be detected in nervous tissue. While the abundance of myosins is comparable to that of kinesins and dyneins, many questions remain about the function and even the distribution of this class of motor molecules in neurons.

Thick filaments in smooth and skeletal muscle comprise myosin II heavy chains and associated light chains [11,11a], some of which are also present at significant levels in nervous tissues. The light chains of nonmuscle myosin II are distinct from muscle light chains, but all are thought to be important for regulation of myosin function. Myosin II heavy chains form dimers that interact with other myosin dimers to generate bipolar filaments. Under some conditions, bundles of actin microfilaments in nonmuscle cells may exhibit myosin II with a characteristic distribution into sarcomere-like structures. Many types of cellular contractility appear to involve myosin II, including the contractile ring in mitosis. Although brain myosin II is relatively abundant [11,11a], relatively little is known about myosin II function in neurons.

The second class, myosin I, was first described in protists and has recently been identified in brain [12,12a]. Myosin I proteins have a single, smaller heavy chain containing an actin-activated ATPase domain highly homologous to myosin II. The myosin I tails diverge from myosin II and do not appear able to form dimers or filaments. An exciting aspect of myosin I is the ability to interact with membrane surfaces. As a result, myosin I may generate movements of plasma membrane components or intracellular organelles. Both myosins (I and II) have been proposed to have a role in the motility of growth cones [11–13].

Even more recently, a third class of myosins has been recognized differing from both myosins I and II. The murine coat color mutant *dilute* turned out to involve a gene with the sequence of novel myosin heavy chain. There are complex neurological deficits associated with the *dilute* mutation [12,12a], suggesting that the different forms of myosin may have narrowly defined functions. Despite intensive study, relatively little is known about neuronal functions for the myosins. Axonal transport of myosin-like proteins has been described, which suggests that they may play a role in slow axonal transport [8]. Myosins are likely to be involved in growth cone motility, synaptic plasticity, and neurotransmitter release.

Molecular motors have identifying hallmarks

There are few instances in which we understand fully the roles played by molecular motors in a neuronal function. The proliferation of different motor molecules and isoforms raises the possibility that some physiological activities may involve multiple classes of motor molecule. The process of matching motors to physiological functions has proven to be a difficult one. In most respects, the three classes of motor are similar in their biochemical and pharmacological sensitivity [8]. For example, myosin, dynein, and kinesin all remain in a bound rigor state without nucleotides. However, some hallmarks do exist that may be used to identify a motor. In the case of kinesin, the most distinctive characteristic is stabilization of binding to microtubules by AMP-PNP [1,8,22,33,33a]. The affinities of myosin for microfilaments and of dynein for microtubules are weakened by treatment with either ATP or AMP-PNP. As a result, if a process is frozen in place by AMP-PNP, then kinesin is likely to be involved. If kinesin is not involved in a process that requires MTs, then cytoplasmic dyneins are likely to be involved. Similarly, movement along MFs is presumed to involve one of the myosin motors. Development of new pharmacological and immunochemical probes specific for different motors should facilitate studies on the motors and motile activities in the future.

CONCLUSIONS

The functional architecture of neurons comprises many specializations in cytoskeletal and membranous components. Each of these specializations is dynamic, constantly changing, and being renewed at a rate determined by the local environment and cellular metabolism. The processes of axonal transport represent the key to neuronal dynamics. Recent advances have provided important insights into the molecular mechanisms underlying axonal transport, although many questions remain. Continued exploration of these phenomena will provide a basis for understanding neuronal dynamics in development, regeneration, and neuropathology.

ACKNOWLEDGMENTS

The collaborative efforts in preparing this chapter were supported by grants to S.T.B. from the NIH (NS23320 and NS23868), the Council for Tobacco Research (3258), and the Robert Welch Foundation (I-1077); to J.L.C. from the Eloise Gerry Fellowships Fund of Sigma Delta Epsilon/Graduate Women in Science, Inc.; and to R.H. from the NIH (NS27173 and HD26956).

REFERENCES

1. Brady, S., Lasek, R., and Allen, R. Fast axonal transport in extruded axoplasm from the squid giant axon. *Cell Motil. Cytoskeleton* 3 [Videodisk Suppl. 1]: Side 2, track 2, 1983.
1a. Brady, S., Lasek, R., and Allen, R. Video microscopy of fast axonal transport in extruded axoplasm: A new model for study of molecular mechanisms. *Cell Motil. Cytoskeleton* 5: 81–101, 1985.
2. Hirokawa, N. Quick-freeze, deep-etch visualization of the axonal cytoskeleton. *Trends Neurosci.* 9:67–71, 1986.
3. Brady, S. T. Axonal dynamics and regeneration. In A. Gorio (ed.), *Neural Regeneration.* New York: Raven Press, 1992, pp. 7–36.
4. Fliegner, K. H., and Liem, R. K. H. Cellular and molecular biology of neuronal intermediate filaments. *Int. Rev. Cytol.* 131:109–167, 1991.
5. Lasek, R. J. Studying the intrinsic determi-

nants of neuronal form and function. In R. J. Lasek, M. M. Black (ed.), *Intrinsic Determinants of Neuronal Form and Function.* New York: Alan R. Liss, Inc., 1988, pp. 1–60.

6. Sullivan, K. F. Structure and utilization of tubulin isotypes. *Annu. Rev. Cell Biol.* 4:687–716, 1988.

6a. Matus, A. Microtubule-associated proteins: their potential role in determining neuronal morphology. *Annu. Rev. Neurosci.* 11:29–44, 1988.

7. Brady, S. T. Cytotypic specializations of the neuronal cytoskeleton and cytomatrix: Implications for neuronal growth and regeneration. In B. Haber, A. Gorio, J. D. Vellis, and J. R. Perez-Polo (ed.), *Cellular and Molecular Aspects of Neural Development and Regeneration.* New York: Springer-Verlag, 1988, pp. 311–322.

8. Brady, S. T. Molecular motors in the nervous system. *Neuron* 7:521–533, 1991.

9. Steward, O., and Banker, G. A. Getting the message from the gene to the synapse: sorting and intracellular transport of RNA in neurons. *Trends. Neurosci.* 15:180–186, 1992.

10. Tanaka, E. M., and Kirschner, M. Microtubule behavior in the growth cones of living neurons during axon elongation. *J. Cell Biol.* 115:345–364, 1991.

10a. Reinsch, S. S., Mitchison, T. J., and Kirschner, M. Microtubule polymer assembly and transport during axonal elongation. *J. Cell Biol.* 115:365–380, 1991.

11. Korn, E. D., and Hammer, J. A. Myosins of nonmuscle cells. *Annu. Rev. Biophys. Biophys. Chem.* 17:23–45, 1988.

11a. Cheney, R. E., Riley, M. A., and Mooseker, M. S. Phylogenetic analysis of the myosin superfamily. *Cell Motil. Cytoskeleton* 24:215–223, 1993.

12. Mercer, J. A., Seperack, P. K., Strobel, M. C., Copeland, N. G., and Jenkins, N. A. Novel myosin heavy chain encoded by murine dilute coat colour locus. *Nature* 349:709–713, 1991.

12a. Pollard, T. D., Doberstein, S. K., and Zot, H. G. Myosin-I. *Annu. Rev. Physiol.* 53: 653–681, 1991.

13. Smith, S. J. Neuronal cytomechanics: the actin-based motility of growth cones. *Science* 242: 708–715, 1988.

14. Oblinger, M., and Lasek, R. J. Axotomy-induced alterations in the synthesis and transport of neurofilaments and microtubules in dorsal root ganglion cells. *J. Neurosci.* 8: 1747–1758, 1988.

15. Grafstein, B., and Forman, D. S. Intracellular transport in neurons. *Physiol. Rev.* 60: 1167–1283, 1980.

16. Lasek, R. J., and Brady, S. T. The axon: a prototype for studying expressional cytoplasm. *Cold Spring Harb. Symp. Quant. Biol.* XLVI: 113–124, 1982.

17. Hammerschlag, R., and Stone, G. C. Membrane delivery by fast axonal transport. *Trends Neurosci.* 5:12–15, 1982.

18. Kelly, R. B. Pathways of protein secretion in eukaryotes. *Science* 230:25–32, 1985.

19. Donaldson, J. G., Kahn, R. A., Lippincott-Schwartz, J., and Klausner, R. D. Binding of ARF and β-COP to Golgi membranes: possible regulation by a trimeric G protein. *Science* 254:1197–1199, 1991.

20. Stone, G. C., Hammerschlag, R., and Bobinski, J. A. Involvement of coated vesicles in the initiation of fast axonal transport. *Brain Res.* 291:219–228, 1984.

21. Smith, R. S. The short term accumulation of axonally transported organelles in the region of localized lesions of single myelinated axons. *J. Neurocytol.* 9:39–65, 1980.

21a. Tsukita, S., and Ishikawa, H. The movement of membranous organelles in axons. Electron microscopic identification of anterogradely and retrogradely transported organelles. *J. Cell Biol* 84:513–530, 1980.

22. Lasek, R. J., and Brady, S. T. AMP-PNP facilitates attachment of transported vesicles to microtubules in axoplasm. *Nature* 316:645–647, 1985.

23. Sahenk, Z., and Lasek, R. J. Inhibition of proteolysis blocks anterograde-retrograde conversion of axonally transported vesicles. *Brain Res.* 460:199–203, 1988.

23a. Schroer, T. A., Brady, S. T., and Kelly, R. Fast axonal transport of foreign vesicles in squid axoplasm. *J. Cell Biol.* 101:568–572, 1985.

24. Stoeckel, K., and Thoenen, H. Retrograde axonal transport of nerve growth factor: Specificity and biological importance. *Brain Res.* 85:337–341, 1985.

24a. Kristersson, K. Retrograde transport of macromolecules in axons. *Annu. Rev. Pharmacol. Toxicol.* 18:97–110, 1987.

25. Hammerschlag, R. How do neuronal proteins know where they are going? Speculations on the role of molecular address markers. *Dev. Neurosci.* 6:2–17, 1983.

25a. Kelly, R. B., and Grote, E. Protein targeting in the neuron. *Annu. Rev. Neurosci.* 16:95–127, 1993.

26. Dotti, C. G., and Simons, K. Polarized sorting of viral glycoproteins to the axon and dendrites of hippocampal neurons in culture. *Cell* 62:63–72, 1990.

27. de Camilli, P., Benfenati, F., Valtorta, F., and Greengard, P. The synapsins. *Annu. Rev. Cell Biol.* 6:433–460, 1990.

28. McGuinness, T. L., Brady, S. T., Gruner, J., Sugimori, M., Llinas, R., and Greengard, P. Phosphorylation-dependent inhibition by synapsin I of organelle movement in squid axoplasm. *J. Neurosci.* 9:4138–4149, 1989.

29. Lasek, R. J., Garner, J., and Brady, S. Axonal transport of the cytoplasmic matrix. *J. Cell Biol.* 99:212s–221s, 1984.

30. Oblinger, M. M., Brady, S. T., McQuarrie, I. G., and Lasek, R. Differences in the protein composition of the axonally transported cytoskeleton in peripheral and central mammalian neurons. *J. Neurosci* 7:453–462, 1987.

31. Aguayo, A. J., Rasminsky, M., Bray, G. M., Carbonetto, S., McKerracher, L., Villegas-Perez, M. P., Vidal-Sanz, M., and Carter, D. A. Degenerative and regenerative responses of injured neurons in the central nervous system of adult mammals. *Philos. Trans. Soc. Lond. [Biol.]* 331:337–343, 1991.

31a. Schnell, L., and Schwab, M. Axonal regeneration in the rat spinal cord produced by an antibody against myelin associated neurite growth inhibitors. *Nature* 343:269–272, 1990.

32. Garner, J. A. Differential turnover of tubulin and neurofilaments in central nervous system neuron terminals. *Brain Res.* 458:309–318, 1988.

32a. Roots, B. Neurofilament accumulation induced in synapses by leupeptin. *Science* 221:971–972, 1983.

33. Brady, S. T. A novel brain ATPase with properties expected for the fast axonal transport motor. *Nature* 317:73–75, 1985.

33a. Vale, R. D., Reese, T. S., Sheetz, M. P. Identification of a novel force-generating protein, kinesin, involved in microtubule-based motility. *Cell* 42:39–50, 1985.

34. Goldstein, L. S. B. The kinesin superfamily: tails of functional redundancy. *Trends Cell Biol.* 1:93–98, 1991.

35. Vallee, R. B., Shpetner, H. S. Motor proteins of cytoplasmic microtubules. *Annu. Rev. Biochem.* 59:909–932, 1990.

CHAPTER 28

Development of the Nervous System

ALARIC T. ARENANDER AND JEAN DE VELLIS

FUNDAMENTAL CONCEPTS UNIFYING DEVELOPMENTAL DIVERSITY

Development is the study of the principles and processes that underlie growth and evolution of a biological organism. Most developmental research has been devoted to studying the early periods of intense and extensive transformations that are associated with the unfolding of an organism from a single fertilized egg, through embryogenesis,

Basic Neurochemistry: Molecular, Cellular, and Medical Aspects, 5th Ed., edited by G. J. Siegel et al. Published by Raven Press, Ltd., New York, 1994. Correspondence to Alaric T. Arenander, Departments of Anatomy and Psychiatry, Mental Retardation Research Center, Brain Research Institute, School of Medicine, University of California, Los Angeles, California 90024.

to postnatal maturation. During this period, the immense diversity of neural phenotype emerges [1,2]. What are the mechanisms that regulate the systematic and highly coherent series of events that fashion the vast neural circuitry? In this chapter, we will examine the molecular and cellular processes during these developmental periods in neural tissue that give rise to the brain's enormous phenotypic diversity.

Two fundamental concepts mold our perspective of how the nervous system develops and functions: the dynamic interdependencies of the genes and environment, and that of neuronal and neuroglial cells. During development, the systematic expression of the genetic blueprint creates and continuously molds the environment at all levels of its hierarchical organization, extending from the level of the single cell to the surroundings of the organism. The genetic machinery, in turn, relies on feedback from the environment to function properly. This interaction creates a highly integrated, self-referential process that links the genetic information with the multitude of influences existing at all the different layers of the environment [3]. Great progress has been made in the systematic dissection of individual linear pathways of environmental-genetic connections. For example, a growth factor and its receptor activate an intracellular signaling pathway to induce the expression of a specific gene. In this way, many environmental signals and numerous cell processes have been correlated with the appearance of different neural phenotypes.

The presumption behind these research studies is that knowledge of these single linear paths of environment-genetic linkage will provide a satisfying understanding of the basis of phenotypic diversity. As we have discovered and examined the function of more and more extracellular factors, receptors, and signaling pathways impinging upon an extensive genetic network functioning in a highly complex, combinatorial fashion, our research perspective is being transformed from a simple linear to a more realistic and integrated parallel model (Fig. 1). Multiple families of extracellular factors influence many receptors and intracellular signaling pathways which exhibit considerable interaction or "cross-talk." In addition, a network of transcription factors is being elucidated. This network is characterized by extensive inter- and intra-family interaction contributing to multiple levels of control over the expression and functional activity of transcription factors responsible for differential gene expression. Thus, in contrast to the linear model, neural phenotypic diversity arises from highly integrated networks of intracellular processes linked to environmental signals.

Biological interdependency in neural development is also dramatically displayed in the relationship of neuronal cells and neuroglial (or glial) cells [3–6]. The intimate coupling of these two types of cells is a major locus of genetic and epigenetic interaction in determining the functioning and the morphological, chemical, and electrical development of the nervous system. Students have traditionally learned that the neuronal cell represents the *structural* unit of the nervous system, relegating glia to the status of passive packaging. This narrow perspective has now been replaced by the accumulated evidence for glial cell regulation of nearly every aspect of neuronal development and function, supporting the premise that the fundamental *functional* unit of the nervous system is the dynamic interaction of neuronal and glial cells.

CELL CULTURE TECHNIQUES ALLOW EXPERIMENTAL CONTROL OF DEVELOPMENTAL EVENTS

Cell culture techniques provide a powerful means of systematically studying complex nervous systems [3,4,7,8]. The development of simple *in vitro* systems has had a great impact on neurochemistry, since it enables researchers to exert greater control over the chemical and cellular complexity of the ner-

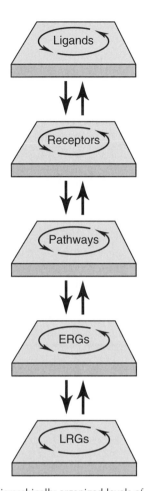

FIG. 1.   Hierarchically organized levels of information processing underlying the generation of neural phenotypic diversity. The enormous phenotypic diversity of the nervous system requires a mechanism that can generate increasing degrees of restriction in cell phenotype, such as cell shape and neurotransmitter expression. The original, simple linear perspective of an extracellular factor acting through its receptor directing the expression of phenotypic characteristics is now being replaced by the recognition that each level of information processing is itself a complex domain of interacting components. In this view, many families of signaling molecules or factors bind to a growing number of interacting receptors, with overlapping specificity and component makeup, to activate many different, interacting intracellular signaling pathways leading to the complex expression pattern of early response genes *(ERGs)*. These ERGs, many of which function as transcription factors, in turn, interact to regulate the final expression of late response genes *(LRGs)*, encoding proteins that are phenotypic determinants. Thus, from this perspective, each cell's developmental fate is determined by the sum total of all the multiple signals and combinatorial intracellular processes.

vous system [1,6,7]. Many cell culture preparations of developing neural cells from vertebrate and invertebrate species are now available. As a result, the neurochemical dissection of development has greatly improved, revealing a growing spectrum of regulatory molecules and mechanisms that participate in neural development.

Vertebrate cell culture was developed in 1907 by Harrison. By placing fragments of frog embryo nervous tissue in a drop of clotted lymph, he was able to demonstrate that each nerve axon or dendrite is the extension of the neuronal cell body. This simple observation supported the neuronal doctrine at the expense of opponents who had claimed that nerve fibers were the product of fusion of many cells. Harrison's experiment was the prototype of the *explant cell culture* technique. In the 1960s, a second system, the *dissociated cell culture*, was introduced. In this method the tissue is dissociated mechanically or enzymatically to yield a suspension of single cells. The dispersed cells are usually cultured on the pretreated surface of a culture dish. A third system, *reaggregate cell culture*, was initiated by Moscona to provide a tissue-like environment for the cells. A few hours after dissociated cells are placed in a rotating flask, small, round aggregates are found floating in the media. These three systems, in which cultures are prepared directly from the tissues of an organism, are collectively termed primary cultures. It is possible to remove the primary neural tissue cells from the culture dish and establish secondary cultures and thus expand the population. Such cell preparations, e.g., of glia, can usually be passed successfully only a limited number of times owing to either dedifferentiation or terminal differentiation of cells. A fourth system is that of *clonal cell culture* lines, established by culturing the progeny of a single cell. Neural cell lines come from endogenous tumors or from chemically or virally transformed cells. The tumorigenic properties of these cell lines present obvious limitations to their usefulness.

Control of the physicochemical environment of the cells is possible *in vitro*. Substances can be added to or withdrawn from the culture medium, allowing precise temporal analysis of the sequence of events that occur, for example, in hormone action. Tissue culture also circumvents the problem of the blood-brain barrier and thus removes the endocrine and other signaling agents endogenous to the central nervous system. Furthermore, it also allows the study of a discrete nervous system area isolated from the normal *in vivo* homeostatic mechanisms.

Each of the tissue culture systems described offers particular advantages [8]. Dissociated cell cultures allow the visualization of individual living cells that can be monitored morphologically and electrophysiolog-

ically. It is possible to obtain and correlate biochemical, morphological, and electrophysiological data from a single cell. An alternative to observing and quantitating parameters at the single cell level is to separate the cell types either prior to primary culturing if possible or after the culture is established. Ingenious methods developed in different laboratories now make it possible to obtain cultures of all the cell types listed in Table 1 enriched 90 to 99 percent in one cell type. These pure cultures have become the system of choice for many neurochemists.

An advantage of using reaggregate cultures rather than dissociated cultures is the ability to provide a more structured, three-dimensional extracellular space that more

TABLE 1. Cell markers for identifying major cell types

Neuroepithelial stem cells	Schwann cells
Nestin	Galactocerebroside (GC)
Vimentin (VIM)	Glial fibrillary acidic protein (GFAP)
Neuronal cells	Laminin
α-Internexin	Myelin basic protein (MBP)
Enolase (γ/γ isozyme)	NGFR (p75, 217c)
Neurofilament	O4
Oligodendrocytes	Sulfatide (SULF)
Carbonic anhydrase II (CA)	S100
Cholesterol ester hydrolase (CEH)	Ependymal cells
Cyclic nucleotide phosphohydrolase (CNP)	Cilia
GD3 ganglioside (GD3)	Epen-1
Galactocerebroside (GC); 01	Ran-2
Glutathione-S-transferase (GST, Pi class)	Macrophages (microglia)
Glycerolphosphate dehydrogenase (GPDH)	ED1
Myelin-associated glycoprotein (MAG)	Labeled latex beads
Myelin basic protein (MBP)	MAC-1
O4	MAC-3
O10	Nonspecific esterase
POA	Vault
Proteolipid protein (PLP)	Meningeal cells
Sulfatide (SULF)	Epen-1
Transferrin (Tf)	Fibronectin
Astrocytes	Ran-2
Carbonic anhydrase II (CA)	Fibroblasts
Glial fibrillary acidic protein (GFAP)	Fibronectin
Glutathione-S-transferase (GST, Mu class)	Thy-1
Ran-2	
S-100 protein	

Most of the markers listed are available as both monoclonal and polyclonal antibodies. Since the antibodies are generated in different species, double and triple immunofluorescent labeling of cells is possible. Cell surface cilia of ependymal cells represent another type of marker. Macrophages readily phagocytose fluorochrome-labeled latex beads, which then can be detected by fluorescence.

closely approximates the *in vivo* conditions for cell growth and development. Such conditions may reduce the dilution of secreted cellular factors and increase the opportunity for morphological and biochemical differentiation to proceed more like *in vivo* events. The cells inside an aggregate are first distributed at random. They then sort out into patterns often resembling the organization seen *in vivo*. The importance of cell contact and histotypic organization is illustrated by the observation that glutamine synthetase, a marker of retinal glial Müller cells, is inducible by glucocorticoids in reaggregate but not dissociated cell cultures. Some laboratories are now using three-dimensional matrix cultures made form natural components, such as collagen and fibronectin, to obtain similar biological advantages.

Clonal cell lines of tumoral origin have provided useful knowledge in neurochemistry over the past two decades. They provide homogeneous cell populations in large quantities in a very reproducible manner. The cell lines of choice are those that continue to express in culture the differentiated properties of their normal cell counterparts. The first such clonal cell line was the C6 glioma cell line established from a chemically induced tumor in an adult rat; C6 cells possess differentiated properties of both astrocytes and oligodendrocytes. Like oligodendrocytes *in vivo* or in primary culture, C6 cells express glucocorticoid-inducible glycerolphosphate dehydrogenase and the myelin component 2′,3′-cyclic nucleotide phosphohydrolase. They also display glucocorticoid-inducible glutamine synthetase and glial fibrillary acidic protein (GFAP), characteristic properties of astrocytes. C6 cells have been shown to possess many of the regulatory control mechanisms and differentiated properties of glial cells and to provide large numbers of cells for experiments studying molecular mechanisms. The PC12 clonal cell line was established from a rat pheochromocytoma, an adrenal medullary tumor. PC12 cells have many properties in common with primary sympathetic neuron and chromaffin cell cultures. In response to nerve growth factor (NGF), they extend neurites and increase tyrosine hydroxylase (TH) activity. Useful clonal cell lines have also been established from mouse and human neuroblastoma. These cell lines express several neurotransmitter-synthesizing enzymes, which makes them good candidates for the study of regulation of gene expression as well as for the establishment of cDNA libraries.

The generation of cell lines devoid of tumoral properties has been achieved by the use of retroviral vectors for transferring oncogenes to glial or neuronal progenitor cells in culture. These cell lines display properties of their normal cell counterparts. For instance, a *v-myc* immortalized sympathoadrenal progenitor cell line, the *MAH* cell line, differentiates into neurons upon exposure to FGF. Other cell lines displaying glial progenitor properties have been established using the polyoma large T or the adenovirus E1A genes. More recently, astroglial and neuronal cell lines have been established from transgenic mice carrying targeted constructs of the polyoma large T or SV40 large T genes.

Cultured cells were originally maintained in the presence of biologically derived media, such as fetal calf serum. Chemically defined media are produced by replacing serum with pure growth factors, hormones, and adhesion molecules. These media have overcome the troublesome, uncontrollable, and undefined nature of sera and permitted the examination of the requirement of each cell type for survival, growth, and differentiation in culture. This has led not only to the discovery of the various target cells for different factors, but also of many new target cell-derived factors.

MOLECULAR MARKERS ENABLE PRECISE IDENTIFICATION OF CELL TYPES

Cell culture techniques in neurobiology expanded during the 1970s and increased the need for cell-type specific markers that would unambiguously identify all the cell types present in dissociated primary culture of neural tissue [4,7,8]. The problem was most acute in developing systems because of the multiplicity of cell lineages and developmental stages, as well as the inadequacies of morphological criteria to identify population subsets. To develop neural cell markers, several neurobiologists turned to immunological approaches that were successful in analyzing lymphocyte subpopulations. Many cell markers are immunogenic molecules present in or on a single cell type and that can be detected with specific monoclonal or polyclonal antibodies.

General immunological markers used to identify each major cell type (Table 1) reflect the varying physiology of each cell type. The difference in the protein composition of intermediate filaments among cells gave rise to the usefulness of the antibody to GFAP in the identification of astrocytes and of the antibody to one of the neurofilament proteins to mark neurons. Embryonic cells of all classes have vimentin, which is retained only in adult radial glia, such as Müller cells in the retina and Bergmann glia in cerebellum. Because oligodendrocytes largely lack intermediate filaments, but produce abundant myelin, specific myelin-associated proteins and lipids provide numerous markers. Schwann cells placed in culture rapidly lose their myelin-associated markers. These cells were originally identified by the polyclonal antibody RAN-1, which is no longer available. Fortunately, the monoclonal antibody 217c, now known to recognize the low-affinity nerve growth factor receptor $p75^{NGFR}$, has replaced it as a Schwann cell marker.

Functional or developmental specific sublets of neuronal populations require an array of appropriately restricted markers. Neurotransmitters, neurotransmitter-synthesizing enzymes, and neuropeptides have provided a great diversity of markers to identify specific neuronal subpopulations and to map neuronal networks. As more antibodies become available, multiple double- and tri-ple-labeling immunohistochemical studies will enhance our ability to identify subpopulations of neurons and to delineate developmental cell lineages. In addition, novel approaches using molecular biological techniques promise to increase the specificity of cell lineage analysis. One such method consists of using a retrovirus vector construct as a means of introducing foreign marker genes, such as LacZ, into cells at some stage of development and then examining the time course of development and phenotype of the clonal progeny.

GENERAL DEVELOPMENT OF THE NERVOUS SYSTEM

Genetic information contained in the single fertilized cell is capable of giving rise to the billions of neurons in the adult vertebrate nervous system. Underlying the great diversity in the final neural design, arising from variability in genetic and epigenetic interaction, are basic transforming steps common to all vertebrates (Fig. 2). Early in embryogenesis, a sequence of events transforms the zygote into a unilaminar sheet of ectoderm cells. A trilaminar embryo then appears that possesses the three primary "germ" layers: ectoderm, endoderm, and mesoderm. Neural ectoderm is then induced by interaction of the mesoderm with the overlying ectoderm. This neural plate is committed to develop into neural tissue, as can be demonstrated by transplantation experiments in which neural ectoderm surgically placed in other parts of the embryo produces auxiliary neural tissue. In addition, local areas of the plate along its anterior-posterior axis are predestined to develop into specific brain regions.

The next major step is characterized by migration of neural plate cells toward the midline and the acquisition of different cell shapes. Differential changes in cell morphology result in the edges of the neural plate folding in to form the neural groove, the

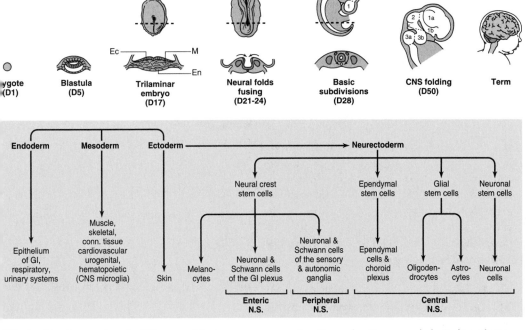

FIG. 2.   Morphogenesis and cell lineages of the human nervous system. **Top series:** Gross morphological transformations. On Day 1 (D1), the fertilized egg (the zygote) begins the process of sequential transformations that lead to a trilaminar embryo by Day 17. The D17 embryo is shown in both dorsal view (**top,** 2–3 mm in length) and, at the level of the *dashed line,* in cross-section. The three primary germ layers are labeled: ectoderm *(Ec)*, mesoderm *(M)*, and endoderm *(En)*. By Day 21, the neural folds begin to fuse to form the neural tube. The "zipping up" of the tube begins at the middle of the embryo and proceeds anteriorly and posteriorly until the tube is completely sealed. By the end of the 1st month, the anterior bulging of the tube forms the major subdivisions (length about 4–5 mm) and the neural crest cells are migrating *(arrows)*. By the end of the 2nd month (25–31 mm), the basic folding pattern of the CNS has appeared, setting the stage for the extensive cell proliferation and process outgrowth that greatly expands the size of the brain by term (not drawn to scale). **Bottom series:** Lineages derived from the primary germ layers. All the cells of the CNS and PNS, except the microglial cells, which are of mesodermal origin, are derived from the neuroectoderm. The neural crest cells leave the dorsal aspect of the neural tube and take their migratory pathways to innervate the body and its organs as the various components of the enteric and peripheral nervous systems. The stem cells of the neural tube proliferate and give rise to committed progenitor cells for different lineages which, in turn, give rise to cells committed to each sublineage shown. See subsequent figures for more detailed information related to each of the main lineages. (Illustration by Sharon Belkin, Media Unit, MRRC, UCLA.)

edges of which eventually contact and adhere. Thus, the groove "zips up" to form a tube of cells surrounding a central fluid space, creating the neural tube. At the same time, cells on the margins of the plate migrate into the region between the surface ectoderm and the dorsal aspect of the neural tube and become the cells of the neural crest (NC). The pseudostratified epithelial cells of the neural tube continuously and rapidly proliferate. Increasing fluid pressure within the central canal leads to "ballooning" of the rostral end of the tube to form the three brain vesicles that define the major divisions of the brain: forebrain, midbrain, and hindbrain.

Neuroepithelium initially contains only one undifferentiated population of stem cells. With time this gives rise to all the cells committed to the two main lineages, neuronal and glial stem cells, and subsequently the many sublineages of the stem cell type

[6], described in the last section of this chapter. The neuronal stem cells continue to proliferate until unknown signals induce them to exit from the mitotic cycle. These postmitotic cells lose contact with the ventricular surface and migrate, forming the mantle layer of cells. The accumulation of postmitotic neuronal cells results in the progressive thickening of the neural tube destined to become the future central nervous system (CNS), the spinal cord, and brain. Although neuroepithelial cells give rise to neuronal cells and glia at about the same time, neuronal proliferation ceases early in embryogenesis, whereas glial cells continue to divide, even into postnatal periods of development. The mechanisms controlling population size and a cell's exit from the mitotic cycle are not understood.

During this same period, cells from the NC continue to profilerate even as they disperse by various migratory routes to their final target sites to form the sensory and autonomic ganglia of the peripheral nervous system (PNS) as well as non-neural cells such as skin melanocytes, endocrine cells, and part of the muscles and bones of the face.

DEVELOPMENTAL PROCESSES: ENVIRONMENTAL FORCES MOLDING GENETIC POTENTIAL

Developing cells of the nervous system are embedded in complex fields of mechanical tension, biochemical signals, and electrical current. This constantly changing pattern of spatial and temporal information for each cell is created, in large part, by the chemistry of the nerve cells themselves and represents the major environmental forces that drive the sequence of developmental processes. The dynamic interaction between these environmental influences and the machinery of nerve cells force the cells to undergo considerable transformation during periods of growth and survival, migration and sorting, and morphological and biochemical differentiation [9,10].

Selective cell survival and proliferation determine the number of each type of nerve cell

A basic tactic in creating complex biologic systems is to generate an excess of elements and then, through a set of selective processes, determine which elements will remain to participate in the final organizational pattern. This strategy is widely used in the construction of the vertebrate nervous system. During development, the interaction between genetic and epigenetic forces is expressed, in part, as the balance between cell survival and cell death [11]. Intimately linked to this balance is the control of cell proliferation.

For invertebrate development genetic instructions are the prime controller of population size and diversity. Because of the short life span and the relatively simple nervous system necessary to control the organism in a relatively constant ecological niche, the most reliable and economical approach is to rapidly generate simple, preprogrammed neuronal/glial circuitry. The development of the nematode *Caenorhabditis elegans* is an example of cell lineage generated independent of the environment. Precursor cells undergo cycles of stereotyped divisions, creating a number of restricted, preprogrammed cellular lineages. Even the little amount of cell death appears to be due to intrinsic instructions that select specific pathways to terminate in senescence.

Vertebrate development reflects the other extreme of the genetic/epigenetic continuum—unlike invertebrates, numerous environmental cues are employed to direct lineage decisions, including the decisions for survival, division, or death. Prolonged gestation and the plasticity inherent in allowing outside influences to guide developmental decisions permit the construction of large-scale, highly interconnected, activity-dependent circuitries.

Early experiments demonstrated that the presence and size of the target tissue are critical in determining the number and functions of the surviving neuronal cells [12]. Removal of limb buds or transplantation of an extra limb bud results in predictable decreases or increases, respectively, of the innervating motor and sensory neurons. Each set of neuronal cells exhibits a characteristic degree of target-dependent cell death during development: some groups remaining quite stable in number, while others lose up to two-thirds of the cell's progeny. What are the factors that influence the balance between cellular survival and death? The nature of the microenvironment of the cell soma as well as the environment into which the cell process grows are both important. Critical factors produced in the innervated target tissue contribute to the regulation of cell survival: Limited amounts of soluble factor(s) released by target cells lead to competition among cells dependent on the factor. Thus, during specific periods of early cell development, factors are necessary for survival.

Specific paths of cell migration to final target environments are controlled by gradients of diffusible and substrate-bound neurochemical signals

Migration of cells plays a significant role in brain morphogenesis. Most neurons travel long distances through the complex extracellular terrain of the developing embryo to reach their final position. What mechanisms are used by neurons to move along the path, and what are the signals that are used to guide them? The most common mechanism for cell translocation is a combination of (a) the extension of a cell process and its attachment to the substratum followed by (b) the pulling of the entire cell toward the point of attachment by means of contractile proteins associated with an intracellular network of microfilaments.

Directional control of cell movement appears to be of two types: (a) cells moving along other "guide" cells arranged as scaffolding, and (b) cells moving across a multicellular terrain guided by a concentration gradient. For example, small molecules diffusing through or attached to the extracellular matrix can alter a cell's behavior. In the complex neuropil of the cerebral cortex, molecular signals undoubtedly permit neurons to distinguish radial glial processes along which they travel from the other neuronal, glial, and endothelial surfaces.

Neural crest (NC) cell movement is another model of molecular control of cell migration and contrasts with the work from the cortical systems. Since there are no glial cells to create highways for the crest cells, the migration of these cells into the spaces surrounding the neural tube depends on the nature of the extracellular matrix. In order to migrate to specific destinations, a number of signals must be regulated in a coordinated fashion both temporally and spatially. Nearly all of the major components of the matrix—collagen, fibronectin, laminin, proteoglycans, and hyaluronic acid—regulate NC cell migration. For example, NC cell migration correlates with the appearance of high levels of hyaluronic acid.

A variety of substrate- and cell-attached factors influence neural development by regulating adhesion properties of cells. Interactions occur directly between cells or between a cell and the extracellular matrix of the microenvironment. The molecules mediating these interactions have been implicated in regulating the specificity and timing of cell-cell adhesion and the consequences on cell morphology and physiology. Hence, they influence the ability of cells not only to migrate, but to sort themselves out, and to stabilize spatial relationships considered important for the process of differentiation. These molecules have names such as cell adhesion molecules (CAMs), intercellular adhesion molecules (I-CAMs), integrins and cadherins [13,14].

CAMs are a family of high-molecular-weight glycoproteins that possess morphoregulatory properties during neural development. There are five well-characterized members of this family of cell surface glycoproteins important in brain development: neural CAM (N-CAM), neuronal-glial CAM

(Ng-CAM; also called NILE or L1), TAG-1, tenascin (also known as cytotactin or J1), and adhesion molecule on glia (AMOG/beta 2 isoform of the membrane Na, K-ATPase pump). The most thoroughly examined N-CAM is detected early in embryogenesis and throughout the development of the nervous system in both glia and neuronal cells. It is a cell surface glycoprotein of the immuno-globulin (Ig) superfamily mediating Ca^{2+}-independent homophilic binding and aggregation of neuronal cells. N-CAM may contribute to a variety of developmental processes, such as glial guidance of axonal processes, neurite fasciculation, axon-target cell interaction, and the creation and stabilization of cell position relationships (see also Chap. 29). A-CAM, also known as N-cad-herin, is a member of a family of non-Ig glycoproteins that are important in cell-cell interaction functioning in a Ca^{2+}-dependent fashion.

L1 also displays Ca^{2+}-independent binding, is found only on neuronal cells, and is involved in heterotypic binding between neuronal and neuroglial cells. In culture, NGF and TGF-β1 and TGF-β2 increase the expression of L1 on immature astrocytes, while the TGFs, but not NGF, lead to decreases in N-CAM expression. The increase in L1 correlates with increased neurite outgrowth of dorsal root ganglion neuronal cells on these astrocytes. In contrast, PDGF and FGF have no effect on astrocyte CAMs. The transient expression of TAG-1 on the surface of a subset of neuronal cells in the CNS is correlated with neurite extension promotion and is considered to play a role in the initial stage of axonal growth and guidance over terrains of neuroepithelial cells. The loss of TAG-1 expression coincides with the onset of L1 expression, associated with axon-axon homophilic interaction and the process of fasciculation. Tenascin is a large extracellular matrix protein with restricted neural expression during embryogenesis. Tenascin is composed of 6 subunits which possess repeating domains similar to epidermal growth factor (EGF) and fibronectin.

This glycoprotein has been implicated in cell proliferation and neural cell attachment. The later data suggest a role in neurite outgrowth and cell migration, which helps determine synaptic architecture and boundary formation in the developing PNS and CNS. Tenascin is one of many factors controlling neural crest migration and differentiation. In the adult PNS, tenascin is found confined in the extracellular matrix at the node of Ranvier and the perineurium.

Integrins are members of a large family of membrane receptors. The multiple subtypes forming homo- and hetero-dimers with distinct ligand specificity provide a complex receptor system mediating attachment to extracellular matrices and cell-cell adhesion events. I-CAMs and other matrix components such as collagen, laminin, and fibronectin function as integrin ligands. Adhesive properties of cells can vary by either selective expression of different integrins or by altering the binding properties of existing integrins. In the latter case, the state of molecular activation or inhibition determines whether an integrin binds its respective ligands. Integrin activation can not only lead to rapid changes in cell adhesion properties in the local microenvironment but can also trigger intracellular events. As signaling receptors, integrins can encode environmental information and interact with intracellular transduction cascades modulated by other extracellular ligands such as growth factors and neurotransmitters. Thus, these receptors provide the developing neural cells a system capable of linking adhesion/migration information with other development signals controlling proliferation and differentiation.

In summary, interactions of cells with each other and with the extracellular matrix during development depend on a multifactorial, complex array of molecular interactions and signaling events that are constantly being integrated by the cell to produce behavior appropriate for the developmental time and position.

Cell process outgrowth determines the cytoarchitecture and circuitry of the nervous system

Cell process elongation and branching determine the cell's final morphological phenotype and its participation in the local and global neural circuitries [15–17]. On the average, each of the billions of neuronal cells forms more than 10,000 specific interconnections. This process of morphological differentiation requires the directed growth of a considerable number of cell processes to multiple specific targets, often at great distances from the cell body. Control over the active elongation of a cell process creates the final size and geometry of the neuronal axon and dendritic tree. What are the molecular mechanisms that control the progressive elongation of a cell process? What environmental signals are present to guide the processes through a complex, three-dimensional, multicellular terrain? What are the processes that determine the time and place of branching? Are the molecules implicated in regulating cellular migration involved in controlling neurite outgrowth? In general, many of the same soluble and matrix components that regulate cell proliferation, survival, and migration have been shown to also mediate process outgrowth *in vivo* and *in vitro*.

Growth cones are located at the leading edge of a neurite and display two types of motile structures: long spike-like structures called filopodia and thin, broad sheets of membrane called lamellipodia. These delicate structures are important in pathfinding and outgrowth branching. Growth cone movement can be influenced by small soluble factors. Local concentration gradients of NGF and/or FGF can initiate and direct growth and movement. Specific neurotransmitters, such as serotonin and dopamine, can also alter neurite elongation and growth cone movement. For example, serotonin inhibits neuronal outgrowth of specific subsets of neurons. Inhibition of neurite outgrowth can also be suppressed by electrical activity.

Adhesion molecules, either on the cell or in the extracellular matrix, may also play an important role in neurite outgrowth, since these molecules mediate neurite-neurite and neurite-glial interactions. The probability of outgrowth initiation, rate of elongation, and degree of branching of neurites are strongly influenced by the adhesive quality of the cells' substrata. Adhesion of growth cone structures may stabilize extensions. Growth cones may follow the path of greatest adhesiveness, leading to directional control over neurite outgrowth. The glycoprotein laminin, found in the extracellular matrix and on the surface of Schwann cells, can accelerate neurite outgrowth.

Neuronal-glial interaction may also be involved in outgrowth. Sympathetic neurons grown in the absence of Schwann cells extend unbranched, axon-like neurites; in the presence of glial cells, however, process outgrowth is extensively branched and dendrite-like in form. In CNS preparations, this interaction is further characterized by the specificity of the astrocytic environment—glia from local homotopic regions give rise to branched neurites, and glia from heterotopic regions induce unbranched neurites.

Intracellular pathways are involved in the regulation of neurite outgrowth. cAMP and inositol phospholipids have been implicated as intracellular regulators, and work on the control of Ca^+ influx has proved to be successful in helping to establish a causal relationship with neurite outgrowth: Ca^{2+} influx can regulate both neurite elongation and growth cone movements. Studies of invertebrate neurons and isolated growth cones suggest that in the presence of various agents that inhibit neurite outgrowth, e.g., serotonin and electrical activity, the level of free cytoplasmic Ca^{2+} is closely correlated with neurite outgrowth. Further support of Ca^{2+}-mediated control of neurite growth has been obtained from studies under conditions in which neurite outgrowth and Ca^{2+} influx could be directly manipulated. Data suggest that specific levels of Ca^{2+} influx promote normal neurite elongation and growth cone movements.

The basic cytoarchitecture of the cortex is a result of a plastic process of process outgrowth as discussed above relying on adhesion factors and control of terminal arborization, which can be dependent on neuronal activity. The final lattice-like pattern of complex cortical circuitry and its computational capacity arise from a combination of selective and nonselective process outgrowth and synapse formation coupled to regressive events including selective cell death, process elimination, and synapse elimination. These events can be activity-dependent and/or -independent processes. For example, the vertical connections in the cortex arise with little dependence on neuronal activity during development, whereas the horizontal connecting outgrowth is clearly regulated by evoked or spontaneous neural activity. Thus, the formation of cortical clusters is dependent upon patterned visual activity; binocular deprivation can eliminate the clustered organization of the horizontal connections. In the case of cortical cluster organization, selective elimination of collaterals, and not cell death, is the essential molding parameter.

In summary, a number of parameters of outgrowth initiation, elongation, branching, and cessation combine to generate axonal or dendritic geometry. These components can be modulated *in vitro* by a variety of soluble and substrate-bound factors, suggesting that, *in vivo*, control over morphological differentiation is multifactorial.

MOLECULAR MECHANISMS OF DEVELOPMENT

Environmental factors control developmental decisions made by cells of each lineage

Diffusible growth factors control the processes of proliferation and differentiation [6,12]. The discovery of nerve growth factor in the early 1950s began an era of remarkable success in developmental neurochemistry. NGF is abundant in male mouse salivary gland from which it can be purified as a complex of three dissimilar subunits, one of which, the β subunit, appears to be the only neuroactive component. The NGF gene, which codes for the pro-β-NGF protein precursor, is highly conserved across species.

NGF influences are thought to be initiated by the formation of NGF-receptor complexes on the cell surface and subsequent translocation of the complex into the cytoplasm. Responsive cells possess both high- and low-affinity receptors. Low-affinity receptors in the presence of NGF may cooperatively interact, cluster together, and be converted to high-affinity receptors as part of the biological response. In sympathetic nerve cells possessing axonal processes, NGF binds selectively to receptors at the axonal terminals, where it is internalized and transported retrogradely along the axon to the cell body. Following NGF treatment, a cascade of cytoplasmic and nuclear events occur within a temporal sequence ranging from seconds to days. NGF treatment of PC12 cells, for example, leads to increased formation of cyclic AMP (cAMP) and hydrolysis of phosphoinositides, induction of Na^+ influx, and membrane ruffling. Within minutes there are changes in protein phosphorylation and increased gene transcription. Intermediate events include increases in ornithine decarboxylase, choline acetyltransferase, and acetylcholinesterase activity; initial process outgrowth; and a second round of gene expression leading to changes in the levels of about 5% of cellular proteins. Late events are represented by extensive neurite outgrowth and the formation of functional synapses.

Physiological effects of NGF can be classified as (a) an essential neurotrophic or nourishing influence during early development resulting in selective neuronal survival; (b) a potent influence on neuron differentiation; or (c) a strong neurotropic or guiding influence on direction of neurite growth. The main experimental strategy employed over the years to demonstrate the presence of the different activities of NGF has been to either block (via specific antibodies or drugs) or enhance (via addition of exogenous NGF) its actions.

A recent breakthrough of major importance to elucidate the molecular mechanisms of NGF action is the discovery that NGF binds to two cell surface receptors, $p75^{NGFR}$ and the *trk* proto-oncogene (p^{140trk}) with a similar low-affinity Kd, but that both are required to obtain high-affinity NGF binding and to generate a specific physiological response.

NGF binding to $p140^{trk}$ results in activation of its intrinsic tyrosine kinase activity, resulting in Trk autophosphorylation. Tyrosine phosphorylation seems to be a key initial event in signal transduction that via an intracellular cascade of events leads to neurite extension and neuronal differentiation.

Although the sequence of NGF has been known for 22 years, no related members had been positively identified until 3 years ago when brain-derived neurotrophic factor (BDNF) was sequenced and it became apparent that it had 50% sequence homology with NGF. This finding rapidly led to the identification of other numbers of this family by using the polymerase chain reaction and hybridization screening. These new members of the NGF family now called the neurotrophins have been designated neurotrophins 3, 4, and 5 (NT3, 4, 5). Interestingly, all five members of the neurotrophin family bind to the $p75^{NGFR}$. The specificity of the response to ligand binding seems to reside in the members of the *trk* receptor family. NGF binds to Trk A, BDNF to Trk B, and NT-3 preferentially to Trk C and to a lesser extent to Trk A and B. NT 4 and 5 stimulate Trk B, but it is not yet known if they affect the other members of the *trk* family. The specificity of target cell response (Table 2) seems to depend on the type of *trk* receptor expressed. For instance, PC12 cells only express Trk A

TABLE 2.   Neurons responsive to neurotrophins

	NGF	BDNF	NT-3
PNS			
Dorsal root sensory neurons	+	+	+
Sympathetic neurons	+	−	Weak
Nodose neurons	−	+	+
PC12 cells	+	−	−
CNS			
Cholinergic neurons	+	+	Weak
Dopaminergic neurons	−	+	+
Retinal ganglion cells	−	+	ND

+, Survival or differentiation or both; −, no response; ND, not determined.

and dorsal root sensory neurons express either Trk A or Trk B. Sympathetic neurons express Trk A.

The survival and differentiation influences of NGF are not unique. In the past decade, the existence of many other such factors has been reported.

FGFs were discovered by high-affinity binding to heparin. Initially two molecules, acidic (aFGF) and basic (bFGF), were described. Now the family members number seven and may increase. Many studies have reported the existence of growth factors with trophic or tropic activities on neuronal and glial cells. Many of these factors are now recognized to be members of the FGF family. In addition to its possible influence during brain angiogenesis, FGF appears to act as an inducing factor during early embryonic transformations, a survival and neurite-promoting agent for central neurons, and a mitogen for astrocytes and oligodendrocytes. bFGF can increase transcriptional activity such as increased levels of ornithine decarboxylase, process outgrowth and decrease protein phosphorylation in PC12 cells, actions similar to those reported for NGF. In fact, recent reports suggest that both FGFs may mimic all the short- and long-term influences of NGF on PC12 cells.

Epidermal growth factor (EGF) is another small but potent polypeptide mitogen isolated originally from male mouse salivary glands. EGF is a potent mitogen for many cells in culture, including astroyctes, and can also stimulate glial differentiation. Its effects are not limited to mitotic control. EGF can directly influence neuronal cell development. The survival and process outgrowth of cerebral neurons in culture, for example, are enhanced by EGF. In PC12 cells, EGF induces tyrosine phosphorylation, Na^+/H^+ exchange-mediated K^+ influx, membrane ruffling, and cell division. *In vivo* and *in vitro* studies demonstrate that EGF or EGF-like activity and its receptor can be found during embryonic development. EGF stimulates, for example, proliferation of neural crest cells and increases their release of hyaluronic acid and production of proteoglycans. These results suggest that EGF, by regulating the composition of the extracellular matrix and thereby influencing migration, may play a role in the morphogenesis of the neural crest.

Recently a large superfamily of neural cytokines has been delineated acting not only on the developmental processes of neuronal cells but of glial cells as well.

Two neurotrophic factor activities, the cholinergic differentiation factor (CDF) and the ciliary neurotrophic factor (CNTF), that were extensively studied for a decade were recently molecularly characterized [18]. CDF was first identified as cell culture conditioned media activity that induces cholinergic phenotype in sympathetic neurons. The amino acid sequence of CDF revealed a complete homology to leukemia inhibitory factor (LIF) purified on the basis of its ability to induce macrophage characteristics in a myeloid cell line. CDF/LIF have effects on many of the cell types, including oligodendrocyte lineage cells, liver, bone, fat, kidney, and various embryonic cells. CNTF activity was identified by its ability to support survival of parasympathetic ciliary neurons. Although CNTF is molecularly distinct from CDF/LIF, it displays many of the differentiative effects of CDF/LIF on sympathetic neurons. Among the large family of interleukins (IL1 to IL-10), IL-6 has functional overlaps with CDF/ LIF. These functional overlaps by factors collectively referred to as cytokines may be explained by sequence elements and structural themes common among their respective receptors. The sections of this chapter on cell lineages will illustrate the rapidly growing importance of cytokines in neural cell development.

Genetic networks and neural development

One of the most fascinating and rapidly growing fields of research is the elucidation of the complex network of genetic information that controls development. The immense phenotypic diversity of the nervous system reflects the coordination of the numerous genetic programs that regulate cell-type specific gene expression. How does a cell become responsive to a given set of environmental signals, encode this information into specific channels of intracellular transduction, and regulate differential gene expression? The answer lies, in part, in the complex world of transcriptional regulators. It is estimated that 5% of the mammalian genome, about 5,000 genes, encode for transcription factors (Fig. 3). Of these, up to one-half are anticipated to have expression restricted to the nervous system. The large number of transcription factors can be subdivided into families whose members all share a conserved amino acid sequence responsible for DNA-binding and dimerization. At present, 12 distinct motifs have been identified. Four classes are illustrated in Fig. 4. Research demonstrates that members of these and other classes can function as transcriptional regulators exerting control over developmental processes of proliferation and differentiation [19].

Levels of integration within the transcriptional regulator network

Part of the complexity of control lies in the large number of different factors available to generate cell-type specific transcriptional

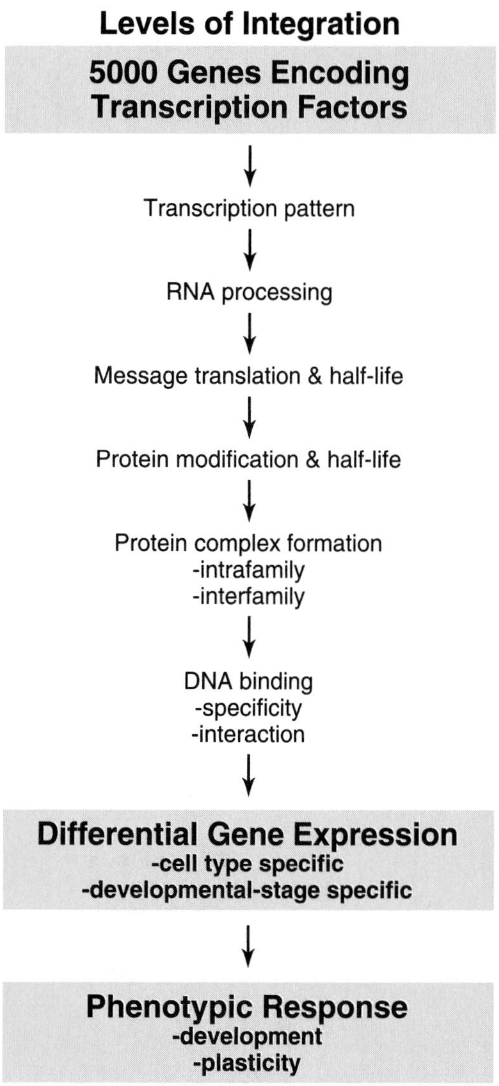

Levels of Integration

5000 Genes Encoding Transcription Factors

↓

Transcription pattern

↓

RNA processing

↓

Message translation & half-life

↓

Protein modification & half-life

↓

Protein complex formation
-intrafamily
-interfamily

↓

DNA binding
-specificity
-interaction

↓

Differential Gene Expression
-cell type specific
-developmental-stage specific

↓

Phenotypic Response
-development
-plasticity

FIG. 3. Levels of integration within the transcription factor network. Of the estimated 5,000 genes in the human genome encoding for transcription factors, perhaps half will exhibit expression specific to the nervous system. This predicted restriction in expression is considered to reflect the need to generate the combinatorial control mechanisms necessary to create the enormous phenotypic diversity unique to neural development. Listed are the various levels of processing whereby complex interactions among many factors and many events are integrated to carry out the critical task of differential gene expression that determines the unique phenotypic response during development and adult plasticity.

regulation. More importantly, the control over the expression and functional state of these numerous transcription factors is a source of considerable complexity and opportunity for combinatorial integration. Figure 3 illustrates the many points or levels of control that can be exerted over these developmental regulators. For example, the ability to alter the transcriptional expression of these factors is an initial and key point of control. As shown, other classical levels of control such as translation, are expected to add levels of complexity. Because the activity of most of these transcriptional regulators can be controlled by phosphorylation and dimerization, the number of permutations of interactive modes expands rapidly. Heterodimer formation can determine whether a transcriptional regulator is functionally active or not.

Thus, at any point of time in the life of a given cell, the sum total of activity at all the levels of integration will be reflected by the nature of the genetic program that is read. This program creates not only the new cell phenotype, but also sets the stage for the next round of developmental decisions, in part due to the alteration in the pattern of expression of transcriptional regulators now unleashed to reverberate in the cell physiology.

Early response genes as development control signals

How do epigenetic influences participate in decision making? Environmental influences come in the form of growth factors, neurotransmitters, and other ligands that are linked to changes in membrane receptors and intracellular signaling pathways, and agents or fields capable of altering membrane electrical properties. Most extracellular signals trigger a change in cell physiology that can last for several days. How do these changes come about? In particular, how can environmental factors "start the ball rolling" and trigger a new wave of genomic activ-

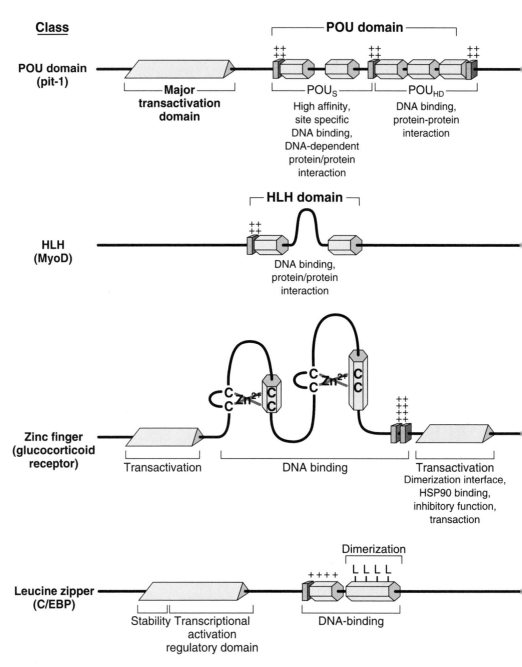

FIG. 4.   Major classes of transcription factors. Twelve distinct families of transcription factors have been classified by their DNA-binding motifs. Four examples of these transcription factors implicated in the control of cell proliferation and differentiation are depicted here. Conserved regions unique to each family include regions of basic amino acids functioning as DNA-binding sites *(solid rectangles)* and putative helical regions associated with DNA-binding or dimerization *(cylinders)* are shown. Transcriptional activation domains *(solid triangles)* are generally not conserved even within a family generating considerable diversity of functional transactivation among interacting family members. Each family has at present more than half a dozen members. The classes shown possess a *POU domain* (Pituitary-1, *pit-1*), *basic helix-loop-helix domain* (*HLH;* MyoD), nuclear receptor type of *zinc finger domain* (glucocorticoid receptors), or the *basic region/leucine zipper domain* (*bZIP;* CCAAT/enhancer binding proteins, *C/EBP*). (Modified from He and Rosenfeld [19].)

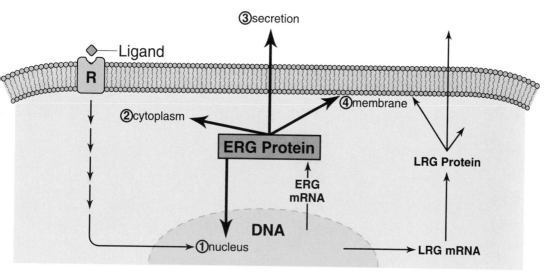

③secretion

Ligand

R

④membrane

②cytoplasm

ERG Protein

LRG Protein

ERG
mRNA

DNA

①nucleus

LRG mRNA

FIG. 5.   Early response genes. This figure illustrates the four major classes of early response gene (ERG) products serving as either (1) nuclear transcription factors (e.g., FOS and JUN), (2) cytoplasmic enzymes (e.g., nitric oxide synthetase and prostaglandin synthetase II) or structural components (e.g., actin), (3) membrane receptors (e.g., nerve growth factor receptor), or (4) secreted factors (e.g., IL-6 and other cytokines). All of these ligand-inducible ERGs are considered to play a role in regulating developmental events. Of particular importance are the ERGs encoding transcription factors which have the ability to regulate the genomic response of neural cells to extracellular signals. The characteristic rapid and transient induction of this class of ERG mRNAs and proteins represents a self-referral loop of genetic control, whereby genetic information is rapidly expressed only to return to the nucleus and directly participate in the subsequent combinatorial control of late response gene (LRG) transcription and phenotypic alterations. Thus, the cell-type specific, differential control of ERG and LRG expression may be closely coupled. (Modified from Arenander and de Vellis, *Prog. Brain Res.* 94:177–188, 1992.)

ity? Recently, researchers have found that li-gand-induced changes result in very rapid gene expression that is independent of any protein synthesis [20]. This large class of genes can be expressed within minutes of cell activation. Because of the very rapid onset of expression, these genes are referred to as early response genes (ERGs) or primary response genes (Fig. 5).

Ligand-activated intracellular signaling pathways induce the transcription of ERGs that encode for four categories of cell proteins: (1) transcription factors, (2) cytoplasm enzymes and structural components, (3) secreted cytokines, and (4) membrane proteins. Each category represents developmentally important factors, such as IL-6, and the NGF receptors. Most of the known transcription factors, including members of the

families illustrated in Fig. 4, are ERGs. Therefore, transcriptional regulation of many transcriptional regulators is under tight and rapid control by environment agents. In addition, since a developing cell is normally exposed to many different signals at a given movement, the ligand-mediated, rapid, and transient induction of ERGs represents a tightly controllable, complex mode of encoding environmental information to carry out developmental decisions (Fig. 6). A number of ERG transcription factors have already been shown to play important roles in regulating cell proliferation and differentiation. For example, combinatorial activity of the leucine zipper transcription factor superfamily, including members of the *fos* and *jun* families, are necessary for a cell to respond to a mitogen and enter the cell cycle. Thus, neu-

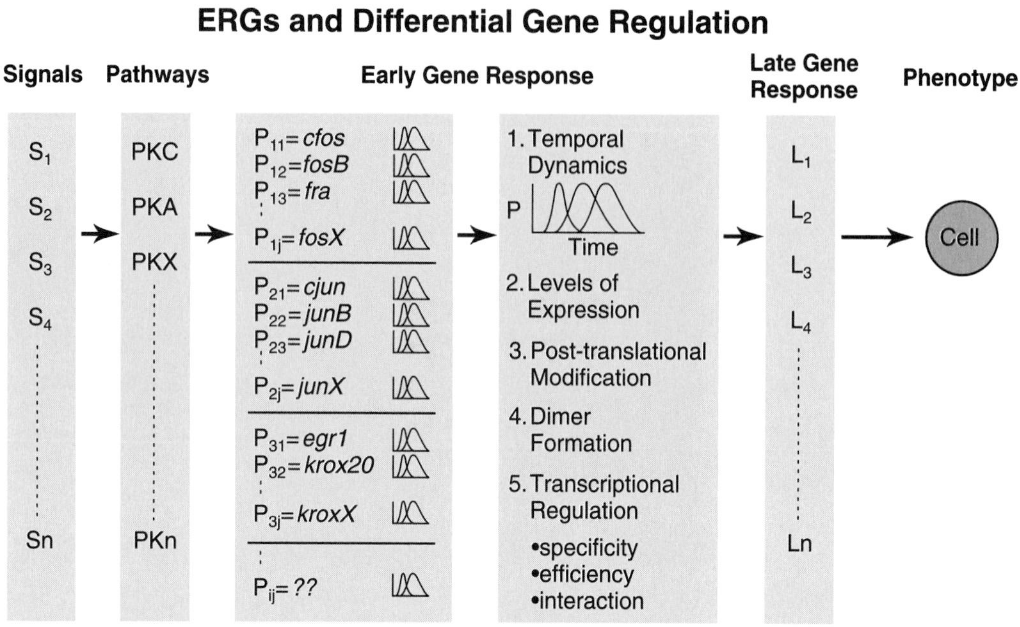

ERGs and Differential Gene Regulation

FIG. 6. The early response gene network and phenotypic diversity. This figure emphasizes the complexity of ERG transcription factor interaction during neural development. The level and kinetics of expression of ERG mRNAs and the subsequent dynamics of interaction among ERG proteins are shown. A wide range of environmental signals (S_1, S_2, ... S_n) can influence a cell by activating intracellular pathways, indicated here by specific protein kinases (PKs), such as protein kinase C *(PKC)* and A *(PKA)*, ... *(PKn)*. These kinases are considered to activate target transcription factors capable of inducing the expression of a constellation of ERG families, depicted as P_1, P_2, ... P_i with family members such as *cfos (P_{11})*, *fosB (P_{12})*, *fra1 (P_{13})*, ... *fosX (P_{1j}, hypothetical)*. The total number of ERGs is equal to (i) × (j) = P_{ij}, estimated to be several hundred. Each pathway induces a largely overlapping subset of ERGs, each displaying its own characteristic kinetics and levels of mRNA accumulation, denoted by the small generic graphic symbol inserted to the right of each ERG. The next level of potential complexity is evident in the five main properties summarized for ERG proteins synthesis, modification, and interaction which together serve to orchestrate the late gene response (L_1 ... L_n). The concept of combinatorial control suggests that, in addition to the complexity of both ligand-receptor coupling and interaction among signaling pathways responsible for transcriptional activation, the various members of different families of ERG transcription factors extensively interact during the process of transcriptional control of late response genes exerting a primary role in determining phenotypic diversity. (Modified from [31].)

ral phenotypic diversity can be explained in terms of the history of expression of transcriptional regulators, some members changing rapidly (ERGs), some slowly. Together, they exert a combinatorial hold on the cell's genetic programs and physiology and determine cell fate.

Transcriptional regulator networks functioning in invertebrate development

Our understanding of the genetic network orchestrating neural development in mam-

mals is rapidly increasing, due in large part to the considerable advancement in developmental research of the fly. As part of the genetic network in *Drosophila*, a large number of genes encoding transcription factors and proteins for cell-cell communication help define cell lineages. Most transcription factors perform more than one function during development. For example, many participate during early segmental processes as well as in the later development of the neural, sexual, and bristle components. Figure 7 illustrates how four major groups of genes interact during development to create the primary body axis and segmentation pattern of the embryo. For example, four maternal effect proteins (e.g., *bicoid* and *dorsal*) are active in the unfertilized egg. Upon fertilization, these genes establish anterior-posterior concentration gradients that lead to differential effects on the expression of a variety of other genes encoding transcription factors, such as gap genes, which, in turn, organize the anterior-posterior axis of the embryo. Thus, a maternal effect mutant has no head and two caudal regions. Gap genes (e.g., *Krüppel*) help define the middle segment and to activate the expression of pair-rule

(e.g., *hairy, fushi tarazu*), segment polarity (e.g., *engrailed*), and homeotic genes (see below). Mutations of gap genes produce embryos with deleted middle segments. Homeotic genes (named for the homeobox DNA-binding sequence) specify the identity of each segment. For example, mutation of the *Antennapedia* gene results in the antenna on the head being replaced by a leg! A similar regulatory cascade of transcription factors organizes the dorsal-ventral axis (Fig. 8).

Our understanding of gene regulation of neural development in *Drosophila* is most complete for the embryonic sensory nervous system [21]. The entire sensory system appears within 5 and 9 hours after fertilization and is known in detail. Five sets of genes have been described that progressively determine the structure and function of this system. The first set are known as *prepattern genes,* described above, that set up the anterior-posterior and dorsal-ventral body axis and segmentation. Many of these genes contain homeodomains and serve multiple roles during different developmental events, e.g., the pair-rule gene, *fushi tarazu,* later controls the development of the fly CNS. Following the establishment of the body coordinates, *proneural gene* expression makes cells competent to become neural precursors. All the proneural genes encode HLH transcriptional regulators. The *achaete-scute complex* (AS-C) is a set of four proneural genes required for sensory organ formation. Mutations lead to no or very few neuronal precursors. *Daughterless (da)* expression is necessary for sensory organ precursors to appear. Because *AS-C* and *da* genes code for bHLH transcription factors, these two gene products can interact to form heterodimers capable of regulating specific target genes. Two additional HLH proteins interact to expand and further refine the complexity of combinatorial control exerted by these transcription factors. *Hairy* (*h*, named for mutants with ectopic bristles) and *extramacrochaete (emc)* can interact to form heterodimers with *AS-C* and *da,* but since *h* and *emc* are HLH proteins lacking functional basic DNA-binding do-

Genetic Network Cascade in *Drosophila* Segment Development

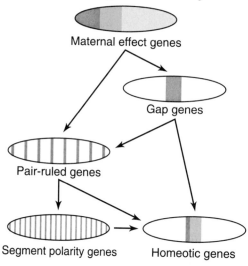

Maternal effect genes

Gap genes

Pair-ruled genes

Segment polarity genes   Homeotic genes

FIG. 7.   Genetic network cascade in early *Drosophila* development. Body segmentation in the *Drosophila* embryo results from the sequential and spatially localized expression of specific genes. During early development, maternal effect genes set up the anterior-posterior orientation of the oblong embryo. Within a very short time, four different groups of genes depicted here that encode for transcription factors are expressed and function to regulate not only each other's expression, but also many other genes whose products are necessary for proper sequential transformation of linear positional information into a periodic pattern. Note the alternating patterns of gene expression (*red* versus *white* areas) that establish boundaries necessary for proper segmentation. (Modified from Wilkinson and Krumlauf [32].)

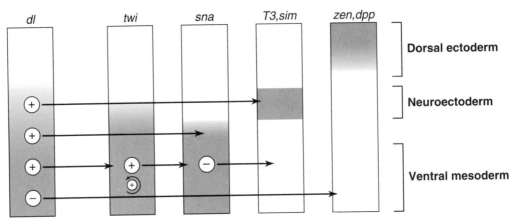

FIG. 8.   Dorsal-ventral morphogenesis in *Drosophila:* TF regulatory cascade. The generation of the dorsal-ventral axis is dependent upon a network of transcription factors (TF). The key nuclear morphogen is *dorsal (dl)*, a member of the *rel/NFkappaB* TF family, whose shallow gradient in early embryo nuclei **(left box:** a schematic sideview section representation of the embryo, dorsal is at top, ventral at bottom) is based upon a gradient in nuclear translocation: nuclear localization of TF in ventral nuclei *(red),* both nuclear and cytoplasmic localization in lateral regions *(pink),* and only cytoplasmic localization in dorsal regions *(white)* where it remains inactive. *dl* creates, in turn, the expression gradient of at least six other TFs (see **four boxes to right**). *dl* activates the expression of *twist (twi),* an HLH TF, and *snail (sna),* a zinc-finger TF. The combined expression of *twi* and *sna* lead to induction of the ventral mesoderm. In addition, the combination of *twi* positive autoregulation *(small circular arrow)* and *dl's* ability to activate *sna* along with *twi,* creates a relatively steep gradient of *sna* expression that creates, in turn, a sharply bound domain of inhibition of T3, one of the members of the *AS-C* HLH TF family and *single-minded (sim),* a HLH TF. Thus, the activation of T3 and *sim* by *dl (top long arrow)* is limited to a narrow lateral band of nuclei that become cells of the neuroectoderm that form the nervous system. The dorsal ectoderm cells arise from the control of *zerknüllt (zen)* and *decapentaplegic (dpp),* both homeobox TFs. Since *dl* exerts a strong inhibitory influence over *zen* and *dpp (bottom long arrow),* the gradient of these TFs **(last box)** is the inverse of *dl.*

mains, the heterodimers formed are inactive. In this way, *h* and *emc* negatively regulate *AS-C* and *da* with the resulting loss of neural tissue.

Neuronal precursors then express the third set of genes, *neurogenic genes,* represented by HLH transcription factors like the *enhancer of split (E[spl])* complex and membrane proteins such as *mastermind (mam).* This set of genes mediate lateral inhibition among cells in proneural cell clusters. Mutations lead to lack of suppression, causing all cells in a cluster to enter the neural lineage. The fourth set are *neuronal type selector genes,* controlling the type of sensory neurons that a precursor becomes and hence the type of sensory organ that forms. The *cut* gene product is a homeodomain transcription factor

that controls cell-type specific gene expression and organ type. Finally, cells express *cell lineage genes* that determine the phenotypic makeup of the cells in the sensory organ. Two genes in particular decide the identity of the final cell phenotypes and hence determine how many neurons and glia will be in each organ. In *numb* mutations (loss of a zinc-finger transcription factor), all progeny become socket or hair cells with the loss of neuronal and glial cells. Another gene, *oversensitive,* has the opposite effect: all neurons and glia and no socket or hair cells. Thus, PNS development relies on the sequential expression of HLH, homeobox, and zinc finger classes of transcription factors that participate in a complex combinatorial network to progressively determine neural cell fate.

Transcriptional regulator networks functioning in vertebrate development

The remarkably similar mechanisms of genetic and developmental control between invertebrates and vertebrates stand in contrast to the timing and form of development in phylogenetically distant species. Similarities include the existence of highly conserved families of HLH and homeobox transcriptional regulators specifying cell fate. In mammalian development, a genetic regulatory network seems to be functioning analogous to that described for *Drosophila*. Recent studies demonstrate that in the developing mammalian CNS, homologous sets of homeobox, HLH, and zinc finger genes are expressed, representing a genetic network regulating the development of the hindbrain segments, termed rhombomeres (Fig. 9). It is important to note that rhombomere boundaries correspond to domains of cell lineage restriction. Figures 9 and 10 show the spatial pattern of expression of the mammalian *Hox* genes, homologous to the homeotic *Antennapedia* and *bithorax* complexes in *Drosophila*. Note that rhombomere 4 corresponds to a region of overlap and boundaries of expression of at least five different genes. *krox20* is a ligand-inducible, zinc finger ERG transcription factor named for the conserved DNA sequence found in the *Drosophila* gap gene *Krüppel* (*Krüppel*box) whose expression appears prior to rhombomeres and the *Hox* genes in a transient stripe pattern. Segment-restricted gene expression suggests these ERG and homeobox gene products control segmentation and neuronal phenotypic diversity. Recent evidence confirms that *krox20* is part of the upstream transcriptional cascade directly controlling the expression of the transcriptional regulator, *HoxB2*. Thus, a cascade of regulatory interactions within the transcription factor network critically directs mammalian neural development.

Another example of advancement from application of *Drosophila* genetic mechanisms is the identification of a phylogeneti-

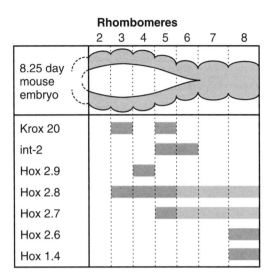

Rhombomeres

FIG. 9. Segmentally restricted hindbrain gene expression. Vertebrate rhombomeres are analogous to the *Drosophila* segments and are shown in this schematic of the anterior neural tube and forebrain expansion. Below the neural tube are shown the expression pattern (*red*, strong expression; *pink*, weak expression; no bar, no expression). Note that each member of the *HoxB* (known previously as *Hox2*) gene family, the *int-2* gene, and the *krox* gene are expressed in a spatially restricted manner. These overlapping expression domains create unique combinations of transcription factors within each rhombomere which are considered, in turn, to regulate the phenotype of the cells in each hindbrain region. In addition, research demonstrates that the zinc finger transcription factor, *Krox20*, is part of the transcriptional cascade that regulates the segmental expression of *HoxB2* (old name, *Hox2.8*). (Modified from Wilkinson and Krumlauf [32].)

cally highly conserved *POU* domain of approximately 150 amino acids possessed by a large family of transcription factors that are expressed during embryonic development of the nervous system [22]. Unlike most homeodomain proteins, restricted to the spinal cord and/or hindbrain, *POU* proteins are expressed in the developing forebrain and midbrain (Fig. 10). *POU*-domain proteins function as positive or negative transcription factors with highly divergent transactivation domains. Each gene in the family exhibits a distinct pattern of brain expression, most

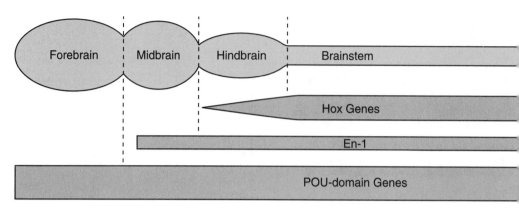

FIG. 10. Developmental expression patterns of Hox and POU-domain genes. During embryonic development, Hox and POU-domain gene families exhibit different anterior boundaries of expression, as depicted in the length and shape of the *red bar*. As such, they are considered to regulate the spatial patterning of neural growth and differentiation of each region of the CNS during embryogenesis. Note that the POU-domain genes are expressed in the forebrain. (Modified from Treacy and Rosenfeld [22].)

likely related to the regulation of different cell lineages. *Pit-1* is found expressed in the anterior pituitary and is a tissue-specific activator of the pituitary-specific genes, prolactin and growth hormone. Like its predecessor, *unc-86*, required for the commitment of several neuronal lineages in *C. elegans*, *Pit-1* is a control gene determining three of the five cell lineages in the anterior pituitary. The other *POU*-domain proteins are anticipated to play similar roles in regulating neuronal and glial lineage decisions in the forebrain and thus contribute to the generation of neural diversity. The *POU*-domain early response gene, *SCIP*, is discussed later in the context of glial cell development.

CELL LINEAGES OF THE NERVOUS SYSTEM

The neural crest lineage

The developmental fate of most cells is not fixed initially, but becomes progressively restricted by epigenetic and genetic interactions (Fig. 2). Work on molecular mechanisms in CNS neuronal lineage development is just beginning. In contrast, we have considerable information about the multipotent NC cells and how they become progressively restricted to specific sublineages [23–25]. NC cells migrate from the neural tube along specific pathways to their peripheral destinations. At these target sites, the NC cells differentiate into a diverse number of cell types including Schwann cells and neuronal cells of the PNS, pigment cells, endocrine cells, and cells forming connective tissue of the face and neck (Fig. 11). Although the anatomical and temporal developmental pathways have been extensively described, the molecular mechanisms responsible for the progressive restriction are just now being discovered.

A basic property of differentiated neuronal cells is the expression of one classical neurotransmitter and several neuropeptides. *In vivo* studies with NC cells first demonstrated that the choice of neurotransmitter phenotype could be altered by the environment. In these studies, NC cells were examined by means of chimera transplantation. Two of the final NC cell phenotypes are sympathetic (mainly adrenergic) and parasympathetic (cholinergic) cells. Presumptive adrenergic neurons transferred to the presumptive cholinergic region of young embryos migrated along the path of vagal neural crest cells and became cholinergic instead of sympathetic. The nature of the environment could thus switch neurotransmitter phenotype. The inverse experiment also worked: Presumptive cholinergic cells become adrenergic when transferred to the adrenergic region. Thus, premigratory NC cells from different axial levels share some common developmental potential and differentiate in a manner appropriate for their final position. These transplantation experiments using heterogeneous cell populations, however, could be interpreted as evidence for selective or instructive processes: selective cell elimination of an inappropriate phenotype or environmental instructions of appropriate cell phenotype.

Environmental Factors Control Lineage Decisions of Neural Crest Cells

Several experimental approaches have shown that environmental factors are critical in determining neurotransmitter phenotype by altering existing cell properties and not by selecting different hypothetical subpopulations of neural crest cells. For example, during normal postnatal development, the innervation of the sweat glands of the foot pads of cats and rats switches from noradrenergic to cholinergic. Research shows that environmental cues of the target tissue specify both early and late neurotransmitter phenotypes. Cross-innervation studies provide further evidence that the target can retrogradely specify neurotransmitter properties

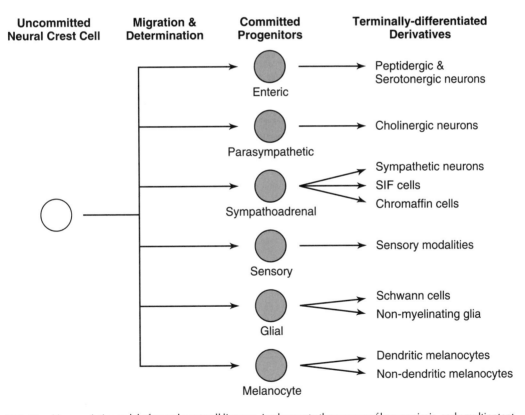

FIG. 11.   Neuropoietic model of neural crest cell lineage. Analogous to the process of hemopoiesis, early multipotent neuropoietic stem cells undergo extensive migration along complex pathways to different embryonic environments. Committed progenitor cells (enteric, parasympathetic, etc.) generate restricted sublineages under the influence of environmental growth factors. These cell populations expand in number and undergo terminal differentiation to the final adult phenotypes. (Modified from Anderson, *Neuron* 3:1–12, 1989.)

of the neuron that innervates it. Neurons that ordinarily provide noradrenergic innervation of hairy skin become cholinergic and peptidergic when induced to innervate sweat glands. Converse experiments give expected results.

The cellular and molecular mechanisms that specify neurotransmitter phenotype have been described by culture experiments (Fig. 12). Polypeptide growth factors such as NGF, bFGF, and IL-6 appear to be the primary controllers of neuronal differentiation of the sympathoadrenal progenitor cells. Research findings demonstrate that bFGF promotes the proliferation and initial differentiation of the sympathoadrenal precursor. For example, bFGF leads to increased neurite outgrowth and upregulation of neuronal-specific genes. The survival of these committed neuronal precursor cells, however, ultimately depends upon NGF-responsiveness and NGF availability. bFGF can upregulate the NGF receptor (p75^{NGFR}), and cell depolarization induces *trk* genes, which together, can produce high-affinity, functional NGFRs, providing trophic responsiveness.

A number of cytokines appear to control the final stage of differentiation of the sympathetic neuronal lineage. Long ago, it was found that individual sympathetic neurons grown on heart-cell monolayers modify their biochemical, pharmacological, and electrical properties and shift from adrenergic to cholinergic phenotypes. Growing the neurons in heart-cell conditioned medium produces similar results, suggesting that non-neuronal cells, e.g., heart myoblasts or glial cells, release a soluble factor, now termed cholinergic differentiation factor (CDF, also known as LIF, leukemia inhibitory factor) that is responsible for the developmental switch. CNTF (ciliary neurotrophic factor), belonging to the same cytokine subfamily as CDF/LIF, also increases cholinergic and decreases noradrenergic properties. While promoting the cholinergic phenotype, CNTF and CDF also inhibit sympathetic neuroblast proliferation. Thus, non-neuronal cells are a source of many molecules that can influence the choice of neurotransmitter and neuropeptide in cultured sympathetic neurons,

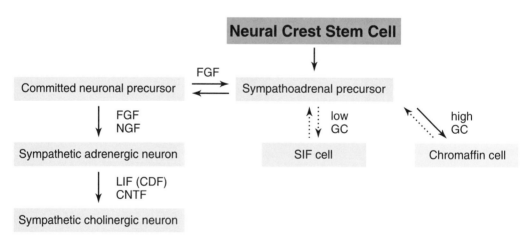

FIG. 12.   Growth factor control of neural crest lineage decisions. Regional and temporal differences in environmental factors influence the final phenotype of neural crest progeny. A number of environmental factors influence the committed precursors that give rise to the final four mature phenotypes of the sympathoadrenal lineage. Under conditions of low or high concentrations of glucocorticoids *(GC),* the sympathoadrenal precursors become either small, intensely fluorescent *(SIF)* cells of the sympathetic ganglia or chromaffin cells of the adrenal medulla, respectively. In environments containing high levels of *FGF* and *NGF* and little or no GC, committed neuronal precursors appear which terminally differentiate into either sympathetic adrenergic neuronal cells, or, under the influence of cholinergic differentiation factor *(CDF;* also known as leukemia inhibitory factor, *LIF)* and ciliary neuronotrophic factor (CNTF) switch neurotransmitter phenotype and become sympathetic cholinergic neuronal cells.

suggesting that the spatiotemporal differential expression of a variety of cytokines helps determine the diversity of cell fate.

One more key player is known to participate in sympathoadrenal lineage fate. The presence and levels of glucocorticoid (GC) strongly influence lineage decisions. Since sympathetic ganglia cells normally grow *in vivo* in the presence of glial cells and become predominantly adrenergic, a second factor was sought in order to explain the discrepancy with the *in vitro* switch studies showing the appearance of the cholinergic phenotype. Studies showed that physiological levels of GC can modulate biochemical differentiation by blocking the shift from adrenergic to cholinergic phenotype. CDF effects can also be blocked by conditions that mimic neuronal activity such as elevated potassium levels. In addition, the level of GC is an important determinant of the path of the sympathoadrenal precursor: Low levels generate SIF cells and high levels generate chromaffin cells.

Recent research has begun to identify the intracellular signaling pathways activated by environmental factors that lead to the induction of developmental control genes in NC cells and their derivatives. For example, developmental restriction of melanogenesis normally occurs before day 5 in the embryonic quail. This process can be altered by treating day 9 embryonic dorsal root ganglion cells with phorbol ester, which activates protein kinase C (PKC). Schwann cell precursors, which normally lack melanogenic activity, undergo a metaplastic transformation into melanocytes when PKC activity is reduced. This suggests that environmental signals capable of altering levels of PKC regulate lineage decisions in NC cells.

Transcriptional Regulation of the Neural Crest Lineage

A number of candidate control genes have been characterized that could give rise to progressive restriction in migrating behavior and control over proliferation and differentiation. Several newly discovered genes appear to underlie cell lineage commitment, while other genes appear important as mediators of the ligand-dependent switch of neurotransmitter phenotype in committed neuronal cells. In mammalian development, a gene analogous with the *AS-C* genes in *Drosophila*, which determine whether a cell becomes a neuronal precursor, has been described. The *MASH1* gene (mammalian achaete-scute homolog-1) is transiently expressed by spatially restricted subsets of early CNS neuroepithelial and PNS neural crest cells. The precursors of sympathetic and enteric neurons express this bHLH transcription factor just prior to the onset of cell-type specific gene expression such as tyrosine hydroxylase, suggesting that *MASH1* is a marker of cells as they enter the sympathoadrenal lineage. It is likely that *MASH1* is a neural crest control gene determining the commitment step of lineage development. It is expected that *MASH1*, like the activity of *AS-C* genes, will be regulated by a number of other HLH gene families homologous to *da (E12), emc (Id), h (HES)*, by way of alternative HLH pairing—heterodimerization leading to either enhanced or inhibited function in the differentiating mammalian NC cells and CNS.

Once the cells are committed to the sympathoadrenal lineage, a choice of neurotransmitter phenotype must take place. The developmental switch between chromaffin and neuronal phenotype is associated with changes in cell-type specific gene expression, which requires the differential control of neural crest genetic programs. The molecular mechanism at work integrating the influences of these two types of environmental signals, peptide growth factors and glucocorticoids, involves, in part, the antagonistic interaction of transcription factors. Culture work demonstrates that FGF and NGF are antagonistic to GC in their abilities to upregulate chromaffin-specific genes. The opposite control is also true. Two classes of transcription factors, FOS (as part of the peptide-inducible AP-1 complex) and GC receptors (see Fig. 5), have been shown to interact in a similar, reciprocal inhibitory fashion. This suggests that, as part of the combinatorial control process, interaction between these different families of transcription factors represents a probable molecular mechanism of reciprocal inhibition exerted by environmental factors.

Glial cell development

Our understanding of glial cell development in the CNS has advanced rapidly in the last decade [24]. The discovery and initial characterization of the oligodendrocyte-type 2 astrocyte (O-2A) cell lineage now represents the most extensively characterized cell lineage system available to study nervous system development. A variety of cellular and molecular approaches have provided us with a preliminary understanding of the environmental signals and the phenotypic responses that are of importance *in vitro*. The current success in cell identification, using antibodies against glial-specific antigens and molecular probes for detecting cell-type specific mRNAs, has led to a rapid increase in our understanding of the key environmental agents that regulate the rate and direction of glial cell differentiation along specific lineage pathways.

The Oligodendrocyte Lineage In Vitro

Oligodendrocytes (OLs) are generated postnatally and pass through a series of cell phenotypes from undifferentiated stem cells to mature myelin-forming cells. This sequential process of maturation of OLs can be reproduced in culture (Fig. 13). In the rat, four main stages of development *in vitro* have been delineated. The oligodendroblast (also referred to as the oligodendrocyte-type 2 astrocyte bipotential progenitor cell, O-2A cell) is a proliferating, bipolar cell. These cells, when cultured in chemically defined medium containing 0.5% (low) serum to enhance survival, rapidly differentiate in a relatively synchronous manner into mature oli-

godendrocytes over a 3- to 5-day period. In contrast, under high serum conditions, many cells become GFAP$^+$/O4$^-$ cells called type 2 astrocytes (AIIs). This cell type is controversial, perhaps being an artifact of tissue culture or a "reactive" oligodendrocyte. Bipolar oligodendroblast cells become multipolar, O4$^+$ "pre-OL" cells. These O4$^+$/GC$^-$ cells become "immature-OLs" with the appearance of GC expression. The "mature-OL" phenotype is identified by the sequential appearance of additional myelin-specific antigens, proteolipid protein (PLP) and then myelin basic protein (MBP). Thus, immunostaining with glial-specific markers, defines seven phenotypically distinct cell types *in vitro*, six of which compose the oligodendrocyte lineage: oligodendrocyte precursors, oligodendroblast cells, pre-OL cells, immature-OL cells, and mature-OL cells, and multipolar AII cells (A2B5$^+$/GFAP$^+$) and flat AI cells (A2B5$^-$/GFAP$^+$). This classification scheme can be used to monitor the rate, direction and extent of OL cell differentiation.

Oligodendrocyte Lineage In Vivo

Preliminary descriptions of the patterns of gliogenesis in the forebrain subcortical white matter using immunocytochemical probes are available and closely resemble the *in vitro* data. Similar findings are reported for the cerebellum. The subventricular zones (SVZ) covering portions of the lateral ventricles are considered the origin of progenitor cells that multiply and eventually migrate to and differentiate within the overlying white and gray matter. The separation of OL and AI lineage is considered to occur during embryonic development based on retroviral studies and double labeling, ultrastructural localization, and cell morphology.

A number of glial markers provide static, yet overlapping, information concerning OL lineage development. Small, proliferating GD3$^+$, undifferentiated "neuroectodermal" cells are observed densely packed in the embryonic SVZ. Starting at E16, and

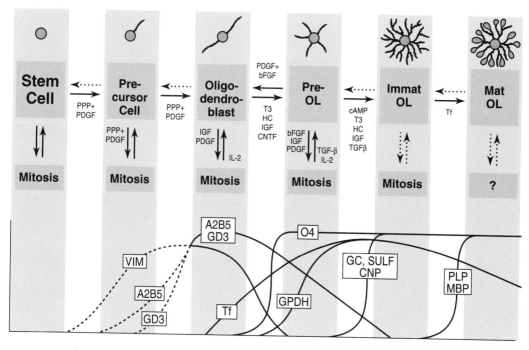

FIG. 13. The oligodendrocyte lineage. The figure illustrates the characteristics that accompany the sequential differentiation within the oligodendrocyte lineage beginning from very early stem cells to the mature oligodendrocyte. This version depicts six cell phenotypes based on morphology, proliferative regulation, and immunological determinants defined primarily from *in vitro* data. The various growth factors listed have been shown to regulate cell proliferation and/or differentiation. *Dashed arrows* indicate a particular direction may be possible, but without clear experimental support. The time course of expression of cell-type specific markers is shown at the bottom. Note that each main stage of lineage development displays not only a different morphology but also a unique antigen profile. Growth factors include *bFGF* (basic fibroblast growth factor), *cAMP* (cyclicAMP), *CNTF* (ciliary neurotrophic factor, *HC* (hydrocortisone), *IGF* (insulin-like growth factor), *IL-2* (interleukin-2), *PPP* (platelet-poor plasma), *PDGF* (platelet-derived growth factor), *Tf* (transferrin), *TGFβ* (transforming growth factor beta), *T3* (triiodothyronine). Cell markers (*dotted lines* indicate unresolved expression pattern): *A2B5* (ganglioside), *CNP* (2,3-cyclic nucleotide-3-phosphohydrolase), *GD3* (ganglioside), *GPDH* (glycerolphosphate dehydrogenase), *GC* (galactocerebroside glycolipid), *O4* (ganglioside), *PLP* (proteolipid protein), *MBP* (myelin basic protein), *SULF* (sulfatide), *VIM* (vimentin).

continuing to 7–10 days postnatal, larger, GD3+/CA+ "progenitor" cells appear in the SVZ, many of which are A2B5+ and may be similar to the oligodendroblasts described *in vitro* above (CA, carbonic anhydrase). These cells migrate into the overlying subcortical white matter. By the end of the 1st postnatal week, the GD3+/CA− cells diminish in number while O4+ and GC+/CA+ cells rapidly increase in number in the white matter tracts. Thus, early stages of OL differentiation appear to occur in the SVZ, which contains a heterogeneous population of "progenitor"

phenotypes. The subsequent development of O4+ progenitors into GC+ "immature" OLs and MBP+ "mature" OLs occurs in the white and gray matter and not the SVZ or neighboring subcortical regions.

Growth Factor Regulation of Oligodendrocyte Development

The oligodendrocyte cell lineage culture is an excellent system to study the influence of growth factors on cell lineage development. Each of the four main stages of OL lineage progression can be identified by its characteristic markers and, through the use of growth factors, experiments can be designed to increase or decrease the degree of proliferation and/or block, delay, or accelerate maturation of developing precursor cells. Although research shows that OL differentiation is a "default" pathway, occurring in serum-free medium, in the absence of environmental signals, a number of studies demonstrate that OL development is more complex and is responsive to numerous environmental signals. For example, OL lineage cells continue to proliferate for extended periods *in vivo*, in contrast to *in vitro* studies. In addition, treatment of OL progenitor cells with growth factors known to be present in the developing CNS yields a complex set of ligand-dependent, phenotypic responses.

bFGF and PDGF are two of the key molecular signals controlling OL cell development (Fig. 14). In the presence of PDGF, OL progenitor cells are stimulated to divide with a short cell cycle length of 18 hr, are highly motile and bipolar, and differentiate in a synchronous, symmetrical clonal fashion with a time course similar to that *in vivo*. In the presence of bFGF, however, progenitor cells are stimulated to divide with a longer cell cycle length (45 hr), become nonmotile pre-OLs, with a multipolar shape and are inhibited from expressing GC, PLP, or MBP. Progenitor cells treated with both bFGF and PDGF exhibit a third phenotypic response, remaining motile, bipolar progenitor cells that do not differentiate and divide indefinitely. This ligand-dependent, conditional "immortalization" can greatly expand the OL progenitor cell population over extended periods of time. Upon removal of bFGF or both mitogens, the progenitor cells differentiate along the OL lineage.

The source of PDGF appears to be AI cells. From *in situ* hybridization data, PDGFα-receptor is expressed only in GC-negative OL lineage cells and not in identifiable astrocytes or neuronal cells. In addition, bFGF appears to upregulate the PDGF α-receptor in OL progenitor cells. By altering

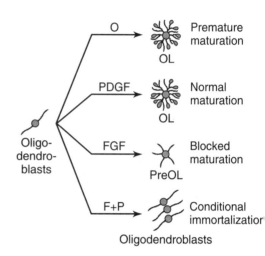

FIG. 14. Growth factor control of oligodendrocyte lineage decisions. *In vitro* studies have demonstrated that the developmental fate of O-2A progenitor cells in culture can be regulated by environmental factors. Progenitor cells cultured in the absence of either *bFGF* (basic fibroblast growth factor) or *PDGF* (platelet-derived growth factor), develop to mature oligodendrocytes *(OL)*, but do so on a timetable more rapid than *in vivo*. The addition of PDGF stimulates several rounds of cell division, slowing/delaying the time of development to mature OLs that more closely resembles the normal *in vivo* timecourse. In contrast, FGF stimulates continual proliferation while blocking phenotypic development at the preOL (O4⁺/GC⁻) cell stage. Evidence suggests that FGF can lead to downregulation of cell surface GC and simplification of morphology indicating possible "dedifferentiation" or plasticity of the GC⁺ cell phenotype. The combination of both factors leads to a stable condition of the immature O-2A phenotype exhibiting continual proliferation. Upon removal of the either FGF or both factors, cells leave the state of "conditional" immortalization and proceed to differentiate normally.

the responsiveness of these cells to PDGF, bFGF and PDGF together maintain the "proliferative" state. These studies indicate that (1) there is no obligatory relationship between cell proliferation and differentiation, (2) different environmental signals lead to different behavioral responses, and (3) cooperation between extracellular signals can generate additional, unique phenotypes. In addition, both diffusible (CNTF) and nondiffusible (extracellular matrix-bound) components act directly on OL progenitor cells to inhibit OL differentiation and/or induce the AII phenotype. Thus, cell-cell interaction in the developing CNS in the form of diffusible and nondiffusible factors modulate normal OL development including commitment to OL (or AII) cell fate, the extent of cell division, and the timing and rate of cell differentiation.

Transferrin is an iron carrier protein that acts as a trophic factor for neurons, astrocytes, and oligodendrocytes [26]. As the brain barrier gets established during development, neural cells become dependent on transferrin produced by oligodendrocytes and choriod plexus epithelial cells (Fig. 15). The production and secretion of transferrin by oligodendrocytes is the major source of transferrin in the CNS. It suggests an impor-

tant function for oligodendrocytes in addition to myelination of axonal tracts. Transferrin concentration in cerebrospinal fluid is highest at the time of peak myelination. Oligodendrocytes, myelin, and several areas of the brain contain higher levels of iron than the liver, presumably in the form of ferritin-bound iron.

Schwann Cell Lineage in the PNS

The Schwann cell lineage is also characterized by the sequential and overlapping expression of many stage-specific markers. Expression patterns of antigens allows delineation of at least six developmental stages both *in vivo* and *in vitro* that give rise to two types of Schwann cells in the adult (Fig. 16). The appearance of S100 and O4 defines the

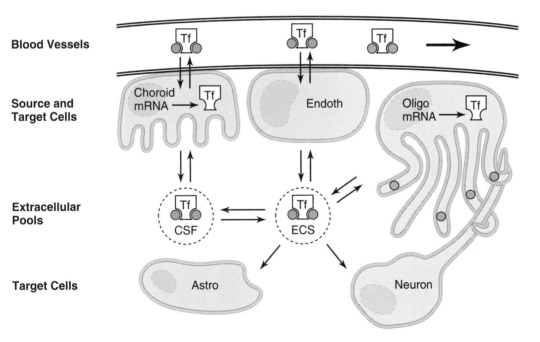

FIG. 15. Regulation of transferrin in the CNS. Transferrin *(Tf)* is an important molecule regulating the movement and storage of iron in the nervous system. Although blood-borne Tf is exchanged by choroidal epithelia cells and the endothelial cells of the capillary beds in the brain, only the oligodendrocytes and choroid cells in the brain can produce Tf *in vivo*. Each Tf molecule can bind two atoms of iron *(red balls)* that in the brain are distributed between the two large pools, the cerebrospinal fluid *(CSF)* and the extracellular space *(ECS)*. Astrocytes and neurons are considered to be completely dependent upon these pools and, in turn, upon the oligodendrocytes, choroidal cells, and the body for Tf.

immature Schwann cell stage. Then, a non-myelinating Schwann cell type can be defined by the appearance of galactocerebroside and association with axons. These cells also express N-CAM and L1 recognition molecules. Note the curious combination of antigens in nonmyelinating Schwann cell: O4 and GC indicative of the CNS OL phenotype and GFAP and S100 found in CNS astrocytes. From this stage, cells move along one of two possible paths. In the PNS, the ensheathing glial cells, depending upon the size of the

axons they are associated with, either remain at the nonmyelinating stage (small axons) or begin to produce myelin-associated proteins and the sheath (large axons; see Fig. 17). The latter developmental path involves the appearance of proliferative, premyelinating Schwann cells that express myelin genes, such as Po, MBP, and MAG. These cells then lose GFAP, NGFR, N-CAM and L1, while producing myelin membrane as myelinating Schwann cells.

Cyclic AMP in culture can mimic most

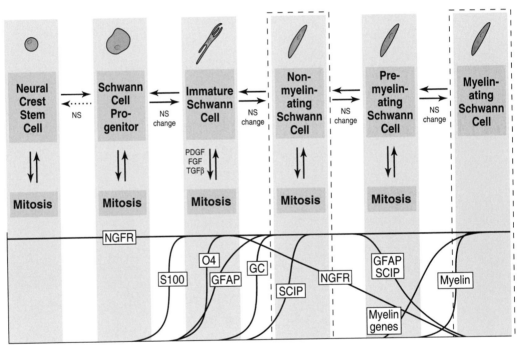

FIG. 16.   The Schwann cell lineage. The Schwann cell is the axon-ensheathing cell of the PNS and thus displays many properties and developmental processes similar to CNS oligodendrocytes. The figure illustrates the sequential differentiation of Schwann cells from early, uncharacterized neural crest stem cell to the final two mature phenotypes (surrounded by *dashed boxes*): the nonmyelinating and the myelinating Schwann cells of the adult, based on the size of the axons they ensheath (see Fig. 17 for developmental anatomy of these two mature phenotypes). Unlike the CNS, the vast majority of Schwann cells do not become myelin producing cells. This 6-stage version of Schwann cell development is based upon cell morphology, proliferative potential, and, most importantly, the expression of stage-specific antigens (appearance and/or disappearance of specific markers; **bottom**), derived from both *in vivo* and *in vitro* data. It appears that upon reaching the nonmyelinating phenotype **(box 4 from left)**, cells are fated to either remain in this state and represent the adult population of nonmyelinating cells or to differentiate further, expressing myelin-associated genes. The premyelinating phenotype then become myelinating cells of the PNS (stage 6). See Fig. 14 for abbreviations of antigens and growth factors. Cell markers include *NGFR* (nerve growth factor receptor), *S100* (monoclonal antibody against a soluble cytoplasmic protein), *GFAP* (glial fibrillary acidic protein), and *SCIP* (suppressed cyclic AMP-inducible POU domain transcription factor).

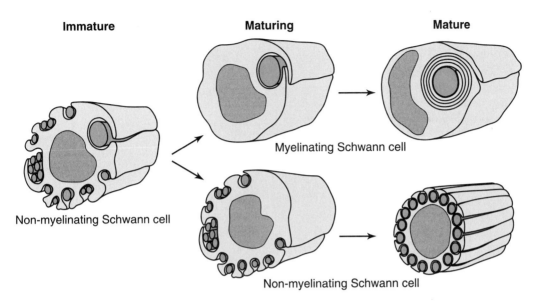

Immature   **Maturing**   **Mature**

Myelinating Schwann cell

Non-myelinating Schwann cell

Non-myelinating Schwann cell

FIG. 17.   Schwann cell development and axonal sorting. Immature O4-positive Schwann cells can be found to take one of two paths of differentiation. Initially, both large and small (usually <1 μm diameter) caliber axons are found embedded in furrows along the surface of a chain of immature Schwann cells. This illustration shows a cross section through a single cell. During the period of cell proliferation and axonal sorting, large axons that require myelin laminar ensheathment separate, by some undefined process of axonal/Schwann cell interaction, from smaller caliber axons that require only a simple, nonmyelin ensheathment. In maturing myelinating Schwann cells, single axons are enveloped by the lips of the trough on the cell surface, one of which elongates to create the myelin wrapping as the number of turns of membrane increase, and the lamellae become more compact as the cytoplasmic content is lost. In maturing nonmyelinating Schwann cells, no myelin membrane is formed, but many small caliber axons remain completely embedded within separate furrows in each cell. Thus, the adult nerve contains two Schwann cell phenotypes, nonmyelinating and myelinating. (Modified from A. Peters, S. Palay, and H. de Webster, *The Fine Structure of the Nervous System: Neurons and Their Supporting Cells,* 3rd Edition, 1991.)

of the effects of axons, including expression of early progenitor antigens, suggesting that a cyclic AMP trigger drives most of Schwann cell development *in vivo*. For example, cell proliferation by bFGF or PDGF requires the presence of high levels of intracellular cyclic AMP. The role of cyclic AMP may be to upregulate mitogen membrane receptors. Thus, in the developing nerve, axon-associated factors elevate cyclic AMP, which is responsible for inducing two key events. The first event is the expression of O4 antigen and the responsiveness to mitogens in immature progenitors and nonmyelinating Schwann cells. The second event is the further differentiation into premyelinating and myelinating Schwann cells, if the suppression of proliferation takes place owing to

some secondary permissive signal associated with the ensheathed large caliber axons.

Of great interest is the expression pattern of SCIP (suppressed cyclic AMP-inducible POU domain protein). SCIP is a member of the POU family of transcription factors with characteristics of an early response gene. POU proteins are usually considered to function as transcriptional activators of cell-type specific genes and determine cell fate. In CNS and PNS myelinating cells, SCIP is found expressed at high levels only during a very narrow window of development and to act as a repressor of myelin-specific genes. In Schwann cells, SCIP is expressed in the progenitors, but not more mature, myelinating Schwann cells (see Fig. 16). In these proliferating nonmyelinating and premyelinating Schwann cells, SCIP acts on promoters of myelin-associated genes, such as Po and MBP, as a repressor. Thus, SCIP expression is found in cells with elevated levels of cyclic AMP to be correlated with rapid down regulation of the ERG *cjun* transcription factor and the onset of rapid proliferation and repression of myelin genes. In response to denervation, SCIP is rapidly and transiently re-expressed during the period of rapid cell proliferation of premyelinating Schwann cells and considered to antagonize the expression of myelin-specific genes.

CONCLUSIONS

Most development focuses on the formation of the complexity of neural tissue during embryonic and postnatal development. These changes provide a basis for later juvenile and adult stages of growth, in which the dynamic interaction between the genes and the environment continues. Although development is now less dramatic, environmental signals continue to produce lasting changes in neural structure and function in the adult nervous system. Genetic-epigenetic interaction is now associated with physiological and behavioral learning. It is likely that the main elements employed during early development that allows a cell to "learn" to participate in the system are the same elements used during the continual process of learning and corresponding plastic modification of the nervous system across the life span of the organism. Learning during the life of the organism is correlated with changes occurring at every level of the hierarchy of information flow (Fig. 1) leading to the continued expression and refinement of neuronal/glial networks. External and internal events continue to regulate gene expression, and neuronal and glial cells continue to interact metabolically. In its broadest sense, development continues during adulthood. Since neural plasticity can be defined as the long-lasting changes in neural structure and func-

tion following environmental perturbation, the term is applicable to adult development. The molecular and cellular basis of adult neural plasticity has focused on environment-induced changes in neurotransmitter metabolism, synaptic structure and function, and local circuits. Three experimental models have proved to be most successful in helping to delineate the molecular basis of plasticity: environmental control over catecholamine biosynthesis [28], long-term potentiation, and experience-dependent alterations in brain structure and function. In this summary, we will highlight the first research area.

Neurotransmitters serve to transduce electrical information from one cell to another, participating in the pattern of information flow in the nervous system. States of altered neurotransmitter metabolism can lead to changes in neuronal processing and physiological and behavioral control. Since the level of neurotransmitters in synaptic terminals is partly determined by the activity of rate-limiting synthesizing enzymes, which in turn depends on appropriate activity of signal pathways, transcription factors, and of mRNA transcription, environmental change of short duration can lead to significant, long-lasting alterations in brain function [29,30]. For example, brief, excitatory perturbation of sympathetic neurons via electrical, pharmacological, or behavioral input can, for example, lead to long-term changes in the levels of neurotransmitters. These perturbing signals all lead to cell depolarization, which may be linked to the later events of enhanced transcriptional rates of tyrosine hydroxylase (TH), the rate-limiting enzyme in the synthesis of catecholamines and decreased transcriptional rates for the polypeptide precursor for substance P, a small putative peptide neurotransmitter colocalized with catecholamines. Thus, not only do neurotransmitter levels undergo long-lasting alterations following brief environmental stimulation, but neurotransmitters are differentially regulated by the same external stimuli.

CNS neurons show similar responsiveness, suggesting that the phenomenon is widespread and of fundamental importance in the control of adult function. *In vivo* and *in vitro* experiments demonstrate that a single, brief stimulation of the locus coeruleus (LC), leading to cell depolarization, results in increased amounts of mRNA and activity of TH. Increases in TH can still be observed for several weeks. It has been suggested that another, more subtle, consequence of environmental perturbation could be detected based on the unique, extensive axonal domain of the LC. Since TH is synthesized in the cell body, the influence of induced levels of TH will be determined in part by the distance traversed by TH to reach the synaptic terminal and thus influence synaptic function. Because of the variable axonal path length and constant rate of axoplasmic flow, the initial environmental stimulation will result in maximal elevations of TH activity in the LC by 2 days; neurotransmitter activity, however, will peak in the cerebellum at 4 days, and in the frontal cortex at 12 days. In this way, the genomic activation in a single location is expressed in an anatomically dispersed temporal sequence. Since the LC has extensive and diffuse axonal projections that are involved in controlling shifts in states of arousal, vigilance, and attention, brief environmental stimulation of PNS and CNS neurons in the adult nervous system can lead to gene activation and long-lasting patterns of altered synaptic function.

In the future, rapid advances in molecular biology, cell culture, and grafting will further our understanding of how the abstract genetic intelligence becomes progressively and continually transformed into the hierarchically organized dynamic networks of information and structure. Throughout the life span of an organism, environmental perturbation leads to alterations in neural structure and function. Therefore development can be viewed as a continual process of short- and long-term information storage whereby genetic and epigenetic interaction, at every step of development, becomes represented in the evolving structural and functional design of the nervous system. The nervous system is always adapting and we are always learning.

ACKNOWLEDGMENTS

The authors thank Sharon Belkin and Carol Gray of the Mental Retardation Research Center for help in preparing the illustrations. The authors' research was supported by NICHD grant 2P01-HD06576-18, Department of Energy contract DE-FC03-87-ER60615 and NIH grant 1RO1-NS29220-01.

REFERENCES

1. Purves, D., and Lichtman, J. W. *Principles of Neural Development*. Sunderland, MA: Sinauer Associates, 1985.
2. Smythies, J. R., and Bradley, R. J. (eds.). *International Review of Neurobiology*. New York: Academic Press, 1992.
3. Arenander, A. T., and de Vellis, J. Frontiers of glial physiology. In R. Rosenberg (ed.), *The Clinical Neurosciences*. New York: Churchill Livingstone, 1983, pp. 53–91.
4. Fedoroff, S., and A. Vernadakis (eds.). *Astrocytes*. Orlando: Academic Press, 1987, Vol. 2.
5. Lauder, J., and McCarthy, K. Neuronal-glial interactions. In S. Federoff and A. Vernadakis (eds.), *Astrocytes*. Orlando: Academic Press, 1987, Vol. 2, pp. 295–314.
6. Jacobson, M. *Developmental Neurobiology*. New York: Plenum Press, 1991.
7. Saneto, R. P., and de Vellis, J. Neuronal and glial cells: Cell culture of the central nervous system. In A. J. Turner and H. S. Bachelard (eds.), *Neurochemistry—A Practical Approach*. Washington, DC: IRL Press, 1987, pp. 27–63.
8. Shahar, A., de Vellis, J., Vernadakis, A., and Haber, B. (eds.). *A Dissection and Tissue Culture Manual of the Nervous System*. New York: Alan R. Liss, Inc., 1989.
9. Patterson, P. H. Process outgrowth and the specificity of connections. In Z. W. Hall (ed.), *An Introduction to Molecular Neurobiology*. Sunderland, MA: Sinauer Associates, 1992, pp. 388–427.

10. McConnell, S. K. The generation of neuronal diversity in the central nervous system. *Annu. Rev. Neurosci.* 14:269–300, 1991.

11. Oppenheim, R. W. Cell death during development of the nervous system. *Annu. Rev. Neurosci.* 14:453–501, 1991.

12. Patterson, P. H. Neuron-target interactions. In Z. W. Hall (ed.), *An Introduction to Molecular Neurobiology.* Sunderland, MA: Sinauer Associates, 1992, pp. 428–459.

13. Cunningham, B. A., Hemperly, J. J., Murray, B. A., Prediger, E. A., Brackenbury, R., and Edelman, G. M. Neural cell adhesion molecule: structure, immunoglobulin-like domains, cell surface modulation, and alternative RNA splicing. *Science* 236:799–806, 1987.

14. Reichardt, L. F., and Tomaselli, K. J. Extracellular matrix molecules and their receptors: functions in neural development. *Annu. Rev. Neurosci.* 14:531–570, 1991.

15. Shankland, M., and Macagno, E. R. (eds.). *Determinants of Neuronal Identity.* New York: Academic Press, 1992.

16. Mattson, M. P. Cellular signaling mechanisms common to the development and degeneration of neuroarchitecture. A review. *Mech. Aging Dev.* 50:103–157, 1989.

17. Katz, L. C., and Callaway, E. M. Development of local circuits in mammalian visual cortex. *Annu. Rev. Neurosci.* 14:31–56, 1992.

18. Patterson, P. H. The emerging neuropoietic cytokine family: first CDF/LIF, CNTF and IL-6; next ONC, MGF, GCSF? *Curr. Opin. Neurobiol.* 2:94–97, 1992.

19. He, X., and Rosenfeld, M. G. Mechanisms of complex transcriptional regulation: implications for brain development. *Neuron* 7:183–196, 1991.

20. Arenander, A. T., and Herschman, H. R. Primary response gene expression in the nervous system. In S. Loughlin and J. Fallon (eds.), *Neurotrophic Factors.* New York: Academic Press, 1992, pp. 89–128.

21. Jan, Y. N., and Jan, L. Y. Genes required for specifying cell fates in *Drosophila* embryonic sensory nervous system. *TINS* 13:493–498, 1990.

22. Treacy, M. N., and Rosenfeld, M. G. Expression of a family of POU-domain protein regulatory genes during development of the central nervous system. *Annu. Rev. Neurosci.* 15:139–165, 1992.

23. Anderson, D. J. Molecular control of neural development. In Z. W. Hall (ed.), *An Introduction to Molecular Neurobiology.* Sunderland, MA: Sinauer Associates, 1992, pp. 355–387.

24. Hatten, M. E., Kettenmann, H., and Ransom, B. R. (eds.). *Glial Cell Lineage,* Glia 4:124–243, 1991.

25. Anderson, D. J. Molecular control of cell fate in the neural crest: the sympathoadrenal lineage. *Annu. Rev. Neurosci.* 16:129–158, 1993.

26. Espinosa de los Monteros A., Peña, L. A., and de Vellis, J. Does transferrin have a special nervous system? *J. Neurosci. Res.* 24:125–136, 1989.

27. Kaas, J. H. Plasticity of sensory and motor maps in adult mammals. *Annu. Rev. Neurosci.* 14:137–167, 1991.

28. Teyler, T. J., and DiScenna, P. Long-term potentiation. *Annu. Rev. Neurosci.* 10:131–161, 1987.

29. Black, I. B., Adler, J. E., Dreyfus, C. F., Friedman, W. F., LaGamma, E. F., and Roach, A. H. Biochemistry of information storage in the nervous system. *Science* 236:1263–1268, 1987.

30. Black, E. B., Adler, J. E., Dreyfus, C. F., Jonakait, G. M., Katz, D. M., et al. Neurotransmitter plasticity at the molecular level. *Science* 225:1266–1279, 1984.

31. Arenander, A. A., deVellis, J. Early response gene expression signifying functional coupling of neuroligand receptor systems in astrocytes. In S. Murphy (ed.). *Astrocytes.* New York: Academic Press, 1993, pp. 109–136.

32. Wilkinson, D. G., Krumlauf, R. Molecular approaches to the segmentation of the hindbrain. *TINS* 13:335–339, 1990.

CHAPTER 29

Neural Plasticity and Regeneration

CARL W. COTMAN, FERNANDO GÓMEZ-PINILLA, AND
JENNIFER S. KAHLE

Basic Neurochemistry: Molecular, Cellular, and Medical Aspects, 5th Ed., edited by G. J. Siegel et al. Published by Raven Press, Ltd., New York, 1994. Correspondence to Carl W. Cotman, IRU in Brain Aging, University of California, Irvine, California 92717-4550.

In this chapter the major principles of neural plasticity and advances in this field are reviewed and discussed. The term *plasticity*, in the most general sense, refers to changes observed in the nervous system or in behavior. In 1890, William James [1] first introduced the term *behavioral plasticity* to describe any meaningful change in behavior. *Neural plasticity* refers to changes observed in the function or structure of the nervous system at a cellular level that serve behavioral plasticity. As early as 1928, Ramón y Cajal had already recognized the importance of change in the CNS, "to impede or moderate the gradual decay of neurons to overcome the almost invincible rigidity of their connections and to reestablish normal nerve paths when disease has severed centers that were intimately associated" [2] (see also Chap. 50).

Recent research has shown that the brain has a remarkable capacity for plastic responses throughout life: immediate functional plasticity coupled with long-lasting structural change. For example, in the last few years it has been shown that the healthy nervous system exhibits subtle and specific neural plasticity in response to stimuli such as learning a new task, environmental enrichment, or cycles in hormone levels. In addition, recent research has shown that the brain has the capability to repair itself after cell loss due to injury or neurodegenerative disease. The study of plasticity in animal models, coupled with current methods, has advanced to the point where it is realistic to examine the principles learned from basic research and apply them to the human brain and clinical interventions. In fact, several experimental paradigms that have emerged in the past decade have proven to be excellent models in which to test possible therapies. For example, tissue transplantation and manipulation of neurotrophic factors either by themselves or in combination are now therapeutic strategies being evaluated for disorders such as Parkinson's disease.

In the first section of this chapter we will discuss synaptic remodeling in the normal mature brain, then discuss recent data on synaptic growth after injury. We will also discuss how transplants can replace lost neurons, rebuild circuitry to a degree, and replace neurotransmitters and/or regulators. The major challenge in the field is how to enhance and focus the basic plastic substrates of the CNS to direct recovery of function and decrease neuronal degeneration.

NORMAL REMODELING OF SYNAPTIC CONNECTIONS

It has been well established that during early development there is continuous growth and modification of connections between neurons and their targets. While it is generally appropriate to distinguish events that occur during development from those in the mature CNS, recent studies show that remodeling of synaptic connections also occurs in the brain during adult life. Remodeling of synaptic connectivity can occur in response to sensory stimuli, in learning a new task, and is associated with cyclic changes in the physiological status of the organism.

Changes in environment evoke plastic responses

Changes in the environment with which the organism interacts can produce changes in various aspects of cellular morphology in the brain, presumably via novel or increased sensory activation. A well-characterized example of this is the differences in the cortex seen when animals are raised in increasingly more complex environments. After time-periods as short as 4 days, the cortex of rats living in environmentally enriched conditions (e.g., with other rats and continually changing objects) exhibit several plastic changes including expanded cortical thickness, greater cell body size, more complex dendritic branching, and increased number of glial cells [3,4].

Long-term synaptic plasticity and structural changes

Learning and memory formation have been thought to involve permanent changes in the brain, but the mechanisms underlying these processes remain elusive. The hippocampus is a structure in the CNS that has been determined to play an important role in learning and memory formation. Several types of synaptic plasticity have been described in the hippocampus. One long-lasting functional change that has been associated with learning is called long-term potentiation (LTP). After a series of short high-frequency synaptic bursts, the amplitude of the synaptic response increases and can be maintained at the increased level for days or weeks. Several mechanisms participate in this long-term change, including specific structural changes and possibly the formation of new synapses. For example, after a burst of synaptic activity that produces LTP, the associated dendritic spines change shape and there are greater numbers of synapses on the dendritic shafts in the region (Fig. 1A,B). These changes persist, lasting at least 8 hours after the onset of LTP [5] (see Chap. 50).

Normal hormone-induced structural changes

It is well established that circulating hormones in the body are able to elicit specific behaviors (see also Chap. 49). Recent evidence demonstrates that changes in hormonal levels are able to induce changes in neuronal morphology in the CNS [6]. For example, in the normal rodent brain the development of the synaptic density in the CA1 region of the hippocampus depends on the availability of androgens. In addition, it appears that removal of circulating gonadal steroids by ovariectomy causes a decrease in dendritic spine density in the CA1 region of

the female adult rat. These changes are observed a short time after treatment, raising the possibility that there are hormone-induced changes in the synaptic density during the normal estrous cycle. Quantitative electron microscopic analysis has confirmed that dendritic spines on neurons in the CA1 hippocampal region and the ventromedial hypothalamus undergo cyclic changes during the estrous cycle of the rat. Specifically, during estrus the spine density is significantly lower than the spine density during proestrus (Fig. 1C,D).

Steroid hormones can also influence neuronal activity by regulating the expression of various neurotransmitter receptors. For example, studies of the hypothalamus of the rat have shown that serotonin receptors in the preoptic area are up-regulated by androgens and oxytocin receptors in the ventromedial nucleus are up-regulated by estrogens.

Taken together, the results of these studies suggest that new synapse formation occurs normally in several areas of the CNS throughout life. In addition, as discussed in the next section, the CNS has the ability to regrow and form new synaptic connections in response to traumatic stimuli, possibly employing some of the same mechanisms. One such mechanism involves neurotrophic factors, as will be discussed below.

REACTIVE SYNAPTOGENESIS

Depending on the context, several modalities of neural plasticity following injury can be described, including regeneration, axon sprouting, and reactive synaptogenesis. Generally, when the damaged axons themselves regrow and reestablish their original connections, the process is known as *regeneration.* *Axon sprouting* refers to the process whereby axons from undamaged neurons form new branches. Synapse formation that occurs in reaction to a stimulus (e.g., entorhinal cor-

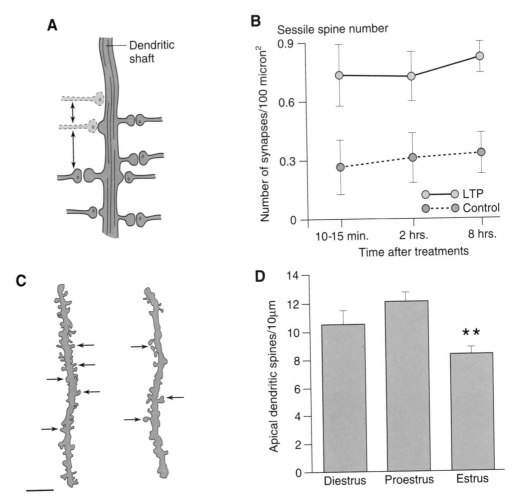

FIG. 1. Structural changes in neuronal dendrites correlated with long-term potentiation (LTP) and hormonal cycles. **A:** LTP-dependent increase in sessile spine synapses may involve an increase in synaptic formation on pyramidal neurons possibly through a shaft to sessile spine to spine transition. **B:** Increases in sessile spine synapses persist for at least 8 hours. Each data point is mean ± S.E.M. (*n* = 5 slices). **C:** Dendrites exhibit changes in spine numbers depending on the phase of the estrous cycle. Camera lucida drawings of apical dendrites of CA1 pyramidal neurons in the hippocampus. The left dendrite was measured during proestrus. The right dendrite has fewer spines and was measured during estrus. The *arrows* indicate dendritic spines. Scale bar, 10 μm. **D:** Spine density was significantly lower during estrus. The *asterisks* denote a significant difference from proestrus (*P* < 0.01). (Reproduced with permission from Chang and Greenough, *Brain Res.* 309:35, 1984, and Woolley et al., *J. Neurosci.* 10:4035, 1990.)

tex lesions, not normal development) is called *reactive synaptogenesis.* The term reactive synaptogenesis applies here only to situations in which synapses have been formed and makes no assumptions as to the driving stimulus or the type of sprouting involved [7].

The response of the hippocampus to the unilateral removal of the entorhinal cortex provides an illustration of the general principles of reactive synaptogenesis

One of the best illustrations of the general principles and mechanisms of reactive synaptogenesis is represented by the response of the hippocampus to the unilateral removal of the entorhinal cortex input. Fibers of the entorhinal cortex represent a major input to the dentate gyrus and terminate in the outer two-thirds of the dentate gyrus molecular layer. This circuitry is of particular interest because of its critical role in higher cognitive functions such as learning and memory (see Chap. 50) and its vulnerability to degeneration in Alzheimer's disease (see Chap. 45) and to a lesser degree during the course of aging (see Chap. 30). Thus, this system is an excellent model not only for minor cell loss, but for changes triggered by significant injury to the brain. These studies also provide insight into the mechanisms underlying sub-

tler events, such as learning, that occur over much longer time periods.

Following unilateral ablation of the entorhinal cortex, over 80% of the synapses degenerate and the cholinergic projections from the medial septum and hippocampal hilus sprout in the denervated molecular layer. Another source of sprouting fibers is the commissural-associational pathway. The projections from the ipsilateral and contralateral CA4 neurons normally terminate in the inner one-third of the dentate gyrus molecular layer. Following entorhinal lesions, these fibers sprout into the denervated zone, eventually occupying the inner one-half of the molecular layer (Fig. 2).

Fibers from the contralateral entorhinal

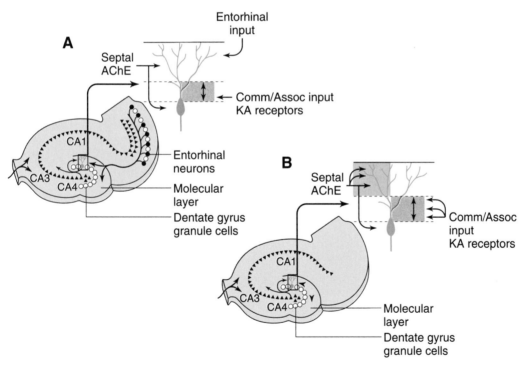

FIG. 2.   Changes in the dentate gyrus molecular layer following a unilateral entorhinal lesion. **A:** Normal distribution of entorhinal inputs to the outer two-thirds of the molecular layer, commissural/associational (Comm/Assoc) inputs, and kainic acid (KA) receptors in the inner one-third of the molecular layer. Cholinergic inputs, visualized with acetylcholinesterase (AChE) histochemistry, occupy the outer molecular layer as well as a thin band of fibers in the supragranular zone. **B:** Following an entorhinal ablation, the cholinergic afferents sprout and AChE staining intensifies in the outer molecular layer. Comm/Assoc afferents sprout and expand outward into the denervated zone. This is accompanied by an expansion of KA receptor distribution. (Reproduced from Cotman and Anderson. In Waxman (ed.), *Physiological Basis for Functional Recovery in Neurological Disease.* New York: Raven Press, 1988, p. 313.)

cortex, normally sparse in the molecular layer, also sprout extensively in the denervated zone after a unilateral lesion. Since this input is essentially homologous to the lost entorhinal input, the sprouted fibers may participate in the recovery of function following unilateral entorhinal ablation. Consistent with this idea, studies show that a unilateral entorhinal lesion causes temporary deficits in spontaneous or reinforced alternation tasks, and the rate of behavioral recovery corresponds to the rate of sprouting of the homologous contralateral fibers [8].

To some extent remodeling in the normal, healthy brain may involve processes that parallel those involved in remodeling that occurs after injury [9]. It appears that the brain has some intrinsic capabilities for plasticity, and these are enhanced when the homeostasis of the brain is challenged. It is interesting, in this respect, that following injury, regions not primarily associated with the lesion also exhibit synaptic density changes and subsequent recovery of control levels over a long period of time. The synaptic changes occur despite the absence of degenerating terminals within these zones. Thus, pronounced transneuronal changes may occur after major trauma to the CNS, suggesting that reactive synaptogenesis may adjust the functional integrity of complex circuitry in areas with and without a primary lesion [10].

Cytoskeletal protein levels increase after lesions

Several investigators hypothesize that sprouting in the CNS may involve a reactivation of mechanisms that primarily operate during development. There are many examples of developmentally regulated genes, including those encoding cytoskeletal proteins normally expressed during development. For example, the fetal form of α-tubulin, referred to as Tα1 in the rat, is expressed at high levels in the fetal brain during development of neuronal processes, and its expression is normally greatly reduced in the mature brain.

Other examples are tau and MAP-2 proteins, two of the major microtubule-associated proteins which form the cytoskeleton of neurons in the vertebrate nervous system. MAP-2 and tau proteins promote the assembly and integrity of microtubules in axons and dendrites, suggesting a major role in the determination of neuronal morphology.

In mature neurons, altered gene expression and increased synthesis of microtubules and associated proteins are observed during periods of neurite outgrowth. For example, following entorhinal cortex lesions in adult rats there is an increase in levels of MAP-2 protein in the processes of sprouting neurons in the outer molecular layer of the dentate gyrus [11]. Furthermore, following axonal injury to the mature nervous system, the fetal form of α-tubulin, Tα1, is rapidly reinduced and maintained at high levels during axon outgrowth [12]. These results support the idea that the neuronal cytoskeleton is dynamically modified in response to lesions and may involve the re-expression of mechanisms normally activated during development.

The hippocampus in Alzheimer's disease shows plasticity similar to that observed in the rodent brain

One of the goals of modern neurochemistry is to employ the findings from basic research and animal models to predict and evaluate mechanisms in human disease. Alzheimer's disease causes extensive neuronal degeneration in select brain areas including the entorhinal cortex, the origin of the major excitatory projection to the hippocampus. The course of degeneration is such that the neurons of the entorhinal cortex (layers II and III) projecting into the hippocampus are among the first affected. But while degeneration is a prominent feature of Alzheimer's disease, reactive growth in both neurons and glial cells is exhibited in this disease as well (see Chap. 45).

In the dentate gyrus of the normal brain there is a light cholinergic input, whereas in

Alzheimer brains the cholinergic input is increased in the denervated zone, as predicted from the animal models discussed earlier [13]. The fetal forms of several cytoskeletal proteins are also re-expressed in Alzheimer brains. As predicted from entorhinal cortex lesion models, the message for the developmental form of the cytoskeletal protein α-tubulin is present in Alzheimer brains at high levels [12]. These results suggest that as neurons are lost in the early period of the disease, the remaining cells sprout and form new synapses to compensate for lost connections and maintain neuronal circuitry.

NEUROTROPHIC FACTORS AND BRAIN PLASTICITY

Injury to the nervous system triggers an increase in the activity of several neurotrophic factors. Neurotrophic factors are a special class of endogenous signaling proteins that promote the survival, division, and growth, as well as regulate the differentiation and morphological plasticity of neural cells (Table 1). Some neurotrophic factors regulate all such functions in select neural populations while other factors regulate select functions.

After brain injury, extracts of both tissue and fluid around the injury show increased trophic factor activity [14]. The increase in trophic factor production and growth capabilities of cells in the CNS after cell loss is generally interpreted as a natural response of the CNS to compensate for damage. When damaged, neurons appear to react in a manner dependent on the type of injury. For example, neurons that are axotomized generally dedifferentiate and degenerate while the remaining healthy neurons may undergo a sprouting reaction. Neurotrophic factors may participate in this response to injury by triggering growth and preventing degeneration. These injury-induced factors appear to participate in axon and dendritic sprouting as well as mitosis of non-neuronal cells such as astrocytes and microglia.

TABLE 1. Examples of growth factor molecules with neurotrophic activity[a]

Neurotrophin family
  Nerve growth factor (NGF)
  Brain-derived neurotrophic factor (BDNF)
  Neurotrophin-3 (NT-3)
  Neurotrophin-4 (NT-4)
  Neurotrophin-5 (NT-5)

Ciliary neurotrophic factor (CNTF)

Fibroblast growth factor family (FGF)
  Acidic fibroblast growth factor (aFGF or FGF-1)
  Basic fibroblast growth factor (bFGF or FGF-2)
  Int-1 or FGF-3, hst-1 or FGF-4, FGF-5, FGF-6, FGF-7

Interleukin 1

Interleukin 3

Interleukin 6

Insulin-like growth factor (IGF)

Epidermal growth factor (EGF)

Platelet-derived growth factor (PDGF)

Transforming growth factor α (TGFα)

Transforming growth factor β (TGFβ)

[a] Some of these growth factors have direct neurotrophic actions as well as indirect actions via the regulation of the production and effectiveness of other growth factors. These actions are often coordinated in molecular cascades as is discussed in the text. (For a recent review of these growth factors and their actions, see Loughlin and Fallon (eds.), *Neurotrophic Factors.* San Diego: Academic Press, 1993.)

The best-characterized neurotrophic factor is nerve growth factor (NGF), first described by Levi-Montalcini and Hamburger in 1953 [15], now considered a member of the neurotrophin family of growth factors. Besides neurotrophins, there are several other growth factor families, such as the fibroblast growth factor (FGF) family, which includes basic FGF (FGF-2). Studies of neurotrophins and FGFs can illustrate the principles of neurotrophic factor function in general. Both neurotrophins and FGFs play important roles during the development of the CNS; however, in this chapter we will focus on the actions of trophic factors on differentiated cells.

Properties of NGF and FGF

NGF, NT-3, NT-4, NT-5, and brain-derived neurotrophic factor (BDNF) are members of the neurotrophin family of growth factors. NGF, originally purified from the mouse submandibular gland, can be isolated in two distinct forms known as 7S and 2.5S. The 7S NGF contains two copies of three types of polypeptides designated α, β, and γ, and the 2.5S NGF is biologically and immunologically indistinguishable from the β subunit. The neurotrophins possess a strictly conserved domain that determines their basic structure, and exhibit approximately 50% amino acid homology. However, the variable domain is sufficient to determine their specificity via recognition by particular high-affinity receptors. A human proto-oncogene member of the *trk* tyrosine kinase type of receptors is the high-affinity receptor, originally predicted by kinetic studies [16]. The receptor subtype that specifically recognizes NGF is known as *trk*^{A}. Two other similar receptors subtypes, *trk*^{B} and *trk*^{C}, recognize BDNF and NT-3, respectively. Besides *trk* receptors, the neurotrophins share a common receptor subunit that binds all of them with similar low affinity. A variety of studies support the notion that the low- and high-affinity receptors are interconvertible; however, this issue is still controversial.

NGF is considered to be a target-derived growth factor that influences presynaptic neurons where its receptors are located. Under specific conditions, NGF is also synthesized by non-neuronal cells such as astrocytes, suggesting that the action of NGF can be local as well as target derived. In the CNS, NGF appears to act on cholinergic neurons.

FGFs are protein mitogens originally identified as promoters of fibroblast division in culture. The FGF family has seven structurally related growth factors with diverse effects in various tissues. The best-characterized members of the FGF family are acidic and basic fibroblast growth factors (FGF-1 or aFGF and FGF-2 or bFGF) [17] which together with their receptors are present in the brain. FGF-2 is a single chain protein of 146 amino acids with an approximate molecular weight of 16.5 kDa.

Similar to NGF, FGF-1 and FGF-2 possess low-affinity and high-affinity receptors. The low-affinity receptor appears to be a cell-surface heparin sulfate proteoglycan (HSPG). It appears that the low affinity receptor must be bound before the high affinity receptor can be bound and trigger a biological action. A large body of evidence indicates that HSPG stores, protects, and potentiates the action of FGF-2. There are at least three high-affinity receptors that have been described and are known as *flg* (type I), *bek* (type II), and *cek* (type III). FGF-2 undergoes both anterograde and retrograde transport by neurons and appears to have effects on the local cell environment as well as on target neurons. FGF-2 appears to exert trophic actions on a variety of CNS cell types including astrocytes and most populations of neurons studied to date.

Neurotrophic factors can rescue damaged neurons

Recent studies have shown that select neurotrophic factors can rescue damaged neurons and promote neuronal survival. When FGF-2 is added in small quantities to cultured hippocampal cells, there is an increase in neuronal survival and in the number of process-bearing neurons (Fig. 3A). The effect of FGF-2 lasts for several days, and many types of CNS neurons are supported by FGF-2. Further work has demonstrated that glycosaminoglycans (i.e., heparin and heparan sulfate) interact synergistically with FGF-2 to increase process outgrowth [18].

Studies on cells in culture predict that FGF-2 may promote neuronal survival and growth *in vivo*. Disruption of the cholinergic septal projection to the hippocampus causes a loss of trophic support provided to the septal cells by the hippocampal neurons resulting in the subsequent degeneration of septal neurons. However, when the septal-hippocampal projection was transected and FGF-2 was infused into the ventricles, FGF-2 enhanced the survival of cholinergic septal neu-

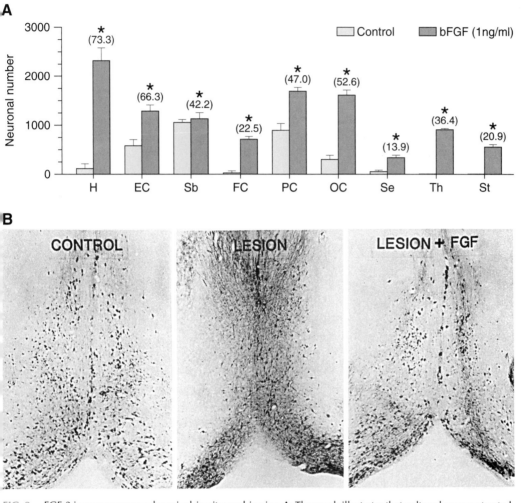

FIG. 3.   FGF-2 increases neuronal survival *in vitro* and *in vivo*. **A:** The graph illustrates that cultured neurons treated with FGF-2 (bFGF) survive longer than controls. At day 6 *in vitro* there were significantly (*; $P < 0.01$) more surviving neurons in cultures treated with FGF-2 (1 ng/ml). H, hippocampus; EC, entorhinal cortex; Sb, subiculum; FC, frontal cortex; PC, parietal cortex; OC, occipital cortex; Se, septum; Th, thalamus; St, striatum. *Bars* are means + SEM for six duplicate cultures. Numbers in *parentheses* are percentages of neurons present after 24 hr surviving to 6 days in the presence of FGF-2. (Adapted with permission from Walicke, *J. Neurosci.* 8:2618, 1988.) **B:** Photomicrographs of acetylcholinesterase-stained neurons taken from an unlesioned control animal *(CONTROL)*, a lesion control animal *(LESION)*, and an animal with a lesion that had received an infusion of FGF *(LESION + FGF)*. Unilateral fimbria-fornix transections were performed in the lesioned animals. Brain slices were prepared 12 days post-lesion and are shown with the lesion side on the left. Note the prominent unilateral loss of neurons in the lesion subject. In the FGF-treated animals, neuronal death was prevented. (Reproduced with permission from Cotman and Anderson. In Siegel et al. (eds.), *Basic Neurochemistry,* 4th Ed. New York: Raven Press, 1989, p. 519.)

rons in young and old rats (Fig. 3B). These findings *in vitro* and *in vivo* indicate that neurotrophic factors can rescue damaged neurons [19].

Besides FGF-2, NGF and other members of the neurotrophin family have also been shown to be effective in protecting axotomized septal neurons. Studies have shown that long-term chronic infusion of NGF can completely restore the septo-hippocampal projection [20]. Furthermore, the same type of results have been observed using implants of cells that were genetically engineered to synthesize NGF (as discussed below). However, the question remains whether growth factors are helpful in restoring the normal physiological function of the damaged circuitry.

FGF-2 is induced in the dentate gyrus following entorhinal cortex lesions

After a unilateral entorhinal cortex lesion, the hippocampus ipsilateral to a lesion shows an enhancement of FGF-2 immunoreactivity as well as extensive fiber sprouting and reactive synaptogenesis in the outer two-thirds of the dentate gyrus molecular layer where the entorhinal fibers normally terminate. The increase in FGF-2 parallels the time course for sprouting [21]. Basic FGF is also increased in the processes and cell bodies of astrocytes surrounding lesion areas. There is also an increase in FGF-2 in the extracellular matrix of the dentate gyrus on the lesion side, which suggests that FGF-2 may be released from astrocytes and becomes available to other neural elements (Fig. 4).

FGF-2 and NGF are not the only growth factors that are up-regulated after injury. In fact, several other growth factors or their receptors have been shown to increase under similar lesion paradigms, i.e., interleukin-1 (IL-1) and epidermal growth factor receptor. These observations support the idea that growth factors work in concert, coordinating their actions in molecular cascades.

Molecular cascades involving cytokines, FGF-2, and NGF appear to regulate the growth response

Increasing evidence indicates that the biological role of growth factors exceeds that of simply promoting cell growth and indeed they have major roles as physiological regulators. Even though growth factors generally promote growth, depending on interactions with other molecules, they can also inhibit growth. Recent studies *in vitro* and *in vivo*

demonstrate that there are physiological interactions between various growth factors, consistent with the idea that multiple growth factors coordinate their actions in molecular cascades.

Following brain injury, several cellular and molecular events occur nearby the injury site that determine the physiological response of the remaining cells and appear to be associated with the action of growth factors. After injury, one of the earliest cellular responses appears to involve microglia. This is followed by increases in astrocyte reactivity. This cellular sequence has led to various investigations examining possible cascades of growth factors involving these cells. Indeed, glial cells such as microglia and astrocytes are common sources of growth factors and play a determinant role in the injury response [22]. One such cascade is illustrated in Fig. 5. Microglia release cytokines such as IL-1 that induce reactive astrocytes. In this process, IL-1 promotes the release of other growth factors such as IL-6 and NGF by astrocytes. Reactive astrocytes also secrete FGF-2 and IL-1, which may play an autocrine role for astrocytes [23]. Microglia also release transforming growth factor β1, which regulates the action of FGFs on cells and protects and strengthens the extracellular matrix. Extracellular matrix components such as proteoglycans, in turn, potentiate the action of growth factors such as FGF-2 (see above). As growth factors are released into the extracellular fluid they become available to other cells such as neurons, which also produce growth factors such as NGF. Not only do these growth factors work in concert to regulate growth factor production but also some growth factors increase the responsiveness of cells to other growth factors. For example, studies have shown that cells in culture cannot respond to NGF until they are primed with FGF-2 [24]. In this case, FGF-2 induces receptors for NGF in cells preparing them for the action of NGF. Thus, it is highly likely that growth factors are organized in molecular cascades to act as major regulators of cell development and plasticity.

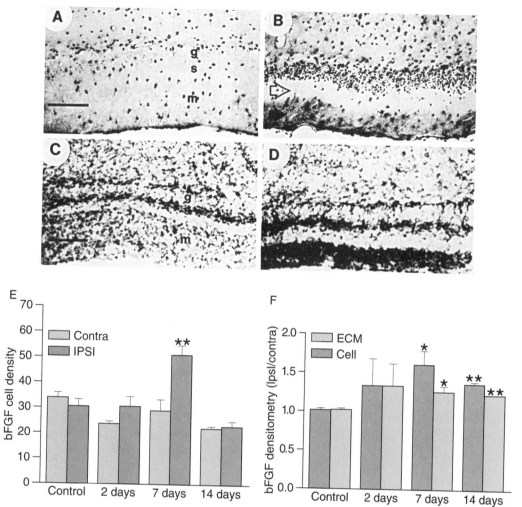

FIG. 4. FGF-immunoreactivity increases 7 days after lesions. The outer molecular layer of the dentate gyrus ipsilateral to a unilateral entorhinal cortex lesion exhibits an increase in FGF-2 immunoreactivity **(B)** as compared to the contralateral (control) dentate gyrus **(A)**. The *solid arrow* indicates dense FGF-2 staining in the outer molecular layer and the *open arrow* indicates a clear zone in the inner molecular layer. Entorhinal cortex lesions increase the number of FGF-2 astrocytes and FGF-2 immunoreactivity in the outer molecular layer of the dentate gyrus. AChE histochemistry on the control side **(C)** versus the lesion side **(D)** shows that the increase of FGF-2 immunoreactivity displays a similar pattern to sprouting **(D)** of cholinergic fibers in the dentate gyrus outer molecular layer. The photograph was taken from a rat killed 2 days after lesion. g, granule cell layer of the dentate gyrus; s, supragranular layer of the dentate gyrus; m, molecular layer of the dentate gyrus. Scale bars, 200 μm. **E:** The graph shows the average ratio of FGF-2-immunoreactive astrocytes observed under camera lucida on the ipsilateral side versus the contralateral side. On the ipsilateral side, the number of FGF-2 cells is increased by 2 days after entorhinal cortex lesion, reaches significance by postlesion day 7 (**; $P < .01$), and returns to normal levels by postlesion day 14. The data are expressed as mean (+SEM) number of cells per 100 μm^2 of tissue sample. **F:** Computer densitometry readings were taken from individual astrocytes and the surrounding extracellular matrix (ECM) from the immunohistochemical material. The graph shows the ratio of optical density on the ipsilateral side versus the contralateral side. There is an increase in FGF-2 immunoreactivity in astrocytes and ECM by postlesion day 7 (*; $P < .05$) and remaining through day 14 (**; $P < .01$). (Reprinted with permission from Gómez-Pinilla et al., *J. Neurosci.* 12:345, 1992.)

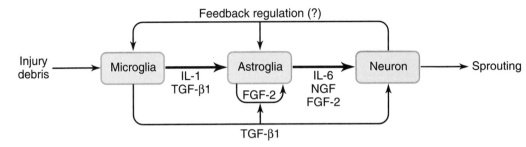

FIG. 5. Simplified mechanism by which growth factors may regulate neuronal plasticity following injury to the CNS. Primed by the original insult, microglia, astroglia, and neurons interact with each other by releasing growth factors to the extracellular space. The actions of growth factors are organized in molecular cascades in which one growth factor affects the release or action of another growth factor. This generally results in increased cell survival and/or sprouting. IL-1, interleukin-1; IL-6, interleukin-6; TGF-β1, transforming growth factor β1; FGF-2, fibroblast growth factor 2; NGF, nerve growth factor.

Select neurotrophic factors and their receptors are regulated in an activity-dependent manner

Increasing evidence indicates that growth factors are not solely regulated by mechanisms such as injury or denervation but also by neuronal activity. Recent studies have shown that the expression of NGF is significantly altered after seizures. Within 1 hour after the onset of limbic seizures in rats, the level of messenger RNA for NGF dramati-

TABLE 2. Neurotrophic factor mRNA levels regulated by activation and inhibition of excitatory (glutamate) and inhibitory (γ-amino butyrate; GABA) transmitter receptors[a]

	Percent of control mRNA levels	
	BDNF	NGF
Glutamate activation (kainate; 25 μM)	1,350	850
Non-NMDA inhibition (NBQX; 1 mM)	75	70
NMDA inhibition (MK-801; 10 μM)	50	35
GABA activation (muscimol; 2 mg/kg)	40	55
GABA inhibition (bicuculline; 50 μM)	375	ND

[a] Increased excitation via glutamate receptors or block of GABA receptors results in increased levels of BDNF and NGF mRNA levels. Decreased excitation via GABA receptors or block of glutamate receptors results in decreased levels of BDNF and NGF mRNA levels. (From Zafra *et al., Proc. Natl. Acad. Sci. U.S.A.* 88:10037, 1991, and Zafra *et al., EMBO J.* 9:3545, 1990.)

cally increases in the dentate gyrus. Increases are also observed in the neocortex and olfactory forebrain, within several hours after seizures [25].

Levels of NGF and BDNF can also be regulated by the differential activity of various neurotransmitter systems that project to a particular region. Levels of NGF and BDNF mRNA are increased via the excitatory neurotransmitter glutamate, and down-regulation occurs via the inhibitory neurotransmitter GABA (Table 2). For example, treatment with the non-NMDA glutamate agonist kainate results in an increase in BDNF mRNA, whereas treatment with the GABA system activator muscimol results in a decrease in BDNF mRNA [26].

The regulation of trophic molecules by neuronal activity suggests that the function of trophic factors exceeds that of regulation of differentiation and survival of neurons. Indeed, growth factors are excellent candidates for roles in the regulation of injury-induced circuit reorganization and modulation of normal neural remodeling.

REGENERATION

Peripheral nerve and Schwann cells promote regeneration

The processes involved in CNS axon regeneration are best illustrated by recent work on the visual system [27]. Transection of the mammalian optic nerve results in the death of retinal ganglion cells and in the failure of the surviving cut axons to regenerate. When a cut optic nerve is sutured to a portion of autologous peripheral nerve, fewer retinal ganglion cells degenerate and optic nerve axons will grow into the peripheral nerve graft (Fig. 6A). As much as one-fifth of the surviving retinal ganglion neurons will grow

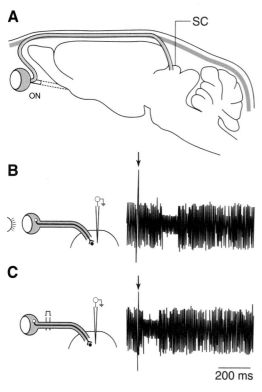

FIG. 6. Transected optic nerve can regenerate through a peripheral nerve graft and form functional synapses within the superior colliculus. **A:** Diagram of adult rat brain in sagittal section showing peripheral nerve grafts (○) used to replace the transected optic nerve (ON). One end of an autologous peroneal nerve graft was attached to the orbital stump of the ON transected close to the eye. The distal end of the graft was inserted into the superior colliculus (SC). **B:** Inhibition of ongoing activity of an SC neuron by light flash. **C:** Inhibition of spontaneous activity of the same neuron after electrical stimulation of the peripheral nerve graft. (Each trace represents 25 superimposed sweeps.) Stimuli were delivered at arrows. (Adapted with permission from Vidal-Sanz et al., *J. Neurosci.* 7:2894, 1987, and Keirstead et al., *Science* 246:255, 1989; © 1989 by the AAAS.)

axons into the graft. The regenerating fibers can grow for distances of up to 4 cm (double that of the normal retinotectal projection) at rates of 1–2 mm/day. As fibers regenerate, axonal transport of cytoskeletal proteins such as tubulin, neurofilament, and actin changes to resemble transport of these proteins in the developing optic nerve [28] (see Chap. 7). Analysis of the constituents of the peripheral nerve graft revealed that the presence of Schwann cells or their extracellular matrix in the graft promotes CNS fiber regeneration. Adhesion molecules on the surface of Schwann cells and specific extracellular matrix proteins, such as laminin, influence axonal outgrowth. If these molecules are bound with antibodies that inhibit their function, fiber regeneration is also inhibited.

Regenerating axons can form synapses

Using electrophysiological techniques, it was demonstrated that the regenerated axons can respond to light in a manner similar to intact retinal ganglion cells, indicating that, functionally, the regenerated axons behave like native fibers. Illuminating the retina within discrete fields produces a discharge of ganglion cells that have regenerated into the graft. The onset or cessation of light is followed by changes in spontaneous electrical activity characteristic of normal retinal responses. The optic nerve normally sends projections to the superior colliculus. If the free end of a peripheral nerve graft to the optic nerve is placed in the superior colliculus of the host, the regenerated axons will arborize in the superior colliculus and penetrate it for distances of up to 500 μm. The new axons will form functional synapses on neuronal elements within the superior colliculus. The newly formed synapses are well differentiated in both morphology and function. Illumination of specific regions of the retina produces either excitatory or inhibitory responses in post-synaptic superior collicular neurons similar to the ON and OFF cells described in the normal superior colliculus (Fig. 6B,C).

Axons retain the propensity to regenerate in adult animals

When CNS axons are severed, local connectivity may be reestablished by the growth of damaged cell processes or the extension of collateral sprouts from adjacent undamaged neurons. Whereas cut axons will regrow for long distances in the peripheral nervous system or in the CNS of fish and invertebrates, mammalian CNS axons rarely grow for more than a few millimeters through the injured area. The failure of CNS axons to regrow for long distances has been attributed to several

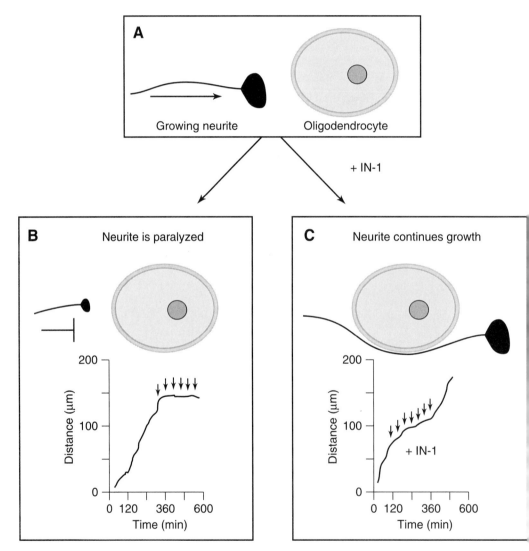

FIG. 7.   Neutralization of growth inhibitor proteins associated with oligodendrocytes promotes the growth of neurites near oligodendrocytes. **A:** Dorsal root ganglion neuronal process with growth cone growing on laminin in the presence of NGF makes contact with an oligodendrocyte. **B:** Growth cone subsequently collapses (60 min later) and remains paralyzed. Velocity plot shows arrest of growth cone upon encounter with oligodendrocyte. Contact is indicated by *arrows.* **C:** No growth arrest occurs in the presence of IN-1 antibodies neutralizing NI-35/250. Velocity plot shows continued growth despite contact with oligodendrocyte *(arrows).* (Adapted with permission from Schwab [30].)

factors. One example is proteoglycan growth inhibitors associated with astrocytic "glial scars," which form after injury [29]. A growth inhibitor associated with glial scars is thought to include the carbohydrate component of putative heparin-sulfate proteoglycans.

Another factor is myelin-associated neurite growth inhibitors produced by oligodendrocytes [30]. Researchers have known from cell culture studies that growing neurites normally avoid rat oligodendrocytes and myelin, but the mechanism has been unclear. It appeared that there were inhibitory factors associated with oligodendrocytes that were not metabolites of these cells but part of the cellular membrane because oligodendrocyte membranes also inhibit neurite growth. Recent studies show that oligodendrocytes express two cell surface proteins of 35 kDa (NI-35) and 250 kDa (NI-250) and two glycoproteins of the J1 family (160 and 180 kDa) that inhibit neurite outgrowth. Neurites will not normally grow over oligodendrocytes, but will grow over them in the presence of antibodies against oligodendrocyte-associated growth-inhibitory proteins (Fig. 7). Inhibition of these glial-produced growth inhibitors also results in expanded regeneration of transected CNS axons—up to distances of 1 cm within 2 weeks. Some of these proteins may have a critical role in the normal development of circuitry by directing the growth of developing projections into the proper areas [30]. These results also indicate that axons retain the ability to regenerate in adult mammals, but are suppressed by growth inhibitors on nearby oligodendrocytes.

Mammalian CNS axons have the ability to elongate for surprising distances when presented with the appropriate cellular milieu. Severed central axons will grow for long distances when attached to a portion of peripheral nerve, suggesting that axon regeneration depends more on the non-neuronal environment of the growing fibers than on the origin of the parent cell bodies. This observation illustrates the influence of extrinsic conditions, such as growth factors and basal lamina, on the developing or regenerating axon.

BRAIN TRANSPLANTS

The cell replacement strategy of brain transplantation has been developed in an attempt to overcome the intrinsic limitation of neurons to divide and replace lost cells. Through successful cell replacement, the damaged brain can be reconstructed, to a certain extent, in order to compensate for neuronal loss. Partial survival of brain tissue implants in rats was first reported by Elizabeth Dunn in 1917 [31]. There has been great progress in this area in the last decade mainly because of the advancement of cellular and molecular approaches. Poor integration of the implanted tissue with the host tissue and lack of control of the activity of host cells versus implanted cells have restrained the advancement in this field. Progress in the field corresponds to a better understanding of the optimal conditions for survival and integration of the implanted cells. Two critical variables that have been defined are the types of cells used and the developmental stage of those cells. In general, brain tissue implants can be performed with two different objectives: 1) to restore a cell population and its connectivity that has been damaged, and/or 2) to provide a new or additional source of the product of a particular cell population that is no longer functional.

Neural transplants integrate into brain circuitry and restore function

Proper integration of the implanted tissue with host tissue is a major requirement for successful transplantation therapy. One reason for poor integration has been the low viability of the implanted cells in the host tissue. Therefore, current investigation is focused on intervention procedures that can enhance the survival of implanted cells. Provision of a supply of growth factors with the graft appears to be a potential solution. Availability of growth factors appears to play an important role in the integration and functionality of the transplant. Growth factors help in the integration of implanted cells and also help maintain the functional status of the remaining endogenous cells.

A large body of evidence indicates that the age of the donor tissue is a key factor in the integration, survival, and functionality of the implant. Studies suggest that younger implanted cells have better chances for integration. In fact, transplants of embryonic tissue in animal models exhibit a remarkable capacity to overcome most of the limitations outlined above. It is well established that the symptoms of Parkinson's disease are the result of an almost complete loss of the neurotransmitter dopamine, which is normally provided by neurons in the substantia nigra. Therapeutic replacement of striatal dopamine (e.g., administration of L-DOPA) reverses the symptoms of Parkinsonism; however, long-term drug treatment has not been successful for diverse reasons. Thus, a large body of research has been devoted to finding ways to replace the cells that no longer release dopamine in the striatum.

Embryonic mesencephalic tissue grafting in mammalian models of Parkinson's disease has been shown to restore dopaminergic transmission and reverse sensorimotor deficits [32]. These results have prompted the use of similar approaches in clinical trials in human subjects affected by Parkinson's disease. Following tissue grafting, patients have shown moderate improvement of motor symptoms. PET scan assessment has shown that the tissue graft appears to have survived and grown [33] (see Chap. 44). A major limitation of tissue grafting approaches is that Parkinson's disease is a progressive disorder; therefore, any long-term positive effect owing to the graft is counteracted by further degeneration of endogenous dopaminergic neurons. In light of this, cell replacement strategies that consider delivery of both dopamine and growth factors

that keep the endogenous cells functional are realistic approaches for the future.

Results similar to those obtained for Parkinson's disease have been obtained in tissue transplantation approaches in experimental models of other neurodegenerative diseases such as Huntington's disease, amyotrophic lateral sclerosis, and hereditaria ataxia. However, inputs to the graft are usually limited and tissue grafts are restricted to simple cell replacement, not rebuilding of complete circuits. Although some conditions that facilitate successful results have been identified, more research is needed to clarify the optimal conditions for survival and performance of the grafted cells. Recent advances in the fields of molecular biology and genetics have provided new possibilities for brain tissue implant approaches, such as the genetic modification of graft cells, involving both neurons and non-neuronal cells.

Genetically engineered cells allow specific manipulation of the brain microenvironment

Recently there has been rapid progress in gene mapping, in particular those genes linked to diseases. This information has aided in the development of new therapeutic strategies for some diseases by manipulating the genome. Some of these molecular approaches have been used to incorporate new genetic information to modify the expression of a resident defective gene *in vivo*. This type of gene transfer therapy has been used to treat enzyme deficiencies such as adenosine deaminase deficiency in human subjects [34]. The results of clinical trials are encouraging and may help stimulate gene therapy approaches to treat similar disorders affecting the CNS.

Another type of gene therapy with strong potential of application to CNS diseases has been generated by a combination of advances in brain tissue transplantation, growth factors, and gene transfer technology. In this case, cells are genetically modified to deliver discrete substances into the

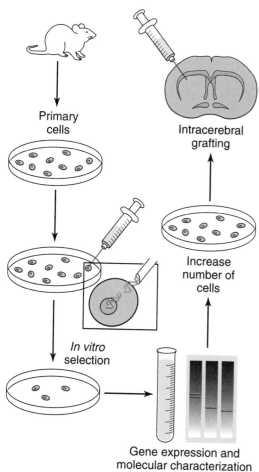

Primary
cells

Intracerebral
grafting

Increase
number of
cells

In vitro
selection

Gene expression and
molecular characterization

FIG. 8.   A schematic illustration of the gene transfer-intracerebral grafting technique. Primary cells (e.g., skin fibroblasts) are obtained from a donor biopsy and maintained under standard culture conditions. When a sufficient number of cells have grown, the cells are then genetically modified using one of a number of techniques (the lipofection method is shown here). After selection to determine successful incorporation of the transgene, transgene expression is assessed. The population of modified cells is grown to a desired number and implanted within the brain of the donor animal (autologous grafting). (Reprinted with permission from Gage et al., *TINS* 14:328, 1991.)

host tissue. Modified lines of fibroblast cells in which genes encoding growth factors such as NGF or FGF-2 have been inserted into the genome (Fig. 8). Grafts of fibroblasts engineered to deliver NGF have been shown to be effective in saving axotomized septal neu-

rons, which are responsive to NGF. Grafts of genetically engineered cells that synthesize and secrete growth factors is a realistic approach that in the near future may be used to combat neuronal degenerative diseases such as Parkinson's, Alzheimer's, and Huntington's diseases. The same gene transfer techniques may be used to treat deficiencies, such as dopamine deficiency in Parkinson's disease, by directly supplying neurotransmitters or other substances to regions of the brain where levels are low.

ADAPTIVE VERSUS PATHOLOGICAL PLASTICITY

Plasticity may become pathological after breakdown of brain homeostasis such as in aged-related dementias: plaque biogenesis

One of the neuropathological hallmarks of Alzheimer's disease is the presence of senile plaques. They appear to form along the areas of interface between degeneration and neuronal sprouting. We have suggested that there is an abortive turning of the sprouting reaction into plaque formation [13].

In the earlier literature, some reports suggested that sprouting occurred around plaques. In fact, Ramón y Cajal in 1928 [2] had suggested that sprouting fibers were attracted to plaques by some neurotrophic factor, which was a remarkable insight considering that at the time there was little knowledge regarding the role of neurotrophic factors in the brain. Plaques located along the sprouting zone in the dentate gyrus are FGF-2 immunoreactive, as is the area surrounding them. Double-label immunocytochemistry shows that FGF-2 immunostaining is associated with astrocytes. Denervation may serve to trigger a molecular cascade that causes astrocytes to synthesize FGF-2. Thus, it appears that within this microenvironment glial cells are stimulated to produce increased levels of FGF-2 that may, in effect, "trick" fibers into growing into plaques (Fig. 9).

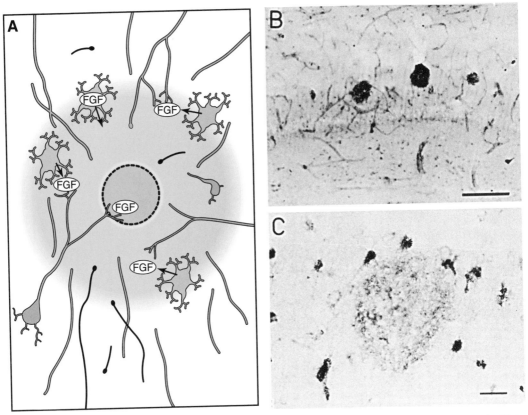

FIG. 9.   FGF-2 is present in the senile plaque environment. **A:** The diagram illustrates the potential sites of FGF-2 involvement in plaque formation and misdirected plasticity. **B:** Basic FGF-immunoreactivity detects senile plaques located in the dentate gyrus molecular layer of Alzheimer brains (scale bar = 100 μm). **C:** The photomicrograph illustrates the presence of FGF-2-immunoreactive astrocytes surrounding a FGF-2-immunoreactive senile plaque (scale bar = 10 μm). (Reprinted with permission from Cotman et al. [26].)

It is well known that HSPG can bind to FGF-2 and can act synergistically with FGF-2 to stimulate neuritic growth in culture. HSPG within plaques may accumulate FGF-2 produced by local cellular reactions. Thus, in at least some plaques, the potential exists for misdirected neuronal growth, since there exist both neurotrophic factor(s) and suitable substrate(s) for sprouting axons.

It is ironic that the initial and/or subsequent mechanisms that promote growth and slow degeneration may in certain circumstances contribute to the disorganization of the environment. Basic FGF in plaques may activate a number of other growth-promoting processes, some of which may further add to the growth of plaques [35]. For example, it appears that FGF-2 can enhance the production of the amyloid precursor protein in C6 glioma cells and in primary cultures of astrocytes. Further, it appears that β-amyloid can increase the production of FGF-2 by astrocytes. Such feedback cycles may produce molecular cascades that enhance the progression of pathology.

CONCLUSIONS

Research over the past decade has shown that the brain is highly plastic at the level of its circuitry. It is clear that there is sprouting and synaptic reorganization during normal development and throughout adult life in response to stimuli such as changes in neuronal activity and hormonal cycles. In addition, the brain has a remarkable potential to rebuild circuitry in response to injury or neurodegenerative disease. Many of these plastic responses appear to involve common mechanisms for normal remodeling and for repair after injury. One such mechanism involves neurotrophic factors, which are regulated by both neuronal activity and injury, acting in concert as part of molecular cascades. Research in this area is rapidly expanding with the characterization of pharmacology of activity-dependent regulation, the identification of key control points in molecular cascades, and the development of various new methods such as transfected cells. However, growing evidence suggests that, ironically, normal repair mechanisms can also contribute to the development of pathology if the natural plastic responses are overstimulated or deregulated, as seen in the development of senile plaques in Alzheimer's disease. As the neurochemistry and molecular regulation of sprouting and reactive synaptogenesis are characterized, it not only provides an opportunity to understand normal brain plasticity mechanisms but also to develop strategies to regulate these mechanisms and help prevent brain injury and stimulate recovery.

REFERENCES

1. James, W. *The Principles of Psychology.* New York: Holt, 1890.
2. Cajal, R. S. *Degeneration and Regeneration of the Nervous System.* Oxford: Oxford University Press, 1928.
3. Diamond, M. C. Aging and environmental influences on the rat forebrain. In A. B. Scheibel and A. F. Wechsler (eds.), *The Biological Substrates of Alzheimer's Disease.* Orlando, FL: Academic Press, 1986, pp. 55–63.
4. Wallace, C. S., Kilman, V. L., Withers, G. S., and Greenough, W. T. Increase in dendritic length in occipital cortex after 4 days of differ-

ential housing in weanling rats. *Behav. Neural Biol.* 58:64–68, 1992.
5. Lee, K. S., Schottler, F., Oliver, M., and Lynch, G. Brief bursts of high-frequency stimulation produce two types of structural change in rat hippocampus. *J. Neurophysiol.* 44:247–258, 1980.
6. McEwen, B. S. Steroid hormones in the brain. In B. Smith and G. Adelman (eds.), *Neuroscience Year, Supplement 2 to the Encyclopedia for Neuroscience.* Boston, MA: Birkhauser, 1992, pp. 144–146.
7. Nieto-Sampedro, M., and Cotman, C. W. Synaptic plasticity. In G. Adelman (ed.), *Encyclopedia of Neuroscience.* Boston, MA: Birkhauser, 1987, pp. 1166–1167.
8. Scheff, S. W., and Cotman, C. W. Recovery of spontaneous alternation following lesions of the entorhinal cortex in adult rats: possible correlation to axon sprouting. *Behav. Biol.* 21: 286–293, 1977.
9. Purves, D. *Body and Brain.* Cambridge, MA: Harvard University Press, 1988.
10. Hoff, S. F., Scheff, S. W., Kwan, A. Y., and Cotman, C. W. A new type of lesion induced synaptogenesis: I. Synaptic turnover in non-denervated zones of the dentate gyrus in young adult rats. *Brain Res.* 222:1–13, 1981.
11. Cáceres, A., Busciglio, J., Ferreira, A., and Steward, O. An immunohistochemical and biochemical study of the microtubule-associated protein MAP-2 during post-lesion dendritic remodeling in the central nervous system of adult rats. *Mol. Brain Res.* 3:233–246, 1988.
12. Cotman, C. W., Geddes, J. W., and Kahle, J. S. Axon sprouting in the rodent and Alzheimer's disease brain: a reactivation of developmental mechanisms? In J. Storm-Mathisen, J. Zimmer, and O. P. Ottersen (eds.), *Prog. Brain Res.* Amsterdam: Elsevier Science Publishers B.V., 1990, pp. 427–434.
13. Geddes, J. W., Monaghan, D. T., Cotman, C. W., Lott, I. T., Kim, R. C., and Chui, H. C. Plasticity of hippocampal circuitry in Alzheimer's disease. *Science* 230:1179–1181, 1985.
14. Nieto-Sampedro, M., and Cotman, C. W. Growth factor induction and temporal order in central nervous system repair. In C. W. Cotman (ed.), *Synaptic Plasticity.* New York: Guilford Press, 1985, pp. 407–455.
15. Levi-Montalcini, R., and Hamburger, V. A diffusible agent of mouse sarcoma producing

hyperplasia of sympathetic ganglia and hyper-neurotization of viscera in the chick embryo. *J. Exp. Zool.* 123:321–361, 1953.

16. Hempstead, B. L., Martin-Zanca, D., Kaplan, D. R., Parada, L. F., and Chao, M. V. High-affinity NGF binding requires coexpression on the *trk* proto-oncogene and the low-affinity NGF receptor. *Nature* 350:678–683, 1991.

17. Baird, A., and Bohlen, P. Fibroblast growth factors. In M. B. Sporn and A. B. Roberts (eds.), *Peptide Growth Factors and Their Receptors I.* New York: Springer-Verlag, 1991, pp. 369–418.

18. Gospodarowicz, D., and Cheng, J. Heparin protects basic and acidic FGF from inactivation. *J. Cell Physiol.* 128:475–484, 1986.

19. Anderson, K. J., Dam, D., and Cotman, C. W. Basic fibroblast growth factor prevents death of cholinergic neurons in vivo. *Nature* 332: 360–361, 1988.

20. Tuszynski, M. H., Buzsaki, G., and Gage, F. H. Nerve growth factor infusions combined with fetal hippocampal grafts enhance reconstruction of the lesioned septohippocampal projection. *Neuroscience* 36:33–44, 1990.

21. Gómez-Pinilla, F., Cummings, B. J., and Cotman, C. W. Induction of basic fibroblast growth factor in Alzheimer's disease pathology. *NeuroReport* 1:211–214, 1990.

22. Patel, A. J., Kiss, J., and Gray, C. Organization of septo-hippocampal neurons and their regulation by trophic factors produced by astrocytes. In A. J. Hunter and M. Clark (eds.), *Neurodegeneration.* London: Academic Press, 1992, pp. 59–80.

23. Yoshida, K., and Gage, F. H. Fibroblast growth factors stimulate nerve growth factor synthesis and secretion by astrocytes. *Brain Res.* 538: 118–126, 1991.

24. Cattaneo, E., and McKay, R. Proliferation and differentiation of neuronal stem cells regulated by nerve growth factor. *Nature* 347: 762–765, 1990.

25. Gall, C. M., and Isackson, P. J. Limbic seizures increase neuronal production of messenger RNA for nerve growth factor. *Science* 245: 758–761, 1989.

26. Cotman, C. W., Cummings, B. J., and Pike, C. J. Molecular cascades in adaptive versus pathological plasticity. In A. Gorio (ed.), *Neuroregeneration.* New York: Raven Press, Ltd., 1993, pp. 217–240.

27. Aguayo, A. J., Rasminsky, M., Bray, G. M., Carbonetto, S., McKerracher, L., Villegas-Perez, M. P., Vidal-Sanz, M., and Carter, D. A. Degenerative and regenerative responses of injured neurons in the central nervous system of adult mammals. *Philos. Trans. R. Soc. Lond. [Biol.]* 331:337–343, 1991.

28. McKerracher, L., Vidal-Sanz, M., and Aguayo, A. J. Slow transport rates of cytoskeletal proteins change during regeneration of axotomized retinal neurons in adult rats. *J. Neurosci.* 10:641–648, 1990.

29. Bovolenta, P., Wandosell, F., and Nieto-Sampedro, M. CNS glial scar tissue: a source of molecules which inhibit central neurite outgrowth. In A. C. H. Yu, L. Hertz, M. D. Norenberg, E. Sykova, and S. G. Waxman (eds.), *Prog. Brain Res.* Amsterdam: Elsevier Science Publishers B.V., 1992, pp. 367–379.

30. Schwab, M. E. Myelin-associated inhibitors of neurite growth and regeneration in the CNS. *TINS* 13:452–456, 1990.

31. Bjorklund, A. Brain implants, transplants. In G. Adelman (ed.), *Encyclopedia of Neuroscience.* Boston, MA: Birkhauser, 1987, pp. 165–167.

32. Dunnett, S. B. Transplantation of embryonic dopamine neurons: what we know from rats. *J. Neurol.* 238:65–74, 1991.

33. Sawle, G. V., Wroe, S. J., Lees, A. J., Brooks, D. J., and Frackowiak, R. S. The identification of presymptomatic parkinsonism: clinical and [18F]dopa positron emission tomography studies in an Irish kindred. *Ann. Neurol.* 32: 609–617, 1992.

34. Miller, D. A. Human gene therapy comes of age. *Nature* 357:455–460, 1992.

35. Cotman, C. W., and Gómez-Pinilla, F. Basic fibroblast growth factor in the mature brain and its possible role in Alzheimer's disease. *Ann. N.Y. Acad. Sci.* 638:221–231, 1991.

CHAPTER 30

Biochemistry of Aging in the Mammalian Brain

Caleb E. Finch

Basic Neurochemistry: Molecular, Cellular, and Medical Aspects, 5th Ed., edited by G. J. Siegel et al. Published by Raven Press, Ltd., New York, 1994. Correspondence to Caleb E. Finch, Neurogerontology Division, Andrus Gerontology Center and Department of Biological Sciences, University of Southern California, Los Angeles, California 90089-0191.

OVERVIEW ON AGING

Despite taxonomic diversity, canonical changes can be shown in short- and long-lived mammals

Most animals manifest a *canonical* pattern of aging in the brain and other organs (Tables 1,2), which implies strong underlying genetic controls. Nonetheless, there are important individual variations in the trajectory of aging. Among canonical aging changes of mammals are the accumulation of lipofus-cins or aging pigments in nondividing cells, the decrease of striatal dopamine receptors, and the proliferation of smooth muscle cells in blood vessels in many organs [1].

There are, however, important species differences among brain aging changes in mammals. In older humans, with Alzheimer's disease (AD), neurons accumulate neurofibrillary tangles and extracellular senile plaques with deposits of the βA4 amyloid fragment (see Chap. 45). In contrast, laboratory rodents show neither change. Table 1

TABLE 1. Comparative brain aging in mammals: general characteristics[a]

	Age-related changes of mammals scaled on a unit lifespan: a sampling	
	Mid-life	*Senescence*
Reproduction	Menopause or total infertility in females, in association with imminent depletion of ovarian oocytes (C, D, Hm, H, P, M, Op, R, Wh)	Decreased male fertility (H, P, M, R)
Tumors	Many endocrine-related tumors of reproductive organs (H, P, M, R, D)	
Growth hormone		Decreased frequency of pulses: smaller amplitude (H, P, R)
Thermoregulation		Impaired responses to cold (H, M, R) Impaired febrile response (H, P)
Coronary and cerebral arteries	Early atherosclerotic lesions (H, M, R)	Widespread atherosclerosis (H, P, D, R, Rb, M)
Immune functions	Slow decline in humoral antibody production (H, P, R, M)	
Bone	Onset of osteoporosis in female (H, P, R, Rb, M)	Female osteoporosis > male (H, P, R, Rb, M)
Joints		Arthritic changes very common (C, D, H, M, R)
Reaction times		Generally slowed (H, R)
Vision		Universally decreased accommodation of eye (presbyopia) (H, P)
Hearing		Sporadic loss (H)
Striatal dopaminergic neurons	Onset of D-2 receptor decline (H, M, P, R, Rb)	Dopamine conc. decline (H, M, R, Rb)
Large neurons		Heterogeneous changes; some show increased size and dendritic complexity; others show atrophy and dendritic withering (H, R, M)
Cerebrovascular βA4		Widespread in absence of Alzheimer's disease (H, P, D)

Excerpted with permission of University of Chicago Press, from Finch [1], pp. 154–155.
[a] Onset of senescence in population (usual age, in years): C, cattle = 15–25; D, dog = 10–15; H, human = 60–80; Hm, golden hamster = 2–3; M, mouse = 2–3; Op, opossum = >2; P, (rhesus) monkey = 20–30; R, rat = 2–3; Rb, rabbit = 4–6; Wh, pilot whale = >40??

outlines these and other comparisons of brain aging between mammalian species. Although the focus here is on brain aging in mammals, readers will find a short discussion of aging in other animals later in this chapter.

Aging in species with different life spans is often compared in proportion to the maximum life spans, not absolute age, which implies assumptions about "the rate of aging." One might suppose that the 3-fold greater glucose oxidation and protein synthesis/gram brain in rats than in humans and macaques (see [1], p. 264) is due to a greater rate of neuronal metabolism and hence neuronal aging. However, oxygen consumption per neuron differs by <10% between rat and human. Thus, species differences in whole brain metabolism may reflect neuron density more than biosynthesis rates. Moreover, the old correlations between brain size, basal metabolism, and life span in different orders of mammals are not supported (see [1] pp. 251, 276–8).

Gene-environmental interactions in aging changes

Aging processes are difficult to resolve into tractable hypotheses that can be experimentally tested. The brain, like all other organs, develops complex age-related changes that arise from gene-environment interactions across the life span. Aging seems unlikely to result from a single molecular process throughout all organs, at least in part, because genotypic determinants of brain aging are subject to diverse environmental influences. For example, humans show increased risk of depression and mortality after death of a spouse; the impact from death of long-term cage mates among rodents housed in multiples is unknown. It is therefore important in experimental design to account for individual changes during aging. Yet, some brain aging processes show trends that are general enough for molecular and genetic

analysis. Overall, the nervous system shows a remarkable ability to compensate for minor changes or even major injury throughout life.

CELL NUMBERS

The distinction between neuron loss and neuron atrophy is a major issue

Most brain neurons in mammals are postmitotic and thus at risk for irreversible damage that will be more long-lasting to organ function than in organs with cell replacement, such as liver or skin. The old tenet of massive neocortical neuron loss during aging is not supported by rigorous analyses of individuals with defined health status [2]. Because cell counts are biased toward larger neurons, atrophy can be misinterpreted as cell loss. Many early studies on brain aging changes were confounded by unrecognized pathological lesions. The distinction between aging and disease in the brain as in other organs is often subtle.

As examples that irreplaceable cells need not be lost during aging, the GnRH-containing neurons in the hypothalamus that drive the ovulatory surges of gonadotropins show no evidence of loss during the loss of estrous cycles in reproductively senescent mice. The inferior olive also shows no neuron loss even in the tenth decade of humans (Monagle and Brody, 1981, cited in [2]).

Neuron atrophy during aging is generally reported as a decrease of mean perikaryal area. However, a few studies have shown that the mean perikaryal area decrease is the result of an increase of small neurons at the expense of the large (Fig. 1). By microspectrophotometry, brains from normal, elderly individuals and those with AD often show nucleolar shrinkage or loss of cell body RNA in large neurons [Terry, 1987, cited in Fig. 1 legend]. Nucleolar shrinkage probably represents reduced ribosomal RNA synthesis. In some specimens, the losses may represent early stages of AD and

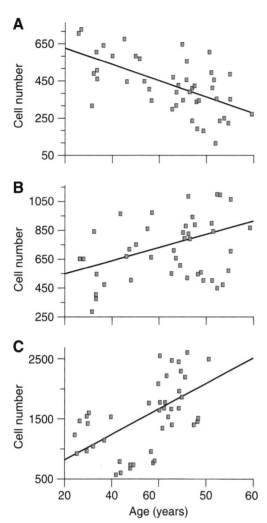

FIG. 1. Aging leads to alterations in neuronal and glial cell populations. Brains from a group of 51 individuals with normal cognitive function were used in this study. The brains were fixed and sectioned at 20 μm. After staining with cresyl violet, cortical cells were counted with a Quantimet 920. **A:** Large neurons (>90 μm) show a strong negative correlation with aging in all midfrontal, superior temporal, and inferior parietal areas of the neocortex. **B:** Small neurons (<90 μm but >40 μm) increase in number with advancing age. **C:** Glial cells (<40 μm) increase with advancing age. (Data redrawn from Terry et al., *Ann. Neurol.* 21:530–539, 1987.)

other diseases, which were not severe enough to be diagnosed. However, some neurons show hypertrophy during normal aging, e.g., in human and primate basal forebrain cholinergic neurons [2] which con-

trasts with atrophy of these neurons in rodents [5].

Very long-term responses to 6-OHDA are a model for neuron atrophy during aging and in Parkinson's disease (PD)

During PD, nucleoli shrink in the remaining neurons of the substantia nigra compacta (SNC) (work of D. Mann, reviewed in [2,4]). This is puzzling, because SNC lesions induced dopaminergic (DAergic) hyperactivity in young rats, e.g., increased synthesis/release of dopamine (DA) at the terminals, or increased tyrosine hydroxylase (TH) (see Chap. 12). A lesion model shows PD-like atrophy of SNC neurons and also enhanced synthesis in the striatal terminals, in which adult rats were given unilateral injections of the neurotoxin 6-hydroxydopamine (6-OHDA) and sacrificed 9 months later. Striatal DA was initially depleted on the lesioned side, with increased DOPAC/DA ratios; this latter change indicates increased DA release at the remaining striatal terminals. SNC DAergic cell bodies that survived the 6-OHDA lesion showed cell atrophy, with 30% shrinkage of cell bodies, nuclei, and nucleoli of tyrosine hydroxylase (TH)-immunoreactive neurons than in the contralateral (non-lesioned) side; similar atrophy occurs during PD. The nucleolar shrinkage implies decreased synthesis of ribosomes, which would be consistent with loss of neuronal RNA in the substantia nigra during PD. Moreover, the striatum was the only major brain region to show a loss of bulk RNA during normal aging [3]. By *in situ* hybridization, TH-mRNA decreased by an extent >80% on the lesioned side. The SNC of PD also showed a similar loss of TH-mRNA [2]. Despite the 80% loss of nigral TH-mRNA 9 months after lesioning, the striatum showed complete recovery of TH protein concentration and enzyme activity. These slowly developing changes suggest a need for prolonged studies to model human neurologic diseases spanning a decade or more.

Glial hyperactivity is generally observed during aging and may not always be associated with irreversible neurodegeneration

Astrocytic hyperactivity may be a canonical age change in healthy humans and laboratory rodents, with 10–30% increases in astrocyte volume with age [3,6]. Aging rodent and human brains show progressive increases in astrocyte-specific glial fibrillary acidic protein (GFAP) and GFAP mRNA in rodents and humans [7]. While astrocytes can proliferate in the adult brain as well as immigrate from other brain regions, in the hippocampus of aging rats the numbers of astrocytes change much less than the increases in GFAP [6].

It is unclear if the astrocytic hyperactivity of aging is caused by neurodegenerative events, since the onset of astrocytic hyperactivity can be detected by middle age in rodents when there is little evidence for neurodegeneration. Thus, the specificity of age changes in glia is a major question. However, even if "nonspecific aging" proves to be a general cause of astrocytic hyperactivity, this would nonetheless be important as a substrate for changes in AD and other neurodegenerative processes with more anatomical specificity, that are age-related. Other astrocytic changes may be related to hormones [6].

Microglia are of interest because of their link as a cell type to bone marrow-derived macrophages and because of their increase in degenerating regions during PD and AD. Microglia, like astrocytes, are clustered around the amyloid-containing senile plaques, which suggest their participation in inflammatory processes [8]. Moreover, resident microglia contain mRNA for C1q, a complement protein [9]. The numbers of microglia also increase during normal aging in rat neocortex.

PLASTICITY AND AGING

How aging may impair neural plasticity is one of the major themes in the neurobiology of aging, which is pertinent to changes in memory during usual aging, as well as to the extreme deficits in AD. Sprouting is one measure of plasticity. Some neurons retain considerable capacity for sprouting, as shown by aberrant sprouting responses during AD, wherein abnormal-looking neurites appear in senile plaques and neurons sprout in response to the loss of afferents (see Chaps. 29, 45).

Receptor supersensitization shows impairment in old rodents, whereas desensitization is not impaired

Several approaches showed age changes in neuronal plasticity. The supersensitization (up-regulation) of receptors in response to chronic treatment with antagonists was smaller in aging rodents in three systems: striatal D_2 receptors, in response to haloperidol; pineal β-adrenergic receptors in response to reserpine or constant light (Randall et al., 1981, cited in [1]); and cortical muscarinic receptors in response to oxotremorine (Pedigo and Polk, 1985, cited in [37]). In contrast to impaired supersensitization, receptor down-regulation by agonists showed no age changes. Effects of aging on the regulation of receptor genes are unclear.

Aging impairs collateral sprouting in the rat hippocampus

Responses to deafferenting lesions may show age changes that are specific for brain regions and genotype or species. In view of the extensive sprouting observed in Alzheimer's disease (see Chap. 45), it is unlikely that the basic mechanics of sprouting are impaired during aging in the hippocampus. Although aging male rats show slower responses in collateral sprouting after lesions of entorhinal cortex or septum that deafferented the hippocampus (heterotypic and homotypic reinnervations), in most studies, 2-year-old rats eventually recovered as many synapses as the young after 3–6 months (see Chap. 29) [10]. Larger impairments of plasticity are shown by the superior cervical ganglia (SCG), in which explants from young rats showed 5-fold increases of substance P, whereas those from 2-year-old rats showed no elevations [11]. Autonomic changes are also shown by the impaired regulation of HSP-70 responses in blood vessels and adrenals of old rats during restraint stress [12]. Extensive heterogeneity in sprouting responses among individual old rats could be a consequence of differences in age-related disorders, such as pituitary tumors and kidney lesions, among individuals [1].

Hormonal changes are implicated in delayed responses

Many other adaptive cellular responses are slowed during aging, including induction of liver enzymes during metabolic stresses (see [1], pp. 373–377). Several genes have altered expression in liver because of age changes in the hormonal regulation, rather than through fundamental impairments in the genomic apparatus. By analogy, we may consider age changes in circulating hormones as well as locally acting paracrine and autocrine growth factors as causes of slowed sprouting responses.

One candidate is corticosterone, which slows the rate of synaptic replacement [13]. Most rat strains show a strong trend for increased blood corticosterone during aging [6,14]. In contrast, little or no change is seen in C57BL/6J mice. Gonadal steroids have complex effects on sprouting, with gender differences and interactions with adrenal steroids. Deficits of testosterone, which are common in old rats with testicular tumors, may explain the loss of vasopressin fibers in many limbic regions. The loss could be reversed in limbic regions within a month by testosterone implants [15].

NEUROTRANSMITTERS AND RECEPTORS

Brain changes in cholinergic functions are regionally specific

Age-related changes in synaptic chemistry and physiology are emerging as robust phenomena in a few neural systems, in which the scheme from gene expression to synaptic functions is partly mapped for aging changes (see Table 3). Hippocampus (HC), striatum (ST), and neuromuscular junction (NMJ) of aging rodents show different features of cholinergic aging, in conjunction with changes in anatomy and other neurotransmitters, particularly DA (Table 1). Cholinergic functions, which are quantitatively minor among other brain neurotransmitters, are intensively studied because of cholinergic hypotheses of memory deficits during normal aging and during AD.

In general, aging changes in neurotransmitters and receptors are selective in rodents and neurologically normal humans. Many changes are not consistent even in the same species, e.g., whether cholinergic forebrain neurons atrophy or hypertrophy or both (Table 2). The largest age changes,

TABLE 2. Cell atrophy and neuropathology

Age-related change	Laboratory rodents	Dog	Primate	Normal human
Cholinergic forebrain neuron				
Atrophy	++/−		0	+
Hypertrophy	+/−		+	+
Neurofibrillary tangles (NFT) in cholinergic forebrain neurons	0	0	0	+
Senile plaques with β/A4 amyloid	0	+	+	+
Cerebrovascular amyloid	0	+	++	++
Cerebrovascular arteriosclerosis	+/−	+	++	+++

TABLE 3.   Age changes in rodent striatum, hippocampus, and neuromuscular junction[a]

	Region		
	Striatum (ST)	Hippocampus (HC)	Neuromuscular junction (NMJ) (diaphragm)
A. *Neuron loss*			
Intrinsic neurons	−20% AChergic	−20% pyramidal (cholinoceptive)	
Afferent projections	−35 to 0% Nigro-striatal	−20 to 0% forebrain AChergic	negligible
B. *Dopamine system*			
Dopamine conc.	0 to −20%		
D_2R mRNA	−20%		
D_2 receptor	−10 to −50%		
DA uptake	−25 to 0%		
DA release			
K^+ induced	0		
muscarinic (M_2)	Less sensitive		
D_2	0		
C. *Cholinergic system*			
ChAT		−50 to +35%	
AChE		−25 to 0%	+35%
Muscarinic receptor			
M_1	0	0	
M_2	−40%	−50%	
M_1 mRNA	0	0	
Nicotinic receptor	−40%	−50%	+35%[b]
Choline uptake	−20 to 0%	−20 to 0%	+35%
ACh release, basal	0	0	
depolarization by K^+	−30%	−30%	
Nicotinic		Less sensitive	
M_2-autoreceptor	More sensitive	Less sensitive	
MEPP[c]			0

See [36–40] for HC and ST and [41–44] for NMJ.
[a] Data from literature compare changes in 24- to 30-month-old (life span) vs. 3- to 6-month-old (young adult) male rats and mice.
[b] α-bungarotoxin binding.
[c] Miniature end plate potentials.

however, are relatively modest by comparison with the major (>90%) loss of basal ganglia DA during PD and the variable (25–90%) loss of choline acetyltransferase (ChAT) and other cholinergic markers during AD. A key point is that receptor affinity as measured by ligand binding does not change. This implies that synaptic age changes are due to altered relative amounts of particular proteins, rather than to the ichnographic "fundamental molecular aging."

The striatum (ST) has some of the most consistent neurochemical aging changes in mammals. Progressive declines of dopamine-2 receptors (D_2-R) are shown by ligand binding in mice, rats, rabbits, and human brain and by positron emission tomographic (PET) imaging in humans. These declines can be detected during midlife, when they are not confounded by age-related pathology, and appear to be progressive, reaching net decreases of 20–40% by the life span. DA loss is smaller and more controversial in rodents than in humans, and far less than in

PD. The loss of D_2-R is paralleled by a decrease of D_2-R mRNA in aging rodents. These changes are attributed to two causes: a 20% loss of intrinsic striatal cholinergic neurons, which are a major location of the D_2 receptor, and a slowed synthesis of the D_2-R. Despite their 10–50% decrease, D_2-Rs show no age-related dysfunctions in the sensitivity of DA release to haloperidol in perfused slices. Impairments in DA-activated adenylyl cyclase are consistently reported, but there is no consensus on age changes in D_1-R.

Cholinergic controls over transmitter release show marked, but selective impairments of DA and acetylcholine (ACh) release in ST and of ACh release in hippocampus (HC) of aging rats. Most reports agree on sizable decreases in nicotinic and muscarinic M_2 binding sites in both HC and ST. Although no age changes are found in mRNAs for some M_1, M_3, M_4 in ST or in other brain regions, the mRNA for the M_2-R has not been resolved for possible effects of age. Major impairments were identified with the M_2 control of DA release. Muscarinic control of ACh release, presumably via M_2 autoreceptors, had a different pattern, with no age change in ST, but marked impairments in HC and neocortex (Fig. 2). These regional differences imply that the M_2 sites lost with aging in ST are not on local cholinergic neurons.

Postsynaptic receptor defects are implicated in several aging changes in HC and ST. Unit recordings show a repeatable decrease in sensitivity of HC neurons to ACh *in vivo* and *in vitro*. The low-affinity GTPase activity stimulated by carbachol or oxotremorine was impaired by $\geq$30% in HC and ST. Of the many G proteins, only the GTP-binding subunits $G_{\alpha i}$ and $G_{\alpha o}$ have been assayed; these

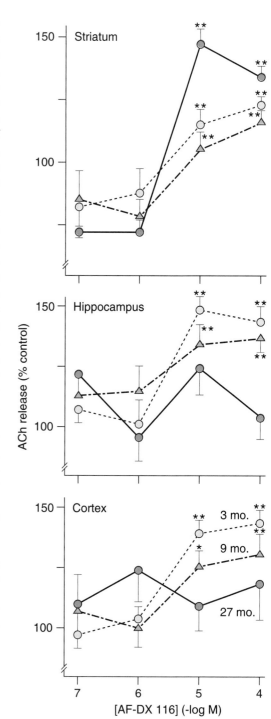

FIG. 2. ACh release by brain slices at increasing concentrations of the muscarinic agonist AF-DX 116, relative to controls (100%). Slices were taken from the indicated brain regions of male rats at the indicated ages. In cortex and hippocampus, slices from the 27-month-old rats showed no enhancement of ACh release by AF-DX 116, whereas the striatum became more sensitive. (Redrawn from Araujo et al. [36].)

showed no age change in ST or HC. In ST, in contrast to the reduced sensitivity to muscarinic agonists, the calcium ionophore A23087 or the signal transducer IP_3 (see Chap. 20) showed no age impairment in enhancing the K^+-stimulated DA release. An impairment of Ca^{2+} regulation is implied at the ligand-muscarinic receptor interface.

Moreover, there are age-related changes of intraneuronal Ca^{2+} metabolism in HC and elsewhere. For example, Ca^{2+}-dependent, K^+-mediated after-hyperpolarization increases by 50% with age, as measured in HC slices [16]. Hormonal changes in corticosteroids and other hormones may contribute to disturbances in local or even systemic Ca^{2+} and P_i homeostasis during normal aging and AD [17,18]. Renal lesions and elevations of parathyroid and calcitonin hormones are common in aging rats (see [1], pp. 516–519) and may interact with brain aging.

Recall from above that NGF treatment partially reversed the perikaryal atrophy in cholinergic projections to the HC in aging rats and also improved learning performance [5]. ChAT in the rat ST retains responsiveness to NGF throughout the life span, and may even become more sensitive [2]. In view of the lack of change in NGF mRNA in aging rats or in AD, aging in these systems may not be attributed to deficits of NGF.

The neuromuscular junction (NMJ) shows changes that vary with the muscle target and that are distinct from disuse atrophy

During aging in rats, the NMJ shows different effects of aging in the diaphragm than in a leg muscle, the extensor digitorum longus (EDL); age changes in the EDL are consistent with disuse atrophy (Table 3) [41–44]. The diaphragm shows about 35% increases in the numbers of motoneuron terminals during aging, which account for increased ACh release (spontaneous and induced), choline uptake, and expanded ACh receptor fields. The miniature end-plate potential (MEPP) firing rates did not change. The causes of increased presynaptic terminal arborization are unknown.

However, the EDL shows another type of synaptic plasticity during aging. Ultraterminal sprouts emanating from the end-plate that terminate on neighboring muscle fibers increased 4-fold during aging. Ultraterminal sprouting is characteristic of disuse atrophy and may have reached its ceiling by 2 years. Unlike the diaphragm, MEPP rates increased with age in EDL. The neurite outgrowth activity from old rats, assayed *in vitro* with chick motoneurons, was greater than from younger rats; denervation of the young EDL yielded the same activity as in the old; and denervation of the old EDL did not increase activity further.

Regionally selective receptor changes during aging show the value of resolving the types of cells and processes that may account for the local biochemical-physiological aging changes. Progress may depend on anatomic and electrophysiological data on the same rodent genotypes and genders. While impairment of synaptic plasticity may vary between neural systems with aging, the compensatory mechanisms in general preserve neural functions to a remarkable degree, despite some slowed processing of information.

AGING PIGMENTS AND MEMBRANES

Intracellular pigments (lipofuscins and neuromelanins) show cell-type specificity and little relation to neuron death

The accumulation of aging pigments or lipofuscin was historically one of the first brain aging changes to be established. These heterogeneous intracellular depots include complex lipids, lysosomal-type hydrolases, and other proteins. They slowly accumulate in myocardium and neurons throughout the body, at rates that are cell-specific (see [1], pp. 409–412). Aging pigments have a notable autofluorescence (430–470 nm) and may be an iminopropene. Despite the limited biochemistry, most distinguish *lipofuscin* aging pigments from *neuromelanins*. Neuromelanin granules accumulate from birth onward in the substantia nigra and certain other neurons of humans; in contrast, laboratory rodents do not have neuromelanins. Aging pigments show little toxicity. In the human inferior olivary nucleus, the aging pigment depots grow large enough at late ages to displace the cell nucleus. Yet, the inferior olive shows no neuron loss (see p. 629).

The accumulation rate of aging pigment may be related to cell activity. For example, in a 71-year-old woman who lost one eye when 16 years old, the alternate layers of the lateral geniculate differed in aging pigment, corresponding to the separation of optic fibers from each eye (see [1], p. 410). The protease inhibitor leupeptin rapidly causes pigment accumulation in brain and retina [19], which implicates inefficient protein degradative pathways. This fits with DeDuve's lysosomal hypothesis about the origin of aging pigments. Conversely, aging pigment accumulation is inhibited in rodents by diet restriction, vitamin E, and ergots (see [1], p. 411).

Brain membrane compositional changes may influence membrane fluidity

Membranes in many cell types are reported to show trends for complex changes in composition and biophysical properties [20,21]. Of potential importance are the "lipid substitution groups" defined by G. Rouser; e.g., cerebrosides and sphingomyelin increase at the expense of phosphatidyl choline in human brain during aging. Oligodendroglia may be a source of increased myelin, since the myelin around the pyramidal tracts continues to thicken long after maturation. A little explored issue is brain membrane fluidity, which may decrease with aging and influence receptors.

Vascular membrane changes: a relation to microperfusion?

Vascular membrane changes may also contribute to brain age changes. Cerebrovascular atherosclerosis is ubiquitous to some degree in humans, but is not recognized as a dysfunctional lesion in aging rodents. However, the microvasculature shows a general trend for increased hyalinization and PAS staining in normal human and rodent brain (Sobin, et al., 1992, cited in [2]). These histochemical changes imply alterations in basement membrane carbohydrates, which might alter local microperfusion without much change in regional blood flow.

ENERGY METABOLISM

Humans are the best characterized for resting brain metabolism during aging [22]. In neurologically normal individuals, basal cerebral glucose and oxygen consumption show modest declines of 10–30% over the life span. These decreases are in the range of decreases in cerebral blood flow and of parenchymal atrophy. Overall, age contributes much less to the total variance than intersubject variations. However, correlations in metabolism between cortical regions may be stronger in young adults than in the elderly, which implies decreased integration of cortical functions and which would be consistent with the subtle age-related alterations in cognitive functions. These changes of normal aging are clearly distinct from the larger decreases of AD.

GENE EXPRESSION

New evidence for DNA instability revives an old hypothesis

The decades-old hypothesis that aging is caused by DNA damage has not been supported by direct evidence until recently. Accumulating somatic mutations are plausible factors in age-related abnormal growths, e.g., mutations in oncogenes. Recent discoveries show two types of DNA damage in the brain: I-spots which are chemically modified DNA bases (see [1], p. 435); and mitochondrial DNA deletions (see [1], p. 447–448; (Soong, et al. *Nature Genetics* 2:318–323, 1992). Neither lesion was detected in fetal brain, and they appear to accumulate slowly during adult life. I-spots in DNA from the cell nucleus result from treatment with chemical carcinogens in tissues with dividing cells. Mitochondrial DNA deletions cause some degenerative diseases of muscle, e.g., Kearne-Sayers disease, through inhibiting oxidative phosphorylation (see Chap. 34). It is not known how either type of DNA lesion is distributed among types of brain cells.

The Brattleboro rat strain has well-known deficiencies of vasopressin, which result from a frame shift mutation that prevents intracellular processing through the translated, but abnormal C-terminal glycoprotein. However, from birth onward, the Brattleboro hypothalamus shows an increased number of solitary neurons with normal vasopressin and C-terminal glycoprotein [23]; these cells are hemizygous for the mutant and revertant protein (Fig. 3). cDNA cloned by PCR from older Brattleboro rats showed clusters of frame shift revertant cells (F. van Leewen, *personal communication*). These remarkable findings imply the reverse process through which normal genes could become damaged at a slow rate to yield hemizygous mutant neurons or glia.

Demethylation of the rare nuclear DNA dinucleotide ^{Me}CpG during aging may be important in changes in gene expression. Loss of ^{Me}C in many vertebrate cells during differentiation is often correlated with increased gene expression. Several reports show age-related loss of methylation from nuclear DNA (see [1], pp. 369–370). A comparison of brain DNA demethylation in two species showed progressive loss of ^{Me}C that was faster in laboratory mice, which live half as long as *Peromyscus leucopus* (white-footed mice). Age-related loss of ^{Me}C could alter transcription by changing interactions of ^{Me}C-containing sequences with DNA-binding proteins.

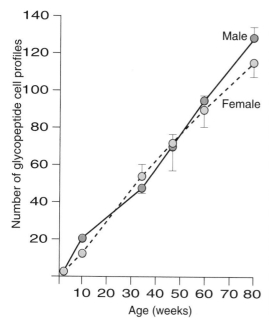

FIG. 3.   The age-related increase of vasopressin-immunopositive hypothalamic neurons of Brattleboro rats, which have a frame-shift mutation in the vasopressin gene. Immunopositive neurons are represented by an increase of glycopeptide. All profiles on the ordinate axis. (Redrawn from van Leewen et al. [23].)

mRNA synthesis shows cell-type selectivity

The evidence for selectivity in neuron atrophy strongly argues against major impairment of transcription during aging. In fact, the evidence is now very strong that most changes in transcription are highly selective and differ between cell types. The contrary belief was fairly general in the recent past, which we challenged by assaying the sequence complexity of brain polysomal poly-(A)RNA populations. Assay by saturation hybridization of mRNA to single copy DNA estimates the number of different mRNA types (complexity). During development, brain and other organs show major shifts in mRNA subsets. However, we did not detect changes in whole brain mRNA mass or complexity during the life span of two rat strains [24]. Moreover, most brain cells appear unchanged even in advanced AD, where only a minor fraction of neurons degenerate. Cell-type specifying mRNAs must persist to maintain the proteins upon which cytoarchitectonics depend. Two examples of mRNA changes are discussed.

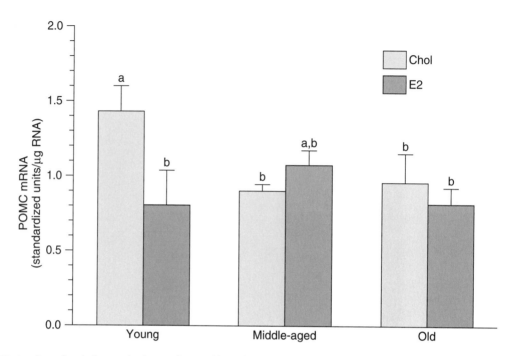

FIG. 4. Age-related changes in the regulation of hypothalamic POMC mRNA by E2. Ovariectomized C57BL/6J mice of 3 ages (young, 4 mos.; middle-aged, 13 mos.; old, 25 mos.) were given 3 days of implants with *CHOL* (cholesterol) or *E2* (estradiol; physiological levels). The middle-aged and old mice had lower levels of POMC mRNA and that did not decrease further with E2. (Redrawn from Karelus and Nelson [25].)

POMC is of interest as a hormonally regulated neuropeptide precursor that decreases with aging in mice and rats [25]. Because estrogen influences POMC transcription and because of decreased ovarian estrogen production during aging (see pp. 628–629), it was necessary to control for changes in hormone status. Hypothalamic POMC mRNA responsiveness to estrogen is lost at middle-age (Fig. 4), when hypothalamic controls on the pituitary-ovary axis are also impaired (see [1], pp. 182–185). These data also show the importance of including intermediate ages to resolve whether the age change was progressive, related to maturation, or to old age.

In contrast to the decline of POMC mRNA, recall from the section entitled "Aging impairs collateral sprouting in the rat hippocampus" (p. 631) that GFAP mRNA increases with age in hippocampus. The cause here is in association with the as-

trocytic hyperactivity of aging. Hormones may have a role here as in POMC, since GFAP expression is influenced by sex steroids, adrenal steroids, and TGF (transforming growth factor)-β1. These steroids show changes with age in rodents and/or humans, while TGFβ-1 mRNA increases with aging in hippocampus (Nichols, N.R., Johnson, S.A., Finch, C.E. *Soc. Neurosci. Abstr.* 18:1486, 1992).

Steroid receptor regulation may be a factor in neuroendocrine changes

Age changes in gene expression may involve alteration in sex steroid receptors and other nuclear proteins that bind to specific DNA sequences as trans-acting regulators of transcription. Estrogen receptors (E_2-R) consistently decrease in number in the hypothalamus of aging female rodents [25,26]. A 35% loss of neurons containing β-endorphin suggests that neuron loss could be a factor, since these neurons also contain E_2-R. Moreover, the nuclear retention of E_2 is shorter in middle-aged female mice, which suggests the hypothesis that altered nuclear receptor dynamics cause the failure of E_2 to induce POMC (Fig. 4). In turn, dysregulation of POMC could impair the LH surge in middle-aged rats.

The two receptors for adrenal steroids are being studied during aging: type I, mineralocorticoid receptor; type II, glucocorticoid receptor. Both types show fairly consistent 35% decreases in hippocampus of aging male rats [14,27,28]. The loss of receptors may be greatest in the pyramidal layers, which also show neuron loss. In the male rat hypothalamus, type II receptors are also lost [28]. Major open questions in transcriptional regulation in the brain during aging are the contributions of neuron loss to receptor decreases and whether there are age changes in the interactions of receptors and DNA response elements.

PROTEINS

Altered proteins may increase through oxidative damage

Oxidation of proteins is emerging as prominent in aging. In mammals, flies, and nematodes, a portion of cellular enzymes becomes oxidized and inactive, although immunologically detectable (see [1], pp. 398–400; [29]). Free radical-mediated oxidation may inactivate enzymes in brain and other tissues. Moreover, PBN, a free radical quencher, reversed protein oxidation in brains of middle-aged gerbils and also improved learning [30]. The cause of oxidation and other post-translational modifications during aging is unknown, but may include altered intracellular redox environment and slowed protein synthesis.

Slowing of protein synthesis could be a factor in slowed axoplasmic flow

Many studies conclude from the incorporation of amino acids that protein synthesis is slowed with age in brain and other organs of rodents by 20–50% (see [1], pp. 370–373). The slowed axoplasmic transport in the sciatic nerve [31] is also generally consistent with slowed protein synthesis. However, because few brain mRNAs or enzymes show decreases with age, the rates of degradation must also be slowed to maintain steady state. Another outcome of slowed turnover might be the accumulation of intraneuronal proteins, such as neurofibrillary proteins in AD.

EXPERIMENTAL MANIPULATIONS OF BRAIN AGING

Diet restriction and hypophysectomy delay aging in many organs of rodents

Diet has major influences on aging in rodents, as represented by slowed aging in many peripheral tissues from chronic hypophysectomy or diet restriction (see [1], Chap. 10; [32]). In brain, diet restriction slowed the loss of D_2-R in aging rats. Both diet restriction and hypophysectomy also slow a demyelinating disease of spinal roots in aging rats (radiculoneuropathy) that may cause hind limb paralysis. Diet restriction also reduces the amount of oxidized enzymes and increases the life span (see [1], pp. 512–535; [32]). The mechanisms are unclear, but could arise from common effects of hypophysectomy and diet restriction on glucose metabolism.

Some hypothalamic and hippocampal aging changes are linked to steroid exposure

Two steroids are also implicated in region-specific physiological and anatomical changes during aging in rodents: estradiol and corticosterone. In the hypothalamus of female mice and rats, chronic exposure to endogenous ovarian steroids, presumably estrogens, impairs the preovulatory gonadotropin surge in association with the loss of estrous cycles at midlife (see [1], pp.

543–545). Ovariectomy of young rodents slows many hypothalamic and pituitary age changes, most of which can also be prematurely induced by chronic exposure of young rodents to exogenous estradiol. We do not know the cell type(s) that mediate these effects of estradiol and the role of neuron death vs. synaptic remodeling. There is no clear analog of estrogen-dependent hypothalamic aging in women, since a preovulatory-like surge can be induced in postmenopausal women.

Certain features of hippocampal aging show adrenocorticosteroid-dependent aging with similar bidirectional responses to experimental manipulations. Pyramidal neuron damage and astrocytosis during aging in male rats is slowed by adrenalectomy and conversely is accelerated by exposure to stress or glucocorticoids [6,14]. As in the effects of estradiol in the hypothalamus, we do not know which hippocampal cells mediate these effects of stress or corticosterone. However, adrenalectomy partly reduced the Ca^{2+}-dependent afterhyperpolarization in pyramidal neurons [14]. This and other findings suggest that corticosteroids could interact with cytotoxic effects of Ca^{2+} [6,14]. The role of life-long exposure to endogenous corticosteroids is further shown by the improved cognitive performance and lesser neuron loss during aging in rats that were neonatally handled and that also had lower basal blood corticosterone (see Chap. 49).

MAMMALS ARE NOT THE ONLY ANIMAL MODELS FOR AGING!

Mammals are not the only animals to show defined aging changes. Domestic fowl show aging in neuroendocrine functions in which hypothalamic changes are implicated [33]; genotypic influences on reproductive decline and altered monamine metabolism are topics of interest for comparison with mammals. There are also major opportunities for studies on invertebrates that show evidence

for aging in the nervous system: *Drosophila* (life span 2 months), soil nematodes (*Caenorhabditis,* life span, 1 month), and molluscs (*Aplysia californica,* life span 9–12 months; *Lymnaea stagnalis* [pond snail], life span 24–30 months). Much is known about neural changes with aging in molluscs. *Aplysia* shows major changes in reproduction and in behavior, during which the mRNA for egg-laying hormone (ELH) increased 25-fold in abdominal ganglia, while that for FMRFamide may decrease; in motor systems, neurons that show the least decrement during aging are also those that are the least plastic in young animals [34]. *Lymnaea* also has aging changes in neuroendocrine functions (see [1], pp. 131–132).

Although little is known about neural aging in *Drosophila,* its superb genetics are helping to analyze the functions of the β-amyloid precursor protein (β-APP): A gene knockout of a related protein gave viable flies with changed phototaxis that was reversible by the human APP_{695} [35]. Moreover, the flies can be selected for life span on the basis of the reproductive schedule (work of M. Rose, reviewed in [1]). Nematodes also offer superb genetics of life spans; again, virtually nothing is known about cellular aging (T. Johnson, in [1], pp. 300–304). Both flies and nematodes show marked changes in locomotion at later ages.

In choosing a mammalian model, one must keep in mind that rodents and primates represent different evolutionary selections for reproductive schedules. Additionally, there are 30–40 millions of years since the divergence of mice from rats, or of rhesus from humans. The neuropathology of aging differs among mammals (Table 2). Although rodents are well justified as short-lived models by practicality, the genetic differences between rodents and humans could cause many species differences in responses to interventions.

Many argue for inbred strains of mice or rats to minimize the risk that the young and old individuals represent slightly different genotypes. Moreover, inbred strains favor replication of results between laboratories. Few brain age changes have been verified by different laboratories using the same rodent genotype. There is reason to extend findings from inbreds to hybrids and outbreds, to avoid bias by one genotype. The NIA provides investigators with several different common strains and F1 hybrids from mice and rats; adult ages across the life span are provided at a subsidized cost.

The largest variety of genotypes is available in mice, which continues to be the favored mammalian model for genetic approaches. The life span of most "normal" strains is 24–36 months; anything less than 20 months indicates specific pathology, not accelerated aging. The differences between genotypes mostly influence the type or rate of progression of pathological lesions, such as benign tumors, kidney diseases, ectopic calcification, and organ amyloid deposits (see [1], Chaps. 6 and 10). No genotype shows a uniform acceleration of aging processes. Similarly, the progerias in humans represent genetic disorders with segmental

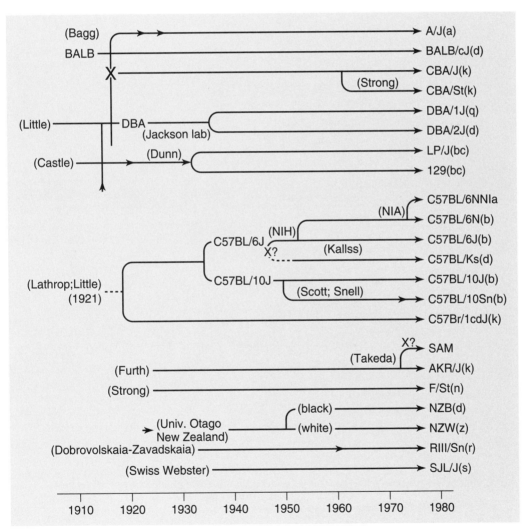

FIG. 5.   Origins of mouse strains that are commonly used for studies of aging. The histocompatibility allele set (H-2 haplotype) is given in parenthesis on the right margin. (Reproduced with permission of the University of Chicago Press, from Finch [1].)

or mosaic features of aging. Senescence-accelerated mice (SAM) develop systemic amyloid deposits in the liver with no relation to the amyloid of AD, periodic acid-Schiff-positive deposits in the hippocampus, and behavioral change during their 1 year life spans; SAM mice have a mutant serum lipoprotein (see [1], pp. 334–335). Lineages of mouse strains commonly used for studies on aging are in Fig. 5.

The growing interface between research on the immune and nervous systems is beginning to impact on the neurobiology of aging, e.g., in the recognition that complement and other inflammatory mediators are present in lesions of AD [8,9] and that the main histocompatibility complex (MHC) influences age changes in reproduction and immune functions (see [1], Chap. 6). Use of inbred mice that were developed for immunogenetics could help in analyzing inflammatory features of normal and pathological aging and the many interactions of glycoproteins encoded in the MHC.

PROSPECTS

The neurobiology of aging offers many emerging questions for biochemical and molecular biology studies. There is now a database of independently replicated observations for a wide range of animal models. The approaching avalanche of information on genes expressed in nervous tissues will yield much to analyze for mechanisms of aging. These molecular approaches should reveal the circuits of gene regulation which determine for a given genotype which cells are destined to degenerate, as well as the physiological circuits that maintain brain functions throughout the life span.

REFERENCES

1. Finch, C. E. *Longevity, Senescence, and the Genome.* Chicago: University of Chicago Press, 1990.

2. Finch, C. E. Neuron atrophy during aging: programmed or sporadic. *Trends Neurosci.* 16:104–111, 1993.

3. Finch, C. E., and Morgan, D. G. RNA and protein metabolism in the aging brain. *Annu. Rev. Neurosci.* 13:75–87, 1990.

4. Pasinetti, G. M., Osterburg, H. H., Kelly, A. B., Kohama, S., Morgan, D. G., Rheinhard, J. F. Jr., Stellwagen, R. H., Finch, C. E. Slow changes of tyrosine hydroxylase gene expression in dopaminergic neurons after neurotoxin lesioning: a model for neuron aging. *Mol. Brain Res.* 13:63–73, 1992.

5. Fischer, W., Bjorklund, A., Chen, K., and Gage, F. H. NGF improves spatial memory in aged rodents as a function of age. *J. Neurosci.* 11:1889–1906, 1991.

6. Landfield, P. W., Waymire, J. L., and Lynch, G. Hippocampal aging and adrenocorticoids: quantitative correlations. *Science* 202:1098–1102, 1978.

7. Day, J. R., Laping, N J., Johnson, S. A., Finch, C. E. GFAP mRNA increases with age in rat and human brain. *Neurobiol. Aging* 14 [*in press*], 1993.

8. McGeer, P. L., and Rogers, J. Anti-inflammatory agents as a therapeutic approach to Alzheimer's disease. *Neurology* 42:447–449, 1992.

9. Johnson, S. A., Lampert-Etchells, M., Rozovsky, I., Pasinetti, G. M., Finch, C. E. Complement mRNA in the mammalian brain: responses to Alzheimer's disease and experimental lesions. *Neurobiol. Aging* 13:641–648, 1992.

10. Anderson, K. J., Scheff, S. W., and DeKosky, S. T. Reactive synaptogenesis in hippocampal area CA1 of aged and young adult rats. *J. Comp Neurol.* 252:374–384, 1986.

11. Adler, J. E., Black, I. B. Plasticity of substance P in mature and aged sympathetic neurons in culture. *Science* 225:1499–1500, 1984.

12. Blake, M. J., Udelsman, R., Feulner, C. J., Norton, D. D., Holbrook, N. J. Stress-induced HSP-70 expression in adrenal cortex: a glucocorticoid sensitive, age-dependent response. *Proc. Natl. Acad. Sci. USA* 88:9873–9877, 1991.

13. Scheff, S. W., Hoff, S. F., and Anderson, K. J. Altered regulation of lesion-induced synaptogenesis by adrenalectomy and corticosterone in young adult rats. *Exp. Neurol.* 93:456–470, 1986.

14. Sapolsky, R. M. *Stress, the Aging Brain, and the Mechanisms of Neuron Death.* Cambridge, MA: MIT Press, 1992.

15. Goudsmit, E., Fliers, E., and Swaab, D. F. Testosterone supplementation restores vasopressin innervation in the senescent rat brain. *Brain Res.* 473:306–313, 1988.

16. Kerr, S. D., Campbell, L. W., Hao, S.-Y., and Landfield, P. W. Corticosteroid modulation of hippocampal potentials: increased effect with aging. *Science* 245:1505–1509, 1989.

17. Landfield, P. W., Applegate, M. D., Schmitzer-Osborne, S. E., and Naylor, C. E. Phosphate/calcium alterations in the first stages of Alzheimer's disease: implications for etiology and pathogenesis. *J. Neurol. Sci.* 106:221–229, 1991.

18. Landfield, P. W. Calcium homeostasis in brain aging. *Diagnosis and Treatment of Senile Dementia.* In Bergener, M., Reisberg, B. (eds), Berlin: Springer-Verlag, 1989, pp. 276–287.

19. Ivy, G. O., Schottler, F., Wenzel, J., Baudry, M., and Lynch, G. Inhibitors of lysosomal enzymes: accumulation of lipofuscin-like dense bodies in the brain. *Science* 226:985–987, 1984.

20. Naeim, F., and Walford, R. L. Aging and cell membrane complexes: The lipid bilayer, integral proteins, and cytoskeleton. In C. E. Finch and E. L. Schneider (eds.), *Handbook of the Biology of Aging,* 2d Ed. New York: Van Nostrand, 1985, pp. 272–289.

21. Finch, C. E. Neuroendocrine and autonomic aspects of aging. In C. E. Finch and L. Hayflick (eds.), *Handbook of the Biology of Aging.* New York: Van Nostrand, 1977, pp. 262–280.

22. Grady, C. L., and Rapoport, S. I. Cerebral metabolism in aging and dementia. In J. E. Birren, R. B. Sloane, and G. D. Cohen (eds.), *Handbook of Mental Health and Aging,* 2nd Ed. New York: Academic Press, 1992, pp. 201–228.

23. van Leewen, F., van der Beek, E., Seger, M., Burbach, P., and Ivell, R. Age-related development of a heterozygous phenotype in solitary neurons of the homozygous Brattleboro rat. *Proc. Natl. Acad. Sci. U.S.A.* 86:6417–6420, 1989.

24. Colman, P. C., Kaplan, B. B., Osterburg, H. H., and Finch, C. E. Brain poly(A)RNA during aging: stability of yield and sequence complexity in two rat strains. *J. Neurochem.* 34:335–345, 1980.

25. Karelus, K., and Nelson, J. F. Aging impairs estrogenic suppression of hypothalamic pro-opiomelanocortin mRNA in the mouse. *Neuroendocrinology* 55:627–633, 1992.

26. Wise, P. M., and Parsons, B. Nuclear estradiol and cytosol progestin receptor concentrations in the brain and pituitary gland and sexual behavior in ovariectomized estradiol-treated middle-aged rats. *Endocrinology* 115:810–816, 1984.

27. Van Eekelen, J. A. M., Rots, N. Y., Sutanto, W., Oitzl, M. S., and DeKloet, E. R. Brain corticosteroid receptor gene expression and neuroendocrine dynamics during aging. *J. Steroid Biochem. Mol. Biol.* 40:679–683, 1991.

28. Eldridge, C. J., Fleenor, D. G., Kerr, S. D., and Landfield, P. W. Impaired up-regulation of type II corticosteroid receptors in hippocampus of aged rats. *Brain Res.* 478:248–256, 1989.

29. Stadtman, E. R. Protein oxidation and aging. *Science* 257:1220–1224, 1992.

30. Floyd, R. A. Oxidative damage to behavior during aging. *Science* 254:1597, 1991.

31. McQuarrie, I. G., Brady, S. T., and Lasek, R. J. Retardation in the slow axonal transport of cytoskeletal elements during maturation and aging. *Neurobiol. Aging* 10:359–365, 1989.

32. Weindruch, R. H., and Walford, R. L. *The Retardation of Aging and Disease by Dietary Restriction.* Springfield, IL: CC Thomas, 1986.

33. Ottinger, M. A. Neuroendocrine and behavioral determinants of reproductive aging. *Crit. Rev. Poultry Biol.* 3:131–142, 1991.

34. Kindy, M. S., Srivatsan, M., and Peretz, B. Age-related differential expression of neuropeptide mRNAs in Aplysia. *NeuroReport* 2:465–468, 1991.

35. Luo, L., Tully, T., and White, K. Human amyloid precursor protein ameliorates behavioral deficit of flies deleted for *Appl* gene. *Neuron* 9:595–605, 1992.

36. Araujo, D. M., Lapchak, P. A., Meany, M. J., Collier, B., and Quirion, R. Effects of aging on nicotinic and muscarinic autoreceptor function in the rat brain: relationship to presynaptic cholinergic markers and binding sites. *J. Neurosci.* 10:3069–3078, 1990.

37. Decker, M. W. The effects of aging on hippocampal and cortical projections of the forebrain cholinergic system. *Brain Res. Rev.* 12:423–438, 1987.

38. Joseph, J. A., Roth, G. S., and Strong, R. The striatum, a microcosm for the examination of age-related alterations in the CNS: a selected review. *Rev. Biol. Res. Aging* 4:181–199, 1990.

39. Joseph, J. A., and Roth, G. S. Loss of muscar-

inic regulation of striatal dopamine function in senescence. *Neurochem. Int.* 20[Suppl.]: 237S–240S, 1992.

40. Morgan, D. G., and May, P. C. Age-related changes in synaptic neurochemistry. In E. L. Schneider and J. W. Rowe (eds.), *Handbook of the Biology of Aging,* 3rd Ed. San Diego: Academic Press, 1990, pp. 219–254.

41. Randall, P. K., and Fahim, M. A. Model systems in electrophysiological aging research. *Rev. Biol. Res. Aging* 2:211–226, 1985.

42. Smith, D. O. Muscle-specific decrease in pre-synaptic calcium dependence and clearance during neuromuscular transmission in aged rats. *J. Neurophysiol.* 59:1069–1082, 1988.

43. Smith, D. O. Acetylcholine synthesis and release in the extensor digitorum longus muscle of mature and aged rats. *J. Neurochem.* 54: 1433–1439, 1990.

44. Smith, D. O., and Emmerling, M. Biochemical and physiological consequences of an age-related increase in acetylcholinesterase activity at the rat neuromuscular junction. *J. Neurosci.* 8:3011–3017, 1988.

CHAPTER 31

Circulation and Energy Metabolism of the Brain

DONALD D. CLARKE AND LOUIS SOKOLOFF

Basic Neurochemistry: Molecular, Cellular, and Medical Aspects, 5th Ed., edited by G. J. Siegel et al. Published by Raven Press, Ltd., New York, 1994. Correspondence to Donald D. Clarke, Chemistry Department, Fordham University, Bronx, New York 10458.

The biochemical pathways of energy metabolism in the brain are in most respects like those of other tissues, but special conditions peculiar to the central nervous system *in vivo* limit full expression of its biochemical potentialities. In no tissue are the discrepancies between *in vivo* and *in vitro* properties greater, or the extrapolations from *in vitro* data to conclusions about *in vivo* metabolic functions more hazardous. Valid identification of the normally used substrates and products of cerebral energy metabolism, as well as reliable estimations of their rates of utilization and production, can be obtained only in the intact animal; *in vitro* studies serve to identify pathways of intermediary metabolism, mechanisms, and potential rather than actual performance.

Although it is sometimes stated that the brain is unique among tissues in its high rate of oxidative metabolism, the overall cerebral metabolic rate for O_2 ($CMRO_2$) is of the same order as the unstressed heart and renal cortex [1]. Regional metabolic fluxes in brain may greatly exceed $CMRO_2$, however, and these are closely coupled to fluctuations in metabolic demand.

INTERMEDIARY METABOLISM

ATP production in brain is highly regulated

Oxidative steps of carbohydrate metabolism normally contribute 36 of the 38 high-energy phosphate bonds (~P) generated during the aerobic metabolism of a single glucose molecule. Approximately 15 percent of brain glucose is converted to lactate and does not enter the Krebs (citric acid) cycle. There are indications, however, that this might be matched by a corresponding uptake of ketone bodies. The total net gain of high-energy phosphate (~P) is 33 equivalents per mole of glucose utilized. The steady-state level of adenosine triphosphate (ATP) is high and represents the sum of very rapid synthesis and utilization. On average, half of the terminal phosphate groups turn over in approximately 3 sec; in certain regions, turnover is probably considerably faster [2]. The level of ~P is kept constant by regulation of adenosine diphosphate (ADP) phosphorylation in relation to ATP hydrolysis. The active adenylate kinase reaction, which forms equivalent amounts of ATP and adenosine monophosphate (AMP) from ADP, prevents any great accumulation of ADP. Only a small amount of AMP is present under steady-state conditions; consequently, a relatively small percentage decrease in ATP may lead to a relatively large percentage increase in AMP. Since AMP is a positive modulator of several reactions that lead to increased ATP synthesis, such an amplification factor provides a sensitive control for maintenance of ATP levels [3]. Between 37° and 42°C, brain metabolic rate increases at a rate of approximately 5 percent per degree.

The level of creatine phosphate in brain

is even higher than that of ATP, and creatine phosphokinase is extremely active. The creatine phosphate level is exquisitely sensitive to changes in oxygenation, providing ~P for ADP phosphorylation and thus maintaining ATP levels. The creatine phosphokinase system may also function in regulating mitochondrial activity. In cells with a very heterogenous mitochondrial distribution, such as neurons, the creatine phosphate shuttle may play a critical role in energy transport [4]. The BB isoenzyme of creatine kinase is characteristic of, but not confined to, brain. Thus the presence of BB in body fluids does not necessarily indicate disruption of neural tissue.

Glycogen is a dynamic, but limited, energy store in brain

Although present in relatively low concentration in brain (3.3 mmol/kg brain in rat), glycogen is a unique energy reserve that requires no energy (ATP) for initiation of its metabolism. As with glucose, glycogen levels in brain appear to vary with plasma glucose concentrations. Brain biopsies have shown that human brain contains much higher glycogen levels than rodent brain, but the effects of anesthesia and pathological changes in the biopsied tissue may have contributed to these high levels. Glycogen granules have been seen in electron micrographs of glia and neurons of immature animals but only in astrocytes of adults. Barbiturates decrease brain metabolism and increase the number of granules seen, particularly in astrocytes of synaptic regions; however, biochemical studies show that neurons do contain glycogen and that enzymes for its synthesis and metabolism are present in synaptosomes. Astrocyte glycogen may form a store of carbohydrate made available to neurons by still undefined mechanisms. Associated with the granules are enzymes concerned with glycogen synthesis and, perhaps, degradation. The increased glycogen found in areas of brain injury may be due to glial changes or to decreased utilization during tissue preparation.

The accepted role of glycogen is that of a carbohydrate reserve utilized when glucose falls below need. However, there is a rapid, continual breakdown and synthesis of glycogen (19 μmol/kg/min). This is approximately 2 percent of the normal glycolytic flux in brain and is subject to elaborate control mechanisms. This suggests that, even under steady-state conditions, local carbohydrate reserves are important for brain function. If glycogen were the sole supply, however, the normal glycolytic flux in brain would be maintained for less than 5 min.

The enzyme systems that synthesize and catabolize glycogen in other tissues are also found in brain, but their kinetic properties and modes of regulation appear to differ [5]. Glycogen metabolism in brain, unlike in other tissues, is controlled locally. It is isolated from the tumult of systemic activity, evidently because of the blood-brain barrier (BBB). Although glucocorticoid hormones that penetrate the BBB increase glycogen turnover, circulating protein hormones and biogenic amines are without effect. Beyond the BBB, cells are sensitive to local amine levels; drugs that penetrate the BBB and modify local amine levels or membrane receptors thus cause metabolic changes (see Chap. 32).

Separate systems for the synthesis and degradation of glycogen provide a greater degree of control than would be the case were glycogen degraded by simply reversing the steps in its synthesis (Fig. 1). The level of glucose-6-phosphate, the initial synthetic substrate, usually varies inversely with the rate of brain glycolysis because of greater facilitation of the phosphofructokinase step relative to transport and phosphorylation of glucose. Thus a decline in glucose-6-phosphate at times of energy need decreases glycogen formation.

The glucosyl group of uridine diphosphoglucose (UDP-glucose) is transferred to the terminal glucose of the nonreducing end of an amylose chain in an α-1,4-glycosidic

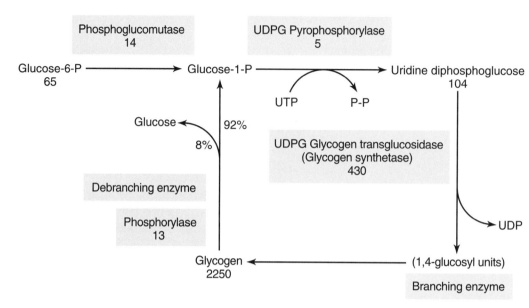

FIG. 1.   Glycogen metabolism in brain. Enzyme data from mouse brain homogenates. Numerals below each enzyme represent V_{max} at 38°C (in mmol/kg wet weight/min); metabolite levels from quick-frozen adult mouse brain in μmol/kg wet weight; (P-P) pyrophosphate. (Metabolic data from J. V. Passoneau et al., *J. Biol. Chem.* 244:902, 1969; enzyme data from B. M. Breckenridge and P. D. Gatfield, *J. Neurochem.* 3:234, 1961.)

linkage (Fig. 1). This reaction is catalyzed by glycogen synthetase and is the rate controlling reaction in glycogen synthesis [5]. In brain, as in other tissues, glycogen synthetase occurs in both a phosphorylated (D) form, which is dependent for activity on glucose-6-phosphate as a positive modulator, and a dephosphorylated, independent (I) form sensitive to, but not dependent on, the modulator. Although in brain the independent form of the glycogen synthetase requires no stimulator, it has a relatively low affinity for UDP-glucose. At times of increased energy demand, not only is there a change from the dependent to the independent form, but also an independent form with even lower affinity for the substrate develops. The inhibition of glycogen synthesis is enhanced, and this increases the availability of glucose-6-phosphate for energy needs. Goldberg and O'Toole [5] hypothesize that the independent form in brain is associated with inhibition of glycogen synthesis under conditions of energy demand, whereas the dependent form is responsible for a relatively small regu-

lated synthesis under resting conditions. Regulation of the dependent form may be responsible for reducing the rate of glycogen formation in brain to approximately 5 percent of its potential rate. In liver, where large amounts of glycogen are synthesized and degraded, the independent form of the synthetase is associated with glycogen formation. At the present time, it appears that the two tissues use the same biochemical apparatus in different ways in relation to differences in overall metabolic patterns.

   Under steady-state conditions, it is probable that less than 10 percent of phosphorylase in brain (Fig. 1) is in the unphosphorylated *b* form (requiring AMP), which is inactive at the very low AMP concentrations present normally. When the steady state is disturbed, there may be an extremely rapid conversion of the enzyme to the *a* form, which is active at low AMP levels. Brain phosphorylase *b* kinase is indirectly activated by cAMP and by the micromolar levels of Ca^{2+} released during neuronal excitation (see Chap. 22). Endoplasmic reticulum of brain, like that in muscle, is capable of taking up Ca²⁺ to terminate its stimulatory effect. These reactions provide energy from glycogen during excitation and when cAMP-forming systems are activated. It has not been possible to confirm directly, however, that the conversion from phosphorylase *b* to *a* is a control point of glycogenolysis *in vivo*. Norepinephrine and, probably, dopamine activate glycogenolysis through cAMP; but epinephrine, vasopressin, and angiotensin II do so by another mechanism, possibly involving Ca²⁺ or a Ca²⁺-mediated proteolysis of the phosphorylase kinase.

Hydrolysis of the α-1,4-glycoside linkages leaves a limit dextrin that turns over at only half the rate of the outer chains (see also Chap. 34). The debrancher enzyme that hydrolyzes the α-1,6-glycoside linkages may be rate limiting if the entire glycogen granule is to be utilized. Because one product of this enzyme is free glucose, approximately one glucose molecule for every eleven of glucose-6-phosphate is released if the entire glycogen molecule is degraded (Fig. 1). α-Glucosidase (acid maltase) is a lysosomal enzyme whose precise function in glycogen metabolism is not known. In Pompe's disease (the hereditary absence of α-glucosidase), glycogen accumulates in brain as well as elsewhere (Chap. 34). The steady-state level of glycogen is regulated precisely by the coordination of synthetic and degradative processes through enzymatic regulation at several metabolic steps [6].

Brain glycolysis is regulated mainly by hexokinase and phosphofructokinase

Aerobic and anaerobic glycolysis have been historically defined as the amount of lactate produced under conditions of "adequate" oxygen and no oxygen, respectively. More recently, glycolysis refers to the Embden-Meyerhoff glycolytic sequence from glucose (or glycogen glucosyl) to pyruvate. Glycolytic flux is defined indirectly—It is the rate at which glucose must be utilized to produce the observed rate of ADP phosphorylation.

Figure 2 outlines the flow of glycolytic substrates in brain. Glycolysis first involves phosphorylation by hexokinase. The reaction is essentially irreversible and is a key point in the regulation of carbohydrate metabolism in brain. The electrophoretically slow-moving (type I) isoenzyme of hexokinase is characteristic of brain. In most tissues, hexokinase may exist in the cytosol (soluble), or it may be firmly attached to mitochondria. Under conditions in which no special effort is made to stop metabolism while isolating mitochondria, 80 to 90 percent of brain hexokinase is bound. In the live steady state, however, when availability of substrate keeps up with metabolic demand and end products are removed, an equilibrium exists between the soluble and the bound enzyme. Binding changes the kinetic properties of hexokinase and its inhibition by glucose-6-phosphate, so that the bound enzyme on mitochondria is more active. The extent of binding is inversely related to the ATP/ADP ratio, so that conditions in which energy utilization exceeds supply shift the solubilization equilibrium to the bound form and produce a greater potential capacity for initiating glycolysis to meet the energy demand. This mechanism allows ATP to function both as the substrate of the enzyme and, at another site, as a regulator to decrease ATP production through its influence on enzyme binding. It also confers preference on glucose in the competition for the MgATP²⁻ generated by mitochondrial oxidative phosphorylation. Thus a process that will sustain ATP production continues at the expense of other uses of energy. Because energy reserves are rapidly exhausted postmortem, it is not surprising that brain hexokinase is found to be almost entirely bound.

The significance of reversible binding of other enzymes to mitochondria is not clear. The measured glycolytic flux, when compared with the maximal velocity of hexokinase, indicates that, in the steady state, the hexokinase reaction is 97 percent inhibited. Brain hexokinase is inhibited by its product glucose-6-phosphate, and to a lesser extent

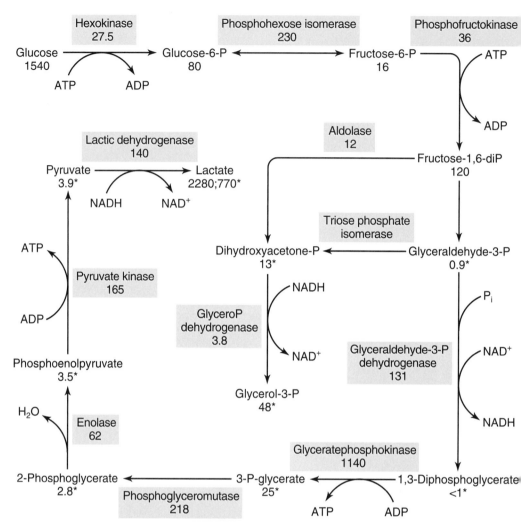

FIG. 2. Glycolysis in brain. Enzyme and metabolic data expressed as in Fig. 1; (*) 10-day-old mouse brain (Matchinski, 1970). (Data from H. McIlwain, *Biochemistry and the Central Nervous System,* Boston: Little, Brown, 1966, pp. 1–26; F. M. Matchinski, *Adv. Biochem. Psychopharmacol.* 2:217–243, 1970.)

by ADP and allosterically by 3-phosphoglycerate and several nucleoside phosphates, including cAMP and free ATP^{4-}. The ratio of ATP to Mg^{2+} may also have a regulatory action. In addition to acting on enzyme kinetics, glucose-6-phosphate solubilizes hexokinase, thus reducing the enzyme's efficiency when the reaction product accumulates. The sum total of these mechanisms is a fine tuning of the activity of the initial enzyme in glycolysis in response to changes in cellular environment. Glucokinase (low-affinity hex-

okinase), a major component of liver hexokinase, has not been found in brain.

Glucose-6-phosphate represents a branch point in metabolism because it is a common substrate for enzymes involved in glycolytic, pentose phosphate shunt and glycogen-forming pathways. There is also slight, but detectable, glucose-6-phosphatase activity in brain, the significance of which is not clear. The liver requires this enzyme to convert glycogen to glucose. The differences between liver and brain hexokinase and the differences between modes of glycogen metabolism of these two tissues can be related to the function of liver as a carbohydrate storehouse for the body, whereas brain metabolism is adapted for rapid carbohydrate utilization for energy needs. In glycolysis, glucose-6-phosphate is the substrate of phosphohexose isomerase. This is a reversible reaction (small free energy change) whose 5:1 equilibrium ratio in brain favors glucose-6-phosphate.

Fructose-6-phosphate is the substrate of phosphofructokinase, a key regulatory enzyme controlling glycolysis [3]. The other substrate is $MgATP^{2-}$. Like other regulatory reactions, it is essentially irreversible. It is modulated by a large number of metabolites and cofactors whose concentrations under different metabolic conditions have a great effect on glycolytic flux. Prominent among these are availability of ~P and citrate levels. Brain phosphofructokinase is inhibited by ATP, Mg, and citrate and is stimulated by NH_4^+, K^+, PO_4^{3-}, 5'-AMP, 3',5',-cyclic AMP, ADP, and fructose-1,6-bisphosphate.

When oxygen is admitted to cells metabolizing anaerobically, utilization of O_2 increases, whereas utilization of glucose and production of lactate drop (Pasteur effect). Modulation of the phosphofructokinase reaction can account directly for the Pasteur effect. In the steady state, ATP and citrate levels in brain apparently are sufficient to keep phosphofructokinase relatively inhibited as long as the level of positive modulators (or disinhibitors) is low. When the steady state is disturbed, activation of this enzyme produces an increase in glycolytic flux that takes place almost as fast as events changing the internal milieu.

Fructose-1,6-bisphosphate is split by brain aldolase to glyceraldehyde-3-phosphate and dihydroxyacetone phosphate. Dihydroxyacetone phosphate is the common substrate for both glycerophosphate dehydrogenase, an enzyme active in NADH oxidation and lipid pathways (see Chap. 5), and triose phosphate isomerase, which maintains an equilibrium between dihydroxyacetone phosphate and glyceraldehyde-3-phosphate; the equilibrium strongly favors accumulation of dihydroxyacetone phosphate.

After the reaction with glyceraldehyde-3-phosphate dehydrogenase, glycolysis in the brain proceeds in the usual steps. Brain enolase (D-2-phosphoglycerate hydrolyase), which catalyzes dehydration of 2-phosphoglycerate to phosphoenolpyruvate, is present as two related dimers, one of which (γ) is specifically associated with neurons and the other (α) with glia. The neuronal subunit is identical to the neuron-specific protein 14-3-2. Immunocytochemical determination of the enolases makes them useful in determining neuron/glia ratios in tissue samples, but neuron-specific enolase is not confined to neural tissue. Brain phosphoenolpyruvate kinase controls an essentially irreversible reaction that requires not only Mg^{2+} (as do several other glycolytic enzymes) but also K^+ or Na^+. This step also may be regulatory.

Brain tissue, even when it is at rest and well oxygenated, produces a small amount of lactate, which is removed in the venous blood, accounting for 13 percent of the pyruvate produced by glycolysis. The measured lactate level in brain depends on the success in rapidly arresting brain metabolism prior to tissue processing. Five lactate dehydrogenase isoenzymes are present in adult brain; of these, the one that moves electrophoretically most rapidly toward the anode (band 1) predominates. This isoenzyme is generally higher in those tissues that are more dependent on aerobic processes for energy; the slower moving isoenzymes are relatively higher in tissues such as white skeletal muscle, which is better adapted to function at suboptimal oxygen levels. The distribution of lactate dehydrogenase isoenzymes in various brain regions, layers of the retina, brain neoplasms, and brain tissue cultures and during development indicates that their synthesis might be controlled by tissue oxygen levels. Lactate dehydrogenase functions in the cytoplasm as a means of oxidizing NADH, which accumulates as a result of the activity of glyceraldehyde-3-phosphate dehydrogenase in glycolysis. It thus permits glycolytic ATP production to continue under anaerobic conditions. Lactate dehydrogenase also functions under aerobic conditions because NADH cannot easily penetrate the mitochondrial membrane. The oxidation of NADH in the cytoplasm depends on this reaction and on the activity of shuttle mechanisms that transfer reducing equivalents to the mitochondria.

Glycerol phosphate dehydrogenase is another enzyme indirectly associated with glycolysis that participates in cytoplasmic oxidation of NADH. This enzyme reduces dihydroxyacetone phosphate to glycerol-3-phosphate, oxidizing NADH in the process. Under hypoxic conditions, levels of α-glycerophosphate and lactate increase initially at comparable rates, although the amount of lactate produced greatly exceeds that of α-glycerophosphate. The relative levels of the oxidized and reduced substrates of these reactions indicate much higher local levels of NADH in brain than are found by gross measurements. In fact, the relative proportions of oxidized and reduced substrates of the reactions that are linked to the pyridine nucleotides may be a better indicator of local oxidation-reduction states (NAD^+/NADH) in brain than is provided by the direct measurement of the pyridine nucleotides themselves [3,7].

An aspect of glucose metabolism that has led to much confusion among neurochemists is the observation that labeled glucose appears in carbon dioxide much more slowly than might be suggested from a cursory examination of the glycolytic pathway plus the citric acid cycle [8]. Glucose flux is 0.5 to 1.0 μmol/min/g wet weight of brain in a variety of species. The level of glycolytic plus Krebs cycle intermediates is 2 μmol/g. Hence, these intermediates might be predicted to turn over every 2 to 4 min, and $^{14}CO_2$ production might be predicted to reach a steady state in 5 to 10 min. This is not observed experimentally. In addition, large quantities of radioactivity are trapped in amino acids related to the Krebs cycle (70 to 80 percent) from 10 to 30 min after a glucose injection. This is due to the high activity of

transaminase in comparison with flux through the Krebs cycle, and the amino acids developed by transamination behave as if they are part of the cycle. When the pools of these amino acids (~20 μmol/g) are added to the levels of the Krebs cycle components plus glycolytic intermediates, the calculated time for $^{14}CO_2$ evolution is increased by a factor of 10, which agrees with the values observed experimentally.

In contrast, in tissues such as liver, the amino acids related to the Krebs cycle are present at much lower steady-state values, and approximately 20 percent of the radioactivity from administered glucose is trapped in these amino acids at short times after injection. As a result, ignoring the radioactivity trapped in amino acids has a relatively small effect on estimates of glycolytic fluxes in liver but makes an enormous difference in brain. Immature brain more nearly resembles liver in this respect. The relationship of the Krebs cycle to glycolysis undergoes a sharp change during development, coincident with the metabolic compartmentation of amino acid metabolism characteristic of adult brain.

The pyruvate dehydrogenase complex plays a key role in regulating oxidation

Pyruvate dehydrogenase (14 nmol/min/mg protein in rat brain), which controls the entry of pyruvate into the Krebs cycle as acetyl coenzyme A (acyl CoA), is actually a mitochondrial multienzyme complex that includes the enzymes pyruvate dehydrogenase (decarboxylase), lipoate acetyltransferase, and lipoamide dehydrogenase; the coenzymes thiamine pyrophosphate, lipoic acid, CoA, and flavine; and nicotinamide adenine dinucleotides. It is inactivated by being phosphorylated at the decarboxylase moiety by a tightly bound $MgATP^{2-}$-dependent protein kinase and activated by being dephosphorylated by a loosely bound Mg^{2+}- and Ca^{2+}-dependent phosphatase. About half the brain enzyme is usually active. Pyruvate protects the complex against inactivation by inhibiting the kinase. ADP is a competitive inhibitor of Mg^{2+} for the inactivating kinase. Under conditions of greater metabolic demand, increases in pyruvate and ADP and decreases in acyl CoA and ATP make the complex more active. Pyruvate dehydrogenase is inhibited by NADH, decreasing formation of acyl CoA during hypoxia and allowing more pyruvate to be reduced by lactate dehydrogenase, thus forming the NAD^+ necessary to sustain glycolysis. Several investigators have reported abnormalities of the complex (particularly lipoamide dehydrogenase) in hereditary ataxias, but not all studies have confirmed these findings, and the relationship remains tenuous. Pyruvate dehydrogenase defects do occur in several of the mitochondrial enzyme deficiency states (see below and Morgan-Hughes [9]; these are also described in Chap. 34).

Although acetylcholine synthesis is normally controlled by the rate of choline uptake and choline acetyltransferase activity (see Chap. 11), the supply of acyl CoA can be limiting under adverse conditions. Choline uptake is, however, independent of acyl CoA concentration. A cytoplasmic pyruvate dehydrogenase specifically associated with acetylcholine synthesis has been suggested, but there is little evidence in support of such a hypothesis. The mitochondrial membrane is not permeable to the acyl CoA produced within it, but there is efflux of its condensation product citrate. Acyl CoA can then be formed from citrate in the cytosol by ATP citrate lyase. The acetyl moiety of acetylcholine is formed in a compartment, presumably the synaptosome, with rapid glucose turnover. The cytosol of cholinergic endings is reported to be rich in citrate lyase, and it is possible that citrate shuttles the acyl CoA from the mitochondrial compartment to the cytosol. During hypoxia or hypoglycemia, acetylcholine synthesis can be inhibited by failure of the acyl CoA supply.

Energy output and oxygen consumption are associated with high levels of enzyme activity in the Krebs cycle

The actual flux through the Krebs cycle depends on glycolysis and acyl CoA production, which can "push" the cycle, the possible control at several enzymatic steps of the cycle, and the local ADP level, which is known to be a prime activator of the mitochondrial respiration to which the Krebs cycle is linked. The steady-state level of citrate in brain is about one-fifth that of glucose. This is relatively high compared with levels of glycolytic intermediates or with that of isocitrate.

As in other tissues, there are two isocitrate dehydrogenases in brain. One is active primarily in the cytoplasm and requires nicotinamide-adenine dinucleotide phosphate ($NADP^+$) as cofactor; the other, bound to mitochondria and requiring NAD^+, is the enzyme that participates in the citric acid cycle. The NAD^+-linked enzyme catalyzes an essentially irreversible reaction, has allosteric properties, is inhibited by ATP and NADH, and may be stimulated by ADP. The function of the cytoplasmic $NADP^+$ isocitrate dehydrogenase is uncertain, but it has been postulated that it supplies NADPH necessary for many reductive synthetic reactions. The relatively high activity of this enzyme in immature brain and white matter is consistent with such a role. α-Ketoglutarate dehydrogenase, which oxidatively decarboxylates α-ketoglutarate, requires the same cofactors as does the pyruvate decarboxylation step.

Succinate dehydrogenase, the enzyme that catalyzes the oxidation of succinate to fumarate, is tightly bound to the mitochondrial membrane. In brain, succinate dehydrogenase may also have a regulatory role when the steady state is disturbed. Isocitrate and succinate levels in brain are little affected by changes in the flux of the citric acid cycle as long as an adequate glucose supply is available. The highly unfavorable free energy change of the malate dehydrogenase reaction is overcome by the rapid removal of oxaloacetate, which is maintained at low concentrations under steady-state conditions by the condensation reaction with acyl CoA [6].

Malic dehydrogenase is one of the several enzymes in the citric acid cycle that is present in both cytoplasm and mitochondria. The function of the cytoplasmic components of these enzyme activities is not known with certainty, but they may assist in the transfer of hydrogen equivalents from cytoplasm into mitochondria.

The Krebs cycle functions as an oxidative process for energy production and as a source of various amino acids, for example, glutamate, glutamine, γ-aminobutyrate, aspartate, and asparagine. To export net amounts of α-ketoglutarate or oxaloacetate from the Krebs cycle, the supply of dicarboxylic acids must be replenished. The major route for this seems to be the fixation of CO_2 to pyruvate or other substrates at the three-carbon level. Thus the rate of CO_2 fixation sets an upper limit at which biosynthetic reactions can occur. This has been estimated as 0.15 μmol/g wet weight brain/min in studies of acute ammonia toxicity in cats, or approximately 10 percent of the flux through the citric acid cycle (see below). Liver, on the other hand, seems to have ten times the capacity of brain for CO_2 fixation, as is appropriate for an organ geared to making large quantities of protein for export [10]. In brain, pyruvate carboxylase, which catalyzes CO_2 fixation, appears to be largely an astrocytic enzyme. Pyruvate dehydrogenase seems to be the rate-limiting step for the entry of pyruvate into the Krebs cycle from glycolysis.

The pentose shunt (hexose monophosphate pathway) is active in brain

Under basal conditions at least 5 to 8 percent of brain glucose is likely to be metabolized via the pentose shunt in the adult monkey, and 2.3 percent in the rat [8]. Both shunt enzymes and metabolic flux have been found in isolated nerve endings. The pentose pathway has relatively high activity in developing brain, reaching a peak during myelination. Its main contribution is probably to produce the NADPH required for reductive reactions necessary for lipid synthesis (see Chap. 5). Shunt enzymes and metabolic flux are found in synaptosomes. Although the capacity of

the pathway (as determined using nonphysiological electron acceptors) remains constant throughout the rat life span, activity with physiological acceptors could not be detected in middle-aged (18-month) and older animals. It is possible that the shunt serves as a reserve pathway for use under such stresses as the need for increased lipid synthesis, repair, or reduction of oxidative toxins. The shunt pathway also provides pentose for nucleotide synthesis; however, only a small fraction of the activity of this pathway would be required. As with glycogen synthesis, turnover in the pentose phosphate pathway decreases under conditions of increased energy need, for example, during and after high rates of stimulation. Pentose phosphate flux apparently is regulated by the concentrations of glucose-6-phosphate, $NADP^+$, glyceraldehyde-3-phosphate, and fructose-6-phosphate. Since transketolase, one of the enzymes in this pathway, requires thiamine pyrophosphate as a cofactor, poor myelin maintenance in thiamine deficiency may reflect the failure of this pathway to provide sufficient NADPH for lipid synthesis [6].

Glutamate in brain is compartmented into separate pools

The pools that subserve different metabolic pathways for glutamate equilibrate with each other only slowly. This compartmentation is a vital factor in the separate regulation of special functions of glutamate (see Chap. 17) and γ-aminobutyrate (see Chap. 18), such as neurotransmission, and general functions, such as protein biosynthesis. Glutamate metabolism in brain is characterized by the existence of at least two distinct pools; in addition, the Krebs cycle intermediates associated with these pools are also distinctly compartmented. A mathematical model to fit data from radiotracer experiments that require separate Krebs cycles to satisfy the hypotheses of compartmentation has been developed. A key assumption of the current models is that γ-aminobutyrate is metabolized at a site different from its synthesis. The best fit of kinetic data is obtained when glutamate from a small pool that is actively converted to glutamine flows back to a larger pool (8 μmol/g) that is converted to γ-aminobutyrate. Of possible relevance to this is the finding that glutamic acid decarboxylase (GAD) is localized at or near nerve terminals, whereas γ-aminobutyrate transaminase, the major degradative enzyme, is mitochondrial.

Evidence points to an inferred small pool of glutamate (2 μmol/g) as probably glial. Glutamate released from nerve endings appears to be taken up by glia and by presynaptic and postsynaptic terminals (see Chap. 3), converted to glutamine and recycled to glutamate and γ-aminobutyrate (see Chaps. 17 and 18). Various estimates of the proportion of glucose carbon that flows through the GABA shunt have been published, but the most definitive experiments show the value to be approximately 10 percent of the total glycolytic flux. Although this may seem small, that portion of the Krebs cycle flux that is used for energy production (ATP synthesis, maintenance of ionic gradients) does not require CO_2 fixation, but the portion used for biosynthesis of amino acids does. By recycling the carbon skeleton of some of the glutamate released during neurotransmission through glutamine and γ-aminobutyrate to succinate, the need for dicarboxylic acids to replenish intermediates of the Krebs cycle is diminished when export of α-ketoglutarate takes place.

It is difficult to get good estimates of the extent of CO_2 fixation in brain, but estimates of the maximum capability obtained under conditions of ammonia stress, when glutamine levels increase rapidly, suggest that CO_2 fixation occurs at 0.15 μmol/g/min (in cat) and 0.33 μmol/g/min (in rat), that is, at about the same rate as for the GABA shunt.

For comparison, it should be pointed out that only approximately 2 percent of the glucose flux in whole brain goes toward lipid synthesis, and approximately 0.3 percent is used for protein synthesis. Thus the turnover of neurotransmitter amino acids is a major biosynthetic activity in brain.

Metabolic compartmentation of glutamate is usually observed when labeled ketogenic substrates are administered to animals. It is interesting that acetoacetate and β-hydroxybutyrate do not show this effect, apparently because ketone bodies are a normal substrate for brain and are taken up in all kinds of cells. Acetate and similar substrates, which are not taken up into brain efficiently, appear to be more readily taken up or activated, or both, in glia. This is believed to lead to the abnormal glutamine/glutamate ratio that is observed. Similarly, metabolic inhibitors like fluoroacetate appear to act selectively in glia and produce their neurotoxic action without marked inhibition of the overall Krebs cycle flux in brain. This difference in behavior has led to suggestions that acetate and fluoroacetate may be useful markers for the study of glial metabolism by the technique of autoradiography [11].

A nonuniform distribution of metabolites in living systems is a widespread occurrence. Steady-state levels of γ-aminobutyrate are well documented to vary over a fivefold range in discrete brain regions (2 to 10 mM), and it has been estimated that γ-aminobutyrate may be as high as 50 mM in nerve terminals. Observations in brain indicate the existence of pools of metabolites with half-lives of many hours for mixing, which is most unusual. The discovery of subcellular morphological compartmentation—different populations of mitochondria in cerebral cortex that have distinctive enzyme complements—may provide a somewhat better perspective by which to visualize such separation of metabolic function [12].

In addition to the phasic release of both excitatory and inhibitory transmitters, there may be a continuous tonic release of GABA, dependent only on the activity of the enzyme responsible for its synthesis and independent of the depolarization of the presynaptic membrane. Such inhibitory neurons could act tonically by constantly maintaining an elevated threshold in the excitatory neurons so that the latter would start firing when a decrease occurred in the continuous release of GABA acting on them. This is consistent with a known correlation between the inhibition of GAD and the appearance of convulsions after certain drug treatments. GABA levels have been observed to be depleted by some convulsant drugs and elevated by others.

DIFFERENCES BETWEEN *IN VITRO* AND *IN VIVO* BRAIN METABOLISM

In addition to the usual differences between *in vitro* and *in vivo* studies that pertain to all tissues, there are two unique conditions that pertain only to the central nervous system. First, in contrast to cells of other tissues, individual nerve cells do not function autonomously. They are generally so incorporated into a complex neural network that their functional activity is integrated with that of various other parts of the central nervous system and with somatic tissues as well. Any procedure that interrupts the structural and functional integrity of the network would inevitably alter quantitatively and, perhaps, even qualitatively, its normal metabolic behavior. Second, the phenomenon of the BBB selectively limits the rates of transfer of soluble substances between blood and brain (see Chap. 32). This barrier discriminates among various potential substrates for cerebral metabolism. The substrate function is confined to those compounds in the blood that are not only suitable substrates for cerebral enzymes but can also penetrate from blood to the brain at rates adequate to support the brain's considerable energy demands. Substances that can be readily oxidized by brain slices, minces, or homogenates *in vitro* and that are effectively utilized *in vivo* when formed endogenously within the brain are often incapable of supporting cerebral energy metabolism and function when present in the blood because of restricted passage through the BBB. The *in vitro* techniques establish only the existence and potential capacity of the enzyme systems required for the utilization of a given substrate; they do not define the extent to which such a pathway is actually utilized *in vivo*. This can be done only by studies in the intact animal, and it is this aspect of cerebral metabolism with which this chapter is concerned.

CEREBRAL ENERGY METABOLISM *IN VIVO*

A variety of methods have been used to study the metabolism of the brain *in vivo*; these vary in complexity and in the degree to which they yield quantitative results. Some require such minimal operative procedures on the laboratory animal that no anesthesia is required, and there is no interference with the tissue except for the effects of the particular experimental condition being studied. Some of these techniques are applicable to normal, conscious human subjects, and consecutive and comparative studies can be made repeatedly in the same subject. Other methods are more traumatic and either require the animal to be killed or involve such extensive surgical intervention and tissue damage that the experiments approach an *in vitro* experiment carried out *in situ*. All, however, are capable of providing specific and useful information.

Behavioral and central nervous system physiology are correlated with blood and cerebrospinal fluid chemical changes

The simplest way to study the metabolism of the central nervous system *in vivo* is to correlate spontaneous or experimentally produced alterations in the chemical composition of the blood, spinal fluid, or both, with changes in cerebral physiological functions or gross central nervous system-mediated behavior. The level of consciousness, the reflex behavior, or the electroencephalogram (EEG) is generally used to monitor the efects of the chemical changes on the functional and metabolic activities of the brain. For example, such methods first demonstrated the need for glucose as a substrate for cerebral energy metabolism; hypoglycemia produced by insulin or other means altered various parameters of cerebral function that could not be restored to normal by the administration of substances other than glucose.

The chief virtue of these methods is their simplicity, but they are gross and nonspecific and do not distinguish between direct effects of the agent on cerebral metabolism and those secondary to changes produced initially in somatic tissues. Also, negative results are often inconclusive, for there always remain questions of insufficient dosage, inadequate cerebral circulation and delivery to the tissues, or impermeability of the BBB.

Brain samples are removed for biochemical analyses

The availability of analytical chemical techniques makes it possible to measure specific metabolites and enzyme activities in brain tissue at selected times during or after exposure of the animal to an experimental condition. This approach has been very useful in studies of the intermediary metabolism of the brain. It has permitted the estimation of the rates of flux through the various steps of established metabolic pathways and the identification of control points in the pathways where regulation may be exerted. Such studies have helped to define more precisely the changes in energy metabolism associated with altered cerebral functions produced, for example, by anesthesia, convulsions, or hypoglycemia. Although these methods require killing the animal and analyzing tissue samples, they are *in vivo* methods in effect since they attempt to describe the state of the tissue while it is still in the animal at the moment of killing. These methods have encountered their most serious problems with regard to this point. Postmortem changes in

brain are extremely rapid and are not always completely retarded even by the most rapid freezing techniques available. These methods have proved to be very valuable, nevertheless, particularly in the area of energy metabolism.

Radioisotope incorporation can identify and measure routes of metabolism

The technique of administering radioactive precursors followed by the chemical separation and assay of products in the tissue has added greatly to the armamentarium for studying cerebral metabolism *in vivo*. Labeled precursors are administered by any one of a variety of routes; at selected later times the brain is removed, the precursor and the various products of interest are isolated, and the radioactivity and quantity of the compounds in question are assayed. Such techniques facilitate the identification of metabolic routes and the rates of flux through various steps of the pathway. In some cases, comparison of the specific activities of the products and precursors has led to the surprising finding of higher specific activities in the products than in the precursors. This is conclusive evidence of the presence of compartmentation. These methods have been used effectively in studies of amine and neurotransmitter synthesis and metabolism, lipid metabolism, protein synthesis, amino acid metabolism, and the distribution of glucose carbon through the various biochemical pathways present in the brain.

Radioisotope incorporation methods are particularly valuable for studies of intermediary metabolism that generally are not feasible by most other *in vivo* techniques. They are without equal for the qualitative identification of the pathways and routes of metabolism. They suffer, however, from a disadvantage: Only one set of measurements per animal is possible because the animal must be killed. Quantitative interpretations are often confounded by the problems of compartmentation. Also, they are all too frequently misused; unfortunately, quantitative conclusions are often drawn on the basis of radioactivity data without appropriate consideration of the specific activities of the precursor pools.

Oxygen utilization in the cortex is measured by polarographic techniques

The oxygen electrode has been employed for measuring the amount of oxygen consumed locally in the cerebral cortex *in vivo* [13]. The electrode is applied to the surface of the exposed cortex, and the local partial pressure for oxygen (PO_2) is measured continuously before and during occlusion of the blood flow to the local area. During occlusion, the PO_2 falls linearly as oxygen is consumed by tissue metabolism, and the rate of fall is a measure of the rate of oxygen consumption locally in the cortex. Repeated measurements can be made successively in the animal, and the technique has been used to demonstrate the increased oxygen consumption of the cerebral cortex and the relation between the changes in the EEG and the metabolic rate during convulsions [13]. The technique is limited to measurements in the cortex and, of course, to oxygen utilization.

Arteriovenous differences identify substances consumed or produced by brain

The primary functions of the circulation are to replenish the nutrients consumed by the tissues and to remove the products of their metabolism. These functions are reflected in the composition of the blood traversing the tissue. Substances taken up by the tissue from the blood are higher in concentration in the arterial inflow than in the venous outflow, and the converse is true for substances released by the tissue. The convention is to subtract the venous concentration from the arterial concentration so that a positive arteriovenous difference represents net uptake and a negative difference means net release. In nonsteady states, as after a perturbation, there may be transient arteriovenous differences that reflect changes in tissue concentrations and re-equilibration of the tissue with the blood. In steady states, in which it is presumed that the tissue concentration remains constant, positive and negative arteriovenous differences mean net consumption or production of the substance by the tissue respectively. Zero arteriovenous differences indicate neither consumption nor production. This method is useful for all substances in blood that can be assayed with enough accuracy, precision, and sensitivity to enable the detection of arteriovenous differences. The method is useful only for tissues from which mixed representative venous blood can be sampled. Arterial blood has essentially the same composition throughout and can be sampled from any artery. In contrast venous blood is specific for each tissue, and to establish valid arteriovenous differences the venous blood must represent the total outflow or the flow-weighted average of all the venous outflows from the tissue under study, uncontaminated by blood from any other tissue. It is not possible to fulfill this condition for many tissues.

The method is fully applicable to the brain, particularly in humans, in whom the anatomy of venous drainage is favorable for such studies. Representative cerebral venous blood, with no more than approximately 3 percent contamination with extracerebral blood, is readily obtained from the superior bulb of the internal jugular vein in humans. The venipuncture can be made percutaneously under local anesthesia, and the measurements can therefore be made during the conscious state undistorted by the effects of general anesthesia. Using this method with the monkey is similar, although the vein must be surgically exposed before puncture. Other common laboratory animals are less suitable because extensive communication between cerebral and extracerebral venous beds is present, and uncontaminated representative venous blood is difficult to obtain from the cerebrum without major surgical intervention. In these cases, one can sample blood from the confluence of the sinuses (torcular herophili) even though it does not contain fully representative blood from the brainstem and some of the lower portions of the brain.

The chief advantages of these methods are their simplicity and applicability to unanesthetized humans. They permit the qualitative identification of the ultimate substrates and products of cerebral metabolism. They have no applicability, however, to those intermediates that are formed and consumed entirely within the brain without being exchanged with blood, or to those substances that are exchanged between brain and blood with no net flux in either direction. Furthermore, they provide no quantification of the rates of utilization or production because arteriovenous differences depend not only on the rates of consumption or production by the tissue but also on blood flow (see below). Blood flow affects all the arteriovenous differences proportionately, however, and comparison of the arteriovenous differences of various substances obtained from the same samples of blood reflects their relative rates of utilization or production.

Combining cerebral blood flow and arteriovenous differences permits measurement of rates of consumption or production of substances by brain

In a steady state the tissue concentration of any substance utilized or produced by the brain is presumed to remain constant. When a substance is exchanged between brain and blood, the difference in its steady state of delivery to the brain in the arterial blood and removal in the venous blood must be equal to the net rate of its utilization or production by the brain. This relation can be expressed as follows:

$$CMR = CBF \ (A - V)$$

where $(A - V)$ is the difference in concentration in arterial and cerebral venous blood,

CBF is the rate of cerebral blood flow in volume of blood per unit time, and CMR (cerebral metabolic rate) is the steady-state rate of utilization or production of the substance by the brain.

If both the rate of cerebral blood flow and the arteriovenous difference are known, then the net rate of utilization or production of the substance by the brain can be calculated. This has been the basis of most quantitative studies of the cerebral metabolism *in vivo.*

The most reliable method for determining cerebral blood flow is the inert gas method of Kety and Schmidt [see ref. 14]. It was originally designed for use in studies of conscious, unanesthetized humans, and it has been most widely employed for this purpose; but it also has been adapted for use in animals. The method is based on the Fick principle (i.e., an equivalent of the law of conservation of matter), and it utilizes low concentrations of a freely diffusible, chemically inert gas as a tracer substance. The original gas was nitrous oxide, but subsequent modifications have substituted other gases, such as ^{85}Kr, ^{79}Kr, or hydrogen, that can be measured more conveniently in blood. During a period of inhalation of 15 percent N_2O in air, for example, timed arterial and cerebral venous blood samples are withdrawn and analyzed for their N_2O contents. The cerebral blood flow (in ml per 100 g of brain tissue per minute) can be calculated from the equation:

$$CBF = 100 \ \lambda \ V(T) / \int_0^T [A(t) - V(t)] \ dt$$

where $A(t)$ and $V(t)$ are the arterial and cerebral venous blood concentrations of N_2O, respectively, at any time t; $V(T)$ is concentration of N_2O in venous blood at end of period of inhalation, i.e., time, T; λ is partition coefficient for N_2O between brain tissue and blood; t is variable time in minutes; T is total period of inhalation of N_2O, usually 10 min or more; and $\int_0^T [A(t) - V(t)] \ dt$ is integrated arteriovenous difference in N_2O concentrations over total period of inhalation.

The partition coefficient for N_2O is approximately 1 when equilibrium has been achieved between blood and brain tissue; at least 10 min of inhalation is required to approach equilibrium. At the end of this interval the N_2O concentration in brain tissue is about equal to the cerebral venous blood concentration. Because the method requires sampling of both arterial and cerebral venous blood, it lends itself readily to the simultaneous measurement of arteriovenous differences of substances involved in cerebral metabolism. This method and its modifications have provided most of our knowledge of the rates of substrate utilization or product formation by the brain *in vivo*.

REGULATION OF CEREBRAL METABOLIC RATE

Brain consumes about one-fifth of total body oxygen utilization

The brain is metabolically one of the most active of all the organs in the body. This consumption of oxygen provides the energy required for its intense physicochemical activity. The most reliable data on cerebral metabolic rate have been obtained in humans. Cerebral oxygen consumption in normal, conscious, young men is approximately 3.5 ml/100 g brain/min (Table 1); the rate is similar in young women. The rate of oxygen consumption by an entire brain of average

TABLE 1. Cerebral blood flow and metabolic rate in a normal young adult man[a]

Function	Per 100 g of brain tissue	Per whole brain (1,400 g)
Cerebral blood flow (ml/min)	57	798
Cerebral O_2 consumption (ml/min)	3.5	49
Cerebral glucose utilization (mg/min)	5.5	77

[a] Based on data derived from the literature, in Sokoloff [16].

weight (1,400 g) is then about 49 ml O_2/min. The magnitude of this rate can be more fully appreciated when it is compared with the metabolic rate of the body as a whole. The average man weighs 70 kg and consumes about 250 ml O_2/min in the basal state. Therefore, the brain alone, which represents only approximately 2 percent of total body weight, accounts for 20 percent of the resting total body oxygen consumption. In children the brain takes an even larger fraction, as much as 50 percent in the middle of the first decade of life [15].

Oxygen is utilized in the brain almost entirely for the oxidation of carbohydrate [16]. The energy equivalent of the total cerebral metabolic rate is, therefore, approximately 20 W or 0.25 kcal/min. If it is assumed that this energy is utilized mainly for the synthesis of high-energy phosphate bonds, that the efficiency of the energy conservation is approximately 20 percent, and that the free energy of hydrolysis of the terminal phosphate of ATP is approximately 7 kcal/mol, this energy expenditure can then be estimated to support the steady turnover of close to 7 mmol or approximately 4×10^{21} molecules of ATP per minute in the entire human brain. The brain normally has no respite from this enormous energy demand. The cerebral oxygen consumption continues unabated day and night. Even during sleep there is only a relatively small decrease in cerebral metabolic rate; indeed, it may even be increased in rapid eye movement (REM) sleep (see below).

What are the energy-demanding functions of the brain?

The brain does not do mechanical work, like that of cardiac and skeletal muscle, or osmotic work as the kidney does in concentrating urine. It does not have the complex energy-consuming metabolic functions of liver, nor, despite the synthesis of some hormones and neurotransmitters, is it noted for its biosynthetic activities. Recently, considerable emphasis has been placed on the extent of macromolecular synthesis in the central nervous system, an interest stimulated by the recognition that there are some proteins with short half-lives in the brain. These represent relatively small numbers of molecules, and, in fact, the average protein turnover and the rate of protein synthesis in the mature brain are slower than most other tissues except, perhaps, muscle. Clearly, the functions of nervous tissues are mainly excitation and conduction, and these are reflected in the unceasing electrical activity of the brain. The electrical energy is ultimately derived from chemical processes, and it is likely that most of the brain's energy consumption is used for active transport of ions to sustain and restore the membrane potentials discharged during the process of excitation and conduction (see Chap. 3).

Not all of the oxygen consumption of the brain is used for energy metabolism. The brain contains a variety of oxidases and hydroxylases that function in the synthesis and metabolism of a number of neurotransmitters. For example, tyrosine hydroxylase is a mixed-function oxidase that hydroxylates tyrosine to 3,4-dihydroxyphenylalanine (DOPA), and dopamine-β-hydroxylase hydroxylates dopamine to form norepinephrine. Similarly, tryptophan hydroxylase hydroxylates tryptophan to form 5-hydroxytryptophan in the pathway of serotonin synthesis. These enzymes are oxygenases, which utilize molecular oxygen and incorporate it into the hydroxyl group of the hydroxylated products. Oxygen is also consumed in the metabolism of these monoamine neurotransmitters, which are oxidatively deaminated to their respective aldehydes by monoamine oxidases. All of these enzymes are present in brain, and the reactions catalyzed by them utilize oxygen. When, however, the total turnover rates of the neurotransmitters and the sum total of the maximal velocities of all the oxidases involved in their synthesis and degradation are considered, it is clear that the oxygen consumed in the turnover of the neurotransmitters can account for only a very small, possibly immeasurable, fraction of the total oxygen consumption of the brain.

Continuous cerebral circulation is absolutely required to provide sufficient oxygen

Not only does the brain utilize oxygen at a very rapid rate, but it is absolutely dependent on continuously uninterrupted oxidative metabolism for maintenance of its functional and structural integrity. There is a large Pasteur effect in brain tissue, but even at its maximum rate anaerobic glycolysis is unable to provide sufficient energy to meet the brain's demands. Since the oxygen stored in the brain is extremely small compared with its rate of utilization, the brain requires the continuous replenishment of its oxygen by the circulation. If cerebral blood flow is completely interrupted, consciousness is lost within less than 10 sec, or the amount of time required to consume the oxygen contained within the brain and its blood content. Loss of consciousness as a result of anoxemia, caused by anoxia or asphyxia, takes only a little longer because of the additional oxygen present in the lungs and still-circulating blood. There is evidence that the average critical level of oxygen tension in the brain tissues, below which consciousness and the normal EEG pattern are invariably lost, lies between 15 and 20 mmHg. This appears to be so whether the tissue anoxia is achieved by lowering the cerebral blood flow or the arterial oxygen content. Cessation of cerebral blood flow is followed within a few minutes by irreversible pathological changes within the brain, readily demonstrated by microscopic anatomical techniques. It is well known, of course, that in medical crises, such as cardiac arrest, damage to the brain occurs earliest and is most decisive in determining the degree of recovery.

The cerebral blood flow must be able to maintain the brain's avaricious appetite for oxygen. The average rate of blood flow in the human brain as a whole is approximately

57 ml/100 g tissue/min (see Table 1). For the whole brain this amounts to almost 800 ml/min or approximately 15 percent of the total basal cardiac output. This level must be maintained within relatively narrow limits, for the brain cannot tolerate any major drop in its perfusion. A fall in cerebral blood flow to half of its normal rate is sufficient to cause loss of consciousness in normal, healthy young men. There are, fortunately, numerous reflexes and other physiological mechanisms to sustain adequate levels of arterial blood pressure at the head level (e.g., baroreceptor reflexes) and to maintain the cerebral blood flow, even when arterial pressure falls in times of stress (e.g., autoregulation). There are also mechanisms to adjust the cerebral blood flow to changes in cerebral metabolic demand.

Regulation of the cerebral blood flow is achieved mainly by control of the tone or the degree of constriction or dilation of the cerebral vessels. This, in turn, is controlled mainly by local chemical factors, such as P_aCO_2, P_aO_2, pH, and still unrecognized factors. High P_aCO_2, low P_aO_2, and low pH—products of metabolic activity—tend to dilate the blood vessels and increase cerebral blood flow; changes in the opposite direction constrict the vessels and decrease blood flow [17]. Cerebral blood flow is regulated through such mechanisms to maintain homeostasis of these chemical factors in the local tissue. The rates of production of these chemical factors depend on the rates of energy metabolism, and cerebral blood flow is, therefore, also adjusted to the cerebral metabolic rate [17].

Local rates of cerebral blood flow and metabolism can be measured by autoradiography and are shown to be coupled to local brain function

The rates of blood flow and metabolism presented in Table 1 and discussed above represent the average values in the brain as a whole. The brain is not a homogeneous organ, however; it is composed of a variety of tissues and discrete structures that often function independently or even inversely with respect to one another. There is little reason to expect that their perfusion and metabolic rates would be similar. Indeed, experimental evidence clearly indicates that they are not. Local cerebral blood flow in laboratory animals has been determined from the local tissue concentrations, measured by a quantitative autoradiographic technique, and from the total history of the arterial concentration of a freely diffusible, chemically inert, radioactive tracer introduced into the circulation [18]. The results reveal that blood-flow rates vary widely throughout the brain with average values in gray matter approximately four to five times those of white matter [18].

A method has been devised to measure glucose consumption in the discrete functional and structural components of the brain in intact conscious laboratory animals [19]. This method also employs quantitative autoradiography to measure local tissue concentrations but utilizes 2-deoxy-D-[^{14}C]glucose as the tracer. The local tissue accumulation of [^{14}C]deoxyglucose as [^{14}C]deoxyglucose-6-phosphate in a given interval of time is related to the amount of glucose that has been phosphorylated by hexokinase over the same interval, and the rate of glucose consumption can be determined from the [^{14}C]deoxyglucose-6-phosphate concentration by appropriate consideration of (a) the relative concentrations of [^{14}C]deoxyglucose and glucose in the plasma; (b) their rate constants for transport between plasma and brain tissue; and (c) the kinetic constants of hexokinase for deoxyglucose and glucose. The method is based on a kinetic model of the biochemical behavior of 2-deoxyglucose and glucose in brain. The model (diagrammed in Fig. 3) has been mathematically analyzed to derive an operational equation that presents the variables to be measured and the procedure to be followed to determine local cerebral glucose utilization.

To measure local glucose utilization, a

A

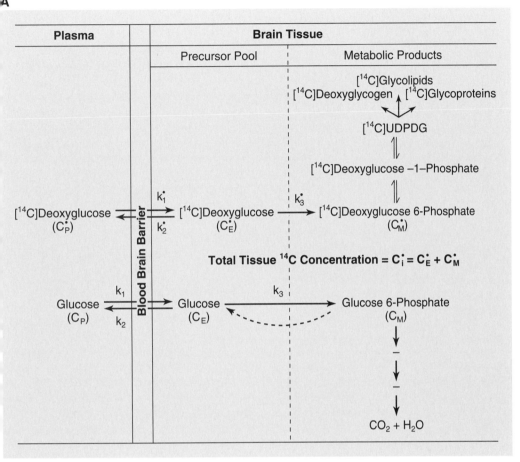

Plasma		Brain Tissue	
		Precursor Pool	Metabolic Products

[¹⁴C]Glycolipids
[¹⁴C]Deoxyglycogen ↖ ↗ [¹⁴C]Glycoproteins

[¹⁴C]UDPDG

[¹⁴C]Deoxyglucose –1–Phosphate

k_1^*

[¹⁴C]Deoxyglucose
(C_P^*) ⇄ [¹⁴C]Deoxyglucose
(C_E^*) $\xrightarrow{k_3^*}$ [¹⁴C]Deoxyglucose 6-Phosphate
(C_M^*)

k_2^*

Blood Brain Barrier

Total Tissue ¹⁴C Concentration = $C_i^* = C_E^* + C_M^*$

k_1

Glucose
(C_P) ⇄ Glucose
(C_E) $\xrightarrow{k_3}$ Glucose 6-Phosphate
(C_M)

k_2

$CO_2 + H_2O$

FIG. 3. Theoretical basis of radioactive deoxyglucose method for measurement of local cerebral glucose utilization. **A:** Theoretical model. C_i^* represents the total ¹⁴C concentration in a single homogeneous tissue of the brain. C_p^* and C_p represent the concentrations of [¹⁴C]deoxyglucose and glucose in the arterial plasma, respectively; C_E^* and C_E represent their respective concentrations in the tissue pools that serve as substrates for hexokinase. C_M^* represents the concentration of [¹⁴C]deoxyglucose 6-phosphate in the tissue. The constants k_1^*, k_2^*, and k_3^* represent the rate constants for carrier-mediated transport of [¹⁴C]deoxyglucose from plasma to tissue, for carrier-mediated transport back from tissue to plasma, and for phosphorylation by hexokinase, respectively. The constants k_1, k_2, and k_3 are the equivalent rate constants for glucose. [¹⁴C[Deoxyglucose and glucose share and compete for the carrier that transports them both between plasma and tissue and for hexokinase, which phosphorylates them to their respective hexose 6-phosphates. The dashed arrow represents the possibility of glucose 6-phosphate hydrolysis by glucose-6-phosphatase activity, if any. UDPDG, UDP-deoxyglucose.

pulse of [¹⁴C]deoxyglucose is administered intravenously at zero time, and timed arterial blood samples are then drawn for the determination of the plasma [¹⁴C]deoxyglucose and glucose concentrations. At the end of the experimental period, usually about 45 min, the animal is decapitated, the brain is removed and frozen, and brain sections, 20 μm in thickness, are autoradiographed on X-ray film along with calibrated [¹⁴C]methylmethacrylate standards. Local tissue concentrations of ¹⁴C are determined by quantitative densitometric analysis of the autoradiographs. From the time courses of the arterial

B

General equation for measurement of reaction rates with tracers:

$$\text{Rate of reaction} = \frac{\text{Labeled Product Formed in Interval of Time, 0 to T}}{\left[\begin{array}{c}\text{Isotope effect}\\\text{correction factor}\end{array}\right]\left[\begin{array}{c}\text{Integrated specific activity}\\\text{of precursor}\end{array}\right]}$$

Operational equation of $[^{14}C]$deoxyglucose method:

Labeled Product Formed in Interval of Time, 0 to T

$$R_i = \frac{\overbrace{\underbrace{C_i^*(T)}_{\substack{\text{Total } ^{14}\text{C in tissue}\\\text{at time T}}} - \underbrace{k_1^* e^{-(k_2^*+k_3^*)T} \int_0^T C_p^* e^{(k_2^*+k_3^*)t}\,dt}_{\substack{^{14}\text{C in precursor}\\\text{remaining in tissue at time T}}}}{\underbrace{\left[\frac{\lambda \cdot V_m^* \cdot K_m}{\Phi \cdot V_m \cdot K_m^*}\right]}_{\substack{\text{Isotope effect}\\\text{correction}\\\text{factor}}}\underbrace{\left[\underbrace{\int_0^T \left(\frac{C_p^*}{C_p}\right)dt}_{\substack{\text{Integrated plasma}\\\text{specific activity}}} - \underbrace{e^{-(k_2^*+k_3^*)T}\int_0^T \left(\frac{C_p^*}{C_p}\right)e^{(k_2^*+k_3^*)t}\,dt}_{\substack{\text{Correction for lag in tissue}\\\text{equilibration with plasma}}}\right]}_{\text{Integrated precursor specific activity in tissue}}}$$

FIG. 3.   *(continued).* **B:** Functional anatomy of the operational equation of the radioactive deoxyglucose method. T represents the time at the termination of the experimental period; λ equals the ratio of the distribution space of deoxyglucose in the tissue to that of glucose; ϕ equals the fraction of glucose that, once phosphorylated, continues down the glycolytic pathway; K_m^* and V_m^* and K_m and V_m represent the familiar Michaelis-Menten kinetic constants of hexokinase for deoxyglucose and glucose, respectively. Other symbols are the same as those defined in A. (From Sokoloff et al. [19].)

plasma $[^{14}C]$deoxyglucose and glucose concentrations and the final tissue ^{14}C concentrations, determined by the quantitative autoradiography, local glucose utilization can be calculated by means of the operational equation for all components of the brain identifiable in the autoradiographs. The procedure is so designed that the autoradiographs reflect mainly the relative local concentrations of $[^{14}C]$deoxyglucose-6-phosphate. The autoradiographs are therefore pictorial representations of the relative rates of glucose utilization in all the structural components of the brain.

Autoradiographs of the striate cortex in monkey in various functional states are illustrated in Fig. 4. This method has demonstrated that local cerebral consumption of glucose varies as widely as blood flow throughout the brain (Table 2). Indeed, in the normal animals there is remarkably close correlation between local cerebral blood flow and glucose consumption [20]. Changes in functional activity produced by physiological stimulation, anesthesia, or deafferentation result in corresponding changes in blood flow and glucose consumption [21] in the structures involved in the functional change. The $[^{14}C]$deoxyglucose method for the measurement of local glucose utilization has been used to map the functional visual pathways and to identify the locus of the visual cortical representation of the retinal "blind spot" in the brain of the rhesus monkey [21] (Fig. 4). These results establish that local energy metabolism in

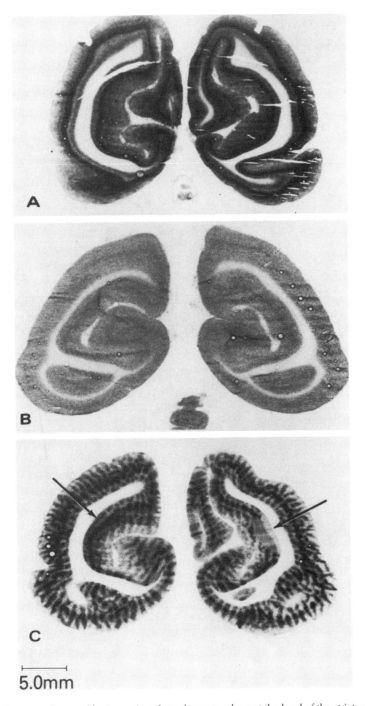

5.0mm

FIG. 4. Autoradiograms of coronal brain sections from rhesus monkeys at the level of the striate cortex. **A:** Animal with normal binocular vision. Note the laminar distribution of the density; the dark band corresponds to layer IV. **B:** Animal with bilateral visual deprivation. Note the almost uniform and reduced relative density, especially the virtual disappearance of the dark band corresponding to layer IV. **C:** Animal with right eye occluded. The half-brain on the left side of the photograph represents the left hemisphere contralateral to the occluded eye. Note the alternate dark and light striations, each approximately 0.3 to 0.4 mm in width, representing the ocular dominance columns. These columns are most apparent in the dark lamina corresponding to layer IV but extend through the entire thickness of the cortex. The *arrows* point to regions of bilateral asymmetry, where the ocular dominance columns are absent. These are presumably areas that normally have only monocular input. The one on the left, contralateral to the occluded eye, has a continuous dark lamina corresponding to layer IV that is completely absent on the side ipsilateral to the occluded eye. These regions are believed to be the loci of the cortical representations of the blind spots. (From Sokoloff [21].)

TABLE 2.   Representative values[a] for local cerebral glucose utilization in the normal conscious albino rat and monkey (μmol/100 g/min)

Structure	Albino rat[b]	Monkey[c]
GRAY MATTER		
Visual cortex	107 ± 6	59 ± 2
Auditory cortex	162 ± 5	79 ± 4
Parietal cortex	112 ± 5	47 ± 4
Sensory-motor cortex	120 ± 5	44 ± 3
Thalamus: lateral nucleus	116 ± 5	54 ± 2
Thalamus: ventral nucleus	109 ± 5	43 ± 2
Medial geniculate body	131 ± 5	65 ± 3
Lateral geniculate body	96 ± 5	39 ± 1
Hypothalamus	54 ± 2	25 ± 1
Mammillary body	121 ± 5	57 ± 3
Hippocampus	79 ± 3	39 ± 2
Amygdala	52 ± 2	25 ± 2
Caudate putamen	110 ± 4	52 ± 3
Nucleus accumbens	82 ± 3	36 ± 2
Globus pallidus	58 ± 2	26 ± 2
Substantia nigra	58 ± 3	29 ± 2
Vestibular nucleus	128 ± 5	66 ± 3
Cochlear nucleus	113 ± 7	51 ± 3
Superior olivary nucleus	133 ± 7	63 ± 4
Inferior colliculus	197 ± 10	103 ± 6
Superior colliculus	95 ± 5	55 ± 4
Pontine gray matter	62 ± 3	28 ± 1
Cerebellar cortex	57 ± 2	31 ± 2
Cerebellar nuclei	100 ± 4	45 ± 2
WHITE MATTER		
Corpus callosum	40 ± 2	11 ± 1
Internal capsule	33 ± 2	13 ± 1
Cerebellar white matter	37 ± 2	12 ± 1
WEIGHTED AVERAGE FOR WHOLE BRAIN		
	68 ± 3	36 ± 1

[a] The values are the means plus or minus standard errors from measurements made in ten rats or seven monkeys.
[b] From Sokoloff and co-workers [19].
[c] From Kennedy and co-workers [22].

brain is coupled to local functional activity and also confirm the long-held belief that local cerebral blood flow is adjusted to metabolic demand in local tissue. The method has been applied to humans by the use of 2-[^{18}F]fluoro-2-deoxy-D-glucose and positron emission tomography, with similar results (see Chap. 46).

SUBSTRATES OF CEREBRAL METABOLISM

Normally, the substrates are glucose and oxygen, and the products are carbon dioxide and water

In contrast to most other tissues, which exhibit considerable flexibility with respect to the nature of the foodstuffs extracted and consumed from the blood, the normal brain is restricted almost exclusively to glucose as the substrate for its energy metabolism. Despite long and intensive efforts, the only incontrovertible and consistently positive arteriovenous differences demonstrated for the human brain under normal conditions have been for glucose and oxygen [16]. Negative arteriovenous differences, significantly different from zero, have been found consistently only for carbon dioxide, although water, which has never been measured, is also produced. Pyruvate and lactate production have been observed occasionally, certainly in aged subjects with cerebral vascular insufficiency, but irregularly in subjects with normal oxygenation of the brain.

It appears, then, that in the normal *in vivo* state, glucose is the only significant substrate for the brain's energy metabolism. Under normal circumstances no other potential energy-yielding substance has been found to be extracted from the blood in more than trivial amounts. The stoichiometry of glucose utilization and oxygen consumption is summarized in Table 3. The normal, conscious human brain consumes oxygen at a rate of 156 μmol/100 g tissue/min. Carbon dioxide production is the same, leading to a respiratory quotient of 1.0, further evidence that carbohydrate is the ultimate substrate for oxidative metabolism. The O_2 consumption and CO_2 production are equivalent to a rate of glucose utilization of 26 μmol glucose/100 g tissue/min, assuming 6 μmol of O_2 consumed and CO_2 produced for each micromole of glucose completely oxidized to CO_2 and H_2O. The glucose utilization actually measured is, how-

TABLE 3.   Relationship between cerebral oxygen consumption and glucose utilization in a normal young adult man

Function	Value[a]
O_2 consumption (μmol/100 g brain tissue/min)	156
Glucose utilization (μmol/100 g brain tissue/min)	31
O_2/glucose ratio (mol/mol)	5
Glucose equivalent of O_2 consumption (μmol glucose/100 g brain tissue/min)	26[b]
CO_2 production (μmol/100 g brain tissue/min)	156
Cerebral respiratory quotient (R.Q.)	0.97

From Sokoloff [16].
[a] Values are the median of the values reported in the literature.
[b] Calculated on the basis of 6 mol of O_2 required for complete oxidation of 1 mol of glucose.

ever, 31 μmol/100 g/min, which indicates that glucose consumption is not only sufficient to account for total O_2 consumption, but is in excess by 5 μmol/100 g/min. For the complete oxidation of glucose, the theoretical ratio of O_2/glucose utilization is 6.0; the excess glucose utilization is responsible for a measured ratio of only 5.5 μmol O_2/ μmol glucose. The fate of the excess glucose is unknown, but it is probably distributed in part in lactate, pyruvate, and other intermediates of carbohydrate metabolism, each released from the brain into the blood in insufficient amounts to be detectable as significant arteriovenous differences. Some of the glucose must also be utilized not for the production of energy but for the synthesis of the chemical constituents of the brain.

Some oxygen is known to be utilized for the oxidation of substances not derived from glucose, as, for example, in the synthesis and metabolic degradation of monoamine neurotransmitters, as mentioned above. The amount of oxygen utilized for these processes is, however, extremely small and is undetectable in the presence of the enormous oxygen consumption used for carbohydrate oxidation.

The combination of a cerebral respira-

tory quotient of unity, an almost stoichiometric relationship between oxygen uptake and glucose consumption, and the absence of any significant arteriovenous difference for any other energy-rich substrate is strong evidence that the brain normally derives its energy from the oxidation of glucose. In this respect, cerebral metabolism is unique because no other tissue, except for the testis [23], has been found to rely only on carbohydrate for energy. This does not imply that the pathways of glucose metabolism in the brain lead, like combustion, directly and exclusively to production of carbon dioxide and water. Various chemical and energy transformations occur between the uptake of the primary substrates, glucose and oxygen, and the liberation of the end products, carbon dioxide and water. Various compounds derived from glucose or produced through the energy made available from glucose catabolism are intermediates in the process. Glucose carbon is incorporated, for example, into amino acids, protein, lipids, and glycogen. These are turned over and act as intermediates in the overall pathway from glucose to carbon dioxide and water. There is clear evidence from the studies with [^{14}C]glucose that the glucose is not entirely oxidized directly and that at any given moment some of the carbon dioxide being produced is derived from sources other than the glucose that enters the brain at the same moment or just prior to that moment. That oxygen and glucose consumption and carbon dioxide production are essentially in stoichiometric balance and no other energy-laden substrate is taken from the blood means, however, that the net energy made available to the brain must ultimately be derived from the oxidation of glucose. It should be noted that this is the situation in the normal state; as is discussed later, other substrates may be used in special circumstances or in abnormal states.

In brain, glucose utilization is obligatory

The brain normally derives almost all of its energy from the aerobic oxidation of glucose, but this does not distinguish between preferential and obligatory utilization of glucose. Most tissues are largely facultative in their choice of substrate and can use them interchangeably more or less in proportion to their availability. This does not appear to be so in brain. The present evidence indicates that, except in some unusual and very special circumstances, only the aerobic utilization of glucose is capable of providing the brain with sufficient energy to maintain normal function and structure. The brain appears to have almost no flexibility in its choice of substrates *in vivo*. This conclusion is derived from the following evidence.

Effects of glucose deprivation

It is well known clinically that a fall in blood glucose content, if of sufficient degree, is rapidly followed by aberrations of cerebral function. Hypoglycemia, produced by excessive insulin or occurring spontaneously in hepatic insufficiency, is associated with changes in mental state ranging from mild, subjective sensory disturbances to coma, the severity depending on both the degree and the duration of the hypoglycemia. The behavioral effects are paralleled by abnormalities in EEG patterns and cerebral metabolic rate. The EEG pattern exhibits increased prominence of slow, high-voltage δ rhythms,

and the rate of cerebral oxygen consumption falls. In studies of the effects of insulin hypoglycemia in humans [24], it was observed that, when the arterial glucose concentration fell from a normal level of 70 to 100 mg/100 ml to an average level of 19 mg/100 ml, the subjects became confused and their cerebral oxygen consumption fell to 2.6 ml/100 g/min, or 79 percent of the normal level. When the arterial glucose level fell to 8 mg/100 ml, a deep coma ensued and the cerebral oxygen consumption decreased even further to 1.9 ml/100 g/min (Table 4).

These changes are not caused by insufficient cerebral blood flow, which actually increases slightly during the coma. In the depths of the coma, when the blood glucose content is very low, there is almost no measurable cerebral uptake of glucose from the blood. Cerebral oxygen consumption, although reduced, is still far from negligible, and there is no longer any stoichiometric relationship between glucose and oxygen uptakes by the brain—evidence that the oxygen is utilized for the oxidation of other substances. The cerebral respiratory quotient (RQ) remains approximately 1, however, indicating that these other substrates are still carbohydrate, presumably derived from the brain's endogenous carbohydrate stores. The effects are clearly the result of hypoglycemia and not some other direct effect of

TABLE 4.   Effects of insulin hypoglycemia on cerebral circulation and metabolism in humans[a]

	Control	Insulin-induced hypoglycemia without coma	Insulin-induced hypoglycemic coma
ARTERIAL BLOOD			
Glucose concentration (mg%)	74	19	8
O_2 content (vol%)	17.4	17.9	16.6
Mean blood pressure (mmHg)	94	86	93
CEREBRAL CIRCULATION			
Blood flow (ml/100 g/min)	58	61	63
O_2 consumption (ml/100 g/min)	3.4	2.6	1.9
Glucose consumption (mg/100 g/min)	4.4	2.3	0.8
Respiratory quotient	0.95	1.10	0.92

[a] From Kety et al. [24].

TABLE 5.   Effectiveness of various substances in preventing or reversing the effects of hypoglycemia or glucose deprivation on cerebral function and metabolism[a]

Effectiveness	Substance	Comments
Effective	Epinephrine	Raises blood glucose concentration
	Maltose	Converted to glucose and raises blood glucose level
	Mannose	Directly metabolized and enters glycolytic pathway
Partially or occasionally effective	Glutamate	Occasionally effective by raising blood glucose level
	Arginine	
	Glycine	
	p-Aminobenzoate	
	Succinate	
Ineffective	Glycerol	Some of these substances can be metabolized to various
	Ethanol	extents by brain tissue and could conceivably be effective
	Lactate	if it were not for the blood-brain barrier
	Glyceraldehyde	
	Hexosediphosphates	
	Fumarate	
	Acetate	
	β-Hydroxybutyrate	
	Galactose	
	Lactose	
	Insulin	

[a] Summarized from the literature, in Sokoloff [16].

insulin in the brain. In all cases, the behavioral, functional, and cerebral metabolic abnormalities associated with insulin hypoglycemia are rapidly and completely reversed by the administration of glucose. The severity of the effects is correlated with the degree of hypoglycemia and not the insulin dosage, and the effects of the insulin can be completely prevented by the simultaneous administration of glucose with the insulin.

Similar effects are observed in hypoglycemia produced by other means, such as hepatectomy. The inhibition of glucose utilization at the phosphohexose isomerase step with pharmacologic doses of 2-deoxyglucose also produces all the cerebral effects of hypoglycemia despite an associated elevation in blood glucose content.

Utilization of substrates other than glucose in hypoglycemia

The hypoglycemic state provides convenient test conditions to determine whether a substance is capable of substituting for glucose as a substrate of cerebral energy metabolism.

If it can, its administration during hypoglycemic shock should restore consciousness and normal cerebral electrical activity without raising the blood glucose level. Numerous potential substrates have been tested in humans and animals. Very few can restore normal cerebral function in hypoglycemia, and of these all but one appear to operate through a variety of mechanisms to raise the blood glucose level rather than by serving as a substrate directly (Table 5).

Mannose appears to be the only substance that can be utilized by the brain directly and rapidly enough to restore or maintain normal function in the absence of glucose [25]. It traverses the BBB and is converted to mannose-6-phosphate. This reaction is catalyzed by hexokinase as effectively as the phosphorylation of glucose. The mannose-6-phosphate is then converted to fructose-6-phosphate by phosphomannose isomerase, which is active in brain tissue. Through these reactions mannose can enter directly into the glycolytic pathway and replace glucose.

Maltose also has been found to be effective occasionally in restoring normal behavior and EEG activity in hypoglycemia, but only by raising the blood glucose level through its conversion to glucose by maltase activity in blood and other tissues [16]. Epinephrine is effective in producing arousal from insulin coma, but this is achieved through its well-known stimulation of glycogenolysis and the elevation of blood glucose concentration. Glutamate, arginine, glycine, p-aminobenzoate, and succinate also act through adrenergic effects that raise the glucose concentrations of the blood [16].

It should be noted, however, that failure to restore normal cerebral function in hypoglycemia is not synonymous with an inability of the brain to utilize the substance. Many of the substances that have been tested and found ineffective are compounds normally formed and utilized within the brain and are normal intermediates in its intermediary metabolism. Lactate, pyruvate, fructose-1, 6-bisphosphate, acetate, β-hydroxybutyrate, and acetoacetate can all be utilized by brain slices, homogenates, or cell-free fractions, and the enzymes for their metabolism are present in the brain. Enzymes for the metabolism of glycerol or ethanol, for example, may not be present in sufficient amounts. For other substrates, for example, D-β-hydroxybutyrate and acetoacetate, the enzymes are adequate, but the substrate is not available to the brain because of inadequate blood levels or restricted transport through the BBB.

Nevertheless, nervous system function in the intact animal depends on substrates supplied by the blood and no satisfactory, normal, endogenous substitute for glucose has been found. Glucose must therefore be considered essential for normal physiological behavior of the central nervous system.

Brain utilizes ketones in states of ketosis

In special circumstances, the brain may fulfill its nutritional needs partly, although not completely, with substrates other than glucose. Normally there are no significant cerebral arteriovenous differences for D-β-hydroxybutyrate and acetoacetate, which are "ketone bodies" formed in the course of the catabolism of fatty acids by liver. Owen and co-workers [26] observed, however, that when human patients were treated for severe obesity by complete fasting for several weeks, there was considerable uptake of both substances by the brain. If one assumed that the substances were completely oxidized, their rates of utilization would have accounted for more than 50 percent of the total cerebral oxygen consumption—more than that accounted for by the glucose uptake. D-β-hydroxybutyrate uptake was several times greater than that of acetoacetate, a reflection of its higher concentration in the blood. The enzymes responsible for their metabolism, D-β-hydroxybutyrate dehydrogenase, acetoacetate-succinyl-coenzyme A (CoA) transferase, and acetoacetyl-CoA-thiolase, have been demonstrated to be present in brain tissue in sufficient amounts to convert them into acyl CoA and to feed them into the tricarboxylic acid cycle at a sufficient rate to satisfy the brain's metabolic demands [27].

Under normal circumstances, when there is ample glucose and the levels of ketone bodies in the blood are very low, the brain apparently does not resort to their use in any significant amounts. In prolonged starvation, the carbohydrate stores of the body are exhausted, and the rate of gluconeogenesis is insufficient to provide glucose fast enough to meet the requirements of the brain; blood ketone levels rise as a result of the rapid fat catabolism. The brain then apparently turns to the ketone bodies as the source of its energy supply.

Cerebral utilization of ketone bodies appears to follow passively their levels in arterial blood [27]. In normal adults, ketone levels are very low in blood, and cerebral utilization of ketones is negligible. In ketotic states resulting from starvation, fat-feeding or ketogenic diets, diabetes, or any other condition that accelerates the mobilization and catabolism of fat, cerebral utilization of ketones is increased more or less in direct proportion to the degree of ketosis [27]. Significant utilization of ketone bodies by brain is, however, normal in the neonatal period. The newborn infant tends to be hypoglycemic but becomes ketotic when it begins to nurse because of the high fat content of the mother's milk. When weaned onto the normal, relatively high carbohydrate diet, the ketosis and cerebral ketone utilization disappear. The studies have been carried out mainly in the infant rat, but there is evidence that the situation is similar in the human infant.

The first two enzymes in the pathway of ketone utilization are D-β-hydroxybutyrate dehydrogenase and acetoacetyl-succinyl-CoA transferase. These exhibit a postnatal pattern of development in brain that is well adapted to the nutritional demands of the brain. At birth, the activity of these enzymes in brain is low; they rise rapidly with the ketosis that develops with the onset of suckling, reach their peak just before weaning, and then gradually decline after weaning to normal adult levels of approximately one-third to one-fourth the maximum levels attained [27,28].

It should be noted that D-β-hydroxybutyrate is incapable of maintaining or restoring normal cerebral function in the absence of glucose in the blood. This suggests that, although it can partially replace glucose, it cannot fully satisfy the cerebral energy needs in the absence of some glucose consumption. One possible explanation may be that the first product of D-β-hydroxybutyrate oxidation, acetoacetate, is further metabolized by its displacement of the succinyl moiety of succinyl CoA to form acetoacetyl CoA. A certain level of glucose utilization may be essential to drive the tricarboxylic cycle and provide enough succinyl CoA to permit the further oxidation of acetoacetate and hence pull along the oxidation of D-β-hydroxybutyrate.

AGE AND DEVELOPMENT INFLUENCE CEREBRAL ENERGY METABOLISM

Metabolic rate increases during early development

The energy metabolism of the brain and the blood flow that sustains it vary considerably from birth to old age. Data on the cerebral metabolic rate obtained directly *in vivo* are lacking for the early postnatal period, but the results of *in vitro* measurements in animal brain preparations and inferences drawn from cerebral blood flow measurements in intact animals [29] suggest that the cerebral oxygen consumption is low at birth, rises rapidly during the period of cerebral growth and development, and reaches a maximal level at about the time maturation is completed. This rise is consistent with the progressive increase in the levels of a number of enzymes of oxidative metabolism in the brain. The rate of blood flow in different structures of the brain reach peak levels at different times, depending on the maturation rate of the particular structure. In the structures that consist predominantly of white matter, the peaks coincide roughly with the times of maximal rates of myelination. From these peaks, blood flow and, probably, cerebral metabolic rate decline to the levels characteristic of adulthood.

Metabolic rate declines and plateaus after maturation

Reliable quantitative data on the changes in cerebral circulation and metabolism in humans from the middle of the first decade of life to old age are summarized in Table 6. By 6 years of age, the cerebral blood flow and oxygen consumption have already attained their high levels, and they decline thereafter to the levels of normal young adulthood [15]. Cerebral oxygen consumption of 5.2 ml/100 g brain tissue/min in a 5- to 6-year-old child corresponds to total oxygen consumption by the brain of approximately 60 ml/min, or more than 50 percent of the total

TABLE 6.   Cerebral blood flow and oxygen consumption in man from childhood to old age and senility[a]

Life period and condition	Age (years)	Cerebral blood flow (ml/100 g/min)	Cerebral O_2 consumption (ml/100 g/min)	Cerebral venous O_2 tension (mmHg)
Childhood	6[b]	106[b]	5.2[b]	—
Normal young adulthood	21	62	3.5	38
Aged				
Normal elderly	71[b]	58	3.3	36
Elderly with minimal arteriosclerosis	73[b]	48[b]	3.2	33[b,c]
Elderly with senile psychosis	72[b]	48[b,c]	2.7[b,c]	33[b,c]

[a] From Sokoloff [15,30].
[b] Statistically significant difference from normal young adult ($p < 0.05$).
[c] Statistically significant difference from normal elderly subjects ($p < 0.05$).

body basal oxygen consumption, a proportion markedly greater than that occurring in adulthood. The reasons for the extraordinarily high cerebral metabolic rates in children are unknown, but presumably they reflect the extra energy requirements for the biosynthetic processes associated with growth and development.

Tissue pathology but not aging produces secondary change in metabolic rate

Despite reports to the contrary, whole brain cerebral blood flow and oxygen consumption normally remain essentially unchanged between young adulthood and old age. In a population of normal elderly men in their eighth decade of life—who were carefully selected for good health and freedom from all disease, including vascular disease—both blood flow and oxygen consumption were not significantly different from those of normal young men 50 years younger (see Table 6) [30]. In a comparable group of elderly subjects, who differed only by the presence of objective evidence of minimal arteriosclerosis, cerebral blood flow was significantly lower. It had reached a point at which the oxygen tension of the cerebral venous blood declined, which is an indication of relative cerebral hypoxia. Cerebral oxygen consumption, however, was still maintained at normal levels through extraction of larger than normal proportions of the arterial blood oxy-

gen. In senile psychotic patients with arteriosclerosis, cerebral blood flow was no lower, but cerebral oxygen consumption had also declined. These data suggest that aging *per se* need not lower cerebral oxygen consumption and blood flow but that, when blood flow is reduced, it is probably secondary to arteriosclerosis, which produces cerebral vascular insufficiency and chronic relative hypoxia in the brain, or secondary to other tissue pathology that decreases function, as in dementia (see Chap. 45). Because arteriosclerosis and Alzheimer's disease are so prevalent in the aged population, most individuals probably follow the latter pattern. However, age-related changes in local regulation are possible and are the subject of research (see Chap. 30).

CEREBRAL METABOLIC RATE IN VARIOUS PHYSIOLOGICAL STATES

Cerebral metabolic rate is determined locally by functional activity in discrete regions

In organs such as heart or skeletal muscle that perform mechanical work, increased functional activity clearly is associated with increased metabolic rate. In nervous tissues outside the central nervous system, the electrical activity is an almost quantitative indicator of the degree of functional activity, and in structures such as sympathetic ganglia and postganglionic axons, increased electrical activity produced by electrical stimulation is definitely associated with increased utilization of oxygen. Within the central nervous system, local energy metabolism is also closely correlated with the level of local functional activity. Studies using the [^{14}C]deoxyglucose method have demonstrated pronounced changes in glucose utilization associated with altered functional activity in discrete regions of the central nervous system specifically related to that function [21]. For example, diminished visual or auditory input depresses glucose utilization in all components of the central visual or auditory pathways, respectively (Fig. 4). Focal seizures increase glucose utilization in discrete components of the motor pathways, such as the motor cortex and the basal ganglia (Fig. 5).

Convulsive activity, induced or spontaneous, has often been employed as a method of increasing electrical activity of the brain (see Chap. 43). Davies and Remond [13] used the oxygen electrode technique in the cerebral cortex of cat and found increases in oxygen consumption during electrically induced or drug-induced convulsions. Because the increased oxygen consumption either coincided with or followed the onset of convulsions, it was concluded that the elevation in metabolic rate was the consequence of the increased functional activity produced by the convulsive state (see Chap. 43).

Metabolic rate and nerve conduction are directly related

Studies using the [^{14}C]deoxyglucose method have defined the nature and mechanisms of the relationship between energy metabolism and functional activity in nervous tissues. Studies in the superior cervical ganglion of the rat have shown almost a direct relationship between glucose utilization in the ganglion and spike frequency in the afferent fibers from the cervical sympathetic trunk [31]. A spike results from the passage of fi-

nite current of Na$^+$ into the cell and K$^+$ out of the cell, ion currents that degrade the ionic gradients responsible for the resting membrane potential. Such degradation can be expected to stimulate Na,K-ATPase activity to restore the ionic gradients to normal, and such ATPase activity would, in turn, stimulate energy metabolism. Indeed, Mata et al. [32] have found that, in the posterior pituitary *in vitro*, the stimulation of glucose utilization due either to electrical stimulation or opening of Na$^+$ channels in the excitable membrane by veratridine is blocked by ouabain, a specific inhibitor of Na,K-ATPase activity (see Chap. 3). Most, if not all, of the stimulated energy metabolism associated with increased functional activity is confined to the axonal terminals rather than to the cell bodies in a functionally activated pathway (Fig. 6) [33].

It is difficult to define metabolic equivalents of consciousness, mental work, and sleep

Mental Work

Convincing correlations between cerebral metabolic rate and mental activity have been obtained in humans in a variety of pathological states of altered consciousness [34]. Regardless of the cause of the disorder, graded reductions in cerebral oxygen consumption are accompanied by parallel graded reductions in the degree of mental alertness, all the way to profound coma (Table 7). It is difficult to define or even to conceive of the physical equivalent of mental work. A common view equates concentrated mental effort with mental work, and it is also fashionable to attribute a high demand for mental effort to the process of problem solving in mathematics. Nevertheless, there appears to be no increased energy utilization by the brain during such processes. From resting levels, total cerebral blood flow and oxygen consumption remain unchanged during the exertion of the mental effort required to solve complex arithmetical problems [34].

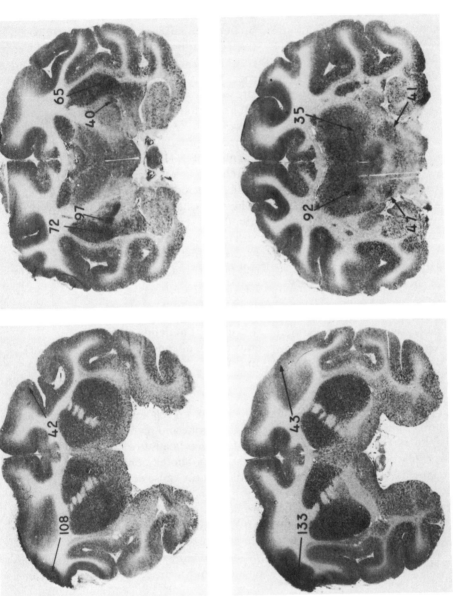

FIG. 5. Local glucose utilization during penicillin-induced focal seizures. The penicillin was applied to the hand and face area of the left motor cortex of a rhesus monkey. The left side of the brain is on the left in each of the autoradiograms in the figure. The numbers are the rates of local cerebral glucose utilization in μmol/100 g tissue/min. Note the following: *upper left,* motor cortex in region of penicillin application and corresponding region of contralateral motor cortex; *lower left,* ipsilateral and contralateral motor cortical regions remote from area of penicillin applications; *upper right,* ipsilateral and contralateral putamen and globus pallidus; *lower right,* ipsilateral and contralateral thalamic nuclei and substantia nigra. (From Sokoloff [21].)

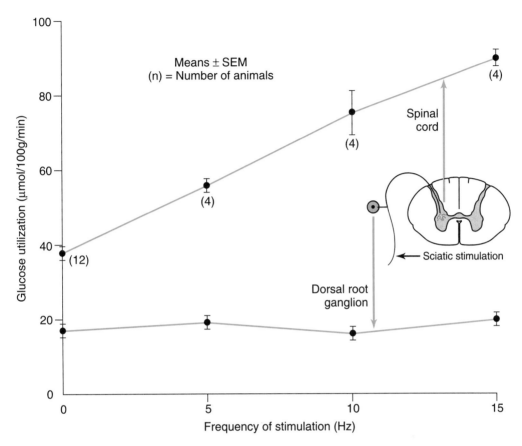

FIG. 6. Effects of electrical stimulation of sciatic nerve on glucose utilization in the terminal zones in the dorsal horn of the spinal cord and in the cell bodies in the dorsal root ganglion. (From Kadekaro et al. [33].)

TABLE 7. Relationship between level of consciousness and cerebral metabolic rate[a]

Level of consciousness	Cerebral blood flow (ml/100 g/min)	Cerebral O_2 consumption (ml/100 g/min)
Mentally alert Normal young men	54	3.3
Mentally confused Brain tumor Diabetic acidosis Insulin hypoglycemia Cerebral arteriosclerosis	48	2.8
Comatose Brain tumor Diabetic coma Insulin coma Anesthesia	57	2.0

[a] From Sokoloff [34].

It may be that the assumptions that relate mathematical reasoning to mental work are erroneous, but it seems more likely that the areas that participate in the processes of such reasoning represent too small a fraction of the brain for changes in their functional and metabolic activities to be reflected in the energy metabolism of the brain as a whole.

Sleep

Sleep is a naturally occurring, periodic, reversible state of unconsciousness, and the EEG pattern in deep slow-wave sleep is characterized by high-voltage slow rhythms very similar to those often seen in pathological comatose states. As found in the pathological comatose states, cerebral glucose metabolism is depressed more or less uniformly throughout the brain of rhesus monkeys in stages 2 to 4 of normal sleep studied by the [^{14}C]deoxyglucose method [35]. There are no comparable data available for the state of paradoxical sleep (REM sleep) or for normal sleep in humans.

CEREBRAL ENERGY METABOLISM IN PATHOLOGICAL STATES

The cerebral metabolic rate of the brain as a whole is normally fairly stable and varies over a relatively narrow range under physiological conditions. There are, however, a number of pathological states of the nervous system and other organs that affect the functions of the brain either directly or indirectly, and some of these have profound effects on the cerebral metabolism.

Psychiatric disorders may produce effects related to anxiety

In general, disorders that alter the quality of mentation but not the level of consciousness (e.g., the functional neuroses, psychoses, and psychotomimetic states) have no apparent effect on the average blood flow and oxygen consumption of the brain as a whole. Thus, no changes in either function are observed in schizophrenia [34] or LSD intoxication (Table 8) [34]. There is still uncertainty about the effects of anxiety, mainly because of the difficulties in evaluating quantitatively the intensity of anxiety. It is generally believed that ordinary degrees of anxiety or "nervousness" do not affect the cerebral metabolic rate, but severe anxiety or "panic" may increase cerebral oxygen consumption [34]. This may be related to the level of epinephrine circulating in the blood. Small doses of epinephrine that raise heart rate and cause some anxiety do not alter cerebral blood flow and metabolism, but large doses that are sufficient to raise the arterial blood pressure cause significant increases in the levels of both.

Coma and systemic metabolic diseases depress brain metabolism

Coma is correlated with depression of cerebral oxygen consumption; progressive reductions in the level of consciousness are paralleled by corresponding graded decreases in the cerebral metabolic rate (see Table 7). There are almost innumerable derangements that can lead to depression of consciousness. Table 9 includes only a few typical examples that have been studied by the same methods and by the same or related groups of investigators. Metabolic encephalopathy is discussed in detail in Chapter 40.

Inadequate cerebral nutrient supply leads to decreases in the level of consciousness, ranging from confusional states to coma. The nutrition of the brain can be limited by lowering the oxygen or glucose levels of arterial blood, as in anoxia or hypoglycemia, or by impairment of their distribution to the brain through lowering cerebral blood flow, as in brain tumors. Consciousness is then depressed, presumably because of inadequate supplies of substrate to support the energy metabolism necessary to sustain function of the brain.

In a number of conditions, the causes of depression of both consciousness and the cerebral metabolic rate are unknown and must, by exclusion, be attributed to intracellular defects in the brain. Anesthesia is one example. Cerebral oxygen consumption is always reduced in the anesthetized state regardless of the anesthetic agent used,

TABLE 8.   Cerebral blood flow and metabolic rate in schizophrenia and in normal young men during LSD-induced psychotomimetic state[a]

Condition	Cerebral blood blow (ml/100 g/min)	Cerebral O$_2$ consumption (ml/100 g/min)
Normal	67	3.9
LSD intoxication	68	3.9
Schizophrenia	72	4.0

[a] From Sokoloff [34].

TABLE 9.   Cerebral blood flow and metabolic rate in humans with various disorders affecting mental state[a]

Condition	Mental state	Cerebral blood flow (ml/100 g/min)	Cerebral O_2 consumption (ml/100 g/min)
Normal	Alert	54	3.3
Increased intracranial pressure (brain tumor)	Coma	34[b]	2.5[b]
Insulin hypoglycemia Arterial glucose level			
74 mg/100 ml	Alert	58	3.4
19 mg/100 ml	Confused	61	2.6[b]
8 mg/100 ml	Coma	63	1.9[b]
Thiopental anesthesia	Coma	60[b]	2.1[b]
Postconvulsive state			
Before convulsion	Alert	58	3.7
After convulsion	Confused	37[b]	3.1[b]
Diabetes			
Acidosis	Confused	45[b]	2.7[b]
Coma	Coma	65[b]	1.7[b]
Hepatic insufficiency	Coma	33[b]	1.7[b]

[a] All studies listed were carried out by Kety and/or his associates, employing the same methods. For references, see Sokoloff [15,34].
[b] Denotes statistically significant difference from normal level ($p < 0.05$).

whereas blood flow may or may not be decreased and may even be increased. This reduction is the result of decreased energy demand and not insufficient nutrient supply or a block of intracellular energy metabolism. There is evidence that general anesthetics interfere with synaptic transmission, thus reducing neuronal interaction and functional activity and, consequently, metabolic demands.

Several metabolic diseases with broad systemic manifestations are also associated with disturbances of cerebral function. Diabetes mellitus, when allowed to progress to states of acidosis and ketosis, leads to mental confusion and, ultimately, to deep coma, with parallel proportionate decreases in cerebral oxygen consumption (see Table 9) [36]. The abnormalities are usually completely reversed by adequate insulin therapy. The cause of the coma or depressed cerebral metabolic rate is not known. Deficiency of cerebral nutrition cannot be implicated because the blood glucose level is elevated and cerebral blood flow and oxygen supply are more than adequate. Neither is insulin defi-ciency, which is presumably the basis of the systemic manifestations of the disease, a likely cause of the cerebral abnormalities, since no absolute requirement of insulin for cerebral glucose utilization or metabolism has been demonstrated. Ketosis may be severe in this disease, and there is disputed evidence that a rise in the blood level of at least one of the ketone bodies, acetoacetate, can cause coma in animals. In studies of human diabetic acidosis and coma, a significant correlation between the depression of cerebral metabolic rate and the degree of ketosis has been observed, but there is an equally good correlation with the degree of acidosis [36]. Hyperosmolarity itself may also cause coma. It is possible that ketosis, acidosis, hyperosmolarity, or a combination may be responsible for the disturbances in cerebral function and metabolism.

Coma is occasionally associated with severe impairment of liver function, or hepatic insufficiency (see Chap. 40). In human patients in hepatic coma, cerebral metabolic rate is markedly depressed (see Table 9). Cerebral blood flow is also moderately depressed but not sufficiently to lead to limiting supplies of glucose and oxygen. The blood ammonia level is usually elevated in hepatic coma, and significant cerebral uptake of ammonia from the blood is observed. Ammonia toxicity has therefore been suspected as the basis for cerebral dysfunction in hepatic coma. Because ammonia can, through glutamic dehydrogenase activity, convert α-ketoglutarate to glutamate by reductive amination, it has been suggested that ammonia might thereby deplete α-ketoglutarate and thus slow the Krebs cycle (see Chaps. 39 and 40). The correlation between the degree of coma and the blood ammonia level is far from convincing, however, and coma has, in fact, been observed in the absence of an increase in blood ammonia concentration. Although ammonia may be involved in the mechanism of hepatic coma, the mechanism remains unclear, and other causal factors are probably involved.

Depression of mental functions and the cerebral metabolic rate has been observed in association with kidney failure, i.e., uremic coma (see Chap. 40). The chemical basis of the functional and metabolic disturbances in the brain in this condition also remains undetermined.

In the comatose states associated with these systemic metabolic diseases, there is depression of both the level of conscious mental activity and cerebral energy metabolism. From the available evidence, it is impossible to distinguish which, if either, is the primary change. It is more likely that the depressions of both functions, although well correlated with each other, are independent reflections of a more general impairment of neuronal processes by some unknown factors incident to the disease.

Measurement of local cerebral energy metabolism in humans

Most of the *in vivo* measurements of cerebral energy metabolism described above, and all of those in humans, were made in the brain as a whole and represent the mass-weighted average of the metabolic activities in all the component structures of the brain. The average, however, often obscures transient and local events in the individual components, and it is not surprising that many of the studies of altered cerebral function, both normal and abnormal, have failed to demonstrate corresponding changes in energy metabolism (see Table 8). The [^{14}C]deoxyglucose method [19] has made it possible to measure glucose utilization simultaneously in all the components of the central nervous system, and it has been used to identify the regions with altered functional and metabolic activities in a variety of physiological, pharmacological and pathological states [21]. As originally designed, the method utilized autoradiography of brain sections for localization, which precluded its use in humans. However, later developments with positron emission tomography [37] made it possible to adapt it for human use, which is described fully in Chapter 46.

REFERENCES

1. Maker, H. S., and Nicklas, W. Biochemical responses of body organs to hypoxia and ischemia. In E. D. Robin (ed.), *Extrapulmonary Manifestations of Respiratory Disease.* New York: Dekker, 1978, pp. 107–150.
2. Gatfield, P. D., et al. Regional energy reserves in mouse brain and changes with ischaemia and anaesthesia. *J. Neurochem.* 13:185–195, 1966.
3. Lowry, O. H., and Passoneau, J. V. The relationships between substrates and enzymes of glycolysis in brain. *J. Biol. Chem.* 239:31–32, 1964.
4. Meyer, R. A., and Sweeney, H. L. A simple analysis of the "phospho creatine shuttle." *Am. J. Physiol.* 246:365–377, 1984.
5. Goldberg, N. D., and O'Toole, A. G. The properties of glycogen synthetase and regulation of glycogen biosynthesis in rat brain. *J. Biol. Chem.* 244:3053–3061, 1969.
6. Lehninger, A. L. *Biochemistry.* New York: Worth, 1982.
7. Stewart, M. A., and Moonsammy, G. I. Sub-

strate changes in peripheral nerve recovering from anoxia. *J. Neurochem.* 13:1433–1439, 1966.

8. Gaitonde, M. K., Evison, E., and Evans, G. M. The rate of utilization of glucose via hexose-monophosphate shunt in brain. *J. Neurochem.* 41:1253–1260, 1983.

9. Morgan-Hughes, J. A. Mitochondrial disease. *Trends Neurosci.* 9:15–19, 1986.

10. Waelsch, H., Berl, S., Rossi, C. A., Clarke, D. D., and Purpura, D. P. Quantitative aspects of CO_2 fixation in mammalian brain *in vivo*. *J. Neurochem.* 11:717–728, 1964.

11. Clarke, D. D. Fluoroacetate and fluorocitrate: mechanism of action. *Neurochem. Res.* 16: 1055–1058, 1991.

12. Leong, S. F., Lai, J. C. K., Lim, L., and Clark, J. B. The activities of some energy metabolizing enzymes in non synaptic (free) and synaptic mitochondria derived from selected brain regions. *J. Neurochem.* 42:1308–1312, 1984.

13. Davies, P. W., and Remond, A. Oxygen consumption of the cerebral cortex of the cat during metrazole convulsions. *Res. Publ. Assoc. Nerv. Ment. Dis.* 26:205–217, 1946.

14. Kety, S. S., and Schmidt, C. F. The nitrous oxide method for the quantitative determination of cerebral blood flow in man: Theory, procedure, and normal values. *J. Clin. Invest.* 27:476–483, 1948.

15. Kennedy, C., and Sokoloff, L. An adaptation of the nitrous oxide method to the study of the cerebral circulation in children; normal values for cerebral blood flow and cerebral metabolic rate in childhood. *J. Clin. Invest.* 36: 1130–1137, 1957.

16. Sokoloff, L. The metabolism of the central nervous system *in vivo*. In J. Field, H. W. Magoun, and V. E. Hall (eds.), *Handbook of Physiology–Neurophysiology*. Washington, D.C.: American Physiological Society, 1960, Vol 3, pp. 1843–1864.

17. Sokoloff, L., and Kety, S. S. Regulation of cerebral circulation. *Physiol. Rev.* 40(Suppl. 4): 38–44, 1960.

18. Freygang, W. H., and Sokoloff, L. Quantitative measurements of regional circulation in the central nervous system by the use of radioactive inert gas. *Adv. Biol. Med. Phys.* 6: 263–279, 1958.

19. Sokoloff, L., Reivich, M., Kennedy, C., Des Rosiers, M. H., Patlak, C. S., Pettigrew, K. D., Sakurada, O., and Shinohara, M. The [^{14}C]deoxyglucose method for the measurement of local cerebral glucose utilization: Theory, procedure, and normal values in the conscious and anesthetized albino rat. *J. Neurochem.* 28:897–916, 1977.

20. Sokoloff, L. Local cerebral energy metabolism: Its relationships to local functional activity and blood flow. In M. J. Purves and L. Elliott (eds.), *Cerebral Vascular Smooth Muscle and Its Control* (Ciba Foundation Symposium 56). Amsterdam: Elsevier/Excerpta Medica/North Holland, 1978, pp. 171–197.

21. Sokoloff, L. Relation between physiological function and energy metabolism in the central nervous system. *J. Neurochem.* 29:13–26, 1977.

22. Kennedy, C., Sakurada, O., Shinohara, M., Jehle, J., and Sokoloff, L. Local cerebral glucose utilization in the normal conscious Macaque monkey. *Ann. Neurol.* 4:293–301, 1978.

23. Himwich, H. E., and Nahum, L. H. The respiratory quotient of testicle. *Am. J. Physiol.* 88: 680–685, 1929.

24. Kety, S. S., Woodford, R. B., Harmel, M. H., Freyhan, F. A., Appel, K. E., and Schmidt, C. F. Cerebral flow and metabolism in schizophrenia. The effects of barbiturate semi-narcosis, insulin coma, and electroshock. *Am. J. Psychiatry* 104:765–770, 1948.

25. Sloviter, H. A., and Kamimoto, T. The isolated, perfused rat brain preparation metabolizes mannose but not maltose. *J. Neurochem.* 17:1109–1111, 1970.

26. Owen, O. E., Morgan, A. P., Kemp, H. G., Sullivan, J. M., Herrera, M. G., and Cahill, G. F., Jr. Brain metabolism during fasting. *J. Clin. Invest.* 46:1589–1595, 1967.

27. Krebs, H. A., Williamson, D. H., Bates, M. W., Page, M. A., and Hawkins, R. A. The role of ketone bodies in caloric homeostatis. *Adv. Enzyme Regul.* 9:387–409, 1971.

28. Klee, C. B., and Sokoloff, L. Changes in D(−)-β-hydroxybutyric dehydrogenase activity during brain maturation in the rat. *J. Biol. Chem.* 242:3880–3883, 1967.

29. Kennedy, C., Grave, G. D., Jehle, J. W., and Sokoloff, L. Changes in blood flow in the component structures of the dog brain during postnatal maturation. *J. Neurochem.* 19: 2423–2433, 1972.

30. Sokoloff, L. Cerebral circulatory and metabolic changes associated with aging. *Res. Publ. Assoc. Nerv. Ment. Dis.* 41:237–254, 1966.

31. Yarowsky, P., Kadekaro, M., and Sokoloff, L. Frequency-dependent activation of glucose utilization in the superior cervical ganglion by electrical stimulation of cervical sympathetic trunk. *Proc. Natl. Acad. Sci. U.S.A.* 80:4179–4183, 1983.

32. Mata, M., Fink, D. J., Gainer, H., Smith, C. B., Davidsen, L., Savaki, H., Schwartz, W. J., and Sokoloff, L. Activity-dependent energy metabolism in rat posterior pituitary primarily reflects sodium pump activity. *J. Neurochem.* 34:213–215, 1980.

33. Kadekaro, M., Crane, A. M., and Sokoloff, L. Differential effects of electrical stimulation of sciatic nerve on metabolic activity in spinal cord and dorsal root ganglion in the rat. *Proc. Natl. Acad. Sci. U.S.A.* 82:6010–6013, 1985.

34. Sokoloff, L. Cerebral circulation and behavior in man: Strategy and findings. In A. J. Mandell and M. P. Mandell (eds.), *Psychochemical Research in Man.* New York: Academic, 1969, pp. 237–252.

35. Kennedy, C., Gillin, J. C., Mendelson, W., Suda, S., Miyaoka, M., Ito, M., Nakamura, R. K., Storch, F. I., Pettigrew, K., Mishkin, M., and Sokoloff, L. Local cerebral glucose utilization in non-rapid eye movement sleep. *Nature* 297:325–327, 1982.

36. Kety, S. S., Polis, B. D., Nadler, C. S., and Schmidt, C. F. Blood flow and oxygen consumption of the human brain in diabetic acidosis and coma. *J. Clin. Invest.* 27:500–510, 1948.

37. Reivich, M., Kuhl, D., Wolf, A., Greenberg, J., Phelps, M., Ido, T., Casella, V., Fowler J., Hoffman, E., Alavi, A., Som, P., and Sokoloff, L. The [^{18}F]fluoro-deoxyglucose method for the measurement of local cerebral glucose utilization in man. *Cir. Res.* 44:127–137, 1979.

CHAPTER 32

Blood-Brain–Cerebrospinal Fluid Barriers

A. Lorris Betz, Gary W. Goldstein, and Robert Katzman

Basic Neurochemistry: Molecular, Cellular, and Medical Aspects, 5th Ed., edited by G. J. Siegel et al. Published by Raven Press, Ltd., New York, 1994. Correspondence to A. Lorris Betz, Departments of Pediatrics, Surgery, and Neurology, University of Michigan, D3227 Medical Professional Building, Ann Arbor, Michigan 48109–0718.

CONSTANCY OF THE BRAIN'S INTERNAL ENVIRONMENT

In no other organ is constancy of the internal environment more important than in the brain. Elsewhere in the body, the extracellular concentrations of hormones, amino acids, and potassium undergo frequent fluctuations, particularly after meals and exercise or during times of stress. In the central nervous system a similar change in the composition of the interstitial fluid could lead to uncontrolled brain activity because catecholamines and certain amino acids are centrally acting neurotransmitters and potassium influences the threshold for activation of synapses. Consequently, the cerebrospinal fluid (CSF) concentrations of many solutes are maintained lower than their concentrations in plasma (Table 1). The blood-brain-CSF barriers isolate brain cells from the normal variations in body fluid composition and regulate the composition of the brain's extracellular fluid in order to provide a stable environment for nerve cell interactions.

DEVELOPMENT OF THE CONCEPT OF BLOOD-BRAIN–CEREBROSPINAL FLUID BARRIERS

The concept of the blood-brain-CSF barriers was developed in the late nineteenth century when Ehrlich observed that vital dyes administered intravenously stained all organs except the brain. He concluded that the dyes had a lower affinity for binding to brain than to other tissues. In 1913, however, Goldmann disproved the binding hypothesis by administering trypan blue dye directly into the CSF. By this route, the dye readily stained the entire brain substance but was restricted to the brain and spinal cord and did not enter the bloodstream to reach other organs. The studies with vital dyes agreed well with the parallel work of Biedl and Kraus in 1898 with bile acids and of Lewandowsky in 1900 with ferrocyanide. These compounds were not neurotoxic when administered by vein

but caused seizures and coma when injected directly into the brain. These experiments established that the central nervous system is separated from the bloodstream by blood-brain and blood-CSF barriers. The cellular basis for these barriers was not established until 50 years later, when the development of electron microscopy permitted examination of the ultrastructure of the brain's microvasculature and the choroid plexus.

MEMBRANE TRANSPORT PROCESSES

Contemporary research has focused on how selected molecules are able to enter and leave the brain and how CSF is formed. This work has led to an appreciation of the important role played by membrane transport processes in the function of the blood-brain-CSF barriers [1,2]. Monographs about the blood-brain and blood-CSF barriers are available for those readers interested in a more complete review of these subjects [3,4].

Physical and biological processes determine molecular movement across membranes of the blood-brain-CSF barriers

The processes that determine molecular movement across membranes are diffusion, pinocytosis, carrier-mediated transport, and transcellular transport [5]. The types of carrier-mediated transport are described in Chap. 3.

Diffusion

Diffusion is the process by which molecules in solution move from an area of higher to one of lower concentration. With this type of transport, the net rate of solute flux is directly proportional to the difference in concentration between the two areas. In biologic systems, this process is an important mechanism for the movement of molecules within a fluid compartment; however, diffusion across a lipid membrane, (e.g., the cell membranes of the blood-brain barrier) is only

TABLE 1.   Typical cerebrospinal fluid (CSF) and plasma concentrations of various substances[a]

Substance	CSF	Plasma	CSF/plasma ratio
ELECTROLYTES (mEq/l)			
Na	138	138	1.0
K	2.8	4.5	0.6
Cl	119	102	1.2
HCO_3	22	24	0.9
Ca	2.1	4.8	0.4
Mg	2.3	1.7	1.4
PO_4	0.5	1.8	0.3
METABOLITES (mM)			
Glucose	3.3	5.0	0.7
Lactate	1.6	1.0	1.6
Pyruvate	0.08	0.11	0.7
Urea	4.7	5.4	0.9
Creatinine	0.09	0.14	0.7
AMINO ACIDS (μM)			
Alanine	26.0	350	0.1
Arginine	22.4	80.9	0.3
Aspartic acid	0.2	2.0	0.1
Asparagine	13.5	112	0.1
Glutamic acid	26.1	61.3	0.4
Glutamine	552	641	0.9
Glycine	5.9	283	0.02
Histidine	12.3	79.8	0.2
Isoleucine	6.2	76.7	0.1
Leucine	14.8	155	0.1
Lysine	20.8	171	0.1
Methionine	2.5	27.7	0.1
Ornithine	3.8	73.5	0.1
Phenylalanine	9.9	64.0	0.2
Phosphoethanolamine	5.4	5.1	1.0
Phosphoserine	4.2	8.3	0.6
Serine	29.5	140	0.2
Taurine	7.6	77.2	0.1
Threonine	35.5	166	0.2
Tyrosine	9.5	73.0	0.1
Valine	19.9	309	0.1
PROTEINS (mg/l)			
Total protein	350	70,000	0.005
Albumin	155	36,600	0.004
Transferrin	14.4	2,040	0.007
IgG	12.3	9,870	0.001
IgA	1.3	1,750	0.001
IgM	0.6	700	0.001

[a] Values are from Fishman [1].

possible when the solute is lipid soluble or when the membrane contains specialized channels. Diffusion is the primary mechanism for blood-brain exchange of respiratory gases and other highly lipid-soluble compounds.

Pinocytosis

In the process of pinocytosis, extracellular fluid is engulfed by invaginating cell membranes, forming a vesicle that then separates from the membrane. This vesicle may move through the cell cytoplasm and release its contents on the other side of the cell layer by means of exocytosis. Under normal conditions, pinocytosis is thought to contribute little to the transport of solutes across the blood-brain barrier. Instead, the few vesicles that are observed within brain capillary endothelial cells are probably destined to fuse with lysosomes. Nevertheless, some proteins may traverse the brain endothelial cell through a process that has been called absorptive-mediated transcytosis [6].

Transcellular Transport

Transport across a layer of cells requires the presence of carrier or channel molecules on luminal and antiluminal sides of the cells. Facilitated and active transport are defined in Chap. 3. In transcellular facilitated diffusion, the carriers on opposite sides of the cell are usually similar, and solutes are not moved against concentration gradients. Active transport across a cell layer, however, requires a special arrangement of transport proteins within the plasma membranes. The active transport system is found on only one side of the cell and is usually associated with a nonactive transport system on the other side of the cell. With this arrangement, a solute accumulates within the cell by active transport through one membrane and subsequently leaves the cell by a channel or facilitated transport process through the opposite membrane. When plasma membranes of two surfaces of a cell have different properties, that cell is said to be *polar*. Cellular polarity

underlines active transcellular transport and secretion of fluid by epithelial cells in the choroid plexus.

When fluid is secreted at one site and absorbed at another, there is bulk flow of fluid. This means that solutes of various sizes move together with the solvent as a bulk liquid. This process is important in the circulation and absorption of CSF, which is secreted by the choroid plexus, circulated through the ventricular and subarachnoid spaces, and absorbed through arachnoid villi into the bloodstream.

Transport processes combine to provide stability for constituents of CSF and brain extracellular fluid

Bradbury and Stulcová [7] defined stability of the blood-CSF systems as follows. If a substance is present in CSF at concentration C_{CSF} and in plasma at concentration C_{pl}, stability occurs when, as a result of a change in plasma concentration, a new steady state is reached so that

$$\Delta C_{CSF} < \Delta C_{pl}$$

At steady state, the flux of this substance from plasma to CSF, J_{in}, must equal its flux out, J_{out}, so that for any change in plasma concentration, ΔC_{pl}, stability of CSF will occur when

$$\Delta J_{in}/\Delta C_{pl} < \Delta J_{out}/\Delta C_{CSF}$$

where J_{in} and J_{out} represent transport processes that need not be identical. For instance, one might be passive and one active. If the carrier involved in J_{in} is saturated at the usual plasma concentration, then the ratio $\Delta J_{in}/\Delta C_{pl}$ will approach zero. Such carrier-mediated transport is probably the most common mechanism controlling the flow of water-soluble substances from the capillary lumen to the brain, but carrier systems have also been found to operate for outward flux. Here, the greatest stability is achieved when the carrier system operates well below saturation, so that the ratio $\Delta J_{out}/\Delta C_{CSF}$ is a positive number. Such asymmetrical carrier mechanisms have been implicated in the maintenance of a stable K^+ concentration in CSF and may also exist for some amino acids and organic acids.

BLOOD-BRAIN BARRIER

Endothelial cells in brain capillaries are the site of the blood-brain barrier

Studies of Reese and Karnovsky and Brightman and Reese demonstrated that brain endothelial cells differ from endothelial cells in capillaries of other organs in two important ways [8]. First, continuous tight junctions are present between the endothelial cells that prevent transcapillary movement of polar molecules varying in size from proteins to ions. Second, there are no detectable transendothelial pathways. Thus, there is an absence of transcellular channels and fenestrations as well as a paucity of plasmalemmal and intracellular vesicles. As a result of these special anatomical features, the endothelial cells in brain provide a continuous cellular barrier between the blood and the interstitial fluid (Fig. 1).

Not all areas of the brain contain capillaries that produce a barrier. In these nonbarrier regions, the morphologic features of the capillaries are similar to those of systemic microvascular beds. Thus, the tight junctions are discontinuous, there are more plasmalemmal vesicles, and some endothelial cells even exhibit fenestrations. Table 2 lists

TABLE 2.   Areas of brain without a blood-brain barrier

Pituitary gland
Median eminence
Area postrema
Preoptic recess
Paraphysis
Pineal gland
Endothelium of the choroid plexus

the brain regions that contain capillaries of this type. The absence of a blood-brain barrier in many of these regions may relate to their feedback role in the regulation of peptide hormone release.

Surrounding the capillary endothelial cell is a collagen-containing extracellular matrix. Embedded within this basement membrane are contractile pericytes. These cells may regulate endothelial cell proliferation and, under certain pathological conditions, take on phagocytic functions. Almost the entire outer surface of the basement membrane is covered with foot processes from astrocytes. This close association suggests an interaction between astrocytes and endothelial cells that is important for the function of the blood-brain barrier. Support for this hypothesis is found in brain tumors and nonbarrier regions of the brain, where the absence of intimate astrocyte-endothelial cell contact is associated with the absence of a blood-brain barrier.

Substances with a high lipid solubility may move across the blood-brain barrier by simple diffusion

Diffusion is the major entry mechanism for most psychoactive drugs. As shown in Fig. 2, the rate of entry of compounds that diffuse into the brain depends on their lipid solubility, as estimated by oil/water partition coefficients. For example, the permeability of very lipid soluble compounds, such as ethanol, nicotine, iodoantipyrine, and diazepam, is so high that they are completely extracted from the blood during a single passage through the brain. Hence, their uptake by brain is limited only by blood flow, and this provides the basis for use of iodoantipyrine to measure cerebral blood flow rate. In contrast, polar molecules, such as glycine and catecholamines, enter the brain only slowly, thereby isolating the brain from neurotransmitters in the plasma. The brain uptake of some compounds (e.g., phenobarbital and phenytoin) is lower than predicted from

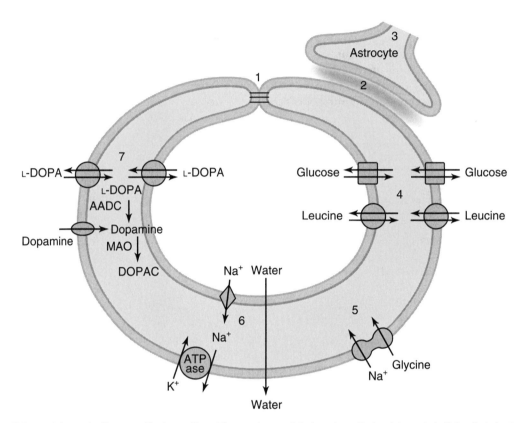

FIG. 1. Schematic diagram of brain capillary. The continuous tight junctions **(1)** that join endothelial cells in brain capillaries limit the diffusion of large and small solutes across the blood-brain barrier. The basement membrane **(2)** provides structural support for the capillary and, along with the astrocytic foot processes **(3)** that encircle the capillary, may influence endothelial cell function. Transport carriers **(4)** for glucose and essential amino acids facilitate the movement of these solutes into brain, while secondary transport systems **(5)** appear to cause the efflux of small, nonessential amino acids from brain to blood. Sodium ion transporters on the luminal membrane and Na,K-ATPase on the antiluminal membrane **(6)** account for the movement of sodium from blood to brain, and this may provide an osmotic driving force for the secretion of interstitial fluid by the brain capillary. The enzymatic blood-brain barrier **(7)** consists of the uptake of neurotransmitter precursors such as L-DOPA into the endothelial cells via the large neutral amino acid carrier, and their subsequent metabolism to 3,4-dihydroxyphenylacetic acid (DOPAC) by aromatic amino acid decarboxylase (AADC) and monoamine oxidase (MAO) present within the endothelial cell. Neurotransmitters in the interstitial fluid may also be accumulated and metabolized by the brain capillary.

their lipid solubility as a result of binding to plasma proteins.

Water

Water readily enters the brain by diffusion. Using intravenously administered deuterium oxide as a tracer, the measured half-time of exchange of brain water varies between 12 and 25 sec, depending upon the vascularity of the region studied. Although this rate of exchange is rapid compared with the rate of exchange of most solutes, it is limited both by the permeability of the capillary endothelium and by the rate of cerebral blood flow. In fact, the calculated permeability constant of the cerebral capillary wall to the diffusion of water is about the same as that estimated for its diffusion across lipid membranes (Fig. 2).

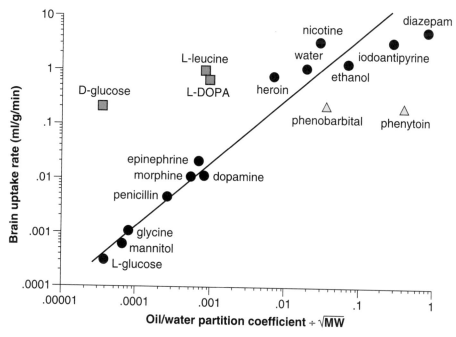

FIG. 2. Relationship between lipid solubility and brain uptake of selected compounds. The distribution into octanol relative to water for each test substance serves as a measure of its lipid solubility. This value is adjusted for differences in molecular weight (MW) and plotted on the x-axis. The brain uptake rate for radiolabeled solutes, measured as the product of the blood-brain barrier permeability and surface area (PS product), is plotted on the y-axis. In general, the higher the oil-water partition coefficient, the greater the brain uptake (●). Uptake of the two anticonvulsants phenobarbital and phenytoin is lower than predicted from their lipid solubility partly because of their binding to plasma proteins (△). Uptake of D-glucose, L-leucine, and L-DOPA is greater than predicted by their lipid solubility because specific carriers facilitate their transport across the brain capillary (■). Data are estimates based on several sources [9–14].

As a consequence of its high permeability, water moves freely into or out of the brain as the osmolality of the plasma changes. This phenomenon is clinically useful, since the intravenous administration of poorly permeable compounds such as mannitol (Fig. 2) will osmotically dehydrate the brain and reduce intracranial pressure. For example, when plasma osmolality is raised from 310 to 344 mOsm, a 10 percent shrinkage of the brain will result, with half of the shrinkage taking place in 12 min.

Gases

Gases, such as CO_2, O_2, N_2O, and Xe, and volatile anesthetics diffuse rapidly into brain. As a consequence, the rate at which their concentration in brain comes into equilibrium with the plasma is limited primarily by the cerebral blood flow rate. Hence, the inert gases (e.g., N_2O and Xe) can be used to measure cerebral blood flow.

An interesting contrast is found between CO_2 and H^+ with regard to their effects on brain pH. Since the blood-brain barrier permeability of CO_2 greatly exceeds that of H^+, the pH of the brain interstitial fluid will reflect blood pCO_2 rather than blood pH. Consequently, in a patient with a metabolic acidosis and a compensatory respiratory alkalosis, the brain is alkalotic.

Carrier-mediated transport enables molecules with low lipid solubility to traverse the blood-brain barrier

Although D-glucose and L-glucose are stereoisomers, the brain extraction of D-glucose is

TABLE 3.   Transport systems that operate from blood to brain

Transport system	Typical substrate	Transport rate[a]
METABOLIC SUBSTRATES		
Hexose	Glucose	700
Monocarboxylic acid	Lactate	60
Large neutral amino acid	Phenylalanine	12
Basic amino acid	Lysine	3
Acidic amino acid	Glutamate	0.2
Amine	Choline	0.2
Purine	Adenine	0.006
Nucleoside	Adenosine	0.004
Saturated fatty acid	Octanoate	
VITAMINS AND COFACTORS		
Thiamine	Thiamine	
Pantothenic acid	Panthothenic acid	
Biotin	Biotin	
Vitamin B_6	Pyridoxal	
Riboflavin	Riboflavin	
Niacinamide	Niacinamide	
Carnitine	Carnitine	
Inositol	myo-Inositol	
ELECTROLYTES		
Sodium	Sodium	200
Potassium	Potassium	12
Chloride	Chloride	140
HORMONES		
Thyroid hormone	T_3	
Vasopressin	Arginine vasopressin	
Insulin	Insulin	
OTHER PEPTIDES		
Transferrin	Transferrin	
Enkephalins	Leu-enkephalin	

[a] Transport rates (nmol/g/min) are estimated from experimentally determined uptake rates [14–16] and the normal plasma concentrations of the typical substrate.

more than 100-fold greater than that of L-glucose (Fig. 2). This apparently anomalous relationship is also observed for other metabolically essential compounds (Table 3). The high permeability of these polar compounds is mediated by specific transport proteins (see Chap. 3) in the plasma membranes of the endothelial cells (Fig. 1).

Glucose

Glucose is the primary energy substrate of the brain, and its metabolism accounts for nearly all of the brain's oxygen consumption (see Chap. 31). Since entry of glucose into the brain is critical, mechanisms for glucose transport across the blood-brain barrier have been particularly well studied [17]. Stereo-specific, but insulin-independent, GLUT-1 glucose transporters are highly enriched in brain capillary endothelial cells (Fig. 3) and mediate the facilitated diffusion of this polar substrate through the blood-brain barrier [18]. The activity of these transporters is sufficient to transport two to three times more

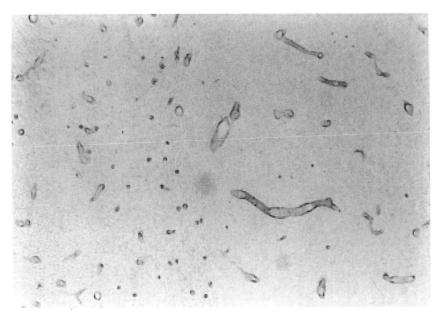

FIG. 3.   Expression of glucose transporter (GLUT-1) in microvessels of rat brain. Using a rabbit polyclonal antibody generated against the C terminus of the rat brain/human erythrocyte GLUT-1 protein, 5-μm thick sections of rat cerebral cortex embedded in paraffin blocks were stained for expression of the transporter. Biotinylated goat antirabbit immunoglobulin was used to demonstrate the distribution of the primary antibody. The selective staining of brain microvessels is consistent with their role in the passage of glucose through the blood-brain barrier. (GLUT-1 antibody obtained from Dr. L. R. Drewes.)

glucose than is normally metabolized by the brain.

The stereospecificity of the glucose transport system permits D-glucose, but not L-glucose, to enter the brain. Hexoses such as mannose and maltose are also transported rapidly into the brain; the uptake of galactose is intermediate, whereas fructose is taken up very slowly. 2-Deoxyglucose is taken up quickly and will competitively inhibit the transport of glucose. Once within neurons and glia, 2-deoxyglucose is phosphorylated but not further metabolized. If 2-deoxyglucose is used in tracer quantities, the amount of the phosphorylated tracer in the brain reflects the rate of glucose metabolism (see Chaps. 31 and 46).

Monocarboxylic Acids

Monocarboxylic acids, including L-lactate, acetate, pyruvate, and ketone bodies, are transported by a separate stereospecific system [15]. The rate of entry of these substances is significantly lower than that of glucose; however, they may become important metabolic substrates during starvation.

Neutral L-Amino Acids

The rate of movement of neutral L-amino acids into brain is variable [14,15]. Phenylalanine, leucine, tyrosine, isoleucine, valine, tryptophan, methionine, histidine, and L-DOPA may enter as rapidly as glucose. These essential amino acids cannot be synthesized by the brain and, therefore, must be supplied from protein breakdown and diet (see Chap. 39). Several are precursors for neurotransmitters synthesized in the brain (see Chaps. 12–14). The transport of these large neutral amino acids into brain is inhibited by the synthetic amino acid 2-aminonorbornane-2-carboxylic acid (BCH), but not by 2-(methylamino)-isobutyric acid (MeAIB); hence, the transport system in the blood-brain barrier is similar to the leucine-preferring (L) transport system defined by Christensen (see Kotyk and Janacek [5]). Since a single type of transport carrier mediates the transcapillary movement of structurally related amino acids, these compounds compete with each other for entry into the brain. Therefore, an elevation in the plasma level of one will inhibit uptake of the others (Fig. 4). This may be important in certain metabolic diseases such as phenylketonuria (PKU), where high levels of phenylalanine in plasma reduce brain uptake of other essential amino acids (see Chap. 39).

Small neutral amino acids such as alanine, glycine, proline, and γ-aminobutyric (GABA) are markedly restricted in their entry into the brain (e.g., glycine in Fig. 2). These amino acids are synthesized by the brain, and several are putative neurotransmitters (see Chap. 18). This restriction is consistent with the inability of MeAIB to inhibit brain uptake of amino acids and suggests that the alanine-preferring (A) transport system [5] is not present on the luminal surface of the blood-brain barrier. In contrast, these small neutral amino acids appear to be transported out of the brain across the blood-brain barrier, suggesting that the A-system carrier is present on the antiluminal surface of the brain capillary [20]. This may explain why the CSF/plasma concentration ratios are particularly low for these amino acids (Table 1). Thus, essential amino acids that serve as precursors for catecholamine and indoleamine synthesis are readily transported into brain (L system), whereas amino acids synthesized by brain, including those amino acids that act as neurotransmitters, not only are limited in their entry but also are actively transported out of the brain (A system).

In addition, there are distinct transport systems that facilitate the brain uptake of

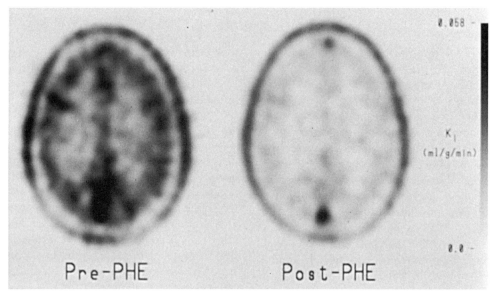

FIG. 4. Competitive inhibition of amino acid transport in human brain. Regional brain uptake of the neutral amino acid analog ^{11}C-aminocyclohexane carboxylic acid (ACHC) was determined in a normal volunteer using positron emission tomography (see Chap. 46) before (Pre-PHE) and after (Post-PHE) oral ingestion of phenylalanine. Higher values for the influx rate constant (K_i) are noted by darker shading. Note the marked reduction of ACHC uptake rate in brain following ingestion of phenylalanine. In contrast, there is little or no effect on ACHC entry into the scalp or the ACHC present in cerebral veins (*dark spots at top and bottom of image*). The reduced uptake of ACHC after ingestion of phenylalanine indicates that phenylalanine competes with ACHC for transport into the brain. For more details on methodology, see Koeppe et al. [19].

basic and acidic amino acids (Table 3). Lysine and arginine are essential amino acids, and, therefore, they must be provided from the blood. The acidic amino acids glutamate and aspartate are both important metabolic intermediates as well as neurotransmitters (see Chap. 17). While the brain content of these amino acids is maintained primarily by *de novo* synthesis, they can also be transported into brain at a slow rate across the blood-brain barrier.

Choline

Choline enters the central nervous system through a carrier-mediated transport process that can be inhibited by molecules such as dimethyl aminoethanol, hemicholinium, and tetraethyl ammonium chloride. Since choline cannot be synthesized by brain, it has been proposed that blood-brain barrier transport may regulate the formation of acetylcholine in the central nervous system [21].

Vitamins

Vitamins are, by definition, substances that cannot be synthesized by mammalian organisms but are required in small amounts to support normal metabolism. Since vitamins cannot be synthesized by brain, they must be obtained from the blood. Thus, specific transport systems are present in the blood-brain barrier for most vitamins (Table 3) [22]. These transport systems generally have a low transport capacity, since the brain requires only small amounts of the vitamins and efficient homeostatic mechanisms preserve brain vitamin content without the need for a rapid influx from the blood. Nevertheless, dietary deficiencies of some vitamins can produce neurological disease (see Chap. 35).

Metal ions are exchanged between plasma and brain very slowly compared with other tissues

Intravenously administered $^{42}K^+$, for example, exchanges with muscle K^+ in 1 hr, but K^+ exchange in brain is only half completed in 24 to 36 hr. Na^+ exchange is somewhat faster, with half-exchange into brain occurring in 3 to 8 hr. Despite its relatively slow entry into the brain, Na^+ exchange across the blood-brain barrier appears to occur by mediated transport [16]. This occurs, in part, through brain capillary Na,K-ATPase (see Chap. 3), which is primarily located on the antiluminal membrane of the endothelial cell (Fig. 1). Na,K-ATPase in the brain capillary may also mediate removal of interstitial fluid K^+ from brain and thereby maintain a constant brain K^+ concentration in the face of fluctuating plasma concentrations. In addition, the antiluminal location of Na,K-ATPase may underlie the proposed role of the brain capillary in secretion of interstitial fluid, an extrachoroidal source of CSF.

Some proteins cross the blood-brain barrier by binding to receptors or by absorption on the endothelial cell membrane

Receptor-Mediated Transcytosis

Most proteins in the plasma are not able to cross the blood-brain barrier because of their size and hydrophilicity. Consequently, the concentrations of plasma proteins in brain are very low (Table 1). However, the brain levels of certain proteins (e.g., insulin and transferrin) vary as the plasma levels change and the brain uptake of these peptides is greater than expected based on their size and lipid solubility. Furthermore, the brain uptake of some proteins is saturable. These properties suggest the presence of a specific transport process. It is now believed that proteins such as insulin, transferrin, insulin-like growth factors, and vasopressin cross the blood-brain barrier by a process called receptor-mediated transcytosis [6]. The brain capillary endothelial cell is highly enriched in receptors for these proteins and, following binding of protein to the receptor, a portion of the membrane containing the protein-receptor complex is endocytosed into the endothelial cell to form a vesicle. Although the subsequent route of passage of the protein through the endothelial cell is not known, there is eventual release of intact protein on the other side of the endothelial cell.

Absorptive-Mediated Transcytosis

Polycationic proteins and lectins cross the blood-brain barrier by a similar, but nonspecific process called absorptive-mediated transcytosis [6]. Rather than binding to specific receptors in the membrane, these proteins absorb to the endothelial cell membrane based on charge or affinity for sugar moieties of membrane glycoproteins. The subsequent transcytotic events are probably similar to receptor-mediated transcytosis; however, the overall capacity of absorptive-mediated transcytosis is greater because it is not limited by the number of receptors that are present in the membrane. Thus, cationization may provide a mechanism for enhancing brain uptake of almost any protein.

Metabolic processes within the brain capillary endothelial cells are important to blood-brain barrier function

Most neurotransmitters present in the blood do not enter the brain because of their low lipid solubility and lack of specific transport carriers in the luminal membrane of the capillary endothelial cell. This is illustrated for dopamine in Fig. 2. In contrast, L-DOPA, the precursor for dopamine, has affinity for the large neutral amino acid transport system and more easily enters brain from blood than would be predicted by its lipid solubility (Figs. 1 and 2). This is why patients with Parkinson's disease are treated with L-DOPA rather than with dopamine (see Chap. 44); however, the penetration of L-DOPA into the brain is limited by the presence of the enzymes L-DOPA decarboxylase and monoamine oxidase within the capillary endothelial cell [23]. This "enzymatic blood-brain barrier" limits transendothelial passage of L-DOPA into brain and explains the need for

large doses of L-DOPA in the treatment of Parkinson's disease. Therapy is currently enhanced by concurrent treatment with an inhibitor of peripheral L-DOPA decarboxylase.

Intracapillary monoamine oxidase may also play a role in the inactivation of neurotransmitters released by neuronal activity, since monoamines are actively accumulated and metabolized by brain capillaries [23]. The fact that monoamines show very little uptake when presented from the luminal side suggests that the uptake systems are present only on the antiluminal membrane of the brain capillary endothelial cell (Fig. 1).

The brain capillary contains a variety of other neurotransmitter-metabolizing enzymes such as cholinesterases, GABA transaminase, aminopeptidases, and endopeptidases. In addition, several drug- and toxin-metabolizing enzymes that are typically found in the liver are also found in brain capillaries [24]. Thus, the "enzymatic blood-brain barrier" protects the brain not only from circulating neurotransmitters but also from many toxins.

Blood-brain barrier undergoes development

Many of the features of the blood-brain barrier, including the presence of tight junctions in the capillary endothelium and the exclusion of protein molecules, are present in newborn animals [25]. In addition, the relationship between lipid solubility and barrier penetration is similar in adults and newborns.

Even after achieving an adult-like "tightness," the immature blood-brain barrier exhibits a greater than expected permeability to certain solutes such as organic acids, essential amino acids, adenine, choline, and potassium as the result of an increase in the transport capacity for these compounds. The selective increase in permeability to these substances undoubtedly relates to an increased need to support rapid brain growth. Thus, even in the immature animal, the blood-brain barrier is specialized to match the brain's requirements.

BLOOD-CEREBROSPINAL FLUID BARRIER

CSF is formed by active transport of solutes across the epithelial cells in the choroid plexus

Since the concentrations of several constituents are maintained at levels different in CSF from those in plasma (Table 1), CSF is not simply a protein-free ultrafiltrate of plasma. The functional unit of the choroid plexus, composed of a capillary enveloped by a layer of differentiated ependymal epithelium, is diagrammed in Fig. 5. In normal subjects, the rate of CSF secretion is 0.3 to 0.4 ml/min, about one-third the rate at which urine is formed. Although the total volume of CSF cannot be precisely measured, it is estimated

to be 100 to 150 ml in normal adults. This means that the CSF is totally replaced three or four times each day.

The major site of CSF formation is the choroid plexus present in all cerebral ventricles (Fig. 6). This conclusion was first deduced from the observation that fluid accumulates and enlarges the ventricles if the aqueduct of Sylvius is obstructed. Furthermore, neurosurgeons have reported seeing drops of fluid form on the surfaces of the choroid plexus. Through histochemical and ultrastructural investigations, we now know that the choroid plexus epithelial cells have morphological features similar to those of other secretory cells, and there is abundant physiological data indicating that the choroid plexus is the primary site of CSF formation. However, extrachoroidal formation of CSF has also been demonstrated, and this may be the result of ion transport by brain capillaries, as discussed above.

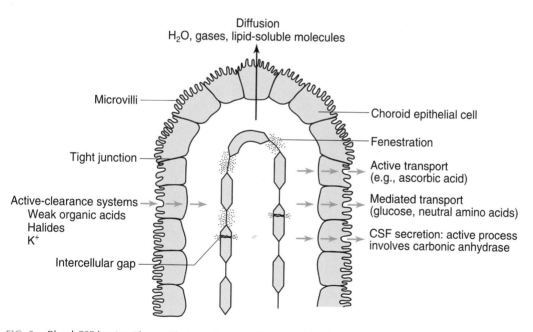

FIG. 5. Blood-CSF barrier. The capillaries in the choroid plexus differ from those of the brain in that there is free movement of molecules across the endothelial cell through fenestrations and intercellular gaps. The blood-CSF barrier is at the choroid plexus epithelial cells, which are joined together by tight junctions. Microvilli are present on the CSF-facing surface. These greatly increase the surface area of the apical membrane and may aid in fluid secretion. Diffusion, facilitated diffusion, and active transport into CSF, as well as active transport of metabolites from CSF to blood, have been demonstrated in the choroid plexus.

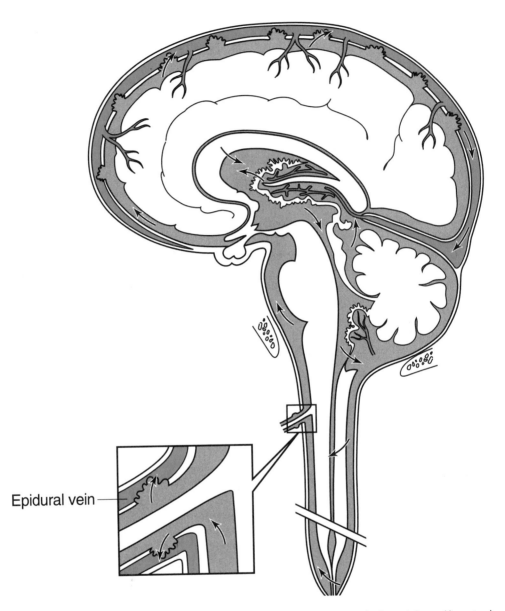

FIG. 6.   Circulation of CSF. CSF is secreted by the choroid plexus present in the cerebral ventricles and by extracho-roidal sources. It subsequently circulates through the ventricular cavities and into the subarachnoid space. Absorption into venous blood occurs through the arachnoid granulations in the superior sagittal sinus and along the spinal nerve root sheaths (inset). (From Fishman [1].)

Rate of formation of CSF can be measured by various means

A simple method of measuring the rate of formation of CSF is to measure the time it takes CSF pressure to recover after a known volume of CSF is removed. The rate in humans is 0.35 ml/min. A more accurate method of measuring CSF formation involves perfusion between the ventricle and the cisterna magna with a simulated CSF containing inulin. Because inulin diffuses very slowly into tissue during such a perfusion, the dilution of inulin is taken as a measure of the rate of formation of new CSF. Such perfusions have been carried out in a wide variety of species. Typical rates of CSF formation are as follows: rabbit, 0.001 ml/min; cat, 0.02 ml/min; rhesus monkey, 0.08 ml/min; and goat, 0.19 ml/min. In humans, the average value is 0.37 ml/min, and this corresponds rather closely to the value determined from drainage experiments.

By use of the ventriculocisternal perfusion method, it has been found that CSF formation decreases very little as intracranial pressure increases. Moreover, CSF is formed at a normal rate and osmolality, even when the fluid perfused through the ventricle is moderately hypertonic or hypotonic. When the perfused fluid is very hypotonic, however, CSF formation may cease. CSF formation is also reduced if serum osmolality is raised.

Carrier-mediated transport drives secretion of CSF

The movement of substances from the blood into CSF is, in many ways, analogous to that from blood into brain. There is free movement of water, gases, and lipid-soluble compounds from the blood into the CSF. Substances important for brain metabolism and maintenance of CSF electrolytes, such as glucose, amino acids, and cations, are transported by saturable carrier-mediated processes. Macromolecules such as proteins and most small polar molecules do not enter the CSF (Fig. 5).

The most important transport systems in the choroid plexus epithelial cells are those responsible for CSF secretion (Fig. 7). In most fluid-secreting epithelial tissues, transcellular movement of water is driven by active transport of Na^+ and Cl^-. The choroid plexus epithelium is no exception [26]; however, in contrast to the basolateral localiza-

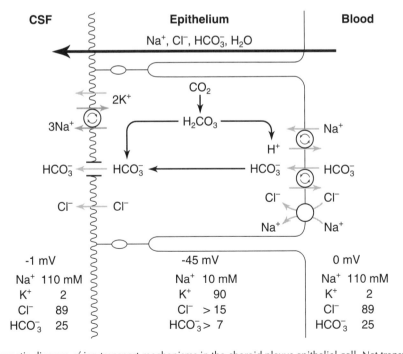

FIG. 7. Schematic diagram of ion transport mechanisms in the choroid plexus epithelial cell. Net transport of Na^+, Cl^-, and HCO_3^- across the choroid plexus epithelium results in the secretion of CSF. (From Saito and Wright [26]).

tion of Na,K-ATPase in other epithelia, this cation pump is found on the apical microvilli of the choroid plexus [27]. By pumping Na^+ out of the epithelial cell into the CSF, Na,K-ATPase maintains a low intracellular Na^+ activity. The active extrusion of Na^+ is associated with the downhill movement of Na^+ across the basolateral membrane mediated by both a coupled Na^+-Cl^- symport system and a Na^+-H^+ antiport system (see Chap. 3). In addition, carrier-mediated exchange of HCO_3^- for Cl^- is an important step in the movement of anions from blood to CSF; by producing intracellular HCO_3^-, carbonic anhydrase within the choroid plexus epithelial cell also strongly influences secretion of CSF. The importance of these transport systems in CSF secretion was determined through the use of specific inhibitors such as ouabain for Na,K-ATPase, furosemide for the coupled Na^+-Cl^- symport, acetazolamide for carbonic anhydrase, and 4-acetamide-4′-isothiocyano-2,2′-disulfonic stilbene for the Cl^- – HCO_3^- antiport. Acetazolamide and furosemide are used therapeutically to decrease the rate of CSF formation in hydrocephalus. Because CSF secretion results from the active transport of ions, it is influenced very little by changes in intracranial pressure.

Other active transport systems in the choroid plexus are linked to the efflux of specific solutes [28]. For example, iodide and thiocyanate are transported from the CSF by saturable carrier mechanisms that can be competitively inhibited by perchlorate. This system must be active because transport can be carried out against unfavorable electrochemical gradients. Another important transport system removes weak organic acids from the CSF. Among the molecules cleared by this mechanism are penicillin and neurotransmitter metabolites, such as homovanillic acid and 5-HIAA. This clearance system, which transports against an unfavorable CSF to blood gradient, is saturable and inhibited by probenecid. Clearance of organic acids by a probenecid-sensitive transport mechanism may also occur

across the blood-brain barrier in brain capillaries.

CSF circulates through the ventricles and over the surface of the brain

Choroid plexus pulsations are transmitted throughout the CSF and can be seen on the manometer at the time of lumbar spinal tap. The fluid circulation is from the lateral ventricles through the foramina of Monro into the third ventricle, the aqueduct of Sylvius, and then into the fourth ventricle. The fluid passes from the fourth ventricle through the foramina of Luschka and Magendie to the cisterna magna and then circulates into the cerebral and spinal subarachnoid spaces (Fig. 6). If obstructions are placed at the foramina between these ventricles, the ventricle upstream from the obstruction will enlarge significantly, producing obstructive hydrocephalus. Thus, if a foramen of Monro is obstructed, the ipsilateral ventricle will enlarge. If the aqueduct is obstructed, both lateral ventricles and the third ventricle will enlarge.

Occasionally, disease processes affect CSF removal. For example, obliteration of the subarachnoid space by inflammation or thrombosis of the sinuses will prevent clearance of fluid. When this occurs, CSF pressure increases, and hydrocephalus develops without obstruction of the ventricular foramina. This is called communicating hydrocephalus.

CSF is removed at villi and granulations over the large venous sinuses in the skull and at the cranial and spinal nerve root sheaths

There is evidence that absorption of CSF by the arachnoid villi occurs by a valve-like process, permitting the one-way flow of CSF from the subarachnoid spaces into the venous sinuses. CSF absorption does not occur until CSF pressure exceeds the pressure within the sinuses. Once this threshold is reached, the rate of absorption is proportional to the difference between CSF and sinus pressures. A normal human can absorb CSF at a rate up to six times the normal rate of CSF formation with only a moderate increase in intracranial pressure.

The combination of bulk absorption of solute and solvent by the arachnoid villi and the selective removal of molecules by the choroid plexus is termed the sink function of the CSF. This implies that molecules reaching the interstitial fluid of the brain may diffuse into CSF and then be removed by bulk absorption or active transport, or by both mechanisms. This sink action helps to maintain the low concentration of many substances in both brain and CSF compared with plasma concentrations.

CEREBROSPINAL FLUID-BRAIN INTERFACE

The absence of tight junctions between some ependymal and pial cells permits diffusion of proteins and other hydrophilic molecules from the CSF into the interstitium of the brain, and vice versa. However, large molecules such as proteins and inulin penetrate poorly.

Quantitative studies of the movement of substances between CSF and brain suggest that the concentration of ions in extracellular fluid in brain should be the same as that in CSF. This relationship has been directly demonstrated for K^+ using ion-specific electrodes placed in the brain's interstitial space. Brain interstitial K^+ concentration is approximately 3 mM, similar to that of CSF, and independent of the plasma K^+ concentration [29].

BYPASSING THE BARRIERS WITH DRUGS

A number of agents of potential therapeutic importance do not readily enter the brain because they have low lipid solubility and are not transported by the specific carriers present in the blood-brain barrier or choroid plexus. To overcome this limitation, schemes have been developed to enhance drug entry into the central nervous system.

The most obvious method of circumventing the barriers is to inject the agents directly into the CSF. Although ventricular or cisternal access sites may be used, intrathecal administration of antineoplastic agents is usually accomplished by intralumbar injection. Because of limited drug penetration into brain substance, these routes are most often used in patients who have a disease process such as chronic meningitis or leukemia in the CSF.

Enhanced delivery of drug into brain can be accomplished by raising its concentration in the blood, but this approach is often limited by the occurrence of systemic side effects. It is possible to achieve similar high concentrations of drug in the brain vasculature by infusing the drug directly into the carotid artery. In this way, the same total systemic dose produces a much higher concentration gradient across the blood-brain barrier and leads to a greater uptake by the brain.

Another way to enhance delivery is to increase the permeability of the blood-brain barrier. The disease itself may produce this effect, and this is why the rate of penicillin passage into brain is highest early in the course of meningitis; however, when the capillaries are intact some intervention is necessary to open the barrier. The infusion of hyperosmolar solutions into the carotid circulation alters blood-brain barrier permeability in laboratory animals [30] and has been used in the treatment of patients with brain tumors. The change in permeability appears to be caused by separation of the tight junctions that normally seal together the endothelial cells in brain capillaries.

Designing drugs with high blood-brain barrier permeability is a more selective way to improve delivery into brain. In fact, most neuroactive drugs are effective because they dissolve in lipid and easily enter the brain. A good example of the importance of structure and lipid solubility is provided by comparison of the brain uptake of heroin and morphine [9]. These compounds are very similar in structure except for two acetyl groups that make heroin more lipid soluble. This greater lipid solubility of heroin explains its more rapid onset of action. Once within the brain the acetyl groups on heroin are removed enzymatically to produce morphine, which only slowly leaves the brain. By analogy, it would seem ideal to develop new therapeutic drugs that readily enter and then are trapped within the central nervous system.

A similar strategy for enhancing brain uptake of drugs involves producing prodrugs that have affinity for one of the blood-brain barrier transport systems. For example, the large neutral amino acid system appears to tolerate a considerable range of side-chain structures [14]. The attachment of drugs to proteins to form chimeric peptides that enter brain by receptor- or absorptive-mediated endocytosis may also prove to be a useful and flexible approach [6]. Clearly an understanding of transport processes is crucial to development of the next generation of drugs useful in treating various brain diseases.

ACKNOWLEDGMENTS

This work was supported by grants NS-23870, HL-18575, NS-15655, ES-02380, and EY-03772 from the National Institutes of Health.

REFERENCES

1. Fishman, R. A. *Cerebrospinal Fluid in Diseases of the Nervous System.* Philadelphia: W. B. Saunders, 1980.
2. Goldstein, G. W., Betz, A. L. The blood-brain barrier. *Sci. Am.* 254:74–83, 1986.
3. Spector, R., Johanson, C. E. The mammalian choroid plexus. *Sci. Am.* 261:68–74, 1989.
4. Bradbury, M. *The Concept of a Blood-Brain Barrier.* Chichester: Wiley, 1979.
5. Kotyk, A., Janácek, K. *Cell Membrane Transport.* New York: Plenum, 1975.
6. Pardridge, W. M. *Peptide Drug Delivery to the Brain.* New York: Raven, 1991.
7. Bradbury, M. W. B., Stulcová, B. Efflux mechanism contributing to the stability of the potassium concentration in cerebrospinal fluid. *J. Physiol. (Lond.)* 208:415–430, 1970.
8. Brightman, M. W. Morphology of blood-brain interfaces. *Exp. Eye Res. (Suppl.)* 25:1–25, 1977.
9. Oldendorf, W. H. The blood-brain barrier. *Exp. Eye Res (Suppl.)* 25:177–190, 1977.
10. Oldendorf, W. H. Clearance of radiolabeled substances by brain after arterial injection using a diffusible internal standard. In N. Marks, R. Rodnight (eds.), *Research Methods in Neurochemistry.* New York: Plenum, 1981, Vol. 5, pp. 91–112.
11. Fenstermacher, J. D. Drug transfer across the blood-brain barrier. In Breimer, D. D., Speiser, P. (eds.), *Topics in Pharmaceutical Sciences 1983.* Amsterdam: Elsevier Science, 1983, pp. 143–154.
12. Cornford, E. M., Braun, L. D., Oldendorf, W. H., Hill, M. A. Comparison of lipid-mediated blood-brain-barrier penetrability in neonates and adults. *Am. J. Physiol.* 243:C161–C168, 1982.
13. Hironaka, T., Fuchino, K., Fujii, T. Absorption of diazepam and its transfer through the blood-brain barrier after intraperitoneal administration in the rat. *J. Pharmacol. Exp. Ther.* 299:809–815, 1984.
14. Smith, Q. R., Momma, S., Aoyagi, M., Rapoport, S. I. Kinetics of neutral amino acid transport across the blood-brain barrier. *J. Neurochem.* 49:1651–1658, 1987.
15. Pardridge, W. M. Brain metabolism: A perspective from the blood-brain barrier. *Physiol. Rev.* 63:1481–1535, 1983.
16. Schielke, G. P., Betz, A. L. Electrolyte transport. In M. W. B. Bradbury (ed.), *Physiology and Pharmacology of the Blood-Brain Barrier.* Heidelberg: Springer-Verlag, 1992.
17. Lund-Anderson, H. Transport of glucose from blood to brain. *Physiol. Rev.* 59:305–352, 1979.
18. Kalaria, R. N., Gravina, S. A., Schmidley, J. W., Perry, G., Harik, S. I. The glucose transporter of the human brain and blood-brain barrier. *Ann. Neurol.* 24:757–764, 1988.
19. Koeppe, R. A., Mangner, T., Betz, A. L., et

al. Use of [^{11}C[aminocyclohexanecarboxylate for the measurement of amino acid uptake and distribution volume in human brain. *J. Cereb. Blood Flow Metab.* 10:727–739, 1990.

20. Betz, A. L., Goldstein, G. W. Polarity of the blood-brain barrier: Neutral amino acid transport into isolated brain capillaries. *Science* 202:225–227, 1978.

21. Cohen, E., Wurtman, R. J. Brain acetylcoline synthesis: Control by dietary choline. *Science* 191:561–562, 1976.

22. Spector, R. Micronutrient homeostasis in mammalian brain and cerebrospinal fluid. *J. Neurochem.* 53:1667–1674, 1989.

23. Hardebo, J. E., Owman, C. Barrier mechanisms for neurotransmitter monoamines and their precursors at the blood-brain barrier. *Ann. Neurol.* 8:1–11, 1979.

24. Minn, A., Ghersi-Egea, J. F., Perrin, R., Leininger, B., Siest, G. Drug metabolizing enzymes in the brain and cerebral microvessels. *Brain Res. Rev.* 16:65–82, 1991.

25. Johanson, C. E. Ontogeny and phylogeny of the blood-brain barrier. In E. A. Neuwelt (ed.), *Implications of the Blood-Brain Barrier and Its Manipulation.* New York: Plenum, Vol. 1, pp. 157–198, 1989.

26. Saito, Y., Wright, E. M. Bicarbonate transport across the frog choroid plexus and its control by cyclic nucleotides. *J. Physiol. (Lond.)* 336:635–648, 1983.

27. Ernst, S. A., Palacios, J. R., Siegel, G. J. Immunocytochemical localization of Na$^+$,K$^+$-ATPase catalytic polypeptide in mouse choroid plexus. *J. Histochem. Cytochem.* 34:189–195, 1986.

28. Lorenzo, A. V. Factors governing the composition of the cerebrospinal fluid. *Exp. Eye Res. (Suppl.)* 25:205–228, 1977.

29. Jones, H. C., Keep, R. C. The control of potassium concentration in the cerebrospinal fluid and brain interstitial fluid of developing rats. *J. Physiol.* 383:441–453, 1987.

30. Rapoport, S. I., Fredericks, W. R., Ohno, K., Pettigrew, K. D. Quantitative aspects of reversible osmotic opening of the blood-brain barrier. *Am. J. Physiol.* 238:R421–R431, 1980.

PART FIVE

Medical Neurochemistry

CHAPTER 33

The Muscle Fiber and Disorders of Muscle Excitability

Basic Neurochemistry: Molecular, Cellular, and Medical Aspects, 5th Ed., edited by G. J. Siegel et al. Published by Raven Press, Ltd., New York, 1994. Correspondence to Robert L. Barchi, Institute of Neurological Sciences, University of Pennsylvania School of Medicine, Philadelphia, Pennsylvania 19104-6074.

Normal contraction of skeletal muscle requires that electrical signals originating in a motor nerve be transmitted across the neuromuscular junction, disseminated along the muscle surface membrane, propagated into the fiber interior along the T-tubular system, and finally coupled to Ca^{2+} release from the sarcoplasmic reticulum and ultimately cause actin-myosin interaction. Failure at any one of these steps will result in muscle weakness or paralysis even in the presence of a normal contractile apparatus. First, the molecular aspects of normal muscle contraction and of the membrane systems that link contraction to nerve excitation are briefly considered. Then some of the pathobiological processes that can affect excitation in skeletal muscle are explored.

MUSCLE FIBERS ARE ORGANIZED IN REPEATING UNITS

Light microscopists have long recognized that the physiological unit of muscle, the cell or fiber, contains repeating structures known as sarcomeres that are separated from each other by dark lines called Z disks. Within each sarcomere, the A and I bands are seen; the A band, lying between two I bands, occupies the center of each sarco-

mere and is highly birefringent. Within the A band is a central lighter zone, the H band, and in the center of the H band is the darker M band. Z disks are at the centers of the I bands (Fig. 1).

The electron microscope reveals two sets of filaments

This striation pattern of voluntary muscle is due to a regular arrangement of two sets of filaments (Fig. 1). The thin filaments (diameter ~80 Å) appear to be attached to the Z bands and are found in the I band and occupy part of the A band. The thick filaments

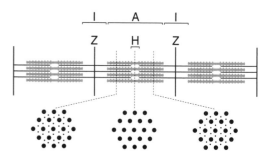

FIG. 1.   Schematic representation of the structure of striated muscle. Actin-containing thin filaments originate at Z lines. Note thick myosin-containing filaments that bear cross-bridges. The M disk lies in the center of the H band (see text). (From H. E. Huxley, The mechanism of muscle contraction. *Science* 164:1356, 1969.)

(diameter ~150 Å) occupy the A band and are connected crosswise by material in the M band. In cross section, the thick filaments are arranged in a hexagonal lattice: The thin filaments occupy the centers of the triangles formed by the thick filaments.

Contraction is due to the relative sliding of the filaments

With the identification of two sets of discontinuous filaments in the sarcomere came the recognition that (a) the two kinds of filaments become crosslinked only on excitation and (b) contraction of muscle does not depend on shortening the length of the filaments but rather on the relative motion of the two sets of filaments (sliding-filament mechanism). Thus, the length of the muscle depends on the length of the sarcomeres, and in turn variation in sarcomere length is based on variation in the degree of overlap between the thin and thick filaments. High-resolution electron micrographs have shown that cross-bridges emanate from the thick filaments, and it is thought that, in active muscle, these structures are responsible for the links with thin filaments.

Other proteins are found in the two sets of filaments

Myosin is the chief constituent of thick filaments and actin the chief constituent of thin filaments. Tropomyosin and a complex of three subunits collectively called troponin are present in the thin filaments and play an important role in the regulation of muscle contraction. Although the proteins constituting the M and the Z bands have not been fully characterized, they include α-actinin and desmin as well as the enzyme creatine kinase. A continuous elastic network of proteins such as connectin surround the actin and myosin filaments, providing muscle with a parallel passive elastic element.

MEMBRANE SYSTEMS COUPLE NERVE EXCITATION TO MUSCLE CONTRACTION

The neuromuscular junction connects nerve to muscle

Synaptic transmission at the neuromuscular junction (NMJ) requires the integrated activity of complex macromolecular systems at both the presynaptic and the postsynaptic level (Fig. 2). Defects in any of the elements can cause degradation in synaptic efficiency and block transmission of information. The outcome of synaptic failure at the NMJ is easily detected as muscle weakness, fatigability, or paralysis. In many respects, synaptic transmission at the NMJ resembles that at other peripheral and central nerve synapses; molecular details of this process are provided in Chapter 9.

Terminal elements of motor nerves form specialized structures at their point of contact with muscle that constitute the NMJ. The distal arborizations of the motor neuron form enlarged presynaptic terminals containing large numbers of acetylcholine-packed vesicles. These terminals lie in depressions called gutters in the postsynaptic sarcolemma.

The postsynaptic membrane at the NMJ is highly specialized; it is organized into deep transverse folds under the nerve terminal. The crests of these folds contain a high density of nicotinic acetylcholine receptors (see Chap. 11). Acetylcholinesterase, the enzyme that terminates neurotransmitter action by hydrolyzing acetylcholine to choline and acetate, is present in the basal lamina that coats the postsynaptic membrane.

The machinery for neurotransmitter release in the presynaptic terminal is also highly organized and is oriented with respect to the transverse folds of the postsynaptic membrane. A small fraction of the synaptic vesicles in the terminal are found associated with regions of increased membrane density called release zones. These zones are located precisely over the infoldings of the postsy-

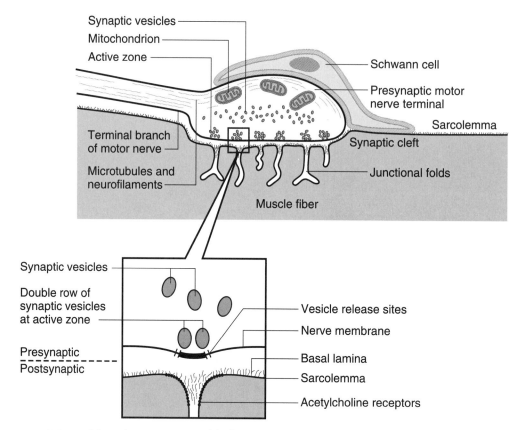

Synaptic vesicles
Mitochondrion
Active zone
Schwann cell
Presynaptic motor nerve terminal
Sarcolemma
Terminal branch of motor nerve
Synaptic cleft
Microtubules and neurofilaments
Junctional folds
Muscle fiber

Synaptic vesicles
Double row of synaptic vesicles at active zone
Vesicle release sites
Nerve membrane
Presynaptic
Postsynaptic
Basal lamina
Sarcolemma
Acetylcholine receptors

FIG. 2. Schematic representation of the key presynaptic and postsynaptic elements at the NMJ.

naptic membrane. Following nerve stimulation, vesicles at these sites fuse with the plasma membrane and release their content of acetylcholine directly over the postsynaptic receptor molecules on the folds below.

The muscle sarcolemma spreads the message

The muscle cell is surrounded by a plasma membrane that, together with the various connective tissue elements and collagen fibrils, forms the sarcolemma. The interior of the resting cell is maintained by pumps and channels in the plasma membrane at an electrical potential about 80 mV more negative than the exterior. Unlike membranes of nerves, muscle membranes have a high conductance to chloride ions in the resting state; G_{Cl} accounts for about 70 percent of the total membrane conductance. Potassium conductance accounts for most of the remainder, and the membrane potential is normally close to the Nernst potential for these two ions (Chap. 4). Asymmetrical concentration gradients for sodium and potassium ions are maintained at the cost of energy by the membrane Na,K,-ATPase.

During the generation of an action potential, a rapid and stereotyped membrane depolarization is produced by an increase in sodium conductance mediated by voltage-dependent sodium channels [1]. The conductance increase is self-limited, and membrane repolarization is assisted by the delayed opening of a potassium conductance pathway. Action potentials originating at the NMJ spread in a nondecremental fashion over the entire surface of the muscle.

The transverse tubular system and sarcoplasmic reticulum combine to link electrical signals to Ca²⁺ release

Depolarization of the sarcolemma penetrates the interior of the muscle cell along transverse (T) tubules that are continuous with the outer membrane (Fig. 3). These tubules are seen as openings on the surface of the muscle cell either at the level of the Z bands or at the junction of the A and I bands, depending on the species, and the depolarization of the membrane spreads activity along the tubules to the interior of the fiber. As this T-tubular network courses inward, close associations are formed with specialized terminal elements of the sarcoplasmic reticulum (SR). At the electron microscope level, the structure formed by a single tubule interposed between two terminal SR elements is called a triad. The SR stores Ca²⁺ in relaxed muscle and releases it into the sarcoplasm on depolarization of the cell membrane and the T-tubular system.

A great deal of work has focused on the proteins present in the T-tubule/SR junction. These proteins may be the molecular counterpart of the so-called foot processes seen in electron micrographs by Franzini-Armstrong [2]. One protein, an integral component of the T-tubular membrane, is a form of L-type dihydropyridine-sensitive voltage-dependent calcium channel [3]. Another protein in the junctional region is a large protein associated with the SR membrane that may couple conformational changes in the Ca²⁺ channel protein induced

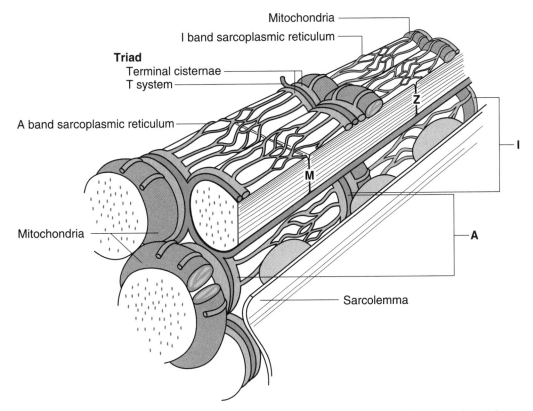

FIG. 3. A schematic drawing of part of a mammalian skeletal muscle fiber showing the relationship of the SR, terminal cisternae, T system, and mitochondria to a few myofibrils. (From B. R. Eisenberg, A. E. Kuda, and J. B. Peter, Stereological analysis of mammalian skeletal muscle. I. Soleus muscle of the adult guinea pig. *J. Cell. Biol.* 60:732, 1974.)

by T-tubular depolarization to Ca^{2+} release from the SR [4].

A Ca^{2+} channel protein is needed for coupling at the triad

The skeletal muscle T-tubular system contains a dihydropyridine-binding form of voltage-dependent calcium channel. On biochemical analysis, this protein contains five subunits: a large α_1-subunit that contains the binding site for the dihydropyridines, a large glycosylated α_2-subunit, and smaller β-, γ-, and δ-subunits [1]. The α_1-subunit bears strong sequence homology to the voltage-dependent sodium channel. It is organized into four internal repeat domains, each containing six to eight transmembrane α helices. The fourth helix in each domain contains the identifying K/R-X-X repeating motif that is the signature of voltage-dependent ion channels. This subunit by itself is capable of forming voltage-dependent ion channels when expressed in appropriate cell systems.

Skeletal muscle contains higher concentrations of this L-type Ca^{2+} channel than can be accounted for on the basis of measured voltage-dependent Ca^{2+} influx. It is now clear that much of the Ca^{2+} channel protein in the T-tubular membrane does not actively gate calcium movement, but rather acts as a voltage transducer that links depolarization of the T-tubular membrane to Ca^{2+} release through a receptor protein in the SR membrane.

Sarcoplasmic reticulum Ca^{2+} release is mediated by a large protein that binds ryanodine

The bar-like structures that connect the terminal elements of the SR with the T-tubular membrane in the triad are formed by a large protein that is the principal pathway for Ca^{2+} release from the SR [5]. This protein, which binds the plant alkaloid ryanodine with high affinity, is a huge homotetramer of a 565-kDa polypeptide. The purified complex exhibits Ca^{2+} channel activity in planar bilayers that

is modulated by ATP, Ca^{2+}, and Mg^{2+}. The manner in which activation of the ryanodine receptor complex is coupled to events at the T-tubular membrane is not yet clear, although evidence now points to a direct mechanical linkage through a conformational change in the dihydropyridine receptor protein.

Ca^{2+} is stored in elements of the sarcoplasmic reticulum

The SR maintains the low intracellular Ca^{2+} concentration of resting muscle by means of an ATP-dependent Ca^{2+} pump, the Ca-ATPase, located in the SR membrane (see Chap. 3). The free energy of ATP hydrolysis is utilized for the uptake of Ca^{2+} into the SR vesicle via a phosphorylated enzyme intermediate (see Chap. 3). Other SR proteins assist in Ca^{2+} uptake and storage. Phospholamban is prominent in cardiac muscle and slow-twitch muscle, where its phosphorylation participates in the control of Ca-ATPase and Ca^{2+}-uptake activity. Another protein, calsequestrin, contains numerous low-affinity Ca^{2+} binding sites; it is present in the lumen of the SR and is thought to participate in the Ca^{2+} storage function. Fast-twitch muscle contains a soluble Ca^{2+}-binding protein, parvalbumin, which is structurally related to troponin-C. Parvalbumin may play a role in regulating the Ca^{2+} level in the initial stages of relaxation.

THE CONTRACTILE PROTEINS GENERATE FORCE

Actin forms the backbone of the thin filaments

The thin filaments of muscle are linear polymers of slightly elongated, bilobar actin subunits, each about 4×6 nm, arranged in a helical fashion, with their longer dimension roughly at right angles to the filament axis [6]. Each monomer has a molecular weight of about 42 kDa and contains a single nucleotide binding site. On addition of salts to a solution of actin monomers a drastic change in viscosity results, and negatively stained electron micrographs reveal the presence of double-helical filaments that are essentially identical to the thin filaments in appearance. The two physical states of actin characterized by low and high viscosity are called, respectively, globular (G) and fibrous (F). The nucleotide in G-actin is ATP, that in F-actin ADP. The transformation of ATP to ADP takes place during polymerization but is not involved in muscle contraction. This reaction presumably takes place when actin filaments are laid down in the course of development, growth, or regeneration.

A wide variety of proteins interact with actin in both muscle and nonmotile cells. They may affect the polymerization-depolarization of actin and are involved in the attachment of actin to other cellular structures, including the Z disks in muscle as well as membranes both in muscle and nonmuscle cells. The protein interacting with actin in the Z disk, α-actinin, is also a component of the rod-like bodies found in nemaline myopathy.

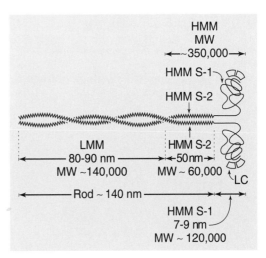

FIG. 4. Schematic representation of the structure of the myosin molecule. (S. Lowey, H. S. Slayter, A. G. Weeds, and H. Baker, Substructure of the myosin molecule. I. Subfragments of myosin by enzymatic degradation. *J. Mol. Biol.* 42:1, 1969.) The rod portion of the molecule has a coiled α-helical structure. Hinge regions postulated in the mechanism of contraction are at the junction of HMM S-1 and HMM S-2 and of HMM S-2 and LMM. It should be noted that HMM S-1 has one chief polypeptide chain, whereas other fragments have two. Note the light chains (LC) in the head region. The scheme suggests the presence of two different subunits in each HMM S-1.

Myosin, the chief constituent of thick filaments, is a multisubunit protein

Myosin is a highly asymmetrical molecule with an overall length of about 150 nm and a molecular weight of about 500 kDa (Fig. 4). Its width varies between about 2 and 10 nm. In contrast to actin, myosin consists of several peptide subunits. Each myosin molecule contains two heavy chains (MW ~200 kDa) that extend the length of the molecule. Over most of their length the two chains are intertwined to form a double α-helical rod; at one end they separate, each forming an elongated globular portion. The two globular portions contain the sites responsible for the ability of myosin to hydrolyze ATP and to combine with actin.

In addition to the two heavy chains, each myosin molecule contains four light chains with molecular weights of about 20 kDa. Fast-twitch muscle contains three types of light chains, designated LC_1, LC_2, and LC_3, in order of increasing speed of migration on sodium dodecyl sulfate-polyacrylamide gel electrophoresis (SDS-PAGE). LC_1 and LC_3 are also referred to as A1 and A2, respectively. Myosin in cardiac and slow-twitch muscle contains only two types of light chains, whose mobilities are similar but not identical to those of LC_1 and LC_2 of fast-twitch muscle myosin.

Each myosin molecule contains two LC_2-type light chains that are related by their ability to undergo phosphorylation by a kinase whose activator is the ubiquitous Ca^{2+}-binding protein calmodulin (see Chap. 22). Some fast-twitch fiber myosin molecules contain pairs of either LC_1 or LC_3; others contain one LC_1 and one LC_3. In slow-twitch and cardiac muscle myosin, there are a pair of LC_1 and a pair of LC_2 light chains per molecule.

Myosin self-assembles into thick filaments

Myosin molecules form end-to-end aggregates involving their rod-like ends, which then grow into larger structures (the thick filament) [7]. The polarity of the myosin molecules is reversed on either side of the central portion of the filament. The globular ends of the molecules form projections ("cross-bridges") on the aggregates, although the central 0.2-μm portion of the thick filament is devoid of these cross-bridges. Electron microscopic and X-ray data suggest that the globular cross-bridges are attached to the filaments by means of flexible hinges. Physicochemical studies have provided direct evidence for segmental flexibility within the myosin molecule. The cross-bridges on the thick filaments are arranged in a helical fashion, emerging at levels separated by 14.3 nm.

Actin activates myosin ATPase

The ATPase activity of myosin itself is stimulated by Ca^{2+} and is low in Mg^{2+}-containing media. If purified actin is added to myosin at low ionic strength in the presence of Mg^{2+}, considerable activation of the myosin ATPase takes place. This activation is accompanied by a remarkable change in the physical state of the system. Turbidity increases and, depending on the concentration, superprecipitation results.

Myosin-catalyzed hydrolysis of ATP occurs in several steps [8]. Binding of ATP to myosin is the first step. This is followed by the rapid formation of tightly bound ADP and inorganic phosphate (P_i). The ADP · P_i complex of myosin undergoes a relatively slow transformation that is followed by the release of the products. In the presence of actin similar complexes are formed, but the rate of the conformational change is accelerated. Tension development occurs following release of P_i. The precise details of the con-

formational changes accompanying the hydrolysis of ATP and details of the mechanism by which the free energy of ATP is converted into mechanical work have not yet been fully elucidated.

Tropomyosin and troponin regulate the interaction of actin and myosin

Tropomyosin and troponin are proteins located in the thin filaments that, together with Ca^{2+} ions, regulate the interaction of actin and myosin (Fig. 5) [9]. Tropomyosin is an α-helical protein consisting of two polypeptide chains; its structure is similar to that of the rod portion of myosin. Troponin is a complex of three proteins. If the tropomyosin-troponin complex is present, actin cannot stimulate the ATPase activity of myosin unless the concentration of free Ca^{2+} exceeds about 10^{-6} M while a system consisting solely of purified actin and myosin does not show Ca^{2+} dependence. Thus the actin-myosin interaction is controlled by Ca^{2+} in the presence of the regulatory troponin-tropomyosin complex. Of the three proteins in troponin, one, TnT, anchors it to tropomyosin; another, TnC, is responsible for combination with Ca^{2+}; and the third, TnI, binds to a site

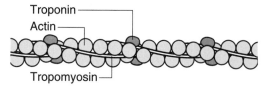

FIG. 5. Model of arrangements of actin, tropomyosin, and troponin in the thin filament. Note that troponin itself is a complex of three proteins. Tropomyosin is close to the groove of the actin filaments in relaxed muscle. Note that according to current views, the actin subunits are bilobar with their long axis more or less perpendicular to the filament axis [E. H. Egelman. The structure of F-actin. *J. Muscle Res. Cell Motility* 6:129–151, 1985.]. The troponin complex also appears more elongated along the filament. (After G. N. Phillips, J. P. Fillers, and C. Cohen, Tropomyosin crystal structure and muscle regulation. *J. Mol. Biol.* 192:111, 1986; from S. Ebashi, M. Endo, and I. Ohtsuki, Control of muscle contraction. *Q. Rev. Biophys.* 2:351, 1969.)

made up of actin and tropomyosin when Ca^{2+} is absent. Troponin C (TnC), which binds Ca^{2+}, is closely related in structure to calmodulin, which regulates cellular functions in many tissues, including the nervous system (see Chap. 22). When Ca^{2+} binds to TnC, TnI is released, and tropomyosin changes its position within the thin filament to permit the combination of myosin with actin.

DEFECTS IN NEUROMUSCULAR TRANSMISSION CAN INTERRUPT NORMAL MUSCLE FUNCTION

Since the NMJ represents the ultimate link between the central nervous system and the initiation of motor activity, diseases that affect its function can have profound clinical consequences. It also provides an "Achilles heel," an optimal target for toxins produced by predators whose intent is to immobilize their prey. An unusual number of plant products and animal toxins affect the NMJ (Table 1). In many cases, research into the pathophysiology of diseases and toxins affecting the junction has shed light on the underlying normal physiologic mechanisms as well as on the clinical conditions themselves.

Events in synaptic transmission proceed in an orderly fashion from the depolarization of the presynaptic nerve terminal membrane through transmitter release and interaction with the postsynaptic membrane, to the modulation of postsynaptic events (see Chap. 9). In considering pathological events at the NMJ, the same conceptual sequence will be followed: toxins and disorders interfering with presynaptic mechanisms will be considered first, followed by a discussion of those targeting events at the postsynaptic level.

Botulinum toxin blocks the release of synaptic vesicles from the presynaptic nerve terminal

Botulism is the clinical disorder that results from exposure to one of a family of exotoxins produced by strains of the bacterium *Clostridium botulinum* [10]. It usually results from the ingestion of foods contaminated with the anaerobic *Clostridium* organisms, but can be produced by contamination of a deep penetrating wound with toxin-producing bacterium. The botulinum exotoxin is one of the most toxic substances known; a dose of less than 50 μg can be lethal in humans. This toxin specifically blocks neuromuscular transmission. If not treated rapidly, ingestion of the toxin can result in widespread weakness and ultimately in death due to paralysis of the muscles of respiration. In addition, botulinum toxin interferes with transmission at cholinergic parasympathetic terminals, producing autonomic symptoms.

At least eight closely related forms of botulinum toxin have been identified. Although these toxins appear to be produced by the *Clostridium* bacteria, they are in fact the result of a lysogenic infection of the bacterium with a phage containing the genetic information encoding the toxin molecule. Individuals exposed to botulinum toxin develop progressive failure of neuromuscular transmission characterized by an abnormally small electrical response in muscle after maximal stimulation of the motor nerve, although activation and conduction in the motor nerve itself are normal. Repeated

---

TABLE 1.   Some toxins and diseases affecting the neuromuscular junction[a]

PRESYNAPTIC ACTION

Botulinum toxin

Black widow spider venom

Snake β-neurotoxins

Lambert-Eaton syndrome

JUNCTIONAL ACTION

Inhibitors of AChE

Congenital AChE deficiency

POSTSYNAPTIC ACTION

Snake α-neurotoxins

Myasthenia gravis

Congenital defects of ACh receptor structure

[a] (AChE) acetylcholinesterase; (ACh) acetylcholine.

stimulation of the motor nerve leads to an increase in the amplitude of the muscle response, in contrast to the decremental response seen in patients with myasthenia gravis (see below). These clinical findings point to a defect in the release of acetylcholine from the presynaptic terminal, which is overcome in part by the elevated levels of intraterminal Ca^{2+} that are produced by repetitive depolarizations.

Botulinum toxin is synthesized as an inactive protomer of ~150 kDa, which must be cleaved into two fragments of ~100 kDa and 50 kDa before it becomes biologically active [11]. These two components, designated the heavy and light chains, are joined by a disulfide bridge; both are needed for toxicity.

The initial step in toxin action involves the binding of the disulfide-linked light chain–heavy chain complex to specific receptors on the presynaptic membrane. Molecules of toxin bound to the surface membrane are then internalized in membrane vesicles that ultimately discharge their contents into lysosomes. The toxin must then cross the lysosomal membrane and enter the cytoplasm before it can interfere with transmitter release. Here the amino terminal portion of the heavy chain plays a unique role (Fig. 6). It can form a transmembrane channel in a lipid bilayer that is large enough to allow an extended peptide chain to pass. In artificial bilayers, channel-forming activity is pH dependent; it is most prominent when the side of the bilayer corresponding to the intralysosomal surface is at low pH (about 4.5) while the cytoplasmic face is neutral (pH 7.0), corresponding to the conditions that prevail *in vivo*.

The toxicity of botulinum toxin ultimately involves the action of the 50-kDa light chain after it is released into the cytoplasm of the presynaptic terminal. A very small number of toxin molecules, probably fewer than 20, are capable of completely blocking all stimulus-induced transmitter release from a synapse, suggesting that an amplification step is involved. The possibility that the toxin light chain is actually an enzyme such as a

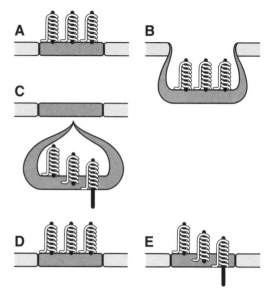

FIG. 6.   Proposed mechanism for the translocation of botulinum toxin into presynaptic nerve terminals. The toxin binds to a specific class of receptors on the plasma membrane of cholinergic nerve terminals (**A**). The toxin is then internalized by the process of receptor-mediated endocytosis (**B**). The endocytotic vesicles become progressively more acidic as they approach the lysosome, and the fall in pH triggers a conformational change in the toxin molecule. A portion of the molecule, probably the N terminus, partitions into the membrane and forms a channel. The light chain may then pass through this channel to reach the ultimate cytoplasmic site of action of the toxin (**C**). In an alternative mechanism, binding of the toxin complex to receptors on the cell surface (**D**) may lead directly to endocytosis when the tissue is exposed to a medium with low pH, triggering pH-dependent channel formation in the plasma membrane (**E**). (From L. L. Simpson [11].)

kinase that covalently modifies a specific protein involved in transmitter release is attractive. The ultimate site of action for this toxin may be the synaptic vesicle release site itself.

Black widow spider venom stimulates abnormal release of acetylcholine

The bite of the black widow spider initially produces an increase in neuromuscular activity that leads to painful skeletal muscle spasms and rigidity. This phase of hyperexcitability is rapidly followed by progressive failure of neuromuscular transmission and paralysis. The venom induces a transient but dramatic increase in spontaneous quantal release of acetylcholine, followed by a progressive decline and failure of both spontaneous and induced transmitter release.

The toxic component of the venom of the female spider is a 130-kDa protein called α-latrotoxin; it has no known enzymatic activity [12]. When applied to planar lipid bilayers, purified latrotoxin forms an ion channel with a conductance in excess of 100 pS that is permeant to Na^+, K^+, and Ca^{2+} but not to anions [13]. If α-latrotoxin has a similar effect on the presynaptic membrane, the result will be membrane depolarization and Ca^{2+} ion influx; the depolarization alone could activate voltage-dependent Ca^{2+} channels, further adding to the influx of Ca^{2+} ions. The net effect would be the triggering of synaptic vesicle fusion and transmitter release on a massive scale and eventually depletion of the neurotransmitter stores in the terminal. Although other mechanisms of action may be involved, the ionophore activity of the toxin provides an attractive hypothesis to explain its effects.

If α-latrotoxin can produce cation channels in artificial lipid bilayers, how is its activity confined so exquisitely to the presynaptic nerve terminal *in vivo*? The answer may lie in the presence of specific receptors for the polypeptide in the presynaptic membrane. α-Latrotoxin appears to bind to these molecules in the presynaptic terminal membrane and then insert into the membrane to form a cation-specific ion channel.

Some snake venoms contain β-toxins that interrupt presynaptic events

Many snake venoms contain polypeptide toxins that act on the neuromuscular junction (NMJ). Some α-toxins act by interfering with the function of acetylcholine receptors in the postsynaptic membrane; these toxins will be considered later in this chapter. A second group, the β-toxins, interfere with neuromuscular transmission through actions on

the presynaptic nerve terminal. Although β-toxins are produced by a variety of crotalids, the β-bungarotoxin found in the venom of the krait *Bungarus multicinctus* is the best-studied of this group.

β-Bungarotoxin, a protein of 20.5 kDa, is a heterodimer of a 13.5-kDa A chain and a 7-kDa B chain linked by at least one disulfide bond [14]. About 25 ng of this toxin is lethal to a mouse. The toxin inhibits the release of synaptic vesicles from motor nerve terminals and from some cholinergic autonomic terminals. Its onset of action is rather slow.

All of the presynaptically acting snake venoms exhibit phospholipase A_2 (PLA_2) activity [15]. This activity is abolished by treatment with *p*-bromophenacyl bromide (BPB), which specifically modifies histidine residue 48 in the A chain. The A chain exhibits extensive sequence homology with other enzymes with PLA_2 activity, especially those from the porcine pancreas. The β-bungarotoxin B chain has sequence homology with a number of protease inhibitors.

After exposure of an isolated nerve-muscle preparation to β-bungarotoxin, there is first a slight reduction in end-plate potential (EPP) amplitude. This is followed over the next hour by an augmentation of EPP amplitude, and finally by a slow but progressive decrease in amplitude that ends in complete block of stimulated transmitter release. During the second stage, there is also a transient increase in the frequency of miniature EPPs (MEPPs) consistent with an increase in intraterminal free Ca^{2+}. These effects require intact PLA_2 activity.

Autoimmune diseases can interfere with neurotransmitter release

Some patients with carcinoma, especially small-cell carcinoma of the lung, develop an unusual syndrome of muscle weakness associated with autonomic dysfunction called the Lambert-Eaton myasthenic syndrome (LEMS). Complaints often begin with progressive proximal muscle weakness and fatigue; unlike myasthenia gravis, bulbar involvement is usually mild and respiratory compromise is unusual. Autonomic complaints can include dry mouth, impotence, and orthostasis.

These patients demonstrate a remarkable reduction in the amplitude of the compound muscle action potential produced by single supramaximal stimulus to the motor nerve of a resting muscle [16]. Repeated stimulation of the same nerve, however, results in progressive improvement in response amplitude, often returning to nearly normal levels. These clinical findings are indicative of a defect in presynaptic neurotransmitter release.

When analyzed at the single cell level, LEMS is characterized by a dramatic reduction in the mean quantal content of the EPP, often to 10 percent or less of normal values. The amplitude of spontaneous MEPPs is normal, as is the MEPP frequency, but the MEPP frequency does not increase normally with increasing extracellular Ca^{2+}. Repetitive stimulation causes a progressive increase in quantal content of the EPP, consistent with the improvement seen in the compound muscle action potential.

LEMS is an autoimmune disease. The salient features of the disease can be passively transferred to mice by injection of IgG from patients who have the disorder. The target of the autoimmune reaction may be a 58-kDa synaptic membrane protein called synaptotagmin that is associated with presynaptic voltage-dependent Ca^{2+} channels. Like serum from LEMS patients, antibodies against synaptotagmin are able to precipitate the Ca^{2+} channel from solubilized membrane preparations. In freeze-fracture images of presynaptic membranes, the normal organization of the large intramembranous particles that form the double rows of the active zones is disrupted. These particles are thought to represent Ca^{2+} channels associated with specific release sites for synaptic vesicles. The number of arrays is reduced, with many particles found instead in irregular aggregates. Mice treated with IgG from

LEMS patients demonstrate the same changes in intramembranous particle distribution. It may be the cross-reactivity between a synaptotagmin-like molecule in the tumor cell and the related molecule in the normal presynaptic membrane that leads to the generation of symptoms at this seemingly unrelated site.

TOXINS AND DISEASES CAN ALSO BLOCK TRANSMISSION AT THE POSTSYNAPTIC LEVEL

Acetylcholine (ACh) released from the nerve terminal interacts specifically with receptor (AChR) molecules in the postsynaptic membrane (see Chap. 11). Molecules of acetylcholinesterase (AChE) in the junctional basal lamina compete for the transmitter and inactivate it by hydrolysis, forming acetate and choline. Successful transmission requires that a significant proportion of the ACh in each quantum reaches receptors in the postsynaptic membrane prior to being hydrolyzed. This in turn depends on the relative number of functional AChR and AChE molecules present as well as their geometric organization in relation to the release zones of the motor nerve terminal. The safety margin of transmission can be adversely affected, and junctional transmission blocked, by factors that modify the number of ACh receptors, their functional ability, or their organization in the synapse, as well as by factors that alter the properties of AChE.

α-Neurotoxins block the activation of nicotinic acetylcholine receptors

Toxins produced by snakes of the families *Elapidae* (cobras, kraits, coral snakes, mambas, and so forth) and *Hydrophidae* (sea snakes) contain potent neuromuscular toxins. A major component in each of these toxins is a curarimimetic α-neurotoxin, which produces a nondepolarizing block of the postsynaptic AChR. When applied to the

NMJ, these related small proteins block both EPPs and MEPPs. The frequency of MEPPs is not changed by pure α-toxin, although crude venom, which contains β-toxins as well, may have dramatic presynaptic effects. The LD_{50} for these toxins is typically 50 to 150 μg/kg in mice. Exposure of humans to low doses of toxin, which produces partial blockade of junctional receptors, can produce a clinical picture of weakness and fatigability that resembles acquired myasthenia gravis. Higher doses can lead to complete neuromuscular block, paralysis, respiratory failure, and death.

The α-toxins responsible for this postsynaptic curarimimetic activity are low-molecular-weight basic proteins of 7 to 8 kDa [17]. Chemically, they fall into two groups: the long toxins, which have 71 to 74 amino acids and 5 internal disulfide bonds, and the short toxins, with 60 to 62 amino acids and 4 internal disulfide bonds. All the α-toxins have about the same equilibrium dissociation constant for the AChR, but they differ markedly in their binding kinetics. The short toxins bind to and dissociate from the AChR five to nine times faster than the long toxins. Because of this, the binding of the short toxins can be reversed by washing while the long toxins bind essentially irreversibly. The relative irreversibility of the binding of the long α-neurotoxins to the AChR, especially that of α-bungarotoxin from the venom of *Bungarus multicinctus*, has made them valuable tools for the purification and characterization of this ion channel protein.

The α-toxins exhibit a high degree of homology when their primary sequences are aligned with respect to the cysteine residues. Several have been crystallized and their tertiary structure determined. The proteins are concave disks with a small projection at one end. Their elliptical dimensions are approximately 3.8 × 2.8 × 1.5 nm, and for the most part the structure is only a single polypeptide chain thick. The reactive site of the protein is on the concave surface and involves the regions encompassed by residues 32 to 45

and 49 to 56 as well as isolated residues from other regions of the molecule.

The α-neurotoxins bind specifically to sites on the α-subunits of the AChR; there is one binding site per subunit and thus two binding sites per receptor molecule (see Chap. 11). The binding site sterically overlaps that for ACh, and α-bungarotoxin binding prevents the interaction of ACh with the receptor.

In myasthenia gravis, an autoimmune response against the acetylcholine receptor leads to neuromuscular failure

Myasthenia gravis (MG), perhaps the prototypic human disorder of neuromuscular transmission, is an acquired autoimmune disease affecting AChRs on the postsynaptic membrane [18]. Clinically, the disorder is characterized by muscle weakness and abnormal fatigability. Most patients have circulating antibodies against the AChR in their serum.

Patients with MG typically show fluctuating symptoms; weakness and fatigability may be worse in the evenings and usually becomes more severe with exercise. Weakness may involve only the extraocular muscles, producing diplopia, or may be so extensive as to cause quadraparesis and respiratory compromise. Although spontaneous remissions can occur, the untreated disease is often progressive and can eventually lead to death from respiratory failure.

The classic electrophysiological observation in MG is a decrementing response in the extracellularly recorded compound muscle action potential with repeated nerve stimulation (Fig. 7). Using intracellular electrodes, the amplitude of the MEPP is found to be decreased. The quantum content of the EPP is normal, although its amplitude is reduced consequent to a reduction in MEPP amplitude. The decrease in MEPP amplitude is due to a reduction in the number of AChR molecules present in the postsynaptic membrane combined with a pathologic alteration

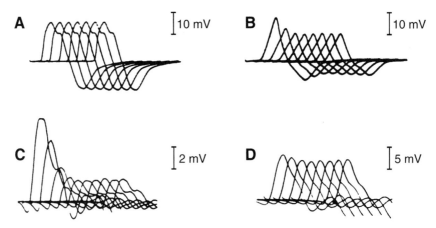

FIG. 7. Compound muscle action potentials recorded from the abductor digiti minimi of human subjects during repetitive stimulation of the ulnar nerve at three stimuli per second. **A:** A recording from a normal individual shows no change in the amplitude of the muscle electrical response during the stimulation interval. **B:** In a patient with MG, the same stimuli produce a 40 percent decrement in response amplitude over the first five stimuli, with a slow partial recovery during subsequent stimulation. Similar studies from a patient with severe MG before (**C**) and 2 min after (**D**) intravenous administration of 10 mg edrophonium. Note the change in amplitude scale between the two recordings and the reversal of the abnormal decrement by this short-acting AChE inhibitor.

in the architecture of the postsynaptic membrane.

The density of receptors in the myasthenic postsynaptic membrane may be as low as 20 percent of normal. In addition, the highly organized architecture of the postsynaptic membrane, with junctional folds immediately subjacent to presynaptic active zones and high densities of ACh receptors at the crests of these folds, is lost. The distance between pre- and postsynaptic membrane is often increased, and the postsynaptic membrane is highly simplified.

The destruction seen at the postsynaptic membrane is mediated by antibodies directed against the AChR [19]. Although it is attractive to postulate that functional block of AChRs by circulating antibodies is the primary mechanism through which transmission failure occurs, this does not seem to be the case. The major effects of anti-AChR antibodies seem to be twofold. First, antibodies cross-link receptor proteins and increase their rate of endocytosis and lysosomal degradation. In the absence of an increased rate of receptor synthesis, this results in a net decrease in receptor density in the postsynaptic membrane. Second, these antibodies target the postsynaptic membrane for complement fixation and activation of the lytic phase of the complement reaction cascade. The presence of lytic C9 in myasthenic postsynaptic membranes has been demonstrated both in humans and in animal models of myasthenia.

Although the mechanism of ongoing neuromuscular damage in this disease has been defined, the nature of the initial triggering event is unclear. One hypothesis involves the role of myocytes, muscle-like cells that occur in the thymus gland. These cells express AChRs on their surface membranes. An initial inflammatory response in the thymus may trigger the generation of cross-reacting antibodies that subsequently target AChRs on muscle. This hypothesis would help to explain the beneficial role of thymectomy in patients with MG. The diversity of predisposing and associated factors, however, suggests that a number of different triggering events may lead to the development of a common clinical picture.

Genetic defects in receptor structure can produce clinical disease

Given the central role of the AChR in neuromuscular transmission, it is reasonable to expect that mutations that affect channel function will also interfere with normal neuromuscular transmission. Defects that render the channel nonfunctional would be lethal, but milder alterations might be compatible with life.

Recently, investigators have described several genetic disorders of neuromuscular transmission that in some ways resemble MG as it is seen in infants. In one of these, an abnormally low density of AChRs was found at the NMJ. In the other, the kinetics of channel opening appeared abnormal, with a marked prolongation of the EPP and MEPP, which was further increased by the addition of AChE inhibitors [20]. Although the quantum content of the EPP was normal, its amplitude was significantly reduced. Activity and kinetic properties of AChE were normal. It is postulated that the defect in this disorder is an abnormally slow closing rate for the channel.

Abnormalities in acetylcholinesterase activity can interfere with neuromuscular transmission

At the NMJ, the duration of neurotransmitter action on the postsynaptic membrane is controlled by the rate of hydrolysis of ACh by AChE (see Chap. 11). This enzyme is associated with the basal lamina between the presynaptic membrane and the muscle plasma membrane. Roughly one-third of the released ACh from each quantum is hydrolyzed before reaching the postsynaptic membrane. The remaining molecules interact with postsynaptic receptors but are rapidly inactivated before having an opportunity for significant lateral spread. Thus, the site of action of released ACh is focused on a small area under the point of release from the presynaptic active zone.

Inhibition of AChE allows ACh to diffuse laterally out of the synapse and to interact with additional receptors along the way. The result is a marked prolongation of the EPP. Also, since receptors are desensitized after exposure to their transmitter, prolonged exposure to ACh eventually leads to reduced sensitivity and to block of neuromuscular transmission. Careful reduction of end-plate AChE activity following administration of AChEs can prolong the action of released ACh sufficiently to increase the amplitude of an abnormally low EPP above that required for successful neuromuscular transmission. It is this effect that allows these agents to be used in the treatment of MG. Too much medication, however, will produce long-term postsynaptic depolarization, receptor inactivation, and transmission block. Irreversible inhibitors of AChE are components of some nerve gases, and accidental poisoning by organophosphate insecticides can be fatal (see Chap. 11).

ABNORMAL EXCITABILITY OF THE SARCOLEMMA CAN AFFECT MUSCLE FUNCTION

Once a signal from a motor neuron has passed the NMJ, it must be spread throughout the muscle fiber as an action potential that is propagated along the sarcolemma and into the T-tubular system. The electrical activity of the sarcolemma must faithfully reproduce the activity of the innervating axon if the resulting contraction is to be of the intensity and duration dictated by the central nervous system. If the sarcolemma responds with multiple action potentials to a single stimulus at the NMJ, prolonged contractions will occur. Conversely, if the sarcolemma fails to respond to a postsynaptic potential of normal size, paralysis of the muscle will ensue. Both of these situations do occur: hyperexcitable states in the myotonic disorders and propagation failure in the periodic paralyses.

Normal excitability in the sarcolemma requires the integrated function of numerous ion channels

Like other excitable membranes, the muscle sarcolemmal membrane potential is produced by asymmetrical distributions of Na^+, K^+, and Cl^- ions in conjunction with varying conductances to these ions that are controlled by specific ion channels (Chap. 4). Action potentials result from a rapid but self-limited increase in Na^+ conductance mediated by voltage-dependent Na^+ channels, while activation of a delayed K^+ channel assists in membrane repolarization. Both channels function in muscle much as they do in nerve membranes (see Chap. 4).

The T-tubular system in muscle, however, imposes some special constraints. Although the amount of K^+ moving outward with each action potential is normally inconsequential with respect to transmembrane concentration gradients when released into the extracellular space outside a neuron or muscle fiber, the same amount of K^+ released into the restricted volume of the tubule can increase the local K^+ concentration by as much as 0.4 mM with each impulse. This K^+ must diffuse out of the tubule, a process that occurs with a time constant of 20 msec or more.

With repeated stimulation of a muscle fiber, K^+ will accumulate in the T-tubular system. If K^+ conductance were the predominant ion conductance in the resting muscle surface membrane, this accumulation would ultimately cause depolarization of the sarcolemma, interfering with normal signal propagation. This effect is minimized in skeletal muscle by the presence of a high resting conductance to chloride ions in the sarcolemma. This shunting conductance normally damps out the effect of T-tubular potassium accumulation on the sarcolemmal membrane potential.

Abnormalities of membrane chloride conductance can induce repetitive firing in the sarcolemma

A number of human muscle diseases are characterized by an abnormality of muscle relaxation called *myotonia*. Myotonia is the persistent contraction of a skeletal muscle following voluntary activation that is associated with repetitive action potential generation in the surface membrane. The most common of these is myotonic muscular dystrophy, which is actually a multisystem disease in which the myotonic feature is a relatively minor component. In two other diseases, myotonia congenita and recessive generalized myotonia, however, myotonia is the major presenting symptom and often the only abnormality found [21]. Patients afflicted with these inherited diseases have trouble relaxing their muscles normally. Doorknobs and handshakes are difficult to release, clumsiness is a problem, and falls often occur.

Years ago, an interesting disease similar to human myotonia congenita was described in a breed of goats [22]. When studied electrically, muscle fibers from these goats generated multiple repetitive action potentials in response to a single stimulus; these persistent runs of action potentials caused a striking delay in relaxation of the muscle after a short stimulus to the motor nerve. Studies of these myotonic goats showed that the sarcolemma in affected animals had a remarkable reduction in membrane chloride conductance, often to less than 20 percent of normal. Blockade of chloride channels in normal goat muscle duplicated both the symptoms and the electrical abnormalities of the myotonic animals. Subsequently, a number of drugs and toxins that caused transient myotonia in animals and humans were found to act by blocking the sarcolemmal chloride channel, eventually leading to the hypothesis that many of the human myotonic disorders were also chloride channel defects (Fig. 8).

The application of molecular genetic approaches to the human myotonic disor-

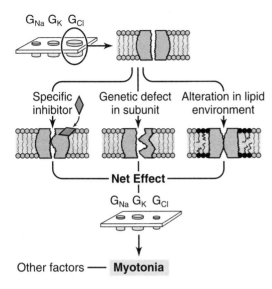

FIG. 8. Myotonia can be produced in skeletal muscle by a variety of factors that block membrane chloride conductance (G_{Cl}). In normal muscle, this can result from exposure to specific inhibitors of the channel or from alterations in the lipid environment. Genetic defects in the channel protein underlie the most common inherited myotonic disorders.

ders has proven very fruitful. Myotonic dystrophy, which produces muscle weakness and wasting, mental retardation, and skeletal and gonadal abnormalities in addition to myotonia, is associated with an expanded trinucleotide repeat mutation at chromosome 19, which appears to affect a form of kinase. The mechanism by which this mutation produces myotonia is as yet unknown. In myotonia congenita and recessive generalized myotonia, in which the muscle myotonic symptoms are the principal expression of the disease, tight linkage has been found to chromosome 7q 35, the site of the gene encoding the human skeletal muscle chloride channel [21]. A unique mutation in the chloride channel coding sequence has been identified in this gene in myotonia congenita.

The role of a chloride channel mutation in producing human myotonia is also supported by work with mouse mutants known as *mto* and *adr*. The phenotypes of both mutants resemble recessive generalized myoto-

nia, and they show the same abnormal electrical activity and low chloride conductance in their muscle membranes. The *adr* mutation is due to a mutation in its skeletal muscle chloride channel gene that is caused by a transposon insertion. This gene is located on a portion of the mouse chromosome that is syntenic with the location of the defective human gene in myotonia congenita and recessive generalized myotonia.

When the sarcolemma is not sufficiently excitable, weakness or paralysis can result

A fascinating group of inherited muscle diseases called the periodic paralyses is characterized by intermittent episodes of skeletal muscle weakness or paralysis that occur in people who usually appear completely normal between attacks [23]. The periods of paralysis are often associated with changes in the serum K^+ concentration; while the serum K^+ concentration can go either up or down, the direction is usually consistent for a particular family and forms one basis for classifying these diseases as either hyperkalemic or hypokalemic periodic paralysis. A variant of periodic paralysis in which spells of weakness are less frequent and in which a form of myotonic hyperexcitability is often seen is called paramyotonia congenita.

Recordings from muscle fibers isolated from patients during an attack of periodic paralysis have shown that the paralytic episodes are associated with acute depolarization of the sarcolemma. In all forms of the disease, this depolarization is due to an increase in membrane conductance to Na^+ ions. In the case of hyperkalemic periodic paralysis and paramyotonia congenita, this abnormal conductance can be blocked by tetrodotoxin, a small polar molecule that is highly specific for the voltage-dependent Na^+ channel. Single channel recordings in hyperkalemic periodic paralysis have revealed that some of the muscle membrane Na^+ channels show abnormal inactivation kinetics, intermittently entering a mode in which they fail to inactivate. These channels will produce a persistent noninactivating Na^+ current that will in turn produce membrane depolarization. Since normal Na⁺ channels enter an inactivated state after depolarization (see Chap. 4), the net result of long-term depolarization will be a loss of sarcolemmal excitability and paralysis.

Na⁺ channel mutations cause periodic paralysis

Since the voltage-dependent Na⁺ channel has been successfully cloned and sequenced from human skeletal muscle and its chromosomal localization determined, it was possible to test the involvement of this channel with the disease through genetic linkage analysis. Measurements in families with both hyperkalemic periodic paralysis and paramyotonia demonstrated a very tight linkage between the adult skeletal muscle Na⁺ channel gene on chromosome 17q23.3–25.1 and the phenotypic expression of the disease [23]. The hypokalemic form of periodic paralysis is not linked to this Na⁺ channel gene.

The voltage-dependent Na⁺ channel in skeletal muscle closely resembles those found in brain and in cardiac muscle [1] (see Chap. 4). The purified protein contains one very large α-subunit of ~260 kDa-MW and one 38-kDa MW β-subunit. The α-subunit is heavily glycosylated. This subunit, which has been cloned, sequenced, and functionally expressed, contains all the elements necessary for a normal ion-selective channel. Its structure resembles that of the α₁-subunit of the voltage-dependent Ca²⁺ channel in having four large internal repeat domains, each encompassing 220 to 300 amino acids. Each

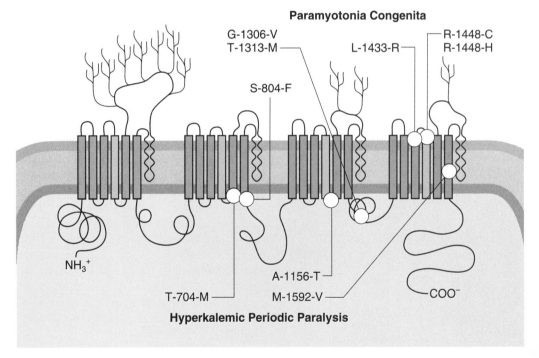

FIG. 9. Point mutations have been identified in the skeletal muscle Na⁺ channel α-subunit of families with hyperkalemic periodic paralysis or paramyotonia congenita. Mutations in hyperkalemic periodic paralysis have been found near the cytoplasmic ends of transmembrane helices in domains 2 and 4. Mutations in paramyotonia congenita involve either the interdomain 2 to 3 region or the region near the extracellular end of the S4 helix in domain 4. Several additional mutations have been identified in families with clinical features that combine elements of both diseases. (From R. L. Barchi, Ion channels and abnormalities of excitation in skeletal muscle. *Curr. Opin. Neurol. Neurosurg.* 6:40, 1993.)

domain contains six to eight transmembrane helices organized compactly in the plane of the membrane. Current models of channel structure propose that the four repeat domains are organized in a ring to form a central ion channel. One helix in each domain, the S4 helix, contains positively charged lysine or arginine residues at every third residue, separated by nonpolar amino acids. This positively charged helix plays a central role in the voltage-sensing function of the channel.

Once the sequence of the normal human skeletal muscle Na+ channel and of the gene that encodes it became available, the door was opened to a direct analysis of defects in the coding sequence that might produce clinical disease. A total of seven different mutations have now been identified in the coding region of the skeletal muscle Na+ channel in different families with hyperkalemic periodic paralysis or paramyotonia congenita [23]. These mutations are distributed throughout the primary sequence of this large protein and do not seem to cluster around one particular region, suggesting that a considerable portion of the channel protein may be involved in some way with the conformational changes associated with inactivation (Fig. 9). In addition to shedding light on the origin of the symptoms of the disease, each mutation provides additional insight into the relationships between structure and function in the normal channel.

DEFECTS AT THE TRIAD CAN ALSO AFFECT MUSCLE FUNCTION

A congenital absence of the L-type calcium channel is fatal

An interesting hereditary disorder of mice, called muscular dysgenesis, has been described in which affected pups exhibit an absence of skeletal muscle movement and die shortly after birth from respiratory failure. Electrophysiological investigation of the defective muscle showed that the fault lay at the level of excitation-contraction coupling. When the muscle was analyzed biochemi-

cally, it was found to be deficient in the L-type voltage-dependent Na+ channel that is thought to link T-tubular depolarization to Ca2+ release from the terminal elements of the sarcoplasmic reticulum.

In an elegant experiment, Beam and his colleagues restored excitation-contraction coupling to dysgenic muscle in culture by introducing a plasmid containing the full-length coding sequence for the dihydropyridine-sensitive Ca2+ channel from skeletal muscle into the nuclei of affected cells [24]. Myotubes treated in this way showed normal contractions in response to electrical stimulation. While never described in humans, it seems likely that mutations affecting this T-tubular protein could have similar profound effects on an affected fetus.

Malignant hyperthermia is linked to mutations in the ryanodine receptor protein

A rare complication of general inhalation anesthesia is a syndrome characterized by muscle stiffness and hyperpyrexia. If untreated, this syndrome, called malignant hyperthermia (MH), can be rapidly fatal. Although the inheritance pattern of the disease is difficult to trace, it is likely to be passed from generation to generation as an autosomal dominant trait. A similar disease occurs in a strain of pigs, and this experimental animal model has proven to be very useful in studying the physiology of the disease.

Measurements on isolated muscle from affected pigs or humans show that the defect is at the level of excitation-contraction coupling. Specifically, the muscles release Ca2+ when exposed to caffeine at levels much lower than does normal muscle. Once released, this Ca2+ produces persistent activation of tropomyosin and sustained contraction, which in turn leads to hypermetabolism and hyperpyrexia.

Once the cDNA encoding the ryanodine receptor protein of the terminal RS had been cloned and sequenced, it became possible to localize the gene encoding this protein to a particular location on the porcine chromosome 6 and to a syntenic region of human chromosome 19. Using restriction-length polymorphisms within this gene, linkage between the gene and the expression of the MH phenotype could then be tested. It rapidly became apparent that in the porcine form of MH, as well as in many of the human families expressing the disease, the phenotype was indeed tightly linked to the ryanodine receptor gene [25].

REFERENCES

1. Catterall, W. A. Structure and function of voltage-sensitive ion channels. *Science* 242:50–61, 1988.
2. Franzini-Armstrong, C. Studies of the triad. I. Structure of the junction of frog twitch fibers. *J. Cell Biol.* 47:488–499, 1979.
3. Catterall, W. A. Excitation-contraction coupling in vertebrate skeletal muscle: A tale of two calcium channels. *Cell* 64:871–874, 1991.
4. Campbell, K. P., Knudson, C. M., Imagawa, T., Leung, A. T., Sutko, J. L., et al. Identification and characterization of the high affinity [³H]ryanodine receptor of the junctional sarcoplasmic reticulum Ca²⁺ release channel. *J. Biol. Chem.* 262:6460–6463, 1987.
5. Wagenknecht, T., Grassucci, R., Frank, I., Saito, A., Inui, M., and Fleischer, S. Three-dimensional architecture of the calcium channel/foot structure of sarcoplasmic reticulum. *Nature* 338:167–170, 1989.
6. Pollard, T. D., and Cooper, J. A. Actin and actin-binding proteins. A critical evaluation of mechanisms and functions. *Annu. Rev. Biochem.* 55:987–1035, 1986.
7. Harrington, W. F., and Rodgers, M. E. Myosin. *Annu. Rev. Biochem.* 53:35–74, 1984.
8. Hibberd, M. G., and Trentham, D. R. Relationships between chemical and mechanical events during muscular contraction. *Annu. Rev. Biophys. Biophys. Chem.* 15:119–161, 1986.
9. Zot, A. S., and Potter, J. D. Structural aspects of troponin-tropomyosin regulation of skeletal muscle contraction. *Annu. Rev. Biophys. Biophys. Chem.* 16:535–560, 1987.
10. Sakaguchi, G. *Clostridium botulinum* toxins. *Pharmacol. Ther.* 19:165–194, 1983.
11. Simpson, L. L. Molecular pharmacology of botulinum toxin and tetanus toxin. *Annu. Rev. Pharmacol. Toxicol.* 26:427–453, 1986.
12. Howard, B. D., and Gunderson, C. B. Jr. Ef-

fects and mechanisms of polypeptide neurotoxins that act presynaptically. *Annu. Rev. Pharmacol. Toxicol.* 20:307–336, 1980.
13. Finkelstein, A., Rubin, L. L., and Tzeng, M. C. Black widow spider venom: Effect of purified toxin on lipid bilayer membranes. *Science* 193:1009–1011, 1976.
14. Kondo, K., Narita, K., and Lee, C. Y. Amino acid sequences of the two polypeptide chains in beta-bungarotoxin from the venom of *Bungarus multicinctus. J. Biochem.* 83:101–115, 1978.
15. Kondo, K., Toda, H., and Narita, K. Characterization of phospholipase A₂ activity of beta-bungarotoxin from *Bungarus multicinctus. J. Biochem.* 84:1291–1300, 1978.
16. Newsome-Davis, J. Lambert-Eaton myasthenic syndrome. *Springer Semin. Immunopathol.* 8:129–140, 1985.
17. Karlsson, E. Chemistry of protein toxins in snake venoms. In C. Y. Lee (ed.), *Snake Venoms.* Berlin: Springer-Verlag, 1979, pp. 159–204.
18. Lisak, R. P., and Barchi, R. L. *Myasthenia Gravis.* Philadelphia: W. B. Saunders Co., 1982.
19. Lindstrom, J. Immunobiology of myasthenia gravis, experimental autoimmune myasthenia gravis, and Lambert-Eaton syndrome. *Annu. Rev. Immunol.* 3:109–131, 1985.
20. Engel, A. G., Lambert, E. H., Mulder, D. M., et al., A newly recognized congenital myasthenic syndrome attributable to a prolonged open time of the acetylcholine-induced ion channel. *Ann. Neurol.* 11:553–569, 1982.
21. Barchi, R. L. The non-dystrophic myotonic syndromes. In R. N. Rosenberg, S. B. Prusiner, S. DiMauro, R. L. Barchi, and L. M. Kunkel (eds.) *The Molecular and Genetic Basis of Neurological Disease.* Philadelphia: Butterworth, 1993, pp. 873–880.
23. Barchi, R. L. Sodium channel gene defects in the periodic paralyses. *Curr. Opin. Neurobiol.* 2:631–637, 1992.
24. Adams, B. A., and Beam, K. G. Muscular dysgenesis in mice: a model system for studying excitation-contraction coupling, *FASEB J.* 4:2809–2816, 1990.
25. MacLennan, D. H., Duff, C., Zorzato, F., Fujii, J., Phillips, M., Korneluk, R. G., Frodis, W., Britt, B. A., and Worton, R. G. Ryanodine receptor gene is a candidate for predisposition to malignant hyperthermia. *Nature* 343:559–561, 1990.

CHAPTER 34

Diseases of Carbohydrate, Fatty Acid, and Mitochondrial Metabolism

SALVATORE DiMAURO AND DARRYL C. DE VIVO

Defects of energy metabolism cause profound disturbances in the function of muscle or brain or both. Such defects may present as a myopathy, encephalopathy, or encephalomyopathy. Clinical features are best appreciated by having an understanding of the preferred oxidizable substrates for brain and muscle.

Muscle in the resting state utilizes fatty acids predominantly. The immediate source of energy for muscle contraction is ATP, which is rapidly replenished at the expense of creatine phosphate by the phosphorylation of ADP by creatine kinase. During exercise of moderate intensity, the fuel choice depends on the duration of work. Initially, glycogen is the main fuel source; after 5 or 10 min, blood glucose becomes the more im-

Basic Neurochemistry: Molecular, Cellular, and Medical Aspects, 5th Ed., edited by G. J. Siegel et al. Published by Raven Press, Ltd., New York, 1994. Correspondence to Salvatore DiMauro, Department of Neurology, College of Physicians and Surgeons, Columbia University, New York, New York 10032.

portant fuel. As work continues, fatty acid utilization increases, and after approximately 4 hr lipids are the primary source of energy. During high-intensity exercise (near-maximal power), additional ATP is generated by the anaerobic breakdown of glycogen and by glycolysis. Intense exercise is performed in essentially anaerobic conditions, whereas mild or moderate exercise is accompanied by increased blood flow to exercising muscles, facilitating substrate delivery, and favoring aerobic metabolism. This adaption is known as the "second-wind" phenomenon [12].

Brain utilizes glucose predominantly in the postabsorptive state, with regional variations of the metabolic rate depending on the mental or motor task being performed [7]. As with muscle, the immediate intracellular energy source is ATP buttressed by the creatine phosphate stores. Glycogen provides very little energy reserve because brain concentrations are extremely low, approximately only one-tenth the amount found in muscle per gram wet weight. Therefore, brain is exquisitely sensitive to fluctuations in the blood glucose concentration. Movement of glucose across the blood-brain barrier is facilitated by a carrier protein (GLUT 1) [2]. The facilitated transport of glucose ensures adequate brain glucose concentrations to meet the needs of cerebral metabolism under normal conditions. During starvation, the brain uses little, if any, fatty acids; however, fatty acids of varying chain lengths may be taken up by the brain, the efficiency of transport across the blood-brain barrier being much greater for short- or medium-chain fatty acids than for long-chain fatty acids. Ketone bodies represent the preferred cerebral fuel source during starvation when glucose supply is limited [1] (these features of brain metabolism are discussed in Chap. 31). Defective fatty acid oxidation may therefore affect muscle directly by blocking oxidation of this substrate and brain indirectly by limiting hepatic ketogenesis. Elevated circulating free fatty acids may also have a direct toxic effect on brain, but the precise mechanisms are poorly understood (see Chaps. 40 and 42).

Energy metabolism has been studied extensively in skeletal muscle, and several metabolic disorders have been documented [5,7]. Comparatively less is known about metabolic defects in cerebral energy metabolism—muscle tissue is more accessible for biochemical analysis, and certain cerebral enzyme defects are presumed lethal.

DISEASES OF CARBOHYDRATE AND FATTY ACID METABOLISM IN MUSCLE

In muscle, disorders of glycogen or lipid metabolism cause two main clinical syndromes:

1. Acute, recurrent, reversible muscle dysfunction, with exercise intolerance and myoglobinuria (with or without cramps) is characteristic of phosphorylase, phosphofructokinase (PFK), phosphoglycerate kinase (PGK), phosphoglycerate mutase (PGAM), and lactate dehydrogenase (LDH) deficiencies among the glycogenoses, and of carnitine palmitoyltransferase (CPT) deficiency and short-chain three-hydroxyacyl CoA dehydrogenase (SCHAD) deficiency among the disorders of lipid metabolism.

2. Progressive weakness is associated with acid maltase, debrancher enzyme, and brancher enzyme deficiencies among the glycogenoses, and with carnitine deficiency, some defects of β-oxidation, and other biochemically undefined lipid storage myopathies among the disorders of lipid metabolism. Figures 1 and 2 illustrate schematically the pathways of glycogen and fatty acid metabolism.

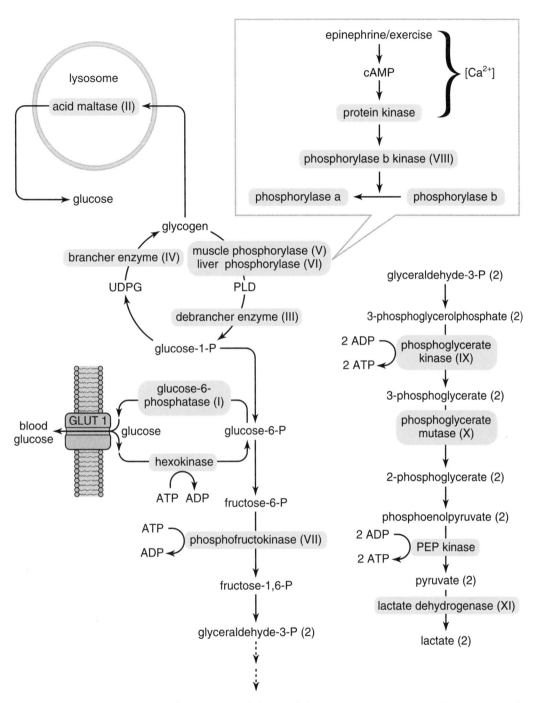

FIG. 1. Schematic representation of glycogen metabolism and glycolysis. *Roman numerals* indicate the sites of identified enzyme defects: (I) glucose-6-phosphatase; (II) acid maltase; (III) debrancher enzyme; (IV) brancher enzyme; (V) muscle phosphorylase; (VI) liver phosphorylase; (VII) phosphofructokinase; (VIII) phosphorylase kinase; (IX) phosphoglycerate kinase; (X) phosphoglycerate mutase; (XI) lactate dehydrogenase. (PLD) phosphorylase-limit dextrin; (UDPG) uridine diphosphate glucose; (P) phosphate.

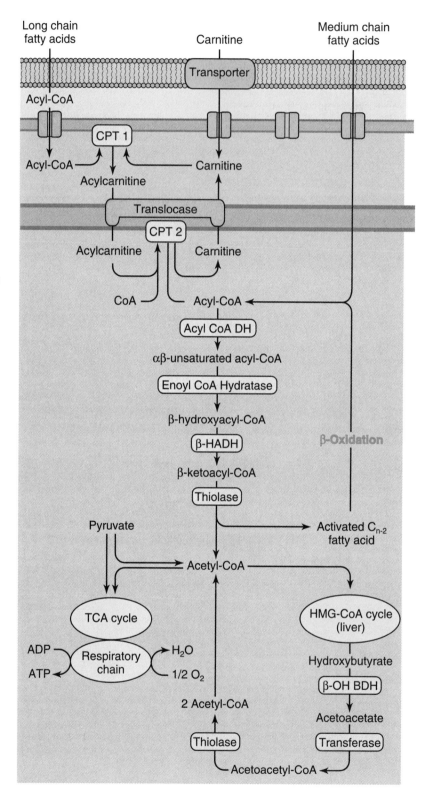

Disorders causing recurrent myoglobinuria and exercise intolerance

Phosphorylase Deficiency (McArdle's Disease; Glycogenosis Type V)

Phosphorylase deficiency is an autosomal recessive myopathy caused by a genetic defect of the muscle isoenzyme of glycogen phosphorylase (Fig. 1). The gene encoding this enzyme has been assigned to chromosome 11. There is a 2:1 predominance of affected males to females. Intolerance of strenuous exercise is present from childhood, but onset is usually in adolescence, with cramps after exercise [5]. Myoglobinuria occurs in about one-half of patients. If they avoid intense exercise, most patients can live normal lives; however, about one-third of them develop some degree of fixed weakness, usually as a late-onset manifestation of the disease. In a few patients, weakness rather than exercise-related cramps and myoglobinuria characterizes the clinical picture.

In patients with myoglobinuria, renal insufficiency is a possible life-threatening complication. Physical examination between episodes of myoglobinuria may be completely normal or show some degree of weakness and, occasionally, wasting of some muscle groups.

Even between episodes, most patients have increased serum creatine kinase (CK) levels; forearm ischemic exercise causes no rise of venous lactate level. This is a useful but nonspecific test in McArdle's disease. The electromyogram (EMG) at rest shows nonspecific myopathic features in about one-half of patients.

Muscle biopsy demonstrates subsarcolemmal blebs that contain periodic acid-Schiff-positive material (glycogen). The histochemical stain for phosphorylase is negative, except in regenerating fibers. Biochemical documentation of the enzyme defect requires muscle biopsy, because the defect is not expressed in more easily accessible tissues (leukocytes, erythrocytes, cultured fibroblasts).

Phosphofructokinase Deficiency (Tarui's Disease; Glycogenosis Type VII)

Phosphofructokinase deficiency is an autosomal recessive myopathy caused by a genetic defect of the muscle (M) subunit of the rate-limiting enzyme of glycolysis, PFK (Fig. 1). The gene encoding PFK-M is on chromosome 1. There is a 2.4:1 predominance of affected males to females. Presenting symptoms are cramps after intense exercise, followed by myoglobinuria in about one-half of patients. A few patients may have mild jaundice, reflecting excessive hemolysis, or typical symptoms and signs of gout. In patients with typical presentation, fixed weakness appears to be less common than in phosphorylase deficiency. On the other hand, in PFK deficiency, as in phosphorylase deficiency, a few patients have only weakness, without cramps or myoglobinuria. In addition to renal insufficiency due to myoglobinuria, other possible complications include renal colic due to urate stones and gouty arthritis [5].

Physical examination may show slight jaundice. Neurological examination is normal. Serum CK level is variably increased in most patients. Forearm ischemic exercise causes no rise of venous lactate level. Serum bilirubin level is elevated in most patients,

---

FIG. 2. Schematic representation of fatty acid oxidation and ketone body synthesis. Fatty acid oxidation is divided between the carnitine cycle and β-oxidation. The carnitine cycle includes four steps: the plasma membrane carnitine transporter; carnitine palmitoyltransferase (CPT) type I; carnitine-acylcarnitine translocase system; and CPT type II. β-oxidation involves four enzymatic steps: acyl CoA dehydrogenase, enoyl CoA hydratase, β-hydroxyacyl CoA dehydrogenase (HADH), and β-ketothiolase. The end product of fatty acid oxidation is the formation of acyl CoA and activated C_{n-2} fatty acid. Acyl CoA may enter the tricarboxylic acid (TCA) cycle or the β-hydroxy-β-methylglutaryl (HMG) CoA cycle. The HMG-CoA cycle forms ketone bodies, β-hydroxybutyrate, and acetoacetate. (CoA) coenzyme A, reduced; (DH) dehydrogenase.

and the number of reticulocytes is increased. Serum uric acid level is also increased in most patients. Electromyogram is usually normal. Muscle biopsy shows focal, mostly subsarcolemmal, accumulation of glycogen. In some patients a small portion of the glycogen is abnormal: By histochemical analysis, it is shown to be diastase resistant; by electron microscopy, it appears finely granular and filamentous in structure. The enzyme defect can be demonstrated by a specific histochemical reaction for PFK. Although a partial defect of PFK activity is manifest in erythrocytes from patients, firm diagnosis usually requires biochemical studies of muscle.

Phosphoglycerate Kinase Deficiency

Phosphoglycerate kinase deficiency is an X-linked recessive disease (type IX, Fig. 1). The most common clinical presentation includes hemolytic anemia with or without central nervous system involvement (see below). Thus far, only three patients have been described with a purely myopathic syndrome, characterized by exercise-induced cramps and myoglobinuria. Between episodes of myoglobinuria, physical and neurological examinations were normal. Forearm ischemic exercise caused contracture and no rise of venous lactate level.

Because the enzyme defect is expressed in all tissues except sperm, diagnosis can be made by biochemical studies of muscle, erythrocytes, leukocytes, and cultured fibroblasts [5,6].

Phosphoglycerate Mutase Deficiency

Phosphoglycerate mutase deficiency is an autosomal recessive myopathy caused by a genetic defect of the muscle subunit of the enzyme PGAM (type X, Fig. 1). Five patients with this enzyme deficiency have been identified thus far.

The clinical picture includes cramps and recurrent myoglobinuria following intense exercise. Aside from episodes of myoglobinuria, none of the patients was weak. Forearm ischemic exercise caused an in-

crease of 1.5 to 2.0 times in venous lactate level, an abnormally low but not absent response. Muscle biopsy showed normal or only moderately increased glycogen concentration. Because other accessible tissues, such as erythrocytes, leukocytes, and cultured fibroblasts, express a different isoenzyme, the diagnosis of PGAM-M subunit deficiency must be established by biochemical studies of muscle [5].

Lactate Dehydrogenase Deficiency

Lactate dehydrogenase deficiency is an autosomal recessive myopathy caused by a genetic defect of the muscle subunit, which is encoded by a gene on chromosome 11 (type XI, Fig. 1). Thus far, two patients with this disease have been described. The clinical picture is characterized by cramps and myoglobinuria after intense exercise.

Forearm ischemic exercise showed a subnormal rise of lactate level, contrasting with an increased rise of pyruvate. The diagnosis can be established by electrophoretic studies of LDH in serum, erythrocytes, and leukocytes, showing lack of subunit M-containing isoenzymes; it should nevertheless be confirmed by biochemical studies of muscle.

Carnitine Palmitoyltransferase Deficiency

Carnitine palmitoyltransferase deficiency is an autosomal recessive myopathy caused by a genetic defect of the mitochondrial enzyme CPT (Fig. 2). The disease has been identified in about 50 patients, with a marked prevalence of affected men (males:female ratio, 5.5:1).

Clinical manifestations are limited to attacks of myoglobinuria, not preceded by contractures, and usually precipitated by prolonged exercise (several hours in duration), prolonged fasting, or a combination of the two conditions. Less common precipitating factors include intercurrent infection, emotional stress, and cold exposure; but some episodes of myoglobinuria occur without any apparent cause. Most patients have two or more attacks, probably because the lack of muscle cramps deprives them of a warning signal of impending myoglobinuria [4,12,15].

For unknown reasons, some women seem to have milder symptoms, such as myalgia, after prolonged exercise without pigmenturia. This has been observed in sisters of men with recurrent myoglobinuria. The only serious complication is renal failure following myoglobinuria.

Physical and neurological examinations are completely normal. Prolonged fasting at rest (to be conducted under close medical observation) causes a sharp rise of serum CK level in about one-half of patients. Also in about one-half of patients, ketone bodies fail to increase normally after prolonged fasting. Forearm ischemic exercise causes a normal increase of venous lactate level. Aside from episodes of myoglobinuria, serum CK level and EMG are normal. A muscle biopsy specimen may appear completely normal or show variable, but usually moderate, accumulation of lipid droplets. Most patients with CPT deficiency benefit from a high-carbohydrate, low-fat diet, and the therapeutic response may serve as an indirect diagnostic clue. Because the enzyme defect appears to be generalized, tissues other than muscle (e.g., mixed leukocytes or isolated lymphocytes or platelets) can be used to demonstrate CPT deficiency, but the diagnosis should be confirmed in muscle.

Immunological studies using antibodies that appear to react specifically to one or the other enzyme have suggested that the myopathic form of CPT deficiency is due to a defect of CPT II. A full-length cDNA for CPT II is now available, and the molecular basis of this disorder is being investigated.

Short-Chain 3-Hydroxyacyl CoA Dehydrogenase Deficiency

Additional defects of β-oxidation have been associated with limb weakness and attacks of myoglobinuria. Three patients have been described with a deficiency of the short-chain isoform for SCHAD. The condition is potentially fatal. Combined skeletal muscle defects of aconitase and succinate dehydrogenase have been described in one patient with limb weakness and myoglobinuria [13,15].

Disorders causing progressive weakness

Acid Maltase Deficiency (Glycogenosis Type II)

Acid maltase deficiency (AMD) is an autosomal recessive disease caused by a genetic defect of the lysosomal enzyme acid maltase, an α-1,4- and α-1,6-glucosidase capable of digesting glycogen completely to glucose (Fig. 1). The gene encoding acid maltase has been localized on chromosome 17. Two major clinical syndromes are caused by AMD: a severe, generalized, and invariably fatal disease of infancy (Pompe's disease) and a less severe neuromuscular disorder beginning in childhood or in adult life. (Other lysosomal disorders are discussed in Chap. 38.)

Infantile, Generalized Cardiomegalic AMD (Pompe's Disease).   Pompe's disease usually becomes manifest in the first weeks or months of life, with failure to thrive, poor suck, generalized hypotonia, and weakness (floppy infant syndrome). Macroglossia is common, as is hepatomegaly, which, however, is rarely severe. There is massive cardiomegaly with congestive heart failure. Weak respiratory muscles make these infants susceptible to pulmonary infection; death usually occurs before age 1 year and invariably before age 2 years [5,7].

Childhood- and Adult-Onset AMD.   The childhood- and adult-onset forms of AMD cause signs and symptoms that are limited to the musculature, with progressive weakness of truncal muscles and of proximal more than distal limb muscles, usually sparing facial and extraocular muscle. In the childhood form, onset is in infancy or childhood, and progression tends to be rapid. In the adult form, onset is usually in the third or fourth decade but occasionally even later, and the course is slower [5].

The clinical picture in male children can closely resemble Duchenne-type muscular dystrophy; in adults it mimics limb-girdle dystrophy or polymyositis. The early and severe involvement of respiratory muscles in most patients with AMD is a distinctive clinical clue. Respiratory failure and pulmonary infection are the most common causes of death.

Serum CK level is consistently increased in all forms of AMD. Forearm ischemic exercise causes normal rise of venous lactate level in patients with childhood or adult AMD. The ECG is altered in Pompe's disease (short P-R interval, giant QRS complexes, and left ventricular or biventricular hypertrophy) but is usually normal in the later onset forms. Electromyogram shows myopathic features and fibrillation potentials, bizarre high-frequency discharges, and myotonic discharges.

Muscle biopsy shows vacuolar myopathy of very severe degree, affecting all fibers in Pompe's disease, but of varying degree and distribution in childhood and adult AMD. In adult AMD, biopsy specimens from unaffected muscles may appear normal by light microscopy. The vacuoles contain periodic acid-Schiff-positive material (glycogen). Electron microscopy shows the presence of abundant glycogen both within membranous sacs (lysosomes) and free in the cytoplasm.

The enzyme defect is expressed in all tissues, and the diagnosis can be made by biochemical analysis of urine, lymphocytes (mixed leukocytes do not give reliable results), or cultured skin fibroblasts. Fibroblasts cultured from amniotic fluid can be used for prenatal diagnosis of Pompe's disease.

Debrancher Enzyme Deficiency
(Glycogenosis Type III, Cori's Disease;
Forbes' Disease)

Debrancher enzyme deficiency is an autosomal recessive disease (Fig. 1). In its more common presentation, debrancher enzyme deficiency causes liver dysfunction in childhood, with hepatomegaly, growth retardation, fasting hypoglycemia, and seizures [7]. Myopathy has been described in about 20 patients [5]. In most, onset of weakness was in the third or fourth decade. Wasting of distal leg muscles and intrinsic hand muscles is common, and the association of late-onset weakness and distal wasting often suggests the diagnosis of motor neuron disease or peripheral neuropathy. The course is slowly progressive. In a smaller number of patients, onset of weakness is in childhood, with diffuse weakness and wasting. The association of hepatomegaly and growth retardation facilitates the diagnosis.

There is no glycemic response to glucagon or epinephrine (see Fig. 1), whereas a galactose load causes a normal glycemic response. Forearm ischemic exercise produces a blunted venous lactate rise or no response. Serum CK activity is variably, often markedly, increased. Electrocardiogram shows left ventricular or biventricular hypertrophy in most patients. Electromyogram may show myopathic features alone or associated with fibrillations, positive sharp waves, and myotonic discharges. This "mixed" EMG pattern in patients with weakness and distal wasting often reinforces the erroneous diagnosis of motorneuron disease. Motor nerve conduction velocities are moderately decreased in one-fourth of patients, suggesting a polyneuropathy.

Muscle biopsy shows severe vacuolar myopathy with glycogen storage. On electron microscopy, the vacuoles correspond to pools of glycogen free in the cytoplasm.

In most patients, the enzyme defect is generalized, and it has been demonstrated in erythrocytes, leukocytes, and cultured fibroblasts. In patients with myopathy, the diagnosis is securely established by measurement of debrancher enzyme activity in muscle biopsy specimens or by studies of iodine adsorption spectra of glycogen isolated from muscle; there is a shift in the spectrum toward lower wavelengths, indicating that the polysaccharide has abnormally short peripheral branches.

Branching Enzyme Deficiency (Glycogenosis Type IV; Andersen's Disease)

Branching enzyme deficiency is an autosomal recessive disease of infancy or early childhood typically causing liver dysfunction with hepatosplenomegaly, progressive cirrhosis, and chronic hepatic failure (Fig. 1). Death usually occurs in childhood. Although muscle wasting and hypotonia are mentioned in several reports, only three patients had severe hypotonia, wasting, contractures, and hyporeflexia, suggesting the diagnosis of spinal muscular atrophy [5].

There are no diagnostic laboratory tests. A muscle biopsy specimen may be normal or show focal accumulations of abnormal glycogen, which is intensely PAS positive and partially resistant to diastase digestion. With the electron microscope, the abnormal glycogen is found to have a finely granular and filamentous structure.

Carnitine Deficiency

Carnitine deficiency is a clinically useful term describing a diversity of biochemical disorders affecting fatty acid oxidation. Carnitine deficiency may be tissue specific or generalized.

Tissue-Specific Carnitine Deficiency. This condition has been previously termed myopathic carnitine deficiency because the patients have generalized limb weakness, starting in childhood. Limb, trunk, and facial musculature may be involved. The course is slowly progressive, but weakness may fluctuate in severity. Laboratory investigations show normal or near-normal serum carnitine concentrations and variably increased serum CK values. Electromyogram shows myopathic features with or without spontaneous activity at rest. Muscle biopsy reveals severe triglyceride storage, best seen with the oil red O stain in frozen sections. This condition is transmitted as an autosomal recessive trait. Originally, it was thought that the primary biochemical defect involved the active transport of carnitine from blood into muscle. However, no defect has ever been documented [8]. Rather, an increasing number of patients have a tissue-specific defect involving the short-chain isoform for acyl CoA dehydrogenase (SCAD). As such, the muscle carnitine deficiency is secondary to a primary enzyme defect.

Generalized Carnitine Deficiency. The only *primary* form of generalized carnitine deficiency, inherited as an autosomal recessive trait, is due to a defect of the specific high-affinity, low-concentration, carrier-mediated carnitine uptake mechanism. Although the defect has been documented only in cultured fibroblasts, the same uptake system is probably shared by muscle, heart, and kidney, thus explaining the lipid storage myopathy and cardiomyopathy. Oral L-carnitine supplementation causes dramatic improvement in cardiac function [16].

Systemic carnitine deficiency was first described in 1975 and thought to represent a defect in the *de novo* biosynthesis of carnitine [8]. However, no defect has been documented. Patients with systemic carnitine deficiency have a generalized decrease in the tissue and plasma concentrations of carnitine and an excessive urinary excretion of carnitine. Many of the patients originally reported to have systemic carnitine deficiency have been reinvestigated and found to have a primary enzyme defect such as medium-chain acyl CoA dehydrogenase deficiency (MCAD). This deficiency is the prototype of a defect in β-oxidation that produces secondary carnitine deficiency. β-Oxidation defects also are associated with dicarboxylic aciduria. This finding is particularly prominent during a metabolic crisis and may be rather inconspicuous between attacks. The differential diagnosis of systemic carnitine deficiency and dicarboxylic aciduria includes other defects of β-oxidation such as deficiencies of the long-chain isoform of acyl CoA dehydrogenase (LCAD), the short-chain isoform of acyl CoA dehydrogenase (SCAD), electron transfer flavoprotein (ETF), and ETF oxidoreductase [3], the long- and short-chain isoforms of 3-hydroxyacyl CoA dehydrogenase (LCHAD, SCHAD), β-ketothiolase, and the newly described trifunctional enzyme protein that includes the catalytic activities of enoyl hydratase, LCHAD, and β-ketothiolase. Cardiac involvement is particularly prominent in those conditions that involve the metabolism of long-chain fatty acids. Other genetically determined biochemical defects involving organic acid metabolism and respiratory chain function may produce secondary carnitine deficiency. Carnitine deficiency also may result from acquired diseases such as chronic renal failure treated by hemodialysis, renal Fanconi's syndrome, chronic hepatic disease with cirrhosis and cachexia, kwashiorkor, and total parenteral nutrition in premature infants [8]. The mechanisms of carnitine depletion in these diverse conditions include excessive renal loss and excessive accumulation of acyl CoA thioesters. These potentially toxic compounds are esterified to acyl carnitines and excreted in the urine, resulting in an excessive loss of carnitine.

The genetically determined defect of membrane carnitine transport is the only known condition that fulfills the criteria for primary carnitine deficiency [16,17]. This condition, like the other conditions involving the carnitine cycle, is not associated with dicarboxylic aciduria. It is transmitted as an autosomal recessive trait and produces a life-threatening cardiomyopathy in infancy or early childhood that is effectively treated with carnitine supplementation. The untreated patient also manifests systemic features of hypotonia, failure to thrive, and alterations of consciousness, including coma. The carnitine concentrations are extremely low in plasma and body tissues, and the excretion of carnitine in the urine is extremely high. The excessive urinary carnitine losses are the result of a defect in renal tubular uptake of filtered carnitine resulting from the primary defect of the plasma membrane carnitine transporter. This condition can be documented by carnitine uptake studies in cultured skin fibroblasts from patients. Uptake studies in parents give intermediate values consistent with a heterozygote state.

One patient has been described with a defect involving the carnitine-acylcarnitine translocase system that facilitates the movement of long-chain acyl-carnitine esters across the inner membrane of the mitochondrion (Fig. 2). This patient had extremely low carnitine concentrations and minimal dicarboxylic aciduria. Investigation of cultured skin fibroblasts from the parents revealed intermediate values, suggesting that this condition is transmitted as an autosomal recessive trait [17].

The carnitine concentrations are normal to high in patients with a primary defect of carnitine palmitoyl transferase, type 1 (CPT 1). Patients with CPT 2 have normal carnitine concentrations. Two clinical syndromes have emerged in relationship to CPT 2. The more common syndrome, as discussed previously, involves recurrent myoglobinuria provoked by fasting or intercurrent infection and later is associated with fixed limb weakness. The less common syndrome involves infants and produces hypoketotic hypoglycemic coma with a Reye-like clinical signature. All cases thought to be recurrent Reye's syndrome should be investigated for defects involving fatty acid oxidation. Low serum carnitine concentrations and increased urinary dicarboxylic acids implicate a biochemical defect of β-oxidation. Low serum carnitine concentrations and normal urinary dicarboxylic acids implicate a defect of the membrane carnitine transporter or the mitochondrial inner membrane carnitine-acylcarnitine translocase system. Normal to high serum carnitine concentrations and no dicarboxylic aciduria suggests a defect of CPT 1 or CPT 2.

Oral administration of L-carnitine is life saving in patients with the genetically determined defect of plasma membrane carnitine transporter [16]. It also is recommended as a supplement in all patients who have documented carnitine deficiency even though clear evidence of benefit is lacking. Medium-chain triglyceride supplementation has proven beneficial in CPT 1 deficiency and should be beneficial also in the other defects of the carnitine cycle. Medium-chain fatty acids cross the plasma membrane and the mitochondrial membranes directly and are esterified to the thioesters in the mitochondrial matrix (see Fig. 2). A ketonemic response to medium-chain triglycerides documents the biological integrity of β-oxidation and implicates a biochemical defect of the carnitine cycle or of β-oxidation involving the metabolism of the longer chain fatty acids.

Pathophysiology of symptoms

Of the nine glycolytic enzyme defects described above, six affect glycogen breakdown or glycolysis (phosphorylase, debrancher, PFK, PGK, PGAM, LDH deficiencies). The impairment of energy production from carbohydrate, which is the common consequence of these defects, should result in similar, exercise-related signs and symptoms [12]. Except for debrancher deficiency, this is the case. Patients with phosphorylase, PFK, PGK, PGAM, or LDH deficiency have exercise intolerance manifested by premature fatigue, cramps, and myoglobinuria. As predicted by the crucial role of glycogen as a fuel source, patients are more prone to experience cramps and myoglobinuria when they engage in isometric exercise, such as lifting weights, or in intense dynamic exercise, such as walking uphill. Energy for these types of exercises derives mainly from anaerobic or aerobic glycolysis. The block of glycogen utilization leads to a shortage of pyruvate and, therefore, of acetyl CoA (Fig. 3), the pivotal substrate of the Krebs cycle, and to a decreased mitochondrial energy output. Moderate exercise typically causes premature fatigue and myalgia, but these symptoms usually resolve after brief rest or slowing of pace; thereafter, patients find that they can resume or continue exercise without problems. This second-wind phenomenon seems to be due to early mobilization of fatty acids

and to increased blood flow to exercising muscles.

Conversely, patients with fatty acid oxidation defects experience myalgia and myoglobinuria after prolonged, though not necessarily high-intensity, exercise. Fasting exacerbates these complaints. Thus, myoglobinuria occurs in CPT deficiency under metabolic conditions that favor oxidation of fatty acids in normal muscle [3,12,15,17]. This observation suggests that impaired cellular energetics are the common cause of myoglobinuria in diverse metabolic myopathies. However, biochemical proof of energy depletion is still necessary. No abnormal decrease of ATP concentration has yet been measured in muscle of patients with McArdle's disease during fatigue (defined as failure to maintain the required or expected force) or during ischemic exercise-induced contracture. It cannot be excluded, however, that contracture (and necrosis) may involve only a relatively small percentage of fibers. Measurements of ATP and phosphocreatine in whole muscle might fail to detect loss of high-energy phosphate compounds in selected fibers. Additionally, ATP deficiency may affect a specific subcellular compartment.

The cause of weakness is also poorly understood. Chronic impairment of energy provision is unlikely because two of the three glycogenoses causing weakness involve a glycogen-synthesizing enzyme (branching enzyme deficiency) and a lysosomal glycogenolytic enzyme (acid maltase deficiency), neither directly involved in energy production [12].

A more likely explanation is that weakness may be due to a net loss of muscle fibers because regeneration cannot keep pace with the rate of degeneration. With fewer functioning fibers, the muscle cannot exert full force. Electromyography reinforces this interpretation: Motor unit potentials are of smaller amplitude and briefer duration than normal, due to loss of muscle fibers from a motor unit. Fibrillations are attributed to areas of focal necrosis of muscle fiber, isolat-

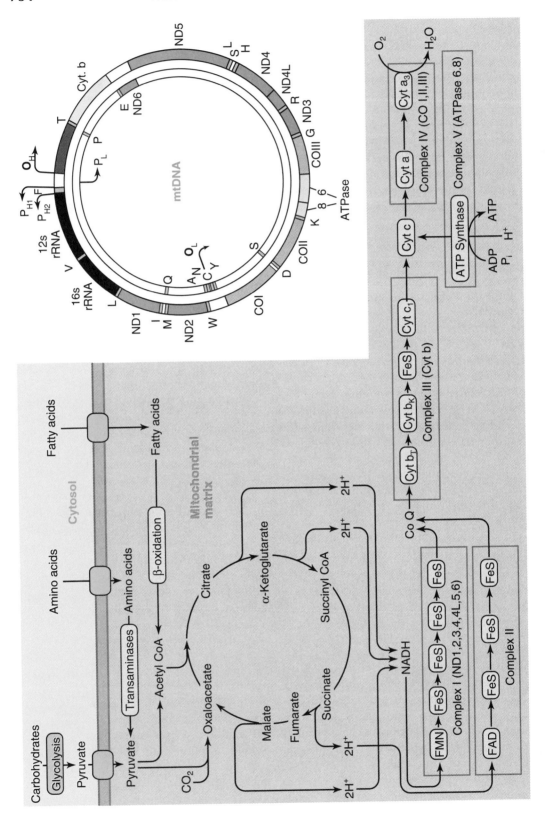

ing areas of the cell from the neuromuscular junction in a form of "microdenervation." Muscle fiber degeneration may be due to excessive storage of glycogen, as in acid maltase and debrancher enzyme deficiency, or lipid droplets, as in carnitine deficiency. In agreement with this hypothesis is the observation that in at least two of the glycogenoses causing weakness, infantile acid maltase deficiency and debrancher enzyme deficiency, glycogen storage is much more severe than in the glycogenoses causing cramps and myoglobinuria. Similarly, lipid storage is much more severe in carnitine deficiency than in CPT deficiency [12].

An additional cause of weakness may be involvement of the anterior horn cells of the spinal cord, which is very conspicuous in infantile acid maltase deficiency. All three glycogenoses causing weakness are in fact due to generalized enzyme defects, but histological signs of denervation are not evident.

DISEASES OF CARBOHYDRATE AND FATTY ACID METABOLISM IN BRAIN

The concentration of glycogen in the brain is small, approximately 0.1 g/100 g fresh tissue, compared with 1.0 g/100 g in muscle and 6 to 10 g/100 g in liver. The functional significance of glycogen in the brain is not completely understood, but it is generally assumed that it represents available energy to be tapped during glucose depletion; however, the limited glycogen reserve renders the brain vulnerable to injury within minutes of onset of hypoglycemia or hypoxia [7].

The role of fatty acids as oxidizable fuels for brain metabolism is negligible, but ketone bodies, derived from fatty acid oxidation, can be utilized, particularly in the neonatal period. Diseases of carbohydrate and fatty acid metabolism may affect the brain directly or indirectly [1,7].

Defective transport of glucose across the blood-brain barrier

Glucose Transporter Protein (GLUT 1) Deficiency

Glucose crosses the blood-brain barrier by a mechanism of facilitated diffusion (Chap. 3 and 32). This stereospecific system has a relatively high K_m for glucose (approximately 6 mM). Normally, the transport of glucose across the blood-brain barrier is not rate-limiting for cerebral metabolism. Recently, two patients were reported with a defect involving the GLUT 1 carrier protein [2]. The clinical presentation was infantile-onset seizures and developmental delay. One patient had deceleration of head growth with resulting microcephaly. The metabolic signature of this condition is a persistent hypoglycorrhachia with low-normal or low cerebral spinal fluid lactate values. The patients responded to a ketogenic diet that was implemented to provide ketone bodies as an alternative fuel source for cerebral metabolism [1,2]. The GLUT 1 protein also is present in erythrocyte membranes. Decreased binding of cytochalasin B was documented in both cases, and decreased uptake of 3-O-methylglucose by freshly isolated erythrocytes was documented in one case. The molecular basis for this newly described condition and

FIG. 3. Scheme of mitochondrial metabolism showing substrate transport, the Krebs cycle, and the respiratory chain. One molecule of mitochondrial DNA (mtDNA) is inserted on the *right*. The 13 structural proteins encoded by mtDNA are located in complexes I, III, IV, and V as indicated in the parentheses. (NADH) nicotinamide adenine dinucleotide, reduced; (FMN) flavin mononucleotide; (FAD) flavin adenine dinucleotide; (FeS) nonheme iron-sulfur protein; (CoQ) coenzyme Q (ubiquinone); (P$_i$) inorganic phosphate. The schematic representation of mtDNA shows the location of the specific tRNA genes *(one-letter code)*. (O$_H$ and O$_L$) origins of replication of the heavy *(external circle)* and light *(internal circle)* strands; PH$_1$, PH$_2$, P$_L$) promoters of transcription; (12S and 16S) ribosomal RNA genes; (ND1–ND6) genes encoding subunits 1 to 6 of NADH-coenzyme Q oxidoreductase (complex I); (COI–COIII) genes encoding subunits I to III of cytochrome *c* oxidase (complex IV); (cyt *b*) cytochrome *b*.

the genetic pattern of inheritance are not known. These patients may be misdiagnosed as examples of cerebral palsy, suspected hypoglycemia, or sudden infant death syndrome.

Diseases With Enzyme Defects Found in Brain

Acid Maltase Deficiency.   Light microscopic studies of the nervous system show large amounts of glycogen in the perikaryon of glial cells in both gray and white matter, whereas cortical neurons contain much smaller quantities of glycogen. In the spinal cord, the neurons of the anterior horn appear ballooned and contain abundant PAS-positive material that is digested by diastase (glycogen). Schwann cells of both anterior and posterior spinal roots and of peripheral nerves also contain excessive glycogen. By electron microscopy, the most striking feature is the presence of glycogen granules within membrane-bound vacuoles. These glycogen-laden vacuoles are particularly abundant in anterior horn cells, in neurons of brainstem motor nuclei, and in Schwann cells, whereas they are scarce in cortical neurons. Glycogen is increased in postmortem brain, and acid maltase activity is undetectable. The severe involvement of spinal and brainstem motor neurons and the massive accumulation of glycogen in muscle contribute to the profound hypotonia, weakness, and hyporeflexia seen in Pompe's disease [7].

Debrancher Enzyme Deficiency.   As mentioned above, the debrancher enzyme defect appears to be generalized. Accordingly, although neither pathology nor debrancher enzyme activity has been reported, increased glycogen concentration has been observed in the brain of a patient. Thus, in debrancher enzyme deficiency, the nervous system seems to be involved biochemically, although clinical signs of brain dysfunction are limited to hypoglycemic seizures in childhood [7].

Branching Enzyme Deficiency.   The branching enzyme also seems to exist as a single molecu-

lar form, and, accordingly, the enzyme defect has been described in multiple tissues, including the brain, from one patient. Although signs and symptoms of brain dysfunction are not prominent in brancher enzyme deficiency, deposits of abnormal polysaccharide, in the form of PAS-positive spheroids, were seen in subpial and perivascular zones of the brainstem and spinal cord but never within neurons. Electron microscopy showed that the spheroids were composed of branched osmiophilic filaments, 600 nm in diameter, and were located within distended astrocytic processes.

Phosphoglycerate Kinase Deficiency.   The most common clinical presentation of phosphoglycerate kinase (PGK) deficiency includes nonspherocytic hemolytic anemia and central nervous system dysfunction. Neurological problems vary in severity. All patients show some degree of mental retardation with delayed language acquisition and behavioral abnormalities, and some have hemiplegia or seizures. The enzyme defect has been directly proved in the brain, and the severe brain involvement can be explained by impairment of the glycolytic pathway. The lack of symptoms of brain dysfunction in some patients with PGK deficiency (e.g., the two patients with recurrent myoglobinuria described above) are probably attributable to the presence of sufficient residual enzyme activity to prevent severe energy shortage.

Lafora and Other Polyglucosan Storage Diseases

In Lafora disease and other polyglucosan storage diseases, there is accumulation of an abnormal glucose polymer resembling amylopectin (polyglucosan) in the central and peripheral nervous systems as well as in other tissues, but the biochemical defect(s) remain unknown [7].

Lafora disease is transmitted as an autosomal recessive trait and is characterized by epilepsy, myoclonus, and dementia. Other neurological manifestations include ataxia, dysarthria, spasticity, and rigidity. Onset is in adolescence, and death occurs in most patients before 25 years of age.

The pathological hallmark of the disease is the presence in the brain of Lafora bodies: round, basophilic, PAS-positive intracellular inclusions varying in size from small "dust-like" bodies less than 3 nm in diameter to large bodies up to 30 nm in diameter. Lafora bodies are typically seen in neuronal perikarya and processes, not in glial cells, and are more abundant in cerebral cortex, substantia nigra, thalamus, globus pallidus, and dentate nucleus. Ultrastructural studies have shown that Lafora bodies consist of two components: amorphous electron-dense granules and irregular branched filaments.

Although the storage material is histochemically and biochemically similar to the polysaccharide that accumulates in branching enzyme deficiency, brancher enzyme activity was normal in brain and muscle from one patient. A different form of polyglucosan body disease was described in patients with a characteristic neurological syndrome consisting of progressive upper and lower motorneuron involvement, sensory loss, neurogenic bladder, and, in one-half of the patients, dementia without myoclonus or epilepsy. Onset is in the fifth or sixth decade, and the course varies between 3 and 30 years. Polyglucosan bodies are disseminated throughout the central and peripheral nervous systems in processes of neurons and astrocytes but not in perikarya. Other tissues are also affected, including liver, heart, and skeletal and smooth muscle. In Ashkenazi Jewish patients with this disorder (but not in patients of different ethnic origins), branching enzyme activity is decreased in leukocytes, peripheral nerve, and, presumably, brain, but is normal in muscle [5]. The molecular basis for the differences in organs affected and clinical course between "typical" branching enzyme deficiency (see above) and polyglucosan body disease remains to be explained. The observation that branching deficiency in polyglucosan body disease is confined to Ashkenazi Jewish patients suggests that this disorder is biochemically heterogeneous.

Systemic metabolic diseases affecting the brain

Hypoglycemia may produce lethargy, coma, seizures, and brain damage in gluconeogenic and glycogen synthetase deficiencies [9].

Glucose-6-Phosphatase Deficiency (Glycogenosis Type I; Von Gierke's Disease)

Glucose-6-phosphatase deficiency results in hypoglycemia and excessive intracellular accumulation of glucose-6-phosphate (Fig. 1). As a result, there is formation of lactic acid, uric acid, and lipids. A second form of the disease (type Ib) has been described. The defect in this form involves the glucose-6-phosphate translocation system that is important in facilitating the movement of the substrate into the microsomal compartment for enzymatic conversion to glucose by glucose-6-phosphatase. The clinical features of type Ia and Ib are similar, but normal enzyme activity is present in type Ib. Hepatomegaly, bleeding diathesis, and neutropenia are present. The neurological signs result from the chronic hypoglycemia. Recent studies indicate that lactate may be used by the brain as an alternative cerebral metabolic fuel when hypoglycemia is associated with lactic acidosis. Nocturnal intragastric feeding and frequent daytime meals ameliorate most of the clinical and metabolic abnormalities of this condition.

Fructose-1,6-Bisphosphatase Deficiency

First described by Baker and Winegrad in 1970, fructose-1,6-bisphosphatase deficiency has now been reported in approximately 30 cases. It is more common in females and is inherited as an autosomal recessive disorder. Initial manifestations are not strikingly dissimilar from those of glucose-6-phosphatase deficiency. Neonatal hypoglycemia is a common presenting feature associated with profound metabolic acidosis, irritability or coma, apneic spells, dyspnea, tachycardia, hypotonia, and moderate hepatomegaly. Lactate, alanine, uric acid, and ketone bodies are elevated in the blood and urine [9]. The enzyme is deficient in liver, kidney, jejunum, and leukocytes. Muscle fructose-1,6-bisphosphatase activity is normal.

Fructose-1,6-bisphosphatase is an important rate-limiting step in gluconeogenesis. This gluconeogenic step antagonizes the opposite reaction that forms fructose-1,6-bisphosphate from fructose-6-phosphate and ATP (see Chap. 31). A futile cycle exists between these two enzymes, one forming fructose-1,6-bisphosphate and the other disposing of this substrate. Hers and associates have shown that small amounts of fructose-2,6-bisphosphate also are formed by the PFK reaction. This metabolite stimulates the PFK reaction and inhibits the fructose-1,6-bisphosphatase reaction. This finding nicely explains the subtle interplay between the key rate-limiting step in glycolysis (PFK) and the rate-limiting step in gluconeogenesis catalyzed by fructose-1,6-bisphosphatase.

Phosphoenolpyruvate Carboxykinase Deficiency

Distinctly rare and even more devastating clinically than deficiencies of glucose-6-phosphatase or fructose-1,6-bisphosphatase, phosphoenolpyruvate carboxykinase (PEPCK) activity is almost equally distributed between a cytosolic form and a mitochondrial form. These two forms have similar molecular weights but differ by their kinetic and immunochemical properties. The cytosolic activity is responsive to fasting and various hormonal stimuli. Hypoglycemia is severe and intractable in the absence of PEPCK [9]. A young child with cytosolic PEPCK deficiency had severe cerebral atrophy, optic atrophy, and fatty infiltration of liver and kidney.

Pyruvate Carboxylase Deficiency

Pyruvate carboxylase (PC) deficiency has been documented in 35 cases [19]. This enzyme, mitochondrial in location, catalyzes the conversion of pyruvate to oxaloacetate and is biotin dependent (Chaps. 35, 39). The first report of PC deficiency involved an infant with subacute necrotizing encephalomyelopathy, or Leigh's syndrome. Subsequent reports have failed to confirm this causal relationship between PC deficiency and the neuropathological features of Leigh syndrome. Leigh syndrome has now been assigned to several other biochemical defects, including pyruvate dehydrogenase deficiency, cytochrome oxidase deficiency, biotinidase deficiency, and defects involving complex I and complex V of the respiratory chain.

Most patients with PC deficiency present with failure to thrive, developmental delay, recurrent seizures, and metabolic acidosis. Lactate, pyruvate, alanine, β-hydroxybutyrate, and acetoacetate concentrations are elevated in blood and urine. Hypoglycemia is not a consistent finding despite the fact that PC is the first rate-limiting step in gluconeogenesis.

Sixteen patients had an associated hyperammonemia, citrullinemia, and hyperlysinemia. This presentation is the most malignant, with death in early infancy. This French phenotype is commonly associated with the absence of any immunological cross-reacting material (CRM) corresponding to the PC apoenzyme protein.

The North American phenotype is associated with the presence of CRM. Possibly as a result, the clinical presentation is less devastating in early infancy, although the outcome is almost invariably fatal in later infancy or early childhood. These patients do not have the associated abnormalities of ammonia metabolism, and the serum aspartic acid concentrations are not as severely depleted. Only one patient has been described with the North American phenotype and a benign clinical syndrome. She has had recurrent episodes of metabolic acidosis requiring hospitalization. Otherwise, her growth and neurological development have been normal.

Prenatal and postnatal diagnoses can be made by enzyme assay of cultured amniocytes, fibroblasts, or white blood cells. Treatment remains symptomatic. Sodium bicarbonate is necessary to correct the acidosis. Aspartic acid supplementation will improve the systemic condition but has no effect on the neurological disturbances. Biotin supplementation is of no value.

Biotin-Dependent Syndromes

Infants may present with developmental delay and may demonstrate laboratory abnormalities resulting from the deficiencies of the four biotin-dependent carboxylases (see Chap. 39). Three of the carboxylases, located in the mitochondria, are involved in organic acid metabolism. Multiple carboxylase deficiency, when present in the newborn period, is the result of a deficiency of holocarboxylase synthetase, the enzyme that catalyzes the binding of biotin to the apocarboxylase. These infants often die shortly after birth. Older infants gradually develop neurological signs, with developmental delay and seizures associated with alopecia, rash, and immunodeficiency. There is a deficiency of biotinidase, the enzyme responsible for the breakdown of biocytin, the lysyl derivative of biotin, to free biotin. Biotinidase deficiency can be recognized at birth by measuring the serum activity. Biotinidase deficiency occurs in 1:41,000 live births, and it is eminently treatable by the oral administration of biotin.

Glycogen Synthetase Deficiency

Glycogen synthetase deficiency has been described in three families. It caused stunted growth and severe fasting hypoglycemia with ketonuria. Mental retardation was reported in the three children who survived past infancy. The liver was virtually devoid of glycogen and showed fatty degeneration in all cases. In two patients, the brain showed diffuse, nonspecific changes in the white matter (presence of reactive astrocytes and increased microglia), which were considered secondary to prolonged hypoglycemia or anoxia. Biochemical studies showed that glycogen synthetase activity was markedly decreased in liver but normal in muscle,

erythrocytes, and leukocytes, suggesting the existence of multiple tissue-specific isoenzymes under separate genetic control. It is not known whether brain glycogen synthetase is different from that in liver.

In *liver phosphorylase deficiency* (glycogenosis type VI; Hers disease; Fig. 1) and in two genetic forms of *phosphorylase kinase deficiency* (one X-linked recessive, the other autosomal recessive), hypoglycemia is either absent or mild. Symptoms of brain dysfunction do not usually occur (type VIII, Fig. 1) [7].

Fatty Acid Oxidation Defects

These metabolic defects often produce recurrent disturbances of brain function. Drowsiness, stupor, and coma occur during acute metabolic crises and mimic the Reye's syndrome phenotype. The neurological symptoms have been attributed to hypoglycemia, hypoketonemia, and the deleterious effects of potentially toxic organic acids. The hypoglycemia results from a continuing demand for glucose by brain and other organs resulting from the primary biochemical defect of fatty acid oxidation (Fig. 2). Avoidance of catabolic circumstances that require the utilization of fatty acids is the basic principle of treatment. L-carnitine supplementation is recommended for all conditions associated with generalized carnitine deficiency. Some patients may benefit from medium-chain triglyceride supplementation, as discussed previously. Certain forms of ETF-oxidoreductase deficiency respond to riboflavin supplementation. The riboflavin-responsive multiple acyl CoA dehydrogenase deficiency represents the milder form of glutaric aciduria type II.

DISEASES OF MITOCHONDRIAL METABOLISM

Mitochondrial dysfunction produces syndromes involving muscle and central nervous system

Although some energy can be quickly obtained from glucose or glycogen through anaerobic glycolysis, most of the energy derives from the oxidation of carbohydrates and fatty acids in the mitochondria. The common metabolic product of sugars and fats is acetyl CoA, which enters the Krebs cycle. Oxidation of one molecule of acetyl CoA results in the reduction of three molecules of NAD and one of FAD. These reducing equivalents flow down a chain of carriers (Fig. 3) through a series of oxidation-reduction events. The final hydrogen acceptor is molecular oxygen, and the product is water. The released energy "charges" the inner mitochondrial membrane, converting the mitochondrion into a veritable biological battery. This oxidation process is coupled to ATP synthesis from ADP and inorganic phosphate (P_i), catalyzed by mitochondrial ATPase [18]. Considering the enormous amount of information collected since 1960 on mitochondrial structure and function, it is surprising that diseases of terminal mitochondrial metabolism (Krebs cycle and respiratory chain) have attracted the attention of clinical investigators only recently [4,6,10,14,21].

Initial clues that some diseases might be due to mitochondrial dysfunction come from electron microscopic studies of muscle biopsies showing fibers with increased numbers of structurally normal or abnormal mitochondria. These fibers have a "ragged red" appearance in the modified Gomori trichrome stain. Because the diagnosis was based on mitochondrial changes in muscle biopsies, these disorders were initially labeled mitochondrial myopathies. It soon became apparent, however, that many mitochondrial diseases with ragged red fibers were not confined to skeletal muscle but were multisystem disorders. In these patients, the clinical picture is often dominated by signs and symptoms of muscle and brain dysfunction, probably due to the great dependence of these tissues on oxidative metabolism. This group of disorders, often called mitochondrial encephalomyopathies, includes three distinctive syndromes (Table 1) [11].

The first, Kearns-Sayre syndrome (KSS), is characterized by childhood onset of progressive external ophthalmoplegia and pigmentary degeneration of the retina. Heart block, cerebellar syndrome, or high cerebrospinal fluid protein may also appear. Almost all cases are sporadic. The second syndrome, myoclonus epilepsy with ragged red fibers (MERRF), is characterized by myoclonus, ataxia, weakness, and generalized seizures. The third syndrome, mitochondrial myopathy, encephalopathy, lactic acidosis, and stroke-like episodes (MELAS), affects young children, who show stunted growth, episodic vomiting and headaches, seizures, and recurrent cerebral insults resembling strokes and causing hemiparesis, hemianopsia, or cortical blindness. Unlike KSS, MERRF and MELAS are usually familial, and analysis of several pedigrees has documented non-Mendelian maternal inheritance [11].

Inheritance of mitochondrial DNA is from the ovum

What makes mitochondrial diseases particularly interesting from a genetic point of view is that the mitochondrion has its own DNA (mtDNA) and its own transcription and translation processes (see Chap. 23). The mtDNA encodes only 13 polypeptides; nuclear DNA (nDNA) controls the synthesis of 90 to 95 percent of all mitochondrial proteins. All known mitochondrially encoded polypeptides are located in the inner mitochondrial membrane as subunits of the respiratory chain complexes (Fig. 3), including seven subunits of complex I, the apoprotein of cytochrome *b*, the three larger subunits of cytochrome *c* oxidase (complex IV), and two subunits of ATPase (complex V).

In the formation of the zygote, almost all the mitochondria are contributed by the ovum. Therefore, mtDNA is transmitted by material inheritance in a vertical, non-Mendelian fashion. Strictly maternal transmission of mtDNA has been documented in humans by studies of restriction-fragment-

TABLE 1:   (KSS) Kearns-Sayre syndrome; (MERRF) myoclonus epilepsy with ragged red fibers; (MELAS) mitochondrial encephalomyopathy, lactic acidosis, and stroke-like episodes; (CSF) cerebrospinal fluid; boxes highlight differential features (see text).

Distinguishing Features of Mitochondrial Encephalomyopathies

Cinical Features	KSS	MERRF	MELAS
ophthalmoplegia	+	−	−
retinal degeneration	+	−	−
heart block	+	−	−
CSF protein > 100 mg/dl	+	−	−
myoclonus	−	+	−
ataxia	+	+	−
weakness	+	+	+
episodic vomiting	−	−	+
cerebral blindness	−	−	+
hemiparesis, hemianopsia	−	−	+
seizures	−	+	+
dementia	+	+	+
short stature	+	+	+
sensorineural hearing loss	+	+	+
lactic acidosis	+	+	+
family history	−	+	+
ragged red fibers	+	+	+
spongy degeneration	+	+	+
mtDNA deletion	+	−	−
mtDNA point mutation	−	tRNA^{lys}	tRNA$^{leu(UUR)}$

length polymorphisms (RFLPs) in DNA from platelets. In theory, diseases caused by mutations of mtDNA should also be transmitted by maternal inheritance: An affected mother ought to pass the disease to all her children (were it not for the "threshold effect"; see later), but only her daughters would transmit the trait to subsequent generations [4,6,14,21]. Characteristics that distinguish maternal from Mendelian inheritance include the following:

1. The number of affected individuals in subsequent generations should be higher (again, were it not for the "threshold effect") than in autosomal dominant disease.

2. Inheritance is maternal as in X-linked diseases, but children of both sexes are affected.

3. Because there are hundreds or thousands of copies of mtDNA in each cell, the phenotypic expression of a mitochondrially encoded gene depends on the relative proportions of mutant and wild-type mtDNAs within a cell ("threshold effect").

4. Because mitochondria replicate more

often than do nuclei, the relative proportion of mutant and wild-type mtDNAs may change within a cell cycle.

5. At the time of cell division, the proportion of mutant and wild-type mtDNAs in the two daughter cells can shift, thus giving them different genotypes and, possibly, different phenotypes, a phenomenon called mitotic segregation.

Maternal inheritance has been documented in diseases due to point mutations of mtDNA, while most diseases due to mtDNA deletions or duplications are sporadic.

Classification of mitochondrial diseases

Two major classifications of mitochondrial diseases have been proposed. One is based on genetics and the other on biochemistry [6]. The genetic classification divides mitochondrial diseases into three groups.

1. Defects of mtDNA, which include point mutations and deletions or duplications. From a biochemical point of view, these disorders will be associated with dysfunction of the respiratory chain because all 13 subunits encoded by mtDNA are subunits of respiratory chain complexes. Diseases due to *point mutations* are transmitted by maternal inheritance, and the number has rapidly increased during the past few years. The main syndromes include MERRF; MELAS (Table 1); Leber's hereditary optic neuropathy (LHON), a disorder causing blindness in young adult males; and NARP (neurogenic atrophy, ataxia, and retinitis pigmentosa), which, depending on the relative proportion of mutant mitochondrial genomes in tissues, can cause a multisystem disorder in young adults or a devastating encephalomyopathy of childhood (Leigh's syndrome). Diseases due to *deletions or duplications* are usually sporadic, for reasons that are not completely clear. They include, besides KSS (Table 1), isolated

progressive external ophthalmoplegia, and Pearson's syndrome, a usually fatal infantile disorder dominated by sideroblastic anemia and exocrine pancreas dysfunction.

2. Defects of nuclear DNA. As mentioned above, the vast majority of mitochondrial proteins are encoded by nDNA, synthesized in the cytoplasm, and "imported" (through a complex series of steps) into the mitochondria. Defects of genes encoding the proteins themselves or controlling the importation machinery will cause mitochondrial diseases, which will be transmitted by Mendelian inheritance. From a biochemical point of view, all areas of mitochondrial metabolism can be affected (see discussion of biochemical classification, below).

3. Defects of communication between nDNA and mtDNA. The nDNA controls many functions of the mtDNA, including its replication. It is, therefore, conceivable that mutations of nuclear genes controlling these functions could cause alterations in the mtDNA. Two human diseases have been attributed to this mechanism [6]. The first is associated with *multiple mtDNA deletions* and is characterized clinically by ophthalmoplegia, weakness of limb and respiratory muscles, and early death. Transmission is usually autosomal dominant, and it is assumed that a mutation in a nuclear gene makes the mtDNA prone to develop deletions. The second disease is associated with *mtDNA depletion* in one or more tissues, more commonly in muscle. Depending on the tissue affected and the severity of the mtDNA decrease, the clinical picture can be a rapidly fatal congenital myopathy, a slightly more benign myopathy of childhood, or a fatal hepatopathy. Transmission appears to be autosomal recessive or dominant, and it is postulated that a nDNA mutation may impair mtDNA replication. As expected, all subunits encoded by

mtDNA are markedly decreased in the affected tissues.

The *biochemical classification* is based on the five major steps of mitochondrial metabolism illustrated in Fig. 3 and, accordingly, divides mitochondrial diseases into five groups:

1. Defects of mitochondrial transport
2. Defects of substrate utilization
3. Defects of the Krebs cycle
4. Defects of oxidation/phosphorylation coupling
5. Defects of the respiratory chain

All disorders except those in group 5 are due to defects of nDNA and are transmitted by Mendelian inheritance. Disorders of the respiratory chain can be due to defects of nDNA, mtDNA, or to defects of intergenomic communication. Usually, mutations of nDNA cause isolated severe defects of individual respiratory complexes, whereas mutations in mtDNA or defects of intergenomic communication cause variably severe multiple deficiencies of respiratory chain complexes. The description that follows is based on the biochemical classification.

Defects of mitochondrial transport

Movement of molecules across the inner mitochondrial membrane is tightly regulated by specific translocation systems. The carnitine cycle is shown in Fig. 2 and is responsible for the translocation of acyl CoA thioesters from the cytosol into the mitochondrial matrix. The carnitine cycle involves four elements: the plasma membrane carnitine transporter system, CPT I, the carnitine-acyl carnitine translocase system in the inner mitochondrial membrane, and CPT II. Genetic defects have been described for each of these four steps, as have been discussed previously [8,16,17].

Defects of substrate utilization

Alterations of pyruvate metabolism may be due to defects of pyruvate carboxylase, as discussed earlier, or the pyruvate dehydrogenase complex (PDHC).

Pyruvate Dehydrogenase Deficiency

Over 100 patients have been described with a disturbance of the pyruvate dehydrogenase complex. The clinical picture includes several phenotypes ranging from a severe, devastating metabolic disease in the neonatal period to a benign recurrent syndrome in older children. There is considerable overlap clinically and biochemically with other disorders (see later).

The PDHC catalyzes the irreversible conversion of pyruvate to acetyl CoA (Fig. 3) and is dependent on thiamine and lipoic acid as cofactors (see Chap. 35). The complex has five enzymes: three subserving a catalytic function and two a regulatory role. The catalytic components include pyruvate dehydrogenase, E_1; dihydrolipoyl transacetylase, E_2; and dihydrolipoyl dehydrogenase, E_3. The two regulatory enzymes include PDH-specific kinase and phospho-PDH–specific phosphatase. The multienzyme complex contains nine protein subunits, including protein X. Protein X serves to anchor the E_3 component to the E_2 core of the complex. The E_1 α-subunit is encoded by a gene on the short arm of the X-chromosome and a gene on chromosome 4. The E_1 β-subunit is encoded by a gene on chromosome 3, and the E_3 component is encoded by a gene on chromosome 7. Biochemical defects have been documented for the E_1 α-subunit, E_2 (one case), E_3, protein X (two cases), and the phospho-PDH–specific phosphatase. The great majority of cases involve a mutation defect of the E_1 α-subunit. Most of these patients are males, reflecting the location of the E_1 α-subunit gene on the X chromosome.

The most devastating phenotype of PDH deficiency presents in the newborn period. The majority of patients are males who are critically ill with a severe metabolic acidosis. There is an elevated blood or cerebrospinal fluid lactate concentration and associated elevations of pyruvate and alanine. These patients have seizures, failure to thrive, optic atrophy, microcephaly, and dysmorphic features. Multiple brain abnormalities have been described, including dysmyelination of the cortex, cystic degeneration of the basal ganglia, ectopic olivary nuclei, hydrocephalus, and partial or complete agenesis of the corpus callosum. A less devastating phenotype presents in early infancy. These patients demonstrate the histopathological features of Leigh's disease. Other patients affected in infancy survive with a chronic neurodegenerative syndrome manifested by mental retardation, microcephaly, recurrent seizures, spasticity, ataxia, and dystonia.

Mutations involving the E_1 α-subunit behave clinically like an X-linked dominant condition. These mutations usually are lethal in the males during early infancy. The clinical spectrum in the heterozygous female is more varied, ranging from a devastating condition in early infancy to a mild chronic encephalopathy with mental retardation. The least symptomatic females may give birth to affected male and female progeny and pose a significant problem in clinical diagnosis and genetic counseling.

Treatment is largely symptomatic, and the prognosis ranges from dismal to guarded. Thiamine, lipoic acid, ketogenic diet, and physostigmine have been tried in different concentrations and doses with equivocal results. Some patients with periodic ataxia resulting from PDHC deficiency may respond to acetazolamide.

Fatty Acid Oxidation Defects

Defects of β-oxidation may affect muscle exclusively or in conjunction with other tissues.

Glutaric Aciduria Type II. Glutaric aciduria type II (multiple acyl CoA dehydrogenase deficiency; Fig. 2) usually causes respiratory distress, hypoglycemia, hyperammonemia, systemic carnitine deficiency, nonketotic metabolic acidosis in the neonatal period, and death within the first week. A few patients with onset in childhood or adult life showed lipid storage myopathy, with weakness or premature fatigue [3,16,17].

Short-Chain Acyl CoA Deficiency. Short-chain acyl CoA deficiency (Fig. 2) was described in one woman with proximal limb weakness and exercise intolerance. Muscle biopsy showed marked accumulation of lipid droplets. Although no other tissues were studied, the defect appeared to be confined to skeletal muscle, suggesting the existence of tissue-specific isozymes [17].

Defects of the Krebs cycle

Fumarase deficiency was reported in three children with mitochondrial encephalomyopathy. Two of them had developmental delay since early infancy, microcephaly, hypotonia, cerebral atrophy; one died at 8 months of age. The third patient was a 3.5-year-old mentally retarded girl. The laboratory hallmark of the disease is the excretion of large amounts of fumaric acid and, to a lesser extent, succinic acid in the urine. The enzyme defect has been found in muscle, liver, and cultured skin fibroblasts [6].

Defects of oxidation-phosphorylation coupling

The best example of a disorder of oxidation-phosphorylation coupling is Luft's disease, or nonthyroidal hypermetabolism. Only two patients with this condition have been reported. Family history was noncontributory in either case. Symptoms started in childhood or early adolescence with fever, heat intolerance, profuse perspiration, resting tachypnea and dyspnea, polydipsia, polyphagia, and mild weakness. The basal metabolic rate was markedly increased in both patients, but all tests of thyroid function were normal. Muscle biopsies showed ragged-red fibers and proliferation of capillaries. Other tissues were morphologically normal. Studies of oxidative phosphorylation in isolated muscle mitochondria from both patients showed maximal respiratory rate even in the absence of ADP, an indication that respiratory control was lost. Respiration proceeded at a high rate independently of phosphorylation, and energy was lost as heat, causing hypermetabolism and hyperthermia [6].

Abnormalities of the respiratory chain

Identification of the different biochemical blocks in the respiratory chain is usually based on polarographic studies showing differential impairment in the ability of isolated intact mitochondria to use different substrates. For example, defective respiration with NAD-dependent substrates, such as pyruvate and malate, but normal respiration with FAD-dependent substrates, such as succinate, suggests an isolated defect of complex I (Fig. 3). However, defective respiration with both types of substrates in the presence of normal cytochrome c oxidase (complex IV) activity localizes the lesions to complex III (Fig. 3).

Polarographic studies can be complemented by measurement of reduced-minus-oxidized spectra of cytochromes, showing decreased amounts of reducible cytochromes a and a_3 in patients with complex IV deficiency, and decreased concentration of reducible cytochrome b in many (but not all) patients with complex III deficiency (Fig. 3). Finally, electron transport through discrete portions of the respiratory chain can be measured directly. Thus, an isolated defect of NADH–cytochrome c reductase activity suggests a problem within complex I, while a simultaneous defect of NADH and succinate–cytochrome c reductase activities points to a biochemical error in complex III (Fig. 3). The function of complex III alone can be tested by measuring the activity of reduced coenzyme Q–cytochrome c reductase.

Defects of Complex I

Defects of complex I have been described in about 25 patients and seem to cause two major clinical syndromes: pure myopathy, with exercise intolerance and myalgia presenting in childhood or adult life; and multisystem disorder. Patients with multisystem disorder are not clinically homogeneous: Some had a fatal infantile form of the disease, causing severe congenital lactic acidosis, hypotonia, seizures, respiratory insufficiency, and death before age 3 months. Others had a less severe encephalomyopathy with onset in childhood or adult life and characterized by the association, in various proportions, of the following signs and symptoms: exercise intolerance, weakness, ophthalmoplegia, pigmentary retinopathy, optic atrophy, sensorineural hearing loss, dementia, cerebellar ataxia, and pyramidal signs [6,10,14]. This clinical heterogeneity is hardly surprising when one considers the large number of proteins comprising complex I, but the molecular defect in most patients is not known (Fig. 3).

Defects of Complex II

In the few reported patients with complex II deficiency, the biochemical defect has not been fully characterized, and the diagnosis has often been based solely on a decrease of succinate–cytochrome c reductase activity (Fig. 3). The clinical picture is characterized by severe infantile myopathy, with lactic acidosis in two cases, and by encephalomyopathy in three cases [6].

Defects of Complex III

As in defects of complex I, the clinical picture of complex III disorders falls into one of two groups: (a) childhood- or adolescent-onset myopathy with or without involvement of extraocular muscles; (b) encephalopathy, with exercise intolerance, fixed weakness, pigmentary degeneration of the retina, sensorineural hearing loss, cerebellar ataxia, pyramidal signs, and dementia [6,10,14].

Biochemically, some patients show lack of reducible cytochrome b, whereas others have normal cytochrome spectra. In the patients with a normal amount of reducible cytochrome *b,* the defect may involve the non-heme iron sulfur protein (Rieske protein) or coenzyme Q (Fig. 3).

In a young woman with complex III deficiency myopathy, the bioenergetic capacity of muscle was studied by [^{31}P]nuclear magnetic resonance (NMR). The ratio of phosphocreatine to inorganic phosphate concentration (PC_r/P_i) was greatly reduced at rest, decreased further with mild exercise, and returned to pre-exercise values very slowly. Treatment with menadione (vitamin K_3) and ascorbate (vitamin C), two compounds whose redox potentials permit them to function between coenzyme Q and cytochrome *c* (Fig. 3), was associated with marked improvement of exercise capacity. NMR showed increased PC_r/P_i ratios at rest and improved rates of recovery after exercise.

Defects of Complex IV

As seen with defects of complexes I and III, the clinical phenotypes of complex IV (cytochrome oxidase [COX]) deficiency fall into two main groups: one in which myopathy is the predominant or exclusive manifestation, and another in which brain dysfunction predominates (Fig. 3). In the first group, the most common disorder is *fatal infantile myopathy,* causing generalized weakness, respiratory insufficiency, and death before age 1 year. There is lactic acidosis and renal dysfunction, with glycosuria, phosphaturia, and aminoaciduria (DeToni-Fanconi-Debre syndrome). The association of myopathy and cardiopathy in the same patient and myopathy and liver disease in the same family has also been described [6].

In patients with pure myopathy, COX deficiency is confined to skeletal muscle, sparing heart, liver, and brain. The amount of immunologically reactive enzyme protein is markedly decreased in muscle by enzyme-linked immunosorbent assay (ELISA) and by immunocytochemistry of frozen sections.

Benign infantile mitochondrial myopathy, in contrast, has been described in a few children with severe myopathy and lactic acido-sis at birth, who then improve spontaneously and are virtually normal by age 2 years. This condition is due to a reversible COX deficiency. The enzyme activity is markedly decreased ($<$19 percent of normal) in muscle biopsies taken soon after birth but returns to normal in the first year of life. Immunocytochemistry and immunotitration show normal amounts of enzyme protein in all muscle biopsies. This finding differs from the virtual lack of CRM in patients with fatal infantile myopathy and may represent a useful prognostic test. The selective involvement of one or more tissues and the reversibility of the muscle defect in the benign form suggest the existence of tissue-specific and developmentally regulated COX isoenzymes in humans [6].

Subacute necrotizing encephalomyelopathy (Leigh's disease) typifyes the second group of disorders of complex IV, dominated by involvement of the central nervous system. Leigh's disease usually starts in infancy or childhood and is characterized by psychomotor retardation, brainstem abnormalities, and apnea [20]. The pathological hallmark consists of focal, symmetrical necrotic lesions from thalamus to pons and involving the inferior olives and the posterior columns of the spinal cord. Microscopically, these spongy brain lesions show demyelination, vascular proliferation, and astrocytosis. In these patients, COX deficiency is generalized, including cultured fibroblasts in most (but not all) cases: This may provide a useful tool for prenatal diagnosis in at least some families. Immunological studies show presence of CRM in all tissues.

Partial defects of COX have been reported in patients with progressive external ophthalmoplegia and proximal myopathy and in patients with encephalomyopathy. However, the precise pathogenic significance of COX deficiency in these disorders remains uncertain.

Defects of Complex V (ATPase)

Two patients with muscle mitochondrial ATPase deficiency have been reported. One was a young woman with congenital, slowly progressive myopathy; the other was a 17-year-old boy who, at age 10 years, was found to have muscle carnitine deficiency [6]. Later he developed a multisystem disorder characterized by weakness, dementia, ataxia, retinopathy, and peripheral neuropathy. In both patients, respiration of isolated mitochondria was decreased with all substrates but returned to normal after addition of the uncoupling agent 1,4-dinitrophenol. This finding suggested that the biochemical defect involved the phosphorylative pathway rather than the respiratory chain. ATPase activity was decreased and responded poorly to dinitrophenol stimulation.

ACKNOWLEDGMENTS

Some of the work discussed in this chapter was supported by USPHS grants NS11766 and NS176965 from the National Institute of Neurological and Communicative Disorders and Stroke, a center grant from the Muscular Dystrophy Association, and a laboratory grant from the Colleen Giblin Foundation for Pediatric Neurology Research. We are grateful to Ms. Alice H. Marti for typing the manuscript.

REFERENCES

1. De Vivo, D. C. The effects of ketone bodies on glucose utilization. In J. V. Passonneau, R. A. Hawkins, W. D. Lust, and F. A. Welsh (eds.), *Cerebral Metabolism and Neural Function.* Baltimore: Williams & Wilkins, 1980, pp. 243–254.

2. De Vivo, D. C., Trifiletti, R. R., Jacobson, R. I., Ronen, G. M., Behmand, R. A., and Harik, S. I. Defective glucose transport across the blood-brain barrier as a cause of persistent hypoglycorrhachia, seizures, and developmental delay. *N. Engl. J. Med.* 325:703–709, 1991.

3. DiDonato, S., Frerman, F. E., Rimoldi, M., Rinaldo, P., Taroni, F., and Wiesmann, U. N.

Systemic carnitine deficiency due to lack of electron transfer flavoprotein: Ubiquinone oxidoreductase. *Neurology* 36:957–963, 1986.

4. DiMauro, S., Bonilla, E., Lombes, A., Shanske, S., Minetti, C., and Moraes, C. T. Mitochondrial encephalomyopathies. *Neurol. Clin.* 8:483–506, 1990.

5. DiMauro, S., and Servidei, S. Glycogen storage diseases. In R. N. Rosenberg, S. B. Prusiner, S. DiMauro, R. L. Barchi, and L. M. Kunkel (eds.), *The Molecular and Genetic Basis of Neurological Disease.* Stoneham, MA: Butterworth-Heinemann, 1992, pp. 93–119.

6. DiMauro, S. Mitochondrial encephalomyopathies. In R. N. Rosenberg, S. B. Prusiner, S. DiMauro, R. L. Barchi, and L. M. Kunkel (eds.), *The Molecular and Genetic Basis of Neurological Disease.* Stoneham, MA: Butterworth-Heinemann, 1992, pp. 665–694.

7. DiMauro, S., and De Vivo, D. C. Disorders of glycogen metabolism. In A. Lajtha (ed.), *Handbook of Neurochemistry.* New York: Plenum, 1985, Vol. 10, pp. 1–13.

8. Engel, A. G. Carnitine deficiency syndromes and lipid storage myopathies. In A. G. Engel and B. Q. Banker (eds.), *Myology.* New York: McGraw-Hill, 1986, pp. 1663–1696.

9. Haymond, M. W. Hypoglycemia. In A. M. Rudolph (ed.), *Pediatrics, 19th ed.* Norwalk, CT: Appleton & Lange, 1991, pp. 323–331.

10. Morgan-Hughes, J. A. The mitochondrial diseases. In F. L. Mastaglia and J. N. Walton (eds.), *Muscle Pathology.* Edinburgh: Churchill Livingstone, 1992, pp. 367–424.

11. Rowland, L. P., Blake, D. M., Hirano, M., DiMauro, S., Schon, E. A., Hays, A. P., and De Vivo, D. C. Clinical syndromes associated with ragged red fibers. *Rev. Neurol.* 147:467–473, 1991.

12. Rowland, L. P., Layzer, R. B., and DiMauro, S. Pathophysiology of metabolic muscle disorders. In A. K. Asbury, G. M. McKhann, and W. I. McDonald (eds.), *Diseases of the Nervous System.* Philadelphia: W. B. Saunders, 1986, pp. 197–207.

13. Schulz, H. Oxidation of fatty acids. In D. E. Vance and J. E. Vance (eds.), *Biochemistry of Lipids and Membranes.* Menlo Park, CA: Benjamin/Cummings, 1985, pp. 116–142.

14. Shoffner, J. M., and Wallace, D. C. Oxidative phosphorylation diseases: Disorders of two genomes. *Adv. Hum. Genet.* 19:267–330, 1990.

15. Tein, I., DiMauro, S., and De Vivo, D. C. Re-

current childhood myoglobinuria. In L. A. Barnes, D. C. De Vivo, G. Morrow, F. Oski, and A. M. Rudolph (eds.), *Advances in Pediatrics.* Chicago: Mosby Year Book, 1990, Vol. 37, pp. 77–119.

16. Treem, W. R., Stanley, C. A., Finegold, D. N., Hale, D. E., and Coates, P. W. Primary carnitine deficiency due to a failure of carnitine transport in kidney, muscle, and fibroblasts. *N. Engl. J. Med.* 319:1331–1336, 1988.

17. Jackson, S., and Turnbull, D. M. Lipid disorders of muscle. In R. N. Rosenberg, S. B. Prusiner, S. DiMauro, R. L. Barchi, and L. M. Kunkel (eds.), *The Molecular and Genetic Basis of Neurological Disease,* Boston: Butterworth-Heinemann, 1993, pp. 651–661.

18. Tzagoloff, A. *Mitochondria.* New York: Plenum, 1982.

19. Van Coster, R., Fernhoff, P. M., and De Vivo, D. C. Pyruvate carboxylase deficiency: A benign variant with normal development. *Pediatr. Res.* 30:1–4, 1991.

20. Van Coster, R., Lombes, A., De Vivo, D. C., Chi, T. L., Dodson, W. E., Rothman, S., Orrechio, E. J., Grover, W., Berry, G. T., Schwartz, J. F., Habib, A., and DiMauro, S. Cytochrome *c* oxidase-associated Leigh syndrome: Phenotypic features and pathogenetic speculations. *J. Neurol. Sci.* 104:97–111, 1991.

21. Wallace, D. C. Diseases of the mitochondrial DNA. *Annu. Rev. Biochem.* 61:1175–1212, 1992.

CHAPTER 35

Vitamin and Nutritional Deficiencies

John P. Blass

That diet affects health has been known since Hippocrates. However, chemical characterization of the major foodstuffs, including the vitamins and other micronutrients, occurred only during the last century. The minimum daily requirements needed to prevent nutritional disorders were defined primarily in healthy young male volunteers. These studies led to such public health triumphs as the erradication of pellagra (see below). Current research in this area includes the effects on nutritional requirements of genetic variations and of environmental stresses, including intercurrent diseases (see also Chaps. 38 and 39).

MACRONUTRIENTS

Macronutrients comprise the quantitatively major portions of the diet: carbohydrates, proteins, fats, and water.

Basic Neurochemistry: Molecular, Cellular, and Medical Aspects, 5th Ed., edited by G. J. Siegel et al. Published by Raven Press, Ltd., New York, 1994. Correspondence to John P. Blass, Department of Neurology, Cornell University Medical College, White Plains, New York 10605.

Protein-calorie malnutrition does not reduce brain/body weight ratios

Even severe deprivation of calories and protein during adult life is widely believed to have few, if any, lasting effects on brain function in survivors. During development, calorie restriction clearly reduces brain size and body size, but brain/body ratios typically increase [1]. The body appears to spare nutrients for development of the brain. Decrease in brain substance may represent in part lack of glia (which typically develop postnatally in the rat) and adaptation to a smaller number of motor units. In laboratory animals, effects of nutritional deprivation on performance appear to relate to motivational and attentional factors at least as much as to diminution in cognitive capacities.

In humans, nutrition during development correlates directly with body size, but there is no evidence that tall people are significantly more intelligent than short ones, within the same gene pool. Children malnourished as a result of specific gastrointestinal disease are often small but are rarely mentally deficient. An approximation of a direct experiment in humans occurred in the Netherlands in 1944, when the Dutch population under the Axis powers starved while that under the Allies was well fed [2]. In the cohort born during that period under Axis occupation, there was a small reduction in height but none in intellectual performance. The incidence of personality problems may have increased slightly. Epidemiological studies of the effects of longer term malnutrition are hard to assess mechanistically because of confounding variables related to poverty.

Moderate caloric restriction during growth and development actually prolongs the lives of laboratory animals [3]. Because the conditions under which rodents and other laboratory animals are reared in captivity are artificial, the effect of restricted calories may result in the prevention of malignant obesity. Optimal nutrition during development is not the same as maximal nutrition.

Dietary variations can alter brain levels of neurotransmitter precursors

Tryptophan

Tryptophan is an obligatory precursor of 5-hydroxytryptamine (serotonin; see Chap. 13). This amino acid also substitutes, inefficiently, for vitamin B_3 (see below). Tryptophan is present in relatively small amounts in most proteins. It crosses the blood-brain barrier, like tyrosine, predominantly by the carrier system for long-chain neutral amino acids (see Chap. 32). As a result, a protein-rich meal can actually reduce the passage of tryptophan into the brain by elevating the levels of other amino acids competing for that carrier. Therapeutically, pure tryptophan has been reported to be useful in treating subgroups of patients with depression, sleeplessness, or hyperactive behaviors. These subgroups have not been characterized by other independent criteria. An outbreak of a neuromuscular disorder associated with large doses of tryptophan appears to have been due to a chemical contaminant in the commercial preparations.

Tyrosine

Tyrosine or its precursor phenylalanine are obligatory precursors of dopamine and norepinephrine (see Chap. 12). Both amino acids are present in relatively large amounts in proteins. Tyrosine has been proposed for the treatment of depression and to damp stress-induced oscillations in blood pressure.

Choline

In mammals, choline synthesis requires a dietary source of one-carbon groups (see Chap. 5). Blood levels of choline normally reflect the amount of choline ingested. Lecithin is an efficient dietary precursor of choline (see Chap. 5). In nutrition, the term lecithin is used for at least two different materials. One is phosphatidylcholine. The other is a mixture of phospholipids, often extracted from soybeans, in which phosphatidylcholine is a component. Increasing dietary lecithin can increase levels of choline in the brain and under restricted circumstances can increase release of acetylcholine.

Carnitine participates in mitochondrial reactions

Carnitine, like choline, can be synthesized by mammals if dietary sources of one-carbon groups are adequate (see Chap. 5). It participates in the transfer of acyl groups across mitochondrial membranes. These include acetyl groups for acetylcholine synthesis. Both carnitine and acetylcarnitine enter the nervous system, but the more lipid-soluble acetyl-L-carnitine has been described as having a variety of effects on the nervous system in experimental animals not seen with carnitine.

Hereditary deficits in the ability to transport carnitine or to synthesize its acyl derivatives have been associated with diseases of skeletal and cardiac muscle and more variably with metabolic encephalopathy (see Chap. 34). Secondary deficiency of carnitine has been described in a number of disorders of mitochondrial oxidation, due in part to the detoxification and urinary excretion of potentially damaging short chain acids as the carnitine derivatives [4]. The anticonvulsant valproic acid can increase carnitine requirements in susceptible individuals [5]. Treatment with acetylcarnitine has been reported to slow the progression of Alzheimer's disease [6].

Essential fatty acid deficiency may not damage the brain

In laboratory animals, diets devoid of essential fatty acids (ω-3 or ω-6 linoleic acid) induce dermatitis without prominent disorder of the nervous system. A syndrome of essential fatty acid deficiency has not been convincingly demonstrated in humans.

MICRONUTRIENTS

Micronutrients are chemicals that must be present in the diet of mammals in small amounts to maintain health. They include vitamins and some minerals. Characterization of each micronutrient has required recognition of a syndrome associated with a deficiency of that nutrient in humans or in laboratory animals in which a model disorder, often neurological, could be standardized as a bioassay system [7].

Thiamine (vitamin B_1) is involved in several neurological disorders

At the turn of the century, brown husks from polished rice were found to cure the neurological syndrome of beri-beri in both birds and humans [7]. Funk introduced the term vitamine when he recognized that the vital factor was an amine.

Biochemistry

Thiamine contains a pyrimidine linked to a thiazole moiety. The biologically active forms are phosphorylated derivatives. The pyrophosphate (TPP) acts as a coenzyme for four enzymes in the nervous system (see Chaps. 31,34). Three are intramitochondrial multienzyme complexes that catalyze the oxidative decarboxylation of α-ketoacids to their respective coenzyme A (CoA) derivatives:

1. Pyruvate to acyl CoA: pyruvate dehydrogenase complex (PDHC)
2. α-Ketoglutarate to succinyl CoA: α-ketoglutarate dehydrogenase complex (KGDHC)
3. α-Ketoacids derived from the branched-chain amino acids into C − 1 CoA derivatives: branched-chain dehydrogenase complex (BCDHC)

These three dehydrogenase complexes share a common enzyme component, namely, lipoamide dehydrogenase. PDHC, which produces acyl CoA used in acetylcholine synthesis, appears to be found in particularly high concentrations in cholinergic neurons. The fourth TPP-requiring enzyme in the brain is transketolase (TK), which carries out rearrangements of sugars (see Chap. 31). A kinase can convert a membrane-bound form of TPP to thiamine triphosphate (TTP), and a specific phosphatase hydrolyzes TTP to the diphosphate. TTP appears to play a role in nerve membrane function, notably in Na⁺ gating. The cDNAs for a number of TPP-requiring enzymes have been obtained, and a TPP-binding motif has been proposed that is partially conserved in yeast, rat, and human (Fig. 1).

Experimental Thiamine Deficiency

Several animal models of thiamine deficiency have been characterized. Thiamine-deficient weakness in chickens and opisthotonic posturing in deficient pigeons were used in the first bioassays. In thiamine-deficient cats, the earliest ultrastructural changes occur in synapses including synaptic mitochondria; dramatic changes in glia follow. Mink develop a thiamine-deficiency syndrome if fed raw fish, which contain a thiaminase; cerebrocortical necrosis in calves is due to dietary thiamine deficiency.

Extensive studies of thiamine deficiency have been done in rats and mice. Dietary thiamine deficiency is now conventionally induced with artificial diets complete in all foodstuffs except thiamine. Since the vitamin deficiency induces loss of appetite, each

control must be "pair fed" the same (weighed) amount that a deficient animal consumes to allow for the general effects of decreased nutrition. Weanling rodents fed a diet devoid of thiamine usually stop gaining weight after about 2 weeks and die after 4 to 5 weeks.

Experimentally, thiamine deficiency is now more frequently induced by the combination of a thiamine-deficient diet and a thiamine antagonist, either pyrithiamine or oxythiamine. However, pyrithiamine can directly inhibit action potentials, and oxythiamine does not enter the brain efficiently. In the pyrithiamine model in mice, abnormal neuropsychological responses develop within five to seven days, gross neurological abnormalities in eight to nine days, and death usually by ten to eleven days. Strain (i.e., genetics) significantly modifies the response to experimental thiamine deficiency in mice (Fig. 2). In rats, abnormalities of motor performance occur by day three, additional neurological symptoms by day twelve, and death within two weeks.

The rodent models exhibit selective vulnerability, i.e., histological changes are relatively localized (see below and Chaps. 40, 42). Biochemical changes are greatest in regions destined to show histological changes. Early neurochemical changes include increases in glucose utilization and lactate pro-

```
Hum  TK     KASYRVYCLLGDGELSEGSVWEAMAFASIYKLDNLGAILDINRLGQSDPAP
Hum  E1k    LLHGDA*AFAGQGIV*YETFH*LSDL*PSYTTHGTVHVVVNNQIGFT*TDP
Hum  E1αp   GKDEVCLTLYGDGAANQGQIFEAYNMAALWKL*PCIFICENNY*GMGTSVE
Hum  E1αb   NANRVVICYFGEGAASEGDAHDGFNFAATLEC*PIIFFCRNN**GYAISTP
Rat  E1αb   NANQIVICYFGEGAASEGDAHAGFNFAATLEC*PIIFFCRNN**GYAISTP
Sac  TK     LSDNYTYVFLGDGCLQEGISSEASSLAGHLKLGNLIAIYDDNKITIDGATS
Sac  E1k    LLHGDA*AFAGQGVV*YETM*GFLTL*PEYSTGGTIHVITNNQIGFT*TDP
Sac  PDC    DPKKRVILFIGDGSL*QLTVQEISTMIRWGLK*PY*LFVLNND*GYTIEKL
```

FIG. 1. Proposed thiamine-binding motif. (Hum) human; (Sac) yeast; (TK) transkelotase; (E1k) the E1 component of KGDHC; (E1αp) the α-peptide of the E1 component of PDHC; (E1αb) the α-peptide of the E1 component of the branched-chain dehydrogenase complex; (PDC) pyruvate decarboxylase. Note the conservation of both a positively charged residue (N) and of a negatively charged residue (D or E) flanked by two G. (Sequence of Hum TK from unpublished studies by Drs. Eun-Hee Jung and K-F.R. Sheu. For references, see Hawkins, C.F., Borges, A., Perham, R.N. A common structural motif in thiamine pyrophosphate-binding enzymes. *FEBS Lett.* 255:77–82, 1989.)

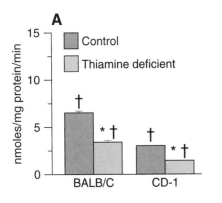 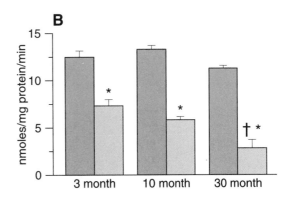

* Denotes a significant effect of thiamine deficiency.
† Denotes a significant effect between strains.

* Denotes a significant effect of thiamine deficiency.
† Denotes a significant effect of aging.

FIG. 2.   Strain and age differences in response to thiamine deficiency in mice. **A:** Transketolase activity in the brains of thiamine-deficient and pair-fed control Balb/C and CD-1 mice. **B:** KGDHC activity in the brains of thiamine-deficient and pair-fed control Balb/C mice of different ages. (Data derived from Freeman et al. [22].)

duction, local decreases in pH, and local increases in intracellular Ca^{2+}. In late stages, decreases in oxidation of glucose can be detected in affected regions in *ex vivo* or *in vivo* studies. Levels of ATP and adenylate energy charge potential (energy charge potential is $[\{ATP\} + \frac{1}{2}\{ADP\}]/[\{ATP\} + \{ADP\} + \{AMP\}]$; see Chap. 40) are maintained until very late stages. In affected areas, blood flow rises, but in animals successfully treated with thiamine it falls below normal.

In experimental thiamine deficiency in rodents, the activities of KGDHC, TK, and perhaps PDHC fall [8]. BCDHC has not been measured directly. Levels of TTP are maintained even in terminal stages. The decrease in KGDHC activity parallels the decrease in glucose oxidation. The fall in TK persists even after successful treatment of symptomatic thiamine deficiency. In rodent models, decreases in PDHC do not seem to occur in preparations in which PDHC is solublized (i.e., mitochondria are lysed), except perhaps in the brainstem of rats with dietary thiamine deficiency [9].

Neuropharmacology

Cholinergic systems are exquisitely sensitive to thiamine deficiency, as they are to other conditions that impair carbohydrate oxidation, perhaps due to alterations in Ca^{2+} release [8]. Deficits in performance in the early stages of thiamine deficiency can be normalized by treatment with central cholinergic agonists. Serotonergic systems, including uptake mechanisms, are impaired in at least the later stages. Catecholaminergic functions are also impaired, as measured physiologically. The levels of glutamate and aspartate decrease, at least in the later stages, whereas decreases in GABA have been more variable.

Human Thiamine Deficiency Diseases

In developed countries, clinically significant thiamine deficiency is rare except as a complication of severe alcoholism or other disorders impairing nutrition [10]. It is more common in developing countries where polished rice is the staple grain. The "TPP effect" is the percentage increase in red cell TK activity on adding exogenous TPP *in vitro* and has been widely used in epidemiological studies of thiamine nutriture.

After five to six days of a diet deficient only in thiamine, healthy young men developed a nonspecific syndrome of lassitude, irritability, muscle cramps, and electrocardiographic changes, which was cured by dietary thiamine.

More prolonged thiamine deficiency frequently leads to damage to peripheral nerves (see Chap. 36). This neuropathy tends to be worse distally than proximally, involves myelin more than axons, and is often painful. The neuropathy may be linked to deficiencies in multiple water-soluble vitamins known for historical reasons as the vitamin B complex.

The Wernicke-Korsakoff syndrome consists of an acute (Wernicke) phase and a chronic (Korsakoff) phase [10]. The acute syndrome consists of staggering gait, paralysis of eye movements, and confusion, associated with small hemorrhages along the third and fourth ventricles and with reduced cerebral metabolic rate as measured by cerebral blood flow. Injections of thiamine can be lifesaving, with clinical improvement often evident within minutes. It is believed that prompt treatment with thiamine can prevent the chronic Korsakoff phase. In Korsakoff's syndrome, a striking loss of working memory accompanies relatively little loss of reference memory (see Chap. 50). Affected patients characteristically make up stories in response to leading questions (confabulate). In this phase, patients do not respond to thiamine treatment. The neuropathological lesions responsible for Korsakoff's syndrome have been debated; recent studies report severe damage to the cholinergic neurones of the nucleus basalis complex.

Thiamine Requirements

Thiamine requirements can be altered genetically or environmentally. Among genetic disorders, thiamine-dependent maple-syrup-urine disease is due to a reduced affinity of BCDHC for TPP (see Chap. 39). A rare form of lactate acidosis is due to reduced affinity of PDHC for TPP (see Chap. 34). Both disorders respond to treatment with very large doses of thiamine. Wernicke-Korsakoff syndrome is associated with a variant form of TK having a decreased affinity for TPP [10].

This variation, which may be more common in chronic alcoholics, put them at risk on a deficient diet. Subacute necrotizing encephalomyelopathy (SNE) of Leigh is an uncommon, autosomal recessive disorder in which the neuropathology resembles Wernicke-Korsakoff syndrome. The role of thiamine in this disorder has been controversial, but patients with SNE have been described in whom a defect in PDHC has been documented at the cDNA level.

Environmentally, a number of dietary constituents are known that impair the absorption of thiamine, including ethanol. Severe illness or injury also has been reported to increase thiamine requirements. Rare patients are intolerant of thiamine, particularly in very large doses.

Niacin (vitamin B_3) is the treatment for pellagra

The deficiency disease pellgra, which includes mental symptoms, was recognized in the eighteenth century, shortly after the introduction of American corn (maize) into Europe [7,11].

Biochemistry

Niacin and niacinamide refer to nicotinic acid and its amide. Although these pyrimidine derivatives can be synthesized from tryptophan in mammals, perhaps at least in part by intestinal bacteria, 60 mg of dietary tryptophan are required to synthesize 1 mg of the vitamin. Niacin is a vitamin because most human diets do not contain enough tryptophan to fulfill the normal human requirement of 10 to 30 mg/day. Brain and other tissues incorporate nicotinic acid into the coenzymes NAD^+, NADH, $NADP^+$, and NADPH. These cofactors participate in multiple oxidation-reduction reactions (see Chap. 31). Cerebral tissues contain an active enzyme that hydrolyzes NAD^+ and $NADP^+$ but not NADH or NADPH. This enzyme, which is inhibited by niacin/niacinamide, may play a role in metabolic regulation.

Experimental Niacin Deficiency

Antiniacin compounds can induce deficiency disorders within days in rodents on an otherwise normal diet [11]. Brain converts 6-aminonicotinamide to the enzymatically inactive NADP analog and N-acetylpyridine to inactive analogs of NAD and NADP. Experimental niacin deficiency has been reported to reduce the levels of NAD and NADP coenzymes in brain by 30 percent or more, with a higher proportion of NAD in the oxidized form and a higher percentage of NADP in the reduced form. Changes in apoenzymes are variable, but may be particularly marked on enzymes of the pentose phosphate pathway. Niacin deficiency, like thiamine deficiency, is a model for selective vulnerability; the inferior olivary nuclei are particularly susceptible to the actions of 3-acetylpyridine, histologically and biochemically.

Neuropharmacology

N-Acetylpyridine poisoning can cause relatively localized decreases in the synthesis of acetylcholine in the brainstem [11].

Human Niacin Deficiency Diseases

A diet high in corn predisposes to niacin deficiency, since the major storage protein of American corn (zein) has relatively little tryptophan relative to other amino acids that compete for the same carrier. Addition of purified niacin to the diet has largely abolished pellagra, which was once a common disease in areas where corn was a dietary staple. Pellagra is associated with the tetrad of dermatitis (particularly in sun-exposed areas), diarrhea, dementia, and death. A chronic toxic delerium which can resemble schizophrenia may be the only clinical abnormality, at least early in the course.

Niacin Requirements

Dietary requirements for niacin, like those for thiamine, can be modified by both genetic and environmental factors. Hartnup's syndrome is a hereditary disorder in which tryptophan transport is impaired and requirements for dietary niacin increase. Phenylketonuria and hyperphenylalaninemia can increase niacin requirements by increasing the levels of amino acids that compete with tryptophan for transport systems (see Chap. 39). As noted above, the proportion of corn in the diet influences the requirement for niacin. Poisoning with vacor, a niacin antagonist, can induce widespread and persistant neurological dysfunction.

Pyridoxine (vitamin B_6) deficiency can induce seizures

Pyridoxine is a vitamin for which deficiency disorders and toxicity affecting the nervous system have been reported.

Biochemistry

Pyridoxine is a pyridine derivative that can exist as an alcohol, amine, or aldehyde. The concentration in brain is normally about 100-fold that in the blood. The active coenzyme is the phosphorylated derivative pyridoxal phosphate, which readily forms Schiff bases. This coenzyme participates in decarboxylation reactions, including those that form the neurotransmitters GABA from glutamate, serotonin (5-hydroxytryptamine) from 5-hydroxytryptophan, and probably DOPA from dihydroxyphenylalanine. It is also involved in transaminations including that converting α-ketoglutarate to glutamate. The conversion of tryptophan to nicotinamide requires pyridoxine as a cofactor, and the excretion of xanthurenic acid after a tryptophan load is widely used to test the adequacy of pyridoxine nutriture.

Experimental Pyridoxine Deficiency

Pyridoxine deficiency states have been induced in at least 12 mammalian species. Newborn animals are more sensitive to the dietary deficiency than are weanlings. Pups born to a rat deficient in pyridoxine show neuropathological damage including impaired synaptogenesis and hypomyelination.

A number of pyridoxine antagonists have been well characterized, including deoxypyridoxine and several hydrazides that can produce deficiency states.

Pyridoxine deficiency reduces cerebral metabolic rate. The activity of decarboxylases falls more than that of transaminases. Glutamic acid decarboxylase activity (GAD) falls by as much as 70 percent.

Rats and dogs fed pyridoxine-deficient diets first develop impairment in learning and conditioning. Irritability, seizures, and gait imbalance (ataxia) then develop, as well as anemia. The intensity of the seizures correlates with the extent of the fall in GAD activity. The ataxia may relate to the demonstrated demyelination in long tracts and peripheral nerves. Antagonists induce more widespread disturbances that nevertheless respond completely to treatment with pyridoxine.

Human Diseases Related to Pyridoxine

Pure pyridoxine deficiency has occurred in human infants fed a formula from which vitamin B_6 had been inadvertently omitted. The prominent finding was intractable seizures, which responded promptly to injections of the vitamin. Deficiency of pyridoxine can contribute to the polyneuropathy of B-complex deficiency. However, *very large* doses of pure pyridoxine can themselves lead to a persistant sensory neuropathy [12].

Pyridoxine Requirements

Like those of other nutrients, pyridoxine requirements can be altered by genetic or environmental factors and are increased in a number of disorders of the nervous system [7,13,14]. Doses of pyridoxine several hundredfold the normal daily requirement prevent the seizures. Maintenance with doses at least tenfold the normal requirement typically permits normal development if irreversible brain damage has not occurred. It has been suggested that mild forms of pyridoxine dependency may be a relatively common cause of intractable seizures and mental retardation, but neurochemical studies of these patients are limited. In one who came to autopsy, there was a diminished ratio of GABA to glutamate, but GAD activity was comparable to that of controls [13]. In another, cerebral metabolic rate for oxygen was reduced approximately 25 percent below normal even during seizures and was restored to normal with B_6 treatment [14]. In homocystinuria and cystothioninuria, two disorders of amino acid metabolism, some patients respond to large doses of pyridoxine. In those patients, the mutations appear to reduce the affinity of the relevant enzymes for the cofactor (see Chap. 39).

Environmentally, hydrazides and oximes can increase pyridoxine requirements. Large doses of pyridoxine are routinely given with the antituberculous medication isonicotinic hydrazide to prevent drug-induced neuropathy.

Biotin is involved in carboxylation reactions

Biotin is a derivative of fused imidazole and thiophene rings [15]. The enzyme holocarboxylase synthetase links biotin covalently onto specific lysine residues of the proteins for which it acts as a coenzyme. Those enzymes carry out carboxylation reactions, including methylmalonyl CoA from propionic acid (propionyl CoA carboxylase), malonyl CoA from acyl CoA (acyl CoA carboxylase), and oxaloacetic acid from pyruvic acid (pyruvate carboxylase). The pyruvate carboxylase reaction is involved in gluconeogenesis in the periphery and in priming the tricarboxylic acid cycle in the brain and other tissues.

Pure dietary deficiency of biotin is unknown, presumably because the intestinal flora of both humans and laboratory animals synthesizes the small amounts required.

Genetic defects in biotin metabolism sometimes respond to large doses of the vitamin [15]. Defects include a form of lactic acidosis, due to deficiency of pyruvate carboxylase; a form of propionic aciduria, due to an anbornamilty in propionyl carboxylase; and a form of multiple carboxylase deficiency, due to a mutation in the holocarboxylase synthetase (see Chap. 34). A child with a proposed defect in intestinal absorption of biotin has also been described.

Addition to the diet of very large amounts of undenatured forms of the egg white protein, avidin, which avidly binds biotin, induces a biotin-responsive syndrome experimentally and clinically. Humans complain of malaise, without prominent neurological signs.

Cobalamin (vitamin B₁₂) deficiency is associated with relatively common neurological syndromes

Biochemistry

The cobalamins are a series of porphyrin-like compounds [16]. The active forms contain a cobalt ion linked to one of the methylene groups. The cobalamins are synthesized by many microorganisms but not by higher plants or animals. The usual dietary source is meat, particularly liver. Effective absorption requires a series of transport proteins, including a glycoprotein *intrinsic* factor secreted by gastric parietal cells. Conversion to the active coenzymes adenosylcobalamin and methylcobalamin requires at least two reductase reactions and an adenosyltransferase step. The reductases are flavoproteins that require NAD^+ as a cofactor. Thus, B_{12} metabolism involves at least three vitamins: B_{12} itself, B_3, and riboflavin. Stores of cobalamins in humans are normally large enough to maintain health for over 2 years without effective absorption from the diet.

Cobalamins have two well-established biochemical functions. Adenosylcobalamin is the cofactor for the mutase that converts methylmalonyl CoA to succinyl CoA (see Chap. 39, Fig. 1, reaction 12). This reaction is part of the pathway of metabolism of propionic acid, which itself derives from the metabolism of odd-chain fatty acids and from certain amino acids.

Methylcobalamin is the cofactor for the methyltransferase that converts homocysteine to the amino acid methionine. This reaction is important in folate metabolism as well. Its impairment appears to foster folate deficiency by an accumulation of N^5-methyltetrahydrofolate in a "folate trap." Deficiency of either cobalamins or folate or of both can restrict the supply of metabolically available one-carbon groups for pathways including those of nucleic acid synthesis.

Experimental Cobalamin Deficiency

Experimental deficiency of cobalamin has been difficult to induce [17]. Poisoning with nitrous oxide or cycloleucine can produce conditions resembling the human disorder. Pigs with dietary deficiency provide another model.

Diseases in Humans

Cobalamin deficiencies are relatively common clinically [16]. Pure dietary deficiency responding promptly to treatment with oral cobalamins has been described in a few children of strict vegan mothers. A more common syndrome is caused by failure of absorption due to an inadequate supply of the glycoprotein intrinsic factor, usually on an autoimmune basis. The most characteristic abnormality is pernicious anemia characterized by abnormal leukocytes called megaloblasts. Neurological symptoms occur in most of these patients and can preceed the hematological changes [18].

Combined system disease is the most common neurological syndrome. These patients develop unpleasant tingling sensations (paresthesias), followed by loss of vibratory sensation particularly in the legs, and spastic weakness. The characteristic neuropathology is a spongy demyelination in the long tracts of the spinal cord, particularly prominent in the posterior columns. Combined system disease responds poorly to treatment with cobalamins.

Cobalamin deficiency is characteristically associated with severe malaise that does respond dramatically to treatment, even before the hematological response is evident. Relatively low serum levels of B_{12} have been reported in subgroups of psychiatric patients including patients with Alzheimer's disease, but responses to treatment with the vitamin have in general not been dramatic. Recent studies indicate that elevated levels of serum or cerebrospinal fluid methylmalonate can identify patients whose neuropsychiatric manifestations benefit from B_{12} treatment even though the levels of the vitamin in their serum are not in the deficient range [18].

Whether the damage to the nervous system relates to decreased activity of the methylmalonyl mutase or of the methyltransferase or of both remains unsettled. Increased excretion of methylmalonate has been reported to be a marker for patients whose neuropsychiatric manifestations improve with treatment with B_{12}, but clinically normal children with pure mutase deficiency are known. Children with homocystinuria and related disorders do not develop the clinical or pathological stigmata of combined system disease (see Chap. 39), and an infant with an apparent reduction in methyltransferase activity was clinically normal when reported at age 1 year. Patients with severe inherited deficiencies in the activites of both enzymes secondary to a defect in the metabolism of the cobalamins do develop profound disease of the nervous system, with some characteristics of combined system disease.

Cobalamin Requirements

As with other nutrients, requirements for cobalamin can be modified by genetic and environmental influences. Genetic factors apparently predispose to intrinsic factor deficiencies with resultant cobalamin deficiency. Furthermore, at least six different inherited methylmalonic acidurias have been described [16]: absence of the mutase; decreased affinity of the mutase for adenosylcobalamin; deficiency of mitochondrial cobalamin reductase; deficiency of a mitochondrial cobalamin adenyltransferase; and

two distinguishable defects associated with abnormal cytosolic metabolism of cobalamine (see Chap. 39). Environmental causes of increased cobalamin requirements include surgical removal of the stomach, excessive destruction of cobalamins in the gut by bacteria in a blind loop, or destruction by certain kinds of intestinal tape worm.

Abnormalities of other vitamins can also damage the nervous system

Folic Acid

Folic acid contains a pterin moiety linked to *para*-amino benzoic acid, which is linked to one or more glutamate residues [19]. It plays a key role in the transfer of one-carbon (active methylene) groups, including the conversion of serine to glycine and the cobalamin-dependent transfer from homocystein to methionine. Dietary deficiency of folate with normal cobalamin leads to anemia without significant neurological signs. On the other hand, both genetic and environmental disorders of folate metabolism have been associated with disease of the nervous system. Genetic defects in the enzyme reactions are discussed further in Chap. 39.

Genetic disorders of folate absorption, intraconversion, and utilization are rare [19]. They have occasionally been associated with phenocopies of well-known psychiatric syndromes. A boy with apparent deficiency of hepatic dihydrofolate reductase was treated with folate and developed a sociopathic personality in his teens. A folate-responsive form of mental retardation with catatonia has been described in an adolescent girl with $N^{5,10}$-methylenetetrahydrofolic acid reductase deficiency. Her younger sister was mentally impaired with "psychosis"; an unrelated boy with a defect of the same emzyme had seizures and proximal muscle weakness without notable pyschiatric problems. Most patients with glutamate formiminotransferase deficiency have had a syndrome of psychomotor retardation in infancy, but a few have been entirely normal clinically.

Environmentally, a number of common medications, including phenytoin and certain antitumor agents, increase requirements for dietary folate. Treatment with folate can mask the hematological signs of cobalamin deficiency without affecting the progressive damage to the nervous system.

Pantothenic Acid

Pantothenic acid is a substituted hydroxybutyric acid that is a constituent of CoA [20]. Experimental induction of pantothenic acid deficiency leads to signs of peripheral nerve damage—demyelination in laboratory animals and paresthesias in humans. Late signs of central nervous system damage in animals may relate as well to the adrenal failure that is a prominent part of the syndrome.

α-Tocopherol (Vitamin E)

α-Tocopherol is an isoprenoid linked to a double-ring system. Deficiency of this lipid-soluble vitamin is typically secondary to malabsorption of fats. The typical syndrome in humans is a spinocerebellar degeneration [21]. α-Tocopherol is an antioxidant. It and its derivatives have been widely tested to treat conditions in which active oxygen radicals are believed to form, including mitochondrial disorders and aging.

Ascorbic Acid (Vitamin C)

Ascorbic acid is an unsaturated sugar derivative that is a potent reducing agent [7]. The uptake of ascorbic acid into synaptosomes requires glucose and oxygen; uptake into the brain appears to be via the cerebrospinal fluid rather than the blood. Fatigue and emotional changes are common in the full-blown disease scurvy, but diffuse disease of the small blood vessels with small hemorrhages is much more striking.

CONCLUSIONS

Development and function of the brain depend on nutrients, both macronutrients and micronutrients. The major nutrients and their neurochemical functions appear to be largely known. The nervous system is a frequent although not invariable site of clinical predilection for nutritional disorders. Nutritional requirements can, as indicated in the discussion above, be modified by both genetic and environmental factors (Table 1). Defining optimal nutritional intake in relation to genetic and environmental variables is an area of current research.

ACKNOWLEDGMENTS

It is a pleasure to thank Dr. Gary Gibson and other co-workers of the Dementia Research Service for helpful comments. This work was supported in part by grants AG03857, AG09014, and AG08702 and by the Will Rogers Institute.

TABLE 1.   Types of nutritional syndromes affecting the nervous system

Type of syndrome	Definition	Applicable nutrients
Deficiency	Intake of specific nutrient inadequate to maintain health in the general population	Thiamine, niacin, pyridoxine, cobalamins
Dependency	Dramatic increase in requirements for *specific* nutrients due to *specific* genetic abnormalities	Thiamine, niacin, pyridoxine, biotin, cobalamins, folate, carnitine
Insufficiency	Increased requirements for *specific* nutrients due to *specific* genetic variations or to environmental factors (including intercurrent disease or medications)	Thiamine, niacin, pyridoxine, biotin, folate, cobalamins, carnitine

REFERENCES

1. Dobbing, J. S. Infant nutrition and later achievement. *Nutr. Rev.* 42:1–7, 1984.
2. Stein, Z., Susser, M., Saenger, G., and Marolla, G. *Famine and Human Development.* New York: Plenum, 1974.
3. Harrison, D. E., and Archer, J. R. Genetic differences in effects of food restriction on aging in mice. *J. Nutr.* 117:376–382, 1987.
4. Stumpf, D. A., Parker, W. D., and Angelini, C. Carnitine deficiency, organic acidemias, and Reyes syndrome. *Neurology* 35:1014–1045, 1985.
5. Triggs, W. J., Bohan, T. P., Lin, S. N., and Willmore, L. J. Valproate-induced coma with ketosis and carnitine insufficiency. *Arch. Neurol.* 47:1131–1133, 1990.
6. Spagnoli, A., Lucca, U., Menasce, G., Bandera, L., Cizza, G. et al. Long-term acetylcarnitine treatment in Alzheimer's disease. *Neurology* 41:1726–1732.
7. McIlwain, H., and Bachelard, H. S. Nutritional factors and the central nervous system. In *Biochemistry and the Central Nervous System.* 5th ed., London: Churchill Livingstone, 1985, pp. 244–281.
8. Sable, H. Z., and Gubler, C. J. (eds.), *Thiamin.* New York: New York Academy of Sciences, 1981.
9. Butterworth, R. F. Cerebral thiamine-dependent enzyme changes in experimental Wernicke's encephalopathy. *Metab. Brain Dis.* 1: 165–175, 1986.
10. Blass, J. P., and Gibson, G. E. Deleterious aberrations of a thiamine-requiring enzyme in four patients with Wernicke-Korsakoff syndrome. *N. Engl. J. Med.* 297:1367–1370, 1977.
11. Gibson, G. E., and Blass, J. P. Oxidative metabolism and acetylcholine synthesis during acetylpyridine treatment. *Neurochem. Res.* 10: 453–467, 1985.
12. Bendich, A., and Cohen, M. Vitamin B_6 safety issues. *Ann. N.Y. Acad. Sci.* 585:321–330, 1990.
13. Lott, I. B., Coulombe, T., DiPaolo, R. V., Richardson, E. P., and Levy, H. L. Vitamin B_6-dependent seizures: Pathology and chemical findings in brain. *Neurology* 28:47–54, 1978.
14. Sokoloff, L., Lassen, N. A., McKhann, G. M., Tower, D. B., and Albers, W. Effects of pyridoxine withdrawal on cerebral circulation and metabolism in a pyridoxine-dependent child. *Nature* 183:751–753.
15. Theone, J., Baker, H., Yoshino, M., and Seetman, L. Biotin-responsive carboxylase deficiency associated with subnormal plasma and urinary biotin. *N. Engl. J. Med.* 304:817–821, 1981.
16. Rosenberg, L. E. Disorders of propionate and methylmalonate metabolism. In J. B. Stanbury, J. B. Wyngaarden, D. S. Fredrickson, J. L. Goldstein, and M. S. Brown (eds.), *The Metabolic Basis of Inherited Disease, 5th ed.* New York: McGraw-Hill, 1976, pp. 474–497.
17. Hakim, A. M., Cooper, B. A., Rosenblatt, D. S., and Pappius, H. M. Local cerebral glucose utilization in two models of B_{12} deficiency. *J. Neurochem.* 40:1155–1160, 1987.
18. Lindenbaum, J., Healton, E. B., Savage, D. G., Brust, J. C., Garret, T. J., Podell, E. R., Marcell, P. D., Stabler, S. P., and Allen, R. H. Neuropsychiatric disorders caused by cobalamin deficiency in the absence of anemia or macrocytosis. *N. Engl. J. Med.* 318:1720–1728, 1988.
19. Erbe, R. W. Inborn errors of folate metabolism. *N. Engl. J. Med.* 293:753–757, 807–812, 1975.
20. Bean, W. B., and Hodges, R. E. Pantothenic acid deficiency induced in human subjects. *Proc. Soc. Exp. Biol. Med.* 86:693–698, 1954.
21. Krendel, D. A., Gilchrist, J. M., Johnson, A. O., and Bossen, E. H. Isolated deficiency of vitamin E with progressive neurologic deterioration. *Neurology* 37:538–540, 1987.
22. Freeman, W. B., Nielson, P. E., and Gibson, G. E. Effect of age on behavioral and enzymatic changes during thiamin deficiency. *Neurobiol. Aging* 8:429–434, 1987.

CHAPTER 36

Biochemistry of Neuropathy

DAVID E. PLEASURE

COMPARISON OF THE PERIPHERAL AND CENTRAL NERVOUS SYSTEMS

Many diseases affect both the peripheral nervous system (PNS) and the central nervous system (CNS). This is to be expected because of the substantial anatomical and molecular overlaps between these two tissues. Somatic motor and sensory neurons that give rise to PNS axons maintain a large fraction of their total protoplasmic bulk within the CNS. Neurons of the enteric plexi and autonomic ganglia resemble various classes of CNS neurons in neurotransmitter specificity and growth factor requirements. Phagocytic PNS microglia-like cells share with CNS microglia a common derivation from bone marrow; common expression of plasma membrane receptors for complement, antibodies, and other extracellular molecules; and similar ca-

Basic Neurochemistry: Molecular, Cellular, and Medical Aspects, 5th Ed., edited by G. J. Siegel et al. Published by Raven Press, Ltd., New York, 1994. Correspondence to David Pleasure, Department of Neurology and Pediatrics, University of Pennsylvania, Philadelphia, Pennsylvania 19104.

pacities to secrete cytokines and other biologically active molecules. Although CNS macroglia develop from the neural tube, and Schwann cells and enteric glia from the neural crest [1,2], some of their functions, such as regulation of conduction and neuronal trophic support, and the means by which these functions are accomplished, e.g., by synthesis of myelin by oligodendroglia and Schwann cells or expression of glutamine synthetase by astroglia and enteric glia, are similar.

Extracellular matrix appears a more important factor in neuronal migration and axonal guidance in PNS than CNS, but these targeting processes employ many cell adhesion molecules in common in the two tissues [3]. Still another resemblance between CNS and PNS is in the regulation of transfer of molecules between the bloodstream and neural extracellular space. The blood-nerve barrier, like the blood-brain barrier, is composed of capillary endothelial cells that, unlike the endothelial cells of capillaries in most other tissues, are linked by tight junctions. Endoneurial capillary endothelial pinocytosis is infrequent, but the cells express specific carriers to facilitate rapid passage of polar substrates and metabolites.

It is important to point out, however, that there are a substantial number of PNS-specific disorders. This selectivity can be attributed to mutations of genes expressed more prominently in PNS than CNS, e.g., the myelin protein PMP-22 [4,5]; immune-mediated diseases involving PNS-characteristic epitopes, e.g., myelin P2 protein and certain sulfated glycolipids [6,7]; regions of incompetence of the blood-nerve barrier that permit entry of neurotoxins; and physical trauma from which the CNS is protected by its bony covering. It should also be emphasized that the PNS has a greater capacity for regeneration than does CNS. For example, whereas oligodendroglia impede axonal regeneration [8], Schwann cells produce cytokines (e.g., ciliary neurotrophic factor) and basal lamina components that support neuronal survival and axonal elongation [9].

After brief consideration of diseases affecting both PNS and CNS, the principal focus of this chapter is on the special features of the PNS that influence both disease susceptibility and regenerative capacity of this tissue.

DISEASES AFFECTING BOTH THE PERIPHERAL AND CENTRAL NERVOUS SYSTEMS

Because of the similarities between the PNS and CNS, it is not surprising that many diseases affect both (see Table 1). It should be noted, however, that the clinical expressions of such diseases are variable and sometimes restricted to the PNS. For example, patients with thiamine deficiency often display symmetrical distal sensorimotor polyneuropathy without accompanying Wernicke's or Korsakoff's syndrome; infection with human immunodeficiency virus (HIV) may cause early chronic demyelinative polyneuropathy, with dementia then appearing months later; tertiary syphilis may destroy dorsal root ganglion sensory neurons (syndrome of tabes dorsalis) without injuring neurons in the cerebral cortex; and sulfatidase deficiency (metachromatic leukodystrophy) may cause polyneuropathy initially, with CNS dysfunction only later. In some instances, this apparent PNS specificity is simply an ascertainment artifact; that is, although both the CNS and PNS are involved, only the PNS component is detectable to the clinician in the early stages. In other cases, subtle host factors or as yet unappreciated etiologic variables dictate the PNS selectivity.

TABLE 1.   Examples of diseases affecting both the PNS and the CNS

Infections (AIDS, syphilis)

Neurotoxins (acrylamide, triorthocresylphosphate)

Vitamin (B_1, B_{12}, E) deficiencies

Hormone deficiencies (hypothyroidism)

Arteritis (periarteritis nodosa)

Familial lipid storage disorders (sulfatidase deficiency, galactocerebrosidase deficiency, adrenoleukodystrophy)

CELLULAR AND MOLECULAR CHARACTERISTICS OF THE PERIPHERAL NERVOUS SYSTEM

The PNS differs from the CNS in cell type and in protein and lipid composition

Support Cells

Whereas in the CNS, oligodendroglia invest large axons in myelin and astroglia regulate ion and metabolite concentrations in neuropil, these functions are the responsibility of Schwann cells in the PNS. Two major Schwann cell phenotypes are recognized in the normal PNS. Myelin-forming Schwann cells ensheath single axons greater than 1 μm in diameter for hundreds of microns and synthesize myelin-specific lipids (e.g., galactocerebroside) and proteins (e.g., myelin P0 glycoprotein). Nonmyelinating Schwann cells invest multiple smaller axons, express surface galactocerebroside but not other myelin lipids or proteins, and contain intermediary filaments composed of peptide subunits that closely resemble glial fibrillary acidic protein (GFAP) [10]. It has been demonstrated that the choice between the myelin-forming and nonmyelinating phenotypes is determined by the caliber of the axons with which the Schwann cells are in contact [11], but recent studies have clearly shown that the Schwann cells also exert reciprocal control over the cytoskeletal organization of the axons they invest and over axonal caliber and axoplasmic flow [12].

When Schwann cell–axonal contact is lost, as occurs in the distal stump of nerves undergoing Wallerian degeneration, Schwann cells briefly reenter the cell cycle, lose expression of myelin components or GFAP, upregulate synthesis and expression of surface low-affinity nerve growth factor receptors (L-NGFR) and neural cell adhesion molecules (N-CAM), and form tubular cellular aggregates (''bands of Bungner''). Myelin-forming and nonmyelinating Schwann cell phenotypes are restored as axonal regeneration progresses through the distal stump.

Enteric glia, neural crest-derived support cells of the myenteric plexi, are process-bearing cells of irregular morphology. Their processes form a partial glial sheath around the enteric ganglia. Groups of their processes also partially enclose axons within the ganglionic neuropil [2]. Like CNS astroglia, enteric glia strongly express GFAP and glutamine synthetase.

Two other supporting elements of the PNS are of mesodermal origin [13]. Perineurium, comprised of flattened, basal lamina-lined cells that delineate nerve fascicles, provides a barrier to movement of ionic compounds and macromolecules between non-neural tissues and the endoneurium. Fibroblasts constitute roughly 10 percent of total cells within endoneurium and are the major cell type in epineurial connective tissue.

PNS Myelin

Peripheral nervous system myelin contains a unique basic protein, P2, distinct from the family of myelin basic proteins shared by the CNS and PNS. Although the function of P2 is not known, it has extensive sequence similarity to low-molecular-weight fatty acid binding proteins expressed in liver and other tissues. Peripheral nervous system myelin contains a lower level of myelin-associated glycoprotein (MAG) than does CNS myelin. This glycoprotein plays an essential role in the initial Schwann cell–axonal interaction that initiates myelination [14]. The major PNS myelin structural protein P0, of much lower M_r (27,000) than MAG (98,000), is also a glycoprotein. P0 is specific to PNS myelin and is preferentially located in compact myelin, where its extracellular domain participates in homophilic interactions that ensure adhesion between intraperiod lines of successive myelin wraps [15]. Proteolipid protein, an acylated protein that appears to play a role in compaction of CNS myelin similar to that of P0 in the PNS, is also synthesized by Schwann cells, but at much lower levels than by oligodendroglia. Yet, it is excluded from PNS myelin [16]. Another recently cloned and sequenced low-molecular-weight PNS myelin protein, PMP-22, shows considerable sequence similarity to a growth arrest-specific protein expressed by resting but not proliferating fibroblasts [17].

The differences between the lipid compositions of CNS and PNS myelins are less profound than the differences in proteins. Molar ratios of cholesterol to phospholipid to galactosphingolipid are similar; however, human PNS myelin contains several sulfated glucuronyl glycolipids not expressed in adult human CNS myelin that cross-react with antibodies against carbohydrate epitopes of MAG [7].

PNS Collagens

The collagens, a family of extracellular structural proteins characterized by a triple α-helical configuration and a high content of hydroxyproline, hydroxylysine, and glycine, are abundant in the PNS but are much rarer in the CNS. In the CNS, collagen is encountered primarily in association with blood vessels and is virtually absent from the remainder of the neuropil. In the PNS, the collagens comprise 30 percent or more of total protein and are present in endoneurium both in the form of interstitial collagen fibrils and as a component of the basal lamina surrounding the processes of Schwann cells and perineurial cells, in addition to lining the outer aspect of endoneurial capillaries. Fibroblasts are responsible for the synthesis of the bulk of the interstitial collagen fibrils, whereas Schwann cells and, probably, perineurial mesothelial cells secrete the more heavily glycosylated basal lamina forms of collagen.

Blood-nerve barrier leaks at PNS nerve terminals and dorsal root ganglia

Both the CNS and PNS demonstrate local regions of incompetence of the respective blood-tissue barrier systems, and in both tissues these regions have specific physiological functions. In the CNS, for example, function of medullary chemosensory nuclei requires free passage of polar molecules from the blood. In the PNS, trophic proteins secreted by target organs gain access to axon terminals that are not invested in a perineurial sheath. Lectins and other proteins useful as anatomical tracers also gain access to the PNS at nerve terminals, and some viruses are able to penetrate at this site. In some species, such as the rabbit, proteins gain access to endoneurium in the region of the dorsal root ganglia as well as at nerve terminals.

The length of PNS axons increases their vulnerability

Peripheral nervous system sensory and motor axons may exceed 1 m in length. Since PNS axons lack ribosomes, the supply of essential structural proteins and enzymes to distal regions derived from the neuronal perikaryon must be transported through the axons for great distances. The proteins that polymerize to form neurofilaments and microtubules, and many enzymes, move centrifugally at 1 to 10 mm/day. Organelles such as neurotransmitter vesicles and mitochondria, which are also derived from the neuronal perikaryon, are transported through axoplasm at velocities of greater than 100 mm/day, by a process involving interactions between kinesin and microtubules. Proteins internalized by the nerve terminal are translocated toward the neuronal perikaryon at approximately 100 mm/day, employing a mechanism in which dynein and microtubules play roles. PNS neurons with long axons are particularly vulnerable to disorders that compromise either perikaryal synthesis of axonal proteins or the local axonal machinery that is responsible for axoplasmic transport (see also Chap. 27).

Long axons are also more likely to sustain localized damage owing to trauma, ischemia, or other noxious influences. Furthermore, since thousands of Schwann cells are required to myelinate such a long axon, the likelihood is high that a pathological process randomly compromising the capacity of Schwann cells to maintain myelin will interfere with saltatory conduction along such a fiber. Nonrandom distal segmental demyelination, owing to diminution in distal axonal caliber ("axonal dwindling"), is also most apt to occur in relation to the longest axons.

The clinical features of most polyneuropathies reflect this heightened vulnerability of the longest fibers. Typically, patients manifest symmetrical distal sensory disturbances, usually first in the feet, weakness of distal more than proximal muscles, and loss of distal prior to proximal tendon reflexes.

Trauma in the PNS leads to Wallerian degeneration and segmental demyelination

Movements of the limbs subject nerves to repeated stretch. Although collagen fibrils afford tensile strength, and there is some waviness in the course of axons that permits a degree of nerve elongation without axonal ripping, stretch that is too great causes axonal disruption. Nerves in exposed regions, e.g., the median nerve at the wrist, the ulnar nerve at the elbow, and the common peroneal nerve at the knee, are vulnerable to compression that, if sufficiently severe, can cause either demyelination or axonal transection. Such compression can also interrupt blood flow, causing nerve infarction. In addition to these mechanical injuries, superficial nerves experience considerable thermal fluctuations that can kill cells directly if sufficiently severe or predispose the nerves to damage by precipitation of cold-insoluble proteins or other mechanisms (for an example, see leprosy, below). A brief review of the responses of PNS to trauma-induced Wallerian degeneration or segmental demyelination will be helpful in suggesting why PNS is in general so much more successful in regenerating than is CNS.

Wallerian Degeneration

Axotomized Schwann cells in the nerve segment distal to a nerve transection manifest a transient phase of intense proliferation and form tubular aggregates. Mononuclear cells from the bloodstream enter the trauma zone and assist resident Schwann cells in catabolizing fragmented myelin. These blood-derived macrophages secrete cytokines (e.g., interleukin-1 and platelet-derived growth factor) that enhance local growth factor production [18] and stimulate Schwann cell mitosis. Distal to the transection, Schwann cell synthesis of myelin proteins and lipids falls dramatically, but Schwann cell expressions of cell surface adhesion molecules and of L-NGFRs are augmented [19]. While the function of Schwann cell L-NGFR and, indeed, of L-NGFR expression by neurons as well, is not known, embryonic stem cell L-NGFR knock-out transgenic mouse experiments indicate that this receptor is necessary for normal development of PNS sensory nerve fibers [20].

Fibroblasts in the traumatized nerve segment and distal to it augment production of interstitial collagen, increasing the tensile strength of the damaged nerve and providing the collagenous framework required for axonal ensheathment by Schwann cells. This extracellular accumulation of collagen in the injured PNS [21] contrasts sharply with the astrogliosis and increased intracellular GFAP elicited by trauma in the CNS.

As regeneration proceeds, axonal growth cones penetrate the scar and extend into the tubular Schwann cell aggregates. Reestablishment of contact with axons downregulates Schwann cell L-NGFR and N-CAM, and, if the axon reaches a diameter sufficient to support myelination, the Schwann cell is induced to synthesize MAG and, later, the structural proteins of compact myelin.

Segmental Demyelination

Schwann cells in nerve segments subjected to repetitive trauma (e.g., the median nerve at the wrist) may lose contact with the axon, proliferate, and participate in the catabolism of myelin fragments. If several successive internodes along an axon are demyelinated, nerve action potentials cannot be transmitted (conduction block). During subsequent remyelination, several Schwann cells usually participate in the remyelination of what was previously the territory of a single Schwann cell, giving rise to shortened internodes. During the initial period of remyelination, when the myelin sheath is very thin and its capacitance very high, the velocity of nerve conduction of action potentials is markedly below normal. Later, as the sheath approaches its normal thickness, conduction velocity rises. Excess Schwann cells generated during the phase of Schwann cell proliferation and not successful in establishing contact with an axon gradually disappear from the nerve. With repeated cycles of demyelination and remyelination, however, as can occur with repeated trauma or, more commonly, in various inherited and acquired demyelinative neuropathies, layers of redundant Schwann cells are generated that encircle demyelinated or partially remyelinated axons, forming "onion bulbs."

PATHOGENESIS OF DISEASES AFFECTING PRINCIPALLY OR SOLELY THE PERIPHERAL NERVOUS SYSTEM

Examples of disorders exclusively or predominantly of the PNS are listed in Table 2. Some of these diseases are quite common, e.g., diabetic neuropathy [22], Guillain-

TABLE 2.　Some diseases affecting only the PNS

Infections (leprosy, diphtheria)

Neurotoxins (pyridoxine, cisplatin, botulism)

Immune-mediated neuropathies (Guillain-Barré syndrome, experimental allergic neuritis, neuropathy with IgM$_k$ antimyelin-associated glycoprotein. Lambert-Eaton syndrome)

Amyloidosis (familial neuropathic and myeloma-associated forms)

Hirschsprung's disease

Refsum's disease

Hereditary motor-sensory neuropathies

Diabetic neuropathy

Neurofibromatosis type I

Barré syndrome, and neurofibromatosis type 1 [23], whereas others are rare, e.g., pyridoxine neuropathy [24], but are cited because they illustrate pathogenetic mechanisms. In some of these disorders, e.g., botulism, in which a bacterial exotoxin impedes release of neurotransmitter vesicles from cholinergic terminals at neuromuscular junctions, both the etiology and pathogenesis are relatively well understood. In others, such as the familial neuropathic amyloids, though the etiology is quite clear (various point mutations [25,26] leading to the accumulation in PNS of insoluble protein aggregates), the mechanisms by which deposition of these proteins in endoneurium elicit PNS degeneration remain obscure.

Infections

The lepromatous form of leprosy is characterized by loss of cutaneous sensibility, a consequence of damage caused by the growth of Hansen's bacilli in Schwann cells in affected cutaneous nerves. Hansen's bacilli, fastidious organisms that proliferate only at temperatures below that maintained by most mammals, are able to grow in subcutaneous Schwann cells because these nerves are in an environment that is often cooler than the CNS and other deeper tissues.

Diphtheria causes a demyelinative neuropathy, initially affecting the cranial nerves and later the nerves to the limbs; whereas segmental demyelination is profound, axons are typically spared. *Corynebacterium diphtheriae*, a bacterium that colonizes the pharynx or, less commonly, the skin secretes a protein exotoxin that gains access to endoneurial fluid both at nerve endings and at the level of the dorsal root ganglia. The exotoxin binds to a Schwann cell plasma membrane receptor and catalyzes ADP-ribosylation and inactivation of an elongation factor required for Schwann cell protein synthesis. Remyelination subsequently occurs, largely owing to the activity of the new Schwann cells generated in the nerve as a consequence of the mitogenic stimulus associated with segmental demyelination.

Polio virus, which multiplies initially in the gut, binds to and selectively infects motor neurons of the anterior horns of the spinal cord and brainstem, producing inflammatory changes within the CNS, Wallerian degeneration of motor axons in the PNS, and motor deficits without accompanying sensory or autonomic dysfunction. Months later, surviving motor neurons reinnervate previously denervated muscle fibers, producing motor units (motor neurons and the muscle fibers that they innervate) that are much larger in size than normal. This reparative process produces partial or complete return of previously lost motor function.

Neurotoxins

Excessive ingestion of pyridoxine (vitamin B_6), usually the result of inappropriate self-medication, causes a progressive, purely sensory axonal polyneuropathy affecting predominantly the largest fibers, attributable to the toxic effect of the vitamin on dorsal root ganglion neurons [24]. A similar purely sensory axonal polyneuropathy with dorsal root ganglion neuronopathy is seen in patients given cisplatin as a chemotherapeutic agent for the treatment of gynecological or bladder carcinoma. In both instances, the toxin, after gaining access to endoneurial fluid, induces damage by binding covalently to macromolecules necessary for neuronal function (pyridoxine to proteins; cisplatin to DNA).

Immune-mediated neuropathies

Experimental Allergic Neuritis

Experimental allergic neuritis (EAN) can be elicited in Lewis rats and monkeys by immunization against myelin P2 basic protein or in rabbits by immunization against the glycolipid galactocerebroside (galC). Although both types of EAN are primarily demyelinative, P2-EAN is mediated by sensitized T lymphocytes [6], whereas galC-EAN is mediated by galC antibodies. The reasons for PNS se-

lectivity of the two EANs are also distinct. Although T lymphocytes can penetrate the CNS as well as PNS, myelin P2 basic protein is restricted to the PNS, and P2-sensitized T-lymphocytes are therefore more likely to set up an inflammatory reaction in the PNS than the CNS. GalC, on the other hand, is a constituent of the plasma membranes of oligodendroglia as well as Schwann cells and of CNS myelin as well as PNS myelin, and PNS selectivity of galC-EAN seems to reflect more ready ingress of complement-fixing galC antibodies to the PNS than the CNS.

Guillain-Barré Syndrome

Guillain-Barré syndrome, or acute idiopathic polyradiculoneuritis, often occurs 1 or 2 weeks after various viral infections. Typically, no virus can be isolated from the PNS. If protected against hypoxemia, most patients recover completely, particularly if treated early in the course by plasmapheresis or immunoglobulin infusion. Guillain-Barré syndrome resembles P2-EAN both clinically and pathologically, being characterized by segmental demyelination and infiltration of endoneurium with lymphocytes and macrophages. Though most likely due to an autoimmune mechanism, the responsible neural antigen has not yet been identified.

IgM_k Paraproteinemia

Elderly men with IgM_k paraproteinemia caused by a plasma cell proliferative disorder occasionally develop a slowly progressive polyneuropathy characterized pathologically by focally abnormal compaction of PNS myelin lamellae. In such cases, the paraproteinemic immunoglobulin has been observed to bind to intact myelin and to MAG. The PNS specificity of this syndrome, despite the greater abundance of MAG in myelin of the CNS than the PNS, may be due to greater penetration of the paraprotein into the PNS than the CNS or, alternatively, to the presence in PNS myelin, but not in adult CNS myelin, of sulfated glucuronyl glycolipids that are recognized by the anti-MAG IgM_k paraprotein [7].

Amyloidosis

Amyloid is the generic term applied to disorders characterized by abnormal deposition of protease-resistant protein aggregates in tissue. The most common type of neural amyloidosis is restricted to the CNS in patients with Alzheimer's disease and is due to accumulation in the neuropil of a fragment of a transmembrane glycoprotein of as yet unknown function. Both acquired and inherited PNS-specific amyloids are also recognized. Aggregates of immunoglobulin light chains accumulate in the nerves of some patients with multiple myeloma and other plasma cell dyscrasias, leading to both compressive neuropathies and selective dysfunction of autonomic and nonmyelinated sensory fibers. Point mutations leading to altered solubility properties of the circulating transport protein transthyretin [25] or of the actin-binding protein gelsolin [26] also lead to accumulation of protein aggregates within nerves and cause dominantly inherited amyloid neuropathies.

Hirschsprung's disease

Hirschsprung's disease presents in infancy with massive segmental dilatation of the colon, the result of absence of intrinsic innervation distal to the affected segment [27]. This is perhaps due to failure of migration of neural crest cells to this portion of the gut or to an abnormal gut wall microenvironment inhospitable to maturation of neural crest cells [2].

Refsum's disease

Refsum's disease is an autosomal recessively inherited peroxisomal defect in the α-oxidation of dietary branched-chain fatty acids, most notably of phytanic acid. Patients with this disease manifest polyneuropathy with enlarged nerves, retinitis pigmentosa, scaly skin, and deafness. The polyneuropathy is largely demyelinative, and the nerve enlargement is due to the accumulation of excess Schwann cells in concentric periaxonal ar-

rays, or "onion bulbs." Myelin isolated from the nerves of such patients contain excess amounts of esterified phytanic acid, and it is presumed that this accumulation causes a decrease in myelin stability. Removal of phytanic acid from the diet yields improvement in the polyneuropathy.

Hereditary motor-sensory neuropathies

Hereditary motor and sensory neuropathy (HMSN) is a heterogeneous group of polyneuropathies with varying patterns of inheritance (dominant, recessive, or X-linked). Some families with HMSN (type 1 and type 3) are characterized by reduced velocity of nerve action potentials, prominent segmental demyelination, Schwann cell proliferation with onion-bulb formation, and distal axonal dwindling; others (type 2) manifest chiefly distal Wallerian degeneration. A partial chromosome 17 duplication involving the PMP-22 PNS myelin protein locus is the cause for human type 1 hereditary sensory-motor neuropathy (type 1 Charcot-Marie-Tooth disease) [5], and a point mutation of the PMP-22 gene is responsible for recessively inherited demyelinative polyneuropathy in the spontaneous mouse mutation trembler [4].

Diabetic neuropathy

Diabetes mellitus is the most common cause of peripheral neuropathy in the United States. The usual clinical pattern is that of a slowly progressive, mixed sensorimotor, and autonomic polyneuropathy. More acute, asymmetrical, motor neuropathies are also seen, particularly in older persons with non-insulin dependent diabetes mellitus [22].

Most of the work on the pathogenesis of diabetic neuropathy has been done with rats that are hyperglycemic because of the administration of the pancreatic islet cell toxin streptozotocin or on a hereditary basis, in particular, the BB strain of rats. In such rats, nerve conduction velocities fall soon after the appearance of hyperglycemia. The relevance of this acute physiological dysfunction to human diabetic neuropathies remains controversial.

Among the pathogenetic mechanisms that have been proposed for diabetic neuropathy are excess glycation of neural proteins; an alteration in nerve polyol metabolism induced by hyperglycemia; and nerve hypoxia. Nonenzymatic glycation of PNS myelin proteins and collagen is accentuated by hyperglycemia. Treatment with aminoguanidine, a glycation inhibitor, diminishes the degree of electrophysiological and histological abnormalities in streptozotocin-diabetic rats [28]. Hyperglycemia causes excess accumulation of sorbitol and fructose within the endoneurium, both in diabetic rats and in diabetic humans, although not to levels likely to cause damage because of osmotic disequilibrium. Hyperglycemia also inhibits carrier-mediated transport of myoinositol into endoneurium. Endoneurial blood flow is diminished in diabetic rats and also in rats rendered hyperglycemic by glucose infusion [29]. The mechanism for hyperglycemia-induced decreased blood flow is unclear. Hypoxia caused by this diminished blood flow could account for the slowing of nerve conduction velocity in these animals. Focal diminution in endoneurial blood flow, presumably the result of local blood vessel pathology, is likely the cause for the scattered infarctions of the proximal regions of peripheral nerves seen at autopsy in some patients with diabetic neuropathy.

Neurofibromatosis

Neurofibromatosis type II (NF II) is a rare, dominantly inherited disease, caused by a chromosome 22 mutation, and characterized by bilateral acoustic nerve Schwann cell tumors. Patients with this condition are also at risk of developing gliomas, meningiomas, and spinal nerve root Schwann cell tumors, but show few of the cutaneous features of neurofibromatosis type 1 (NF I).

NF I (von Recklinghausen's disease) is caused by a variety of mutations in a large, chromosome 17 gene that encodes the GTPase activating protein neurofibromin

[23]. NF I is among the most common genetic neurological diseases, with an incidence of about 1 in 2,000 persons, and is characterized by multiple subcutaneous neurofibromas. Schwann cell tumors infiltrating large nerves and nerve roots also occur in some patients and occasionally undergo malignant transformation. Focal hyperpigmentation of the skin (café-au-lait spots) and iris (Lisch nodules) are also features of NF I and are attributable to abnormalities in migration and proliferation of neural crest-derived pigmented cells.

REFERENCES

1. LeDourain, N. M. Cell line segregation during peripheral nervous system ontogeny. *Science* 231:1515–1522, 1986.
2. Gershon, M. D., and Rothman, T. P. Enteric glia. *Glia* 4:195–204, 1991.
3. Hynes, R. O., and Lander, A. D. Contact and adhesive specificites in the associations, migrations, and targeting of cells and axons. *Cell* 68:303–322, 1992.
4. Suter, U., Weicher, A. A., Oxcelik, T., Snipes, G. J., Kosaras, B., Francke, U., Billings-Gagliardi, S., Sidman, R. L., and Shooter, E. M. *Trembler* mouse carries a point mutation in a myelin gene. *Nature* 356:241–244, 1992.
5. Matsunami, N., Smith, B., Ballard, L., Lensch, M. W., Robertson, M., Albertsen, H., Hanemann, C. O., Muller, H. W., Bird, T. H., White, R., and Chance, P. F. Peripheral myelin protein-22 gene maps in the duplication in chromosome 17p11-2 associated with Charcot-Marie-Tooth 1A. *Nature Genet.* 1:176–179, 1992.
6. Heininger, K., Stoll, G., Linington, C., Toyka, K., and Wekerle, H. Conduction failure and nerve conduction slowing in experimental allergic neuritis induced by P_2-specific T-cell lines. *Ann. Neurol.* 19:44–49, 1986.
7. Chou, D. K. H., Ilyas, A. A., Evans, J. E., Costello, C., Quarles, R. H. and Jungalwala, F. B. Structure of sulfated glucuronyl glycolipids in the nervous system reacting with HNK-1 antibody and some IgM paraproteins in neuropathy. *J. Biol. Chem.* 261:11717–11725, 1986.
8. Caroni, P., and Schwab, M. Codistribution of neurite growth inhibitors and oligodendro-

cytes in rat CNS: Appearance follows nerve fiber growth and precedes myelination. *Dev. Biol.* 136:287–295, 1989.

9. Oppenheim, R. W., Prevette, D., Qin-Wei, Y., Collins, F., and MacDonald, J. Control of embryonic motoneuron survival *in vivo* by ciliary neurotrophic factor. *Science* 251:1616–1618, 1991.

10. Mokuno, K., Kamholz, J., Behrman, T., Black, C., Feinstein, D., Lee, V. and Pleasure, D. Neuronal modulation of Schwann cell glial fibrillary acidic protein (GFAP). *J. Neurosci. Res.* 23:396–405, 1989.

11. Voyvodic, J. T. Target size regulates calibre and myelination of sympathetic axons. *Nature* 346:430–433, 1989.

12. de Weegh, S. M., Lee, V. M., and Brady, S. T. Local modulation of neurofilament phosphorylation, axonal caliber, and slow axonal transport by myelinating Schwann cells. *Cell* 68:451–463, 1992.

13. Bunge, M. B., Wood, P. M., Tynan, L. B., Bates, M. L., and Sanes, J. R. Perineurium originates from fibroblasts: Demonstration *in vitro* with a retroviral marker. *Science* 213: 229–231, 1989.

14. Owens, G. C., and Bunge, R. P. Schwann cells infected with a recombinant retrovirus expressing myelin-associated glycoprotein antisense RNA do not form myelin. *Neuron* 7: 565–575, 1991.

15. D'Urso, D., Brophy, P. J., Staugaitis, S. M., Gillespie, C. S., Frey, A., Stempack, J., and Colman, D. R. Protein zero of peripheral myelin: biosynthesis, membrane insertion, and evidence for homotypic interactions. *Neuron* 4:449–460, 1990.

16. Kamholz, J., Sessa, M., Scherer, S., Vogelbacker, H., Mokuno, K., Baron, P., Wrabetz, L., Shy, M., and Pleasure, D. Structure and expression of proteolipid protein in the peripheral nervous system. *J. Neurosci. Res.* 31: 231–244, 1992.

17. Welcher, A. A., Suter, U., De Leon, M., Snipes, G. J., and Shooter, E. M. A myelin protein is encoded by the homologue of a growth arrest-specific gene. *Proc. Natl. Acad. Sci. U. S. A.* 88:7195–7199, 1991.

18. Heumann, R., Lindholm, D., Bendtlow, C., Meyer, M., Radeke, M. J., Misko, T. P., Shooter, E., and Thoenen, H. Differential regulation of mRNA encoding nerve growth factor and its receptor in rat sciatic nerve dur-

ing development, degeneration, and regeneration: role of macrophages. *Proc. Natl. Acad. Sci. U. S. A.* 81:8735–8739, 1987.

19. Daniloff, J. K., Levi, G., Grumet, M., Rieger, F., and Edelman, G. M. Altered expression of neuronal cell adhesion molecules induced by nerve injury and repair. *J. Cell. Biol.* 103: 929–945, 1986.

20. Lee, K.-F., Li, E., Huber, L. J., Landis, S. C., Sharpe, A. H., Chao, M. V., and Jaenisch, R. Targeted mutation of the gene encoding the low affinity NGF receptor p75 leads to deficits in the peripheral sensory nervous system. *Cell* 69:737–750, 1992.

21. Eather, T. F., Pollock, M., and Myers, D. B. Proximal and distal changes in collagen content of peripheral nerve that follow transection and crush lesions. *Exp. Neurol.* 92: 299–310, 1986.

22. Dyck, P. H., Thomas, P. K., Asbury, A. K., Winegrad, A. I., and Porte, D., Jr. (eds.), *Diabetic Neuropathy.* Philadelphia: W. B. Saunders, 1987.

23. Gutmann, D. H., Wood, D. L., and Collins, F. S. Identification of the neurofibromatosis type 1 gene product. *Proc. Natl. Acad. Sci. U. S. A.* 88:9658–9662, 1991.

24. Xu, Y., Sladky, J., and Brown, M. J. Dose-dependent expression of neuronopathy after experimental pyridoxine intoxication. *Neurology* 39:1077–1083, 1989.

25. Holt, I. J., Harding, A. E., Middleton, L., Chrysostomou, G., Said, G., King, R. H., and Thomas, P. K. Molecular dynamics of amyloid neuropathy in Europe. *Lancet* 1:524–526, 1989.

26. Haltia, M., Levy, E., Maretoje, J., Fernandez Madrid, I., Koivunen, O., and Frangione, B. Gelsolin gene mutation—at codon 187—in familial amyloidosis, Finnish: DNA-diagnostic assay. *Am. J. Med. Genet.* 12:357–359, 1992.

27. Howard, E. R. Muscle innervation of the gut: Structure and pathology. *J. R. Soc. Med.* 77: 905–908, 1984.

28. Yagihashi, S., Kamijo, M., Baba, M., Yagihashi, N., and Nagain, K. Effect of aminoguanidine on functional and structural abnormalities in peripheral nerve of STZ-induced diabetic rats. *Diabetes* 41:47–52, 1992.

29. Cameron, N. E., Cotter, M. A., and Low, P. A. Nerve blood flow in early experimental diabetes in rats: Relation to conduction defects. *Am. J. Physiol.* 261:E1–8, 1991.

CHAPTER 37

Diseases Involving Myelin

RICHARD H. QUARLES, PIERRE MORELL, AND DALE E. McFARLIN*

GENERAL CLASSIFICATION / 772

A deficiency of myelin can result either from failure to produce the normal amount of myelin during development (hypomyelination) or from myelin breakdown after it is formed (demyelination) / 772

Biochemical changes in brain are similar in demyelinating diseases regardless of etiology / 773

ACQUIRED DISORDERS OF MYELIN HAVING AN ALLERGIC AND/OR INFECTIOUS BASIS / 773

Nervous system damage in many acquired allergic and infectious demyelinating diseases is specifically directed against myelin or myelin-forming cells with relatively little damage to other parenchymal elements / 773

Multiple sclerosis is the most common demyelinating disease of the central nervous system in man / 773

Biochemical analyses of MS lesions reveal an increase of catabolic enzymes and a severe loss of myelin proteins and lipids / 775

Although the cause of MS is unknown, genetic, immunological, and environmental factors are believed to contribute to its pathogenesis / 776

Experimental allergic encephalomyelitis is an animal model of autoimmune demyelination / 778

Guillain-Barré syndrome is an acute, monophasic, inflammatory demyelinating disease of the peripheral nervous system, often preceded by a viral infection / 781

Carbohydrate epitopes on the myelin-associated glycoprotein and/or other glycoconjugates are targets for autoimmune demyelination of the peripheral nervous system occurring in association with paraproteinemia / 781

Other acquired demyelinating diseases in humans may be secondary to viral infections, neoplasia, or immunosuppressive therapy / 782

A number of animal diseases caused by viruses involve primary demyelination and are often associated with inflammation / 783

GENETICALLY DETERMINED DISORDERS OF MYELIN / 783

The leukodystrophies are a large group of inherited disorders of central nervous system white matter characterized by a diffuse deficiency of myelin / 783

A growing number of mutations that lead to hypomyelination in mice and other experimental animals have been identified and are of particular value to neurochemists because of insights that they give with regard to the structure and assembly of myelin / 785

TOXIC AND NUTRITIONAL DISORDERS OF MYELIN / 787

Basic Neurochemistry: Molecular, Cellular, and Medical Aspects, 5th Ed., edited by G. J. Siegel et al. Published by Raven Press, Ltd., New York, 1994. Correspondence to Richard H. Quarles, NIH, 9000 Rockville Pike, Park Bldg./Rm. 429B, Bethesda, Maryland 20892.
* Deceased.

The integrity of myelin sheaths is dependent on the normal functioning of myelin-forming oligodendrocytes in the central nervous system and Schwann cells in the peripheral nervous system as well as on the viability of the axons that they ensheath. Neuronal death inevitably leads to subsequent degeneration of both axons and the myelin surrounding them. The title of this chapter was chosen to emphasize that myelin cannot be considered an isolated entity in considering disease processes. Deficiencies of myelin can result from a multitude of causes, including viral infections, inherited disorders, toxic agents, malnutrition, and mechanical trauma that affect myelin, myelin-supporting cells, or myelinated neurons.

GENERAL CLASSIFICATION

A deficiency of myelin can result either from failure to produce the normal amount of myelin during development (hypomyelination) or from myelin breakdown after it is formed (demyelination)

An impediment of normal myelin formation is referred to as hypomyelination or, in some cases, as dysmyelination. According to the definition of Poser, dysmyelination is a genetically determined disorder of myelinogenesis in which "myelin initially formed was abnormally constituted, thus inherently unstable, vulnerable, and liable to degeneration" [1]. Diseases involving loss of normal myelin after it is formed, i.e., demyelination, can be subdivided into primary and secondary categories on the basis of morphological observations. Primary demyelination involves the early destruction of myelin with relative sparing of axons; subsequently, other structures may be affected. Secondary demyelination includes those disorders in which myelin is involved after damage to neurons and axons. The classification used in this chapter is based on etiology as well as comparative neuropathology. Disorders causing hypomyelination and demyelination are both included in four categories: (a) acquired allergic and infectious diseases; (b) genetically determined disorders, (c) toxic and nutritional disorders, and (d) disorders primarily affecting neurons with secondary involvement of myelin.

Biochemical changes in brain are similar in demyelinating diseases regardless of etiology

The most pronounced changes occur in white matter where there is a marked increase in water content, a decrease of myelin proteins and lipids, and, in many cases, the appearance of cholesterol esters and/or glial fibrillary acidic protein (GFAP) [1]. Particularly noteworthy with regard to lipids are dramatic decreases in galactocerebroside, ethanolamine plasmalogens, and cholesterol, all of which are enriched in myelin membranes (see Chap. 6). The major structural proteins of central nervous system myelin, myelin basic protein and proteolipid protein, are also invariably decreased. These changes can be explained by the breakdown and gradual loss of myelin (which is relatively rich in solids) and its replacement by extracellular fluid, astrocytes, and inflammatory cells (that are more hydrated, relatively lipid poor, and free of myelin-specific constituents). The frequent appearance of cholesterol esters in demyelinating diseases is apparently related to the fact that cholesterol is not readily degraded and is esterified by phagocytes, often remaining at the site of the lesion for some time. Since cholesterol esters are essentially absent from normal mature brain, their presence in myelin disorders is indicative of inflammation and recent demyelination. Such compounds are also responsible for the neutral fat staining (sudanophilia) demonstrated histochemically in many demyelinating diseases. In the central nervous system, GFAP is specific to astrocytes, and an increase of this protein during demyelination is due to reactive astrocytes associated with the pathology (see Chap. 1). The magnitudes of the changes mentioned above vary considerably from disease to disease, and from specimen to specimen in the same disease, depending on the severity, location, duration, and activity of the pathological processes.

ACQUIRED DISORDERS OF MYELIN HAVING AN ALLERGIC AND/OR INFECTIOUS BASIS

Nervous system damage in many acquired allergic and infectious demyelinating diseases is specifically directed against myelin or myelin-forming cells with relatively little damage to other parenchymal elements

In most of these disorders (except where noted otherwise), the lesions are disseminated in the nervous system and are characterized by perivenular demyelination and inflammation, macrophage activity, sudanophillic deposits consisting of myelin degradation products, and relative sparing of axons. The extent to which these criteria are fulfilled depends on the particular type and phase of disease. Furthermore, it is not always clear whether the immunological activity is autoimmune in nature or is related primarily to an antecedent viral infection; nor is the amount of damage directly caused by the virus always clear. The clinicopathologic aspects of the diseases discussed here are reviewed in detail elsewhere [1,2].

Multiple sclerosis is the most common demyelinating disease of the central nervous system in man

The clinical aspects of multiple sclerosis (MS) are highly variable both in symptoms and clinical course. The most typical form of the disease begins in the third or fourth decade of life and is manifested by exacerbations and remissions over many years. As time passes, the disease enters a chronic phase and slowly progresses over years. In other patients, the disease is slowly progressive from the beginning. An acute form of MS which rapidly progresses over weeks and months to death within a year occurs in a small number of patients. The reader is referred to other texts [1–4] for additional clinical and pathological details of this major demyelinating disease in humans.

Lesions in the white matter can now be visualized and monitored by magnetic resonance imaging (MRI) in living patients. Chronic lesions are easily detected on T-2-weighted sequences. In most patients, MRI studies show a number of clinically silent lesions. Early in the formation of MS lesions, there is a breakdown of the blood-brain barrier (BBB). This can be detected by the systemic administration of gadolinium (Gd), a paramagnetic substance that enhances the lesion in regions of increased permeability. This enhancement can easily be visualized on T-1-weighted MRI sequences. Sequential studies of acute enhancing MS lesions indicate that the BBB breakdown persists for four to eight weeks. Afterwards, a few lesions completely disappear, but most persist and can be identified on T-2-weighted studies. Evidence of subclinical demyelinating lesions can also be obtained by electrophysiological studies. The diagnosis of MS is based on classical clinical criteria, but MRI, electrophysiological studies, and cerebrospinal fluid abnormalities can be useful [2].

The characteristic lesion in MS is the plaque, which is the macroscopic appearance of a demyelinating lesion. These can be identified grossly at autopsy (Fig. 1) and are sharply demarcated from the surrounding tissue. Plaques occur throughout the white matter, but areas of predilection such as the periventricular white matter are well known. Microscopic examination characteristically shows loss of myelin with preservation of axons (primary demyelination) and viable oligodendrocytes. In chronic lesions, some axonal destruction and loss of oligodendrocytes occur. Plaques develop around venules, and early lesions contain many lymphocytes,

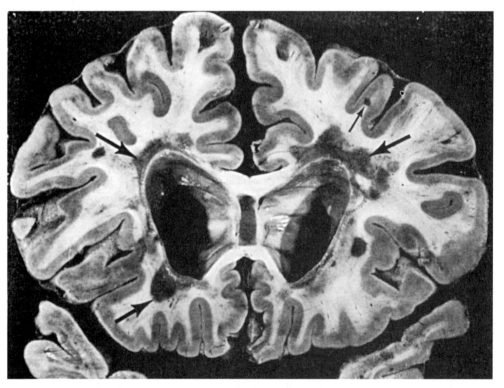

FIG. 1. Coronal slice of brain from a patient who died with MS. Demyelinated plaques are clearly visible in white matter (*large arrows*). Small plaques are also observed at the boundaries between gray and white matter (*small arrows*). (From Raine in ref. [1].)

plasma cells, and macrophages. Reports on the phenotypes of the T-cell infiltrate have varied, with some investigators reporting an overrepresentation of the CD8+ subset while others have observed a predominance of the CD4+ subset at the edge of lesions and in the surrounding parenchyma. The greatest cellularity is found at the margins of acute lesions, which are believed to be the locations at which occur the earliest changes associated with myelin loss.

Electron microscopy of early lesions indicates that a major mechanism for myelin destruction is the direct removal of myelin lamellae from the surface of intact sheaths by macrophages. This involves the attachment of superficial lamellae to coated pits at the macrophage surface, implying the presence of receptors that bind to a ligand on the myelin. The Fc receptors on the macrophages may bind to immunoglobulins attached to the myelin, but this has not been established. For many years there has been discussion about whether the primary pathological effect in this disease is directed at oligodendrocytes or myelin sheaths. Although this question may not be totally resolved, recent observations of apparently healthy oligodendrocytes in areas of active demyelination suggest that myelin sheaths themselves are the primary targets. Old, chronic lesions in contrast to early lesions, are sharply defined and contain bare, nonmyelinated axons and many fibrous astrocytes.

Biochemical analyses of MS lesions reveal an increase of catabolic enzymes and a severe loss of myelin proteins and lipids

Affected areas of MS white matter have the expected decrease of myelin constituents and a buildup of cholesterol esters [1]. For example, polyacrylamide gel electrophoresis of homogenates of macroscopically normal-appearing white matter, outer periplaque, inner periplaque, and plaque show a graded decline of myelin basic protein (MBP) and proteolipid protein (PLP) in sequential samples from the normal-appearing white matter to the center of the plaque in both chronic and acute lesions (Fig. 2). In the center of the chronic plaque, there is a virtual absence of these myelin proteins and an accumulation of GFAP indicative of astrogliosis (Fig. 2B). A plaque from an acute lesion is not completely demyelinated, as indicated by the presence of some MBP and PLP, and shows no accumulation of GFAP (Fig. 2C). The acute plaque contains albumin due to breakdown of the blood-brain barrier. Immunocytochemical and quantitative biochemical analyses of myelin proteins have revealed that myelin-associated glycoprotein (MAG) is often decreased to a greater extent than other myelin proteins at the periphery of plaques. This fact suggests that MAG is affected early in the pathological process [5]. A number of biochemical studies have indicated that myelin constituents are significantly reduced even in some areas of macroscopically normal-appearing white matter of MS brain in comparison to control white matter [1]. This is most likely explained by the presence of microlesions throughout the affected brain. Although the yield of myelin from MS tissue is reduced, most studies indicate that there is no compositional difference between isolated MS and control myelin, suggesting that the etiology of MS is unlikely to be due to an underlying defect in myelin composition.

Plaque formation in MS tissue is thought to involve proteases and other catabolic enzymes [1]. Myelin basic protein is highly susceptible to proteases even when present in myelin membranes. A neutral protease released by stimulated macrophages catalyzes the conversion of plasminogen to plasmin that rapidly degrades MBP. Acid proteinase and other acidic degradative enzymes, presumably lysosomal and of macrophage origin, are elevated in affected MS tissue and are likely to be involved in breakdown of myelin proteins and lipids. In addition, protease activities intrinsic to myelin sheaths (such as Ca^{2+} activated neutral

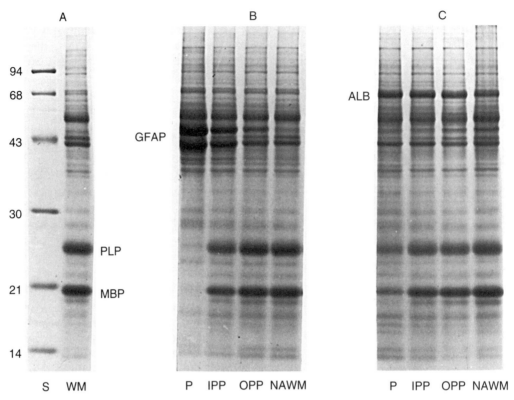

FIG. 2.   Polyacrylamide gel electrophoresis of proteins in control and MS tissue. Total proteins of the tissue samples were solubilized with a detergent (sodium dodecyl sulfate) and electrophoresed on a polyacrylamide gel system that separates proteins according to their size. After electrophoresis, the proteins were stained with Coomassie brilliant blue dye. **A:** Molecular weight standards (S) labeled according to their molecular mass in kiloDaltons and the proteins of control white matter (WM). **B:** Samples from the region of a chronic MS plaque. **C:** Samples from the region of an acute MS plaque. **Tissue samples:** (P) plaque center; (IPP) inner periplaque; (OPP) outer periplaque; (NAWM) macroscopically normal-appearing white matter near the plaque. **Proteins:** (PLP) proteolipid protein; (MBP) myelin basic protein; (GFAP) glial fibrillary protein; (ALB) serum albumin. (From Johnson, D., Sato, S., Quarles, R. H., Inuzuka, T., Brady, R. O., and Tourtellotte, W. W. Quantitation of myelin-associated glycoprotein in human nervous tissue from controls and multiple sclerosis patients. *J. Neurochem.* 46:1086–1093, 1986.)

protease) may facilitate myelin destruction [5,6]. Immunologically reactive, proteolytic fragments of MBP appear in the cerebrospinal fluid of MS patients during exacerbations of the disease [1,2] and presumably reflect myelin breakdown. However, the presence of this material in the CSF is not specific for MS since it occurs in other conditions with myelin damage such as cerebral infarction and encephalitis. Nevertheless, measurements of MBP-related material in CSF may be useful in addition to MRI, in monitoring the course of disease activity in patients.

Although the cause of MS is unknown, genetic, immunological, and environmental factors are believed to contribute to its pathogenesis

Two types of studies have provided data that favor a genetic component [3,4]. The prevalence of MS varies among ethnic groups, with the disorder being very rare among Bantu, Yakutes, Hutterites, and Innuits and low in Hungarian gypsies, Chinese and Japanese. In addition, the frequency is lower in first-generation Japanese Americans than in whites living in the same region of the United States. Also, the occurrence of MS in families is well-known, and there is increased risk among first-degree relatives of individuals with the disease. This risk approaches 20 percent in British Columbia. Twin studies have shown a higher concordance in monozygotic twins than dizygotic twins. These observations have led to two general conclusions. First, a significant genetic component is operative in the pathogenesis; second, two or more genes are involved.

Because immunopathologic factors are operative in MS, as discussed below, studies of candidate genes have focused on those related to human immune reactivity. Considerable emphasis currently is being placed on the trimolecular complex involved in antigen recognition by T cells. Advances in molecular immunology over the past decade have established that T cells recognize processed antigen that is presented by major histocompatibility complex (MHC) molecules. In humans, these HLA molecules (human leukocyte antigen system) are encoded by genes on chromosome 6, and the T-cell receptor (TCR) for antigens consists of α- and β-chains that are encoded on chromosomes 14 and 7, respectively. The knowledge that genes on three chromosomes are involved in antigen recognition by T cells and that MS has a genetic component provides the rationale for an extensive amount of research currently in progress.

Epidemiological studies have provided data that support an environmental factor, possibly an infectious agent. The prevalence of MS is known to vary in different regions. A high prevalence is found above 40° north latitude, and a low prevalence is found below 12°. Migrants from areas of different risk assume the risk of the region to which they migrate provided the age of migration is prior to 15 years. After this age, the migrant essentially has the risk of the original area. This would be consistent with the involvement of an infectious agent acquired early in life. Finally, clusters of MS cases are well described. The best example is in the Faroe

Islands where there were no reports of MS prior to World War II. Clustering of cases after this time suggests that an environmental agent, possibly infectious and related to the arrival of the British troops, was important.

A viral etiology for MS has been proposed and debated for decades [1–4]. Several indirect lines of evidence support this possibility. First, as indicated above, the data suggesting an environmental factor are consistent with its being a virus and suggest that the disease is related to childhood exposure followed by a long latency. Second, there are a number of naturally occurring and experimental disorders in animals in which clinical disease caused by viruses have long incubation periods and evoke primary demyelination with sparing of axons (see below). Although the rationale for a possible viral etiology has stimulated an extensive amount of research, a definite causative agent has not been identified. Efforts to confirm a virus in the central nervous system of MS patients have included morphological studies and numerous attempts at isolation as well as transmission. To date, at least 15 agents have been proposed as candidates; a human retrovirus has been the most recent addition [4]. An agent of the latter type is attractive as a hypothetical cause because retroviruses characteristically produce persistent infection and use virus-coded DNA polymerase (reverse transcriptase) to become incorporated into the host genome where, as such, they hide in the cell. This possibility attracted considerable attention from the observation that a chronic myelopathy known as HTLV-I-associated myelopathy/tropical spastic paraparesis (HAM/TSP) is related to a retrovirus. Patients with HAM/TSP have certain clinical and MRI features that resemble those in some MS patients. However, the pathology is different, and extensive searching for evidence of HTLV-1 involvement has been negative in most MS patients.

Immunological mechanisms have been implicated in the pathogenesis of MS for many reasons [1–4]: (a) the perivenular infiltration of inflammatory cells seen in pathology specimens; (b) the similarity of the pathology to immune-mediated postvaccinal encephalomyelitis and experimental allergic encephalomyelitis (EAE) (see next section); (c) increase of immunoglobulin synthesis in the central nervous system of MS patients that results in oligoclonal bands in the CSF; (d) association with certain HLA types that are linked to immune-response genes; (e) a variety of abnormalities of cellular immune function; and (f) beneficial clinical responses seen after the administration of pharmacological agents that downregulate immune function, as well as the increased disease activity observed after administration of interferon-γ that has the capacity to upregulate the immune system.

It should be emphasized that the above evidence suggesting an immune pathogenesis for MS does not exclude the likelihood of a viral etiology. It may be that an infectious agent somehow elicits an immune reaction that is responsible for the demyelination. For example, an epitope on a viral protein might mimic some structural feature of the myelin sheath and thus induce an autoimmune reaction. However, in spite of the indications that immunological mechanisms are involved in the demyelination of MS, numerous attempts to identify a viral or brain antigen that is the target of a strong and meaningful humoral or cellular immune response in this disease have been unsuccessful. Thus, although it is widely thought that MS is an autoimmune disease instigated by an infectious agent, the putative antigen(s) and virus remain elusive.

Experimental allergic encephalomyelitis is an animal model of autoimmune demyelination

Shortly after Pasteur introduced rabies virus vaccination, it was noted that a small minority of individuals receiving this treatment developed an encephalomyelitis. Autopsy of fatal cases showed widespread lesions in the white matter that were somewhat similar to those in MS and quite distinct from features usually observed in rabies. Production of the vaccine involved growing the virus in central nervous system tissue, and this disorder was reproduced in monkeys by Rivers and co-workers with multiple injections of normal central nervous system tissue. This animal model for postvaccinal encephalomyelitis became known as EAE [1–3]. It has subsequently been produced in many species, including monkeys, rabbits, guinea pigs, rats, and mice. A number of forms of EAE that vary clinically and pathologically have been described. The age and species of the animals being studied, the inoculum, and the use of various adjuvants are important variables that may influence the clinical and pathological aspects as well as pathogenetic mechanisms.

Following the introduction of adjuvants by Freund, it was possible to produce this experimental model, EAE, with a single injection of central nervous system tissue. This prompted an extensive search for the responsible antigen(s) with the hope of developing desensitization techniques that might be efficacious in the treatment of MS. Myelin basic protein was soon found and documented to be an encephalitogen by Einstein, Kies, and co-workers. Nevertheless, it was widely suspected that immune reactivity against other myelin antigens could also contribute to the pathogenesis of demyelination. However, because of the sticky nature of myelin components and particularly MBP, some doubt about efforts to establish this point experimentally remained. It was only recently that the primary amino acid sequences of other myelin proteins were determined, leading to the testing of synthetic peptides for encephalogenicity. Almost 40 years after MBP was discovered, the encephalogenicity of PLP was unequivocally established. It is likely that immune reactivity to other central nervous system components may also be important.

Myelin basic protein is a major component of myelin of all mammals (see Chap.

6), although there are some amino acid sequence differences among species, and MBP exists in a number of molecular isoforms within any one species. In describing particular amino acid sequences in MBP as epitopes, it is important to note that some variations in numbering of residues are found in the literature, and it is helpful to use the numbering of porcine MBP that is the longest (172 amino acids) as a reference. Much is known about the encephalitogenic epitopes of MBP that may vary in different species and even in different inbred strains of a given species. For example, residues 115–123, which cause EAE in strain 13 guinea pigs, are conserved among various species. Consequently EAE can easily be produced in guinea pigs with MBP from virtually any vertebrate. However, the major encephalitogen for Lewis rats resides in amino acids 71–90, and there are variations in this region of the MBP sequence among species. Therefore, the source of MBP is a critical variable in studies of EAE in Lewis rats. In SJL mice, two overlapping portions of the molecule, 9–102 and 95–108, cause EAE, while in some other strains, exemplified by PL mice, the encephalitogenic epitope resides in the first nine N-terminal amino acids, including the terminal acetyl group.

Although proteolipid protein (PLP) has been studied much less than MBP, at least three encephalitogenic epitopes for mice have been identified [3], and it is apparent that these vary among different murine strains. For example, two epitopes residing in residues 139–151 and 141–151, respectively, produce disease in SJL mice, whereas an encephalitogenic epitope for SWR mice is contained in residues 103–116. It seems likely that additional sites that produce EAE will be identified on PLP as it is studied more extensively. In addition, immune responses to other components of the oligodendrocyte/myelin membrane may be involved in autoimmune demyelination. For example, antibodies to galactocerebroside and the myelin-oligodendrocyte glycoprotein (MOG), both of which are on the external surfaces of myelin sheaths and oligodendrocytes, have been implicated in the pathogenesis of some forms of EAE [2,7].

Pathogenetic mechanisms responsible for autoimmune disorders have been investigated in EAE [3]. Patterson demonstrated that the disease could be transferred from affected animals to normal animals with immune cells but not with serum from affected animals. It has been established that the CD4$^+$ subpopulation of T lymphocytes transfers the disease in mice, rats, and guinea pigs. This subset recognizes antigen in association with class II major histocompatibility molecules (la). Both these molecules and the TCR are under genetic control and vary among different murine strains. Analysis of the molecular components involved in T-cell recognition of encephalitogenic antigen has led to a number of strategies for modifying EAE. Some of these approaches alter antigen presentation while others interfere with T-cell function. Much information has been obtained from detailed study of specific forms of EAE such as those in individual murine strains; however, the lessons learned are believed to have application to the disease in general and possibly to human demyelinating disorders.

Treatment with antibody to class II MHC molecules prevents EAE, presumably by altering presentation of encephalitogenic peptides. Another approach has been to treat with nonencephalitogenic peptides that closely correspond to encephalitogenic peptides. For example, it is possible to synthesize peptides, with single amino acid substitutions, that can bind to class II MHC molecules but that are not encephalitogenic in PL mice because they are not recognized by the T cells. Treatment of the PL mice with one of these peptides blocked adoptive transfer of EAE by peptide-specific clones, apparently by competition for class II MHC molecules. This approach is under investigation.

For decades it has been known that EAE can be modified by immunosuppression through a variety of approaches. Over two decades ago, treatment with antilymphocyte serum was shown to be effective. More recently, when CD4$^+$ cells were shown to mediate the disease, the administration of antibodies against this subset was also shown to reverse the disease. Treatment with antisera against T cells potentially leads to general immunosuppression, but knowledge of TCR usage by encephalitogenic cells has resulted in the development of more specific therapeutic strategies. For example, encephalitogenic T-cell clones in PL and B10.PL mice predominately use the Vβ8.2 subfamily of TCR to recognize the peptide responsible for disease. Treatment with a monoclonal antibody specific for Vβ8.2 both prevents the adoptive transfer of EAE and reverses disease in progress. In other studies designed to circumvent the necessity for administering exogenous antibody, Cohen and co-workers demonstrated that vaccination of Le rats with disease-producing T-cell lines (so called T-cell vaccination) could effectively prevent EAE in these animals. Furthermore, vaccination with synthetic peptides corresponding to sequences in specific TCR β-chains that are involved in encephalitogen recognition has also prevented EAE in some rodent models.

The highly specific forms of treatment outlined above are effective in the specific animal models in which they were developed. Alternative approaches have been to induce tolerance by coupling encephalitogenic molecules to immune autologous T cells or by feeding myelin or encephalitogenic proteins (oral tolerance). In addition, considerable attention is being focused on the use of cytokines that regulate immunity. One of these, transforming growth factor-β, has recently been shown to be quite effective in the treatment of EAE. It is critical to identify the mechanisms responsible for T-cell migration to the central nervous system and to determine where antigen recognition occurs and how this produces demyelination. Most workers agree that demyelination is largely mediated by macrophages as origi-

nally described by Lampert. Electron microscopy of demyelinating lesions in EAE has shown the presence of macrophages binding myelin via coated pits in a manner indistinguishable from that occurring in MS, but the underlying mechanisms that direct macrophages to myelin are unknown.

Chronic EAE and chronic relapsing EAE have been produced [1–3] and differ from classic acute EAE by exhibiting closer resemblance to MS with regard to both the clinical course of the disease and the extent of demyelination that occurs. Such models are important in the investigation of immune regulation, the pathogenesis of lesions in white matter, and the use of experimental treatments for modification of disease. Initially, Stone, Raine, Wisniewsky, and colleagues showed that chronic relapsing EAE could be produced in guinea pigs by the injection of whole central nervous system tissue in contrast to injection with MBP. These findings have led to speculation that the chronic disease was in part due to immune reactivity against components of myelin other than MBP. This is supported by the recent demonstrations that PLP is encephalitogenic and that antibodies to MOG can contribute to the pathogenesis of this disease. However, in some species, including rats, monkeys, and mice, chronic relapsing disease has been produced by the adoptive transfer of cells sensitized to MBP, and Zanvill and co-workers have produced chronic relapsing EAE in PL mice after transfer of T-cell clones that react with a single epitope of MBP.

The studies on chronic relapsing EAE illustrate two important points: (a) Immune reactivity to components other than MBP may significantly contribute to the clinical and pathological findings in some models and (b) a clonal T-cell response to MBP is sufficient to give rise to chronic relapsing disease, at least in mice. While the underlying mechanisms are not known, it is possible that the initial disease produced by T-cell reactivity to MBP leads to sensitization against other myelin components.

With regard to Guillain-Barré syndrome (GBS) and other demyelinating diseases of the peripheral nervous system [1,2,8,9], it should be kept in mind that, although peripheral and central nervous system myelin are morphologically similar, they differ significantly in chemical composition, especially in protein constituents (see Chaps. 6 and 36). Immunocytochemical studies have indicated that the peripheral nervous system myelin proteins (P0, P1, P2, and MAG) are decreased or absent in demyelinated regions of nerve obtained at biopsy or autopsy from persons with GBS. Cumulative evidence suggests that nerve injury is mediated by immunological mechanisms, but, as in MS, the role of the patients' cell-mediated and humoral responses in causing the demyelination has not been fully defined. A role of humoral immunity in the disease is suggested by findings that sera from GBS patients cause demyelination in appropriate test systems and that plasmapheresis is an effective therapy in many of these patients.

Although experimental allergic neuritis (EAN) is often considered to be a good animal model of GBS in humans and the P2 myelin protein is implicated as an important antigen in this model (see Chap. 36), neither cellular nor humoral immunity to P2 or other myelin proteins has been detected consistently in GBS. Similarly, although antibodies to galactocerebroside have been shown to cause peripheral demyelination in experimental animals, evidence for significant levels of antibodies to this glycolipid in GBS is lacking. Antibodies to more complex glycolipids, including gangliosides, have been detected in some GBS patients [8,9], and antibodies to G_{M1} ganglioside are particularly associated with a severe form of GBS following *Campylobacter* infection.

In addition to GBS, which is by definition acute and monophasic, there are also chronic relapsing forms of inflammatory demyelinating neuropathy. Antibodies to gangliosides and other glycolipids have been detected in some of these patients as well. However, it remains to be established whether the antiglycolipid antibodies are directly relevant to the pathology in acute and chronic inflammatory polyneuropathies. In general, although immune mechanisms often triggered by viral agents are thought to be very important in these conditions, the situation is similar to that of MS affecting the central nervous system, in that no single antigen has been shown to be a target for autoimmune attack in most patients.

In contrast to the inability to demonstrate a strong immune response against a known myelin antigen in MS or most GBS patients, the presence of antibodies reacting with a myelin protein have been demonstrated clearly in a rarer form of demyelinating peripheral neuropathy (see also Chap. 36). This type of neuropathy occurs in association with paraproteinemia (also called gammopathy), which results from the expansion of a clone of plasma cells leading to large amounts of a monoclonal antibody in the patient's serum. About one-half of the monoclonal IgM antibodies occurring in patients with this type of neuropathy have been shown to bind to MAG [5,9,10]. All of these human anti-MAG monoclonal antibodies bind to an antigenic determinant in the carbohydrate part of the MAG molecule. This carbohydrate antigen is also present on some glycolipids and other glycoproteins that are present in the peripheral nervous system but generally absent from the central nervous system. The principal antigenic glycolipid has been identified as sulfate-3-glucuronyl paragloboside (SGPG). There are also 19- to 28-kDa glycoproteins of peripheral nervous system myelin in humans and some other species that express the reactive epitope. The specificity of these human antibodies is very similar to that of the HNK-1 antibody, which reacts with a number of adhesion proteins in the nervous system (see Chap. 6).

Several animal models involving administration of the human antibodies and/or immunization with the glycolipid antigen strongly suggest that this disease is caused by the antibodies. However, the relative importance of MAG, glycolipids, or other glycoproteins as target antigens responsible for the pathology has not been determined. Reduction of the circulating antibody levels by plasmapheresis or other methods has been shown to be beneficial to some, but not all, of these patients.

In other patients with demyelinating neuropathy in association with paraproteinemia, in which the monoclonal IgM antibodies do not react with MAG and SGPG, the antibodies often react with various ganglioside antigens of nerve [10]. However, a causal relationship between these antiganglioside antibodies and the demyelination also remains to be established. Nevertheless, it may be significant that antibodies reacting with acidic glycolipid antigens are relatively common in patients with demyelinating neuropathies, including those with IgM paraproteinemia and monoclonal antibodies to SGPG (and MAG) or gangliosides, as well as some with inflammatory demyelinating neuropathies and polyclonal antibodies to gangliosides (see previous section).

Other acquired demyelinating diseases in humans may be secondary to viral infections, neoplasia, or immunosuppressive therapy

Acute disseminated encephalomyelitis, also called postinfectious or postimmunization encephalitis, represents a group of disorders of usually mixed viral-immunological etiol-ogy. The condition is most commonly related to a spontaneous viral infection of which major examples are measles, smallpox, or chickenpox [1,2]. The demyelination occurring in these conditions is likely to be mediated at least in part by immune mechanisms, since T cells sensitized to MBP are detected in many of these patients [3].

There is currently much interest in the prominent neural pathology that occurs in a high proportion of patients with acquired immunodeficiency syndrome (AIDS) [11]. Abnormalities related to myelin include a generalized myelin pallor observed histologically, vacuolar myelopathy, and focal demyelination. The biochemical changes associated with pallor and vacuolar myelopathy are unknown, but currently under investigation. It is of some interest that the surface GP120 protein of the human immunodeficiency virus (HIV), which binds to the CD4 receptor during cellular infection, also binds to galactocerebroside with high affinity [12]. Also, antibodies to this glycolipid inhibit viral internalization in two CD4$^-$ neural cell lines, suggesting that galactocerebroside may mediate an interaction of the virus with oligodendrocytes. However, HIV infection in the nervous system *in vivo* is generally believed to be restricted to macrophages and microglia. It is thought that myelin damage associated with HIV may be mediated by cytokines released by infected macrophages or lymphocytes (see section on toxins below).

Progressive multifocal leukoencephalopathy (PML) is historically a rare demyelinating disease that is usually associated with disorders of the reticuloendothelial system, neoplasia, and immunosuppressive therapy [1,2]. However, it is becoming increasingly important in clinical medicine because it is frequently seen as one of the opportunistic secondary infections associated with immunocompromised persons with AIDS. Progressive multifocal leukoencephalopathy is characterized by focal lesions that are noninflammatory and are caused by infection of oligodendrocytes with the JC papovavirus.

A number of animal diseases caused by viruses involve primary demyelination and are often associated with inflammation

Diseases involving demyelination and inflammation are studied as animal models that may provide clues about how a viral infection could lead to the immune-mediated demyelination that is believed to occur in MS [1–4]. Canine distemper virus causes a demyelinating disease, and the lesions in dog brain show a strong inflammatory response with some similarities to acute disseminated encephalomyelitis in man [1]. Visna is a slowly progressive demyelinating disease of sheep caused by a retrovirus [1,2,4]. Interest in this animal model has increased as a result of the myelin pathology in neuroAIDS and recent interest in the possible involvement of a retrovirus in multiple sclerosis. Border disease is another disorder of myelin in sheep and results from prenatal infection with a pestivirus [1]. However, in contrast to the other viral diseases described here that cause demyelination, this is a condition in which the virus interferes with developmental myelinogenesis resulting in a hypomyelination similar to that in the genetic mutants discussed later.

Two neurotropic viruses of mice are of particular interest with regard to how immune-mediated demyelination of the central nervous system can be induced by a viral infection. JHM virus is a neurotropic strain of mouse hepatitis virus in the coronavirus family that infects oligodendrocytes and produces acute and chronic inflammatory demyelination in rodents [1–4]. The acute phase is probably a direct cytopathic effect from the infection of oligodendrocytes, but the chronic phase appears to involve immune mechanisms directed against myelin. Rats infected with JHM virus develop T-cell sensitization to both viral antigens and MBP and lymphocytes from these animals produce typical EAE when transferred to normal recipients. Theiler's virus encephalomyelitis is a chronic, picornavirus-induced disease of the central nervous system in which many cell types are infected [2–4]. Although there are inflammatory demyelinating lesions in this disease, the immune response does not appear to be directed against myelin itself, but rather against viral antigens, some of which may be expressed on the surfaces of infected oligodendrocytes.

GENETICALLY DETERMINED DISORDERS OF MYELIN

The leukodystrophies are a large group of inherited disorders of central nervous system white matter characterized by a diffuse deficiency of myelin

Some of the common diseases in humans, with onset usually prior to 10 years of age, are summarized in Table 1. Included among them are sphingolipidoses in which a specific lipid accumulates due to a genetic lesion in an enzyme that is involved in its catabolism, e.g., Krabbe's disease and metachromatic leukodystrophy (MLD). More details about the histology and enzymology of these diseases are given in Chap. 38. The composition of myelin in the genetically determined disorders can be normal, have a specific alteration reflecting the genetic lesion, or show a nonspecific pathological composition that is found in many myelin disorders. The composition of the small amount of myelin isolated from Krabbe's disease is normal, and the hypomyelination is believed to be caused by the accumulation of galactosylsphingosine (psychosine), which has a cytotoxic effect on myelin forming cells. By contrast, myelin isolated from postmortem MLD brain is enriched in sulfatide (Table 2). It is not known for certain if the myelin formed in MLD is unstable because of the excess sulfatide and degenerates (thus being a true dysmyelination according to the definition at the beginning of this chapter) or if the excess sulfatide is due to sulfatide-enriched micelles that are co-isolated during the myelin purification.

In some genetic disorders such as adrenoleukodystrophy (ALD) and Canavan's disease (spongy degeneration), as well as in a wide variety of disorders involving secondary demyelination, the myelin preparations have similar, abnormal chemical compositions. This is shown in Table 2 for Canavan's disease and subacute sclerosing panencephalomyelitis. Certain experimental disorders induced in animals by toxic agents show the same type of abnormal myelin. In each case,

the isolated pathological myelin has a generally normal ultrastructural appearance, but has much more cholesterol, less cerebroside, and less phosphatidal ethanolamine than does normal myelin. Myelin with this abnormal composition is referred to as the nonspecific pathological type and probably represents a partially degraded form.

The clinical severity of X-linked ALD

TABLE 1.   Genetically determined disorders affecting myelin in humans

Disorder	Inheritance	Genetic lesion	Comments	Reference
Krabbe's leukodystrophy	AR[a]	Galactocerebroside-β-galactosidase	Globoid cells contain galactocerebroside; see text	1, 2 and Chap. 38
Metachromatic leukodystrophy	AR	Aryl sulfatase A	Accumulation of sulfatide in brain; see text and Table 2	1, 2 and Chap. 38
Refsum's disease	AR	Oxidation of branched-chain fatty acids	Increase of branched-chain phytanic acid; especially prominent in peripheral nervous system myelin	1, 2 and Chap. 38
Adrenoleukodystrophy	X-linked	Peroxidation of very long-chain fatty acids	Increased levels of saturated, very-long-chain fatty acids in brain, adrenal cortex, and other tissues, especially in cholesterol esters and gangliosides; see text and Table 2	1, 2 and 13, and Chap. 38
Canavan's disease (spongy degeneration)	AR	Aspartoacylase	Widespread edema in white matter with diminished myelin; N-acetylaspartic aciduria; see text and Table 2	1, 14 and Chap. 39
Pelizaeus-Merzbacher disease (classic and connatal forms)	X-linked	PLP	Severe hypomyelination due to different mutations in the major structural protein of central nervous system myelin; similar to rodent mutants such as the jimpy mouse	1, 15 and 16
Phenylketonuria	AR	Phenylalanine hydroxylase	White matter is up to 40 percent deficient in myelin; hypomyelination may be caused by inhibition of amino acid transport and/or protein synthesis by the high level of phenylalanine that accumulates	1 and Chap. 39

[a] (AR) autosomal recessive.

TABLE 2.   Human myelin composition in three diseases compared with controls[a]

Lipids[b]	Control	Spongy degeneration	Subacute sclerosing panencephalitis	Metachromatic leukodystrophy
TOTAL LIPID (% of dry weight)	70.0	63.8	73.7	63.2
Cholesterol	27.7	58.0	43.7	21.2
Cerebrosides	22.7	8.0	18.8	9.0
Sulfatides	3.8	2.0	2.8	28.4
TOTAL PHOSPHOLIPIDS	43.1	33.4	36.6	36.1
Ethanolamine phosphatides	15.6	9.8	9.7	8.1
Plasmalogen[c]	12.3		9.1	5.3
Lecithin	11.2	11.3	10.4	10.7
Sphingomyelin	7.9	5.9	8.8	7.1
Serine phosphatides	4.8	5.5	4.6	3.8
Phosphatidylinositol	0.6	0.8	1.4	3.1

[a] Data are from Tables I and II in chapter by Norton and Cammer in ref. [1].
[b] Individual lipids expressed as weight percentage of total lipid; see also Chap. 5.
[c] Most of the plasmalogen is phosphatidal ethanolamine and is also included in the ethanolamine phosphatides column.

(Chap. 38) is very different from patient to patient despite the similar enzymatic defect in the oxidation of very long-chain fatty acids [13]. It can vary from a major neurological problem in the childhood form with a severe deficiency of myelin in the brain to a milder form known as adrenomyeloneuropathy, which occurs in young men and affects primarily spinal cord and peripheral nerve, to less common phenotypes without neurological involvement. Unlike most other lipid storage diseases, active ALD brain lesions are characterized by perivascular accumulation of lymphocytes, and it has been hypothesized that the enzyme defect itself is not sufficient to cause the myelin deficit, but that it is caused by an autoimmune reaction that varies from patient to patient [13]. Since ALD involves inflammation, it is not surprising that substantial amounts of cholesterol ester accumulate in the brain. In ALD and other disorders in which myelin debris is phagocytosed, most of the cholesterol esters are in an abnormal floating fraction of lower density than the isolated myelin when the tissue homogenates are fractionated on sucrose gradients.

A growing number of mutations that lead to hypomyelination in mice and other experimental animals have been identified and are of particular value to neurochemists because of insights that they give with regard to the structure and assembly of myelin

These mutants often have names relating to their characteristic tremor due to the myelin deficit, e.g. shiverer, jimpy, quaking, and trembler mice. Several more detailed reviews of these mutants are available [1,16–19]. Analyses of whole homogenates of central or peripheral nervous system tissue from the mutants generally reveal a deficiency of all characteristic myelin lipids (e.g., galactocerebroside and phosphatidal ethanolamine) and proteins, even when the genetic defect only directly affects one of the myelin proteins (see chapter by Quarles in ref. [17]). This implies that there is a coordinated expression of myelin lipids and proteins that is interrupted when one component is abnormal. The magnitude of the deficiencies varies with the severity of the hypomyelination. Generally, the deficiencies of MBP, PLP, and P0 glycoprotein are greater than those of the myelin-associated enzyme 2′, 3′-cyclic nucleoside-3′-phosphodiesterase (CNPase) and MAG, presumably because the mutants exhibit a greater deficiency of compact myelin than of associated oligodendroglial or Schwann cell membranes in which the latter components are localized (see Chap. 6). Although some of the mutants have been studied for many years [1], it is only recently that recombinant DNA techniques have lead to identification of their primary genetic defects.

Mutation of Genes for the Major Proteins of Central Nervous System Myelin, e.g., Shiverer and Jimpy Mice

Mutation of either of the major structural proteins of CNS myelin can lead to a severe dysmyelination: MBP in shiverer and myelin-deficient (mld) mice [18] and PLP in jimpy mice, myelin-deficient (md) rats and shaking dogs [16,17,19]. Ultrastructural abnormalities in the small amount of myelin that is formed by these mutants have been informative with regard to the structural roles of these proteins in compact myelin. Thus the cytoplasmic surfaces of the spiralled oligodendrocyte membranes do not compact to form a major dense line in the absence of MBP in shiverer mutants, and the intraperiod line is abnormal in jimpy mice and md rats, which have little or no PLP (see Chap. 6). The ultrastructure of peripheral nervous system myelin is normal in both of these mutants, since PLP is not in peripheral myelin and P0 appears to be capable of stabilizing both the intraperiod and major dense lines of myelin of the peripheral nervous system in the absence of MBP. In addition to the severe deficiency and abnormal structure of central nervous system myelin, jimpy and the other mutants in which PLP is affected also exhibit a profound loss of oligodendrocytes [19]. This has fostered interest in the possibility that, in addition to a function in myelin structure, PLP or its DM20 isoform may have another essential role in cellular differentiation such as intercellular signaling or functioning as a channel.

The shiverer phenotype can be corrected by introducing normal MBP into transgenic mutant mice resulting in almost complete correction of the shivering, early death, and failure of central nervous system myelin compaction [18]. The gene for PLP is on the X chromosome, so all of the mutants in which PLP is altered exhibit sex-linked inheritance. Most cases of human leukodystrophy diagnosed as congenital Pelizaeus-Merzbacher disease (see Table 1) are also due to mutations of the PLP gene [15,16].

Mutations of Genes Encoding Proteins Different From the Major Structural Components of Myelin, e.g., Quaking and Trembler Mice

The autosomal recessive quaking mutation in mice results in a hypomyelination of both the central and nervous systems [1]. Unlike the shiverer and jimpy mice, which form almost no myelin and die early, quaking mice generate more myelin and live to adulthood. However, the myelin sheaths are thin and poorly compacted, especially in the central nervous system, which is more severely affected than the peripheral nervous system. Although the myelin isolated from the central nervous system of this mutant has all the known myelin proteins, its overall composition resembles that of very immature 7- to 10-day-old normal mice. The identity of the mutated gene in the quaking mouse has not yet been determined, but it is believed to affect the assembly of myelin.

The trembler mutation is autosomal dominant and specific for the peripheral nervous system [1]. Several approaches, including nerve graft experiments, demonstrated that the genetic defect resides in Schwann cells. Cloning experiments determined that a quantitatively minor 22-kDa glycoprotein in peripheral nervous system myelin exhibits point mutations in two allelic forms of this mutant [20], strongly suggesting that this is the cause of the abnormal phenotype. This protein is not specifically associated with peripheral nervous system myelin, since its cDNA had previously been cloned from fibroblasts. The transcribed "growth arrest" mRNA is only expressed when the cells are not dividing. Interestingly, trembler Schwann cells differ from normal Schwann cells by continuing to proliferate after 2 weeks of age, and this mutation could cause prolonged proliferation, thereby preventing sufficient differentiation to allow normal myelination.

TOXIC AND NUTRITIONAL DISORDERS OF MYELIN

Biological toxins that produce myelin loss can be produced by exogenous infectious agents (e.g., diphtheria toxin) or lymphocytes (cytokines)

Diphtheritic neuropathy [1] is a possible complication of *Corynebacterium diphtheriae* infection and is characterized by vacuolation and fragmentation of myelin sheaths in the PNS (see Chap. 36). A similar disorder can be caused by injection of animals with the toxin, which may act by inhibiting protein synthesis in Schwann cells or by binding to myelin and producing channels in the membrane.

Some cytokines released by lymphocytes, such as tumor necrosis factor and lymphotoxin, have been shown to be toxic to oligodendrocytes in culture [21]. As a result there is much ongoing research concerning the role of cytokines in demyelinating diseases, such as multiple sclerosis, that are associated with immune reactions. These toxins could lead to myelin destruction independently of whether the immune reaction is targeted against myelin or an exogenous infectious agent. Damage to myelin by an immune reaction directed to an unrelated antigen is referred to as a bystander effect [4].

Organotin and hexachlorophene cause edematous demyelination with splitting at the intraperiod line and without apparent damage to myelin-forming cells

A number of biochemical studies have been performed with the triethyltin model [1], brought about by the inclusion of this compound in the drinking water of rats. Chronic administration of triethyltin may result in a loss of one-fourth to one-half of the total myelin relative to untreated control animals. The myelin isolated is of the nonspecific pathological type with high cholesterol and low cerebroside, sulfatide, and ethanolamine plasmalogen. The massive myelin loss is not accompanied by inflammatory cells, and the levels of various proteinases are not elevated as they are in such disorders as EAE. The mechanism by which myelin is damaged under these conditions is unknown, although there is evidence suggesting that it may involve inhibition of enzymes and transport mechanisms (see Chap. 3). Nevertheless, the myelin loss clearly contrasts with the situation observed in the allergic and acquired infectious demyelinating disorders. Interestingly, there may be almost complete recovery of myelin after triethyltin is removed from the drinking water. Hexachlorophene is another agent that causes a similar reversible edematous demyelination [1] and that is of clinical significance because it was used as an antiseptic agent for humans.

In neurochemical studies on this type of disorder, loss of myelin is an operational term since part of the myelin is converted to a form with different physical properties that is not isolated with normal myelin. Some of the myelin is converted to an even lighter "floating fraction," containing many myelin components [1]. This fraction probably represents degenerating myelin and does not contain cholesterol esters. It must be emphasized that this type of floating fraction is different from the cholesterol ester-rich floating fractions mentioned earlier that can be isolated in some inflammatory demyelinating diseases.

Lead is a common environmental pollutant that causes hypomyelination and demyelination

Suckling rats exposed to high doses of lead salts fail to myelinate normally in the central nervous system [1] apparently due to retarded growth and maturation of neurons, but the peripheral nervous system is not affected. Trialkyllead administration to animals does not cause edematous demyelination as is seen with trialkyltin, but it does inhibit myelinogenesis in rats when administered to developing animals. In addition, lead can cause segmental demyelination of the peripheral nervous system in rodents. Effects of lead poisoning vary with species, age, dosage, and region of the nervous system.

Tellurium treatment of young rats causes a demyelinating neuropathy

A highly synchronous demyelination and remyelination is produced in rat sciatic nerve that is associated with the inhibition of cholesterol synthesis by some metabolite of this element [22]. It provides an interesting experimental model since it dissociates the axonal signal known to be needed for Schwann cell differentiation from the process of myelin assembly. It is especially interesting that proteins associated with nonmyelinating Schwann cells, such as the nerve growth factor receptor and GFAP, are selectively expressed in internodes undergoing demyelination and are even selectively targeted to particular areas that are undergoing myelin breakdown within one internode.

Undernourishment leads to a preferential reduction in myelin formation

Much of the central nervous system myelin in mammals is formed during a relatively restricted time period of development, corresponding to the final prenatal months and the first few years of postnatal life in humans and 15 to 30 days of postnatal life in rats. Just before this rapid deposition of myelin, there is a burst of oligodendroglial cell proliferation. During these restricted periods of time, a large portion of the brain's metabolic activity and protein and lipid synthetic capacities are involved in myelinogenesis. This developmental phenomenon has practical input for the understanding of hypomyelinating disorders. Any metabolic insult during this "vulnerable period" may lead to a preferential reduction in myelin formation [1].

A model system for such studies is obtained by limiting access of rat pups to the mother and thus inducing undernourishment. Starvation of rats from birth onward leads to a deficit of myelin lipids and proteins and a reduction in the amount of myelin that can be isolated in comparison to normally fed littermate controls. The size of whole brain is also somewhat reduced, but it is clear that the depression of myelin-specific lipids and proteins is greater than that of other brain components. The implication is that there is preferential depression in the synthesis of myelin-specific components during starvation, an interpretation that has been directly demonstrated by *in vivo* isotope incorporation experiments.

Possibly there is not only depression in the amount of myelin deposited (in part due to a lessened number of oligodendroglial cells), but also the developmental program with regard to myelinogenesis is somewhat delayed. The most vulnerable period appears to be the time of oligodendroglia proliferation, since animals deprived in this period have an irreversible deficit of myelin-forming cells and hypomyelination. However, animals deprived at a later age can often demonstrate significant catch-up with regard to the amount of myelin when nutritional rehabilitation is instigated after a period of underfeeding.

Dietary deficiencies of specific substances can cause myelin deficits

Failure to myelinate properly and demyelination are also associated with deficiencies of dietary protein, essential fatty acids, and several vitamins, including thiamine, B_{12}, and B_6 [1] (see also Chap. 35). Hypomyelination also has been shown to be caused by copper deficiency in animals [1], and this model system may be an experimental analog of the sex-linked inherited disorder called Menkes' kinky hair disease in which there appears to be a disorder in copper transport (see Chap. 3).

DISORDERS PRIMARILY AFFECTING NEURONS WITH SECONDARY INVOLVEMENT OF MYELIN

Many insults to the nervous system initially cause damage to neurons but eventually result in regions of demyelination as a consequence of neuronal degeneration. These include mechanical trauma, infarcts, tumors, viral diseases (subacute sclerosing panencephalitis), genetic diseases (Tay-Sachs disease), or diseases of unknown etiology (amyotrophic lateral sclerosis).

The archetypical model for secondary demyelination is Wallerian degeneration

When a nerve (in the peripheral nervous system) or a myelinated tract (in the central nervous system) is cut or crushed, the proximal segment often survives and regenerates [1]. In the distal segment, Wallerian degeneration occurs with both axons and myelin disappearing rapidly (see Chap. 36). Debris is phagocytosed by neural cells and by macrophages. From such experiments, it is clear that the integrity of the myelin sheath depends on continued contact with a viable axon. Any disease that causes injury to neurons may result in axonal degeneration and lead to the onset of myelin breakdown secondary to the neuronal damage.

During Wallerian degeneration in the peripheral nervous system, there is a rapid loss of myelin-specific lipids within a period of a week or two and even more rapid loss of myelin-specific proteins. There is also a concomitant increase in many lysosomal enzymes. Between the second and fourth weeks after nerve section most of the myelin debris has been removed by Schwann cells, and remyelination of regenerating axons begins.

Wallerian degeneration has been studied in the central nervous system by enucleating eyes in rats and examining the optic nerve at different times. The degeneration of myelin in the central nervous system is a much slower process than in the peripheral nervous system and takes place within macrophages (not within the myelin-synthesizing cells, as in the peripheral nervous system). By using this system, it has been demonstrated that the myelin isolated after enucleation, although present in decreasing amounts as degeneration progresses, does not differ significantly in composition from control myelin. It is not of the nonspecific pathological type encountered in other disease processes that lead to secondary demyelination. This may indicate a significant difference from the degenerative demyelination that follows naturally occurring disease processes (also generally referred to as Wallerian degeneration by neuropathological criteria) in which the myelin is of the nonspecific pathological type (see below).

Secondary demyelination occurs in subacute sclerosing panencephalitis and other diseases of the central nervous system

The first human disease to be studied with respect to myelin composition during secondary demyelination was subacute sclerosing panencephalitis, a central nervous system disease caused by a defective measles virus infection [1]. It is probable that this disease involves destruction of both neurons and oligodendroglia. The isolated myelin has a grossly normal ultrastructural appearance and a normal lipid/protein ratio. However, it was found to have the typical nonspecific changes with more cholesterol, less cerebroside, and less ethanolamine phosphatides than normal human myelin (Table

2). No cholesterol esters are found in the myelin, although they are abundant in the white matter. Abnormal myelin of this type has also been isolated from such sphingolipidoses as Tay-Sachs disease, generalized gangliosidosis, and Niemann-Pick disease (see Chap. 38).

REMYELINATION

The capacity for remyelination is much greater in the peripheral nervous system than the central nervous system

Much of this chapter has considered biochemical mechanisms of myelin loss, but the capacity of nervous tissue to repair the damage by remyelination is also an important factor in the eventual clinical outcome of disorders affecting myelin. Following transection of peripheral nerve, as described in the previous section, myelination of the regenerating axons occurs soon after the final clean up of myelin debris by Schwann cells [1]. The Schwann cells that form the new myelin are probably not the same ones that phagocytose the debris, but appear to arise by cell division. As expected, biochemical experiments have shown increased incorporation of radioactive precursors into myelin components during the remyelination phase. The difference in remyelinating ability between the peripheral and the central nervous systems may lie in the nature of the myelinforming cells, i.e., in the requirement for oligodendrocytes to myelinate many axons in contrast to the single segments of myelin formed by Schwann cells. Under some circumstances, such as in EAE and multiple sclerosis, it has been demonstrated that Schwann cells will migrate into the spinal cord and remyelinate demyelinated central nervous system axons.

Remyelination in the central nervous system can be promoted by various treatments, and therapy of human myelin disorders by this approach may be feasible

In spite of the limited remyelination that generally occurs in the central nervous sys-

tem, there has been increased interest recently in the capacity of oligodendrocytes to remyelinate. In part, this has developed in response to observations in experimental animals; e.g., the demonstration that administration of MBP and galactocerebroside to activate suppressor mechanisms in animals with chronic EAE led to both clinical improvement and greater remyelination [2]. In addition, careful observations of acute multiple sclerosis lesions have demonstrated the presence of healthy oligodendrocytes and regeneration of myelin in the presence of myelin breakdown [2]. These lesions contain many cells that appear to be immature oligodendrocytes expressing galactocerebroside and the adhesion-related, HNK-1 carbohydrate epitope that differentiate and begin to remyelinate [23]. Although the remyelination attempt eventually fails and oligodendrocytes are lost from lesions that progress to advanced demyelinated plaques, such observations raise the possibility that management of patients with demyelinating diseases of the central nervous system may eventually involve treatments that stimulate the natural ability of the oligodendrocytes for remyelination.

Remyelination following transient demyelination induced by chemical agents or by murine hepatitis virus in experimental animals is the subject of current research [24]. The results indicate that substantial remyelination occurs, much of it by proliferation and differentiation of O-2A progenitor cells, which are quiescent in normal tissue. *In situ* hybridization studies during remyelination suggest that the differentiating oligodendrocytes recapitulate changes in the expression of mRNAs for myelin proteins observed in normal development. Oligodendrocyte progenitor cells also have been identified in cultures of cells isolated from adult human brain [24]. In addition, there is much interest in growth factors that affect the proliferation and/or differentiation of oligodendrocytes and their progenitors, including insulin-like growth factor, epidermal growth factor, basic fibroblast growth factor, and platelet-derived growth factor [24]. It is feasible that remyelination in patients might be promoted by treatments that increase such factors. Another approach under investigation in experimental models is the capacity of transplants of myelin-forming glial cells to repair demyelinated lesions [25]. Eventually, the treatment of myelin disorders in humans may involve promotion of remyelination as well as prevention of myelin breakdown.

REFERENCES

1. Morell, P. *Myelin* New York: Plenum, 1984.
2. Vinken, P. J., Bruyn, G. W., Klawans, H. L., and Koetsier, J. C. *Handbook of Clinical Neurology, Vol. 47, Demyelinating Diseases.* Amsterdam: Elsevier, 1985.
3. Martin, M., McFarland, H. F., and McFarlin, D. E. Immunological aspects of demyelinating diseases. *Annu. Rev. Immunol.* 10:153–187, 1992.
4. Rodriguez, M. Multiple sclerosis: Basic concepts and hypothesis. *Mayo Clin Proc* 64: 570–576, 1989.
5. Quarles, R. H., Colman, D. R., Salzer, J. L., and Trapp, B. D. Myelin-associated glycoprotein: Structure-function relationships and involvement in neurological diseases. In Martenson, R. E., (ed.), *Myelin: Biology and Chemistry.* Boca Raton, FL: CRC Press, 1992, pp. 413–448.
6. Banik, N. L., Chakrabarti, A. K., and Hogan, E. L. Calcium-activated neutral proteinase in myelin: Its role and function. In Martenson, R. E., (ed.), *Myelin: Biology and Chemistry.* Boca Raton, FL: CRC Press, 1992, pp. 571–598.
7. Gunn, C., Stuckling, A. J., and Linington, C. Identification of a common idiotype on oligodendrocyte-myelin glycoprotein-specific autoantibodies in chronic relapsing experimental allergic encephalomyelitis. *J. Neuroimmunol.* 23:101–108, 1989.
8. Hughes, R. A. C. *Guillain-Barré Syndrome.* Heidelberg: Springer-Verlag, 1990.
9. Asbury, A. K., and Gibbs, C. J. *Autoimmune neuropathies: Guillain-Barré syndrome, Ann. Neurol.* Vol. 27, Supplement. Boston: Little, Brown, 1990.
10. Quarles, R. H. Human monoclonal antibodies associated with neuropathy. *Methods Enzymol.* 179:291–299, 1989.
11. Dubois-Dalcq, M. E., Jordan, C. A., Kelly, W. B., and Watkins, B. A. Understanding HIV1 infection of the brain: A challenge for neurobiologists. *Curr Sci* 4(Suppl.):S67–S76, 1990.
12. Harouse, J. M., Bhat, S., Spitalnik, S. L., Laughlin, M., Stefano, K., Silberberg, D. H., and Gonzalez-Scarano, F. Inhibition of entry of HIV-1 in neural cell lines by antibodies against galactosyl ceramide. *Science* 253: 320–322, 1991.
13. Moser, H. W., and Moser, A. B. Adrenoleukodystrophy (X-linked). In Scriver, C. R., Beaudet, A. L., Sly, W. S., Valle, D. (eds.), *The Metabolic Basis of Inherited Diseases. 6th Ed.* New York: McGraw Hill, 1989, pp. 1511–1532.
14. Matalon, R., Kaul, R., Casanova, J., Michals, K., Johnson, A. B., Rapin, I., Gashkoff, P., and Deanching, M. Aspartoacylase deficiency: The enzyme defect in Canavan disease. *J. Inherit. Metab. Dis.* 12(Suppl. 2):329–331, 1989.
15. Koeppen, A. H. Pelizaeus-Merzbacher disease: X-linked proteolipid protein deficiency in the human central nervous system. In Martenson, R. E. (ed.), *Myelin: Biology and Chemistry.* Boca Raton, FL: CRC Press, 1992, pp. 703–722.
16. Hudson, L. D., and Nadon, N. L. Amino acid substitutions in proteolipid protein that cause dysmyelination. In Martenson, R. E. (ed.), *Myelin: Biology and Chemistry.* Boca Raton, FL: CRC Press, 1992, pp. 677–702.
17. Duncan, I. A., Skoff, R. P., and Colman, D. *Myelination and dysmyelination.* New York: New York Academy of Sciences, 1990.
18. Mikoshiba, K., Aruga, J., Ikenaka, K., and Okano, H. Shiverer and allelic mutant mld mice. In Martenson, R. E., (ed.), *Myelin: Biology and Chemistry.* Boca Raton, FL: CRC Press, 1992, pp. 723–744.
19. Skoff, R. P., and Knapp, P. E. Phenotypic expression of X-linked genetic defects affecting myelination. In Martenson, R. E. (ed.), *Myelin: Biology and Chemistry.* Boca Raton FL: CRC Press, 1992, pp. 653–676.
20. Suter, U., Moskow, J. J., Welcher, A. A., Snipes, G. J., Kosaras, B., Sidman, R. L., Buchberg, A. M., and Shooter, E. M. A leucine to proline mutation in the putative first transmembrane domain of the 22 kDA peripheral myelin protein in the trembler-J

mouse. *Proc. Natl. Acad. Sci. U. S. A.* 89: 4382–4386, 1992.

21. Selmaj, K., Raine, C. S., Farooq, M., Norton, W. T., and Brosnan, C. F. Cytokine cytotoxicity against oligodendrocytes. Apoptosis induced by lymphotoxin. *J. Immunol.* 147: 1522–1529, 1991.

22. Wagner-Recio, M., Toews, A. D., and Morell P. Tellurium blocks cholesterol synthesis by inhibiting squalene metabolism: Preferential vulnerability to this metabolic block leads to peripheral nervous system demyelination. *J. Neurochem.* 57:1891–1901, 1991.

23. Prineas, J. W., Kwon, E. E., Goldenberg, P. Z., Ilyas, A. A., Quarles, R. H., Benjamins, J. A., and Sprinkle, T. J. Multiple sclerosis: Oligodendrocyte proliferation and differentiation in fresh lesions. *Lab. Invest.* 61:489–503, 1989.

24. Dubois-Dalcq, M., and Armstrong, R. The cellular and molecular events of central nervous system remyelination. *BioEssays* 12:569–576, 1990.

25. Blakemore, W. F., and Franklin, R. J. M. Transplanation of glial cells to the CNS. *Trends Neurosci.* 14:323–327, 1991.

CHAPTER 38

Genetic Disorders of Lipid, Glycoprotein, and Mucopolysaccharide Metabolism

Kunihiko Suzuki

Basic Neurochemistry: Molecular, Cellular, and Medical Aspects, 5th Ed., edited by G. J. Siegel et al. Published by Raven Press, Ltd., New York, 1994. Correspondence to Kunihiko Suzuki, Brain and Development Research Center, CB#7250, University of North Carolina School of Medicine, Chapel Hill, North Carolina 27599.

Many neurological disorders occur as the results of genetically determined abnormal metabolism of lipids, the carbohydrate moieties of glycoproteins, or mucopolysaccharides. A majority of them have underlying metabolic abnormalities in the catabolic pathways catalyzed by a group of enzymes commonly referred to as lysosomal enzymes (lysosomal disease). A series of genetic defects of enzymes normally localized in the peroxisome have been attracting increasing attention in recent years (peroxisomal disease). A standard reference volume exists for the biochemical basis of and comprehensive bibliographies for these disorders [1]. Selected citations are listed at the end of this chapter.

LYSOSOME AND LYSOSOMAL DISEASE

The concept of the lysosome as the subcellular organelle responsible for catabolism of cellular constituents was first proposed by de Duve. It contains catabolic enzymes that are generally glycoproteins themselves and have very low pH optima for their function. Defective catalytic activity of any of these enzymes results in a block in the digestive process of the cellular materials essential for normal function. Hers [2] originated the concept of the lysosomal disease in the mid-1960s [2]. Using glycogenosis type II (Pompe's disease) as the model, Hers defined a category of genetic diseases as the "inborn lysosomal disorder" that satisfied two major criteria: (a) an acidic hydrolase normally localized in the lysosome is genetically defective and (b) as the consequence, the substrate of the defective enzyme accumulates abnormally within

pathologically altered secondary lysosomes. Over the years, several important groups of genetic disorders have been identified as belonging to the inborn lysosomal disease. Among them are the sphingolipidoses, mucopolysaccharidoses, and mucolipidoses. These disorders are often referred to as "storage diseases" because the abnormal "storage" of the undigested substrates are often the most conspicuous clinical and pathological manifestations.

PEROXISOME AND PEROXISOMAL DISEASE

The peroxisome is another of the membrane-bound subcellular organelles. It had been known morphologically as microbodies before de Duve characterized it biochemically. Known functions of the peroxisome include metabolism of pipecolic acid, dicarboxylic acids, phytanic acid and very-long-chain fatty acids, biosynthesis of plasmalogens, and biosynthesis of bile acids. Analogous to the lysosomal diseases, a group of inherited disorders are recognized as being caused by genetic defects in the peroxisomes themselves or in one of the enzymes normally localized in the peroxisome. Some of them manifest themselves as primarily neurological disorders and involve metabolic abnormalities in fatty acids.

MOLECULAR GENETICS OF LYSOSOMAL AND PEROXISOMAL DISORDERS

The past several years have witnessed a dramatic transition in studies of lysosomal-

TABLE 1.   Status of cloning of cDNAs and genes

Disease	Enzyme or activator	cDNA/gene
SPHINGOLIPIDOSIS		
Farber (lipogranulomatosis)	Ceramidase	−/−
Niemann-Pick, types A and B	Sphingomyelinase	+/+
Gaucher's	Glucosylceramidase	+/+
Krabbe's (globoid cell leukodystrophy)	Galactosylceramidase	+/−
Fabry's	α-Galactosidase A	+/+
Metachromatic leukodystrophy (MLD)	Arylsulfatase A (sulfatidase)	+/+
G$_{M1}$-gangliosidosis	β-Galactosidase	+/+
Tay-Sachs	β-Hexosaminidase α-subunit	+/+
Sandhoff's	β-Hexosaminidase β-subunit	+/+
MLD variant	Sulfatide activator (SAP-1)	+/+
Gaucher variant	β-Glucosidase activator (SAP-2)	+/+
G$_{M2}$-gangliosidosis AB variant	G$_{M2}$ activator	+/+
Galactosialidosis	Protective protein	+/+
MUCOPOLYSACCHARIDOSIS		
Hurler-Scheie syndrome (MPS I and V)	α-Iduronidase	+/−
Hunter's syndrome (MPS II)	α-Iduronate sulfatase	+/−
Sanfilippo disease (MPS III)		
Type A	Heparan N-sulfatase	−/−
Type B	N-acetyl α-glucosaminidase	−/−
Type C	N-acetyl Co A:α-glucosaminide N-acetyltransferase	−/−
Type D	N-acetyl α-glucosaminide-6-sulfatase	−/−
Morquio's disease (MPS IV)		
Type A	Type A: N-acetyl-galactosamine 6-sulfatase	+/−
Type B	Type B: β-galactosidase	+/+
Maroteaux-Lamy (MPS VI)	Arylsulfatase B	+/+
β-Glucuronidase deficiency (MPS VII)	β-Glucuronidase	+/+
GLYCOPROTEIN STORAGE DISEASE AND MUCOLIPIDOSES		
Sialidosis (Mucolipidosis I)	α-Neuraminidase (sialidase)	−/−
I-Cell disease and pseudo-Hurler polydystrophy (mucolipidoses II and III)	UDP-glcNAc:lysosomal enzyme glcNAc phosphotransferase (see text)	−/−
Mucolipidosis IV	Unknown	—
α-Mannosidosis	α-Mannosidase	−/−
β-Mannosidosis	β-Mannosidase	−/−
α-Fucosidosis	α-Fucosidase	+/+

peroxisomal disorders from those of gene products (enzymes-proteins) to the genes themselves. In most of this group of genetic disorders, the normal cDNAs and the genes responsible for the respective disorders have been isolated and characterized, and in many instances specific mutations identified (Table 1). As expected, information on the gene level is showing highly complex genetic heterogeneity of these diseases, even when they appear homogeneous in clinical manifestations, analytical biochemistry, and enzymatic defects.

Diagnosis may require genetic, enzymatic, and metabolic assays

Earlier, diagnosis of this group of disorders was primarily based on clinicopathological findings and then on identification of abnormally stored materials by analytical biochemistry. The emphasis shifted during the past two decades to enzymatic assays [3]. Enzymatic assays provided relatively easy, noninvasive antemortem diagnosis, because clinically available materials, such as serum, blood cells, cultured fibroblasts, and other biopsied tissues can be used for the purpose. These procedures can generally be used for detection of heterozygous carriers with varying degrees of reliability. Identification of affected fetuses during pregnancy is generally possible with similar procedures. The most commonly used materials for prenatal diagnosis were cultured amniotic fluid cells. In recent years, however, biopsied chorionic villi have gained popularity as the material of choice for prenatal diagnosis, because diagnoses can be achieved immediately after the procedure at a much earlier stage of pregnancy (7 to 8 weeks of gestation *vs.* 18 to 20 weeks with the use of amniocentesis and cell culture).

Unambiguous diagnosis of affected and carrier individuals is possible when specific mutations in the responsible genes are known. However, the DNA diagnosis will not replace earlier procedures, because the DNA diagnosis is too specific. It requires prior information on the nature of the mutations in the family. Negative results for any number of mutations do not exclude the possibility that the patient is affected due to yet-to-be-identified and/or untested mutations. Enzymatic and metabolic procedures have a theoretical advantage in that they test for functionality of a particular metabolic step regardless of the nature of the underlying genetic abnormality.

Treatment is progressing from enzyme or tissue replacement to gene manipulation

Replacement of the defective enzyme with the normal enzyme has been attempted through various routes, including direct injection of purified enzyme or transplantation of various normal organs or bone marrow. Earlier trials have been at best partial successes. Long-term, pragmatic benefits to patients have been variable. In recent years, a more promising outcome has been reported with replacement by enzymes that are modified to minimize undesirable uptake and removal from the circulation. Long-term beneficial effects of bone marrow transplantation is also being reported with increasing frequency. Nevertheless, identification of affected fetuses and termination of pregnancy remain the best that can be offered for a large majority of families with children affected by these devastating genetic neurological disorders. The situation could change dramatically in the next decade or two when and if treatment at the level of genes becomes a reality.

Spontaneous and transgenic animal models are tools for the study of these diseases

Many of the genetic lysosomal diseases in humans have equivalents among other mammalian species [4]. Since most of the human diseases are rare and since there are serious ethical constraints in studying human patients, these "authentic" animal models provide useful tools for studies of all aspects of these disorders, including natural history of the disease processes, pathogenesis, and therapeutic trials. These animal models, particularly those in smaller mammalian species, are expected to be used more extensively in the near future as vehicles for recombinant DNA experiments. In recent years, it has become possible to generate artificial mouse mutant strains with specific gene deficiencies with the homologous recombination and transgenic technology (see Chap. 26 for more details).

LYSOSOMAL DISEASES

Lysosomal diseases are traditionally classified according to the nature of the materials that accumulate abnormally. One should be aware that there are considerable overlaps in substrate specificities of the enzymes and that consequently the classification is merely for the purpose of convenience. For example, genetic β-galactosidase defects can result in primarily G_{M1}-ganglioside accumulation (sphingolipidosis) or bony abnormalities (mucopolysaccharidosis), depending on the nature of mutations. In both instances, degradation of carbohydrate chains of glycoproteins are also impaired (glycoprotein disorder).

SPHINGOLIPIDOSES ARE CAUSED BY GENETIC DEFECTS OF A SERIES OF LYSOSOMAL HYDROLASES INVOLVED IN DEGRADATION OF LIPIDS THAT CONTAIN SPHINGOSINE AS THE BASIC BUILDING BLOCK

Since the nervous system is rich in these lipids (see Chap. 5), many disorders in this category manifest themselves as neurological disorders. Sphingolipids are degraded by sequential removal of the terminal moieties of the hydrophilic chain (sulfate in the case of sulfatide, phosphorylcholine in the case of sphingomyelin, and sialic acid or sugar moieties in others) to ceramide and then to sphingosine and fatty acid (Fig. 1). Genetic disorders are known in humans affecting almost every step of the degradative pathway. The mode of inheritance is Mendelian autosomal recessive for all sphingolipidoses, except for Fabry's disease, which is an X-linked disorder (Table 2).

Farber's disease (ceramidosis, Farber's lipogranulomatosis)

Primary manifestations of Farber's disease are painful, progressively deformed joints, and subcutaneous granulomatous nodules in infants. Nervous system involvement is usually moderate. The nodules, lung, and heart are the main sites of abnormal accumulation of ceramide. However, ceramide levels are also increased in the central nervous system. A mild and probably nonspecific accumulation of simpler gangliosides in the brain is commonly observed. Ceramidase is yet to be cloned, and thus no information on the gene level is available.

Niemann-Pick disease

The disease was traditionally classified into types A, B, C, and D primarily according to clinical phenotypes. However, only types A and B of Niemann-Pick disease are allelic and caused by primary genetic sphingomyelinase deficiency. The designation Niemann-Pick should be used only for these two types. Patients with either type A or type B disease exhibit hepatosplenomegaly and characteristic foamy cells in the bone marrow. Type A disease usually occurs in infants and is characterized by additional severe central nervous system involvement. Patients rarely survive beyond 5 years. On the other hand, type B disease is more slowly progressive, occurring in older age groups. Despite similarly severe organomegaly, type B patients are normal in intellect and free of neurological manifestations. In both types, there is an enormous accumulation of sphingomyelin in the liver and spleen. Although available information is not extensive, a few-fold increase in sphingomyelin appears to occur in the central nervous system only in type A (neuropathic) patients. The degree of the sphingomyelinase deficiency is similar in the two types, and the reason for the dramatically different phenotypes is not known. The human gene coding for sphingomyelinase and its cDNA have been cloned, and a few mutations have been identified [1]. The number of identified mutations is not yet extensive enough for a clear genotype/phenotype correlation.

"Niemann-Pick type C"

The so-called Niemann-Pick types C and D are clinically similar in that patients exhibit

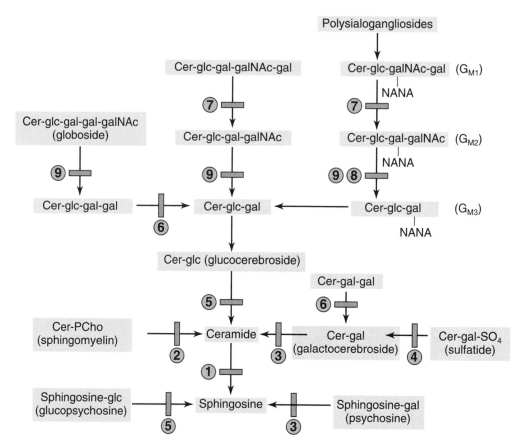

FIG. 1. Chemical and metabolic relationships among the major sphingolipids. Normal catabolic pathways are indicated by *arrows* connecting adjacent compounds. Biosynthesis of these lipids occur in the reverse direction. *Large arrows with numbers* indicate locations of genetic metabolic blocks known in humans. The numbers correspond to those in Table 2. (Cer) ceramide; (PCho) phosphorylcholine.

TABLE 2.   Major sphingolipidoses[a]

Disease	Clinicopathological manifestations	Affected lipids	Enzymatic defects
1. Farber's (lipogranulomatosis)	Mostly infantile disease, tender swollen joints, multiple subcutaneous nodules; later, flaccid paralysis and mental impairment	Ceramide	Acid ceramidase
2. Niemann-Pick	Neuropathic and non-neuropathic forms, hepatosplenomegaly, foamy cells in bone marrow, severe neurological signs in the neuropathic form (type A)	Sphingomyelin	Sphingomyelinase
3. Globoid cell leukodystrophy (Krabbe's)	Almost always infantile disease, white matter signs, peripheral neuropathy, high spinal fluid protein level, loss of myelin, globoid cells in white matter	Galactosylceramide Galactosylsphingosine	Galactosylceramidase

TABLE 2.   (continued)

Disease	Clinicopathological manifestations	Affected lipids	Enzymatic defects
4a. Metachromatic leukodystrophy	Late infantile, juvenile, and adult forms; white matter signs; peripheral neuropathy; high spinal fluid protein level; metachromatic granules in the brain, nerves, kidney, and urine	Sulfatide	Arylsulfatase A ("sulfatidase")
4b. Multiple sulfatase deficiency	Similar to metachromatic leukodystrophy, but additional gray matter signs; facial and skeletal abnormalities; organomegaly similar to mucopolysaccharidoses	Sulfatide, other sulfated compounds (see text)	Arylsulfatases A, B, C (see text)
4c. Sulfatidase activator deficiency	Similar to later onset forms of 4a	Unknown	Sulfatidase activator (SAP-1)
5a. Gaucher's	Neuropathic and non-neuropathic forms, hepatosplenomegaly, "Gaucher's cells" in bone marrow, severe neurological signs in the neuropathic form, also an intermediate form (type III)	Glucosylceramide Glucosylsphingosine	Glucosylceramidase
5b. SAP-2 deficiency	Gaucher-like clinical phenotype	Glucosylceramide	SAP-2 ("Gaucher factor")
6. Fabry's	Primarily adult and non-neurologic, angiokeratoma around buttocks, renal damage, X-linked	Trihexosylceramide (gal-gal-glc-cer) Digalactosylceramide	α-Galactosidase A (trihexosylceramidase)
7a. G_{M1}-gangliosidosis	Slow growth, motor weakness, gray matter signs, infantile form with additional facial and skeletal abnormalities and organomegaly, swollen neurons	G_{M1}-ganglioside Galactose-rich fragments of glycoproteins	G_{M1}-ganglioside β-galactosidase
7b. Galactosialidosis	Similar to late-onset form of 7a	Unknown	"Protective protein" (secondary defect in G_{M1}-ganglioside β-galactosidase and sialidase)
8a. Tay-Sachs disease	Severe gray matter signs, slow growth, motor weakness, hyperacusis, cherry-red spot, head enlargement, swollen neurons	G_{M2}-ganglioside	β-Hexosaminidase A
8b. B1 variant	Commonly later onset, slower progression but otherwise similar to Tay-Sachs disease, milder pathology	G_{M2}-ganglioside	β-Hexosaminidase A (normal against nonsulfated artificial substrates but deficient against G_{M2}-ganglioside and sulfated artificial substrate)
8c. AB variant	Similar to 8a	G_{M2}-ganglioside	G_{M2} activator protein
9. Sandhoff's	Panethnic but otherwise indistinguishable from Tay-Sachs disease	G_{M2}-ganglioside, Asialo-G_{M2}-ganglioside, globoside	β-Hexosaminidase A and B

[a] The numbers correspond to the steps of metabolic blocks in Fig. 1.

organomegaly, slowly progressive central nervous system signs, and abnormal bone marrow cells. Vertical gaze palsy is observed in almost all patients during the course of the disease. Liver and spleen show increased amounts of sphingomeylin. However, there are accompanying and usually even more severe increases in cholesterol and glucosylceramide. Sphingomyelinase activity is often, but not always, significantly lower than normal, but not enough to account for the clinical picture. Fibroblasts of "Niemann-Pick type C" and similar cases have been shown to be defective in esterifying cholesterol added exogenously to the culture medium [5,6]. Accumulation of free cholesterol can be demonstrated also by fluorescent staining with filipin. A large number of patients described in the literature with various diagnoses have been proven to be cases of "Niemann-Pick type C." They include "juvenile dystonic lipidosis," "neurovisceral storage disease with vertical supranuclear ophthalmoplegia," "lipidosis with vertical gaze palsy," "lactosylceramidosis," "maladie de Neville," and "adult neurovisceral lipidosis." These diagnostic procedures have been used successfully for prenatal diagnosis with cultured amniotic fluid cells or with chorionic villi materials. Since the abnormality is observed when cholesterol is given in the form bound to low-density lipoprotein and since direct *in vitro* assays of cholesterol-esterifying enzyme are normal, the defect should be present anywhere between these two steps. It is possible that this is a heterogeneous group of diseases with genetic defects at different steps in cholesterol uptake, intracellular routing, sequestration, and esterification. These new findings clearly argue against the designation Niemann-Pick for this disease. Conceptually, there is no evidence that "Niemann-Pick type C" disease is a sphingolipidosis.

Globoid cell leukodystrophy (Krabbe's disease)

Krabbe's disease and metachromatic leukodystrophy are two of the classic genetic myelin disorders, simply because they involve abnormal degradation of two sphingolipids highly localized in the myelin sheath, galactosylceramide and sulfatide (Fig. 1). The disease is for the most part infantile, although rarer late-onset forms are also known. Clinicopathological manifestations are almost exclusively those of the white matter and the peripheral nerves. The unique globoid cells are hematogenous histiocytic cells that infiltrate the white matter in response to undigested galactosylceramide. Unlike in all other "storage" diseases, the primary natural substrate of the defective enzyme galactosylceramide not only does not accumulate abnormally, but it is almost always much lower than normal because of a rapid and almost complete destruction of the oligodendroglia and the consequent early cessation of myelination. On the other hand, a toxic metabolite, galactosylsphingosine (psychosine) does accumulate and appears to be responsible for the devastating pathology of the disease (the psychosine hypothesis) [7,8]. Effects of psychosine, early cessation of myelination, and possibly overlapping substrate specificities between the two lysosomal β-galactosidases—galactosylceramidase and G_{MI}-ganglioside β-galactosidase—are important in understanding the pathogenesis of this disease.

Metachromatic leukodystrophy

The enzymatic defect in metachromatic leukodystrophy is one step before that in Krabbe's disease (Fig. 1). While these two diseases share many common features, as expected there are significant differences that suggest different pathogenetic mechanisms. Clinically, relatively large proportions of patients with metachromatic leukodystrophy are of juvenile or adult forms. Pathologically, the reduction in the number of oligodendrocytes is less severe. Remaining oligodendrocytes contain acid-phosphatase-positive lamellar inclusions, which on the light microscopic level stain yellow-brown with cresyl violet at acidic pH (metachromasia).

Unlike in globoid cell leukodystrophy, the affected substrate, sulfatide, is always abnormally increased. Both cDNA and the gene coding for the human arylsulfatase A have been cloned, and several mutations causing the clinical disease of metachromatic leukodystrophy have been described [9]. A pseudodeficiency allele is known to occur relatively frequently. Bone marrow transplantation treatment has been tried in patients having late-onset forms of the disease with some degree of positive effects. A metachromatic leukodystrophy-like disorder due to a deficiency in the sulfatidase activator protein is described below.

Multiple sulfatase deficiency

Phenotypically multiple sulfatase deficiency combines features of metachromatic leukodystrophy and mucopolysaccharidoses. In addition to clinical manifestations of metachromatic leukodystrophy, patients present with craniofacial abnormalities, skeletal deformities, and hepatosplenomegaly. There is abnormal urinary excretion of dermatan sulfate and heparan sulfate. Pathological findings are also combinations of the two conditions. Inheritance is Mendelian autosomal recessive. Nevertheless, activities of a series of sulfatases are deficient, including arylsulfatases A, B, and C, steroid sulfatases and sulfatases related to mucopolysaccharide degradation (see mucopolysaccharidoses below). Defective synthesis or instability due to a gene defect that governs all sulfatases needs to be explored. Since some of the sulfatases involved, e.g., arylsulfatase C, are not lysosomal enzymes, and since the primary genetic defect is not known, it is possible that multiple sulfatase deficiency may not be a lysosomal disorder as defined by Hers.

Gaucher's disease

Traditionally Gaucher's disease is classified into three types: type I, mostly adult, non-neuropathic; type II, mostly infantile, severely neuropathic; and type III, intermediate phenotypes. Type I is highly prevalent in the Jewish population, while a large, distinct group of type III patients exist in Scandinavian countries. All types are allelic and are caused by defective glucosylceramidase activity. Glucosylceramide is present in great excess in the enlarged liver and spleen in all types. The brain, in which glucosylceramide is normally almost nonexistent, does not contain increased amounts. Analogous to Niemann-Pick disease, non-neuropathic patients are free of neurological involvement and survive for decades, while type II neuropathic patients die within a few years with severe central nervous system involvement. The difference in the pathogenetic mechanisms in these phenotypes is not known.

Analogous to globoid cell leukodystrophy, glucosylsphingosine (glucopsychosine) may play an important role in the pathogenesis. The degree of central nervous system involvement parallels the amounts of glucopsychosine in the brain. Some of these important questions may be answered in the near future, because normal cDNA and the gene for glucosylceramidase have been cloned and characterized, and several mutations responsible for the disease state have been identified [10].

The most intensive enzyme replacement therapy has been tried in patients with the non-neuropathic form of Gaucher's disease. The recent use of purified enzyme modified at the carbohydrate moiety to increase efficiency of organ targeting and stability has produced encouraging results in some patients. Complete correction of the enzymatic defect was reported in fibroblasts through retrovirus-mediated gene transfer [11]. A line of mice with completely inactivated glucosylceramidase gene has been generated artificially by gene targeting/transgenic technology (see Chap. 26, regarding the technology) [12]. A Gaucher-like disorder due to a natural activator protein deficiency is described below.

Fabry's disease

Unlike most other sphingolipidoses, Fabry's disease is an X-linked disorder, occurring mostly in adults. It is also primarily a systemic disease, and neurological manifestations, when present, are largely secondary. The affected lipids trihexosylceramide (gal-gal-glc-ceramide) and digalactosylceramide are nearly absent in the neural tissues in normal individuals. These lipids accumulate in the brains of patients, where they are derived primarily from the blood vessels. Cerebrovascular pathology commonly results in secondary neurological symptoms. Most patients succumb to renal failure and other vascular diseases. Transplantation of normal kidney has been attempted for treatment, but the results were not encouraging. The enzyme responsible for degradation of these sphingolipids, all with the terminal α-galactose residue, is α-galactosidase A, a mutation of which causes the disease. A normal cDNA coding for α-galactosidase A has been cloned [13], and several mutations have been identified [3].

G_{M1}-gangliosidosis

The infantile form of the disease shows, in addition to psychomotor retardation and other neurological manifestations, mucopolysaccharidosis-like clinical features. The late-onset form is relatively free of systemic signs. Morquio's disease type B is a unique adult form of this disorder, also caused by genetic defects in G_{M1}-ganglioside β-galactosidase (acid β-galactosidase) (see below). These pleomorphic phenotypes are consequences of the wide substrate specificity of the defective enzyme, G_{M1}-ganglioside β-galactosidase, which hydrolyzes not only G_{M1}-ganglioside, asialo G_{M1}-ganglioside, and lactosylceramide, but also terminal β-galactosyl residues of carbohydrate chains of various glycoproteins. Different mutations in the same gene could each specifically inactivate catalytic function for a different substrate. Large accumulations of G_{M1}-ganglioside occur primarily in the brains of patients with the infantile and late-infantile forms of the disease. The major accumulated materials in the systemic organs are fragments of glycopeptides. It is not

known whether G_{M1}-ganglioside accumulates in the brains of patients with Morquio B disease. The human acid β-galactosidase cDNA and the gene have been isolated and characterized, and several mutations have been identified [14]. Within the relatively limited number of patients thus far examined, there appears to be an excellent correlation between the clinical phenotypes and underlying mutations.

Tay-Sachs disease and variants

The classic Tay-Sachs disease prevalent among the Ashkenazi Jewish population is the prototype of human sphingolipidoses. It is caused by a mutation in the β-hexosaminidase α-subunit gene. Normally the hexosaminidase α- and β-subunits form two catalytically active isozymes, β-hexosaminidase A ($\alpha\beta$) and B ($\beta\beta$). A defect in the α-subunit thus results in defective hexosaminidase A with normal hexosaminidase B. Hexosaminidase A can hydrolyze all known natural substrates with terminal β-N-acetylgalactosamine or β-N-acetylglucosamine residues, while hexosaminidase B hydrolyzes all of these substrates *except* G_{M2}-ganglioside. As the result, a relatively specific accumulation of G_{M2}-ganglioside occurs in genetic hexosaminidase α-deficiency states.

A few genetic variants are known on the basis of clinical and enzymatic criteria. Patients with the adult form may not develop clinical symptoms until the second or third decade of life. The enzymologically unique B1 variant is characterized by essentially normal hexosaminidases A and B when assayed with the standard artificial substrates but completely defective hexosaminidase A against the natural substrate, G_{M2}-ganglioside, and recently developed artificial substrates, p-nitrophenyl- or 4-methylumbelliferyl glcNAc-6-sulfate. These enzymatic variants are known to be caused by genetic defects in the hexosaminidase α-subunit gene. In contrast, the AB variant, which is phenotypically indistinguishable from the infantile hexosaminidase α defect, is caused by an entirely different genetic mechanism, a mutation in a specific activator protein (G_{M2} activator protein) (see below).

While all of these phenotypic and enzymological differentiations have been useful, molecular genetic understanding of these diseases is progressing and producing a more complex picture. Normal cDNA and the gene for the hexosaminidase α-chain have been cloned and characterized [15]. It has been known that patients with some forms of the disease lack enzyme activity and immunologically reactive α-subunit, while some patients lack enzyme activity but exhibit immunoreactivity for the α-subunit. Availability of cDNA for the α-subunit has shown that the presence or absence of cross-reactive material largely corresponds to the presence or absence of mRNA for the sub-unit. Both the classic Tay-Sachs disease and the phenotypically indistinguishable disease occurring in the French-Canadian population are mRNA negative, while the B1 variant and some other unusual forms are mRNA positive. Contrary to earlier expectations of a single mutation, two mutations have been identified underlying the classic Jewish infantile form of the disease: a splicing defect and a four-base insertion, the latter accounting for two-thirds to three-fourths of the Jewish infantile alleles [16]. The French-Canadian form showed still another mutation, a major deletion of approximately 7 kb in the 5′ end of the hexosaminidase α-gene. This deletion spans from the putative promoter region beyond the first exon into the first intron.

The first point mutation in the hexosaminidase α-gene was identified in a patient with the B1 variant form of the disease [17]. The normal arginine at residue 178 was substituted by histidine. Computer analysis suggested substantial changes in the secondary structure of the enzyme protein around the mutation, consistent with the unusual enzymological characteristic of this variant. The possible origin of this particular mutation has been traced to Northern Portugal.

During the past five years, more than 50 different mutations have been identified within the β-hexosaminidase α-gene that cause Tay-Sachs disease or its variants. The unexpected complexity of abnormalities at the gene level is likely to render obsolete the traditional clinical and enzymatic classification of the disease.

Sandhoff's disease

When the hexosaminidase β-gene is genetically defective, it results in inactivation of both hexosaminidase A (αβ) and B (ββ). While the typical infantile form of Sandhoff's disease cannot be readily distinguished clinically from an infantile hexosaminidase A defect, histochemical and biochemical studies would disclose accumulation of additional materials other than G_{M2}-ganglioside in the brain. All sphingolipids with the terminal β-hexosamine residue are affected, including G_{M2}-ganglioside, asialo-G_{M2}-ganglioside, and globoside (Fig. 1). Since globoside is primarily a systemic lipid, it does accumulate in systemic organs also.

The cDNA and the gene for the hexosaminidase β-subunit have also been cloned and characterized [18]. It is of interest that, despite the localization on different chromosomes (α on chromosome 15 and β on 5), hexosaminidase α- and β-chains are highly homologous not only in the base and amino acid sequences of cDNAs but also in the gene organization. These two subunit genes, now located on different chromosomes, appear to have been separated from a single gene relatively recently in the evolutionary time scale. Several abnormalities in the β-subunit gene have been identified that are responsible for the infantile and juvenile forms of the disease [1].

Activator deficiencies

In recent years, the concept of sphingolipidoses has been expanded to include a few genetic disorders that affect degradation of sphingolipids but that do not satisfy Hers' original two criteria for the inborn lysosomal disease. Activator protein deficiencies and galactosialidosis are examples of such disorders.

In vivo degradation of the highly hydrophobic lipids often requires, in addition to the specific hydrolases, a third component, commonly referred to as the activator protein. They are generally small glycoproteins localized within the lysosomes, but they are not enzymes themselves. When such an activator is essential for *in vivo* degradation and when it is genetically defective, the end results are very similar to those accompanying deficiency of the enzyme itself. G_{M2}-gangliosidosis AB variant has been well-characterized. It is caused by genetic absence of the activator required for *in vivo* degradation of G_{M2}-ganglioside. The degradative enzyme β-hexosaminidase A is normal in these patients. Conceptually similar diseases have been described in patients who showed metachromatic leukodystrophy-like and Gaucher-like clinical phenotypes and in whom activator proteins, rather than the hydrolases arylsulfatase A and glucosylceramidase, respectively, were genetically defective.

One of the striking genetic characteristics is that both of these activator proteins, the sulfatide activator (SAP-1) and the glucosylceramidase activator (SAP-2), are homologous proteins encoded by a single gene. A single transcript generates a large polypeptide, which is subsequently processed proteolytically into four small, homologous proteins, including the sulfatide activator and the glucosylceramidase activator. *In vitro* evidence suggesting activator protein function has been reported for the remaining two homologous proteins. However, definitive evidence that they are *required* for normal degradation of sphingolipids *in vivo* is still lacking. Several mutations in these activator proteins responsible for the clinical diseases are known [1].

Galactosialidosis ("combined sialidase-β-galactosidase deficiency")

The lysosomal β-galactosidase and sialidase appear to exist as a complex within the lyso-some with a third small protein. This third protein protects the enzymes from being degraded by acid proteases also present in the lysosome, and, when it is absent, both enzymes are degraded rapidly. Genetic abnormality of this protective protein results in deficient activities of both sialidase and β-galactosidase [19]. The protein also possesses carboxypeptidase activity. The disease is generally a slowly progressive neurological disorder, resembling a later onset form of G_{M1}-gangliosidosis. The cDNA and the gene coding for the protective protein have been cloned and characterized [14]. The concept of the protective protein is relatively new. Similar diseases due to defective protective proteins for other lysosomal enzymes may well be discovered in the future.

MUCOPOLYSACCHARIDOSES

Carbohydrate chains of glycosaminoglycans are sequentially degraded by a series of lysosomal enzymes (Table 3). Analogous to sphingolipidoses, genetic enzymatic defects in these degradative steps result in accumulation of undegradable metabolites, causing various forms of mucopolysaccharidoses. These materials are also excreted into urine in massive amounts. The standard classification of mucopolysaccharidoses is based on clinical manifestations and on the nature of the accumulated/excreted materials. The enzymatic classification does not necessarily correspond to the traditional classification; a single classic disease often consists of more than one nonallelic disorder, while two disorders classified earlier to be different may be allelic. All mucopolysaccharidoses are inherited as autosomal recessive traits, except for Hunter's disease, which is X-linked. Studies of mucopolysaccharidoses are now entering the molecular biology era [20].

Hurler's and Scheie's syndromes (mucopolysaccharidoses I and V)

Hurler's syndrome is the prototype of the mucopolysaccharidoses. Scheie's disease,

TABLE 3. Mucopolysaccharidoses

Disease	Clinicopathological manifestations	Affected compounds	Enzymatic defects
Hurler-Scheie (MPS I and V)	Craniofacial abnormalities, cloudy cornea, bone and other mesodermal tissue abnormalities, severe to mild psychomotor retardation, organomegaly, lysosomal storage in mesodermal organs, zebra bodies in neurons	Dermatan sulfate, heparan sulfate	α-L-iduronidase
Hunter's (MPS II)	Generally similar to but milder than Hurler-Scheie, but X-linked, corneal clouding rare	Dermatan sulfate, heparan sulfate	α-Iduronate sulfatase
Sanfilippo's (MPS III)	Four genetically distinct (nonallelic) types, similar clinicopathological manifestations, severe psychomotor retardation, relatively mild bone and other systemic involvement, zebra bodies in neurons	Heparan sulfate	Type A: heparan N-sulfatase Type B: N-acetyl α-glucosaminidase Type C: N-acetyl-CoA: α-glucosaminide N-acetyltransferase Type D: N-acetyl α-glucosaminide 6-sulfatase
Morquio's (MPS IV)	Two nonallelic forms, primarily bone abnormalities, corneal clouding, nervous system involvement secondary to bone changes, type B is allelic to G_{M1}-gangliosidosis	Keratan sulfate	Type A: N-acetyl-galactosamine 6-sulfatase Type B: β-galactosidase
Maroteaux-Lamy (MPS VI)	Severe to mild clinical types, bone and corneal changes, nervous system involvement, generally mild	Dermatan sulfate	Arylsulfatase B (N-acetyl-galactosamine 4-sulfatase)
β-Glucuronidase deficiency (MPS VII)	Organomegaly, bone abnormalities, mild to no psychomotor retardation, inclusions in leukocytes	Dermatan sulfate, heparan sulfate	β-glucuronidase

once considered to be a separate disease and classified as mucopolysaccharidosis V, is now known to be a milder allelic variant of Hurler's syndrome. Neurons in the brain are commonly distended, and they contain characteristic lamellar inclusions, known as zebra bodies. They are the site of abnormal ganglioside accumulation commonly found in this and other mucopolysaccharidoses. While the increase is nonspecific and is mainly in normally minor monosialogangliosides, the degree of the increase is often substantial, ranging from 50 to 100 percent above normal. Polysulfated mucopolysaccharides are inhibitory to some lysosomal enzymes *in vitro*, and similar inhibition *in vivo* might be responsible for the ganglioside increase. Whether the

ganglioside accumulation and neuronal distention contribute to the neurological manifestations of the disease is not known. In recent years, the cDNA and the gene coding for α-iduronidase have been cloned, and information on disease-causing mutations is beginning to appear.

Hunter's syndrome (mucopolysaccharidosis II)

Other than being an X-linked disorder and generally milder and slower in the clinical features and course, patients with Hunter's syndrome resemble closely those with Hunler's syndrome. The responsible enzyme, iduronate sulfatase, has been cloned.

Sanfilippo's disease (mucopolysaccharidosis III)

This is an excellent example of a "disease" identified on the basis of clinicopathological criteria, which has turned out to be a mixture of more than one genetically distinct disease. Four enzymatically different and nonallelic diseases are included under the eponym Sanfilippo's disease. All of the four defective enzymes are involved at different steps of heparan sulfate degradation. Thus the end results are essentially identical. Differential diagnosis cannot be established without appropriate enzyme assays.

Morquio's disease (mucopolysaccharidosis IV)

Unlike other mucopolysaccharidoses, Morquio's disease is primarily a skeletal disorder. Neurological involvement is almost always secondary to skeletal abnormalities. The most common neurological complications are traumatic lesions of the spinal cord at the cervical level due to vertebral deformity. Of the two genetically distinct types—type A (N-acetylgalactosamine 6-sulfatase deficiency) and type B (β-galactosidase deficiency), patients with type A disease are clinically more severely affected. The genetic relationship of type B Morquio's disease to G_{M1}-gangliosidosis has been mentioned above. Since the type B disease is allelic with G_{M1}-gangliosidosis, a mutation responsible for the Morquio B phenotype has been identified in the β-galactosidase gene [14]. N-acetylgalactosamine 6-sulfatase has also been cloned, but no mutation responsible for the type A disease has been described.

Maroteaux-Lamy disease (mucopolysaccharidosis VI)

Maroteaux-Lamy disease is another of the Hurler-like syndromes but can be differentiated from Hurler's syndrome by relatively well-preserved intellectual capacity. Urinary excretion of mucopolysaccharides is predominantly dermatan sulfate. Clinical severity and duration vary among apparently allelic cases. The arylsulfatase B gene has been cloned.

β-Glucuronidase deficiency (mucopolysaccharidosis VII)

This disease is exceedingly rare. The first case was reported by Sly and colleagues in 1973 [21]. While the general clinical picture is that of a mucopolysaccharidosis, the degrees of severity in skeletal abnormalities, organomegaly, and nervous system involvement appear widely variable. β-Glucuronidase is one of the first lysosomal enzymes cloned [22]. Complete "cure" of the disease with restoration of β-glucuronidase activity has been reported in a mutant mouse genetically deficient in glucuronidase activity, when the normal human β-glucuronidase gene was transgenically introduced [23].

GLYCOPROTEIN DISORDERS

Natural substrates of certain lysosomal glycosidases are primarily carbohydrate chains of glycoproteins. When such enzymes are genetically defective, the results are accumulation and urinary excretion of undigested sugar chains and small glycopeptides, since the protein backbone is usually degradable by proteases that are genetically normal in patients (Table 4).

Sialidosis (neuraminidase deficiency; mucolipidosis I)

Apparently, two dissimilar phenotypes result from enzymatic defects in the same lysosomal α-neuraminidase (sialidase). The infantile form had been known as mucolipidosis I because of mucopolysaccharidosis-like appearance of patients. Neurological in-

TABLE 4.   Glycoprotein storage diseases and mucolipidoses

Disease	Clinicopathological manifestations	Affected compounds	Enzymatic defects
Sialidosis (mucolipidosis I)	Two distinct phenotypes, mucolipidosis I (mucopolysaccharidosis-like features, severe to moderate psychomotor retardation) and the cherry-red spot-myoclonus syndrome	Sialyloligosaccharides	α-Neuraminidase (sialidase)
I-Cell disease and pseudo-Hurler polydystrophy (mucolipidoses II and III)	Mucopolysaccharidosis-like features, severe psychomotor retardation, characteristic inclusions in fibroblasts. ML-II is a milder allelic disease	Multiple (see text)	Primary defect in UDP-glcNAc:lysosomal enzyme glcNAc phosphotransferase, secondary abnormality in multiple lysosomal enzymes (see text)
Mucolipidosis IV	Mucopolysaccharidosis-like features, relatively mild central nervous system involvement, conjunctival biopsy for characteristic inclusions can be diagnostic	Unknown	Unknown
α-Mannosidosis	Mucopolysaccharidosis-like features, severe to moderate psychomotor retardation	Oligosaccharides with terminal α-mannose	Acid α-mannosidase
β-Mannosidosis	Infantile and late-onset forms, psychomotor retardation, Sanfilippo-like general clinical features	β-Mannosyl-glcNAc, heparan sulfate?	β-Mannosidase, heparan sulfamidase
α-Fucosidosis	Mucopolysaccharidosis-like features, severe to moderate psychomotor retardation	Fucose-containing oligosaccharides and glycolipids	α-Fucosidase

volvement is severe to moderate, including impaired intellectual capacity. The second type occurs in the juvenile age group. Three findings stand out: typical macular cherry-red spots, intractable myoclonic seizures, and intact intellect. The α-neuraminidase deficient in sialidosis cleaves both α-2,6 and α-2,3 sialyl linkages but is apparently distinct from neuraminidase(s), which hydrolyzes sialic acid from gangliosides. Thus, patients accumulate and excrete excess sialic-acid-containing materials derived from complex carbohydrate chains of glycoproteins, but there is no evidence for increased levels of gangliosides in the brain and elsewhere as the consequence of the genetic defect (see also galactosialidosis, above, and mucolipidosis IV, below)

I-cell disease (mucolipidosis II) and pseudo-Hurler polydystrophy (mucolipidosis III)

Among the disorders primarily affecting glycoprotein metabolism, I-cell disease and pseudo-Hurler's polydystrophy are conceptually unique. These two disorders had been considered to be separate entities on the basis of phenotypic manifestations. However, they are now known to be allelic variants of the same disease. Activities of most, but not all, lysosomal hydrolases are deficient in solid tissues. Notable exceptions are glucosylceramidase and acid phosphatase. On the other hand, their activities are generally much higher than normal in serum and other extracellular fluids, including the culture media in which patients' fibroblasts are grown. The primary genetic cause of the disease is not in any of the individual lysosomal enzymes but in UDP-glcNAc:lysosomal enzyme glcNAc phosphotransferase, which is localized in the Golgi apparatus and is essential for the normal processing and packaging of lysosomal enzymes (see Chap. 2). Without this enzyme, lysosomal enzymes cannot acquire the mannose 6-phosphate recognition marker, which allows them to be properly routed to the lysosome. As the result, lysosomal enzymes are abnormally routed out of the cell. While lack of lysosomal enzyme activities must be primarily responsible for clinicopathological manifestations, this disease does not rigorously satisfy the two classic criteria of Hers for the inherited lysosomal disease.

Mucolipidosis IV

The disease occurs predominantly in Jewish population. The genetic cause has not been unambiguously determined. Earlier, a sialidase deficiency presumably specific for ganglioside degradation was proposed based on moderately abnormal ganglioside patterns in cultured fibroblasts and reduced sialidase activity. The residual activity, however, was nearly half-normal, much higher than usually expected for a disease-causing deficiency. Although two later studies reported much lower residual activities, another laboratory was unable to confirm the result on the same patient. Data have been presented to suggest that at least some of these ambiguities might result from assay procedures that often measure total activity of a mixture of sialidases, only one of which is genetically affected in this disease. Meanwhile questions have been raised as to whether a ganglioside sialidase deficiency is consistent with the phenotypic expression. Accumulation of gangliosides in the tissue seems much milder than expected in a genetic condition in which the ubiquitous ganglioside, G_{M3}, cannot be degraded. Furthermore, if polysialogangliosides cannot be degraded, one would

expect much severer neurological consequences than the relatively mild central nervous system involvement in the disease. More studies are needed to settle these questions.

α-Mannosidosis

α-Mannosidases that participate in processing of carbohydrate chains of glycoproteins are localized in the Golgi apparatus and are genetically intact in α-mannosidosis. The lysosomal α-mannosidase deficient in this disease degrades the carbohydrate chains. Therefore, abnormal accumulations and urinary excretion of undegraded oligosaccharides with terminal α-mannose residues derived from normally synthesized and processed glycoproteins occur as the consequence of the genetic defect. A plant toxin, swainsonine, inhibits α-mannosidases, and its chronic ingestion creates an experimental condition that mimics many aspects of genetic α-mannosidosis. Limitation of this model, however, is that swainsonine inhibits both lysosomal and Golgi α-mannosidases.

β-Mannosidosis

This is the only disorder among those dealt with in this chapter that was discovered first in another mammalian species before an equivalent disease was found in humans. For several years, β-mannosidase deficiency was known in the goat. Affected goats show severe neurological signs almost from birth. The goat disease is rapidly fatal, and almost complete lack of myelination is the unique feature of the neuropathology. Recently, a human patient with β-mannosidase deficiency was reported [24]. Unlike the goat disease, the clinical picture was relatively mild, presenting with Sanfilippo-like features. There was urinary excretion of a disaccharide, β-mannose-glcNAc, and heparan sulfate. The same disaccharide is excreted in the goat disease. It is thought to derive from the innermost mannose in the glycoprotein carbohydrate chains. The parents of the patient had intermediate activities of the enzyme, consistent with the deficiency being the primary genetic defect. There was also a concomitant lack of heparan sulfamidase activity, which was normal in one parent and intermediate in the other. More recently, human β-mannosidosis occurring in infants was also described. The clinical features are more similar to those of the goat disease.

α-Fucosidosis

α-Fucoside residues are present in carbohydrate chains of both sphingoglycolipids and glycoproteins. Fucosylated glycolipids are quantitatively minor but often are functionally important tissue constituents. Many of blood group antigens are fucosylated glycosphingolipids. In patients with genetic α-fucosidase deficiency, accumulations and excretion of fucose-terminated oligosaccharides and fucosylated sphingolipids are observed. Consequences, if any, that result from the genetic α-fucosidase deficiency in individuals with the blood groups expressed by presence of fucosylated glycolipids have not been studied systematically.

PEROXISOMAL DISEASES

A large group of genetic neurological disorders occurs as the result of defects in morphogenesis of peroxisomes or in enzymes that are normally localized in peroxisomes (Table 5). The interested reader is referred to several recent review articles [25]. In the following discussion, only representative disorders will be described.

Zellweger's syndrome (cerebro-hepato-renal syndrome)

Zellweger's syndrome is the classic and the most severe example of genetic disorders

TABLE 5. Major peroxisomal diseases

Disease	Clinicopathological manifestations	Affected compounds	Peroxisomal function
Zellweger's	Craniofacial abnormalities, seizures, psychomotor retardation, severe hypnotic, hepatomegaly, rapid progression to death, hepatic cirrhosis, renal cysts	VLCFA[a], pipecolic acid, bile acid intermediate, phytanic acid, decreased plasmalogen content and synthesis	Absent peroxisomes; all peroxisomal functions defective
Neonatal adrenoleukodystrophy	Zellweger-like clinical features, extensive demyelination in the central nervous system, hepatic cirrhosis, adrenal insufficiency	As in Zellweger disease	Peroxisomes decreased in number and size; all peroxisomal functions defective
X-linked adrenoleukodystrophy	White matter and long tract signs, frequent visual impairment, seizures in late stage, adrenal insufficiency constant but of varying degrees, clinical variant, adrenomyeloneuropathy in older patients, massive central nervous system demyelination, characteristic inclusions	VLCFA in cholesterol esters and in some sphingolipids	Normal peroxisomes in size and number; defect in VLCFA oxidation? Putative gene for transporter protein
Refsum's	Retinitis pigmentosa, cerebellar ataxia, hypertrophic neuropathy, high cerebrospinal fluid protein	Elevated phytanic acid in serum and tissues	Normal peroxisomes in size and number; defect in phytanic acid α-hydroxylase

[a] Very-long-chain fatty acids (greater than C22).

due to peroxisomal dysfunction. The specific genetic defect has not been identified, but the most conspicuous finding is the almost total absence of peroxisomes, particularly in the hepatocytes and the proximal renal tubular epithelium. Consequently, there is a general failure of all metabolic functions normally associated with the peroxisome. The disease occurs early and progresses rapidly. Neurological manifestations are multiple and severe, accompanied by similarly severe systemic signs. A large majority of patients die within several months of birth, but some have survived several years. Consistent with absent peroxisomes, very-long-chain fatty acids, pipecolic acid, intermediates for bile acid biosynthesis, and phytanic acid are all elevated in the tissue, while the plasmalogen content is decreased. All the peroxisomal enzymes examined are deficient in their activities.

Adrenoleukodystrophy (ALD)

The classic form of adrenoleukodystrophy is an X-linked disorder, manifesting itself as a progressive neurological disorder of late infantile to juvenile boys. Severe and often confluent lesions of demyelination in the cerebrum, particularly in the occipital region, are characteristic. There are varying degrees of clinical and pathological signs of adrenal involvement. Most patients die in their adolescent ages. A clinical variant, adrenomyeloneuropathy, occurs in older individuals with predominant spinal cord and peripheral nerve involvement. The clinical course is much slower than the typical adrenoleukodystrophy. Despite the differences in the phenotypes, adrenomyeloneuropathy is probably caused by the same mutation as in the classic adrenoleukodystrophy, since both forms can occur in a single family. A significant proportion of female carriers show varying degrees of clinical signs of the disease.

The most prominent biochemical finding in ALD is increased levels of very-long-chain fatty acids (above C_{22}) in the brain, adrenal gland, plasma cells, red cells, and cultured fibroblasts. These fatty acids are present mostly in the forms of cholesterol esters, cerebrosides, gangliosides, and sphingomyelin. There is no indication of other peroxisomal dysfunction. The biochemical pathogenesis of the massive demyelination is unclear, because, even though the relative increase is large, the absolute amounts of the very-long-chain fatty acids in the tissue are still very small. The putative gene responsible for X-linked ALD has recently been cloned and shown to be a transporter protein [26]. Elucidation of its precise physiological function should provide insight into the pathogenetic mechanism of this disorder.

Neonatal (con-natal, infantile) adrenoleukodystrophy

This disorder is probably distinct genetically from the classic X-linked ALD. Unlike the classic adrenoleukodystrophy, the neonatal form appears to be an autosomal recessive disorder. The disease occurs within one year of birth, and the clinical course rarely exceeds five years. In addition to the clinical and pathological manifestations in common with, but more severe than, X-linked adrenoleukodystrophy, craniofacial dysmorphism reminiscent of Zellweger's syndrome is usually present. Morphologically, peroxisomes are greatly reduced in number and/or size. Consistent with the peroxisome abnormality, biochemical and enzymatic findings are similar to those of Zellweger's syndrome in that there are multiple abnormalities related to peroxisomal functions.

Refsum's disease

The classic form of Refsum's disease occurs in adults of both sexes with hypertrophic polyneuropathy as the most prominent manifestation. There is an abnormal elevation of a methylated fatty acid, phytanic acid, which is exogenously derived from chlorophyll in the food. There is no indication of other peroxisomal dysfunction. Peroxisomes appear morphologically normal in size and number.

Since phytanic acid is exclusively exogenous in origin, chlorophyll-free dietary treatment can be quite effective in alleviating the disease. An exceedingly small number of patients exist who have been reported to have the infantile form of Refsum's disease. Clinical, pathological, and biochemical findings in these patients show substantial overlap with Zellweger's syndrome, as well as with neonatal adrenoleukodystrophy. Whether infantile Refsum's disease represents a genetic entity that is distinct or allelic to either of these diseases is not known (see also Chap. 36).

REFERENCES

1. Scriver, C. R., Beaudet, A. L., Sly, W. S., and Valle, D. (eds.), *The Metabolic Basis of Inherited Disease, 6th Ed.* New York: McGraw-Hill, 1989.
2. Hers, H. G. Inborn lysosomal disease. *Gastroenterology* 48:625–633, 1966.
3. Suzuki, K. Enzymatic diagnosis of sphingolipidoses. *Methods Enzymol.* 138:727–762, 1987.
4. Suzuki, K. "Authentic animal models" for biochemical studies of human genetic diseases. In Arima, M., Suzuki, Y., and Yabuuchi, H. (eds.), *Proceedings of the 4th International Symposium on Developmental Disabilities.* Tokyo: University of Tokyo Press, 1984, pp. 129–138.
5. Pentchey, P. G., Comly, M. E., Kruth, H. S., Vanier, M. T., Wenger, D. A., Patel, S., and Brady, R. O. A defect in cholesterol esterification in Niemann-Pick disease (type C) patients. *Proc. Natl. Acad. Sci. U. S. A.* 82:8247–8251, 1985.
6. Pentchey, P. G., Vanier, M. T., Suzuki, K., and Patterson, M. C. Niemann-Pick disease type C: A cellular cholesterol lipidosis. In Scriver, C. R., Beaudet, A. L., Sly, W. S., and Valle, D. (eds.), *The Metabolic Basis of Inherited Disease, 7th ed.* New York: McGraw-Hill (*in press*).
7. Miyatake T, Suzuki K. Globoid cell leukodystrophy: Additional deficiency of psychosine galactosidase. *Biochem. Biophys. Res. Commun.* 48:538–543, 1972.
8. Svennerholm, L., Vanier, M. T., and Månsson, J. E. Krabbe disease: A galactosylsphingosine (psychosine) lipidosis. *J. Lipid Res.* 21:53–64, 1980.
9. Gieselmann, V., Polten, A., Kreysing, J., Kappler, J., Fluharty, A., and von Figura, K. Molecular genetics of metachromatic leukodystrophy. *Dev. Neurosci.* 13:222–227, 1991.
10. Beutler, E. Gaucher disease: New molecular approaches to diagnosis and treatment. *Science* 256:794–799, 1992.
11. Sorge, J., Kuhl, W., West, C., and Beutler, E. Complete correction of enzymatic defect of type I Gaucher disease fibroblasts by retroviral-mediated gene transfer. *Proc. Natl. Acad. Sci. U. S. A.* 84:906–909, 1987.
12. Tybulewicz, V. L. J., Tremblay, M. L., LaMarca, M. E., et al. Animal model of Gaucher's disease from targeted disruption of the mouse glucocerebrosidase gene. *Nature* 357:407–410, 1992.
13. Bishop, D. F., Calhoun, D. H., Bernstein, H. S., Hantzopoulos, P., Quinn, M., and Desnick, R. J. Human α-galactosidase A: Nucleotide sequence of a cDNA clone encoding the mature enzyme. *Proc. Natl. Acad. Sci. U. S. A.* 83:4859–4863, 1986.
14. Suzuki, K. β-Galactosidase deficiency: GM1 gangliosidosis, Morquio B disease, and galactosialidosis. In Rosenberg, R., Prusiner, S., DiMauro, S., Barchi, R., Kunkel, L. (eds.), *Molecular and Genetic Basis of Neurological Diseases.* Stoneham, MA: Butterworth-Heinemann, 1993, pp. 523–530.
15. Myerowitz, R., Piekarz, R., Neufeld, E. F., Shows T. B., and Suzuki, K. Human β-hexosaminidase α chain: Coding sequence and homology with the β chain. *Proc. Natl. Acad. Sci. U. S. A.* 82:7830–7834, 1985.
16. Suzuki, K. Lysosomal storage disease: Current status with Tay-Sachs disease as a model. In Brosius, J., Fremeau, R. T. (eds.), *Molecular Genetic Approaches to Neuropsychiatric Diseases.* New York: Academic, 81–96, 1991.
17. Ohno, K., and Suzuki, K. The mutation in G_{M2}-gangliosidosis B1 variant. *J. Neurochem.* 50:316–318, 1988.
18. O'Dowd, B. F., Quan, F., Willard, H. F., et al. Isolation of cDNA clones coding for the beta subunit of human β-hexosaminidase. *Proc. Natl. Acad. Sci. U. S. A.* 82:1184–1188, 1985.
19. d'Azzo, A., Hoogeveen, A., Reuser, A. J. J., Robinson, D., and Galjaard, H. Molecular defect in combined β-galactosidase and neuraminidase deficiency in man. *Proc. Natl. Acad. Sci. U. S. A.* 79:4535–4539, 1982.

20. Hopwood, J. J., and Morris, C. P. The muco-polysaccharidoses. Diagnosis, molecular genetics and treatment. *Mol. Biol. Med.* 7: 381–404, 1990.

21. Sly, W. S., Quinton, B. A., McAlister, W. H., and Rimon, D. L. β-Glucuronidase deficiency: Report of clinical, radiologic and biochemical features of a new mucopolysaccharidosis. *J. Pediatr.* 82:249–257, 1973.

22. Catterall, J. F., and Leary, S. L. Detection of early changes in androgen-induced mouse renal β-glucuronidase messenger ribonucleic acid using cloned complementary deoxyribonucleic acid. *Biochemistry* 22:6049–6053, 1983.

23. Kyle, J. W., Birkenmeier, E. H., Gwynn, B., et al. Correction of murine mucopolysaccharidosis VII by a human B-glucuronidase transgene. *Proc. Natl. Acad. Sci. U. S. A.* 87: 3914–3918, 1990.

24. Wenger, D. A., Sujansky, E., Fennessey, P. V., and Thompson, J. N. Human β-mannosidase deficiency. *N. Engl. J. Med.* 315:1201–1205, 1986.

25. Moser, H. W. Peroxisomal disorders. *Biochem. Cell. Biol.* 69:463–474, 1991.

26. Mosser, J., Douar, A.-M., Sarde, C.-O., et al. Putative X-linked adrenoleukodystrophy gene shares unexpected homology with ABC transporters. *Nature* 361:726–729, 1993.

CHAPTER 39

Disorders of Amino Acid Metabolism

MARC YUDKOFF

Basic Neurochemistry: Molecular, Cellular, and Medical Aspects, 5th Ed., edited by G. J. Siegel et al. Published by Raven Press, Ltd., New York, 1994. Correspondence to Marc Yudkoff, Children's Hospital of Philadelphia, 1 Children's Center, Philadelphia, Pennsylvania 19104.

TABLE 1.   Disorders of amino acid metabolism[a]

Disorder	Biochemical derangement	Classical findings
I. Branched-chain amino aciduria (maple syrup urine disease)	Defective branched-chain amino acid breakdown (Fig. 1)	Coma, convulsions, vomiting, respiratory failure in neonate
II. Branched-chain organic acidurias	Failure of organic acid oxidation (Fig. 1) — isovaleric, methylmalonic, propionic, etc.	Similar to above; may be metabolic acidemia and odd odor. Often confused with sepsis of newborn. Urine contains excessive amounts of different organic acids, depending on the nature of the defect. Partial defects may present in later infancy or childhood.
III. Glutaric acidurias	Type I: Primary defect of glutarate oxidation	Type I: Severe basal ganglia/cerebellar disease with macrocephaly. Onset 1–2 years.
	Type II: Defect of electron transfer flavoprotein (ETF)	Type II: Fulminant neurologic syndrome of the neonate. Often with renal/hepatic cysts. Usually fatal.
IV. Phenylketonuria (PKU)	Usually defect of phenylalanine hydroxylase. In rare cases, defect of biopterin metabolism (Fig. 3; reaction 1).	Normal at birth. Mental retardation in untreated children. Avoidable with early institution of diet therapy. Prognosis less favorable in PKU secondary to defect of biopterin metabolism.
V. Non-ketotic hyperglycinemia	Defect of the glycine cleavage system (Fig. 4).	Intractable seizures in neonate. Usually fatal in first few weeks of life.
VI. Homocystinuria	Usually a failure of cystathionine synthase (Fig. 2, reaction 6). Rarely associated with aberrant vitamin B_{12} metabolism (Fig. 2).	Thromboembolic diathesis, marfanoid habitus, ectopia lentis. Mental retardation is frequent.
VII. Urea cycle defects	Failure to convert ammonia to urea via urea cycle (Fig. 5).	Coma, convulsions, vomiting, respiratory failure in neonate. Often mistaken for sepsis of the newborn. Mental retardation, failure to thrive, lethargy, ataxia, and coma in the older child. Associated with hyperammonemia and abnormalities of blood aminogram.
VIII. Defects of biotin metabolism	Failure to "activate" biotin, which is important in carboxylation of organic acids.	Hypotonia, ataxia, acidosis, coma, dermatitis in the neonate. Mental retardation and deafness in older child.
IX. Disorders of glutathione metabolism	Defective synthesis of glutathione, the major intra-cellular anti-oxidant	Spinocerebellar degeneration, mental retardation, cataracts, hemolysis. Severe acidosis in some cases.
X. Disorders of GABA metabolism	Often an absence of succinic semialdehyde dehydrogenase	Hypotonia, ataxia, mental retardation in older child. Increased urine 4-OH-butyric acid.
XI. Canavan's disease	Absence of N-acetylaspartate acylase	Rapidly progressive demyelinating disease of infancy.

[a] For disorders of carbohydrate metabolism and the primary lactic acidoses, see Chap. 34.

Numerous disorders of amino acid metabolism have been described in the eight decades since Garrod introduced the concept of an inborn error of metabolism into medical nosology. Many inborn errors involve an inherited deficiency or altered function of an enzyme or transport system that mediates the disposition of a particular amino acid (Table 1). The results are the accumulation of the amino acid in body fluids and a toxicity syndrome that commonly extends to the central nervous system (CNS). The severity of the clinical syndrome depends on which amino acid accumulates, the duration of such accumulation, and whether other metabolic alterations, e.g., hypoglycemia, accompany the altered amino acid homeostasis.

Neurochemists have long been interested in understanding the relationship between the biochemical derangement and brain injury, since the latter illuminates both the physiology and pathophysiology of brain function. Unfortunately, this relationship is not well understood for any of the aminoacidurias even though some clues have been discovered. Many of these disorders are rare. References may be found in the selected reviews and texts listed in the bibliography.

BIOCHEMISTRY OF THE ORGANIC ACIDURIAS AND UREA CYCLE DEFECTS

All amino acids pursue one of three metabolic fates: (1) incorporation into protein; (2) conversion into "messenger" compounds, e.g., neurotransmitters and hormones; and (3) oxidation to form carbon dioxide, water, energy, and ammonia.

Congenital defects of incorporation into proteins may occur, but they probably are lethal early in development since such lesions have yet to be described. Congenital defects in the synthesis of messenger compounds occur, e.g., the formation of thyroid hormone from tyrosine, but these disorders do not cause the accumulation of the precursor amino acids because only a small portion of total amino acid flux is directed to the production of hormones and neurotransmitters.

Thus, almost all aminoacidurias reflect derangements of the oxidation of amino acids or effects on their transport. The oxidation involves conversion to organic acids prior to their entry into the tricarboxylic acid cycle, where the final oxidation to carbon dioxide, water, and energy is accomplished.

Many forms of organic aciduria have been described (see Table 1). These usually result because of the absence of a specific enzyme of organic acid oxidation. In rare instances, the cause is a failure to activate or transport a water-soluble vitamin that serves as a cofactor for a pathway of organic acid metabolism.

The oxidation of amino acids gives rise to ammonia, which in high concentration is neurotoxic. Most organisms have developed mechanisms for the disposal of this metabolite. In mammals, the urea cycle serves this function, promoting the excretion of 10 to 20 g/day of ammonia in the healthy adult. Congenital deficiencies of the urea cycle (see below) cause hyperammonemia and other evidence of nitrogen accumulation, e.g., elevations in the plasma concentration of glutamine, which is formed from ammonia.

PATHOGENESIS OF THE CLINICAL FEATURES

Infants who succumb in the first days of life commonly manifest neuronal degeneration with a reactive astrogliosis. Evidence of dysmelination is common when the baby survives for a few weeks and cortical atrophy is seen sometimes with long-standing disease. These findings are encountered in many other toxic encephalopathies and are not pathognomonic.

The pathophysiology also may involve competitive inhibition of amino acid transport across the blood-brain barrier. Many amino acids normally are transferred into the CNS from the blood via specialized transport systems, e.g., the L system mediating the uptake of neutral amino acids. Excessive plasma levels of one amino acid, e.g., phenylalanine, may inhibit the transport of others.

An increase in the ratio of the concentration of tryptophan to that of other essential amino acids, a phenomenon that occurs in patients who are treated with low-protein diets, may lead to greater tryptophan entry into the brain and increased synthesis of serotonin.

Decreases of lipids, proteolipids, and cerebrosides have been noted in several of these syndromes, e.g., maple syrup urine disease (MSUD). As noted above, pathological changes in brain myelin are common, especially in infants who die early in life. It is possible that the fundamental lesion involves a failure of myelin protein synthesis as a consequence of the imbalanced amino acid content of the brain tissue.

Finally, in some instances the injury may be referable to the formation of oxygen radicals or to disturbances of ion channel function. Indeed, the probability is high that disordered amino acid metabolism damages the brain by several independent mechanisms, each of which contributes to the final pathophysiology.

DISORDERS OF THE BRANCHED-CHAIN AMINO ACIDS: MAPLE SYRUP URINE DISEASE

The first congenital defect of branched-chain amino acid (BCAA) catabolism to be described was MSUD, a deficiency of branched-chain ketoacid dehydrogenase (Fig. 1, reaction 2), a mitochondrial enzyme. Decarboxylation of the branched-chain ketoacids, which are the transamination products of the BCAAs, proceeds through the dehydrogenase in a reaction for which the cofactors are thiamine pyrophosphate, lipoic acid, nicotinamide-adenine dinucleotide (NAD), flavine adenine dinucleotide (FAD), and coenzyme A (CoA). The ketoacids are freely reaminated to the parent amino acids, the latter being readily measured in the blood and urine. The ketoacids impart to the urine a distinct odor that sometimes is compared with maple syrup or burnt sugar.

The decarboxylase is composed of four subunits: E1-α, E1-β, E2, and E3. A specific kinase and phosphatase mediate the activation and deactivation of the enzyme complex. Most MSUD patients have mutations involving the E1-α subunit that catalyzes the actual decarboxylation of the ketoacid, although defects of the E1-β protein have been also described. Lesions of either the E2 or E3 moieties are extremely rare. The E3 subunit is shared by several enzyme systems, including branched-chain ketoacid decarboxylase, pyruvate dehydrogenase, and 2-oxoglutarate dehydrogenase. Hence, mutations in this protein can cause lactic acidosis and deranged tricarboxylic acid cycle activity as well as an accumulation of the BCAAs.

Infants are protected during gestation because the placenta clears most potential toxins. The classical form of the disease therefore does not become clinically manifest until a few days after birth. Initial periods of alternating irritability and lethargy progress over a few days to frank coma and respiratory embarrassment. Irreversible brain damage is common in babies who survive, particularly those whose treatment is delayed until after the first week of life.

Survivors may suffer a metabolic relapse at any time, particularly when they have an infection that favors the breakdown of endogenous protein by eliciting the secretion of catabolic stimuli like the adrenal stress hormones and leukocyte cytokines. As a consequence, the patient's limited capacity to oxidize BCAAs is overwhelmed and these compounds, together with their cognate ketoacids, accumulate to a toxic level.

Patients with partial enzymatic deficiencies may present later in life with intermittent ketoacidosis, prostration, and recurrent ataxia. The plasma concentrations of BCAAs are elevated during these episodes, but they may be normal or near normal when patients are metabolically compensated.

Rare patients respond to the administration of thiamine in large doses (10–30 mg/day). The clinical course is even more mild than that of patients with intermittent dis-

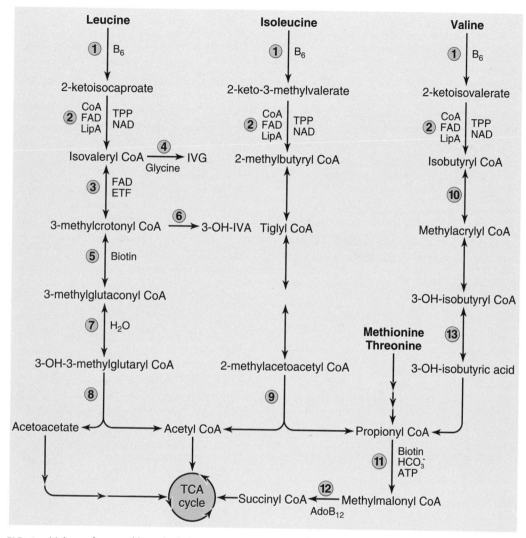

FIG. 1.   Major pathways of branched-chain amino acid metabolism. Maple syrup urine disease is caused by a congenital deficiency of reaction (2). Many of the primary organic acidurias, e.g., isovaleric acidemia and methylmalonic acidemia, are referable to inherited defects of enzymes involved in the oxidation of organic acids derived from the branched-chain amino acids. *Enzymes:* (1) branched-chain amino acid transaminase; (2) branched-chain amino acid decarboxylase; (3) isovaleryl-CoA dehydrogenase; (4) glycine-*N*-acylase; (5) 3-methylglutaconyl-CoA carboxylase; (6) 3-methylglutaconyl-CoA hydroxylase; (7) 3-methylglutaconyl-CoA hydratase; (8) 3-hydroxy-3-methylglutaryl-CoA lyase; (9) 2-ketothiolase; (10) isobutyryl-CoA dehydrogenase; (11) propionyl-CoA carboxylase; (12) methylmalonyl-CoA mutase; (13) 3-hydoxy-isobutyryl-CoA deacylase. (TPP) thiamine pyrophosphate; (LipA) lipoic acid; (ETF) electron-transferring flavoprotein; (AdoB12) adenosylcobalamin; (IVG) isovalerylglycine.

ease. Thiamine is a cofactor for the branched-chain ketoacid dehydrogenase, and the presumed mutation involves faulty binding of the apoprotein to this vitamin.

In many localities, newborn screening has become standard for this disorder, which in the general population has an approximate incidence of 1 in 250,000 live births. Carrier detection is possible, either by measurement of enzymatic activity in cultured fibroblasts or by study of restriction endonuclease fragments of DNA (Southern blotting). Prenatal testing is possible.

Long-term treatment entails dietary restriction of the BCAAs. This is accomplished by administration of a special formula from which these amino acids are removed. The outlook for intellectual development is favorable in youngsters whose diagnosis is made early, and who do not suffer recurrent, severe episodes of metabolic decompensation.

DISORDERS OF ORGANIC ACID METABOLISM

Defects of branched-chain organic acid metabolism

Isovaleric Acidemia

The cause is a congenital deficiency of isovaleryl-CoA dehydrogenase (see Fig. 1, reaction 3), which mediates the formation of 3-methylcrotonyl-CoA from isovaleryl-CoA. Affected patients usually have less than 5 percent of control capacity to oxidize isovaleric acid.

The dehydrogenase is a mitochondrial enzyme (~175,000 Da) composed of four identical subunits that are coded on human chromosome 15. The enzyme first transfers electrons from isovaleryl-CoA to FAD and then to electron-transferring flavoprotein (ETF). A specific ETF-dehydrogenase then shifts the electrons to coenzyme Q in the electron transport chain.

The clinical presentation includes both a fulminant syndrome of neonatal onset and an intermittent disorder that usually becomes manifest in the first year or two of life. In the former instance the baby develops irritability, vomiting, convulsions, and progressive loss of consciousness during the first week. The rancid odor of isovaleric acid, which often is apparent in the urine, saliva, and ear cerumen, accounts for the unusual name "sweaty socks syndrome." Patients frequently exhibit hyperammonemia, ketoaci-

duria, metabolic acidosis, pancytopenia, and hypocalcemia.

Youngsters with the intermittent disease usually present with the characteristic odor, lethargy, ataxia, and vomiting in association with an intercurrent infection or the administration of a relatively large amount of protein. Hyperammonemia is common. A family may have children with both the neonatal and intermittent forms of the disease, suggesting that the clinical presentation may not always correlate well with the genotype.

The hepatic enzyme glycine-N-acylase, which mediates formation of hippuric acid from benzoyl-CoA and glycine, also catalyzes synthesis of isovalerylglycine from glycine and isovaleryl-CoA (K_m ~0.6 mM) (see Fig. 1, reaction 4). Patients excrete isovalerylglycine even when clinically compensated, thereby facilitating diagnosis. Formation of isovalerylglycine also detoxifies isovaleric acid during periods of stress, since the conjugate is hydrophilic and excreted into urine more efficiently than isovaleric acid itself. Indeed, supplementation of the diet with glycine is beneficial, especially during a crisis.

A low-protein diet, to minimize leucine intake, is recommended. Patients usually fare well, and some suffer no relapses at all. The blood carnitine level usually is low, reflecting excessive excretion of isovalerylcarnitine. Carnitine therapy therefore has been suggested, but the utility of this approach still is uncertain.

3-Methylcrotonic Aciduria

3-Methylcrotonic acid is carboxylated in a biotin-dependent reaction to form 3-methylglutaconic acid (see Fig. 1, reaction 5). Isolated carboxylase deficiencies are rare and should be distinguished from 3-methylcrotonic aciduria that occurs secondary to defects of biotin metabolism (see below). Some patients have presented in early infancy with vomiting, metabolic acidosis, hyperlactatemia, convulsions, and coma. Others have remained well for 2 to 5 years, when they have had recurrent vomiting, metabolic acidosis, hypoglycemia, and progressive lethargy leading to coma.

The urine usually contains marked elevations of 3-hydroxyisovaleric acid, which is formed from 3-methylcrotonyl-CoA (see Fig. 1, reaction 6). It should be emphasized that 3-hydroxyisovaleric aciduria can be a nonspecific finding in ketotic patients. Much 3-methylcrotonylglycine also is excreted.

3-Methylglutaconic Aciduria

Deficiencies of 3-methylglutaconyl-CoA hydratase (see Fig. 1, reaction 7), which mediates formation of 3-hydroxy-3-methylglutaryl-CoA, are extremely rare. Patients may present only with delayed speech development or with relatively mild psychomotor retardation. The urine contains increased amounts of 3-methylglutaconate, 3-hydroxyisovalerate, and 3-methylglutarate, the latter presumably being formed from hydrogenation of 3-methylglutaconic acid.

In addition to the hydratase deficiency, several patients now have been described with an autosomal recessive disorder involving 3-methylglutaconic aciduria but with normal hydratase activity. Loading with oral leucine does not increase urinary excretion of 3-methyglutaconate. Most of these children have had a progressive course characterized by neurodegeneration, often beginning in the first few months of life, and death after a few months or years. These patients, unlike those with hydratase deficiency, do not excrete excessive amounts of 3-hydroxyisovaleric acid. The underlying biochemical defect is not yet known.

3-Hydroxy-3-Methylglutaric Aciduria

These patients lack 3-hydroxy-3-methylglutaryl-CoA lyase, which catalyzes conversion of 3-hydroxy-3-methylglutarate to acetoacetate and acetyl-CoA (see Fig. 1, reaction 8). Many patients become ill as neonates, but in others the symptoms are not apparent until 6 to 12 months. The most prominent findings are vomiting, lethargy, coma, convulsions, and metabolic acidosis. An important finding is hypoglycemia without significant ketoaciduria, reflecting the significance of 3-hydroxy-3-methylglutaryl-CoA lyase to the synthesis of ketone bodies. The hypoglycemia may be referable to excessive consumption of glucose in the absence of the capacity to utilize an alternate fuel such as acetoacetate. Hepatomegaly with increased serum transaminases and hyperammonemia can occur and may lead to confusion with Reye's syndrome.

The urine organic acid profile shows increased 3-hydroxy-3-methylglutarate even when patients are stable. Excretion of 3-methylglutaconic acid also is high because the hydratase reaction is reversible (see Fig. 1, reaction 7).

Patients must avoid fasting, which predisposes them both to developing hypoglycemia and, by favoring the synthesis of ketones from fatty acids, to the accumulation of 3-hydroxy-3-methylglutaric acid. Restriction of dietary protein and fat also may have a therapeutic role.

2-Methylacetoacetyl-CoA Thiolase Deficiency

This enzyme mediates the conversion of 2-methylacetoacetyl-CoA to acetyl-CoA and propionyl-CoA (see Fig. 1, reaction 9). It is one of several 3-oxothiolases that catalyze formation of acetyl-CoA and the corresponding acyl-CoA. The reactions usually are reversible, and one such enzyme is a cytoplasmic protein that mediates the condensation of 2 mol of acetyl-CoA to form acetoacetyl-CoA, which then reacts with another mole of acetyl-CoA to generate the 3-hydroxy-3-methylglutaryl-CoA used for cholesterol synthesis.

The mitochondrial thiolase is specific for 2-methylacetoacetyl-CoA. In the liver this enzyme also promotes ketogenesis by catalyzing synthesis of 3-hydroxy-3-methylglutaryl-CoA from acetoacetyl-CoA and acetyl-CoA. It is a tetramer (~170,000 Da) and is stimulated by potassium ion, unlike the cytosolic enzyme.

The inherited disorder, sometimes

termed β-ketothiolase deficiency, causes recurrent acidosis, ketosis, vomiting, and even death. Patients respond to intravenous glucose and bicarbonate. Mental retardation is not unprecedented, but it is exceptional.

Patients commonly excrete large amounts of 2-methyl-3-hydroxybutyric acid, formed via enzymatic reduction of 2-methylacetoacetyl-CoA. Tiglyl-CoA, a precursor to 2-methylacetoacetyl-CoA in the pathway of isoleucine catabolism (see Fig. 1), also accumulates and usually is excreted as tiglylglycine. The ketosis is referable to inhibition of acetoacetyl-CoA metabolism by 2-methylacetoacetyl-CoA. Excretion of these metabolites is variable when patients are not acutely ill.

3-Hydroxyisobutyryl-CoA Deacylase Deficiency

This reaction of valine catabolism involves conversion of 3-hydroxyisobutyryl-CoA to 3-hydroxyisobutyric acid (see Fig. 1, reaction 13). A single patient had multiple congenital anomalies, including tetralogy of Fallot, facial dysmorphism, and dysgenesis of the brain. The infant died at 3 months of age. Methyacrylyl-CoA, a valine metabolite proximal to the site of the metabolic block (see Fig. 1), accumulates and forms ninhydrin-positive conjugates with cysteine and cysteamine that can be detected with amino acid analysis. The urine organic acids are otherwise unremarkable.

Propionic acidemia

Most propionate and methylmalonate are derived from the catabolism of the BCAAs (see Fig. 1). Additional sources are methionine and threonine as well as odd-chain fatty acids and cholesterol. Methylmalonic acid also is derived from the catabolism of thymine.

Children with defects in the oxidation of propionate and methylmalonate may have hyperglycinemia and these disorders once were known as "ketotic hyperglycinemia." As the underlying biochemistry became better understood, this description was discarded in favor of more specific terminology, e.g., propionic acidemia and methylmalonic acidemia.

Propionyl-CoA Carboxylase Deficiency

Essentially all propionyl-CoA is metabolized to methylmalonyl-CoA in a reaction that requires both biotin and ATP (see Fig. 1, reaction 11). The mitochondrial enzyme is a tetramer composed of two α- and two β-subunits (~540,000 Da). The α-subunit has been mapped to human chromosome 13 and the β-subunit to chromosome 3. Leader peptides, facilitating transport of the propeptides into the mitochondria, also have been identified. The α-subunit contains the biotin binding site. A specific enzyme, holocarboxylase synthetase, mediates binding of biotin to propionyl-CoA carboxylase.

Patients with a near-total enzyme deficiency become sick as neonates with dehydration, lethargy progressing to coma, vomiting, ketoaciduria, and hypotonia. The toxicity can extend to the bone marrow, resulting in neutropenia and thrombocytopenia. Hyperammonemia and death from hemorrhage are not unusual. Hyperglycinemia occurs in many cases.

Infants who survive may relapse, particularly in association with an infection. Permanent brain damage, seizures, and mental retardation are frequent. Some patients remain well until later infancy or childhood, when their developmental retardation and failure to thrive are first discovered.

Various mutations have been described. These were formerly classified into two groups, *pccA* and *pccBC*, depending upon the thermostability of the mutant enzyme, its affinity for the effector K^+, and the response to addition of avidin. The *pccA* group, which is more common, has little or no α-chain and the *pccBC* mutants are defective in β-chain activity. Inheritance is autosomal recessive.

Presumptive diagnosis requires demonstration of increased excretion of propionate derivatives, including propionylglycine, 3-hydroxypropionate, tiglylglycine, and methylcitric acid, a condensation product of propionyl-CoA and oxalocacetate. Definitive diagnosis involves the measurement of enzymatic activity in peripheral blood leukocytes. Prenatal diagnosis is feasible.

Treatment entails the restriction of dietary protein to minimize propionate production. Most patients have growth failure. Propionyl-CoA carboxylase is stimulated by biotin, but supplementation with this vitamin is not of documented benefit. Blood carnitine levels are low, probably because of loss as propionylcarnitine, and some evidence points to clinical improvement with carnitine treatment.

Methylmalonic acidemia

Methylmalonyl-CoA Mutase Deficiency

Methylmalonyl-CoA (MMA-CoA) is isomerized to succinyl-CoA via MMA-CoA mutase (see Fig. 1, reaction 12). The enzyme is a dimer (~150,000 Da) made of two identical subunits to which is bound 1 mol of adenosylcobalamin. The gene has been mapped to the short arm of human chromosome 6. Patients can have a complete deficiency of the apoenzyme (mut^0), partial deficiency (mut$^-$), or various defects of vitamin B_{12} metabolism. The latter patients have homocystinuria and hypermethioninemia as well as methylmalonic aciduria.

Patients with the mut^0 lesion present as neonates with vomiting, acidosis, hyperammonemia, hepatomegaly, hyperglycinemia, and hypoglycemia. Neutropenia and thrombocytopenia can occur. Growth failure is very common in children who survive.

The urine contains excessive MMA, even when patients are well. The concentration in the cerebrospinal fluid equals or even exceeds that of the blood.

Treatment involves a diet that is low in the amino acid precursors to MMA. Medical attention should be sought whenever the patient develops an acute infection. Stroke-like episodes and death have occurred during metabolic decompensation. There may be a role for L-carnitine supplementation.

High concentrations of MMA (or propionate) adversely affect oxidative metabolism, resulting in a depletion of ATP. A variety of enzyme systems, e.g., pyruvate carboxylase, are inhibited by these organic acids. In addition, the sequestration of CoA as methylmalonyl-CoA or propionyl-CoA probably causes a depletion of the free CoA pool, which would adversely affect the synthesis of myelin, urea, and glucose.

Vitamin B_{12} is ineffective in patients with either the mut^0 or mut$^-$ lesions, but it may help infants with defects of cobalamin synthesis and/or transport (see below). There is no hazard associated with giving 1 to 2 mg/day of vitamin B_{12}, and this approach is warranted until the results of enzymatic studies are available.

Methylmalonic Aciduria Secondary to Defects of Cobalamin Metabolism

Adenosylcobalamin is a cofactor for the MMA-CoA mutase reaction, and patients with cobalamin deficiency, e.g., pernicious anemia or congenital defects of cobalamin metabolism, may have increased urinary methylmalonate. These children also may have homocystinuria, because methylcobalamin is involved in the remethylation of homocysteine to methionine (Fig. 2, reaction 4; also see section on disorders of sulfur-containing amino acids). Neurological symptoms, frequently of a very severe nature and of onset in early infancy, are common to most of these syndromes (see also Chap. 35).

Intestinal absorption of cobalamin requires intrinsic factor, a glycoprotein that is synthesized in the gastric parietal cells. The cobalamin-intrinsic factor complex is taken up by cells in the ileum, where the complex dissociates. Cobalamin enters the circulation bound to transcobalamin II (TC-II), which also facilitates uptake into tissues. Methylcobalamin is the major circulating form, but the major intracellular form, including within the brain, appears to be adenosylcoba-

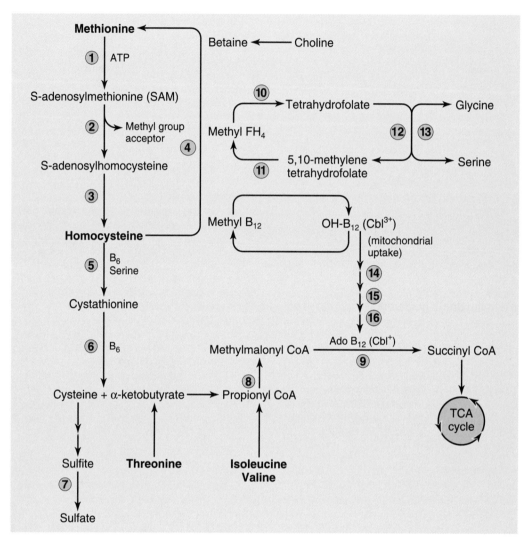

FIG. 2.   The transsulfuration pathway and related metabolic routes. Homocystinuria usually is caused by a congenital deficiency of cystathionine-β-synthase (*reaction 5*). Sometimes homocystinuria is caused by a failure of the remethylation of homocysteine. This may occur because of a failure to generate methylfolate or methylcobalamin. If there is a generalized failure of cobalamin activation or absorption, methylmalonic aciduria as well as homocystinuria may result because cobalamin derivatives are essential to both pathways. *Enzymes:* (1) methionine-activating enzyme; (2) generic depiction of methyl group transfer from *S*-adenosylmethionine; (3) *S*-adenosylhomocysteine hydrolase; (4) homocysteine : methionine methyltransferase; (5) cystathionine-β-synthase; (6) cystathionase; (7) sulfite oxidase; (8) propionyl-CoA carboxylase; (9) methylmalonyl-CoA mutase; (10) homocysteine : methionine methyltransferase (essentially same as reaction 4, in which methyltetrahydrofolate is the methyl donor); (11) $N^{5,10}$-methylenetetrahydrofolate reductase; (12) and (13) glycine cleavage system; (14) and (15) hydroxycobalamin reductases; (16) cobalamin adenosyltransferase. (OH-B12) hydroxycobalamin; (AdoB12) adenosylcobalamin; (Methyl-B12 methylcobalamin; (TCA) tricarboxylic acid.

lamin. The cobalamin-TC-II complex is broken down by a specific lysosomal protease. The free cobalamin then is methylated in the cytoplasm, or it enters the mitochondrion, where, as adenosylcobalamin, it facilitates the MMA-CoA mutase reaction.

Several genetic defects have been identified, including anomalies of cobalamin absorption, cellular uptake, and intracellular handling. Transport defects are represented by inherited deficiency of intrinsic factor (juvenile pernicious anemia), cobalamin malabsorption syndrome, and TC-II deficiency. These patients usually have megaloblastic anemia, methylmalonic aciduria, and homocystinuria. The neurological signs, especially in infants with TC-II deficiency, tend to be quite severe. The CNS lesions probably are caused by the failure to generate from homocysteine an adequate amount of S-adenosylmethionine, the major methyl donor in the developing brain (see section on disorders of sulfur amino acid metabolism).

Primary defects in the synthesis of methylcobalamin and adenosylcobalamin have been described. Patients with methylmalonic aciduria secondary to deranged vitamin B_{12} metabolism can be distinguished from those with the mutase deficiency by their response to pharmacological doses of cyanocobalamin or adenosylcobalamin, which sharply reduces methylmalonate excretion. At least two distinct inherited forms of faulty adenosylcobalamin synthesis, *cblA* and *cblB*, have been identified from clinical findings and complementation analysis in skin fibroblasts. Unlike infants with the mutase deficiency, who present in the first 1 to 2 weeks of life, these patients do not become clinically ill until after the first month of life. They may have ketonuria and metabolic acidemia as well as a severe neurological syndrome involving coma and convulsions. Survivors commonly have mental retardation and microcephaly. Evidence of pathology to the cerebellum and the dorsal columns of the spinal cord is common.

Patients with *cblA* disease have defective adenosylcobalamin synthesis, since the addi-tion of this vitamin to the incubation medium corrects the failure of MMA conversion to succinate. The precise biochemical lesion is not yet known, although patients have normal activity of the adenosyltransferase enzyme, which mediates the formation of adenosylcobalamin from ATP and hydroxycobalamin (see Fig. 2, reaction 16). The patients may lack a specific mitochondrial cobalamin reductase (see Fig. 2, reactions 14 and 15). Patients with *cblB* disease are missing a functional adenosyltransferase enzyme (see Fig. 2, reaction 16).

The diagnosis of defective adenosylcobalamin synthesis should be suggested by methylmalonic aciduria without megaloblastic changes, homocystinuria, or hypomethioninemia. The blood vitamin B_{12} concentration is normal. Prenatal diagnosis is feasible, either through study of the mutase reaction in amniocytes or by quantitation of MMA in amniotic fluid.

More than 90 percent of patients with the *cblA* disease respond favorably to the administration of hydroxycobalamin, which reduces MMA excretion. They have a good prognosis, with most surviving into adulthood in an intact state. Only 40 percent of individuals with *cblB* disease show a positive response. Their prognosis is less sanguine, with neurological impairment often noted among youngsters who survive the initial insult. Protein restriction, which minimizes production of MMA, is also indicated.

Glutaric aciduria

Glutaryl-CoA Dehydrogenase Deficiency

Glutaric acid is an intermediate in the formation of crotonyl-CoA from α-ketoadipic acid, which is derived from the catabolism of lysine, hydroxylysine, or tryptophan:

Lysine/hydroxylysine/tryptophan $\rightarrow\rightarrow$

$$\text{α-ketoadipic acid} \quad 1$$

α-Ketoadipic acid + CoA + NAD $\rightarrow$

$$\text{gluytaryl-CoA} + NADH + H^+ + Co_2 \quad 2$$

Glutaryl-CoA + FAD → crotonyl-CoA +

$$FADH_2 + CO_2 \quad 3$$

Crotonyl-CoA →→ 2 acetyl-CoA   4

Patients with a congenital absence of glutaryl-CoA dehydrogenase seem normal at birth, although they may manifest macrocephaly. Normal development is common for the first 1 to 2 years, when they develop hypotonia, opisthotonus, seizures, rigidity, dystonia, facial grimacing, and seizures. These signs may develop very abruptly, following an intercurrent illness, or in a more gradual manner. Developmental assessment is difficult because of severe motor involvement, but mental retardation may not occur. The neurological syndrome may be progressive, and death may occur during the first decade of life. The diagnostic hallmark is excretion of glutaric acid and 3-hydroxyglutaric acid. Imaging of the brain shows atrophy of the caudate and putamen and a loss of white matter in both frontal and occipital horns. Pathological examination of the brain also shows degenerative changes in the basal ganglia and of the cortical white matter. A special diet low in tryptophan and lysine will reduce excretion of glutaric acid, but it may not improve the clinical status.

Type II Glutaric Aciduria

Oxidation of glutaric acid (reaction 3, above) involves transfer of electrons to FAD, forming $FADH_2$. Type II glutaric aciduria usually is caused by a congenital deficiency of ETF or of ETF : ubiquinone reductase. These proteins, which are encoded by nuclear genes, mediate the transfer of electrons from flavoproteins to the respiratory chain. Other substrates that donate electrons to these proteins are dimethylglycine dehydrogenase and sarcosine dehydrogenase.

Patients often present as neonates with hepatomegaly, hypoglycemia, hypotonia, metabolic acidosis, and a rancid odor to the urine that is similar to that of isovaleric acidemia (see above). The kidneys commonly are enlarged. Cystic changes of both the liver and the kidneys are frequent. Facial dysmorphism also can occur. The outlook is almost uniformly fatal, and the few babies who survive have severely compromised development and a cardiomyopathy that usually causes death. A rare patient does not become symptomatic until after the neonatal period, when hepatomegaly, vomiting, metabolic acidosis, hypoglycemia, and a proximal myopathy become evident.

Pathological examination of the brain reveals dysplasias and other evidence of aberrant neural migration. The gyri of the cortex generally are reduced.

DISORDERS OF PHENYLALANINE METABOLISM: PHENYLKETONURIA

Phenylalanine hydroxylase deficiency

Phenylketonuria (PKU) is among the more common aminoacidurias (~1 in 20,000 live births). The usual cause is a near-complete deficiency of phenylalanine hydroxylase, which converts phenylalanine into tyrosine (Fig. 3, reaction 1). In addition to classical PKU, many youngsters have hyperphenylalaninemia caused by a partial deficiency of the enzyme. They do not suffer mental retardation, but they may have more subtle neurological problems.

The hydroxylase is a trimer (~150,000 Da) of identical subunits. It is located predominantly in the liver. The enzyme has been mapped to human chromosome 12q22-24.1, where the gene is comprised of 13 exons extending over 90 kb of genomic DNA.

Analysis of the gene in peripheral leukocytes means that no longer is it necessary to measure activity in a liver biopsy specimen. Frank deletions in the gene are not common. A frequent cause among northern Europeans (~40 percent) is a G-to-A transition at the 5' donor splice site in intron 12, resulting in absence of the C-terminus. Another relatively common (~20 percent) mutation

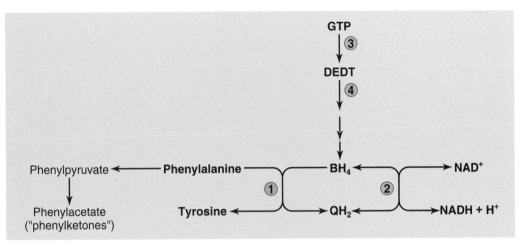

FIG. 3   The phenylalanine hydroxylase (PAH) pathway. Phenylketonuria usually is caused by a congenital deficiency of PAH (reaction 1), but it also can result from defects in the metabolism of biopterin, which is a cofactor for the hydroxylase. *Enzymes:* (1) phenylalanine hydroxylase; (2) dihydropteridine reductase; (3) GTP cyclohydrolase; (4) 6-pyruvoyltetrahydrobiopterin synthase. (QH_2) dihydrobiopterin; (BH_4) tetrahydrobiopterin; (DEDT) D-*erythro*-dihydroneopterin triphosphate.

in northern Europeans involves a C-to-T transition in exon 12, resulting in substitution of a tryptophan for an arginine residue.

Specific mutations have been associated with specific haplotypes, the latter determined by analysis of restriction fragment length polymorphisms. This approach has been utilized for prenatal diagnosis. The study of haplotypes also has revealed that the majority (~75 percent) of northern European patients are compound heterozygotes for a mutation of phenylalanine hydroxylase.

Affected babies are not retarded at birth, but almost all will be impaired if they are not treated by 3 months of age. Mass screening has largely eliminated the untreated PKU phenotype of eczema, poor growth, irritability, a musty odor on the urine and perspiration (caused by phenylacetic acid), and a tendency to self-mutilation. Progressive motor dysfunction has been described in children with long-term hyperphenylalaninemia.

The clinical utility of dietary restriction of phenylalanine (200–500 mg/day of phenylalanine) is clear. Well-controlled patients have normal intelligence, although there ap-pears to be an increased risk of perceptual-learning disabilities, emotional problems, and subtle motor difficulties. Diet therapy probably must be maintained throughout adolescence and, perhaps, indefinitely. Performance may deteriorate after the diet is discontinued.

Exposure to excessive (>1 mM) blood phenylalanine levels in early infancy can impair neuronal maturation and the synthesis of myelin. The responsible factor is hyperphenylalaninemia, not a phenylalanine metabolite or tyrosine deficiency. One hypothesis suggests that excessive phenylalanine levels inhibit the transport of other neutral amino acids across the blood-brain barrier. Conversely, some have proposed that high intracerebral phenylalanine levels impair the transport of tyrosine from the brain to the blood. High brain phenylalanine levels can inhibit synaptosomal Na,K-ATPase activity and the synthesis of neurotransmitters. It also causes disaggregation of brain polysomes, which may explain the dysmyelination that has been described in phenylketonuric brain.

The genotypically normal offspring of

an affected mother untreated during pregnancy may have microcephaly and irreversible brain injury as well as cardiac defects. Scrupulous monitoring of dietary phenylalanine intake in these women has resulted in a much better outcome.

Defects of biopterin metabolism

The electron donor for the hydroxylase is tetrahydrobiopterin (BH_4), which transfers electrons to molecular oxygen to form tyrosine and dihydrobiopterin (QH_2) (see Fig. 3, reaction 2). BH_4 is regenerated from QH_2 in an NADH-dependent reaction (see Fig. 3, reaction 2) that is catalyzed by dihydropteridine reductase (DHPR), which is widely distributed. In the brain this enzyme also mediates hydroxylation of tyrosine and tryptophan. Human DHPR has been mapped to human chromosome 4p15.1-p16.1. The coding sequence shows little homology to other reductases, e.g., dihydrofolate reductase (see Chap. 35).

In rare instances, PKU is caused by defects in the metabolism of BH_4, which is synthesized from GTP via sepiapterin (see Fig. 3, reactions 3 and 4). The BH_4 functions also in hydroxylation of tyrosine and tryptophan.

Even careful phenylalanine restriction fails to avert progressive neurological deterioration because patients are unable to hydroxylate tyrosine or tryptophan, the synthesis of which also requires tetrahydrobiopterin. Thus, neurotransmitters are not produced in sufficient amount (see Chaps. 12 and 13).

Patients sustain convulsions and neurological deterioration. The urine contains low levels of the metabolites of serotonin, norepinephrine, and dopamine. The reductase also plays a role in the maintenance of tetrahydrofolate levels in brain, and some patients have had low folate levels in the serum and brain. Treatment has been attempted with tryptophan and carbidopa (see Chap. 44) to improve serotonin homeostasis, and with folinic acid to replete diminished stores of reduced folic acid. This therapy some-

times is effective. Diagnosis involves assay of DHPR in skin fibroblasts or amniotic cells. Phenylalanine hydroxylase activity is normal.

Other causes of PKU secondary to defective tetrahydrobiopterin synthesis include GTP cyclohydrolase deficiency and 6-pyruvoyltetrahydrobiopterin synthase deficiency. Patients with either defect have psychomotor retardation, truncal hypotonia with limb hypertonia, seizures, and a tendency to hyperthermia. The intravenous administration of BH_4 may lower blood phenylalanine levels, but this cofactor may not readily cross the blood-brain barrier. Treatment with synthetic pterin analogs or supplementation with tryptophan and carbidopa may prove more efficacious, particularly if treatment is started early in life.

DISORDERS OF GLYCINE METABOLISM: NONKETOTIC HYPERGLYCINEMIA

Glycine is essential to the synthesis of creatine, nucleic acids, hemoglobin, glucose, and phospholipids. It also becomes conjugated with bile acids and various medications, e.g., salicylates, in an enzyme-mediated process of detoxification.

Glycine catabolism proceeds primarily via the glycine cleavage system (GCS), a series of mitochondrial proteins that mediate the conversion of glycine to serine (and the reverse reaction as well) (Fig. 4, reaction 1). Pyridoxal phosphate and tetrahydrofolate are cofactors (see Chap. 35). This reaction also provides precursor to the one-carbon pool of folic acid intermediates that is pivotal to many synthetic reactions.

Nonketotic hyperglycinemia (NKH) is caused by a deficiency of the GCS. Affected infants become ill by the first or second day of life. Seizures are very prominent and even may occur *in utero*. The electroencephalogram often displays a hypsarrhythmia or a burst-suppression pattern. Infants regularly display myoclonic jerks, hiccuping, and a

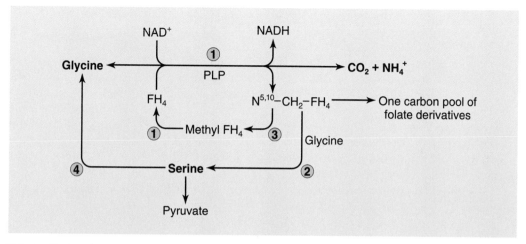

FIG. 4   Glycine cleavage system and some related reactions. Glycine and serine are readily interchangeable. *Enzymes:* (1) glycine cleavage system; (2) and (4) serine hydroxymethyltransferase; (3) $N^{5,10}$-methylenetetrahydrofolate reductase. ($N^{5,10}$-CH_2-FH_4) $N^{5,10}$-methylenetetrahydrofolate; (FH_4) tetrahydrofolic acid.

profound hypotonia. The few patients who survive past the first week of life usually require artificial ventilation and may sustain profound mental retardation and neurological disability. Brain imaging usually shows atrophy and a loss of myelin.

Rare patients present later in life with psychomotor retardation and growth failure. Others have had initially normal development followed by a progressive loss of developmental milestones. Some patients have manifested spinocerebellar degeneration.

Glycine is extremely high in the blood (even >1 mM; normal = 150–350 μM), cerebrospinal fluid, and urine. The glycine concentration in the cerebrospinal fluid is about 100 μM (normal ~10 μM). The ratio of glycine in the cerebrospinal fluid to that in the blood usually is 5 to 10 times the control value (0.02), especially with the classical disease.

The GCS is composed of four distinct subunits: P (pyridoxal-dependent decarboxylase), H (heat-stable, lipoic acid-binding carrier of the aminoethyl group), T (tetrahydrofolate-requiring), and L (lipoamide dehydrogenase). Most infants with the classical disease have had defects either in the P or in the T proteins.

A transient form of NKH, probably reflecting delayed maturation of the GCS, has been described in neonates with seizures but otherwise normal findings on neurological examination. The seizures ceased by 8 weeks of age and did not recur. Glycine concentrations in both the blood and the cerebrospinal fluid were high. Results of urine organic acid analysis were normal.

There is no specific therapy. Exchange transfusion and dialysis may relieve the need for assisted ventilation without altering the progressive neurological deterioration. Sodium benzoate has been administered in the hope that glycine would react with it to form hippuric acid, but this approach is not helpful. Similarly, the restriction of dietary protein and the administration of pyridoxine or choline have not proved useful.

Glycine is a neurotransmitter, having a postsynaptic inhibitory activity in the spinal cord and in some central neurons (see Chap. 18). Therapy with strychnine, which blocks the action of glycine at postsynaptic receptors, has been unavailing. Treatment with diazepam has been attempted because this drug displaces strychnine from its binding sites. The combination of benzoate and diazepam may be more effective, since high doses of the former reduce glycine levels in the CNS, thereby potentiating the ability of strychnine to block the glycine effect.

A few infants have received antagonists of the N-methyl-D-aspartate (NMDA) receptor, an excitatory glutamatergic receptor that is potentiated by glycine (see Chap. 17). Ketamine and dextromethorphan have been used with inconclusive results. Some infants may have had an improvement in the level of their irritability and in their electroencephalogram. One infant, treated with both benzoate and dextromethorphan, was seizure-free by 12 months of age and had only moderately delayed development. However, this favorable experience has not been duplicated at other centers. Treatment with dextromethorphan at the recommended dosage (maximum of 5 mg/kg/day) seems to be well tolerated.

DISORDERS OF SULFUR AMINO ACID METABOLISM: HOMOCYSTINURIA

The transsulfuration pathway (see Fig. 2) entails the transfer of the sulfur atom of methionine to serine with the ultimate formation of cysteine. The first step is the transfer of the adenosyl group of ATP to methionine, yielding S-adenosylmethionine (see Fig. 2, reaction 1), which, as the primary methyl donor in humans, plays a prominent role in the synthesis of several neurotransmitters and of creatine. A portion of the carbon of the polyamines spermidine and spermine is derived from S-adenosylmethionine following the decarboxylation of that compound.

The product of the methyl transfer reaction, S-adenosylhomocysteine, inhibits methyltransferases, a factor that may explain some of the pathology of homocystinuria (see below). S-Adenosylhomocysteine ordinarily is present at a low concentration, since it is cleaved by a specific hydrolase to homocysteine and adenosine (see Fig. 2, reaction 3).

About half of the homocysteine gener-

ated is remethylated to methionine, with either betaine or 5-methyltetrahydrofolic acid (methyl-FH$_4$) serving as methyl donor. The enzyme mediating remethylation, 5-methyltetrahydrofolate-betaine methyltransferase (see Fig. 2, reaction 4), utilizes methylcobalamin as a cofactor. The kinetics of the reaction favor remethylation. A failure of this system can cause one of the homocystinuria syndromes. This occurs because of dietary factors, e.g., vitamin B$_{12}$ deficiency, or because of a congenital absence of the apoenzyme or of the ability to convert folate or vitamin B$_{12}$ to the methylated, metabolically active form (see below).

Homocystinuria usually is caused by a congenital deficiency of cystathionine-β-synthase, a pyridoxine-dependent enzyme that converts homocysteine to cystathionine via condensation with serine (see Fig. 2, reaction 5). This enzyme has been mapped to human chromosome 21. The equilibrium favors cystathionine synthesis. Thus, homocysteine levels normally are very low, since both the remethylation pathway and the cystathionine synthase route efficiently dispose of this amino acid.

Cleavage of cystathionine is accomplished by γ-cystathionase, another pyridoxine-dependent enzyme that is coded on human chromosome 16 (see Fig. 2, reaction 6). The enzyme functions almost entirely to produce cysteine; virtually no reversal of the reaction occurs.

Cystathionine synthase deficiency

Homocystinuria usually is caused by a deficiency of cystathionine-β-synthase. A variety of mutations have been described, including the synthesis of an unstable enzyme; of a protein that loosely binds either pyridoxal phosphate, serine, or homocysteine; or of an enzyme differing in size from the wild strain. Cystathionine synthase is present in many organs, including the brain, and homocystinuric patients typically manifest deficient enzyme activity in these tissues.

Blood homocysteine levels are elevated

(50–200 μM; normal <10 μM) and the blood cysteine concentration tends to be low, reflecting the failure of cysteine synthesis. Increased remethylation of homocysteine that is not converted to cystathionine results in elevated blood methionine, often in excess of 200 μM (normal = 20–40 μM).

Some patients respond to the administration of pharmacological doses of pyridoxine (25–100 mg daily) with a reduction of plasma homocysteine and methionine. Pyridoxine responsiveness appears to be determined by heredity, with siblings tending to show a concordant response. The clinical syndrome is milder in these individuals. Pyridoxine responsiveness usually can be detected with assays of enzyme activity in cultured skin fibroblasts. The precise biochemical mechanism of the pyridoxine effect is not well understood.

About half of individuals who do not respond to pyridoxine will sustain ectopia lentis by age 5 to 10 years. Indeed, the diagnosis commonly is made by an ophthalmologist to whom a child with bilaterally displaced lenses has been referred.

The median IQ score is 78 and 56 for vitamin B_6-responsive and nonresponsive patients, respectively. Some children may come to clinical attention because of psychomotor retardation first noticed at age 1 to 2 years. Other signs are convulsions, which occur in about 20 percent of patients, and psychiatric difficulties, e.g., depression and personality disorders, which occur in about half of cases.

The most striking feature is a thromboembolic diathesis. This can occur in virtually any vessel, with thrombi common in peripheral veins and arteries, the cerebral and renal vasculature, and coronary arteries. Almost 25 percent of pyridoxine nonresponders sustain a major vascular insult during childhood. The comparable risk in untreated pyridoxine-responsive subjects is 25 percent by age 20 years. Vascular insults sometimes occur in association with dehydration secondary to vomiting and diarrhea. The stress of major surgery and anesthesia increases the risk of thrombosis by about 5 percent.

Affected patients commonly manifest a marfanoid habitus with arachnodactyly, high-arched palate, tall stature, and pes cavus. Bony abnormalities are common, with osteoporosis and scoliosis being frequent sources of clinical problems. The orthopedic pathology is more common and severe in vitamin B_6 nonresponders.

Demyelination and spongy degeneration of the white matter have been reported. Infarctions are common in virtually all parts of the brain. The arterial walls show thickening of the intima and splitting of the smooth musculature of the media. The changes are similar to those of atherosclerosis.

The apparent cause of the pathology is homocysteine itself, since hypermethioninemia is not associated with this phenotype. Homocysteine increases the adhesiveness of platelets *in vitro*, perhaps by increasing the synthesis of selected thromboxanes. The administration of homocysteine to rats or baboons can cause endothelial injury. Homocysteine may diminish the mean survival time of peripheral blood platelets, possibly by a direct toxic effect on the vascular endothelium, which becomes denuded and thereby provides an atherogenic nidus. A direct effect of homocysteine on the blood clotting cascade also is possible. The activation of factor V in cultured endothelial cells, resulting in increased conversion of prothrombin to thrombin, has been noted.

Homocysteine also promotes accumulation of copper in the vascular endothelium. This induces the oxidation of ceruloplasmin and the concomitant release of sufficient hydrogen peroxide to injure the endothelium. Supplementation of the medium with catalase was protective, thus confirming the role of oxidant injury.

High levels of homocysteine or one of its metabolites may directly affect brain function. The administration of homocysteine to rats induces grand mal convulsions, a phenomenon that is worsened by either methionine or pyridoxine. Homocysteine-induced blockade of the γ-aminobutyric acid (GABA) receptor (see Chap. 18) may be involved, or the action of homocysteic acid, which has a glutamatergic activity (see Chap. 17).

A high intracerebral concentration of *S*-adenosylhomocysteine may inhibit methylation reactions involving *S*-adenosylmethionine, including the methylation of proteins and of phosphatidylethanolamine as well as catechol-*O*-methyltransferase (see Chap. 12) and histamine-*N*-methyltransferase (see Chap. 14).

Patients who respond to large doses of vitamin B_6 (250–500 mg/day for several weeks) have the best prognosis. This approach is successful if the blood homocysteine and methionine are reduced to normal or near-normal levels. Since supplementation with pyridoxine can cause a deficiency of folic acid, the latter should be given (2–5 mg daily) at the same time. Any patient receiving pyridoxine should be monitored carefully for any signs of hepatotoxicity and for a peripheral neuropathy. Management of the older patient nonresponsive to pyridoxine is difficult. Dietary restriction of methionine would seem logical, but this often is unpalatable to an older patient.

The administration of betaine (6–12 g daily) lowers homocysteine levels by favoring remethylation. A theoretical hazard of betaine treatment is increasing the blood methionine, sometimes to an extravagant degree (~1 mM). Experience to date indicates that betaine administration is safe, with no major side effects except for a fishy odor to the urine.

Other therapeutic approaches have included the administration of salicylate and of dipyridamole to ameliorate the thromboembolic diathesis. Dipyridamole has been effective in animal studies in restoring platelet survival to a near-normal range. Patients also have been treated with dietary supplements of L-cystine, since the block of the transsulfuration pathway in theory could diminish the synthesis of this amino acid.

Remethylation deficiency homocystinuria

Remethylation defects usually are caused by aberrations in the metabolism of methylfo-late or methylcobalamin, the cofactors for the reaction. Patients often present early in life with lethargy, poor feeding, psychomotor retardation, and growth failure. Hematological abnormalities are common, including megaloblastosis, macrocytosis, thrombocytopenia, and hypersegmentation of the leukocytes. Occasional patients are clinically silent until later life, when seizures, dementia, hypotonia, mental retardation, spasticity, or a myelopathy become evident.

Biochemical findings are variable. Interestingly, the blood cobalamin and folate levels often are normal. Many have had homocysteinemia with hypomethioninemia, the latter helping to discriminate this group from homocystinuria secondary to cystathionine-β-synthase deficiency. Urinary excretion of MMA may be high, reflecting the fact that vitamin B_{12} serves as a cofactor for the MMA-CoA mutase reaction (see above).

Methylenetetrahydrofolate reductase deficiency

5,10-Methylenetetrahydrofolate is reduced to methyltetrahydrofolate by a cytoplasmic, NADPH-dependent enzyme, methylenetetrahydrofolate reductase (see Fig. 2, reaction 11). *S*-Adenosylmethionine inhibits the reaction. The enzyme normally is present in human brain, where it may play a role in the reduction of dihydropteridines (see section on disorders of phenylalanine metabolism).

Patients typically present with severe developmental retardation, convulsions, and microcephaly by age 6 to 12 months. A few individuals also have had psychiatric disturbances.

Homocysteinemia (usually ~50 μM) is the rule, with a relatively low (<20 μM) blood methionine. The blood concentration of vitamin B_{12} is normal, and unlike individuals with defects of cobalamin metabolism, these patients manifest neither anemia nor methylmalonic aciduria. The blood folic acid level is usually low.

A thromboembolic diathesis is not unusual, and thromboses have been reported in the brain vasculature. Other pathological changes have included microgyri, demyelination, gliosis, and brain atrophy. Lipid-laden macrophages have been described.

A relatively large number of agents have been utilized to treat this intractable disorder: folinic acid (5-formyltetrahydrofolic acid), folic acid, methyltetrahydrofolic acid, betaine, methionine, pyridoxine, cobalamin, and carnitine. Betaine, which provides methyl groups to the betaine : homocysteine methyltransferase reaction, appears to be a nontoxic approach that lowers blood homocysteine and increases methionine.

Methionine synthase deficiency (cobalamin-E disease)

This enzyme mediates the transfer of a methyl group from methyltetrahydrofolate to homocysteine to yield methionine (see Fig. 2, reaction 4). A cobalamin group bound to the enzyme is converted to methylcobalamin prior to the final formation of methionine.

In cobalamin-E (*cblE*) disease there is a failure of methyl-vitamin B_{12} to bind to methionine synthase. It is not known whether this reflects a primary defect of methionine synthase or the absence of a separate enzyme activity. Patients manifest megaloblastic changes with a pancytopenia, homocystinuria, and hypomethioninemia. There is no methylmalonic aciduria. Patients usually manifest clinically during infancy with vomiting, developmental retardation, and lethargy. They respond well to injections of hydroxycobalamin.

The activity of methionine synthase is restored to normal *in vitro* by addition of large amounts of thiols to the incubation mixture. In contrast, in *cblG* disease, the enzymatic activity remains low even with thiol supplementation of the assay.

Cobalamin-C disease

Complementation analysis allows the classification of patients with primary defects in the metabolism of vitamin B_{12} into one of three groups: *cblC*, *cblD*, and *cblF*. The most common variant is *cblC*. Most individuals become ill in the first few months or weeks of life with hypotonia, lethargy, and growth failure. Optic atrophy and retinal changes can occur. Methylmalonate excretion is excessive, although less than in MMA-CoA mutase deficiency. They do not display ketoaciduria and overwhelming metabolic acidosis.

The fibroblasts do not convert cyanocobalamin or hydroxycobalamin to methylcobalamin or adenosylcobalamin. The activities of both N^5-methyltetrahydrofolate : homocysteine methyltransferase and MMA-CoA mutase are consequently diminished. These biochemical lesions can be rectified by supplementation of the medium with hydroxycobalamin. The precise nature of the underlying defect remains obscure, although it appears to involve a step in the activation of vitamin B_{12}.

The diagnosis should be suspected in a child with homocystinuria, methylmalonic aciduria, megaloblastic anemia, hypomethioninemia, and normal blood levels of folate and vitamin B_{12}. A definitive diagnosis requires demonstration of these abnormalities in fibroblasts. Prenatal diagnosis is possible.

Treatment involves the administration of large doses (as much as 1 mg) of intramuscular hydroxycobalamin. Administration of folate and betaine (see above) may be helpful, as is a reduction of protein intake.

Cobalamin-D disease

This is an extremely rare variant that may become clinically manifest only in later life with mild mental retardation and behavioral abnormalities.

Hereditary folate malabsorption

Most patients present with megaloblastic anemia, seizures, and a progressive syndrome of neurological deterioration (see also Chap. 35). Levels of folate in both the blood and the cerebrospinal fluid have been very low. The anemia is correctable with injections of folate, or with the administration of large oral doses, but the concentration in the cerebrospinal fluid is still low, suggesting that a distinct carrier system mediates folate uptake into the brain and that this system is the same as that facilitating intestinal transport.

THE UREA CYCLE DEFECTS

The urea cycle (Fig. 5) facilitates the removal of waste nitrogen as urea (10–20 g/day in the healthy adult). In the absence of a functioning urea cycle, ammonia and related metabolite accumulation causes encephalopa-

thy and irreversible brain injury (see also Chap. 40). The urea cycle fails either because of acquired disease, e.g., cirrhosis secondary to alcoholism, or because of an inherited defect. The latter usually reflects a congenital enzymopathy.

The initial two steps of the urea cycle are mitochondrial. Carbamyl phosphate synthetase (CPS), which has been mapped to human chromosome 2, mediates the formation of carbamyl phosphate from ammonia (NH_3), HCO_3^-, and ATP (see Fig. 5, reaction 1). *N*-Acetylglutamate (NAG), formed from glutamate and acetyl-CoA via NAG synthetase (see Fig. 5, reaction 12), is an obligatory effector of CPS and is a prominent regulator of ureagenesis. A variety of influences, including dietary protein, arginine, and corti-

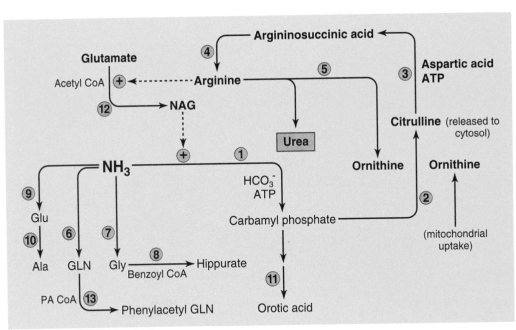

FIG. 5   The urea cycle and related reactions of ammonia metabolism. Congenital hyperammonemia syndromes usually are caused by a deficiency of one of the enzymes of the urea cycle. Ammonia also can be metabolized to glutamate, alanine, glutamine, and glycine. The administration of phenylacetate or of benzoate favors the formation of phenylacetylglutamine and hippurate, respectively, thereby providing an effective antidote to ammonia toxicity. *Enzymes:* (1) carbamyl phosphate synthetase; (2) ornithine transcarbamylase; (3) argininosuccinate synthetase; (4) argininosuccinate lyase; (5) arginase; (6) glutamine synthetase; (7) glycine cleavage system; (8) glycine-*N*-acylase; (9) glutamate dehydrogenase; (10) alanine aminotransferase; (11) the cytosolic pathway of orotic acid synthesis (becomes prominent when there is a block at the level of reaction 2, thus resulting in increased orotic acid excretion); (12) *N*-acetylglutamate synthetase; (13) phenylacetyl-CoA : glutamine transferase. (NAG) *N*-acetylglutamate; (PA-CoA) phenylacetyl-CoA. The plus symbols denote that arginine and NAG are positive effectors for reactions 12 and 1, respectively.

costeroids, augment the concentration of NAG in mitochondria.

Following condensation with ornithine, carbamyl phosphate is converted to citrulline in the ornithine transcarbamylase (OTC) reaction. OTC is coded on band p21.1 of the X chromosome, where the gene contains ten exons and spans 73 kb of DNA. The activity of this enzyme is directly related to dietary protein. There may be "tunneling" of ornithine transported from the cytosol to OTC, with the availability of intramitochondrial ornithine serving to regulate the reaction.

The citrulline is released to the cytosol, where it condenses with aspartate to form argininosuccinate in the argininosuccinate synthetase (AS) reaction (see Fig. 5, reaction 3). This enzyme is coded on human chromosome 9, where a 63-kb gene constituting 14 exons is located. The messenger RNA (mRNA) is markedly increased by starvation or treatment with corticosteroids or dibutyryl cyclic AMP. Citrulline itself is a potent inducer of the mRNA.

Argininosuccinate is cleaved in the cytosol by argininosuccinate lyase (AL), which is coded on human chromosome 7 (see Fig. 5, reaction 4). The products of the reaction are fumarate, which is oxidized in the tricarboxylic acid cycle, and arginine, which is rapidly cleaved to urea and ornithine via hepatic arginase. Both AL and arginase are induced by starvation, dibutyryl cyclic AMP, and corticosteroids. Several isozymes of arginase have been described.

Urea cycle defects in infants are characterized by a severe syndrome of coma, convulsions, and vomiting during the first few days of life. Clinical confusion with septicemia is common, and many infants are treated futilely with antibiotics. Hyperammonemia usually is severe, at a concentration even in excess of 1 mM.

Diagnosis usually is made from the blood aminogram. The plasma concentrations of glutamine and alanine, the major nitrogen-carrying amino acids, usually are high and that of arginine is low. Patients with citrullinemia (deficiency of AS) or argininosuccinic aciduria (deficiency of AL) manifest marked increases of blood citrulline and argininosuccinate levels, respectively.

The infant with either CPS or OTC deficiency may not be distinguished by the blood aminogram. The ornithine level typically is normal in the latter disorder. Urinary orotic acid generally is very elevated in babies with OTC deficiency and normal or even low in the infant with CPS deficiency. Patients with OTC deficiency have increased excretion of orotic acid because carbamyl phosphate spills into the cytoplasm, where it enters the pathway of pyrimidine synthesis. The presence of hyperammonemia, hyperglutaminemia, hyperalaninemia, and orotic aciduria in a critically ill infant affords strong presumptive evidence for OTC deficiency. Conversely, the presence of this pattern on the aminogram in the absence of an untoward orotic aciduria is suggestive of CPS deficiency.

Diagnosis of a urea cycle defect in the older child can be more problematic. Patients may present with psychomotor retardation, growth failure, vomiting, behavioral abnormalities, perceptual difficulties, recurrent cerebellar ataxia, and headache. Thus, it is essential to monitor the blood ammonia level in any patient with unexplained neurological symptoms. The measurement of blood ammonia alone may not be sufficient for diagnosis, since hyperammonemia can be an inconstant finding with partial enzymatic defects. In the latter group, quantitation of blood amino acids and of urinary orotic acid is indicated.

Hyperammonemia also occurs in some organic acidurias, particularly those that affect neonates. Thus, the urine organic acids should be quantitated in all patients with significant hyperammonemia.

A variety of biochemical changes in brain metabolism have been described in experimental models of hyperammonemia. High ammonia levels impair the malate-aspartate shuttle, which mediates the transport of NADH from cytosol to mitochondria.

Changes in the rate of oxidation of glucose and/or pyruvate also occur. The intracellular ATP pool may be depleted, especially in the reticular activating system.

Hyperammonemia also may affect brain volume control through effects on transport. Cell swelling is sometimes observed, perhaps because of the marked increase of brain glutamine. This change probably is most prominent in the astrocytes, where it would be expected to have an osmotic effect. Glial swelling is a common pathological finding in hyperammonemic patients and may be related to glial transport systems (see Chap. 3).

Hyperammonemia also affects neurotransmitter metabolism. Major effects on the metabolism and/or transport of GABA and serotonin have been observed. In the latter instance, a possible mechanism may be increased passage of tryptophan across the blood-brain barrier and consequent increased synthesis of serotonin. Treatment of patients with blockers of serotonergic receptors may alleviate the anorexia that is common.

Ammonia also has been shown in experimental systems to affect ion flux, in particular brain Cl^- flux. This might cause hyperpolarization of membranes.

Surprisingly little is known about the changes in the brain of patients dying with hyperammonemia. Abnormal myelination with cystic degeneration has been described, as has cell swelling, particularly of the astrocytes. Cortical atrophy may occur in youngsters with long-standing disease.

Except for patients with argininosuccinic aciduria, who may demonstrate varying degrees of hepatic fibrosis, there is very little evidence of pathological changes due to hyperammonemia outside of the CNS.

Carbamyl phosphate synthetase deficiency

CPS deficiency is relatively rare. Neonates quickly develop lethargy, hypothermia, vomiting, and irritability. The hyperammonemia typically is severe, at concentrations even in excess of 1 mM. Occasional patients with partial enzyme deficiency have had relapsing lethargy and irritability upon exposure to protein. Brain damage can occur in both neonatal and late-onset groups.

N-Acetylglutamate synthetase deficiency

A deficiency of CPS activity also can arise because of the congenital absence of NAG synthetase, which catalyzes the formation of NAG from glutamate and acetyl-CoA. NAG is an obligatory effector of CPS. The few patients reported have had a malignant course of neonatal onset.

Ornithine transcarbamylase deficiency

This is the most common of the urea cycle defects. Presentation is variable, ranging from a fulminant, fatal disorder of neonates to a schizophrenic-like illness in an otherwise healthy adult. Affected males characteristically fare more poorly than do females with this X-linked disorder. This difference reflects the random inactivation (lyonization) of the X chromosome. If the inactivation affects primarily the X chromosome bearing the mutant OTC gene, then a more favorable outcome can be anticipated. Conversely, if the wild-type X chromosome is inactivated, the female is expected to have a much more active disease.

The human OTC gene spans 73 kb and has 10 exons and nine introns. In the mouse a 750-bp promoter 5′ to the translation initiation codon confers tissue specificity.

The diagnosis has been aided by the use of genetic markers based upon intragenic restriction fragment length polymorphisms. More than 80 percent of carriers can be detected in this manner, and prenatal diagnosis is possible in many cases. Approximately one-third of the mothers of males and two-thirds of the mothers of females have been found to be noncarriers, reflecting the greater propensity for mutation in the male gamete.

Diagnosis of carriers can be made with protein loading tests, in which the excretion of urinary orotic acid has been used as a marker. This approach detects 85 to 90 percent of carriers. A recent elaboration of this test involves the administration of allopurinol to favor orotic acid excretion.

Animal models for OTC deficiency have been developed. These include the sparse fur (spf) mouse and the sparse fur-abnormal skin and hair (spf-ash) mouse. In the former instance a histidine residue replaces an asparagine at position 117 of the gene, resulting in an enzymatic activity that is 15 percent of control. The spf-ash mutation entails a base change in exon 4, resulting in a splicing mutation and a reduction of OTC activity to 5 percent of normal. Both kinds of mutant mice manifest hyperammonemia, orotic aciduria, growth failure, and a very sparse fur.

OTC deficiency must be suspected in any patient, male or female, with unexplained neurological symptoms. The absence of hyperammonemia in a casual sample should not rule out the diagnosis, especially if the history is positive for protein intolerance or an untoward reaction to infections. The family history also may be suggestive. The blood amino acids and urinary orotic acid should be quantitated in such individuals.

Citrullinemia

Neonates with AS deficiency usually die, and most survivors suffer major brain injury. Patients with a partial deficiency may have a milder course, and a few individuals with citrullinemia have been phenotypically normal.

The diagnosis usually is apparent from the hyperammonemia and the extreme hypercitrullinemia. The activity of AS can be determined in both fibroblasts and chorionic villus samples, thus simplifying the problem of prenatal diagnosis.

Argininosuccinic aciduria

These patients excrete an enormous amount of argininosuccinate in their urine. The cere-brospinal fluid also contains this polar molecule in high concentration. Neonates have a stormy clinical course and almost all have died or have sustained severe brain injury.

A peculiar finding in many cases is trichorrhexis nodosa, or dry brittle hair with nodular protrusions that are best visible with light microscopy. The precise cause is unknown.

Arginase deficiency

Most patients are thought to have psychomotor retardation during the first year of life, but the dominant presentation is a progressive, spastic tetraplegia, especially in the lower extremities. Seizures and growth failure may occur, although some patients are of normal size. The motor dysfunction usually comes to clinical attention by age 2 to 3 years. Leukodystrophic changes are seen in the brain. Ammonia levels are elevated in the blood, although not so much as in those disorders that occur in neonates. The plasma arginine concentration usually is two to five times normal. Urine orotic acid excretion is extremely high, perhaps because arginine stimulates flux through the CPS reaction by favoring the synthesis of NAG.

Hyperornithinemia, hyperammonemia, homocitrullinuria syndrome

Affected neonates commonly suffer growth failure and varying degrees of mental retardation. Sometimes symptoms are deferred until adulthood; vomiting, lethargy, and hypotonia are noted after protein ingestion. Recurrent hospitalizations for hyperammonemia are the rule. Some patients have manifested a bleeding diathesis and hepatomegaly. Electron microscopy of the liver has shown irregularities in the shape of the mitochondria.

The underlying biochemical defect is a failure of mitochondrial uptake of ornithine. This results in a failure of citrulline synthesis and a consequent hyperammonemia. Urinary orotic acid is high, presumably because of underutilization of carbamyl phosphate. In contrast, excretion of creatine is low, reflecting the inhibition of glycine transamidinase by excessive levels of ornithine.

Lysinuric protein intolerance

The clinical course in neonates usually is not severe. After weaning or upon exposure to high-protein foods, the infants manifest growth failure, hepatomegaly, splenomegaly, vomiting, hypotonia, recurrent lethargy, coma, abdominal pain, and in rare instances, psychosis. Rarefaction of the bones is common, and both fractures and vertebral compression have been reported. Most patients are not mentally retarded, although this may occur. Some patients have died with interstitial pneumonia that may respond to corticosteroid therapy.

The dibasic aminoaciduria reflects a failure of reabsorption of lysine, ornithine, and arginine by the proximal tubule. There also is a failure to absorb these compounds by the intestinal mucosa. The transport defect occurs at the basolateral rather than the luminal membrane. Hyperammonemia reflects a deficiency of intramitochondrial ornithine. An effective treatment is oral citrulline supplementation, which corrects the hyperammonemia by allowing replenishment of the mitochondrial pool of ornithine.

Management of urea cycle defects

Protein restriction is the mainstay of therapy. In patients with very severe disease, the tolerance of dietary protein may be so poor that it is not possible to feed an amount sufficient to support normal growth.

Treatment with sodium benzoate and sodium phenylacetate favors nitrogen removal by the formation of the amino acid conjugates hippurate and phenylacetylglutamine. Benzoyl-CoA reacts rapidly in the liver with glycine to form hippurate and phenylacetyl-CoA reacts with glutamine to yield phenylacetylglutamine. Excretion of ammonia as phenylacetylglutamine is more effi-

cient than is excretion as hippurate because 2 mol of ammonia is excreted with each mole of phenylacetylglutamine. However, the clinical utility of phenylacetate is limited by its objectionable odor.

Most patients who survive the neonatal period can be successfully maintained on a combination of a low-protein diet and sodium benzoate. A useful adjunct to treatment in cases of citrullinemia and argininosuccinic aciduria is supplementation of the diet with arginine, which enhances the ability to eliminate ammonia as either citrulline or argininosuccinate. In addition, the maintenance of arginine levels in the normal range facilitates protein synthesis.

Liver transplantation now has been utilized in children with urea cycle defects. The long-term utility is still uncertain.

Dialysis, including hemodialysis and peritoneal dialysis, relieves acute toxicity during fulminant hyperammonemia. Exchange transfusions also have been performed, but this technique has not been equally useful in removing ammonia.

DEFECTS OF BIOTIN METABOLISM

Biotin is a cofactor for two steps in amino acid metabolism: the carboxylation of 3-methylcrotonyl-CoA (see Fig. 1, reaction 5) in the pathway of leucine catabolism and the carboxylation of propionyl-CoA to form MMA-CoA (see Fig. 1, reaction 11). It also is a cofactor for the pyruvate carboxylase reaction in the gluconeogenic pathway and for acetyl-CoA carboxylase in the pathway of fatty acid synthesis (see Chap. 5). Hence, dietary deficiencies of biotin or congenital anomalies of biotin metabolism lead to the accumulation of several organic acids.

Biotin is covalently bound to these enzymes via an amide linkage with ϵ-NH$_2$ groups of lysine residues. A specific enzyme, holocarboxylase synthetase, mediates this linkage. Another enzyme, biotinidase, cleaves the biotinyl residues from the enzyme, thereby allowing the recycling of free biotin. Inherited defects of both biotinidase and holocarboxylase synthetase have been described. Prompt clinical recognition of these is essential, because treatment with pharmacological doses of biotin will dramatically improve outcome.

Holocarboxylase synthetase deficiency

Most patients manifest this deficiency early in life, often as neonates, with severe metabolic acidosis, marked tachypnea, hypotonia, vomiting, and seizures. The blood pH is typically quite low (often <7) and the blood lactate level is high. Many infants also have hyperammonemia. Quantitation of urinary organic acids typically shows a marked ketoaciduria with excretion of lactate, 3-methylcrotonylglycine, tiglylglycine, 3-hydroxypropionate, methylcitrate, and 3-hydroxyisovalerate, *inter alia*. If the disorder is not treated promptly, patients can develop a skin rash, alopecia, and varying degrees of psychomotor retardation. The direct assay of holocarboxylase synthetase in fibroblasts is possible. Prenatal diagnosis is feasible, either by determination of enzyme activity or by quantitation of organic acids in the amniotic fluid.

Biotinidase deficiency

Most patients present at 3 to 6 months of age with developmental retardation, hypotonia, seizures, cerebellar signs, alopecia, dermatitis, and conjunctivitis. Hearing loss is common. Quantitation of the urinary organic acids shows increased excretion of lactate, 3-hydroxyisovalerate, methylcitrate, and 3-hydroxypropionate, but this is not observed in every case, and the measurement of biotinidase activity in fibroblasts or peripheral blood cells may be necessary. Biotinidase activity in the serum of affected children usually is less than 10 percent that of control values. Prenatal diagnosis is possible.

Pathological lesions in the brain include cystic changes and demyelination. The cere-

bellum is especially vulnerable. A few patients have manifested changes suggesting meningoencephalitis.

Virtually all patients respond favorably to oral biotin (10–40 mg daily). Many of the clinical findings are reversible, even including some of the neurological abnormalities, although the hearing loss tends to persist.

DISORDERS OF GLUTATHIONE METABOLISM

The tripeptide glutathione (γ-glutamyl-cysteinyl-glycine), which serves as a coreactant in the glutathione peroxidase and glutathione transferase reactions, is the major intracellular antioxidant. It is synthesized according to the following reactions:

$$\text{Glutamate} + \text{cysteine} + \text{ATP} \rightarrow$$
$$\gamma\text{-glutamylcysteine} + \text{ADP} + \text{P}_i \qquad 1$$

$$\gamma\text{-Glutamylcysteine} + \text{glycine} + \text{ATP} \rightarrow$$
$$\text{glutathione} + \text{ADP} + \text{P}_i \qquad 2$$

Glutathione subsequently is metabolized in the γ-glutamyl cycle:

$$\text{Glutathione} + \text{amino acid} \rightarrow$$
$$\gamma\text{-glutamyl-amino acid} + \text{cysteinylglycine} \qquad 3$$

$$\gamma\text{-Glutamyl-amino acid} \rightarrow$$
$$\text{5-oxoproline} + \text{amino acid} \qquad 4$$

$$\text{5-Oxoproline} + \text{ATP} + 2\text{H}_2\text{O} \rightarrow$$
$$\text{glutamate} + \text{ADP} + \text{P}_i \qquad 5$$

$$\text{Cysteinylglycine} \rightarrow \text{cysteine} + \text{glycine} \qquad 6$$

The cycle is renewed after the cysteine formed in reaction 6 and the glutamate derived from reaction 5 are converted to γ-glutamylcysteine via γ-glutamylcysteine synthetase (reaction 1).

The most important congenital defects in glutathione metabolism are glutathione synthetase deficiency (reaction 2), γ-glutamylcysteine deficiency (reaction 1), γ-glutamyltranspeptidase deficiency (reaction 3), and 5-oxoprolinase deficiency (reaction 5).

5-Oxoprolinuria (glutathione synthetase deficiency)

Patients typically have a severe metabolic acidosis caused by excessive formation of 5-oxoproline (pyroglutamic acid). This occurs because the diminution of intracellular glutathione relieves the feedback inhibition on the γ-glutamylcysteine synthetase pathway (reaction 1), thereby augmenting the concentration of γ-glutamylcysteine and the subsequent conversion of this dipeptide to cysteine and 5-oxoproline in the cyclotransferase pathway (reaction 4).

This lesion was discovered in a young adult with mental retardation, severe metabolic acidosis, and evidence of a spastic quadriparesis and cerebellar disease. It also was observed in patients who were first diagnosed in infancy, and who enjoyed a period of normal psychomotor development for several years until late childhood, when a progressive loss of intellectual function became appreciated. Patients also may manifest a mild hemolysis. Pathological changes in the brain have included atrophy of the cerebellum and lesions in the cortex and thalamus.

γ-Glutamylcysteine synthetase deficiency

Patients with this very rare disorder have displayed spinocerebellar degeneration, peripheral neuropathy, myopathy, and an aminoaciduria secondary to renal tubular dysfunction. Psychosis and a hemolytic anemia have been features in some patients.

γ-Glutamyltranspeptidase deficiency

These patients display a marked glutathionuria because of the absence of the major pathway for glutathione utilization. The individuals also have shown varying degrees of mental retardation. The precise relationship

of the neurological signs to the biochemical lesion is problematic. The enzyme is present in the brain, primarily in the capillaries, where it may facilitate amino acid transport.

5-Oxoprolinase deficiency

These patients excrete increased amounts of oxoproline and have a somewhat elevated plasma concentration. They have not had significant neurological symptoms.

DISORDERS OF GABA METABOLISM

GABA is formed via the action of glutamate decarboxylase (see Chap. 18). The metabolism of this neurotransmitter is mediated first by uptake into neurons and glia and subsequent transamination to succinic semialdehyde via GABA transaminase (GABA-T) followed by formation of succinate in the succinic semialdehyde dehydrogenase reaction.

Pyridoxine dependency

The syndrome of pyridoxine dependency is characterized by severe seizure activity of early onset, perhaps even *in utero*. Patients respond dramatically to the parenteral administration of pyridoxine (10–100 mg) with a cessation of convulsive activity and a marked amelioration on the electroencephalogram. Speculation has centered on the possibility that the disease involves faulty binding of pyridoxine, a cofactor in the glutamate decarboxylase reaction, to the enzyme protein.

GABA-transaminase deficiency

Patients with this very rare disorder have severe psychomotor retardation and hyperreflexia. The concentrations of GABA and β-alanine in cerebrospinal fluid and blood are much greater than normal, as is the concentration of homocarnosine in the cerebrospinal fluid. GABA-T activity is much diminished in blood lymphocytes and in the liver. A curious finding is increased stature, perhaps reflecting the ability of GABA to evoke release of growth hormone.

Succinic semialdehyde dehydrogenase deficiency

Affected patients have mental retardation, cerebellar disease, and hypotonia. They excrete large amounts of both succinic semialdehyde and 4-hydroxybutyric acid.

DISORDERS OF *N*-ACETYLASPARTATE METABOLISM: CANAVAN'S DISEASE

Infants seem normal at birth, but a delay in development usually is apparent by 3 months of age. An increased head circumference (>98th percentile) is common, and hydrocephalus sometimes is suspected. Neurological function deteriorates rapidly over the next several months. Optic atrophy ultimately leads to blindness. They manifest minimal interest in their environment. Spasticity is frequent and seizures may occur. Imaging of the brain shows demyelination and brain atrophy with enlargement of the ventricles and widening of the sulci. Pathological examination shows swelling of the astrocytes with elongation of the mitochondria. Vacuoles appear in the myelin sheets.

The excretion of *N*-acetylaspartate is grossly elevated and the concentration of this amino acid in the cerebrospinal fluid may be 50 times control values. The cause is a deficiency of aspartoacylase, which mediates the formation of aspartate and acetyl-CoA from *N*-acetylaspartate. The enzyme normally is found primarily in the white matter, but *N*-acetylaspartate is most abundant in the gray matter. The defect is expressed in cultured skin fibroblasts.

N-Acetylaspartate is among the most abundant amino acids in the brain, although its precise function remains elusive. Putative roles have included osmoregulation and the storage of acetyl groups that subsequently are utilized for myelin synthesis. The relationship of the enzyme defect to the clinical findings remains problematic.

REFERENCES

Bickel, H. Differential diagnosis and treatment of hyperphenylalaninemia. *Prog. Clin. Biol. Res.* 177:93, 1985.

Brusilow, S., Tinker, J., and Batshaw, M. L. Amino acid acylation: A mechanism of nitrogen excretion in inborn errors of urea synthesis. *Science* 207:659, 1980.

Chalmers, R. A., and Lawson, A. M. *Organic Acids in Man, The Analytical Chemistry, Biochemistry and Diagnosis of the Organic Acidurias.* London: Chapman and Hall, 1982.

Eisensmith, R. C., and Woo, S. L. Phenylketonuria and the phenylalanine hydroxylase gene. *Mol. Biol. Med.* 8:3, 1991.

Goodman, S. I., and Markey, S. P. *Diagnosis of Organic Acidemias by Gas Chromatography-Mass Spectrometry. Laboratory and Research Methods in Biology and Medicine.* New York: Allan R. Liss, 1981.

Kikuchi, G. The glycine cleavage system: Composition, reaction mechanism and physiological significance. *Mol. Cell. Biochem.* 1:169, 1973.

Maestri, N. E., Hauser, E. R., Bartholomew, D., and Brusilow, S. W. Prospective treatment of urea cycle disorders. *J. Pediatr.* 119:923, 1991.

Nyhan, W. L. *Diagnostic Recognition of Genetic Disease.* Philadelphia: Lea & Febiger, 1987.

Scriver, C. R., Beaudet, A. L., Sly, W. S., and Valle, D. *The Metabolic Basis of Inherited Disease.* New York: McGraw-Hill, 1989.

CHAPTER 40

Metabolic Encephalopathies and Coma

WILLIAM A. PULSINELLI AND ARTHUR J. L. COOPER

LEVELS OF CONSCIOUSNESS

Metabolic encephalopathy is defined as any disease process that disrupts cerebral metabolism sufficiently to alter consciousness. These may be acute or chronic processes with reversible or irreversible changes, but most if not all metabolic encephalopathies can cause permanent structural injury to the brain if left untreated.

Plum and Posner [1] define consciousness as "the state of awareness of self and

Basic Neurochemistry: Molecular, Cellular, and Medical Aspects, 5th Ed., edited by G. J. Siegel et al. Published by Raven Press, Ltd., New York, 1994. Correspondence to William A. Pulsinelli, Department of Neurology, University of Tennessee, Memphis, The Health Science Center, 855 Monroe Avenue, Room 415, Memphis, Tennessee 38163.

environment'' and describe two essential elements of consciousness: content of the mind and arousal state of the brain. Abstract thinking, attention, language, and memory are examples of the mind's content and collectively represent the brain's higher cognitive functions. The clinical consequences of metabolic encephalopathies on cognitive function range widely from relatively mild changes in attention to severe distortions of abstract thinking and loss of memory.

Arousal of the brain can fluctuate through several levels that are reflected by changes in a person's behavior or "appearance of wakefulness" [1]. Daily, the normal physiological effects of the sleep-wake cycle cause the arousal state of the brain to change from the fully alert to the coma-like state of deep sleep. Disturbances of cerebral metabolism may also affect the arousal state. Progression of such neurochemical abnormalities is associated with an orderly decline in the level of consciousness, with early signs of obtundation followed by signs of stupor and finally coma. The obtunded or lethargic patient is one who appears drowsy, has slowed thinking, and requires mild stimuli to maintain the appearance of wakefulness. The stuporous patient requires repeated, vigorous stimuli to remain awake, and the comatose patient is unarousable even with the most intense sensory stimuli.

Abnormalities of brain chemistry sufficient to cause encephalopathy and coma comprise a large and heterogeneous array of disorders. Vitamin and nutritional deficiencies (Chap. 35), genetic diseases involving lipid (Chaps. 34 and 38), amino acid (Chap. 39), or carbohydrate metabolism (Chap. 34), substrate deficiencies (Chap. 42), and other still unclassified degenerative diseases (Chap. 45) may at an early or late stage disrupt the intricately balanced neurochemistry that subserves the integrative and arousal systems of the brain. It is beyond the scope of this chapter to review the metabolic abnormalities caused by each of these disorders or how such disturbances lead to encephalopathy and coma. In fact, although much is known about the primary neurochemical defects in most of these disorders, there are few definitive studies on how such changes cause altered cognition or arousal. Even in the often studied disorders of hypoxia and ischemia, hypoglycemia, hepatic encephalopathy, and uremia, which are the principal topics of this chapter, the precise pathogenesis of altered consciousness and cognition remains undefined. Accordingly, what follows is a descriptive account of the neurochemical and physiological changes that accompany the alterations of arousal and cognition in the more frequently encountered metabolic encephalopathies.

ANATOMICAL AND PHYSIOLOGICAL SUBSTRATE OF CONSCIOUSNESS

The content of consciousness is a consequence largely of the highly integrative activity of the neocortex. Arousal of the neocortex and other forebrain regions important for cognition is a physiological response mediated by several brainstem nuclei and fiber tracts that together constitute the ascending reticular activating system (ARAS). The anatomical and physiological limits of the ARAS remain undefined, but neurons within the brainstem reticular formation most directly responsible for arousal lie in the midline and extend from the middle of the pons rostrally through the midbrain and into the hypothalamus. Activating pathways ascend from the ARAS through thalamic synaptic relays to the neocortex.

Discrete structural lesions of the forebrain that cause deficits in language, memory, or motor function rarely affect in any clinically important manner the level of arousal unless the lesions are bilateral and involve extensive portions of the neocortex. In contrast, relatively small and localized lesions of the brainstem that interrupt the ARAS or its pathways are capable of altering consciousness through the full spectrum of lethargy to coma. Currently, most metabolic encephalopathies are thought to depress consciousness through diffuse disturbances of brain chemistry that act equally on forebrain and brainstem centers. Thiamine deficiency is one of the few proven exceptions to this general rule. The earliest encephalopathic symptoms of thiamine deficiency are caused by disturbances of specific brainstem, hypothalamic, and thalamic nuclei, which are particularly rich in the thiamine-dependent enzyme pyruvate dehydrogenase (see Chap. 35). Future studies that focus on neurochemical changes in more discrete brainstem nuclei may reveal other metabolic encephalopathies that affect selective brainstem nuclei early in the course of the disease.

The diverse nature and location of the neurons that subserve arousal suggest an equally diverse family of neurotransmitters involved in this complex function. Although details of neurotransmitter physiology and its relationship to arousal mechanisms remain to be clarified, some evidence suggests a role for cholinergic and monoaminergic systems, including norepinephrine, dopamine, and serotonin.

HEPATIC ENCEPHALOPATHY

Human hepatic encephalopathy occurs in two forms. An acute form, fulminant hepatic failure (FHF), is associated with rapid onset of severe inflammatory and necrotic liver disease. The disease is characterized by progression of symptoms from an initial altered mental status and clouded consciousness to coma, usually within a matter of hours or, at most, days. At one time free fatty acids were considered contributors to the disease, but later work discounted this theory. Excessive ammonia may be a factor, but in some patients with FHF the blood ammonia concentration is found to be within normal limits at the onset of neurological symptoms; however, as the crisis progresses, ammonia levels become elevated.

Much more common is chronic cirrhosis or recurrent hepatic encephalopathy, which accompanies chronic disease of the liver. In most cases, the cirrhosis is caused by alcoholism; in some cases, however, the disease may be due to infections, hemochromatosis, drugs, biliary obstruction, cardiovascular disease, genetic factors (see Chap. 39), or excessive exposure to certain organic solvents. Unless certain catastrophes occur, such as gastrointestinal bleeding or the ingestion of a heavy protein load (both of which lead to rapidly elevated blood ammonia levels), episodes of neurological dysfunction most often begin insidiously and develop slowly, nearly always requiring at least several days to reach a peak or to subside. Many patients recover from the neurological symptoms, at least temporarily; repeated bouts are common. Hypertension in the abdominal portal venous system characteristically accompanies chronic liver disease. Extrahepatic venous channels dilate, and the intravascular pressure shunts products of intestinal origin directly around the liver into the systemic circulation, bypassing the detoxification machinery of the liver (hence, the alternative name portal-systemic encephalopathy). In addition to extrahepatic shunting of potential toxins, the toxin-removing machinery of the liver itself may be depressed, further adding to the toxin load of the blood. Indeed, there is evidence that the urea cycle and glutamine synthetase activity may be depressed in cirrhotic livers.

In the following text we critically evaluate the various biochemical abnormalities thought to contribute to hepatic encephalopathy, keeping in mind that symptoms may be due to a combination of biochemical, morphological, energy, and physicochemical changes.

Elevated ammonia produces severe CNS toxicity

Many toxins are considered to contribute to the encephalopathy. These include ammonia, short-chain fatty acids, mercaptans, phenols, middle-molecular-weight compounds (M_r ~2,000), and quinolinic acid. Although there is no doubt that each of these compounds (or class of compounds) at elevated concentrations is toxic to the central nervous system (CNS) and may interact synergistically, much evidence suggests that ammonia is a major toxin in hepatic encephalopathy [2,3]. First, ammonia is a devastating toxin in infants born with defects of the urea cycle; the severity depends on the enzyme lesion. Most affected children must be treated as soon as possible with a regimen designed to lower blood ammonia. Abnormalities visible on computerized brain scans and IQ scores of surviving children correlate with the severity and length of neonatal hyperammonemia. Second, hyperammonemia is sometimes a complicating side effect in the treatment of epilepsy with valproate. In these patients, neurological symptoms occur without obvious liver damage. Third, ammonia is toxic to laboratory animals. However, acute hyperammonemia is somewhat different from that seen in patients with liver disease in that convulsions and hyperkinesia are seen rather than depression of CNS activity. Finally, crises in liver disease patients are induced by the administration of ammonium salts easily tolerated by healthy individuals and by ingestion of meals with a high ammonia-generating potential. Patients often respond, at least temporarily, to therapies designed to lower blood ammonia levels. On the negative side, it has been pointed out that blood ammonia concentrations do not always correlate with the degree of encephalopathy; however, blood ammonia concentration can fluctuate rapidly so that a single determination of the blood level is not necessarily a good predictor of brain ammonia levels. Better correlation exists between the degree of encephalopathy and concentration of glutamine (or its α-keto acid analog, α-ketoglutaramic acid) in the cerebrospinal fluid (CSF) of patients with hepatic encephalopathy.

Abnormalities may involve neurotransmitter amino acids

Ammonia metabolism is linked to the formation and turnover of a number of amino acids, two of which, glutamic and aspartic acids, are putative excitatory transmitters. Brain glutamate and aspartate are consistently lowered in hyperammonemic animals and in animals with experimentally induced liver disease. These changes in whole-brain glutamate and aspartate are usually modest; however, if the changes occur mostly in a select compartment, such as astrocytes or nerve endings, they could have a pronounced physiological effect. Some authors have proposed that glutamate neurotransmitter pools in the nerve endings are poorly repleted in the presence of excess ammonia, possibly by inhibition of glutaminase activity.

One widely publicized theory has suggested that hepatic encephalopathy is related to a defect in brain γ-aminobutyric acid (GABA) metabolism; however, this hypothesis is controversial and is not now widely accepted. GABA levels are usually normal in the brains of animals with experimentally induced liver failure and in biopsy specimens from patients dying with FHF; however, GABA receptor properties and density appear to be altered during hepatic encephalopathy.

The possibility also remains that compounds with GABAergic properties are elevated in the brains of patients with hepatic encephalopathy. Recently, Basile et al. [4] reported that 6 of 11 patients dying of acetaminophen-induced FHF had 2- to 10-fold higher brain concentrations of 1,4-benzodiazepines compared to control subjects. Neither group had received benzodiazepines during the hospital stay. The authors concluded that benzodiazepine antagonists deserve clinical trials in the treatment of hepatic encephalopathy. However, the question remains as to the origin of the benzodiazepines—are they of endogenous or exogenous origin? Moreover, the amounts observed in the brains of the patients were well below the level required to produce coma and almost half of the FHF patients had normal brain levels of benzodiazepines.

Tryptophan, serotonin, and 5-hydroxyindole acetic acid (5-HIAA) are increased in the brains of rats with portacaval shunts. Serotonin and 5-HIAA are elevated in brains, and 5-HIAA is elevated in the CSF of patients with acute and chronic hepatic encephalopathy. Moreover, the serotoninergic receptor properties are altered by excess ammonia.

Fischer [5] advanced the hypothesis that "false neurotransmitters" may contribute to the neurological changes associated with hepatic encephalopathy. False neurotransmitters are structural analogs of naturally occurring neurotransmitters that can occupy receptor sites blocking normal neurotransmitter function. Possible candidates include octopamine, tyramine, and β-phenylethanolamine. Evidence for the false-neurotransmitter hypothesis is as follows:

1. Patients in hepatic coma excrete increased amounts of tyramine and octopamine in their urine.
2. Octopamine and β-phenylethanolamine are increased in brain and CSF of animals with liver failure.
3. L-DOPA may lighten the coma of some patients with hepatic failure.

However, the effect of L-DOPA may be peripheral in that it seems to enhance renal excretion of ammonia. Moreover, dopamine and norepinephrine in postmortem brains of patients with liver cirrhosis are not different from controls. In an experiment in which massive doses of octopamine were administered to rats, brain norepinephrine and dopamine were depleted 86 and 92 percent, respectively, with no discernible untoward effects on behavior.

In various animal models of liver disease, the concentration of tyrosine and phenylalanine is increased in the plasma, whereas the concentration of the branched-chain amino acids (valine, leucine, isoleucine) is depressed. The activity of the carrier of the neutral amino acids across the blood-brain barrier (BBB) is enhanced. These findings prompted Fischer and colleagues [6] to suggest that in liver disease an excessive influx of aromatic amino acids into brain causes an overproduction of monoamines. In patients with hepatic encephalopathy, changes in the plasma branched-chain amino acids (tyrosine and phenylalanine) ratio correlated inversely with the severity of symptoms. Fischer has advocated the administration of mixtures rich in branched-chain amino acids to decrease entry of aromatic amino acids into brain and to redress the imbalance in branched-chain amino acid uptake. Although most reports suggest that the treatment is effective, at least in the short term, some reports suggest no benefit, and the treatment remains controversial.

Hawkins and co-workers [7] investigated the effects of intravenous administration of glucose or glucose plus branched-chain amino acids on the brains of portacaval-shunted rats. Both treatments lowered the high concentration of brain tyrosine, phenylalanine, and tryptophan; neither treatment altered the high level of norepinephrine, but the glucose diet normalized the high level of serotonin and 5-HIAA. Hawkins et al. reported that brain glucose consumption [cerebral metabolic rate for glucose (CMRGlc)] was depressed 25 to 30 percent in all brain regions examined in the portacaval-shunted rat (but see below) and that neither treatment reversed this trend. It seems unlikely that excess monoamine transmitters in the brain are the primary cause of hepatic encephalopathy. One possibility for the beneficial effects of branched-chain amino acids is that they may help to normalize brain glutamate levels.

Abnormalities in protein synthesis are produced by ammonia and liver disease

Ammonia interferes with lysosomal protein degradation in rat hepatocytes and inhibits protein synthesis in brain slices from young rats. In rats 8 weeks after portacaval shunt, an acute ammonia load further depresses the *in vivo* incorporation of lysine into brain proteins; however, *in vivo* incorporation of tracer amounts of labeled leucine or flooding doses of valine into rat brain protein is unchanged 3 to 4 weeks after portacaval shunt. It is not clear whether impaired protein synthesis occurs after 4 weeks or whether rates of protein synthesis vary with different amino acids. There is evidence that the differences in incorporation of labeled amino acids into proteins may be related to the decreased capacity of the basic amino acid carrier of the BBB and the increased capacity of the neutral amino acid carrier in the portacaval-shunted rat. Acute administration of ammonium acetate to rats is associated with a decrease in brain protein. Protein content, particularly in gray matter, is depleted in autopsy specimens from patients dying with liver failure. The loss, which is largely neuronal, may severely compromise normal neuronal function in end-stage liver disease.

Elevated ammonia depresses metabolic energy reserves

In patients with hepatic encephalopathy, the cerebral metabolic rate for oxygen ($CMRO_2$) and cerebral blood flow (CBF) decline roughly in parallel with the decline of neurological function (see Chap. 31). In alert 8-week portacaval-shunted rats with chronic low-grade hyperammonemia, the addition of a superimposed ammonia load, that is, a load easily tolerated by normal animals, promptly led to electroencephalogram (EEG) abnormalities, stupor, and a marked reduction in $CMRO_2$ and CBF. There is some controversy, however, as to whether portacaval shunting raises or lowers CMRGlc of rat brain.

In acute as well as sustained low-level ammonia intoxication in rats, phosphocreatine (PCr) in the brain falls, whereas the adenylate pool (ATP + ADP + AMP) remains unchanged. In more persistent low-grade hyperammonemia, the total adenylate pool declines, but adenylate energy charge (see Chap. 42) remains unaltered. At ammonia levels of 1 to 3 mmol/kg (normal value, ~200

μmol/kg) in the brain, both ATP and adenylate energy charge decline; the decline is especially notable in the brainstem [8].

Ammonia is known to stimulate glycolysis in brain extracts, probably by activating phosphofructokinase. Such stimulation could account for the apparent increase in CMRGlc reported for acutely hyperammonemic animals. Ammonia blocks oxidative metabolism of α-ketoglutarate and pyruvate by brain slices: Ammonia at concentrations of 0.5 to 1.0 mM markedly inhibits rat brain mitochondrial α-ketoglutarate dehydrogenase complex, a rate-limiting step of the tricarboxylic acid (TCA) cycle. Excess ammonia also inhibits isocitrate dehydrogenase in rat liver mitochondria, but its effect on the brain enzyme is unknown.

A theory formulated over 30 years ago proposes that ammonia is deleterious to the CNS because it stimulates reductive amination of α-ketoglutarate, draining TCA carbon. However, in hyperammonemic animals, whole-brain levels of glutamate tend to be depleted, and α-ketoglutarate levels are either normal or elevated. Evidently, inhibition of the TCA cycle is not caused by withdrawal of five-carbon units but is due to a slowing of a key step of the cycle.

Several investigators have suggested that excess ammonia may stimulate glutamine synthetase, thereby draining ATP. This drain is likely to be small, however, and part of the increase in brain glutamine in hyperammonemic animals may be due to decreased glutamine breakdown. Nevertheless, hyperammonemia may cause a depletion of brain energy reserves (Fig. 1). D. D. Clarke (quoted in Berl [9]) pointed out that the diversion of glucose carbon to glutamine could result in a loss of 28 to 38 equivalents of ATP that are potentially available through complete oxidation of glucose to CO_2.

In hyperammonemic rats both the cerebral lactate/pyruvate and cytoplasmic $NADH/NAD^+$ ratios are increased. The mitochondria are impervious to cytoplasmically generated NADH so that the electrons associated with this NADH must cross the inner mitochondrial membrane via a shuttle sys-

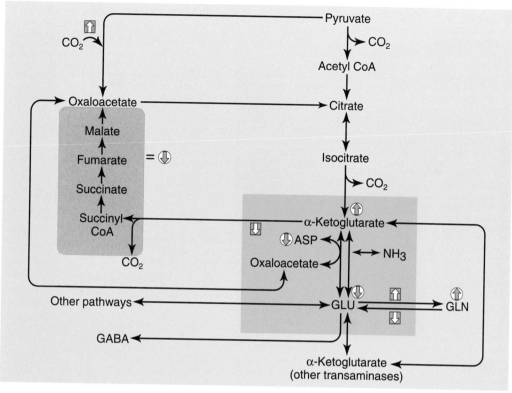

FIG. 1. Effects of excess ammonia on various substrates, TCA cycle, and related enzymes in brain where known. *Boxed arrows* indicate a stimulation or inhibition of an enzymatic reaction. *Encircled arrows* refer to ammonia-induced changes in metabolites. Note that most of the reactions depicted occur in the mitochondria but that changes shown refer to whole-brain metabolites (i.e., cytosol plus mitochondria). Excess ammonia strongly inhibits α-ketoglutarate dehydrogenase complex, impeding flux through the cycle toward malate, but strongly stimulates the anaplerotic pyruvate carboxylase reaction. Stimulation of carbon flow from CO_2 to glutamine will result in loss of ATP by (1) increasing ATP hydrolysis via pyruvate carboxylase and glutamine synthetase; (2) short-circuiting the TCA cycle (from α-ketoglutarate to malate); and (3) bypassing NADH formation at the pyruvate dehydrogenase reaction. Thus, the biochemical derangements induced by excess ammonia can be energetically expensive. (For further details, see text and Berl [9]).

tem. Strong evidence suggests that the malate-aspartate shuttle (MAS) plays a major role in electron translocation in brain. The ammonia-induced changes in the lactate/pyruvate and cytoplasmic NADH/NAD$^+$ ratios suggest a block in the MAS [10], possibly by slowing of the glutamate-aspartate translocator and by decreased activity of the aspartate aminotransferases (Fig. 2). The block in the MAS will further compromise energy metabolism.

Because CO_2 fixation and glutamine synthetase activity in brain are predominantly astrocytic, it is possible that at least a portion of the ammonia-induced cerebral energy deficit is in these cells. This deficit may contribute to the astrocytic pathology (Alzheimer type II changes) characteristic of hepatic encephalopathy in humans and laboratory animals.

Two groups of investigators recently suggested that ammonia per se may not be toxic to the CNS, but that in hyperammonemia the excessive conversion of ammonia to glutamine causes a pathological response [11,12]. One group suggested that excessive conversion of ammonia to glutamine causes an osmotic insult and brain edema [11].

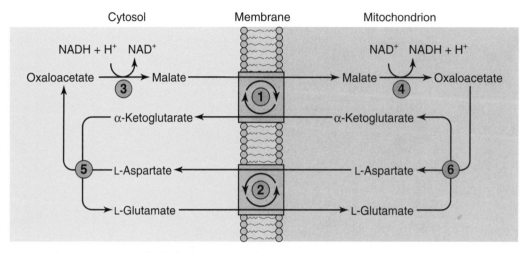

Cytosol   Membrane   Mitochondrion

FIG. 2.   The malate-aspartate shuttle for the transport of reducing equivalents between cytosol and mitochondrion: (1) α-ketoglutarate-malate carrier; (2) glutamate-aspartate carrier; (3) cytosolic malate dehydrogenase; (4) mitochondrial malate dehydrogenase; (5) cytosolic aspartate aminotransferase; (6) mitochondrial aspartate aminotransferase. The enzymatic steps are reversible, but a directionality is imposed via the energy-requiring one-way passage of aspartate from mitochondrion to cytosol. Glutamate and aspartate are consistently lowered in the brains of hyperammonemic animals. These changes may slow both the glutamate-aspartate exchange and flux through the transaminases. The mitochondrial enzyme may be particularly susceptible to changes in glutamate, since its apparent K_m for glutamate has been reported to be approximately 20 mM. (From Cooper and Meister [30]. Copyright © 1985 by John Wiley & Sons, Inc. Reprinted with permission.)

Several groups recently investigated *in vivo* metabolism in the forebrains of acutely and chronically hyperammonemic rats using nuclear magnetic resonance (NMR) techniques (e.g., see [13]). The techniques confirmed the previous observations that glutamate is depressed and glutamine is elevated in the brains of hyperammonemic animals; ATP and PCr levels remain relatively normal at moderate levels of hyperammonemia but fall during severe hyperammonemia. Recent NMR studies of the fate of ^{13}C-labeled glucose showed an increased rate of lactate production and decreased TCA cycle activity in the brains of hyperammonemic rats *in vivo* in accord with the previous predictions outlined above.

HYPOXIC ENCEPHALOPATHY

The metabolic consequences in brain of pure hypoxia as opposed to those of cerebral ischemia are best addressed separately, since

ischemia causes, in addition to a reduced oxygen supply, loss of substrate and impaired removal of metabolic waste products. For a detailed presentation of the metabolic changes that accompany cerebral ischemia, the reader is referred to Chap. 42.

Graded hypoxia produces increasing CNS dysfunction

Pure hypoxic encephalopathy, uncomplicated by the effects of reduced CBF, occurs rarely in humans, since hypoxia-induced cardiac arrhythmias and systemic hypotension cause cerebral hypoperfusion. Hypoxic encephalopathy is encountered in patients who suffer pulmonary disease with ventilation-diffusion-perfusion defects, patients with severe anemia, and in normal individuals who are exposed acutely to high altitudes. In fact, the clinical manifestations of hypoxic encephalopathy in humans are best exemplified in experiments where healthy young individuals are subjected to rapid decompression hy-

TABLE 1.   Hypoxic thresholds for CNS dysfunction[a]

Simulated altitude (ft)	F_iO_2 (%)	PaO_2 (Torr)	Neurological status
Sea level	21	90	Normal
5,000	17	80	Impaired dark vision
8,000–10,000	15–14	55–45	Impaired short-term memory; difficulty learning complex tasks
15,000–20,000	11–9	40–30	Loss of judgment, euphoria, obtundation
>20,000	<9	<25	Coma

[a] Values derived from young volunteers subjected to acute (minutes) decompression hypoxia. (F_iO_2) fractional percentage of ambient oxygen.

poxia over a period of a few minutes. From the results of such experiments it is possible to define the partial pressures of ambient and arterial oxygen (PaO_2) at which neurological impairment occurs (Table 1). However, such PaO_2 threshold values may not directly apply to chronic or slowly developing hypoxia, where multiple compensatory mechanisms have sufficient time to maintain cerebral homeostasis and brain function or where chronic changes have increased vulnerability.

Acute hypoxia, which is induced over a few minutes by breathing air equivalent to that found at approximately 5,000 ft (PaO_2 = 80 Torr), impairs the ability of retinal rods to adapt to the dark. At slightly higher altitudes, between 8,000 and 10,000 ft, which correspond to PaO_2 = 55 to 45 Torr, difficulties with learning complex tasks and impaired short-term memory are encountered. At approximately 15,000 to 20,000 ft, which corresponds to PaO_2 = 40 to 30 Torr, cognitive function becomes more severely impaired, with loss of judgment, a sense of euphoria or delerium, and the onset of muscular incoordination. Acute hypoxia, equivalent to 20,000 ft or above, which corresponds to PaO_2 = 25 to 20 Torr, is associated with rapid loss of consciousness.

Energy failure in moderate hypoxia is not linear with partial pressure of arterial oxygen despite CNS dysfunction

The ultimate cause of encephalopathy associated with severe hypoxia (PaO_2 <25 Torr) is a fall in the partial pressure of tissue oxygen to levels that no longer support mitochondrial respiration. Under such conditions, loss of consciousness is readily explained by a rapid depletion of the high-energy organic phosphates PCr and ATP; however, the neurochemical basis for impaired cerebral function at PaO_2 >25 to 20 Torr is less clear. Experimental studies indicate that energy metabolism remains normal at a time when mild to moderate hypoxia (PaO_2 = 25–40 Torr) has already markedly compromised cognition in human volunteers. Kety and Schmidt [14] and others [15] reported normal $CMRO_2$ in human volunteers at PaO_2 = 25 to 40 Torr; most showed either abnormal mental function or abnormal electrophysiological activity, and a few temporarily lost consciousness despite a normal $CMRO_2$. Graded hypoxia in laboratory animals revealed that ATP levels remained normal above PaO_2 = 20 to 25 Torr [16] (Fig. 3), yet EEG in these animals showed slowing and attenuated sensory evoked responses.

Glycolysis is stimulated to maintain ATP levels under moderate hypoxia

Studies of laboratory animals have demonstrated several important changes in brain chemistry occurring at PaO_2 levels of approximately 50 Torr, an oxygen tension well above that necessary for blocking ATP synthesis. An increase in the cerebral lactate/pyruvate ratio and a decrease in brain tissue pH are the most consistent and earliest changes reported at PaO_2 = 45 to 50 Torr. Consistent with this increase in lactate production is a rise in the CMRGlc, which most certainly in-

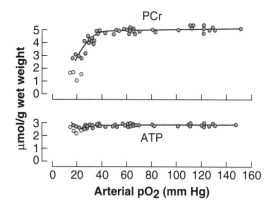

FIG. 3. Brain concentrations of PCr and ATP in rats anesthetized with 70 percent N_2O and subjected to graded hypoxia for periods of 15 to 30 min: (●) animals with $\leq$120 Torr mean arterial pressures; (○), animals with >80 Torr mean arterial pressure. (From Siesjö [16]. Copyright © 1978 by John Wiley & Sons, Inc. Reprinted with permission.)

dicates accelerated glycolysis. The cytosolic redox potential as measured by the NADH/NAD$^+$ ratio shifts toward a more reduced state at approximately this same PaO_2. PCr levels begin to decline slightly at PaO_2 = 45 to 50 Torr; they then fall more rapidly when PaO_2 falls below 20 Torr. The initial decline in PCr is probably related to the early increase in tissue lactic acid and the pH dependency of the creatine kinase equilibrium that favors the conversion of PCr to ATP. The later fall in PCr coincides with the decrease in ATP levels and undoubtedly reflects failure of mitochondrial respiration and oxidative phosphorylation.

To summarize the effects on energy stores, brain tissue oxygen content becomes limiting at PaO_2 in the neighborhood of 45 to 50 Torr. As a consequence, glycolysis is stimulated to a sufficient degree to maintain normal tissue ATP concentrations until the PaO_2 levels fall below 20 Torr. Paradoxically, cerebral dysfunction at 45 to 50 Torr is manifested by abnormal EEG activity and behavior, despite apparently normal energy stores.

Equally as puzzling as the abnormal EEG data is the rise of extracellular K$^+$ concentration at a PaO_2 of approximately 25 to 30 Torr. Since maintenance of Na$^+$ and K$^+$

concentration gradients is thought to rely largely on the activity of Na,K-ATPase, elevation of extracellular K$^+$ implies dysfunction of this enzyme pump or a hypoxic-dependent leakage of K$^+$ through membrane channels (see Chap. 3). In the presence of normal ATP levels, both mechanisms are difficult to understand.

One possible explanation for the early rise of the extracellular K$^+$ concentration is that the microregional concentration of ATP either at the catalytic site of Na,K-ATPase or at the presynaptic ATP-regulated K$^+$ channels is no longer sufficient for critical enzyme/receptor-mediated reactions. Since extracellular ATP normally blocks presynaptic K$^+$ channels, local reduction of extracellular ATP could cause K$^+$ ion leakage, hyperpolarization of presynaptic membranes, and inhibition of synaptic transmission. It is known that hypoxia will induce marked microregional heterogeneity of glucose [17] (Fig. 4) and oxygen [16] metabolism, and

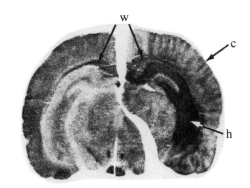

FIG. 4. Carbon-14 autoradiograph of a coronal brain section from a rat subjected to right common carotid artery ligation and hypoxia (PaO_2 = 28–32 Torr). The right cerebral hemisphere is shown on the right side of the photograph. Hypoxia raises CBF to the left hemisphere (patent carotid) to four times normal and to the right hemisphere (ligated carotid) to twice normal values. Note the alternating columns of high and low neocortical (c) metabolism (compared to the contralateral neocortex) and the increased glucose metabolism within the subcortical white matter (w) and hippocampus (h). (From Pulsinelli and Duffy [17]. Copyright © 1979 by the American Association for the Advancement of Science. Reprinted with permission.)

it is possible that measurements of ATP in milligram samples of brain are insensitive to similar microregional changes of ATP. Another possibility is that the available free energy ($\Delta G^{0'}$) of ATP hydrolysis becomes limiting with moderate hypoxia. A shift in the intracellular pH by one unit, that is, pH 7.2 to 6.2, which is fully attainable during hypoxic conditions in brain, will reduce the $\Delta G^{0'}$ of ATP hydrolysis by approximately 0.5 kcal/mol [18]. Although such changes in $\Delta G^{0'}$ appear insignificant in that they represent only 4 percent of the 12.5 kcal available per mole of ATP, it is conceivable that even small reductions in $\Delta G^{0'}$ may further alter the rate of critical enzyme reactions already affected by the hypoxic state.

Neurotransmitter abnormalities are found in moderate hypoxia

Hypoxia-induced changes in neurotransmitter chemistry may contribute in important ways to the symptoms of hypoxic encephalopathy. The synthesis and metabolism of norepinephrine, dopamine, and serotonin are oxygen-dependent (Fig. 5). The rate-limiting reactions of dopamine, norepinephrine, and serotonin synthesis, which are catalyzed by the enzymes tyrosine hydroxylase and tryptophan hydroxylase, require molecular oxygen. Moreover, the conversion of dopamine via the enzyme dopamine-β-hydroxylase to norepinephrine also requires oxygen. The K_m of oxygen for these oxygen-dependent hydroxylases is approximately 12 μM (7 Torr). Brain tissue oxygen content is thought to vary between 2 and 25 μM (1–15 Torr); thus, small changes in tissue oxygen content may reduce monoamine synthesis [19]. At an arterial oxygen concentration of approximately 40 Torr, the turnover of catecholamines and serotonin, which reflect both synthesis and metabolism, is reduced by approximately 25 percent. Values for the tissue concentration of these monoamine neurotransmitters during hypoxia vary from one laboratory to another, and interpretation of these data with regard to the cause of hypoxic encephalopathy is difficult, since both neurotransmitter synthesis and degradation are oxygen-dependent.

The concentration of amino acid neurotransmitters and acetylcholine may also be sensitive to changes in tissue oxygen tension, since synthesis of these neurotransmitters is closely coupled to glycolysis and oxidative metabolism (Fig. 6). Arterial oxygen tensions of 50 to 60 Torr will reduce by 50 percent the incorporation of radiolabeled choline into acetylcholine but will not alter the tissue concentration of this neurotransmitter [20]. At similar arterial oxygen tensions, the incorporation of radiolabeled glucose into γ-aminobutyrate, glutamate, aspartate, serine, and alanine is reduced by approximately 40 to 60 percent, but as with acetylcholine, the tissue concentrations of these amino acids remain unchanged. The significance of these hypoxia-induced changes in the pathogenesis of hypoxic encephalopathy remains problematic. Of note is the finding that alterations in metabolism of acetylcholine, catecholamine, and amino acid neurotransmitters occur at arterial oxygen tensions of 40 to 60 Torr, which are well above those that

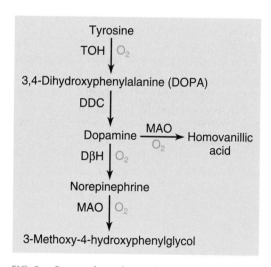

FIG. 5.   Oxygen dependence of dopamine and norepinephrine synthesis and metabolism: (TOH) tyrosine hydroxylase; (DDC) dopamine decarboxylase; (DβH) dopamine β-hydroxylase; (MAO) monoamine oxidase. (Modified from Gibson et al. [19].)

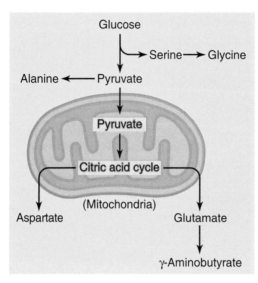

FIG. 6. The relationship between amino acid neurotransmitter synthesis and glycolysis and the TCA cycle. (From Gibson et al. [19].

affect energy metabolism. Such changes may therefore partially explain the early signs and symptoms of hypoxic encephalopathy.

HYPERCAPNIC ENCEPHALOPATHY

Respiratory acidosis causes decreased pH in the CNS

Although CO_2 is a normal metabolite, at elevated concentrations it is toxic; CO_2 is in equilibrium with carbonic acid (H_2CO_3) and bicarbonate (HCO_3^-) which is an important buffer of H^+ ions. Acute pulmonary or ventilatory insufficiency in humans if untreated rapidly leads to alterations in brain function resembling those of acute hypoxia and ischemia. Chronic pulmonary insufficiency is characterized by mild to moderate hypoxemia accompanied by varying degrees of CO_2 retention. Renal conservation of HCO_3^- usually buffers the hypercapnia, and blood pH is usually normal; however, the superpositioning of an added insult, such as infection, ingestion of a sedative, or fatigue, can further compromise lung function, resulting in even greater CO_2 retention and a disruption of the normal buffering mechanisms. The respiratory acidosis associated with CO_2 retention in blood causes an almost proportionate increase in $[H^+]$ in systemic tissues including the CNS.

Hypercapnia produces increased CBF and variable effects on CMRO$_2$

Patients with chronic pulmonary insufficiency may exhibit lethargy, mental confusion, retrograde amnesia, and stupor. The combination of hypoxia and hypercapnia leads to cerebral vasodilation, increased CBF, and sometimes increased intracranial pressure. The associated hypoxemia probably contributes to but is not the underlying cause of the neurological symptoms. Neurological symptoms correlate best with the degree of CO_2 retention. Acute, moderate hypercapnia (5–10 percent CO_2 in the inspired air) produces increased arousal and excitability; higher CO_2 concentrations (>35–40 percent) in the inspired air are anesthetic. Increased CO_2 levels are associated with a number of metabolic changes in the brain. In many studies, the arteriovenous (A-V) difference for oxygen across the brain is generally found to decrease in proportion to increases in CBF, leaving the CMRO$_2$ unchanged. In other studies, however, CMRO$_2$ is reported either elevated or depressed (range, 71–131 percent) [21]. The differences may be due to differences in species and methodology employed in the various studies. It is possible that at moderate concentrations, CO_2 stimulates the catecholamine system, thereby enhancing CMRO$_2$; at very high CO_2 concentrations, or when this system is blocked by drugs, CO_2 becomes a depressant.

In hypercapnia, CMRGlc is depressed, but the magnitude is variable

Some workers have reported a fall in CMRGlc that approximately parallels the fall in $CMRO_2$. Others have shown a proportionately greater decrease in CMRGlc. Glucose is the major fuel for the adult brain under normal circumstances; however, Miller [21] provided evidence that in acute hypercapnia (20 percent CO_2: 26 percent O_2: 54 percent N_2 in the inspired air for 10 min) in the adult rat, $CMRO_2$ is unchanged, but as much as a third of the inspired oxygen is used for the oxidation of other fuels, principally glutamate and lactate. To what extent this could continue in chronic hypercapnia is not known.

Several investigators have shown that acute hypercapnic acidosis results in an increase in cerebral glycolytic intermediates above the phosphofructokinase step and a decrease in metabolites below this step, possibly due to inhibition of phosphofructokinase activity by increased $[H^+]$. Despite continued acidosis and decreased CMRGlc, however, the components of the phosphofructokinase reaction gradually return to near-normal levels. The body temperature of the animals in these experiments was not monitored; it is possible that CMRGlc was decreased because of hypothermia.

Despite decreased CMRGlc during hypercapnia, cerebral ATP levels are generally found to be unaltered. Decreases in cerebral metabolism during hypercapnia are probably a consequence of decreased neuronal activity and not the cause of the encephalopathy. Possible factors contributing to hypercapnic encephalopathy include (1) depleted neurotransmitter glutamate pools, (2) decreased acetylcholine synthesis from pyruvate, (3) ammonia intoxication, and (4) interference with lipid metabolism.

HYPOGLYCEMIC ENCEPHALOPATHY

The large population of insulin-dependent diabetic patients explains the relatively high incidence of encephalopathy caused by hypoglycemia. Many of the earliest signs and symptoms of mild hypoglycemia reflect the workings of physiological protective mechanisms initiated by hypothalamic sensory nuclei and effected through sympathetic and endocrine systems. If these early warning signals, which include diaphoresis, tachycardia, hunger, and anxiety, are unheeded, worsening hypoglycemia will lead to primary CNS symptoms similar to those of hypoxia. Loss of attention, confusion, delerium, seizures, lethargy, stupor, and, finally, coma are the consequences of progressively worsening hypoglycemia.

Less than 30 years ago insulin-induced hypoglycemic coma was an experimental therapy for psychiatric disease. In the course of such therapy Kety and colleagues [22] found that the CMRGlc fell to a greater degree than did $CMRO_2$ in patients subjected to hypoglycemic coma. The disproportionate decrease between $CMRO_2$ and CRMGlc was interpreted as evidence for the metabolism of substrates other than glucose by brain tissue. Experimental animal studies have corroborated the hypothesis that the brain is capable of metabolizing carbon sources other than glucose [23]. Despite the capacity for metabolizing alternative fuels, which include acetoacetate, β-hydroxybutyrate, and several amino acids, cerebral energy metabolism fails, and the concentrations of ATP and PCr fall in the total absence of glucose (see Chap. 31).

Under normal conditions the human brain consumes approximately 10 percent of the glucose delivered to it [24]. As blood glucose concentrations fall below 2.5 mM, CMRGlc and $CMRO_2$ in laboratory animals begin to decline, CMRGlc to a greater degree than $CMRO_2$ [25,26]. At this level of blood glucose, confusion or delerium is the initial sign of hypoglycemia in humans. The EEG initially shows an increase in amplitude and decreased frequency at approximately 2 mM blood glucose, and as the glucose falls further toward 1 mM, EEG amplitude and frequency decrease, and the patient becomes stuporous; below 1 mM, the EEG becomes isoelectric as coma develops.

Generalized energy failure does not account for CNS dysfunction in moderate hypoglycemia

Initially it was assumed that the onset of mental dysfunction and the early EEG changes associated with moderate (blood glucose, 1.5–2.5 mM) hypoglycemia were related to tissue energy failure, especially since they coincided well with changes in CMRGlc and CMRO$_2$. However, many studies involving experimental animals showed that the concentrations of high-energy organic phosphates remain entirely normal during the early stages of symptomatic hypoglycemia [16,26] (Fig. 7). As the blood glucose concentration falls to 1 mM and below, CNS symptoms are readily explained by a rapid decline in high-energy organic phosphates.

Generalized cerebral energy failure cannot account for the early neurological deteri-

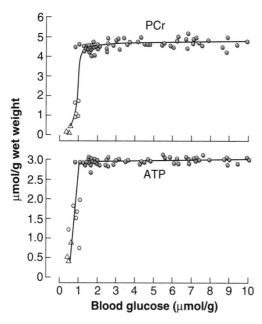

FIG. 7. Neocortical concentrations of PCr and ATP in rats subjected to graded hypoglycemia. Samples of frozen neocortex were used for these measurements. (●) EEG non-isoelectric; (○) EEG isoelectric for 3 min prior to freezing brain; (△) EEG isoelectric for 6 to 28 min prior to freezing brain. (From Siesjö [16]). Copyright © 1978 by John Wiley & Sons, Inc. Reprinted with permission.)

oration associated with moderate hypoglycemia, a situation similar to that encountered in mild symptomatic hypoxia. Since most studies of hypoglycemia correlated EEG activity and neurological behavior with measurements of PCr and ATP from tissue samples of either whole forebrain or neocortex, it is possible that site-specific changes in high-energy phosphates could account for altered consciousness. Indeed, results from McCandless and Abel [25] demonstrated that ATP levels in the reticular formation of the brainstem are decreased by approximately 30 percent and PCr by 55 percent during the precoma stages of hypoglycemia in animals.

Other mechanisms of hypoglycemic encephalopathy

Alternative explanations for the early metabolic encephalopathy associated with hypoglycemia include the accumulation of toxic products of nonglucose metabolism, such as ammonia and free fatty acids. Hypoglycemia enhances the accumulation of toxic levels of brain ammonia possibly derived from glutamate and aspartate, which decrease in hypoglycemia.

Other possible mechanisms that lead to deterioration of mental function during hypoglycemia include impairment of acetylcholine synthesis and changes in the concentrations of other putative neurotransmitters, such as glutamate, aspartate, and GABA [25,27].

UREMIC ENCEPHALOPATHY

Uremic encephalopathy is an acute or subacute syndrome that regularly occurs in patients in whom renal function falls below 10 percent of normal. Neurological symptoms include clouding of consciousness, motor hyperactivity, disturbed sleep patterns, nausea, decreased sexual activity, and bizarre behavior. Many patients suffer from transient hemiparesis and other focal neurological weaknesses. Amaurosis, nystagmus, vertigo, and ataxia are common. Some patients are prone to convulsions. EEG abnormalities occur in animals with experimentally induced uremic encephalopathy and in humans with the disease. Uremia is characterized by retention in the blood of urea, phosphates, proteins, amines, and a number of ill-defined low-molecular-weight compounds. It is interesting that despite acidemia, the pH of brain, muscle, leukocytes, and CSF appears to be normal. Since hemodialysis corrects the encephalopathy, low-molecular-weight compounds may be at least partially responsible. Urea, however, is nontoxic, even at elevated concentrations. In patients with acute renal failure, water, K^+, and Mg^{2+} are normal, whereas Na^+ is slightly decreased, and Al^{3+} increased; Ca^{2+} in the cerebral cortex is almost twice normal [28].

Uremia alters the characteristics of the blood-brain barrier

The permeability of the BBB toward insulin and sucrose is increased. Sodium ion transport is impaired, but potassium ion transport is enhanced; permeability toward weak acids tends to be decreased. The CBF in uremic patients has been reported to be elevated, but $CMRO_2$ and CMRGlc decline. Blood ammonia is normal or only slightly elevated in uremic patients; PCr, ATP, and glucose are increased in the brains of rats with acute renal failure, whereas AMP, ADP, and lactate are decreased. These changes are probably due to a reduction in cerebral energy demands. Osmolality increases to a similar extent in brain, CSF, and plasma (from ~310 to ~350 mOsmol/kg H_2O) in animals with renal failure. In acute renal failure all of the increase in brain osmolality is due to urea, whereas in the chronic model almost half the increase in brain osmolality is due to unknown molecules (idiogenic osmoles). The role of idiogenic osmoles in the uremia-induced encephalopathy is unknown.

Parathyroid hormone may be a factor in uremic encephalopathy and neuropathy

Circulating parathyroid hormone (PTH) (M_r ~10,000) is not removed by hemodialysis. Administration of PTH (but not Ca^{2+} or vitamin D) to normal dogs induces EEG changes comparable to those found in uremic animals, whereas parathyroidectomy prior to induction of uremia prevents the EEG abnormalities and associated hypercalcemia.

Uremia also produces a chronic, peripheral neuropathy, usually in the lower extremities, that is not ameliorated by hemodialysis (see Chap. 36). The neuropathy cannot be attributed to nutritional or other complicating factors. Plasma PTH levels are often elevated in uremic patients, and such patients have significantly lower motor nerve conduction velocities than those of uremic patients with normal or moderately elevated levels of PTH.

Excess PTH in patients with hyperparathyroidism frequently produces psychiatric symptoms and EEG changes similar to those observed in uremic patients. In such patients, parathyroidectomy results in an improvement of both EEG and mental status. As with hyperparathyroid patients, parathyroidectomy or medical suppression of PTH improves the EEG and mental status of uremic patients. Teschan and Arieff [28] concluded that "PTH and/or a high brain calcium content are probably responsible, at least in part, for many of the encephalopathic manifestations of renal failure."

DIALYSIS ENCEPHALOPATHY

Dialysis disequilibrium syndrome

Repeated hemodialysis is now the standard treatment for many patients with chronic renal failure, but some patients develop neurological symptoms as a result of the dialysis. In extreme cases, seizure, coma, and death have resulted, but such incidences are now on the decline. Acute encephalopathy occurs most commonly during rapid removal of blood urea. It was originally thought that the rapid drop of serum osmolality was responsible. It was argued that since osmotically active molecules (including urea) that have accumulated in the brain may be cleared relatively slowly from brain, water will shift from plasma to brain, causing brain swelling; however, Teschan and Arieff [28] cautioned that some of the symptoms may be due to causes other than dialysis disequilibrium. Urea clearance from uremic dog brain parallels that of plasma during rapid hemodialysis. In both uremic dogs and humans, the CSF pH drops during rapid hemodialysis. Arieff suggested that an increase in brain [H+] leads to secondary swelling [28].

Progressive dialysis encephalopathy

In some patients undergoing long-term hemodialysis therapy, a progressive, severe encephalopathy develops, and is almost always fatal. In some cases, a strong correlation exists with increased brain Al^{3+}; in other cases, brain Al^{3+} is not increased. Teschan and Arieff [28] suggested that there may be several etiological agents and recognized three classes:

1. An epidemic form, possibly related to Al^{3+} in the dialysate
2. Spontaneous cases in which Al^{3+} is less likely to be causative
3. Dementia associated with congenital or early childhood renal disease

The last group includes some children who were never dialyzed or exposed to aluminum. Al^{3+} compounds placed on the brain surface are highly toxic. Interesting is the fact that Al^{3+} is increased in the brains of patients with Alzheimer's disease, hepatic encephalopathy, several forms of metastatic cancer, and renal failure. The last group has the highest level of Al^{3+}; Al^{3+} concentration is greater in the brains of patients with chronic renal failure than those with acute renal failure and is greatest in patients with dialysis dementia (11 times normal in one study). Bone and tissues other than brain also contain increased Al^{3+} in uremic patients. Presumably, the source of at least some of this Al^{3+} is the $Al(OH)_3$ given to patients with chronic renal failure to control serum phosphate levels; untreated tap water used to prepare the dialysis fluids for patients on maintenance hemodialysis may be another source of Al^{3+}. The hypothesis that Al^{3+} may be a causative factor is controversial, although recent work by Alfrey [29] suggests that removing Al^{3+} from the dialysate greatly reduces the risk of dialysis encephalopathy.

REFERENCES

1. Plum, F., and Posner, J. B. *The Diagnosis of Stupor and Coma*. Philadelphia: F. A. Davis, 1980.
2. Duffy, T. E., and Plum, F. Hepatic encephalopathy. In I. M. Arias, H. Popper, D. Schachter, and D. A. Shafritz (eds.), *The Liver: Biology and Pathobiology*. New York: Raven Press, 1982, pp. 693–715.
3. Cooper, A. J. L., and Plum, F. Biochemistry and physiology of brain ammonia. *Physiol. Rev.* 67:440–519, 1987.
4. Basile, A. S., Hughes, R. D., Harrison, P. M., Murata, Y., Pannel, L., Jones, E. A., Williams, R., and Skolnik, P. Elevated brain concentrations of 1,4-benzodiazepines in fulminant hepatic failure. *N. Engl. J. Med.* 325:473–478, 1991.
5. Fischer, J. E. False neurotransmitters and hepatic coma. In F. Plum (ed.), *Brain Dysfunction in Metabolic Disorders*. (*Res. Publ. Assoc. Nerv. Ment. Dis., Vol. 53*). New York: Raven Press, 1974, pp. 53–73.
6. James, J. H., Jeppsson, B., Ziparo, V., and Fischer, J. E. Hyperammonaemia, plasma amino acid imbalance, and blood-brain amino acid transport: A unified theory of portal-systemic encephalopathy. *Lancet* 2: 772–775, 1979.
7. Mans, A. M., Davis, D. W., Biebuyck, J. F., and Hawkins, R. A. Failure of glucose and branched-chain amino acids to normalize brain glucose use in portacaval shunted rats. *J. Neurochem.* 47:1434–1443, 1986.

8. Hindfelt, B. Ammonia intoxication and brain energy metabolism. In G. Kleinberger and E. Deutsch (eds.), *New Aspects of Clinical Nutrition*. Basel: Karger, 1983, pp. 474–484.

9. Berl, S. Cerebral amino acid metabolism in hepatic coma. In E. Polli (ed.), *Experimental Biology and Medicine (Neurochemistry of Hepatic Coma, Vol. 4)*. Basel: Karger, 1971, pp. 71–84.

10. Hindfelt, B., Plum, F., and Duffy, T. E. Effects of acute ammonia intoxication on cerebral metabolism in rats with portacaval shunts. *J. Clin. Invest.* 59:386–396, 1977.

11. Takahashi, H., Koehler, R. L., Bruisilow, S. W., and Traystman, R. J. Inhibition of brain glutamine accumulation prevents cerebral edema. *Am. J. Physiol.* 261:H825–H829, 1991.

12. Hawkins, A., and Jessy, J. Hyperammonaemia does not impair brain function in the absence of glutamine synthesis. *Biochem. J.* 277:1697–1703, 1991.

13. Fitzpatrick, S. M., Hetherington, H. B., Behar, K. L., and Schuman, R. G. Effects of acute hyperammonemia on cerebral amino acid metabolism and pH$_i$ in vivo, measured by ^{1}H and ^{31}P nuclear magnetic resonance. *J. Neurochem.* 52:741–749, 1988.

14. Kety, S., and Schmidt, C. F. The effects of altered arterial tensions of carbon dioxide and oxygen on cerebral blood flow and cerebral oxygen consumption of normal young men. *J. Clin. Invest.* 27:484–492, 1948.

15. Cohen, P. J., Alexander, S. C., Smith, T. C., Reivich, M., and Wollman, H. Effects of hypoxia and normocarbia in cerebral blood flow and metabolism in conscious man. *J. Appl. Physiol.* 23:183–189, 1967.

16. Siesjö, B. K. *Brain Energy Metabolism*. New York: Wiley, 1978, pp. 380–446.

17. Pulsinelli, W., and Duffy, T. E. Local cerebral glucose metabolism during controlled hypoxemia in rats. *Science* 204:626–629, 1979.

18. Alberty, R. A. Effect of pH and metal ion concentration on the equilibrium hydrolysis of adenosine triphosphate to adenosine diphosphate. *J. Biol. Chem.* 243:1337–1343, 1968.

19. Gibson, G. E., Pulsinelli, W., Blass, J. P., and Duffy, T. E. Brain dysfunction in mild to moderate hypoxia. *Am. J. Med.* 70:1247–1254, 1981.

20. Gibson, G. E. Hypoxia. In D. W. McCandless (ed.), *Cerebral Energy Metabolism and Metabolic Encephalopathy*. New York: Plenum Press, 1985, pp. 43–78.

21. Miller, A. L. Carbon dioxide narcosis. In D. W. McCandless (ed.), *Cerebral Energy Metabolism and Metabolic Encephalopathy*. New York: Plenum Press, 1985, pp. 143–162.

22. Kety, S. S., Woodford, R. B., Harmel, M. H., Freyhan, F. A., Appel, K. E., and Schmidt, C. F. Cerebral blood flow and metabolism in schizophrenia: The effects of barbiturate semi-narcosis, insulin coma and electroshock. *Am. J. Psychiat.* 104:765–770, 1948.

23. Hawkins, R. Cerebral energy metabolism. In D. W. McCandless (ed.), *Cerebral Energy Metabolism and Metabolic Encephalopathy*. New York: Plenum Press, 1985, pp. 3–23.

24. Plum, F., and Pulsinelli, W. Cerebral metabolism in hypoxic-ischemic brain injury. In A. K. Asbury, G. M. McKhann, and W. Ian McDonald (eds.), *Diseases of the Nervous System*. Philadelphia: W. B. Saunders Co., 1986, pp. 1086–1100.

25. McCandless, D. W., and Abel, M. S. Hypoglycemia in cerebral energy metabolism. In D. W. McCandless (ed.), *Cerebral Energy Metabolism and Metabolic Encephalopathy*. New York: Plenum Press, 1985, pp. 27–41.

26. Ghajar, J. B., Plum, F., and Duffy, T. E. Cerebral oxidative metabolism and blood flow during acute hypoglycemia and recovery in unanesthetized rats. *J. Neurochem.* 38:397–409, 1982.

27. Ghajar, J. B. G., Gibson, G. E., and Duffy, T. E. Regional acetylcholine metabolism in brain during acute hypoglycemia and recovery. *J. Neurochem.* 44:94–98, 1985.

28. Teschan, P. E., and Arieff, A. I. Uremic and dialysis encephalopathies. In D. W. McCandless (ed.), *Cerebral Energy Metabolism and Metabolic Encephalopathy*. New York: Plenum Press, 1985, pp. 263–285.

29. Alfrey, A. C. Dialysis encephalopathy. *Kidney Int.* 29:S53–S57, 1986.

30. Cooper, A. J. L., and Meister, A. Metabolic significance of transaminations. In P. Christen and D. E. Metzler (eds.), *Transaminases*. New York: Wiley, 1985, pp. 534–563.

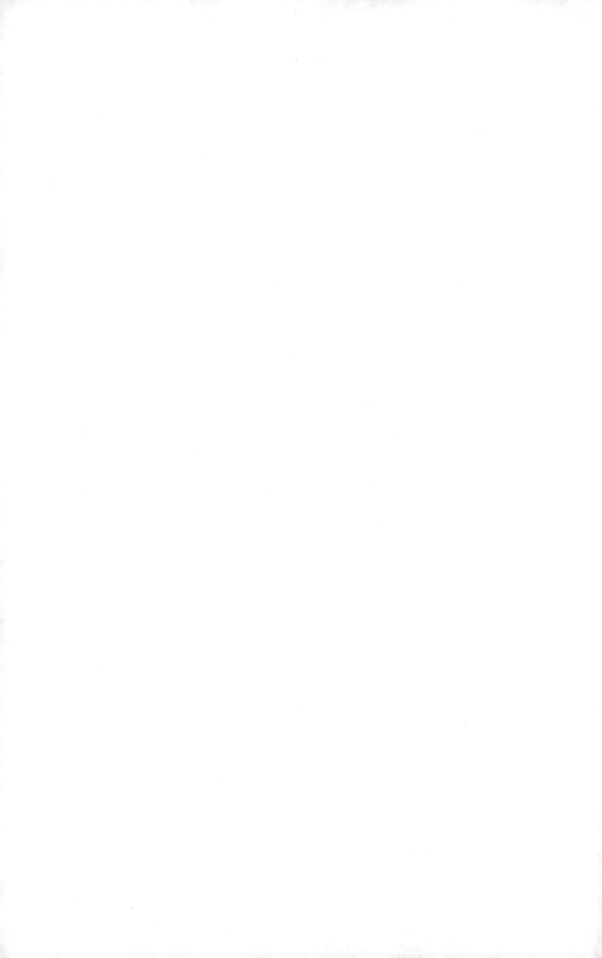

CHAPTER 41

Molecular Targets of Abused Drugs

MICHAEL J. BROWNSTEIN AND TED B. USDIN

Drug abuse imposes an enormous burden on the drug users, their families and friends, and society. In 1980, 69,000 deaths were attributed to alcohol intoxication and 6,000 to the effects of other drugs. In 1983, the estimated cost of alcohol and drug abuse was $177.4 billion, 60 percent of this from lost productivity and unemployment.

While it is true that drug abusers primarily do harm to themselves, they also injure others. Nineteen percent of women diagnosed as having acquired immunodeficiency syndrome (AIDS) by September 1989 were sexual partners of intravenous drug users; 58 percent of children diagnosed as having AIDS by September 1989 were born to mothers who took drugs intravenously or were sexual partners of intravenous drug users.

It is difficult to give a universal definition of drug abuse because different societies condone the use of different drugs and dictate when it is appropriate to use them, the purposes for which they can be used, and the amounts that can be taken. "Abuse," then, is use in excess of the limits imposed by society. The excess can be mild in degree, moderate, or extreme. In the latter case—when the drug consumes the individual completely—the user is referred to as being "addicted." In such a case, he or she may have grown physically or psychologically *dependent* on the drug. That is, discontinuation of the compound (or administration of an antagonist) results in an "abstinence" or "withdrawal syndrome" which consists of drug craving, drug-seeking behavior, plus a variety

Basic Neurochemistry: Molecular, Cellular, and Medical Aspects, 5th Ed., edited by G. J. Siegel et al. Published by Raven Press, Ltd., New York, 1994. Correspondence to Michael J. Brownstein, Laboratory of Cell Biology, National Institute of Mental Health, National Institutes of Health, Bethesda, Maryland 20892.

TABLE 1. Major classes of abused drugs

	Examples	Effects
Opiates	Heroin Morphine Opium Meperidine Methadone	Relief of tension Euphoria Sedation Warm flush and sensation like orgasm with IV use Nausea and vomiting with initial use

CNS depressants
  (sedatives and
  hypnotics)
	Barbiturates—pentobarbital, secobarbital
	Benzodiazepines—diazepam (Valium),
	  triazolam (Halcion), alprazolam (Xanax)
		Sense of well-being
		Reduced anxiety
		Disinhibition (increased sexual interest,
		  aggressive behavior)

Ethanol		Sense of well-being Disinhibition and hyperexcitability
CNS stimulants	Cocaine ("crack") Amphetamines	Mood elevation, euphoria Increased energy, activity, attention Decreased appetite

Psychedelics	Indolealkylamines—lysergic acid
	  diethylamide (LSD), psilocybin,
	  psilocin, dimethyltryptamine
	Phenylethylamines—mescaline, 2,5-
	  dimethoxy-4-methylamphetamine
	  (DOM, "STP")
		Heightened awareness of sights and
		  sounds
		Vivid images and sensory illusions
		Perceived clarity and importance of
		  thoughts
		Mood lability
		Distorted perception of time

Arylcyclohexylamines	Phencyclidine ("angel dust," "PCP")	Mood elevation Sense of intoxication Increased sensitivity to external events Violent behavior Psychosis
Cannabinoids	Δ-9-Tetrahydrocannabinol (marijuana, hashish)	Enhanced perception of color and sound Sense of well-being Drowsiness or buoyant mood Altered sense of time Sense of unreality
Nicotine	(From Tobacco)	Increased heart rate and blood pressure Tremor Slight euphoria Facilitated attentiveness Decreased weight gain

[a] Life-threatening.

Site(s) of action	Toxicity	Withdrawal syndrome	Medical use
μ Opiate receptor (agonist)	Respiratory depression Cardiac arrhythmias Constipation	Drug craving Anxiety Irritability Tearing Runny nose Perspiration Pupil dilation Nausea Vomiting Diarrhea Bone and muscle pain Tremors Weakness	Analgesic
GABA receptor (allosteric facilitator)	Sluggishness Faulty judgment Poor attention Ataxia Respiratory depression and coma	Restlessness Anxiety Tremor Weakness Abdominal cramps Nausea and vomiting Seizure and status epilepticus[a] Delirium tremens[a]	Antianxiety Anticonvulsant Muscle relaxation

Variety of ion channels:
  NMDA receptor (allosteric inhibitor)
  GABA$_A$ receptor (allosteric facilitator)
  5-HT$_3$ receptor (facilitation)
  L-type calcium channel (allosteric inhibitor)
	Ataxia
	Faulty judgment
	Loss of consciousness
	Amnesia
	Coma
	Respiratory depression[a]
		Anxiety
		Tremor
		Seizure and status epilepticus[a]
		Delirium tremens[a]
			None

Cocaine—dopamine transporter (blocker), perhaps norepinephrine and 5-HT transporters Amphetamines—displace catecholamines from synaptic vesicles, catecholamine transporters (blocker)	Tachycardia Hypertension Stroke Arrhythmia Seizure Respiratory depression Cardiovascular collapse Paranoia and hallucinosis	Craving Depression Anxiety Prolonged sleep	Cocaine—local anesthetic Amphetamine—treatment of narcolepsy
5-HT$_2$ receptor (partial agonist)	Confusion and panic		None
NMDA receptor (allosteric inhibitor)	Excitation Incoordination Hypertension Muscular rigidity Cardiac arrhythmias Seizure Coma Protracted psychosis	Fearfulness Tremor Confusion Amnesia	None
Cannabinoid receptor (agonist; site of action of endogenous arachydonyl ethanolamide, "anandamide")			Treatment of nausea—in cancer chemotherapy
Nicotinic cholinergic receptor (initially acts as agonist, then produces depolarization block)	Increased risk of coronary artery disease, chronic respiratory disease, lung cancer, and stroke	Anxiety Malaise	None

of uncomfortable and sometimes life-threatening symptoms. Most, but not all, addicts become physically dependent on the chemicals they abuse; however, it is incorrect to assume that all drugs that induce physical dependency are addictive.

Many of the commonly abused drugs are reinforcing in laboratory animals. Presumably the animals learn to self-administer compounds because their effects are pleasant to experience. Animals can be taught to self-administer other compounds to avoid withdrawal symptoms after they are passively addicted. Like humans, animals induced to press levers to receive drugs can grow *tolerant* to some of their effects and have to get more and more drug to obtain the desired response. Tolerance can result from more rapid metabolism or excretion of a compound or from cellular adaptation to its effects. The adaptive changes may underlie the symptoms associated with drug withdrawal. As one might expect, many of these are just the opposite of the effects caused by the compound itself. Sometimes, one drug can be substituted for another to which a person (or animal) is dependent, preventing the development of the withdrawal syndrome. In this case, the subject is said to exhibit "cross dependence." Similarly, development of tolerance to one compound is often accompanied by development of tolerance to related compounds. This phenomenon is known as "cross tolerance."

In this chapter we mention each of the major classes of abused drugs. Examples of these agents, their "desirable" and toxic effects, the withdrawal syndrome associated with their chronic use, and their molecular targets are summarized in Table 1. By "molecular targets" we mean the most proximal site(s) of a drug's action. Thus, in the case of opiates, the targets are opioid receptors. Since, for the most part, these are discussed in detail elsewhere in this volume, we only identify them and describe them superficially. We cannot elaborate on the regions of the brain responsible for the behavioral effects of each drug or the biochemical alterations that must occur following short- and long-term interactions of the drug with its target. This would require much more space (and, in the case of many of the compounds, a considerable amount of speculation). Likewise, we do not attempt to indicate why it is that some people become addicted while others do not. Data from epidemiological studies suggest genetic contributions to substance abuse, but the genes involved and their relationship to the proximal targets that are the focus of this chapter are unknown. Finally, it is worth noting that most addicts abuse several drugs simultaneously. These contribute in aggregate to the clinical picture presented by any given person.

OPIATES

Opium has been used for millenia as a euphoriant, sedative, and analgesic. It acts on opioid receptors in the brain and spinal cord. Of these, there are three types: μ, δ, and κ (see Chap. 15). To date, one δ [1,2] and one κ receptor have been cloned, but more members of this receptor family are likely to be cloned and characterized in the next few years. The principal site of action of morphine, the active agent in opium, and the other addicting opiates is the μ receptor. The affinity of morphine for this receptor is about 10 times its affinity for δ and κ receptors (which may mediate some of the toxic effects of the drug). The opioid analgesics that are commonly abused exhibit cross tolerance with one another, but they do not exhibit cross tolerance with δ and κ agonists.

Like the δ and κ receptors, the μ receptor appears to be G protein-coupled. Occupation of this receptor by agonists is associated with inhibition of adenylate cyclase and activation of inwardly rectifying potassium channels.

Tolerance to opiate agonists and withdrawal symptoms do not seem to result from a reduction in the number of μ receptors or their affinity for ligands. Instead "counteradaptation'' (and the rebound effects that are seen following withdrawal) may be caused by a long-term increase in the activity of adenylate cyclase, a changed association of the receptors with potassium channels, and a reduction in the production of endogenous peptide agonists (enkephalins).

CENTRAL NERVOUS SYSTEM DEPRESSANTS

The sedatives and anxiolytic agents listed in Table 1 are rather similar in their actions, exhibit cross tolerance with one another (and with ethanol), and share the same target, the γ-aminobutyric acid (GABA$_A$) receptor. This receptor is currently envisioned to be heteromeric, comprised of α, β, and γ (or δ)-subunits. To date, six α-, four β-, two γ-, and one δ-subunits have been cloned. The exact subunit stoichiometry of functional receptors found *in vivo* remains to be determined.

Barbiturates are allosteric enhancers of GABA receptor function. Their actions only require α- and β- subunits, and all of the subunit combinations studied thus far are barbiturate-sensitive [3,4]. This may not be the case *in vivo*, however.

Benzodiazepines also increase GABA-induced chloride currents. Their actions require the presence of the γ-subunit in the receptor complex [5]. It is worth noting that benzodiazepine antagonists and ''inverse agonists'' have been synthesized and identified. The latter are thought to inactivate the GABA receptor; they produce anxiety and decrease seizure threshold.

At high concentrations, both barbiturates and benzodiazepines act on additional targets. Barbiturates, for example, diminish calcium-dependent action potentials and decrease neurotransmitter release. These extra effects may cause toxic symptoms.

ETHANOL

The actions of ethanol are quite similar to those of other central nervous system (CNS) depressants. There is not a clear consensus about its molecular target though. At this point, the safest generalization to make is that ethanol acts on several, somewhat structurally related, ligand-gated and non-ligand-gated ion channels. In nontolerant individuals, a serum ethanol concentration of 10 mM produces a sense of relaxation; 30 mM, 50 mM, 70 mM, and 100 mM concentrations produce moderate intoxications, severe intoxication, coma, and death, respectively. Many of the effects of ethanol discovered in years past were only detected when very high concentrations of the compound were used. Effects on the *N*-methyl-D-aspartate (NMDA) [6] GABA$_A$ [7], and 5-hydroxytryptamine$_3$ (5-HT$_3$) [8] receptors and the L-type calcium channel [9] have been observed at relatively low ethanol concentrations. The dose of alcohol required for half-maximal effects on the NMDA-activated glutamate receptor on adult mammalian neurons, for example, is 10 mM. Somewhat higher levels seem to be needed to potentiate the action of serotonin at 5-HT$_3$ receptors and to enhance the action of GABA at (some but not all) GABA$_A$ receptors [10]. Thus, one might argue that the behavioral disinhibition produced by ethanol is mediated by an action on NMDA receptors and that the ataxia, somnolence, and CNS depression are effected elsewhere. This suggestion remains to be proved.

CENTRAL NERVOUS SYSTEM STIMULANTS

Cocaine and amphetamines act on related targets; they are sympathomimetic. Cocaine blocks the reuptake of dopamine [11–13], norepinephrine [14], and serotonin [15,16] following their release. In this way, it prolongs the actions of the monoamines. Likewise, amphetamines block monoamine reuptake, but they have an another important action as well; they release catecholamines from their intraneuronal stores.

The powerful reinforcing effects of the

CNS stimulants are considered to be due to their actions on dopamine-producing cells in the ventral tegmental area of the midbrain. These project to the nucleus accumbens, ventral pallidum, and frontal cortex. Electrical stimulation of the ventral tegmental area seems to be highly rewarding to animals, but not all drugs that block dopamine reaccumulation are potent reinforcers. One must infer from this that CNS stimulants may not act exclusively on dopaminergic neurons and that their actions on other monoaminergic cells are also important in producing reinforcement. Indeed, the peripheral toxicity of the drugs is almost surely due to effects on norepinephrine-containing sympathetic neurons.

While some tolerance to the effects of cocaine and amphetamines does develop, the abstinence syndrome associated with drug withdrawal is not as severe as that associated with CNS depressant or opiate withdrawal. Cocaine binges, which end when an addict runs out of drug or becomes too disorganized to take any more, are typically followed by a period of anxiety, depression, lifelessness, and deep sleep ("crash"). Despite the lack of physical dependence, the craving for these drugs is extreme and addicts have trouble resisting the temptation to obtain and use more.

PSYCHEDELICS

The psychedelics appear to act as partial agonists on the 5-HT$_2$ receptor, a G protein-linked receptor that mobilizes intracellular calcium [17–19]. The receptor seems to desensitize fairly quickly, and following three to four daily doses of lysergic acid diethylamide (LSD), the drug becomes inactive. Within a week or two, the function of the receptor seems to return to normal and the drug produces its effects once more. LSD shows cross tolerance with mescaline and psilocybin.

ARYLCYCLOHEXYLAMINES

Both phencyclidine and ketamine are arylcyclohexylamines. Members of this drug class are also known as "dissociative anesthetics," so-called because of the feeling of being apart from one's environment that they produce. While ketamine is still used clinically, it causes adverse reactions in as many as half of the adults given it: unpleasant dreams, hallucinations, delirium, and excitement. Phencyclidine, developed and employed in the 1950s as an anesthetic, was soon abandoned because of the above side effects. It gained popularity as a street drug in the 1970s, but recently its use has declined. Unlike LSD, phencyclidine frequently elicits hostile behavior, and unlike the former drug, which is not self-administered by monkeys, phencyclidine is a reinforcer.

There is general agreement that phencyclidine is an allosteric inhibitor of the NMDA-type glutamate receptor [20]. Tolerance develops to some of the behavioral effects of the drug, but there is not a severe abstinence syndrome. Chronic users of the drug do seem to experience long-term toxicity. Their problems include memory loss, withdrawal, nervousness, and depression.

CANNABINOIDS

Cannabinoids, synthesized by the hemp plant, act as agonists on a G protein-coupled receptor. Like the opioid receptors, the cannabinoid receptor is linked to G$_i$, and acts to inhibit the activation of adenylate cyclase [21]. The endogenous ligand for this receptor was recently discovered to be arachydonyl ethanolamide, "anandamide" [22]. The presence of this receptor in the hippocampus may account for the effects of cannabinoids on perception and memory; its presence in the cerebellum and basal ganglia probably underlies the incoordination the drugs produce. Finally, cannabinoid receptors on cells of the ventromedial nucleus of the hypothalamus may be responsible for "the munch-ies," the glucose craving associated with use of marijuana and hashish. It is worth mentioning that cannabinoids produce sleepiness unlike the psychedelics, which cause arousal, and that there is no cross tolerance between cannabinoids and the psychedelics. The withdrawal syndrome seen following protracted use of cannabinoids is relatively mild.

NICOTINE

Nicotine acts on the nicotinic cholinergic receptor [23]. Its effects are quite complicated. Initially it acts as an agonist, stimulating receptors in peripheral sympathetic and parasympathetic ganglia, the adrenal gland, and the brain. Subsequently, it blocks synaptic transmission at these same sites. Thus, its effects represent a summing of positive and negative effects on physiologically competing systems. The most prominent of these effects are an acute increase in heart rate and blood pressure, enhanced attentiveness, and a slight muscle tremor. Habitual users of tobacco products also report that smoking (and administration of nicotine) produces an agreeable sensation. In addition, chronic use of tobacco is associated with reduced weight. Many of the above effects can be reinforcing and contribute to the craving for tobacco products seen when they are withdrawn.

REFERENCES

1. Evans, C. J., Keith, D. E., Jr., Morrison, H., Magendzo, K., and Edwards, R. H. Cloning of a delta opioid receptor by functional expression. *Science* 258:1952–1955, 1992.

2. Kieffer, B. L., Belfort, K., Gavesiaux-Ruff, C., and Hirth, C. G. The δ-opioid receptor: Isolation of a cDNA by expression cloning and pharmacological characterization. *Proc. Natl. Acad. Sci. U. S. A.* 89:12048–12052, 1992.

3. Olsen, R. W., Fischer, J. B., and Dunwiddie,

T. V. Barbiturate enhancement of GABA receptor binding and function as a mechanism of anesthesia. In S. Roth and K. Miller (eds.), *Molecular and Cellular Mechanisms of Anesthetics.* New York: Plenum Publishing, 1986, pp. 165–177.

4. Puia, G., Santi, M., Vicini, S., Pritchett, D. B., Purdy, R. H., Paul, S. M., Seeburg, P. H., and Costa, E. Neurosteroids act on recombinant GABA_A receptors. *Neuron* 4:759–765, 1990.

5. Pritchett, D. B., Sontheimer, H., Shivers, B. D., Ymer, S., Kettenman, H., Schofield, P. R., and Seeburg, P. H. Importance of a novel GABA_A receptor subunit for benzodiazepine pharmacology. *Nature* 338:582–585, 1989.

6. Weight, F. F., Lovinger, D. M., White, G., and Peoples, R. W. Alcohol and anesthetic actions on excitatory amino acid-activated ion channels. *Ann. N.Y. Acad. Sci.* 625:97–107, 1991.

7. Ticku, M. K. Ethanol interactions at the γ-aminobutyric acid receptor complex. *Ann. N.Y. Acad. Sci.* 625:136–143, 1991.

8. Lovinger, D. M., and White, G. Ethanol potentiation of 5-hydroxytryptamine$_3$ receptor-mediated ion current in neuroblastoma cells and isolated adult mammalian neurons. *Mol. Pharmacol.* 40:263–270, 1991.

9. Treistman, S. N., Bayley, H., Lemos, J. R., Wang, X., Nordmann, J. J., and Grant, A. J. Effects of ethanol on calcium channels, potassium channels, and vasopressin release. *Ann. N.Y. Acad. Sci.* 625:249–263, 1991.

10. White, G., Lovinger, D. M., and Weight, F. F. Ethanol inhibits NMDA-activated current in an isolated adult mammalian neuron. *Brain Res.* 507:332–336, 1990.

11. Kilty, J. E., Lorang, D., and Amara, S. G. Cloning and expression of a cocaine-sensitive rat dopamine transporter. *Science* 254:578–579, 1991.

12. Shimada, S., Kitayama, S., Lin, C.-L., Patel, A., Nanthakumar, E., et al. Cloning and expression of a cocaine-sensitive dopamine transporter complementary DNA. *Science* 254:576–578, 1991.

13. Usdin, T. B., Mezey, É., Chen, C., Brownstein, M. J., and Hoffman, B. J. Cloning of the cocaine-sensitive bovine dopamine transporter. *Proc. Natl. Acad. Sci. U.S.A.* 88:11168–11171, 1991.

14. Pacholczyk, T., Blakely, R. D., and Amara, S. G. Expression cloning of a cocaine- and antidepressant-sensitive human noradrenaline transporter. *Nature* 350:350–353, 1991.

15. Blakely, R. D., Berson, H. E., Fremeau, R. T., Caron, M. G., Peek, M. M., et al. Cloning and expression of a functional serotonin transporter from rat brain. *Nature* 354:66–70, 1991.

16. Hoffman, B. J., Mezey, E., and Brownstein, M. J. Cloning of a serotonin transporter affected by antidepressants. *Science* 254:79–80, 1991.

17. Pierce, P. A., and Peroutka, S. J. Antagonism of 5-hydroxytryptamine$_2$ receptor-mediated phosphatidylinositol turnover by d-lysergic acid diethylamide. *J. Pharmacol. Exp. Ther.* 247:918–925, 1988.

18. Sanders-Bush, E., Burris, K. D., and Knoth, K. Lysergic acid diethylamide and 2,5-dimethoxy-4-methylamphetamine are partial agonists at serotonin receptors linked to phosphoinositide hydrolysis. *J. Pharmacol. Exp. Ther.* 246:924–928, 1988.

19. Pritchett, D. B., Bach, A. W. J., Wozny, M., Taleb, O., Dal Toso, R., Shih, J. C., and Seeburg, P. H. Structure and functional expression of cloned rat serotonin 5HT-2 receptor. *EMBO J.* 7:4135–4140, 1988.

20. Wroblewski, J. T., and Danysz, W. Modulation of glutamate receptors: Molecular mechanisms and functional implications. *Annu. Rev. Pharmacol. Toxicol.* 29:441–474, 1989.

21. Matsuda, L., Lolait, S., Brownstein, M. J., Young, A., and Bonner, T. Structure of a cannabinoid receptor: Functional expression of the cloned cDNA. *Nature* 346:561–564, 1990.

22. Devane, W. A., Hanus, L., Breuer, A., Pertwee, R. G., Stevenson, L. A., Griffin, G., Gibson, D., Mandelbaum, A., Etinger, A., and Mechoulam, R. Isolation and structure of a brain constituent that binds to the cannabinoid receptor. *Science* 258:1946–1949, 1992.

23. Claudio, T. Molecular genetics of acetylcholine receptor-channels. In D. M. Glover and B. D. Hames (eds.), *Frontiers in Molecular Neurobiology.* Oxford: IRL Press, 1989, pp. 63–142.

CHAPTER 42

Ischemia and Hypoxia

Akhlaq A. Farooqui, Steven E. Haun, and Lloyd A. Horrocks

Basic Neurochemistry: Molecular, Cellular, and Medical Aspects, 5th Ed., edited by G. J. Siegel et al. Published by Raven Press, Ltd., New York, 1994. Correspondence to Akhlaq A. Farooqui, Department of Medical Biochemistry, 1645 Neil Avenue, Room 479, The Ohio State University, Columbus, Ohio 43210.

THE BRAIN IS ALMOST ENTIRELY DEPENDENT ON AEROBIC METABOLISM

Ischemia or hypoxia may produce brain infarction

Because of the high rate of oxygen metabolism and the lack of tissue oxygen stores, interruption of oxygen delivery to the brain causes immediate cell dysfunction and rapidly leads to cell death. Oxygen delivery to the brain is defined as the product of the oxygen content of arterial blood and the cerebral blood flow (see Chap. 31). Inadequate oxygen delivery (hypoxia) can result from inadequate cerebral blood flow (ischemic hypoxia), inadequate partial pressure of oxygen in arterial blood (hypoxic hypoxia), or inadequate oxygen-carrying capacity of arterial blood (anemic hypoxia). The most common cause of brain hypoxia is ischemia or inadequate cerebral blood flow. The level of cerebral blood flow at which the brain begins to exhibit energy failure is fairly well defined. Reduction of cerebral blood flow below 15 ml/min/100 g of tissue results in failure of electrical activity, and a reduction to less than 10 ml/min/100 g of tissue results in loss of the transmembrane ionic gradient (see Chap. 31). Cellular energy depletion appears to be a triggering event for many of the damaging biochemical processes occurring during ischemia (see below).

Ischemic infarction depends on the vascular distribution and sites of vulnerability

There are many causes of cerebral ischemia in humans, including head trauma, stroke, and cardiac arrest. Cerebral ischemia may be further divided into focal and global categories. In global ischemia, blood supply to the entire brain is interrupted, e.g., cardiac arrest. In focal ischemia, blood supply to a particular region of the brain is interrupted, usually representing the area supplied by a particular vasculature. Cerebral ischemia may also be described as complete or incom-

plete. Complete ischemia is defined as total absence of blood flow to the entire brain or region of the brain. Incomplete ischemia, on the other hand, is defined as a severe reduction of cerebral blood flow in a focal or global pattern. Ischemia may result in reversible cell injury or may be sufficient to cause tissue death (infarction), depending on the duration and severity of ischemia. Not all regions of the brain are affected in the same manner during global ischemia. The most sensitive, i.e., selectively vulnerable, neurons are located in the CA1, CA3, and CA4 regions of the hippocampus, portions of the caudate and cerebellum, and layers 3, 5, and 6 of the neocortex. The mechanisms responsible for this selective vulnerability are not clear [1]. In focal ischemia, the anatomical location and extent of ischemic damage depend on the distribution of the blood vessels whose flow is limited and on the presence of collateral circulation. Damage resulting from focal ischemia commonly occurs in a graded fashion because collateral circulation partially perfuses the area surrounding the ischemic core. This ischemic "penumbra" may receive blood flow that is inadequate to preserve normal cellular function but adequate enough to allow recovery. The concept of the ischemic penumbra is important because the compromised status of these areas may be improved if effective early intervention is achieved.

ANIMAL MODELS OF CEREBRAL ISCHEMIA

Features of the ideal animal model

Animal models are required for detailed study of the pathophysiology of cerebral ischemia. An "ideal" animal model would have the following features:

1. The animal model should closely mimic the development of the clinical insult in humans.
2. The experimental insult should elicit similar responses in each individual ani-

mal tested; i.e., the insult should cause a reproducible injury.

3. The model should be closely physiologically regulated; e.g., temperature, blood glucose, and blood pressure should be tightly controlled.

4. The experimental animal pathology should be similar to that in humans.

Obviously, there are no "ideal" animal models, and it must be clearly understood that no animal model exactly reproduces cerebral ischemia in humans. Animals do not readily develop the cardiovascular disease that commonly underlies stroke, nor do they duplicate the age, nutritional status, or drug history of patients who suffer from stroke or cardiac arrest. Further, animals are usually anesthetized, are paralyzed, and have undergone surgery, particularly craniotomy, all of which may profoundly alter tissue response. Reproducible models are not easily achieved because of anatomical and physiological variability, both within and among species. In addition, lack of strict control of physiological variables, e.g., brain temperature, can lead to misleading results (see below). In spite of these limitations, numerous animal models have been developed and provide meaningful data that can be applied to the understanding of cerebral ischemia in humans.

Experimental ischemia is induced in animals by occluding vessels that perfuse the brain

Many experimental models have been used to study cerebral ischemia in a variety of species including rats, rabbits, gerbils, cats, dogs, goats, pigs, monkeys, baboons, and even humans. Detailed description of the different models of cerebral ischemia and the respective advantages and disadvantages of each is beyond the scope of this chapter. However, models of both focal and global ischemia are described briefly to serve as an introduction to the field of cerebral ischemia. Focal ischemia is modeled by mid-

dle cerebral artery occlusion; in some models this is accompanied by occlusion of the ipsilateral common carotid artery. Models of ischemia can be permanent (no reperfusion) or transient (allowing reperfusion). Rat models of focal ischemia have been extensively developed, and a large base of neurochemical and histopathological data exists for this species [2]. Most models create a fairly reproducible infarct in the ipsilateral hemisphere and provide a clinically relevant approximation of ischemic stroke in humans.

Models of global ischemia are utilized to simulate ischemic injury resulting from cardiac arrest. In large animals, global ischemia has been modeled in numerous ways, including inducing cardiac arrest, using a neck tourniquet, cross-clamping the proximal aorta, and raising the intracranial pressure to levels greater than mean arterial blood pressure. In rats, global ischemia has been modeled primarily by decapitation, two-vessel occlusion, and four-vessel occlusion. Two-vessel occlusion is produced by temporary occlusion of both common carotid arteries combined with systemic hypotension, whereas four-vessel occlusion is produced by electrocoagulation of both vertebral arteries followed by temporary occlusion of both common carotid arteries [2]. Obviously decapitation is permanent global ischemia, but the other models of global ischemia are transient, allowing reperfusion.

Animal models are necessary to study cerebral ischemia, and despite significant shortcomings, animal models have provided and will continue to provide insight into the pathophysiology of cerebral ischemia and may lead to the development of effective pharmacological interventions.

CELL CULTURE MODELS OF ISCHEMIC/HYPOXIC INJURY

Cell culture models are useful tools to study the molecular mechanism of ischemic injury and drug therapy. By controlling the extra-cellular environment, traumatic conditions that are similar but not identical to the insult that occurs *in vivo* can be produced. These conditions permit study of the cellular response to ischemic insult under specified conditions. Measurement of the extracellular pH and ionic environment is much easier in cell culture models than *in vivo*. Furthermore, metabolic products generated by injured cells *in vitro* can be more easily quantified than from tissue *in vivo* [3].

Hypoglycemic and hypoxic injury can be produced easily in cell cultures by reducing the glucose level in the growth media and placing the cultures in an anaerobic incubator, respectively. The most obvious drawback of the *in vitro* cell culture approach is that it categorically lacks ischemia, i.e., reduced blood flow. Although oxygen and glucose deprivations are the major perturbations during ischemic injury *in vivo*, blood contains many other factors that may determine the outcome of the ischemic insult. Furthermore, during ischemia *in vivo*, there is an accumulation of neurotoxic products in the extracellular space. During *in vitro* studies, cell cultures are generally surrounded by excess extracellular medium that attenuates any such accumulation of neurotoxic products [3].

ENERGY FAILURE, LACTIC ACIDOSIS, AND LOSS OF CALCIUM HOMEOSTASIS

The adenylate energy charge drops in ischemic/hypoxic injury

Under normal conditions the brain utilizes glucose and oxygen for ATP production. Ischemia rapidly (within seconds) leads to oxygen depletion and cessation of oxidative phosphorylation (see Chap. 31). Under these conditions, the only source of ATP production is anaerobic glycolysis. Because of a low rate of ATP production, anaerobic glycolysis is not adequate for normal brain func-

tion. Without incoming blood to supply more glucose, the brain is forced to use whatever glucose and glycogen stores it contains. During ischemia these stores are utilized within 2 to 3 min. Brain also contains the enzyme creatine kinase, which catalyzes the conversion of phosphocreatine to ATP. Under anaerobic conditions the brain utilizes this pathway to maintain and stabilize the levels of ATP. However, phosphocreatine stores are consumed in about 1 min. Increases in cytosolic ADP stimulate yet another source of energy, the enzyme adenylate kinase. This reaction results in the conversion of two molecules of ADP to ATP and AMP and may be very important during ischemia. Thus, ATP is depleted within 4 min after the onset of ischemia.

A parameter reflecting the ratio of high-energy phosphate bond production to consumption is the adenylate energy charge (EC):

$$EC = ([ATP] + \tfrac{1}{2}[ADP])/$$
$$([ATP] + [ADP] + [AMP])$$

EC drops during the first minutes of complete ischemia as the levels of ATP and phosphocreatine fall to undetectable levels. The concentration of adenine nucleotides reaches a plateau approximately 10 min after insult, and lactic acid levels reach a maximum at approximately 3 min. It must be noted that energy failure itself is not the determinant of cell degeneration [4]. Other processes such as cellular acidosis, release of glutamate, calcium ion influx, stimulation of membrane phospholipid degradation, and generation of free radicals may play an important role in neurodegeneration during ischemia and reperfusion.

Acidosis is associated with severe brain damage and edema

Lactate accumulation and increased carbon dioxide tension (P_{CO_2}) cause acidosis, which can be severe, reaching pH values of approximately 6.0. Another source of acidosis is intracellular protons, which are generated by ATP hydrolysis according to the following reaction:

$$ATP \rightarrow ADP + P_i \ (inorganic \ phosphate) + H^+$$

When mitochondrial function is compromised by depletion of oxygen supply, the recycling of protons by oxidative phosphorylation declines and the cytosolic proton concentration increases.

Acidosis affects cellular metabolism and function in the following ways. It causes loss of adenine nucleotides from the mitochondria by inhibiting the ATP-Mg^{2+}/inorganic phosphate carrier. It also inhibits the Na^+/Ca^{2+} exchanger at the plasmalemma causing intracellular sequestration of Ca^{2+} (see Chap. 3). It increases the activity of AMP deaminase and the loss of adenine nucleotide precursors from neurons (see Chap. 19). It decreases nicotinamide-adenine dinucleotide (NAD) by acid-catalyzed decomposition, and finally it converts intracellular inorganic phosphate to its inhibitory deprotonated form. Acidosis inhibits the reuptake of neurotransmitters, delocates protein-bound iron and promotes the formation of free radicals, prolongs or prevents the restoration of mitochondrial function, and delays the restoration of the EC. Another major effect of acidosis is enhancement of edema formation. The severity of glial and endothelial cellular edema appears closely related to the degree of acidosis present. Although the specific mechanism is not understood, it is possible that in combination with H^+, Na^+, and other metabolites, lactate increases intracellular osmolarity, thus drawing water from extracellular fluid [4] (see also Chap. 3).

Ischemic/hypoxic injury causes loss of calcium homeostasis

The concentration of cytosolic calcium in neurons is tightly regulated by a variety of membrane pumps and exchange systems (see Chap. 3). Several lines of evidence sug-gest that disruption of calcium homeostasis may be involved in ischemia-induced neuronal degeneration. First, ischemic neurons are known to accumulate abnormally high levels of calcium prior to degeneration. Second, extracellular calcium levels decrease during ischemia, presumably because of calcium influx into injured cells. Third, removal of extracellular calcium from bathing media during the hypoxic insult can prevent hypoxia-induced neuronal degeneration in cell culture models. Finally, the use of calcium channel antagonists and other pharmacological strategies that inhibit the rapid influx of calcium through voltage-gated (see Chap. 4) and N-methyl-D-aspartate (NMDA) receptor-gated (see Chap. 17) calcium channels into injured neurons shows significant protection against neuronal degeneration caused by ischemic injury [5,6].

Calcium is a major second messenger in neurons (see Chaps. 20–23). It plays an important role in the regulation of many enzymic pathways. Of these, four have gained prominence in attempting to explain calcium-mediated cytotoxic effects. They are (a) Ca^{2+}-activated phospholipases, (b) Ca^{2+}-activated proteases, (c) Ca^{2+}-activated protein kinases, and (d) Ca^{2+}-activated phosphatases [7]. In addition, calcium is known to uncouple mitochondrial oxidative phosphorylation. Stimulation of these enzymes, depletion of ATP, and biochemical events involved in reperfusion may be the factors that determine cell death (Table 1).

DEVELOPMENT OF EDEMA

Edema accompanies many injuries and diseases, such as tumors, infections, trauma, and hormonal imbalances as well as ischemia and hypoxia. In any of these conditions, increased intracranial pressure and herniation of portions of the brain through the tentorium or other sites are serious complications. Edema is defined as the increase of tissue volume as the result of an increased water and Na^+ load.

TABLE 1. Major events in brain ischemia

Early changes (sec–min)
  Release of free fatty acids
  Ca^{2+} influx
  Activation of lipolytic enzymes
  Mitochondrial swelling
  Increased NADH
  Increased adenosine

Intermediate changes (<10 min)
  Increased glycolysis
  Decreased glucose, glycogen
  Increased lactate
  Decreased energy charge
  Failure of Na,K-ATPase
  Neurotransmitter release
  Increased cyclic AMP

Late changes (>10 min)
  Decreased protein synthesis
  Increased proteolysis
  Activation of lysosomal enzymes
  Development of edema
  Induction of heat shock proteins
  Induction of c-*fos*
  Induction of ornithine decarboxylase

Cellular (cytotoxic) edema develops almost immediately following vascular occlusion (seconds to minutes) and, provided that circulation is promptly restored, is reversible. In this type of edema, neuronal and glial permeability to ions is increased, but capillary permeability is unchanged. Perivascular and perineuronal astrocytic processes swell, followed by swelling of neurons and endothelial cells. The extracellular space is reduced, and capillary permeability is unchanged. Large amounts of K^+ are lost from neurons to the extracellular fluid, and all cells take up water and sodium chloride (NaCl). Glial cells may have a protective role in this process because they take up large amounts of K^+ as well as Na^+. Cellular edema affects both white and gray matter. The main cause is probably ATP depletion and failure of active transport.

Vasogenic edema develops if reperfusion is delayed or inadequate. It develops within hours to days after the ischemic or hypoxic episode and causes more damage to white matter than to gray. Endothelial damage results in increased capillary permeability, disrupting the blood-brain barrier, and there is extravasation of large proteins and other molecules and plasma filtrate to the extracellular compartment, expanding its size. This type of edema may result in vascular compression, increased intracranial pressure, and herniations of brain tissue. Cellular and vasogenic edema are the most common forms that accompany ischemia and are intrinsic to its pathology. Occasionally, an additional type, interstitial (hydrocephalic) edema, may be observed as a complication of hemorrhagic stroke, in which obstruction of the ventricular system forces cerebrospinal fluid into periventricular areas.

PROTEIN AND NUCLEIC ACID METABOLISM DURING ISCHEMIA

Reduction of protein synthesis and induction of specific proteins

A marked reduction of protein synthesis occurs during ischemia. It is most prominent in the brainstem, including the diencephalon, and in the forebrain, excluding some parts of the telencephalon. There is a general consensus that postischemic inhibition of protein synthesis occurs mainly at the translational level. The most likely mechanism is an inhibition of polypeptide chain initiation because inhibition of protein synthesis is associated with a disaggregation of ribosomes. Normal rates of protein synthesis are observed within 4 hr of recirculation. Ischemia and reperfusion can also induce increased synthesis of a number of specific proteins, despite an overall reduction in the rate of protein synthesis. These proteins are heat shock proteins (HSPs), c-fos protein, and glial fibrillary acidic protein (GFAP). Although the significance and role of induction of the above proteins are not well understood, their induction has been correlated with increased resistance to ischemic injury (HSP), cell activation, differentiation and regeneration (c-fos), and glial response toward the regenerative process (GFAP). Expression of HSP, c-fos, and GFAP may be regulated, in part, by calcium influx through voltage-sensitive channels and the NMDA receptor channel complex and is blocked by the NMDA antagonist MK-801. The mechanism of induction of these proteins may occur by distinct pathways that may not be mechanistically linked. However, these proteins may be good markers for all kinds of trauma [8]. See Chap. 24 for a discussion of gene regulation and transcription.

Protein phosphorylation and ischemic injury

Protein phosphorylation is markedly affected during ischemic injury. At the plasma membrane level, isozymes of protein kinase C perform a variety of functions, including regulation of neurotransmitter release, activation of proton-sodium exchanges, opening of calcium channels, and regulation of gene expression (see Chap. 22). During the very early phases of ischemic injury, both protein kinase C and calcium/calmodulin-dependent kinase are inhibited, while cyclic AMP-dependent protein kinase is not affected (Table 2). The time course of protein kinase C and calcium/calmodulin-dependent kinase closely corresponds with irreversible loss of neurological function, and there is evidence that an endogenous inhibitor of protein kinase C is generated. Another possibility is that the ischemic insult produces the translocation of protein kinase C from cytosol to membrane and the stimulation of Ca^{2+}-induced proteolysis. The membrane-bound protein kinase C is more sensitive to proteolytic digestion than its cytosolic form. Thus, it is possible that ischemia leads to rapid and extensive degradation of membrane-bound protein kinase C with a loss of enzymic function. These observations suggest that protein phosphorylation, particularly by protein kinase C and calcium/calmodulin-dependent kinase, is critical to the maintenance of neurological function during ischemia [9,10].

Effect of ischemia on proteolysis

The activation of the protease calpain by Ca^{2+} during ischemia in gerbils causes the breakdown of the cytoskeletal proteins spectrin and microtubule-associated protein 2 (MAP2), leading to severe cellular damage. *In vitro* the stimulation of calpain after hypoxia can be blocked by calpain inhibitor I. Calpain also induces the conversion of xanthine dehydrogenase to xanthine oxidase and may contribute to the production of free radicals [11].

Ischemic/hypoxic injury markedly affects nucleic acid metabolism

Very little is known about the effects of ischemia on neural cell DNA and RNA. Nucleic acids play a crucial role in the neural cell response to ischemic trauma by directing the synthesis of certain enzymes (ornithine decarboxylase and glutamine synthetase) and a variety of proteins via the production of RNA. Ischemia causes extensive DNA nicks, and chromatin clumping occurs within hours after the insult. It is expected that calcium-dependent endonucleases may be stimulated and may play an important role in neurodegeneration [12].

TABLE 2.   Effect of ischemia on lipolytic enzymes and protein kinases

Enzyme	Effect on activity
Phospholipase A_1	Stimulated
Phospholipase A_2	Stimulated
Phospholipase C	Stimulated
Lysophospholipase	Stimulated
Monoacylglycerol lipase	Not known
Diacylglycerol lipase	Stimulated
Triacylglycerol lipase	Inhibited
Cyclic AMP-dependent protein kinase	No effect
Protein kinase C	Inhibited
Ca^{2+}/calmodulin-dependent protein kinase	Inhibited

PHOSPHOLIPID METABOLISM DURING ISCHEMIA

Ischemia/hypoxia stimulates activities of phospholipases and lipases

Ischemia induces the breakdown of membrane phospholipids (see Chaps. 5 and 20) and the accumulation of free fatty acids including arachidonic and docosahexaenoic acids (see Chap. 23). This release of fatty acids caused by ischemia or electroconvulsive shock was first described by Bazan in 1970 and is thus called the Bazan effect. The breakdown of membrane phospholipids disrupts membrane ionic gradients and may be involved in irreversible injury. The primary sources of free fatty acids are inositol, ethanolamine, and choline glycerophospholipids (see Chap. 5). Three possible processes may be involved in membrane damage caused by ischemia. They are (1) the activation of phospholipases A_1, A_2, and C (see Table 2); (2) the inhibition of phospholipid resynthesis caused by the energy shortage; and (3) changes in membrane integrity that may lead to mechanical rupture.

Calcium influx into the neurons results in stimulation of phospholipases A_1, A_2, and phospholipase C/diacylglycerol lipase pathways. During early stages of ischemia (within 1 min), inositol glycerophospholipids are the main source of the increase in free arachidonic acid and diacylglycerol. This release of arachidonic acid is suggested to be the result of the transneuronal breakdown of inositol glycerophospholipids triggered mainly by the release of glutamate (see Chap. 17) in the synaptic cleft during the ischemic insult [13,14].

Another process that is disrupted during ischemia is phospholipid resynthesis. Under normal conditions, fatty acids and lysophospholipids are recycled through a series of energy-dependent reactions. As a result, the normal phospholipid content of cellular membranes is not altered and intracellular concentrations of free fatty acids, lysophospholipids, and diacylglycerols are maintained at low levels. During ischemia,

stimulation of lipolytic enzymes causes depletion of critical membrane phospholipids, and resynthesis is inhibited because of energy depletion. Thus, ischemia disrupts the balance of the deacylation and reacylation cycle. Ischemic injury also produces physical changes in membrane integrity. These membrane alterations, along with edema, may rupture the cellular membrane.

Ischemia reverses the synthetic reaction for phosphatidylcholine

Another pathway for the release of free fatty acid that may be activated during ischemia is the reversal of choline and/or ethanolamine phosphotransferases (see Chaps. 5 and 20). These enzymes normally produce phosphatidylcholine and phosphatidylethanolamine. During ischemia, however, cytidine 5'-monophosphate (CMP) is not removed because of the lack of ATP production. Thus, the reaction between phosphatidylcholine and CMP (reversal of choline phosphotransferase) produces cytidine 5'-diphosphate (CDP)-choline and diacylglycerol. Similarly, ethanolamine phosphotransferase is also reversed. Diacylglycerol is also produced by the action of phospholipases C and D on phosphatidylcholine. During ischemia, diacylglycerol is not utilized by diacylglycerol kinase for phosphatidic acid production (because of the lack of ATP) but is rapidly hydrolyzed to monoacylglycerol and free fatty acid by a diacylglycerol lipase. The monoacylglycerol is then hydrolyzed by monoacylglycerol lipase. The relative contributions of the phospholipase A_2 and phospholipase C/diacylglycerol pathways in free fatty acid release remain unknown [13,14].

Released fatty acids have several harmful effects

Fatty acids, mostly present in ionized form as soaps, released during ischemia are known to have a variety of detrimental effects on brain structure and function, primarily because of their ability to disrupt cell membranes. Free fatty acids are efficient uncouplers of oxidative phosphorylation and may cause the efflux of ions, such as Ca^{2+} and K^+, stored in the mitochondria. High concentrations of free fatty acids promote the release of glutamate and inhibit its reuptake. Free fatty acids inhibit Na, K-ATPase, and tissue swelling has been observed in brain slices incubated with free fatty acids. Since free fatty acids have detergent properties, they may change the fluidity and permeability of membranes, influencing mechanisms dependent on membrane integrity [13,14].

Arachidonic acid, the substrate for eicosanoid production by monooxygenases (cyclooxygenase and lipoxygenase), is the precursor of several active compounds (details of these reactions are given in Chap. 23). Eicosanoids (prostaglandins, thromboxanes, and leukotrienes) are vasoactive and may be involved in dysautoregulation of the cerebral circulation. They may play a neuromodulatory role, and high levels produced in ischemia may damage cells further in still poorly understood ways. Reaction intermediates in the cyclooxygenase and lipoxygenase pathways that might have deleterious effects on the integrity of cell membrane structure and function include the endoperoxides, prostaglandin G_2 (PGG$_2$) and prostaglandin H_2 (PGH$_2$), and the hydroperoxides. These metabolites have a free radical character and may elicit a cascade of harmful reactions, including (1) peroxidation of polyunsaturated fatty acids in the cell membrane, irreversibly changing their properties; and (2) generation of free radicals in the hydrocarbon core of the cell membrane, possibly cross-linking proteins with phospholipids and altering the microenvironment and structure of proteins in mitochondrial and plasma membranes [13,14].

A significant loss of cholesterol occurs during compression spinal cord trauma; thus, this process may also occur during ischemia. Because the loss of cholesterol is prevented by α-tocopherol, the mechanism may involve free radical lipid peroxidation [15].

In summary, alterations in membrane lipid metabolism and second-messenger systems occur very early after ischemic injury. These changes, i.e., phospholipid hydrolysis, eicosanoid production, and loss of cholesterol, initiate a cascade of pathophysiological events resulting in disruption of membrane structure, permeability, and function, with consequent intracellular-extracellular ionic imbalance, edema, inflammation, and neuronophagia.

ROLE OF GLUTAMATE IN THE PATHOPHYSIOLOGY OF ISCHEMIA

Glutamate accumulates during ischemic/hypoxic injury

Glutamate is a major excitatory amino acid neurotransmitter in the mammalian central nervous system (see Chap. 17). It mediates different cellular responses by interacting with at least five receptor subtypes, namely NMDA, kainate (KA), α-amino-3-hydroxy-5-methyl-4-isoxazole-4-propionate (AMPA), L-2-amino-4-phosphonobutanoic acid (L-AP4), and 1S,3R-*trans*-1-amino-cyclopentyl-1,3-di-carboxylate (*trans*-ACPD) [11]. Excessive amounts of glutamate and other excitatory amino acid neurotransmitters are released into the extracellular space during ischemia and contribute to neuronal injury through overactivation of NMDA, AMPA, KA, and *trans*-ACPD receptors. This process is called excitotoxicity. The best evidence for the role of NMDA receptor stimulation in producing ischemic damage is that neuronal degeneration can be blocked by NMDA receptor antagonists such as 2-amino-5-phosphonovalerate (APV) and MK-801. In specific types of neurons, stimulation of NMDA receptors by glutamate is also associated with an increase in intracellular nitric oxide levels. In normal brain, nitric oxide is nontoxic and acts as a second messenger. However, in the presence of superoxide anion during reperfusion, nitric oxide produces peroxynitrite (see below).

Molecular mechanisms of cell injury caused by glutamate during ischemia are beginning to be discovered. Glutamate-induced neuronal injury may involve two distinct events. First, exposure of neurons to glutamate may cause an acute neuronal swelling resulting from the depolarization-mediated influx of Na$^+$, Cl$^-$, and water (see Chap. 3). This process is reversible if glutamate is removed from the system. The degree to which this event contributes to neuronal injury is unclear, but it has been suggested that water entry causes osmotic lysis, which may disrupt neuronal function.

The second event is characterized by excessive calcium influx primarily via excitatory amino acid receptor channel activation [11]. The elevation of intracellular Ca^{2+} is known to activate lipases, phospholipases, proteases, and protein kinases, each of which, if not properly regulated, can easily be envisioned to produce considerable cellular damage (Fig. 1). A speculative description of glutamate neurotoxicity was recently proposed. Glutamate neurotoxicity may have three stages: first, induction, i.e., overstimu-

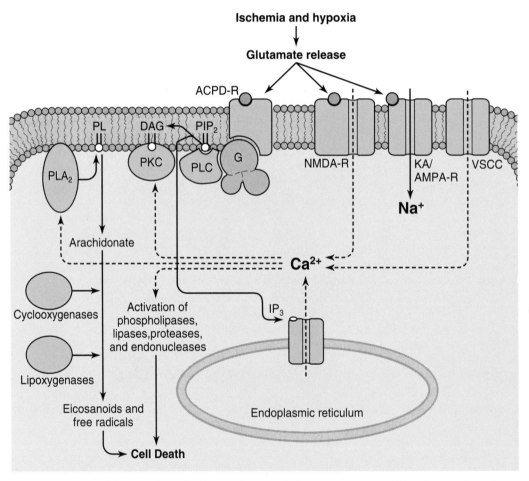

FIG. 1. Hypothetical diagram illustrating the involvement of glutamate receptors, calcium ions, and membrane phospholipid degradation during ischemia. (NMDA-R), N-methyl-D-aspartate receptor; (KA) kainate; (AMPA-R) α-2-amino-3-hydroxy-5-methyl-4-isoxazole-4-propionate receptor; (ACPD-R) 1S,3R-*trans*-1-amino-cyclopentyl-1,3-dicarboxylate receptor; (PL) phospholipids; (PLA$_2$) phospholipase A$_2$; (PIP$_2$) phosphatidylinositol 4,5-bisphosphate; (PLC) phospholipase C; (G) G protein; (DAG) 1,2-diacylglycerol; (PKC) protein kinase C; (IP$_3$) inositol 1,4,5-trisphosphate; (Ca^{2+}) intracellular calcium; (VSCC) voltage-sensitive calcium channels.

lation of glutamate receptors, leading to a set of immediate cellular derangements; second, amplification, i.e., events that intensify these derangements and promote the glutamate involvement of additional neurons; and third, expression, the destruction cascade directly responsible for neuronal cell degeneration [7].

The glutamate hypothesis of neuronal degeneration has some weaknesses. The correlation between density of NMDA receptors and selective neuronal damage after global ischemia is not as tight as originally proposed. Although there is good correlation between the number of NMDA receptors and selective vulnerability of neurons in the CA1 region of the hippocampus, the CA4 region, which has a relatively low density of NMDA receptors, is also vulnerable to neuronal degeneration. In contrast, neurons of the dentate gyrus, which are relatively resistant to ischemia, have a high density of NMDA receptors. Furthermore, it is well known that increases in hydrogen ion concentration inactivate NMDA receptor-mediated calcium currents. Release of glutamate into the extracellular space during ischemia may inactivate the NMDA receptor complex and thereby may have a protective effect on vulnerable neurons. In contrast, extracellular acidosis has a damaging effect on glia [5,7,16].

Glutamate receptors are coupled to phospholipases A_2 and C

NMDA Receptor and Phospholipase A_2

The occurrence of an NMDA-sensitive glutamate receptor that activates the release of arachidonic acid from membrane phospholipids in neuronal preparations obtained from hippocampus, striatum, and hypothalamus is clearly established. Phospholipase A_2 may be the main enzyme responsible for massive arachidonate release in response to stimulation of the NMDA receptor. Unlike the α-adrenergic receptor, which is coupled to phospholipase A_2 through a G protein, in cerebellar granule cells the coupling of NMDA receptors to phospholipase A_2 is not mediated by a G protein. Thus, it seems likely that the elevated intracellular concentration of Ca^{2+} ions, triggered by the opening of NMDA receptor-coupled cation channels, may serve the second-messenger function in activating intracellular phospholipase A_2 directly or through some other signal transduction mechanism [11].

Trans-ACPD Receptor and Phospholipase C

Stimulation of membrane phospholipid degradation by excitatory amino acid agonists has been reported to occur in a variety of neuronal preparations. These include mouse striatal cultures, cerebellar granule cell cultures, rat hippocampus slices, and rat brain synaptoneurosomes. The metabotropic trans-ACPD receptor is involved in the turnover of polyphosphoinositide through the activation of phospholipase C. Thus, in primary neuronal cultures from rat brain, excitatory amino acids stimulate polyphosphoinositide hydrolysis with a rank order of potency as follows: quisqualate > ibotenate > glutamate > kainate, NMDA > AMPA. A similar rank order of potency was also obtained in striatal neurons, but a different rank order of potency (glutamate > quisqualate > kainate) was reported in cerebellar granule cell cultures. These differences in rank order of potencies may be contributed by regional differences in the excitatory amino acid reuptake process and/or regional heterogeneity of excitatory amino acid receptor regulation of phospholipase C [11].

ROLE OF FREE RADICALS IN THE PATHOPHYSIOLOGY OF ISCHEMIA

Free radicals are generated during ischemia and reperfusion

Ischemia and subsequent reperfusion favor the formation of free radicals. A biochemical index of ischemia-induced oxygen radical formation and lipid peroxidation is a reduction in concentrations of the endogenous antioxidants ascorbate, glutathione, ubiquinone, α-tocopherol, and cholesterol (only in mechanical trauma) in brain tissue. Furthermore, the conjugated diene content of brain increases during a 30-min period of severe forebrain ischemia and goes up even more after reperfusion. Postischemic changes also occur in the electron spin resonance spectrum of brain samples from rats pretreated with the oxygen free radical spin trap phenyl-*t*-butyl nitrone, clearly indicating the formation of oxygen radicals during ischemia and reperfusion. All these data suggest that brain antioxidants are consumed in an attempt to quench ischemia and reperfusion-induced free radicals.

The important production sites for superoxide anion ($O_2 \cdot^-$), hydrogen peroxide (H_2O_2), and hydroxyl radical ($OH \cdot$) are the mitochondrial respiratory chain and reaction sequences catalyzed by cyclooxygenase and lipoxygenase. These radicals are also formed during the autooxidation of catecholamines and the xanthine oxidase reaction. The relative importance of each of these pathways has not been determined but all are theoretically capable of producing free radicals upon reperfusion [17].

Recently, another oxygen radical, peroxynitrite anion ($ONOO^-$), was proposed to cause brain injury during ischemia and reperfusion. Nitric oxide synthase, a calcium/calmodulin-dependent enzyme, produces nitric oxide by acting on L-arginine. Nitric oxide has been shown to be an endothelium-derived relaxing factor (EDRF) that mediates the relaxation of blood vessels via generation of cyclic GMP. Nitric oxide synthase is also present in specific neurons of the central nervous system and nitric oxide formed in these neurons and in brain microvascular endothelium may react with oxygen radicals to form peroxynitrite anion in high yield. Peroxynitrite formation may also contribute to the cytotoxic actions of neutrophils and macrophages, which produce significant quantities of superoxide anion. In a proton-

ated form, peroxynitrite decays rapidly to form highly reactive radicals, including hydroxyl radical ($OH \cdot$) and nitrogen dioxide (NO_2). Furthermore, the excess of nitric oxide can itself be toxic to cells. Nitric oxide stimulates ADP ribosyltransferase and binds avidly to iron-sulfur centers of enzymes, including enzymes involved in the mitochondrial electron transport chain, the tricarboxylic acid (TCA) cycle, and DNA synthesis [18].

Superoxide dismutase (SOD), catalase, and glutathione peroxidase are enzymes known to be involved in the defense of the brain against free radicals. Mutations in the copper-zinc form of SOD are linked to familial amyotrophic lateral sclerosis, a degenerative disease of motor neurons in the cerebral cortex, brainstem, and spinal cord [19]. At least in some neurodegenerative diseases, damage caused by free radicals may be linked to defects in a gene that codes for a protein involved in the defense against the oxidation associated with excess free radicals. This supports the hypothesis that an excess of free radicals is involved in cell death and tissue damage during ischemia and reperfusion.

Free radicals may cause cell death and tissue damage

The presence of one or more unpaired electrons in the outer electron orbital makes free radicals extremely reactive intermediates. They can react with lipids, enzymes, or DNA to produce a variety of harmful effects (Table 3). Free radicals can disrupt membrane in-

TABLE 3.   Effects of free radicals on lipid, protein, and nucleic acid metabolism

Target	Effect
Lipids	Peroxidation of fatty acids and cholesterol, alteration in membrane permeability and fluidity
Proteins	Oxidation of SH-groups, stimulation of phospholipases, inhibition of Na,K-ATPase, adenylyl cyclase, and Ca-ATPase
DNA	Strand scission, activation of poly (ADP-ribose) polymerase

tegrity by reacting with proteins and unsaturated lipids in the plasma membrane. These reactions lead to a chemical cross-linking of membrane proteins and lipids and a reduction in membrane unsaturated lipid content. This depletion of unsaturated lipid may be associated with alterations in membrane fluidity and permeability and changes in activities of receptors and membrane-bound enzymes such as Na,K-ATPase and adenylyl cyclase.

Free radical-induced damage to proteins may also result in fragmentation, cross-linking, and aggregation of protein and the induction of autofluorescence that can be measured *in vitro*. This can be manifested by an inactivation of certain enzymes. Extracellular proteins with a large proportion of disulfide bridges appear to be particularly vulnerable to hydroxyl and peroxyl radical attack.

Free radicals also produce damage to nucleic acids by breaking of strands and base modification. Superoxide anion produced from the xanthine/xanthine oxidase system has been shown to cause DNA strand breaks. Hydroxyl radicals react readily with nucleic acids, yielding strand breaks. Strand breaks have important implications for the development of pathological states because DNA strands must be paired for the cell to function properly. Enzymes that repair DNA strand breaks, in general, have decreased fidelity; therefore, there is a higher probability of misincorporating nucleotides into DNA.

In addition to causing neuronal injury, free radicals produced by ischemia and reperfusion may also affect vascular tissue. This is accompanied by damage to vascular endothelium, blood-brain barrier disruption, and vasogenic edema [17].

Free radicals also stimulate the release of glutamate in rat hippocampal slices and neuronal cultures; lazaroids (21-amino steroids), powerful antioxidants, can attenuate the neuronal injury induced by the exogenous application of glutamate or NMDA. This suggests that free radical formation and glutamate release are mutually related and

cooperate in a series of molecular events that link ischemic injury to neuronal cell death [20,21] (see also Chap. 17).

PHARMACOLOGICAL INTERVENTION IN ISCHEMIA

Despite major advancements in our understanding of the biochemical events involved in the pathophysiology of cerebral ischemia, little progress has been made in our ability to arrest, prevent, or reverse ischemic injury. We have realized that the extent of irreversible ischemic damage is governed by both the duration of ischemia and the severity of ischemia (complete versus incomplete). A number of pharmacological agents have been utilized for cerebral ischemia in both animal models and humans (Table 4). No agent has been shown to be of unequivocal value; i.e., there is no effective treatment for cerebral ischemia, presently.

A number of preventive or therapeutic strategies are under investigation

Calcium Channel Blockers

These drugs block the entry of calcium ions into the ischemic neurons. These drugs do not themselves antagonize the effects of calcium ions; instead, they prevent this ion from gaining access to its intracellular site of action. By blocking the entry of calcium ions, they may inhibit the essential role of this cation in the activation of lipolytic enzymes, protein kinases, and phosphatases (see Table 2) during ischemia. Improved cerebral blood flow or no change in cerebral blood flow, improved neurological outcome or no change in neurological outcome, decreased brain lactic acidosis, and decreased infarct size all have been reported following calcium channel blocker treatment in various studies [22].

Vitamin E

α-Tocopherol (vitamin E), a well-known antioxidant, has beneficial effects on brain

TABLE 4. Proposed pharmacological strategies for treatment of cerebral ischemia

Agent	Proposed mechanism of action
CDP-choline	Reverse choline phosphotransferase reaction, decrease production of free fatty acids, induce phospholipid synthesis
CDP-ethanolamine	Reverse ethanolamine phosphotransferase reaction, decrease production of free fatty acids, induce phospholipid synthesis

Ca^{2+} channel blockers
  Lidoflazine
  Flunarizine
  Nimodipine
	Decrease Ca^{2+} entry

Antioxidants/free radical scavengers
  α-Tocopherol
  Ascorbic acid
  Mannitol
  Glutathione
  Catalase
  Superoxide dismutase
  21-Aminosteroids (lazaroids)
	Antioxidant

Opiate antagonists Naloxone	Vasoregulation, antioxidant, anti-GABA activity
Ginkgo biloba derivatives	Platelet-activating factor antagonists, decrease platelet aggregation, decrease Ca^{2+} entry, free radical scavengers
Barbiturates	Membrane stabilizer, free radical scavenger, anticonvulsant, decrease cerebral metabolism
Prostacyclin (PGI$_2$)	Vasodilation, decrease platelet aggregation

Phenothiazines
  Chlorpromazine
  Trifluoperazine
	Inhibition of Ca^{2+}/calmodulin complex

Perfluorocarbons	Hemodilution, increase O$_2$ delivery

Excitotoxic amino acid antagonists
  2-Amino-7-phosphonoheptanoic acid
  LY178002
  MK-801
	Competitive NMDA receptor antagonists
	
	Noncompetitive NMDA antagonist, i.e., blocks NMDA receptor-gated Ca^{2+} channel

Cyclooxygenase inhibitors
  Indomethacin
  Aspirin
	Decrease prostaglandin synthesis

Fibrinolysins
  Streptokinase
  Urokinase
  Tissue plasminogen activator
	Clot dissolution

GM$_1$ ganglioside	Preservation of membrane structure, neuronal regeneration
S-Adenosyl-L-methionine	Improves energy metabolism, reduces brain edema

(CDP) cytidine 5′-diphosphate.

edema and ischemia. It inhibits the activities of phospholipase A$_2$ and lipoxygenase and plays a fundamental role in the stabilization of polyunsaturated fatty acid chains in membrane phospholipids. Vitamin E interacts with cellular membranes and prevents lipid peroxide formation by acting as a hydrogen donor [17,23].

CDP-amines

CDP-amines are key intermediates in the biosynthesis of phosphatidylcholine and phosphatidylethanolamine. The therapeutic actions of CDP-amines are thought to result from restorative effects on phospholipid synthesis in the ischemic brain. CDP-amines attenuate the fatty acid increases and counteract the disruption of cerebral mitochondrial lipid metabolism induced by hypoxia. They have been reported to inhibit the activities of phospholipases A_1 and A_2. CDP-amines have also been reported to increase oxygen consumption and glucose incorporation into amino acids and phospholipids. They improve cerebral blood flow. They may also cause restoration of Na,K-ATPase activity and a decline in lactate production [24].

Glutamate Antagonist MK-801

The use of MK-801 for the treatment of ischemia is controversial. It has been used successfully for the treatment of cerebral ischemia in experimental models. MK-801 may exert its antagonistic effects via a site related to the ion channel (noncompetitive antagonist). The onset of NMDA receptor blockage with MK-801 is more rapid in the presence of glutamate. These two effects may be relevant to the efficacy of MK-801 in cerebral ischemia, which provokes a marked elevation in extracellular concentrations of glutamate. MK-801, in addition to direct receptor blockade, may protect neurons with severe, but not complete, energy failure by preserving ionic gradients across the plasma membrane and enhancing amino acid uptake. Other investigators have been unable to demonstrate neuronal protection with MK-801. Treatment with MK-801 causes a 2 to 3°C decline in body temperature that can last as long as 7 to 8 hr. When body temperature is maintained equally in both placebo- and MK-801-treated animals, the protective effects produced by MK-801 under ambient temperature conditions are lost. The same degree of neuroprotection can be achieved with mild hypothermia. This suggests that the hypothermia, which affects gene expression, rather than NMDA receptor antago-

nism, may be responsible for the neuroprotective effects of MK-801 [25].

GM₁ Ganglioside

Gangliosides have been reported to have a beneficial effect in a variety of central nervous system injuries by increasing central nervous system regeneration, i.e., a neuronotrophic effect. Several studies have utilized GM_1 ganglioside for the treatment of ischemia. GM_1 ganglioside may reduce cerebral edema and ischemic injury by preserving membrane structure, preventing the deterioration of the membrane microenvironment, regulating the activities of lipolytic enzymes and protein kinases, and modulating the influx of calcium ions into neurons [11,26].

U74006F, 21-Aminosteroids (Lazaroids)

U74006F, a nonglucocorticoid 21-aminosteroid, is a potent inhibitor of lipid peroxidation. It has a beneficial effect in animal models of severe head injury, posttraumatic spinal cord ischemia, and cerebral ischemia. The mechanism of 21-aminosteroids is not known, but it may act by inhibiting iron-dependent lipid peroxidation. The 21-aminosteroids significantly reduce Na^+ accumulation, K^+ loss, and water entry into ischemic brain. The effect was most consistent and prominent in tissues surrounding the infarct site [27].

Superoxide Dismutase

SOD has been proposed as a therapeutic agent for reperfusion injury because of its ability to scavenge superoxide anion. However, copper-zinc SOD is a large, water-soluble molecule (molecular mass = 32 kDa) and therefore cannot readily penetrate cell membranes or cross the blood-brain barrier in significant quantities. In addition, SOD has a circulatory half-life of only 8 min in rats. Investigators have tried two different modifications in the delivery of SOD in an effort to increase the intracellular access and circulatory half-life of the intravenously administered enzyme: liposome-entrapped SOD and polyethylene glycol-conjugated SOD. SOD delivered in liposomes has been shown both to increase brain SOD activity and to reduce infarct volume in a rat model of focal cerebral ischemia. In contrast, polyethylene glycol-conjugated SOD does not appear to increase brain SOD activity but has been shown to reduce infarct volume in animal models of focal cerebral ischemia [17].

S-Adenosyl-L-Methionine

S-Adenosyl-L-methionine is the main methyl group donor in transmethylation reactions. In experimental animals, S-adenosyl-L-methionine improves energy metabolism and reduces brain edema. This drug protects the hippocampal CA1 neurons from degeneration and necrosis in a dose-dependent manner.

Platelet-Activating Factor Antagonist

Large amounts of platelet-activating factor (PAF) are produced by brain tissue and endothelial cells in response to ischemia and reperfusion. PAF is a powerful vasoconstrictor and has many cytotoxic properties. PAF antagonists that are present in an extract of *Ginkgo biloba* leaves (ginkgolide B) appear to reduce edema and neuronal damage in several mammalian species [28].

ACKNOWLEDGMENTS

Supported by National Institutes of Health grants PO1 NS10165, RO1 NS29441, and K08 NS01523.

REFERENCES

1. Paschen, W. Molecular mechanisms of selective vulnerability of the brain to ischemia. *Circ. Metab. Cerveau* 6:115–139, 1989.
2. Ginsberg, M. D., and Busto, R. Rodent models of cerebral ischemia. *Stroke* 20: 1627–1642, 1989.
3. Choi, D. W. Limitations of in vitro models of ischemia. In B. S. Meldrum and M. Williams (eds.), *Current and Future Trends in Anticonvulsant, Anxiety, and Stroke Therapy.* New York: Wiley-Liss, 1990, pp. 291–299.
4. Siesjo, B. K. Cerebral circulation and metabolism. *J. Neurosurg.* 60:883–908, 1984.
5. Siesjo, B. K., and Bengtsson, F. Calcium fluxes, calcium antagonists, and calcium-related pathology in brain ischemia, hypoglycemia, and spreading depression: A unifying hypothesis. *J. Cereb. Blood Flow Metab.* 9:127–140, 1989.
6. Meyer, F. B. Calcium, neuronal hyperexcitability and ischemic injury. *Brain Res. Rev.* 14: 227–243, 1989.
7. Choi, D. W. Cerebral hypoxia: Some new approaches and unanswered questions. *J. Neurosci.* 10:2493–2501, 1990.
8. Welsh, F. A., Moyer, D. J., and Harris, V. A. Regional expression of heat shock protein-70 mRNA and c-fos mRNA following focal ischemia in rat brain. *J. Cereb. Blood Flow Metab.* 12:204–212, 1992.
9. Zivin, J. A., Kochhar, A., and Saitoh, T. Protein phosphorylation during ischemia. *Stroke* 21(Suppl. III):III-117–III-121, 1990.
10. Aronowski, J., Grotta, J. C., and Waxham, M. N. Ischemia-induced translocation of Ca^{2+}/calmodulin-dependent protein kinase II: Potential role in neuronal damage. *J. Neurochem.* 58:1743–1753, 1992.
11. Farooqui, A. A., and Horrocks, L. A. Excitatory amino acid receptors, neural membrane phospholipid metabolism and neurological disorders. *Brain Res. Rev.* 16:171–191, 1991.
12. Warnick, C. T., Dierenfeldt, S. M., and Lazarus, H. M. A description of the damaged DNA produced during tissue injury. *Exp. Mol. Pathol.* 41:397–408, 1984.
13. Farooqui, A. A., Hirashima, Y., Farooqui, T., and Horrocks, L. A. Involvement of calcium, lipolytic enzymes and free fatty acids in ischemic brain trauma. In N. G. Bazan, P. Braquet, and M. D. Ginsberg (eds.), *Neurochemical Correlates in Cerebral Ischemia 7.* New York: Plenum Press, 1992, pp. 117–138.
14. Bazan, N. Arachidonic acid in the modulation of excitable membrane function and at the onset of brain damage. *Ann. N.Y. Acad. Sci.* 559:1–16, 1989.

15. Saunders, R. D., Dugan, L. L., Demediuk, P., Means, E. D., Horrocks, L. A., and Anderson, D. K. Effect of methylprednisolone and the combination of α-tocopherol and selenium on arachidonic acid metabolism and lipid peroxidation in traumatized spinal cord tissue. *J. Neurochem.* 49:24–31, 1987.

16. Choi, D. W., Monyer, H., Giffard, R. G., Goldberg, M. P., and Christine, C. W. Acute brain injury, NMDA receptors, and hydrogen ions: Observations in cortical cell cultures. In Y. Ben-Ari (ed.), *Excitatory Amino Acids and Neuronal Plasticity.* New York: Plenum Press, 1990, pp. 501–504.

17. Traystman, R. J., Kirsch, J. R., and Koehler, R. C. Oxygen radical mechanisms of brain injury following ischemia and reperfusion. *J. Appl. Physiol.* 71:1185–1195, 1991.

18. Garthwaite, J. Glutamate, nitric oxide and cell-cell signalling in the nervous system. *Trends Neurosci.* 14:60–67, 1991.

19. Rosen, D. R., et al. Mutations in Cu/Zn superoxide dismutase gene are associated with familial amyotrophic lateral sclerosis. *Nature* 362:59–62, 1993.

20. Pellegrini-Giampietro, D. E., Cherici, G., Alesiani, M., Carla, V., and Moroni, F. Excitatory amino acid release and free radical formation may cooperate in the genesis of ischemia-induced neuronal damage. *J. Neurosci.* 10: 1035–1041, 1990.

21. Monyer, H., Hartley, D. M., and Choi, D. W. 21-Aminosteroids attenuate excitotoxic neuronal injury in cortical cell cultures. *Neuron* 5:121–126, 1990.

22. Wong, M. C., and Haley, E. C., Jr. Calcium antagonists: Stroke therapy coming of age. *Stroke* 21:494–501, 1990.

23. Yoshida, S. Brain injury after ischemia and trauma. The role of vitamin E. *Ann. N.Y. Acad. Sci.* 570:219–236, 1989.

24. Murphy, E. J., and Horrocks, L. A. Mechanisms of action of CDPcholine and CDPethanolamine on fatty acid release during ischemia of brain. In N. G. Bazan (ed.), *New Trends in Lipid Mediators Research.* Basel: S. Karger, 1990, pp. 67–84.

25. Buchan, A. M. Do NMDA antagonists protect against cerebral ischemia: Are clinical trials warranted? *Cerebrovasc. Brain Metab. Rev.* 2: 1–26, 1990.

26. Carolei, A., Fieschi, C., Bruno, R., and Toffano, G. Monosialoganglioside GM$_1$ in cerebral ischemia. *Cerebrovasc. Brain Metab. Rev.* 3: 134–157, 1991.

27. Hall, E. D., Braughler, J. M., and McCall, J. M. Role of oxygen radicals in stroke: Effects of the 21-aminosteroids (lazaroids). A novel class of antioxidants. In B. S. Meldrum and M. Williams (eds.), *Current and Future Trends in Anticonvulsant, Anxiety, and Stroke Therapy.* New York: Wiley-Liss, 1990, pp. 351–362.

28. Braquet, P., Paubert-Braquet, M., Koltai, M., Bourgain, R., Bussolino, F., and Hosford, D. Is there a case for PAF antagonists in the treatment of ischemic states? *Trends Pharmacol. Sci.* 10:23–30, 1989.

CHAPTER 43

Epileptic Seizures

BRIAN MELDRUM

Basic Neurochemistry: Molecular, Cellular, and Medical Aspects, 5th Ed., edited by G. J. Siegel et al. Published by Raven Press, Ltd., New York, 1994. Correspondence to Brian Meldrum, Department of Neurology, Institute of Psychiatry, De Crespigny Park, Denmark Hill, London SE5 8AF, United Kingdom.

EPILEPSY REFERS TO DISORDERS CHARACTERIZED BY SPONTANEOUS RECURRENT SEIZURES

"Epilepsy" refers to an etiologically and clinically diverse group of neurological disorders characterized by spontaneous, recurrent paroxysmal cerebral discharges, called seizures. The latter may have varied subjective, behavioral, or motor manifestations but the common factor has been assumed for the last 100 years to be the paroxysmal, excessive, and synchronous discharge of a group of neurons. Only limited progress has been made in understanding the molecular and cellular basis of either the proneness to epileptic seizures or their acute manifestations (for detailed reviews see [1,2]).

EPILEPTOGENESIS

Epilepsy sometimes has a genetic basis

Some forms of epilepsy in humans appear to have an autosomal dominant inheritance. These include benign familial neonatal convulsions, 2- to 3-Hz spike and wave absence attacks, and juvenile myoclonic epilepsy [3]. Many inborn errors of metabolism are associated with seizures (see section below and Chaps. 38 and 39). Genetic factors contribute also to seizures considered as secondary to some other acquired pathology such as a head injury or a space-occupying lesion.

Inbred strains of chickens, rodents, and primates can show specific types of reflex or sensory epilepsy. Many specific mutations leading to neurological syndromes with seizures are known in mice.

The approximate chromosomal localization for the genes determining epilepsy is known for some of the human and murine epileptic syndromes but in no case has the gene or corresponding protein been identified or sequenced.

Some developmental disorders are associated with epilepsy

The major developmental disorders giving rise to epilepsy are disorders of neuronal mi-gration [4]. These may have genetic or intrauterine causes. Abnormal patterns of neuronal migration through the cortex give rise to various forms of agyria or pachygyria. In type I lissencephaly there is a highly abnormal cortex of four layers and a very high incidence of focal or generalized seizures beginning early in childhood. Lesser degrees of failure of neuronal migration represented by neuronal heterotopia in the subcortical white matter may favor the development of primary generalized or focal epilepsies at later stages in life. Tuberous sclerosis is a developmental disorder with autosomal dominant inheritance, in which disordered neuronal migration and epilepsy are commonly found.

Traumatic injury and focal lesions can be epileptogenic

Epilepsy is commonly a delayed consequence of head injury. It has shown a rather consistent incidence after penetrating head injuries in the major wars of this century. It occurs with a lower incidence after closed head injury. An epileptogenic action of blood or iron may be involved, as may the hyperexcitability that follows cortical de-afferentation. The long latent interval between the injury and the onset of epilepsy indicates that slow processes, possibly of degeneration and regeneration, are involved. Other forms of focal injury, including those produced by benign or malignant tumors, by abscesses, and by parasitoses such as cerebral malaria and cysticercosis, also can lead to focal epilepsy [4].

Kindling, recurrent subconvulsant stimulation, provides an experimental model of epileptogenesis

A brief burst of electrical stimulation sufficient to induce a local afterdischarge but not sufficient to trigger a seizure will eventually trigger a seizure if repeated frequently. This phenomenon is referred to as "kindling" [5]. It can be most readily induced by stimulating the structures that comprise the limbic system. The changes responsible for the low-

TABLE 1. Synaptic functional changes in kindled rats

Enhancement of:
  Voltage-sensitive calcium conductance
  Glutamate metabotropic polyphosphoinositide hydrolysis
  Glutamate release in hippocampus (CA3)
  GABA release in hippocampus (CA1)
  Sensitivity of NMDA receptors in hippocampus (dentate granule cells, CA3 pyramidal cells)
  Protein kinase C activity

Decrease in:
  Calbindin immunoreactivity in the hippocampus
  Type II Ca^{2+}/calmodulin kinase activity

ered seizure threshold occur diffusely in the brain and are permanent. They appear to involve many different neurotransmitter systems including γ-aminobutyric acid (GABA), acetylcholine, and glutamate. Enhanced sensitivity of *N*-methyl-D-aspartate (NMDA) receptors and of glutamate metabotropic receptors (see Chap. 17) is particularly important in facilitating epileptiform discharges [6]. Some of the changes related to synaptic function that have been described in the kindled brain are listed in Table 1.

The kindling process is a model for epileptogenesis and, like long-term potentiation (LTP) (see Chap. 50), it is dependent on activation of NMDA receptors. It can be retarded or prevented by the administration of NMDA receptor antagonists prior to the episodes of kindling stimulation [7].

Metabolic disorders may trigger seizures

Circumstances impairing energy metabolism may produce cerebral seizures of various types when cerebral functions are partially impaired or induce tonic spasms or other forms of brainstem seizures when cortical activity has essentially ceased but some brainstem electrical activity persists. These phenomena are seen in hypoglycemia and cerebral hypoxia, and when oxidative metabolism is poisoned as by cyanide or by fluorocitrate. When seizures are caused by a transient nonrecurrent metabolic disturbance, the disorder is not referred to as epilepsy.

Certain mitochondrial disorders are characterized by myopathy and myoclonus or seizures, such as myoclonus epilepsy with ragged red fibers. The mitochondrial disorders may show maternal transmission. They are biochemically and genetically heterogeneous, but the myopathy and the myoclonus or epilepsy are thought to be directly related to defects in the electron transport chain (see Chap. 34).

A very wide range of other metabolic disorders may show seizures as a secondary feature, ranging from pyridoxine dependency, where a defective synthesis of GABA contributes to the seizures (Chap. 35), to phenylketonuria, where the primary defect is in phenylalanine 4-hydroxylase in the liver (see Chap. 39).

Hyperthermia often lowers the seizure threshold or triggers seizures in human children aged 6 months to 5 years and in young kittens or rodents. The mechanism involved is not known.

BASIC ELECTROPHYSIOLOGY

Macroelectrodes show spikes while intracellular microelectrodes show paroxysmal depolarizing shifts

Macroelectrodes on the scalp, on the cerebral surface, or in the depths of the brain record the net resultant electric potential of many cells around the electrode. These records show high-voltage spikes as the most characteristic feature of epilepsy. These spikes may occur in isolation, in continuous or rhythmic bursts, or may be associated with intervening slow waves. Intracellular records show that corresponding to the macrorecordings of spikes, there occur synchronously in many single cells episodes that look like giant excitatory synaptic potentials. These are referred to as ''paroxysmal depolarizing shifts.'' Intracellular records show a large sustained depolarization of the membrane associated with a burst of action potentials, which are largely Na^+-dependent at the beginning of the burst and Ca^{2+}-dependent at the end (see also Chaps. 9 and 10).

Ionic movements in brain during seizures

Measurements with ion-specific electrodes in brain slices or *in vivo* show that there is a drop in the extracellular concentration of calcium ion, $[Ca^{2+}]e$, that begins at the same time the seizure discharge is recorded. The fall is significant in more or less all types of epilepsy and in some cases can be so marked as to probably prevent presynaptic release of neurotransmitters [8]. Extracellular $[K^+]$ rises, often with a slight delay compared to Ca^{2+}, and reaches a plateau around 10 to 12 mM. There is also a moderate fall in extracellular $[Na^+]$ and a smaller rise in extracellular $[Cl^-]$ (see also Chaps. 3 and 4).

Synaptic synchronization and anatomical networks: the role of inhibition and excitation

Multiple recordings in hippocampus or cortex show that during a seizure many neurons fire synchronously, as a result of synchronous excitatory inputs. This pattern of activity may spread locally by progressive recruitment in the cortex or by spread from CA3 to CA1 subfields in the hippocampus. Spread also occurs by distal recruitment of subcortical or limbic structures. *In vitro* studies with hippocampal or cortical slices showed that the initiation and spread of synchronous discharges can be facilitated by ionic changes such as high $[K^+]e$ or low $[Mg^{2+}]e$, by factors decreasing GABA-mediated inhibition, or by factors enhancing excitation such as the enhanced sensitivity of the NMDA receptor induced by low $[Mg^{2+}]$ (see Chaps. 17 and 18).

CHANGES IN NEUROTRANSMITTER SYSTEMS UNDERLYING EPILEPSY

GABA/benzodiazepine receptors decrease in some conditions

A decrease in the relative proportion of GABAergic terminals has been observed in cor-

tical epileptic foci induced in monkeys with alumina cream. However, there does not appear to be any similar consistent decrease in the temporal lobes of humans with complex partial epilepsy, the principal form of focal epilepsy in humans [9]. It may be that GABAergic interneurons in the hippocampus can become "dormant" through failure of their excitatory input [10] (see Chap. 18).

Decreases in ligand binding to benzodiazepine receptors in the midbrain have been shown by autoradiography in certain rodent species with genetic epilepsy. Patients with complex partial seizures have shown decreases in benzodiazepine receptor density in the temporal lobe as measured by flumazenil binding in positron emission tomography (PET) studies [11] (see also Chap. 46).

Glutamate sensitivity at NMDA receptors may increase

An increased sensitivity to the action of glutamate at NMDA receptors is seen in hippocampal slices from kindled rats and in cortical slices from, or adjacent to, cortical foci in human epilepsy [12]. This leads to an enhanced entry of Ca^{2+} into neurons during synaptic activity that can be detected with ion-specific microelectrodes [13] (see Chap. 17).

Noradrenergic innervation may increase or decrease in rodent models

In various genetically determined rodent models of epilepsy, either excesses or deficiencies of noradrenergic innervation may be found. In the tottering mouse there is an absence-like syndrome consisting of intermittent episodes of behavioral arrest associated with 6- to 7-Hz cortical spike-wave electroencephalographic (EEG) discharges that arise from a noradrenergic hyperinnervation of the forebrain. Selective destruction of the ascending noradrenergic system at birth prevents the onset of the syndrome in the adolescent mouse, implying a causal role for the noradrenergic abnormality.

Opioid peptides have both convulsant and anticonvulsant actions

In experimental studies, opioids and opioid peptides have both convulsant and anticonvulsant actions. Peptides with a μ agonist action given intraventricularly induce hippocampal or limbic seizures, perhaps by inhibiting interneurons. In patients with complex partial seizures, μ receptor density is increased in the temporal cortex as shown by carfentanil binding in PET studies [14]. Opioid receptors are discussed further in Chap. 15.

DRUG-INDUCED CONVULSIONS

Convulsions can be induced by drugs acting on ion channels, or on inhibitory or excitatory neurotransmission

Potassium channel blockers such as 4-aminopyridine are potent convulsant agents (Table 2). Convulsions can also be induced by cholinergic agents, most notably by muscarinic agonists such as pilocarpine and by cholinesterase inhibitors such as physostigmine and diisopropyl fluorophosphonate (see Chap. 11).

Many chemical convulsants impair inhibition mediated by GABA (see Chap. 18). Some do this by blocking its synthesis; 3-mercaptopropionic acid, a competitive inhibitor of glutamic acid decarboxylase, induces seizures with a short latency, consistent with the very rapid turnover of GABA. Compounds that interfere with the synthesis or coenzymic function of pyridoxal phosphate induce seizures by impairing GABA synthesis. Compounds such as bicuculline and benzylpenicillin that compete with GABA for binding at the $GABA_A$ recognition site are powerful convulsants. Convulsions are also produced by compounds that act at the benzodiazepine site on the $GABA_A$ receptor complex to produce an effect opposite to that of benzodiazepines ("inverse agonists"). DMCM, methyl-6,7-dimethoxy-4-ethyl-β-carboline-3-carboxylate, is such an example. Yet other convulsants such as picrotoxin, ethylbicyclo-

TABLE 2.   Biochemical actions of convulsant drugs

Drug	Effect
Drugs that affect ion transport or ionic conductance	
Ouabain	Na,K-ATPase inhibitor
4-Aminopyridine	K^+ channel blocker
Drugs that block energy metabolism	
Fluoroacetate	Inhibits Krebs cycle
Fluorocitrate	Inhibits Krebs cycle
Drugs that block inhibitory transmission	
Strychnine, brucine	Antagonists at glycine receptor in spinal cord
Bicuculline, penicillin	Antagonists at GABA receptor
Convulsant barbiturates (CHEB, DMBB)	Antagonists at GABA complex
Convulsant β-carbolines (DMCM)	Inverse agonists at benzodiazepine site
Allylglycine, 3-mercaptopropionic acid, pyridoxal phosphate antagonists	Block GABA synthesis by inhibiting glutamic acid decarboxylase activity
Tetanus toxin	Blocks GABA release
Drugs that enhance cholinergic excitatory transmission	
Physostigmine, DFP	Anticholinesterases that enhance synaptic acetylcholine concentration
Pilocarpine	Agonist at muscarinic receptor
Drugs that enhance glutamatergic excitatory transmission	
Kainate, domoate	Agonists at kainate receptor
Quisqualate, AMPA	Agonists at AMPA receptor
NMDA, ibotenate, quinolinate	Agonists at NMDA receptor

phosphate, and tetramethylenedisulfotetramine act at the GABA$_A$ receptor complex to block the chloride channel [15].

Agonist compounds acting at glutamate receptors are convulsant following intracerebral or systemic injection. Kainate and domoate (synthesized by marine plants) induce limbic seizures, apparently by acting at high-affinity kainate receptors in the CA3 subfield of the hippocampus. Domoate consumed in mussels has induced limbic seizures acutely in humans with, in some cases, secondary hippocampal pathology and enduring anterograde amnesia. Seizures can also be induced by agonists acting on the other subtypes of ionotropic receptor, i.e., NMDA and quinolinate acting on NMDA receptors and quisqualate or AMPA acting on AMPA receptors (see Chap. 17).

Compounds that act as GABA$_B$ receptor agonists, such as baclofen, facilitate cortical spike and wave discharges of the sort associated with absence attacks. This is seen particularly in the model of absence attacks provided by certain Wistar rats.

ANTICONVULSANT DRUG MECHANISMS

About 14 drugs are in clinical use as antiepileptics. Some are effective predominantly in complex partial seizures and generalized tonic-clonic seizures (phenytoin, barbiturates, carbamazepine); some, in status epilepticus (benzodiazepines); some, predominantly in absence seizures (ethosuximide, trimethadione); and some are broadly active (valproate). These drugs are largely derived from animal screening tests employing acutely induced electrical or chemical seizures. Their mechanisms of action are only partially understood (Table 3). Some act predominantly on ion channels in the neuronal membrane; others act on synaptic transmission [16]. Phenytoin and carbamazepine suppress rapid repetitive firing in cultured neurons by prolonging the inactivation time of Na$^+$ channels. Ethosuximide and related drugs that suppress absence seizures decrease activity in voltage-sensitive Ca^{2+} channels of the T type [17]. Benzodiazepines and barbiturates act to enhance inhibition mediated via GABA/benzodiazepine receptors. Antagonists of excitatory amino acid neurotransmission, acting on glutamate receptors of the NMDA or non-NMDA type, are also anticonvulsant in animal models of epilepsy but their clinical usefulness is not yet identified. Acetazolamide has a modest anticonvulsant action in absence seizures, apparently due to inhibition of carbonic anhydrase activity and resulting changes in pH.

TABLE 3.   Anticonvulsant drugs: mechanisms of action

Drug	Na$^+$ channel[a]	Ca^{2+} channel[b]	GABA[c]	Glutamate[d]
Phenytoin	++			
Carbamazepine	++			
Valproate	++			
Ethosuximide	−	++		
Phenobarbitone	+	−	+	+
Diazepam, clonazepam	+		++	
Vigabatrin			(++)	

[a] Prolonged inactivation of the voltage-dependent Na$^+$ channel.
[b] Blockade of the T calcium current.
[c] Enhancement of GABA-mediated inhibition (by inhibition of GABA-transaminase in the case of vigabatrin).
[d] Antagonist action at the AMPA receptor.
++, strong action at clinically relevant concentration; +, action of possible significance; −, no action.

METABOLIC CONSEQUENCES OF SEIZURES

Energy metabolism in the discharge pathway is massively increased during seizures

During seizure activity there is a greater increase in cerebral metabolic rate than under any other circumstance (see Chap. 31). This is seen in measurements of oxygen consumption ($CMRO_2$) and glucose uptake and metabolism (reviewed by Chapman [18]). It is also reflected in a marked increase in cerebral blood flow (CBF). During seizures there are commonly both an increase in arterial blood pressure and a marked local vasodilation, the latter partly due to local formation of nitric oxide. The increase in CBF often exceeds the increase in $CMRO_2$ so that the oxygen content of the venous blood is increased. Provided that arterial blood pressure, arterial oxygenation, and blood glucose level are maintained, this enhanced level of metabolism can also be maintained. If however the energy supply is diminished, as in hypoglycemia, then the rise in metabolic rate and the severity of the seizure discharge are reduced (Fig. 1).

During seizures, phosphocreatine levels drop in association with a fall in intracellular pH [19] while ATP levels are well maintained (Fig. 2).

Second messengers change rapidly

There are dramatic changes in all the second messengers that reflect increased release of neurotransmitters acting on metabotropic receptors within the first minute of seizure activity (see also Chaps. 10, 20–22). Increases in cyclic AMP levels are partly due to activation of α-adrenergic receptors (see Chap. 12). Increases in cyclic GMP levels are partly due to formation of nitric oxide, following glutamate (NMDA) ionotropic receptor activation. Activation of glutamate, α_1-adrenergic, or muscarinic metabotropic receptors causes phospholipase C activation and phosphoinositide breakdown. The lipase activity

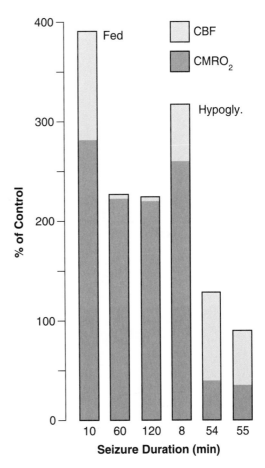

FIG. 1. Overall cerebral blood flow (CBF) and oxygen consumption ($CMRO_2$) during the progression of bicuculline seizures in fed rats and insulin-treated hypoglycemic rats. In the fed rats, burst suppression seizure discharge is maintained throughout the 2-hr period. In the hypoglycemic rats this pattern gives way to single spikes after approx 10 min; their frequency decreases around 55 min. (Modified from Chapman [18].)

results in the formation of diacylglycerol, which activates protein kinase C, and of inositol trisphosphate, which causes release of Ca^{2+} from nonmitochondrial stores (see Chap. 20). There is also a marked increase in intracellular Ca^{2+} concentration, $[Ca^{2+}]i$, due to enhanced Ca^{2+} entry, through receptor and voltage-operated calcium channels (see Chap. 42).

The effects of these changes are to phosphorylate many enzymes, ion channels, and

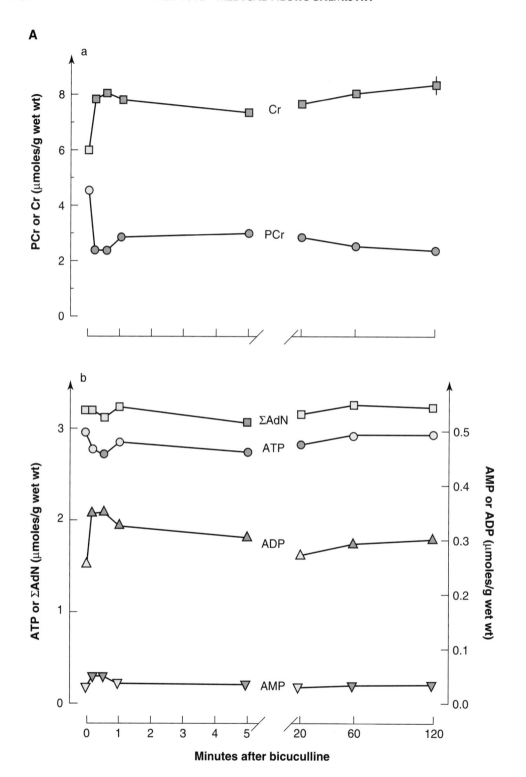

FIG. 2.   Changes in the concentration of various metabolites in the cerebral cortex during maintained seizure activity in paralyzed ventilated rats. **A:** Changes in the concentrations of phosphocreatine (PCr), creatine (Cr), ATP, ADP, AMP, and the sum of adenine nucleotides (ΣAdN).

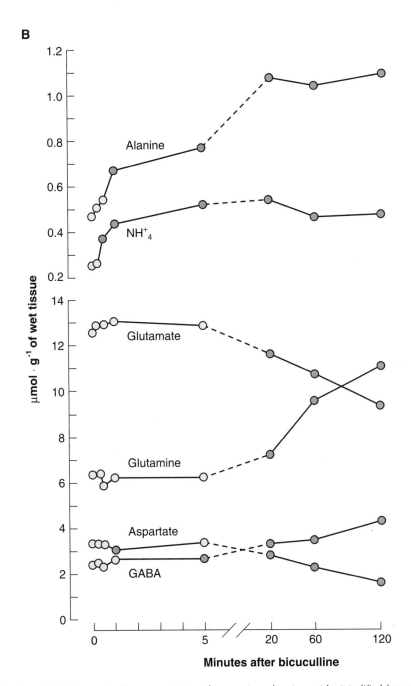

FIG. 2. *(continued).* **B:** Changes in the concentration of ammonia and amino acids. (Modified from Chapman et al. [19].)

TABLE 4.   Increases in cortical free fatty acid and prostaglandin levels at the onset of experimental seizures[a]

Convulsant	FFA	AA	PGF$_{2\alpha}$
Bicuculline	2–4	13–17	
Electroshock	2.5	5–14	18
Picrotoxin			32
Carbachol	1.5	3	70
Pentylenetetrazol	2	3–5	4–150

[a] Data are the ratio of increase to baseline. (FFA) free fatty acids; (AA) arachidonic acid; (PGF$_{2\alpha}$) prostaglandin F$_{2\alpha}$. Modified from Meldrum [15].

cell membrane receptors, and to directly activate calcium-dependent enzymes (see Chap. 22). Among the latter is phospholipase A$_2$, leading to the formation of free fatty acids, in particular arachidonic acid (see below and Chap. 23).

Free fatty acids and prostaglandins increase

Primarily due to activation of phospholipases, free fatty acids are liberated during seizure activity [20]. The greatest increase during seizures induced by electroshock or bicuculline is in the unsaturated fatty acid arachidonic acid (20 : 4), which acts as a precursor for various prostaglandins (Table 4) (see also Chaps. 23 and 42).

Levels of lactate and certain amino acids change rapidly

Seizure activity is associated with a doubling of brain lactate, ammonia, and alanine content within 1 min [19]. The lactate increase occurs in the absence of hypoxia and reflects the relatively greater increase in glycolytic rate than in CMRO$_2$. Glutamate, aspartate, and GABA levels initially remain constant, but if seizure activity is prolonged, glutamate and aspartate levels fall and glutamine and GABA levels rise [19]. Glucose and glycogen levels also fall (see Fig. 2).

The synaptic release of amino acid neurotransmitters was recently studied by *in vivo* microdialysis. In patients with epileptic foci in the temporal lobe, the extracellular concentrations of glutamate and aspartate increase directly prior to or at the moment of seizure onset; the extracellular concentration of GABA rises with a slight delay in both the epileptic focus and the contralateral temporal lobe [21].

Seizures produce changes in gene expression and protein synthesis

Seizure activity has a dramatic effect on gene transcription. This has been studied in rats by *in situ* hybridization with messenger RNA probes (see Chaps. 24 and 25). There are increases in expression of the immediate early genes, c-*fos*, c-*jun*, *jun*B, and tissue plasminogen activator (TPA), in many structures involved in seizure activity, notably in the granule cells of the dentate gyrus. Immunocytochemistry with specific antisera reveals that synthesis of the proteins encoded by the immediate early genes is also enhanced [22].

There are also selective increases in the messenger RNAs for various trophic factors, such as nerve growth factor, brain-derived neurotrophic factor, and neurotrophin 3. These changes have a longer latency (approximately 1 hr) and a longer duration than the changes in the immediate early genes. With a longer latency still, there are increases in the expression of the genes encoding various peptide neurotransmitters and their precursors.

Although the synthesis of some proteins such as those mentioned above and the enzyme ornithine decarboxylase is increased by seizures, the synthesis of most proteins is impaired during or after prolonged seizures in rats or newborn marmosets. When studied with labeled amino acid precursors and autoradiography, protein synthesis is impaired in those regions showing the greatest metabolic activation. The rate of protein synthesis depends on the cellular GDP/GTP ratio, with GDP increases being inhibitory.

PET studies show ictal hypermetabolism and interictal hypometabolism

PET (see Chap. 46) can be used to study the regional metabolism of the human brain during seizures and in the interictal period. Regional glucose uptake can be studied with ^{18}F-fluorodeoxyglucose, and oxygen extraction with oxygen 15. In partial epilepsy, enhanced metabolism is usually seen in the zone of seizure initiation during a seizure. Interictal studies in partial epilepsy commonly show a large zone of hypometabolism, which may be more extensive than the presumed focal zone. Children with absence attacks show a marked diffuse increase in cerebral metabolism during the attack and normal interictal metabolism [2].

PATHOLOGICAL CHANGES SECONDARY TO SEIZURES OR RELATED TO EPILEPTOGENESIS

Status epilepticus causes damage in vulnerable neurons

It has long been known that a very prolonged severe seizure can induce nerve cell death in selectively vulnerable neurons. These are pyramidal neurons in hippocampus CA1; cells in amygdala; small pyramidal neurons in cortical laminae III, V, and VI; cerebellar Purkinje cells; and some thalamic nuclei [4]. Such damage is commonly seen in adolescent or adult humans experiencing status epilepticus lasting more than 2 hr, especially if the body temperature is elevated.

Brain injury of similar nature can be reproduced in rats or baboons by inducing seizures lasting 1.5 to 7.0 hr with chemical convulsants such as bicuculline, allylglycine, kainate, and pilocarpine. The early cellular changes are characteristic of excitotoxic damage (see Chap. 42), i.e., postsynaptic changes involving focal dendritic swelling, mitochondrial dilation, and Ca^{2+} accumulation. Such changes are seen 1 to 4 hr after status epilepticus in most of the selectively vulnerable neurons (e.g., pyramidal cells in the hippocampus, CA1 and CA3 subfields). Subsequently proliferation of astrocytes and microglia may be seen.

Many experimental studies have shown that the selective neuronal death in the hippocampus is related to the local excessive neuronal discharge and not to systemic or local vascular factors. Excessive entry of Ca^{2+} and failure of intracellular calcium buffering and of ATP-dependent Ca^{2+} extrusion (see Chap. 3) are thought to be key events [23]. Activation by Ca^{2+} of proteases (such as calpain), protein kinases, and phospholipases is thought to play a role in determining cell death (see Chap. 42). NMDA receptor antagonists (see Chap. 17) can prevent most of the epileptic damage even when kainate is used to induce seizures and their overall duration is not decreased by the NMDA antagonist [23], indicating that the burst pattern of firing and activation of NMDA receptors plays a crucial role in causing the damage.

Febrile convulsions in early childhood are normally benign. If they are repeated within 24 hr or prolonged more than 30 min, especially if unilateral, they may be associated with a higher incidence in later childhood and adolescence of either primary generalized (tonic-clonic seizures) or complex partial (temporal lobe) seizures. Experimental studies support the concept that prolonged or closely repeated febrile convulsions give rise to cell loss in the hippocampus (CA1 and hilar region) and that this lesion is a cause of focal limbic seizures.

Epileptogenesis is associated with regenerative sprouting in the hippocampus

A regenerative phenomenon referred to as "sprouting" is seen in the kindling model of epilepsy, after focal hippocampal damage following kainate seizures, and in the hippocampi of patients with temporal lobe epilepsy [24,25]. This particularly concerns the mossy fiber system, which contains the axons deriving from the dentate granule cells and that stain for zinc with Timm's stain and for dynorphin by immunocytochemistry. This sprouting becomes prominent in the inner molecular layer of the dentate gyrus and in the dendritic fields of CA1. This axonal sprouting may be in response to enhanced release of growth factors triggered by seizure activity or it may be a response to local degeneration of terminals. The new terminals are excitatory but may be ending on inhibitory interneurons. A loss of certain types of hilar interneurons (those containing somatostatin and neuropeptide Y) may be functionally important, as these normally provide an excitatory feedback to inhibitory interneurons.

The changes following injury that contribute to epileptogenesis are very complex. The precise roles played by particular changes in ion channels, receptors, or neuronal morphology cannot yet be specified.

REFERENCES

1. Delgado-Escueta, A. V., Ward, A. A., Jr., Woodbury, D. M., and Porter, R. J. Basic mechanisms of the epilepsies. *Adv. Neurol.* 44: 3–55, 1986.
2. Engel, J. *Seizures and Epilepsy*. Philadelphia: F. A. Davis, 1989.
3. Noebels, J. L. Molecular genetics and epilepsy. In T. A. Pedley and B. S. Meldrum (eds.), *Recent Advances in Epilepsy*. Edinburgh: Churchill-Livingstone, 1992, Vol. 5, pp. 1–13.
4. Meldrum, B. S., and Bruton, C. J. Epilepsy. In J. Hume Adams and L. W. Duchen (eds.), *Greenfield's Neuropathology*. London: Edward Arnold, 1992, pp. 1246–1283.
5. Wada, J. *Kindling 3*. New York: Raven Press, 1985.
6. Akiyama, K., Daigen, A., Yamada, N., Itoh, T., Kohira, I., Ujike, H., and Otsuki, S. Long-lasting enhancement of metabotropic excitatory amino acid receptor-mediated polyphosphoinositide hydrolysis in the amygdala/pyriform cortex of deep prepyriform cortical kindled rats. *Brain Res.* 569:71–77, 1992.
7. Holmes, K. H., Bilkey, D. K., Laverty, R., and Goddard, G. V. The N-methyl-D-aspartate antagonists aminophosphonovalerate and carboxypiperazinephosphonate retard the development and expression of kindled seizures. *Brain Res.* 506:227–235, 1990.
8. Heinemann, U. Changes in the neuronal microenvironment and epileptiform activity. In H. G. Wieser, E. J. Speckmann, and J. Engel (eds.), *The Epileptic Focus*. London: John Libbey, 1987, pp. 27–44.
9. Babb, T. L. Research on the anatomy and pathology of epileptic tissue. In H. Luders (ed.), *Neurosurgery of Epilepsy*. New York: Raven Press, 1991, p. 719.
10. Sloviter, R. S. Permanently altered hippocampal structure, excitability, and inhibition after experimental status epilepticus in the rat: The "dormant basket cell" hypothesis and its possible relevance to temporal lobe epilepsy. *Hippocampus* 1:41–66, 1991.
11. Savic, I., Widen, L., Thorell, J. O., Blomqvist, G., Ericson, K., and Roland, P. Cortical benzodiazepine receptor binding in patients with generalized and partial epilepsy. *Epilepsia* 31: 724–730, 1990.
12. Hwa, G. G. C., and Avoli, M. Excitatory synaptic transmission mediated by NMDA and non-NMDA receptors in the superficial/middle layers of the epileptogenic human neocortex maintained in vitro. *Neurosci. Lett.* 143:83–86, 1992.
13. Louvel, J., and Pumain, R. N-Methyl-D-aspartate-mediated responses in epileptic cortex in man: An in vitro study. In S. Avanzini, J. Engel, R. Forello, U. Heinemann, (eds.), *Neurotransmitters in Epilepsy*. Amsterdam: Elsevier: 1992, pp. 361–367.
14. Mayberg, H. S., Sadzot, B., Meltzer, C. C., Fisher, R. S., Lesser, R. P., Dannals, R. F., Lever, J. R., Wilson, A. A., Ravert, H. T., Wagner, H. N., Jr., Bryan, R. N., Cromwell, C. C., and Frost, J. J., Quantification of mu and non-mu opiate receptors in temporal lobe epilepsy using positron emission tomography. *Ann. Neurol.* 30:3–11, 1991.
15. Meldrum, B. Epilepsy. In A. N. Davison and R. H. S. Thompson (eds.), *The Molecular Basis of Neuropathology,* London: Edward Arnold, 1981, pp. 265–301.
16. Macdonald, R. L., and Meldrum, B. S. General principles. Principles of antiepileptic drug action. In R. Levy, R. Mattson, B. Meldrum, J. K. Penry, and F. E. Dreifuss (eds.), *Antiepileptic Drugs,* 3rd ed. New York: Raven Press, 1989, pp. 59–83.
17. Coulter, D. A., Huguenard, J. R., and Prince, D. A. Differential effects of petit mal anticonvulsants and convulsants on thalamic neurones: Calcium current reduction. *Br. J. Pharmacol.* 100:800–806, 1990.
18. Chapman, A. G. Cerebral energy metabolism

and seizures. In T. A., Pedley and B. S. Meldrum (eds.), *Recent Advances in Epilepsy*. Edinburgh: Churchill-Livingstone, 1985, Vol. 2, pp. 19–63.

19. Chapman, A. G., Meldrum, B. S., and Siesjo, B. K. Cerebral metabolic changes during prolonged epileptic seizures in rats. *J. Neurochem.* 28:1025–1035, 1977.

20. Bazan, N. G., Birkle, D. L., Tang, W., and Reddy, T. S. The accumulation of free arachidonic acid, diacylglycerols, prostaglandins, and lipoxygenase reaction products in the brain during experimental epilepsy. In A. V. Delgado-Escueta, A. A. Ward, D. M. Woodbury, and R. J. Porter (eds.), *Basic Mechanisms of the Epilepsies*. New York: Raven Press, 1986, p. 879.

21. During, M. S., and Spencer, D. D. Extracellular hippocampal gluamate and spontaneous seizure in the conscious human brain. *Lancet* 341:1607–1610, 1993.

22. Gass, P., Herdegen, T., Bravo, R., and Kiessling, M. Induction of immediate early gene encoded proteins in the rat hippocampus after bicuculline-induced seizures: Differential expression of KROX-24, FOS and JUN proteins. *Neuroscience* 48:315–324, 1992.

23. Meldrum, B. S. Metabolic factors during prolonged seizures and their relation to nerve cell death. In A. V. Delgado-Escueta, C. B. Wasterlain, D. M. Treiman, and R. J. Porter (eds.), *Status Epilepticus Mechanisms of Brain Damage and Treatment*. New York: Raven Press, 1983, p. 261.

24. Clifford, D. B., Zorumski, C. F., and Olney, J. W. Ketamine and MK-801 prevent degeneration of thalamic neurons induced by focal cortical seizures. *Exp. Neurol.* 105:272–279, 1989.

25. Sutula, T., Cascino, G., Cavazos, J., Parada, I., and Ramirez, L. Mossy fiber synaptic reorganization in the epileptic human temporal lobe. *Ann. Neurol.* 26:321–330, 1989.

26. Sutula, T., Xiao-Xian, H., Cavazos, J., and Scott, G. Synaptic reorganization in the hippocampus induced by abnormal functional activity. *Science* 239:1147–1150, 1988.

CHAPTER 44

Neurotransmitters and Disorders of the Basal Ganglia

Irwin J. Kopin

Basic Neurochemistry: Molecular, Cellular, and Medical Aspects, 5th Ed., edited by G. J. Siegel et al. Published by Raven Press, Ltd., New York, 1994. Correspondence to Irwin J. Kopin, National Institute of Neurological Disorders and Stroke, National Institutes of Health, Building 10, Room 5N214, Bethesda, Maryland 20892.

BIOCHEMICAL ANATOMY OF THE BASAL GANGLIA AND ASSOCIATED NEURONAL SYSTEMS

The basal ganglia consist of several large anatomically distinct masses of gray matter situated in the core of the cerebral hemispheres among ascending and descending tracts of white matter and astride the brainstem. These constitute the striatum (caudate and putamen) and the pallidum (internal and external portions of the globus pallidus). The striopallidal system is a complex integrated unit that has many afferent and efferent connections to other parts of the brain, and with several other subcortical structures, constitutes an extrapyramidal system regulating sensorimotor activity, including tone and posture and a frontal cortical-subcortical system implicated in schizophrenia (see Chap. 47). Neurochemical studies have identified the neurotransmitters present in various regions of the brain, described the presence of enzymes involved in the biosynthesis and degradation of many of these transmitters, and demonstrated the presence of uptake sites for inactivation of the transmitters as well as receptors mediating their effects on neuronal activity. To better understand the functional role of the relevant neurotransmitters and neuromodulators, it is important to consider also the neuronal circuits and connections of the basal ganglia.

Identification of neurotransmitter systems in the basal ganglia

A number of important techniques for precise cellular localization of neurotransmitters, enzymes involved in their synthesis or degradation, receptors (and subtypes of receptors), and transporters have been applied to studies of the various neuronal pathways projecting to or arising from the basal ganglia. Catecholamines (dopamine, norepinephrine, and epinephrine) and serotonin can be converted to fluorescent derivatives which can then be used to delineate their distribution in neurons and their processes. Antibodies to neurotransmitters such as γ-aminobutyric acid (GABA) and peptides, as well as against specific proteins, are useful for their immunohistological demonstration in brain. Radiolabeled neurotransmitters and ligands (or blockers) of transporters and receptors have been used for autoradiographic localization of uptake sites and receptor subtypes. The application of *in situ* hybridization using complementary DNA (cDNA) probes for messenger RNAs (mRNAs) that encode peptide precursors, receptors, transporters, biosynthetic enzymes, and specific neuronal proteins has provided a wealth of information regarding neuronal pathways throughout the brain, including the basal ganglia. These techniques provide quantitative as well as anatomical information and, together with biochemical assays, neurophysiologically monitored responses, and behavioral studies, have enormously enhanced understanding of basal ganglia function in health and disease. Some connections between the basal ganglia and associated structures and the involved neurotransmitters are shown in Fig. 1.

The basal ganglia are not homogeneous structures

In the striatum, differences in the intensity of staining with several neuronal markers show that the populations of cells in various regions are not uniform. Compartmentalization was first suggested by differences in the intensity of staining for acetylcholinesterase (AChE). Whereas most of the striatum stains heavily for this enzyme, AChE-poor islands, termed striasomes or patches, constitute 10 to 20 percent of the striatum. The striasomes constitute a labyrinthine mesh embedded in a matrix of AChE-rich striatal tissue. In addition to differences in AChE content, they have been found to differ quantitatively from the remainder of the striatum with respect to the concentration of several other substances (see below); furthermore, the neurons in the striasomes appear to receive distinct cortical input and to project differently from those in the matrix (see [1,2]).

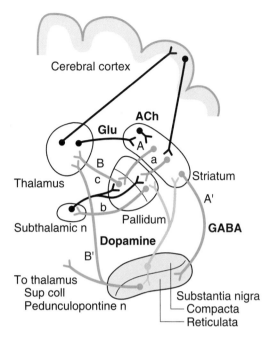

FIG. 1. Major connections and neurotransmitters of the basal ganglia. The major inputs to the striatum are gluta-minergic (Glu) afferents, mostly from the cortex, but with some input from the thalamus. Glutaminergic excitatory and GABAergic inhibitory neurons form two parallel, "direct" and "indirect" pathways from the striatum to the output nuclei of the basal ganglia, the internal layer of the globus pallidus and the substantia nigra reticulata. The direct pathway consists of GABAergic striatal neu-rons which project directly to the GABAergic efferent neurons of the internal layer of the globus pallidus and substantia nigra reticulata. This pathway, which contains two inhibitory synapses (A, A'—striatum to internal layer of the globus pallidus and substantia nigra reticulata B, B'—to thalamus), is believed to be responsible for disin-hibition of the excitatory glutaminergic thalamic input to the sensory, motor, and associated areas of the cortex. The indirect pathway includes a GABAergic projection from the striatum to the external layer of the globus pal-lidus. The external layer of the globus pallidus contains GABA neurons that innervate the subthalamic nucleus. Glutaminergic neurons from the subthalamic nucleus project to the internal layer of the globus pallidus. Thus, the "indirect" pathway contains three inhibitory syn-apses (a—striatum to external layer of the globus pal-lidus; b—external layer of globus pallidus to subthalamic nucleus; c—internal layer of the globus pallidus to thala-mus) resulting in a net inhibition (inhibition of disinhibi-tion) of the excitatory thalamic-cortical connections. The neurons in the thalamus complete the feedback loop by sending their fibers to the cortex. In addition, intrastriatal cholinergic neurons and dopaminergic innervation of the striatum from the substantia nigra compacta are among the most important modulators of these circuits. A variety of peptides, variably colocalized with the four major neu-rotransmitters, modulate basal ganglia function (see text). (ACh) acetylcholine; (Sup Coll) superior colliculus.

Excitatory amino acids provide important afferent input to the basal ganglia

Glutamate and aspartate are excitatory amino acid neurotransmitters that are pres-ent in many neurons throughout the brain. They are involved in basal ganglia afferent, connecting, and output pathways which, with thalamic and subthalamic nuclei, consti-tute feedback circuits that modulate cerebral cortical function. The major afferent neu-ronal pathways to the striatum are from the sensorimotor and other cortical areas and from the thalamus; these fibers release exci-tatory amino acids, mostly glutamate, in syn-apses with dendrites on striatal neurons. Glutamate is also the excitatory neuro-transmitter released from the terminals of the subthalamic neurons projecting to the pallidum, particularly to the internal layer of the globus pallidus, and from the axon terminals of thalamic neurons that send fibers mainly to the cortex. In the stria-tum, release of the excitatory transmitters is modulated by presynaptic receptors for ace-tylcholine, dopamine, GABA, opioids, and adenosine. Also present are many peptides (Table 1) which may have similar modula-tory effects as cotransmitters.

Excitatory amino acid receptors are mainly localized on cells of the striatum

The receptors that respond to excitatory amino acids, particularly to glutamate, regu-late ion channels (ionotrophic), or are cou-pled to G proteins (metabotropic) and exert their effects indirectly, through intracellular second messengers. There are at least three

TABLE 1. Peptides found in the basal ganglia

Substance P (S)[a]	Neuropeptide Y
Substance K	Somatostatin (M)[a]
Cholecystokinin	Dynorphin (S)[a]
Neurotensin (S)[a]	Enkephalin (M)[a]
Neurokinin B	Galinin
Lys[8]-Asn[9]-neurotensin (8–13)	

[a] Preferentially localized in striosomes (S) or matrix (M) as indicated in text.

types of ionotrophic glutamate receptors that can be distinguished by their responses to and binding of selective agonists. These are N-methyl-D-aspartate (NMDA), kainate, and α-amino-3-hydroxy-5-methyl-4-isoxazole-propionate (AMPA) or quisqualate receptors. NMDA receptors appear to be associated with ligand-gated calcium channels, whereas kainate and quisqualate (or AMPA) receptors are associated with ligand-gated K^+/Na^+ channels. A quisqualate-sensitive metabotropic receptor has also been demonstrated. All these excitatory amino acid receptors are demonstrable in the striatum (see Chap. 17 for a more complete description of excitatory amino acid receptors). Since decortication of rats does not diminish significantly the binding of radiolabeled NMDA, AMPA, or kainate in the striatum, whereas destruction of striatal neurons with an excitotoxin (quinolinic acid) strikingly decreases binding of these ligands, it appears that most of these receptors are postjunctional.

GABA is the neurotransmitter of most striatal neurons

The great majority of neurons in the striatum are medium spiny neurons that contain GABA as their neurotransmitter. This was first demonstrated by use of an antibody specific for the enzyme responsible for GABA formation, glutamic acid decarboxylase (GAD). Antibodies to GABA have also been used to locate this neurotransmitter in neurons and their processes. Antibodies to peptide neurotransmitters or probes for mRNA encoding the peptides or their precursors have been used to demonstrate colocalization of these peptides in subpopulations of GABAergic neurons. Some peptides that have been found in the striatum are listed in Table 1. GABAergic neurons of the striatum project to the pallidum and to the substantia nigra. Those that project to the external layer of the globus pallidus often contain enkephalin as a cotransmitter. They synapse on GABAergic neurons which project from the external layer of the globus pallidus to the

glutaminergic neurons in the subthalamic nucleus. The GABAergic striatal neurons that project to the internal layer of the globus pallidus and substantia nigra reticulata often contain substance P and/or dynorphin. GABAergic neurons in the striasomes appear to project to the substantia nigra compacta. Many of these neurons contain neurotensin, tachykinins (substance P or K), and/or dynorphin.

Acetylcholine is the neurotransmitter of striatal interneurons

Acetylcholine is the neurotransmitter contained in many of the large spiny neurons that make up about 5 percent of the striatal neurons. These neurons, which are distinguished by immunoreactivity to choline acetyltransferase (CAT), the enzyme responsible for synthesis of acetylcholine, receive several types of synaptic input: (1) glutaminergic fibers from the cerebral cortex; (2) tyrosine hydroxylase-immunoreactive, presumably dopaminergic, fibers which form small, symmetrical synapses on the soma and proximal dendrites; and (3) substance P-GAD-immunopositive boutons, believed to be axon collaterals from medium spiny neurons. These cholinergic interneurons have relatively short axons that are confined to the striatum and innervate predominantly the medium spiny neurons. Both muscarinic and nicotinic cholinergic receptors are found in the striatum; muscarinic receptors on glutaminergic terminals are thought to inhibit release of the excitatory transmitter, acting as a modulator of glutaminergic stimulation of striatal neurons, whereas nicotinic receptor activation enhances transmitter release.

Dopamine is the neurotransmitter of the nigrostriatal pathway

Cathecholamines are widely distributed throughout the brain, but as shown in Table 2, there are important regional differences in their levels [3]. Such differences in distribution were the first indication of their role

TABLE 2.   Catecholamine content of brain regions[a]

	Dopamine	Norepinephrine	Epinephrine
Frontal cortex	0.2–1.0	2.2–4.1	—
Basal ganglia			
Caudate nucleus	70.5–133.9	1.1–3.1	—
Nucleus accumbens	87.2–100.5	3.6–9.3	—
Globus pallidus	39.6	5.3	—
Amygdala (central nucleus)	15.0–24.1	13.4–17.8	—
Thalamus (anteroventral nucleus)	1.2–7.3	12.7–25.9	—
Hypothalamus			
Paraventricular nucleus	5.8–10.0	49.7–66.6	2.2
Median eminence	44.0–84.0	15.9–41.4	1.8
Locus coeruleus	16.7–23.9	53.1–76.5	0.3–0.6
Cerebellar cortex	0.2–1.3	1.6–2.9	0–0.2
Nucl. solit. tract commissural part	10.1–10.8	38.3–83.0	1.5–2.2

[a] From Palkovits and Brownstein [3].

as brain neurotransmitters. Histofluorescence techniques for visualizing catecholamines and immunohistological localization of tyrosine hydroxylase, the rate-limiting enzyme in catecholamine biosynthesis (see Chap. 12), have been used to define catecholamine-containing neurons and the pathways of their axons to the terminal arborizations at their target regions. The principal dopaminergic fiber systems in brain are the nigrostriatal (from the substantia nigra compacta to the caudate nucleus and putamen), the mesolimbic (from the ventral tegmental area to the nucleus accumbens), the mesocortical (from the ventral tegmental area to the cerebral cortex), and the tuberoinfundibular (from the arcuate nucleus to the median eminence). There are also dopamine-containing neurons and terminals in other brain regions, in the retina, and in the spinal cord. These neurons store dopamine in vesicles within varicosities of the nerve terminals. Intravesicular concentrations of dopamine are maintained at high levels (1–20 mg/g fresh weight). Although dopamine accounts for about half of the total catecholamines in brain, over 80 percent of brain dopamine is in the basal ganglia, and its concentration in the striatum is much greater than that of norepinephrine (see Table 2). Dopamine in the striatum is contained in a dense arborization of fine nerve terminals derived from the dopamine-containing neurons of the substantia nigra compacta. These structures contain tyrosine hydroxylase so that dopamine can be synthesized directly at the terminal varicosities. Tyrosine hydroxylase requires iron and tetrahydropteridine in order to oxidize tyrosine to 3,4-dihydroxyphenylalanine (dopa). Only small amounts of dopa are found in the tissue, however, since it is readily decarboxylated by aromatic amino acid decarboxylase (AADC). This enzyme is present in many tissues including serotonergic neurons where it serves to decarboxylate 5-hydroxytryptophan to form serotonin. Like other amino acid decarboxylases, AADC requires pyridoxyl phosphate as its coenzyme. It is inhibited by many compounds, a few of which have been used therapeutically. The chemical structures of some decarboxylase inhibitors are shown in Fig. 2.

Dopamine synthesis in the nerve terminals is accelerated during depolarization-induced release of the neurotransmitter. This is the result of rapid activation of tyrosine hydroxylase (see Chap. 12). Enhanced release of dopamine results in elevated levels of its metabolites in the tissues and in the surrounding fluids.

Dopamine is metabolized by *O*-methylation and oxidative deamination

The major metabolites of dopamine are products of *O*-methylation and/or oxidative deamination. Major products include 3-methoxytyramine (3-MT), 3,4-dihydroxyphenylacetic acid (DOPAC), and homovanillic acid (HVA, or 4-hydroxy-3-methoxyphenylacetic acid). These are depicted in Fig. 3, which also shows the alternative pathways of metabolism of dopamine (see Fig. 3, Chap. 12 for analogous reactions of norepinephrine). Some of the compounds shown in Fig. 3 are conjugated with sulfate or glucuronate before excretion in the urine or bile. The amine and its *O*-methyl derivative are both subject to the action of monoamine oxidase (MAO), a flavoprotein present in the outer membrane of the mitochondria. MAO exists in two forms: MAO type A (MAO-A) is especially sensitive to inhibition by clorgyline and is present in catecholaminergic neurons and their axons, whereas MAO type B (MAO-B) is inhibited selectively by deprenyl and predominates in serotonin-containing neurons and in astrocytes. Pargyline irreversibly inhibits both MAO-A and MAO-B. The chemical structures of these three propargylamine inhibitors are shown in Fig. 2. Products of the MAO reaction include the aldehyde corresponding to the amine substrate, hydrogen peroxide, and ammonia. Most of the aldehyde undergoes further dehydrogenation

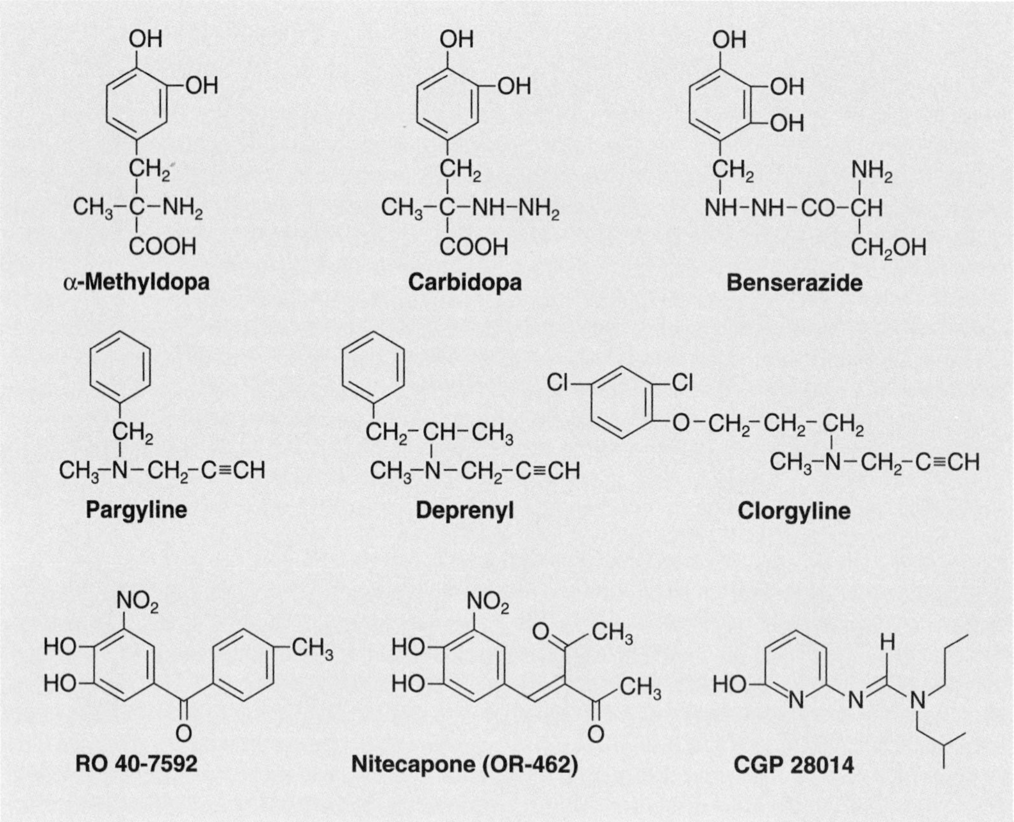

FIG. 2. Inhibitors of enzymes involved in the metabolism of levodopa and of dopamine. Aromatic amino acid decarboxylase (AADC) is inhibited by α-methyldopa, carbidopa, and benserazide. Pargyline inhibits both monoamine oxidase (MAO) subtypes whereas deprenyl is selective for MAO type B and clorgyline for MAO type A. RO 40-7592, nitecapone, and CGP 28014 inhibit catechol-*O*-methyltransferase.

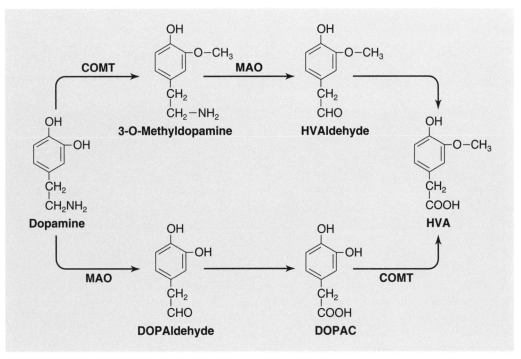

FIG. 3.   Dopamine and its major metabolites. Dopamine is sequentially deaminated and *O*-methylated, or vice versa depending on the site of metabolism (see text). (MAO) monoamine oxidase; (COMT) catechol-*O*-methyltransferase; (HVA) homovanillic acid; (DOPAC) 3,4-dihydroxyphenylacetic acid.

to form, in the case of dopamine, DOPAC, which is a substrate for cathechol-*O*-methyltransferase (COMT), an enzyme that catalyzes the transfer of the methyl group from *S*-adenosylmethionine to the m-hydroxyl group. This process appears to be very efficient in human brain because normally there are only very small quantities of DOPAC in the striatum but substantial amounts of HVA. A portion of the aldehyde undergoes reduction, catalyzed by alcohol dehydrogenase or a similar enzyme, with participation of reduced nicotinamide coenzyme. The alcoholic products that are formed are far less abundant than the acidic metabolites of dopamine, but are major metabolites of norepinephrine.

The black pigment, neuromelanin, which accumulates in the neurons of the substantia nigra compacta, is derived from polymerization of quinones formed from catechols, mostly dopa and dopamine. The function, if any, of neuromelanin is unknown. It may be related to the vulnerability of these neurons to toxic damage or degenerative processes resulting in Parkinson's disease (see below).

Modulation of basal ganglia circuit activities

The basic circuits involving the basal ganglia and the major classical neurotransmitters or neuromodulators involved in their neuronal pathways are depicted in Fig. 1. The basic circuits are regulated by feedback systems and modulatory peptide cotransmitters. Cholinergic and substance P axons terminate on the proximal portions of the dendrites of the medium spiny neurons. The extensive axon collaterals of these neurons release GABA, and probably their peptide cotransmitters, into synapses near or on the cell bodies of other spiny neurons. Interneurons that release acetylcholine also contain somatostatin and neuropeptide Y (NPY), which may modulate striatal neuron activity. Best known and perhaps most important, dopaminergic fibers from the substantia nigra compacta that synapse on the medium spiny neurons, as well as fibers on the more distal parts of their dendritic tree, modulate striatal GABAergic output.

As indicated above, dopaminergic neurons project mainly from the substantia nigra compacta to innervate the striatum, and about 80 percent of the dopamine content in brain is found in the basal ganglia. Dopamine released in the striatum can act at any of several dopamine receptor sites to modulate outflow of GABAergic neurons to the globus pallidus or substantia nigra. There are D_2 receptors on the terminals of corticostriatal projections, enkephalin-containing medium spiny neurons, and cholinergic interneurons and, as autoreceptors, on the dopaminergic neurons on the substantia nigra compacta. D_1 receptors are present on dynorphin-substance P-containing medium spiny neurons and both D_1 and D_2 receptors are present on a subpopulation of striatal neurons. There is considerable evidence that there are important functional interactions between D_1 and D_2 receptors; combined administration of D_1 and D_2 agonists appears to have synergistic biochemical and behavioral effects. The complex array of dopamine receptors on different neurons, the extensive medium spiny neuron axon collateral cross innervation, and the indirect connections via interneurons, as well as striatal neurons that express both receptor subtypes, provide ample opportunity for interactions among D_1 and D_2 receptor-mediated effects. The complexity of interconnections via neuronal networks, feedback circuits, and D_1 and D_2 receptors on the same cell defies simple analysis, but it is evident that the net effects of dopamine deficiency are responsible for striking motor deficits seen in parkinsonian syndromes. Conversely, conditions (genetic, toxic, vascular, tumor, etc.) that cause overactivity of dopamine or the systems normally activated by dopamine result in an array of involuntary dyskinesias. These sometimes appear in association with the hypokinetic features of parkinsonism and are generally attributed to disorders of the basal ganglia and its output pathways. Thus, basal ganglia disorders are associated with parkinsonian hypokinetic as well as a variety of hyperkinetic conditions.

PARKINSONIAN SYNDROMES

Parkinson's disease was first described in a classic monograph, "The Shaking Palsy," published in 1817 by the London physician James Parkinson. The cardinal features of Parkinson's disease are (1) tremor (mainly at rest); (2) muscular rigidity, which leads to difficulties in walking, writing, and speaking and masking of facial expression; (3) bradykinesia, a slowness in initiating and executing movements; and (4) stooped posture and instability. The disease progresses slowly, but may ultimately produce complete akinesia and helplessness. Although the clinical features were well described, the pathological basis of the disease remained unknown for over 100 years. The frequent occurrence of parkinsonism as a sequela to von Economo's encephalitis lethargica, which reached epidemic proportions in 1918 to 1921, led to the discovery that depigmentation of the substantia nigra is a constant feature of parkinsonism, whether as the result of the virus, of exposure to toxins, or from unknown causes. In view of widespread changes elsewhere, there was, however, hesitancy in attributing to so small a brain lesion so extensive a movement disorder.

Chemical pathology of Parkinson's disease: degeneration of nigrostriatal tract and reduced striatal dopamine

Nearly two generations elapsed before the next major advances in understanding Parkinson's disease. In 1958, Carlsson and his co-workers [4] reported on the occurrence of dopamine in the brain (with highest concentrations in the striatum), its depletion by reserpine, and the dramatic effect of dopa in reversing reserpine-induced tranquilization, impoverished motor activity, and ptosis in mice and rabbits. They showed also that pretreatment with an MAO inhibitor potentiated the effects of dopa in reversing reserpine effects. The uneven distribution of catecholamines in brain suggested that these substances may function as neurotransmitters. Two years later, Ehringer and Hornykiewicz [5] noted the greatly reduced (to about one-tenth normal) concentrations of dopamine in the caudate, putamen, and substantia nigra of brains from parkinsonian patients. Shortly thereafter, newly developed histofluorescence techniques demonstrated the previously unknown nigrostriatal dopamine-containing tract with cell bodies in the substantia nigra pars compacta and axonal projections to the striatum. These observations were seminal in understanding the pathophysiology of parkinsonian syndromes.

Diminished formation and metabolism of dopamine are reflected in low postmortem concentrations of DOPAC and HVA in the caudate nucleus and putamen. Since some HVA normally diffuses into the cerebrospinal fluid (CSF), particularly from the caudate nucleus, HVA is readily detectable in CSF [6]. In Parkinson's disease, the CSF concentrations of HVA are far below those found in patients with neurological disorders not involving the basal ganglia, particularly in more severely affected patients. Because HVA is a substrate for the active transport mechanism that removes acidic compounds into the circulation, there is a steep gradient with CSF concentrations of HVA, with highest levels in the lateral ventricles and lowest levels in the lumbar CSF. This acid transport system is inhibited in a dose-dependent manner by probenecid (p-dipropylsulfamylbenzoic acid). Probenecid has been used to differentiate low CSF HVA levels in other disorders of the central nervous system (CNS) from those in Parkinson's disease. Parkinsonian patients given probene-

cid show a lower increase in HVA than do patients with other neurological disorders. Also, it is now possible using positron-emitting analogs of levodopa such as ^{18}F-6-fluorodopa (see Chap. 46) to demonstrate the deficit in forming and storing dopamine in living parkinsonian patients.

Parkinsonian symptoms may occur in association with any disorder that causes damage to the nigrostriatal dopamine neurons or that results in an imbalance diminishing the disinhibition (indirect) circuit. Thus, lesions of the pallidum, as well as those of the substantia nigra compacta, result in the appearance of parkinson-like movement disorders [7]. Neurological disorders such as progressive supranuclear palsy, multiple system atrophy, and the Parkinson-amyotrophic lateral sclerosis (ALS)-dementia complex that include parkinsonian movement abnormalities in addition to other neurological deficits are termed "parkinsonism-plus" syndromes [8]. Infectious diseases, tumors, metabolic disturbances, and toxins may also produce forms of parkinsonism. Those that involve primarily the dopamine system may benefit from therapies aimed at dopamine replacement, whereas those involving other pathways are generally unresponsive to such treatments.

Levodopa treatment of Parkinson's disease

It was long known that dopamine does not penetrate the blood-brain barrier, while its amino acid precursor, levodopa (as indicated by its behavioral effects and by biochemical studies), readily enters the brain and there is decarboxylated to form dopamine. Initial efforts at brain dopamine replacement with dopa failed because of severe side effects, particularly nausea and vomiting. Cotzias et al. [9] gradually increased the doses of levodopa and thereby avoided or reduced adverse side effects, and thus succeeded in administering high doses of dopa, achieving remarkable symptomatic improvement. This established that most of the signs and symptoms of Parkinson's disease were a result of dopamine deficiency. Although there are other biochemical abnormalities in parkinsonian brain, such as diminished levels of serotonin, norepinephrine, GABA, and glutamate decarboxylase, these are not as striking as the loss of dopamine, which appears to be crucial. Strategies were then focused on enhancing the efficacy of levodopa treatment.

Potentiation of levodopa by inhibition of decarboxylation

Passage of levodopa from the intestine into the systemic circulation and into the brain parenchyma entails its absorption from the intestine, passage through the hepatic circulation, and transfer to the brain from blood through the endothelial cells lining the capillaries (see Chap. 32). Considerable AADC activity is present in the intestinal wall, the liver, the kidneys, and the brain capillary endothelium; dopamine formed by decarboxylation of levodopa at these sites is excluded from the brain. Selective inhibition of extracerebral AADC was therefore explored as a means of enhancing levodopa efficacy. The first compound found to inhibit AADC was α-methyldopa (see Fig. 2). This drug inhibits the decarboxylation of levodopa, but is itself a substrate for the enzyme and is converted to α-methyldopamine and α-methylnorepinephrine, which can replace the physiological neurotransmitters. Since they are not as effective in activating receptors, these "false transmitters" reduce catecholaminergic activity. Although α-methyldopa proved useful in treating hypertension, by diminishing brain dopamine, it occasionally results in the appearance of parkinsonian symptoms.

Carbidopa and benserazide (see Fig. 2) can be administered in doses that affect only extracerebral AADC (including that of the brain capillaries) and both have been found to be useful adjuncts to levodopa treatment [10]. These drugs not only enhance the bioavailability of levodopa and have a dopamine-sparing effect, but also inactivate the brain capillary enzymatic barrier to levo-dopa. When levodopa has crossed the blood-brain barrier, aided by an active transport mechanism, it must be converted to dopamine. Some question arises as to the source of the decarboxylase for this, since many of the dopaminergic neurons (including their content of AADC) are absent in the disease. Studies of postmortem striatum, however, have not yet revealed any cases with a total deficiency of AADC in the striatum; there has always been at least a residue of enzyme activity. Moreover, cells of the striatum receive connections from many sources, including serotonin-producing raphe nuclei. Hence, levodopa could also be converted to dopamine by the decarboxylase within those neurons. Dopamine formed would then be available in brain tissue, although its path of diffusion to sensitive receptors might be longer than usual. Untreated parkinsonian patients have elevated densities of D_2 receptors (those that are not linked to inhibition of adenylyl cyclase) in the striatum (see Chap. 21), presumably reflecting a "supersensitive" state in which responses could be elicited by lower dopamine concentrations. Treatment with levodopa lowers the density of D_2 receptors to the level seen in control tissue.

Potentiation of levodopa with MAO-B inhibition

Since dopamine is a substrate for MAO and inhibitors of this enzyme potentiated the effects of dopa in reversing reserpine-induced tranquilization, it was apparent that this might also be true for levodopa used in treating Parkinson's disease. During treatment of depression with MAO inhibitors, however, psychiatric patients who ingested foods (e.g., cheese, wine) rich in tyramine developed acute severe hypertensive reactions. Because similar reactions could occur with concurrent use of levodopa and the MAO inhibitors then in use, these drugs were contraindicated in parkinsonian patients being treated with levodopa.

After the discovery that the hypertensive reactions were due to inhibition of MAO-A and that deprenyl, an irreversible inhibitor of MAO-B, is devoid of the "cheese" effect, this MAO inhibitor was given in combination with levodopa and a peripheral decarboxylase inhibitor to enhance and prolong the effects of levodopa [11]. Unfortunately, both beneficial and adverse effects are similarly affected. Levodopa potentiation by deprenyl may be related not only to its inhibition of dopamine deamination; the drug also inhibits catecholamine uptake and thereby may block inactivation of dopamine as well as prevent the release of norepinephrine by indirectly acting on sympathomimetic amines such as tyramine. Potent blockade of the catecholamine transporters is unusual among MAO inhibitors, and this property of deprenyl may explain its safety with regard to the "cheese reaction." Deprenyl may have additional effects which make it useful in the treatment of Parkinson's disease (see below).

Catechol-O-methyltransferase inhibition

Levodopa is a substrate for COMT, and when decarboxylation is blocked, plasma levels of 3-O-methyldopa (3-OMD) are elevated. Because both levodopa and 3-OMD are absorbed from the intestine and transported into brain by the same saturable carrier system for which many large neutral amino acids (LNAAs) are substrates, 3-OMD and dietary amino acids influence the efficacy of levodopa treatment. Furthermore, 3-O-methylation contributes to the rapid metabolism of levodopa. On the basis of these considerations, attention has been directed at development and testing effects of inhibition of COMT; recently, effects in humans of three relatively nontoxic COMT inhibitors (see Fig. 2) were reported, but the extent of their efficacy in potentiating the effects of levodopa has not yet been established. They do, however, enhance contrast in imaging of brain dopamine neurons during PET scanning with ^{18}F-6-fluorodopa. Nitecapone, a 3-nitrocatechol, does not enter readily into the brain [12], whereas RO 40-7592 (3,4-dihy-

droxy-4-methyl-5-nitrophenone)   inhibits COMT competitively in both the brain and peripheral tissues [13]. CGP 28014, N-(2-pyridone-6yl)-N-N-di- n-propyl-formamidine, which is not a catechol, although a weak inhibitor of COMT in vitro, has been reported to reduce HVA and elevate DOPAC levels in rat striatum.

Alternatives and adjuncts to levodopa treatment of parkinsonian syndromes

The actions of levodopa in Parkinson's disease or of dopamine at receptor sites in the central nervous system are mimicked by a number of compounds. Apomorphine, a semisynthetic catechol alkaloid, has a brief dopaminergic action. It acts both pre- and postsynaptically, the presynaptic autoreceptors being particularly sensitive to this drug. Its best recognized action is at the dopamine receptor sites making up the trigger zone of the emetic center in the area postrema. Like levodopa, apomorphine affects certain neuroendocrine systems. In humans, subemetic doses provoke striking increases in the concentration of growth hormone in the plasma, presumably by acting on cells producing the appropriate releasing factor. In many species it depresses the concentration of serum prolactin by a direct action on D_2 receptors.

Three other dopamine agonists, bromocryptine, lisuride, and pergolide, all of which are ergoline derivatives and act predominantly as D_2 dopamine receptor agonists, have found some practical use in the treatment of early symptoms of Parkinson's disease or as adjuncts to levodopa/carbidopa (or levodopa/benserazide) in later stages of the disease [14]. Amantadine is used in treatment as an adjunctive therapy: Its action favors the release of dopamine from residual intact neurons in much the same way as does amphetamine.

Before the advent of levodopa, anticholinergic agents were among the most commonly used drugs and the therapeutic mainstay in the treatment of Parkinson's disease. They appear to restore the balance that is disturbed when striatal cholinergic neurons have been released from the inhibitory action of dopamine fibers that synapse with them.

Surgical treatments of Parkinson's disease

Prior to the introduction of levodopa, localized lesions in structures associated with the basal ganglia were sometimes effective in relieving some of the motor deficits in severely parkinsonian patients. This is still used in selected refractory patients and may become more prevalent with the demonstration that lesions of the subthalamic nucleus alleviate experimental parkinsonism in monkeys [15], presumably by removing the abnormally predominant inhibition of disinhibition represented by the "indirect" pathway of cortico-striatal-thalamic-cortical feedback, shown in Fig. 1.

A completely novel approach to treatment is based on replacing dopamine-producing tissue in the degenerating striatum. Originally it was hoped that transplants of the patient's own adrenal medullary tissue into the caudate or putamen might supply sufficient dopamine to restore function, but graft survival was poor and the risks outweighed the marginal benefits obtained. Currently attempts are being made to use fetal mesencephalic tissue implants, with reports of some success. Beneficial effects of implanted tissue, however, might be due to stimulation of the patient's residual dopaminergic neurons to develop axonal sprouts that reinnervate the depleted regions, as well as provision of a new source of dopamine-releasing tissue. Mammalian (including human) brain neurons have been shown to have the potential for functionally significant regeneration. Even in severely parkinsonian patients, sufficient numbers of viable dopaminergic neurons remain to support reinnervation and functional improvement. Growth or neurotrophic factors produced by fetal and/or cytokine-stimulated glia may enhance dopaminergic neuronal sprouting. Such sprouting may account for the modest clinical improvement observed after surgical transplantation, even after death of adrenal medullary implants.

MPTP-INDUCED PARKINSONISM

Although many toxins and neurological insults that damage the basal ganglia and/or the substantia nigra result in neurological disorders which include parkinsonian features (see below), one toxin, N-methyl-4-phenyl-1,2,3,6-tetrahydropyridine (MPTP), appears to target relatively specifically those neurons that are involved in Parkinson's disease. This toxin has been used to develop animal models of Parkinson's disease that have proved useful for testing new therapies for the human disease. Investigations of the mechanisms of MPTP toxicity have also provided important insights regarding the possible pathogenesis of Parkinson's disease; they are described in greater detail below.

MPTP

MPTP toxicity was discovered after inadvertent self-administration by drug abusers of a compound produced during illicit synthesis of a narcotic related to meperidine. The users rapidly developed a movement disorder that closely resembles Parkinson's disease, including low levels of HVA in the CSF. MPTP administered to monkeys was found to result in depletion of dopamine in the caudate putamen, destruction of dopaminergic neurons in the substantia nigra, and appearance of a syndrome virtually identical to advanced Parkinson's disease in humans. It was subsequently found that parkinsonism had been encountered previously, as a result of industrial exposure of chemists to MPTP, but the association had not been recognized.

The mechanisms that have been implicated in MPTP toxicity [16] are depicted in Fig. 4. MPTP, which is lipid-soluble, readily penetrates the blood-brain barrier and enters brain cells. Because it is amphophilic

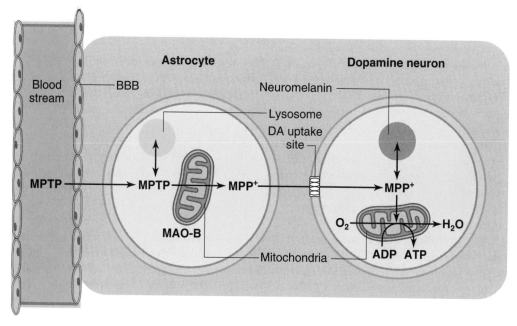

FIG. 4.   Schematic representation of the mechanisms involved in toxicity of MPTP. (BBB) blood-brain barrier; (MPTP) 1-methyl-4-phenyl-1,2,3,6-tetrahydropyridine; (MPP⁺) its four electron oxidation product N-methyl-4-phenylpyridinium.

(having both lipophilic and charged hydrophilic moieties), it is captured into acidic organelles (mostly lysosomes) of astrocytes. MPTP itself does not appear to be toxic, but its oxidized product, 1-methyl-4-phenylpyridinium (MPP⁺), is toxic. Astrocytes (and serotonin neurons) contain MAO-B, which converts MPTP to MPP⁺. The toxic oxidation product reaches the extracellular fluid and then is transported by the dopamine transporter into dopamine nerve terminals. Inhibition of either MAO-B or the dopamine transporter protects against MPTP toxicity. Toxicity of MPP⁺ is dependent upon mitochondrial concentrating mechanisms, as well as upon the plasma membrane uptake system. Energy-driven mitochondrial uptake of MPP⁺ results in sufficiently high concentrations of the toxin to interfere with mitochondrial respiration. The site at which MPP⁺ acts, complex I, appears to be at or near the region at which several other agents, e.g., rotenone, act to block mitochondrial oxidation. Blockade of mitochon-

drial respiration enhances the release from mitochondria of partially reduced oxygen, i.e., the superoxide anion radical (O_2^-), and markedly impairs ATP formation, with resultant failure of energy-dependent ion transport, elevation of cytosolic Ca^{2+} to toxic levels, and disruption of vital cell functions, thereby causing cell death.

Clues to the pathogenesis of Parkinson's disease

The selective vulnerability of nigrostriatal dopamine neurons to MPTP toxicity and the striking resemblance of the resulting clinical syndrome to Parkinson's disease refocused attention to determining etiological factors that contribute to the development of Parkinson's disease. Three separate, but not necessarily exclusive, hypotheses have been explored. The first hypothesis suggests that there are, in the environment, one or more substances that are, at least for vulnerable persons, neurotoxins similar to MPTP. Although there is provocative epidemiological evidence in support of a role for environmental neurotoxins, no such toxin has been identified, and only traces of endogenously produced potential neurotoxins have been demonstrated *in vivo*.

The second hypothesis proposes that a mitochondrial abnormality, possibly genetically determined, increases the vulnerability of some individuals to a destructive process involving the nigrostriatal neurons. In support of this hypothesis are reports of mitochondrial deficits in electron transport at complex I, similar to that caused by MPP^+ in platelets, in muscle, and in substantia nigra of parkinsonian patients [17]. Such putative mitochondrial abnormalities, however, are not necessarily a primary etiological factor; they might be secondary to another metabolic deficit, since free radicals formed during inhibition of complex I appear to inhibit irreversibly electron transport at complex I. Thus, excess free radicals produced from any source might be responsible for the deficiency in complex I activity reported in Parkinson's disease.

The third hypothesis is that oxidative stress or free radical formation, or both, are the bases for damage and death of dopamine neurons [18]. Several special neurochemical characteristics of the substantia nigra might enhance free radical formation and contribute to oxidative stress vulnerability. Autooxidation of catechols to quinones and polymerization of the quinones to neuromelanin may enhance formation of the three reactive oxygen species: O_2^-, hydrogen peroxide (H_2O_2), and the hydroxyl radical ($OH\cdot$). Oxidative deamination of dopamine, by either intraneuronal MAO-A or astrocytic MAO-B, yields H_2O_2 and in regions of high dopamine concentration could result in its formation in excess. Levels of superoxide dismutase, the enzyme that converts O_2^- to H_2O_2, are reported to be elevated in the substantia nigra of parkinsonian patients, suggesting that O_2^- formation and its conversion to H_2O_2 may be greater than normal. H_2O_2 is usually rapidly removed by catalase or peroxidases. Levels of catalase, the enzyme which converts H_2O_2 to water and oxygen, glutathione, and glutathione peroxidase, the enzyme catalyzing the removal of H_2O_2 by oxidation of glutathione, are reported to be low in the substantia nigra of parkinsonian patients. Relatively rapid formation of H_2O_2, coupled with insufficient removal mechanisms, has been proposed as a basis for oxidative damage. Ferric ions catalyze the reaction of H_2O_2 and O_2^- to form hydroxide ions and highly reactive hydroxyl free radicals (Haber-Weiss and Fenton reactions). Proponents of the free radical and related hypotheses cite the high postmortem levels of iron, particularly ferric ion, and increased lipid peroxides, a product of free radical attack, in the substantia nigra of parkinsonian patients as evidence that free radicals produced from iron and H_2O_2 contribute to neuronal death. Others point out that the iron is deposited in astrocytes, macrophages, reactive glia, and nonpigmented neurons and that it is unclear whether iron deposition is a result of the neuronal degeneration or due to an abnormality in iron metabolism.

Neuroprotective strategies

As indicated above, deprenyl, a "safe" MAO-B inhibitor, was found effective in potentiating the antiparkinsonian effects of levodopa. A surprising observation was that levodopa-treated patients receiving deprenyl had a longer life expectancy than did those treated with levodopa alone [19]. The possibility that Parkinson's disease may be related to an MAO-B-activated toxin and/or to oxidative stress (as evidenced by mitochondrial deficiency in electron transport, enhanced lipid peroxidation, high iron content, elevated superoxide dismutase, diminished capacity to remove excess H_2O_2, and the presence of increased iron) exacerbated by H_2O_2 formed during dopamine deamination encouraged trials of deprenyl and/or tocopherol (an antioxidant) as a means for preventing or retarding the degenerative process responsible for Parkinson's disease. In previously untreated parkinsonian patients, deprenyl appeared to delay progression of symptoms and the necessity for initiation of levodopa therapy [20]. Although the findings with deprenyl were dramatic, whether they were the result of symptomatic improvement due to potentiation of endogenous dopamine (by any of several potential mechanisms) or due to a neuroprotective effect is the subject of considerable controversy. The possibility of arresting or retarding the degenerative process responsible for progression of Parkinson's disease remains a subject of intense interest.

DRUG- AND TOXIN-INDUCED MOVEMENT DISORDERS

In addition to MPTP, other drugs that alter the availability of dopamine or affect its actions at receptors may induce movement disorders with parkinsonian features. Some drugs have an opposite effect, producing hyperactive states with involuntary abnormal movements. Indeed, an important and distressing adverse effect of levodopa is the appearance of dyskinesias in some more severely affected parkinsonian patients. Furthermore, the neurons of the basal ganglia and associated structures are peculiarly vulnerable to the effects of a variety of toxins, and this sensitivity plays an important role in the neurological complications that accompany these substances. Generally, toxins produce more extensive neurological damage and a greater variety of clinical deficits than is found in Parkinson's disease. Damage to the nigrostriatal dopaminergic system appears to be responsible for the parkinsonian features that occur after exposure to these toxins, whereas involvement of other basal ganglia or associated systems may be responsible for development of involuntary dyskinesias.

Pharmacological dopamine depletion induces parkinsonism

Reserpine, a natural alkaloid that blocks vesicular transport, depletes stored mono- amines, including dopamine. Dopamine depletion is associated with emergence of a form of parkinsonism and this effect of reserpine and its reversal by treatment with levodopa and/or a MAO inhibitor are among the first clues that parkinsonism is the result of dopamine deficiency. Generally the parkinsonism resulting from reserpine is reversible, presumably because the storage mechanisms blocked by reserpine are restored.

As indicated earlier, α-methyldopa treatment of hypertension sometimes results in the appearance of parkinsonian symptoms. This is presumed to be a consequence of dopamine depletion by replacement of dopamine with a relatively inactive false transmitter, α-methyldopamine, as well as by inhibition of AADC.

Neuroleptics that antagonize dopamine cause not only parkinsonism, but also dyskinesias

Neuroleptics used in the treatment of schizophrenia (see Chap. 47) frequently produced parkinsonian signs as unwanted effects of these drugs [21]. The neuroleptics block the action of dopamine on its receptors and their therapeutic effect seems related to this action. These drugs act on dopamine systems without distinction; for the antischizophrenia effect, however, blockage of specific limbic and cortical dopamine receptor sites alone would probably suffice. Blockade of nigrostriatal dopamine receptors leads to the expression of parkinsonian features. Some newer neuroleptics are more selective. Thioridazine, clozapine, and molindone, for example, have electrophysiological effects in the limbic region of the brain, but little action in the nigrostriatal area. This selectivity may be related to receptor subtype specificity.

Patients who have received neuroleptics for long periods of time may develop a hyperkinetic disorder of the extrapyramidal system characterized by involuntary, purposeless movements affecting many parts of the body. Most commonly these are manifested in a syndrome involving abnormal movements of the tongue, mouth, and masticatory muscles. There are also choreoathetoid movements of the extremities. The mechanism of neurotransmitter disturbance in this tardive dyskinesia remains unknown.

Chronic manganese poisoning

A small proportion of miners exposed to manganese dust develop manganism. Manganese is absorbed from the intestine as well as through the pulmonary alveolar epithelium and once in the systemic circulation, readily enters the brain. After a relatively short interval, i.e., several months, of exposure to high doses of the dust, the disease is ushered in by self-limited psychiatric symptoms. "Manganese madness" is characterized by emotional lability, hallucinations, irritability, and aggressiveness. When the exposure is to low levels of manganese, the behavioral changes may be mild and reversible. After more prolonged exposure, behavioral symptoms are replaced by signs of permanent neurological damage. The manifestations are those of extrapyramidal disease and respond in some measure to treatment with levodopa. The dyskinetic features that do not respond to levodopa treatment are likely the result of more diffuse brain pathology [22]. The globus pallidus is the site of greatest damage, but the striatum, subthalamic nucleus, frontal and parietal cortex, cerebellum, and hypothalamus may also be involved. The mechanism of toxicity is unknown, but trivalent manganese, which efficiently catalyzes catechol autooxidation, thereby increasing the formation of peroxides, superoxides, free radicals, and semiorthoquinones, has been implicated [23]. Oxidative stress causes neuronal damage in cells in which physiological scavenger mechanisms fail; quinones are known cytotoxins.

Carbon disulfide

Carbon disulfide (CS_2) is a volatile, lipid-soluble industrial solvent that enters the body by inhalation or absorption through the skin. The early symptoms of CS_2 poisoning resemble those of manganism; subsequent neurological deficits are widespread and include peripheral neuropathy as well an encephalopathy with memory loss, incoordination, and parkinsonism. Relatively little is known about the pathological changes in humans, but in monkeys exposed to CS_2, damage to the globus pallidus and the substantia nigra suggests that similar pathological changes may account for the parkinsonian features of toxicity in humans.

Carbon monoxide

Inhalation of carbon monoxide, which binds avidly to hemoglobin and to cytochromes, is one of the most common forms of fatal poisoning or suicide. Survivors of acute carbon monoxide poisoning may develop, over several days or weeks, a delayed encephalopathy with memory loss, personality changes, and some parkinsonian movement deficits, presumably associated with damage to the globus pallidus, which has been reported among the pathological features of this syndrome seen at autopsy.

HEPATOLENTICULAR DEGENERATION (WILSON'S DISEASE)

Wilson's disease is an autosomal recessive deficiency in hepatic excretion of copper that may present, usually in the second to fourth decade of life, as a liver, neurological, or psychiatric disorder. Whereas copper is essential for the normal function of a number of enzymes (e.g., as a prosthetic group to tyrosinase, cytochrome oxidase, and superoxide dismutase), excess free copper ions are toxic. Adult humans require about 1 to 2 mg of copper daily. Copper metabolism is regulated by an enterohepatic circulation, with excess copper excreted in the bile and feces. Most copper in plasma is present in ceruloplasmin, which is low in Wilson's disease, and only about 5 percent is present as copper ions bound to protein. In Wilson's disease, toxic accumulations of copper in the liver cause acute fulminant hepatitis or recurrent hepatitis with hepatic cirrhosis of the coarse type; excess copper in the brain produces lesions of the lenticular nucleus (putamen and pallidum) and other brain regions, which result in progressive rigidity, intention tremor, and, ultimately, mental deterioration. In 1921, after recognition of the characteristic pathological changes in the liver and brain, this disease was renamed "hepatolenticular degeneration." In some cases, reduced copper is deposited in the cornea, forming the Kayser-Fleischer ring. This sign is virtually pathognomonic of the disease but appears also in occasional cases of primary biliary cirrhosis. In addition, there may be aminoaciduria, including excretion of some oligopeptides and abnormal excretion of monoamines and their metabolites. Amino acid levels in plasma are normal; thus, the urinary findings may simply result from a renal defect caused by histotoxicity of copper.

In animals administered excess copper, the metal is deposited in the liver, kidney, and other organs, while the brain is spared. Similarly, in genetic disorders of copper metabolism in animals, copper accumulation in peripheral organs is not accompanied by brain copper toxicity. In Wilson's disease, excessive deposition of copper in the basal ganglia presumably is the cause of the neurological syndrome, but it is not known how the metal breaks through the rigorous regulation at the blood-brain barrier and what specific neuronal functions it damages. Now that the gene has been located on the long arm of chromosome 13, there is hope that the molecular basis for the defect may become clear. Therapy of Wilson's disease is directed at removal of copper deposits by judicious use of chelating agents such as penicillamine (3,3-dimethylcysteine) or triethylene tetramine. Recently, zinc acetate was used to block copper absorption, and this avoids copper accumulation [24].

ALS-PARKINSONISM-DEMENTIA OF GUAM

The Chamorro people of Guam have had a very high incidence of a syndrome resembling ALS, with strong elements of parkinsonism and dementia. Positron emission tomographic studies have shown that patients with prominent parkinsonism have greater reductions in striatal [^{18}F]6-fluorodopa uptake than those with mainly ALS [25]. This disease apparently developed prominently during the Second World War when seeds of *Cycas circinalis* (false sago) came into use as a food source. These seeds contain β-*N*-methylamino-L-alanine (BMAA), an amino acid with a predilection for NMDA receptors and which, on chronic administration to monkeys, reproduces some of the features of ALS-parkinsonism-dementia (see Chap. 17). Recent studies of the content of BMAA in flour prepared from the seeds have made it seem very unlikely that sufficient quantities of BMAA could be ingested to cause the widespread neurofibrillary degeneration of nerve cells observed in this disease [26]. Other possible causes are being sought, but fortunately, the disease seems to be disappearing.

HUNTINGTON'S DISEASE

Huntington's disease is characterized by choreiform movements, personality changes, and progressive dementia which usually begin to appear in midlife, although juvenile cases have been reported. The disease is genetically transmitted by an autosomal dominant gene. Using restriction fragment length polymorphism, the gene has been localized, with increasing precision, to a candidate region (4p16.3) close to the telomere on the short arm of chromosome 4. The defective gene was recently identified in a chromosome 4 region between the markers D4S180 and DS182, labeled IT (interesting transcript) 15. Normal IT15 contains 11 to 34 copies of the repeating motif CAG, at the 5' (protein-coding) end, whereas in Huntington's disease, it is present in 42 to 66 copies, with some indication that the length in a given carrier of Huntington's disease is a predictor of the severity (age of onset) of the disease. The sequence of the inferred protein product has no known homology with any currently known protein [27]. By linkage analysis with highly polymorphic DNA markers, it has become possible to identify individuals at high risk for carrying the gene [28], but such predictive testing programs present ethical and legal dilemmas as long as the basic defect remains unknown and preventive treatments are unavailable.

The most consistent postmortem findings are basal ganglia atrophy with neuronal loss and gliosis in the striatum and globus pallidus. The loss of medium spiny GABAergic neurons, with marked reductions in glutamate decarboxylase and in GABA and loss of GABAergic projections from the striatum, is the most characteristic and severe abnormality. Also depleted are receptors (e.g., muscarinic, cholinergic, dopamine, etc.) associated with these neurons.

GABA/enkephalin projections from the medium spiny neurons to the external layer of the globus pallidus (see Fig. 1) degenerate earlier, even before symptoms are apparent, than do GABA/substance P neurons innervating the internal layer of the globus pallidus or substantia nigra reticulata [29]. Other peptidergic neurons, such as those containing somatostatin and NPY, are spared. Basal ganglia concentrations of dopamine and norepinephrine are increased; in the case of dopamine, the increase may represent overactivity of the nigrostriatal fibers. Thus, in at least some respects, Huntington's disease is a biochemical mirror of Parkinson's disease. The early loss of net tonic inhibition (uncontrolled disinhibition) of the subthalamic neurons is believed to be the basis of the chorea. Involvement of the striatal GABA/substance P neurons, which project to the internal layer of the globus pallidus (direct pathway), exaggerates inhibition (loss of disinhibition) and results

in the appearance of bradykinesia and rigidity [30]. Loss of inhibitory projections to the substantia nigra compacta might be responsible for the apparent overactivity of the dopaminergic system. Drugs that interfere with dopaminergic function have an ameliorating effect. Reserpine and α-methyldopa, which lower the amounts of dopamine and some other monoamines in the brain; α-methyl-p-tyrosine, which inhibits the synthesis of catecholamines at the tyrosine hydroxylase step; and neuroleptics, which provide postsynaptic blockade of dopamine receptors, have been found to be efficacious.

Excitotoxin-induced lesions in animals mimic Huntington's disease

Direct injection of excitatory neurotoxins such as kainic acid, a rigid analog of glutamate, into the striatum causes destruction of intrinsic GABA-containing and cholinergic neurons but spares glia and afferent axons [31]. Affected neurons are those which possess receptors for excitatory amino acid neurotransmitters, including NMDA, AMPA, and kainate receptors. Quinolinic acid, a tryptophan metabolite found in brain and other tissues, has a more restricted neurotoxicity. Although quinolinic acid lowers cerebral GABA and substance P, unlike kainic acid, it does not alter the amounts of somatostatin and NPY. Thus, the quinolinic acid-treated animal appears to mimic the chemical pathology of Huntington's disease more precisely. However, the presence of receptors for excitatory amino acid neurotransmitters is insufficient to account for the death of these neurons; neurons bearing such receptors are dispersed widely throughout unaffected regions of the brain. Factors that have been considered but have not been demonstrated to be significant include excess release of an excitatory amino acid neurotransmitter; inadequacy of mechanisms for inactivation of such neurotransmitters; and impaired ability to maintain homeostasis of ions, such as calcium when there is increased excitatory activity, or deficient sequestration of intracellular calcium.

KERNICTERUS

In infants, the predilection of bilirubin for subthalamic and basal ganglia cells may result in kernicterus or jaundice of the nuclei of the brain. The affected babies initially have decreased muscle tone, which after several weeks increases to rigidity. Children who survive often develop choreoathetosis, dystonia, and/or tremors, in addition to the persistent rigidity. Although there is considerable knowledge regarding bilirubin metabolism, the primary molecular target of its toxic effects in brain is not known. Kernicterus appears when the rate of entry into brain of unconjugated bilirubin exceeds the capacity of the brain bilirubin oxidase system to dispose of bilirubin. This may result from hemolysis, a low albumin reserve, low pH, or administration of a displacing drug so that excess free bilirubin is present in plasma and enters brain, or if the brain bilirubin oxidase system is ineffective because of immaturity, birth asphyxia, or other forms of central nervous system injury. Although the mechanism of bilirubin toxicity is not known, removing bilirubin is beneficial and therapy is directed at prevention of high concentrations of bilirubin by exchange transfusion or photoinactivation therapy (blue light).

ACKNOWLEDGMENT

I am grateful to Dr. Theodore L. Sourkes for permission to borrow freely from earlier versions of this chapter in a previous edition of this book.

REFERENCES

1. Graybiel, A. M. Neurotransmitters and neuromodulators in the basal ganglia. *Trends Neurosci.* 13:244–253, 1990.

2. Gerfen, C. R. The neostriatal mosaic: Multiple levels of compartmental organization in the basal ganglia. *Annu. Rev. Neurosci.* 15: 285–320, 1992.

3. Palkovits, M., and Brownstein, M. Catecholamines in the central nervous system. In U. Trendelenberg and N. Weiner (eds.), *Catecholamines II.* Berlin: Springer, 1989, pp. 1–26.

4. Carlsson, A., Lindquist, M., Magnusson, T., and Waldeck, B. On the presence of 3 hydroxytyramine in brain. *Science* 127:471–472, 1958.

5. Ehringer, H., and Hornykiewicz, O. Distribution of noradrenaline and dopamine (3-hydroxytyramine) in the human brain and their behavior in diseases of the extrapyramidal system. *Klin. Wochenschr.* 38:1236–1239, 1960.

6. Sourkes, T. L. On the origin of homovanillic acid in the cerebrospinal fluid. *J. Neural Transm.* 34:153–157, 1973.

7. Sourkes, T. L., and Poirier, L. J., Neurochemical bases of tremor and other disorders of movement. *Can. Med. Assoc. J.* 39:941–951, 1966.

8. Fahn, S. Secondary parkinsonism. In E. S. Goldenson and S. H. Appel (eds.), *Scientific Approaches to Clinical Neurology.* Philadelphia: Lea & Febiger, 1977, pp. 1159–1189.

9. Cotzias, G. C., Papavasilious, P. S., and Gellene, R. Modification of parkinsonism—Chronic treatment with L-dopa. *N. Engl. J. Med.* 280:337–345, 1969.

10. Yahr, M. D., Duvoisin R. C. Drug therapy of parkinsonism. *N. Engl. J. Med.* Jul 6;287(1): 20–24, 1972.

11. Birkmayer, W., Riederer, P., Youdim, M. B. H., and Linauer, W. Potentiation of antikinetic effect after L-dopa treatment by an inhibitor of MAO B, L-deprenil. *J. Neural Transm.* 36:303–323, 1975.

12. Cedarbaum, J. M., Leger, G., and Guttman, M. Reduction of circulating 3-O-methyldopa by inhibition of catechol-O-methyltransferase with OR-611 and OR-462 in cynomologus monkeys: Implications for the treatment of Parkinson's disease. *Clin. Neuropharmacol.* 14: 330–342, 1991.

13. Zurcher, G., Colzi, A., and Da Prada, M. Ro40-7592: Inhibition of COMT in rat brain and extracerebral tissues. *J. Neural Transm. Suppl.* 32:375–380, 1990.

14. Goetz, C. G. Dopamine agonists in the treatment of Parkinson's disease. *Neurology* 40 (Suppl. 3):50–54, 1990.

15. Bergman, H., Wichmann, T., and DeLong, M. R. Reversal of experimental parkinsonism by lesions of the subthalamic nucleus. *Science* 249:1436–1438, 1990.

16. Kopin, I. J. Features of the dopaminergic neurotoxin MPTP. *Ann. N.Y. Acad. Sci.* 648: 96–104, 1992.

17. Schapira, A. H., Cooper, J. M., Dexter, D., Clark, J. B., Jenner, P., and Marsden, C. D. Mitochondrial complex I deficiency in Parkinson's disease. *J. Neurochem.* 54:823–827, 1990.

18. Jenner, P. What process causes nigral cell death in Parkinson's disease? *Neurol. Clin.* 10: 387–403, 1992.

19. Birkmayer, W., Knoll, J., Riederer, P., Youdim, M. B., Hars, V., and Marton, J. Increased life expectancy resulting from addition of L-deprenyl to Madopar treatment in Parkinson's disease: A longterm study. *J. Neural Transm.* 64:113–127, 1985.

20. The Parkinson Study Group. Effect of deprenyl on the progression of disability in early Parkinson's disease. *N. Engl. J. Med.* 321: 1364–1371, 1989.

21. Baldessarini, R. J., and Tarsy, D. Dopamine and the pathophysiology of dyskinesias induced by antipsychotic drugs. *Annu. Rev. Neurosci.* 3:23–41, 1980.

22. Mena, I. Manganese poisoning. In P. J. Vinkeh and G. W. Broyh (eds.), *Handbook of Clinical Neurology.* New York: Elsevier North-Holland, 1977, Vol. 21, pp. 217–327.

23. Archibald, F. S., and Tyree, C. Manganese poisoning and the attack of trivalent manganese upon catecholamines. *Arch. Biochem. Biophys.* 256:638–650, 1987.

24. Brewer, G. J., and Yuzbasiyan-Gurkan, V. Wilson disease. *Medicine (Baltimore)* 71:139–164, 1992.

25. Snow, B. J., Peppard, R. F., Guttman, M., Okada, J., Martin, W. R., Steele, J., Eisen, A., Carr, G., Schoenberg, B., and Calne, D. Positron emission tomographic scanning demonstrates a presynaptic dopaminergic lesion in Lytico-Bodig. The amyotrophic lateral sclerosis-parkinsonism-dementia complex of Guam. *Arch. Neurol.* 47:870–874, 1990.

26. Duncan, M. W., Steele, J. C., Kopin, I. J., and Markey, S. P. 2-Amino-3-(methylamino)-propanoic acid (BMAA) in cycad flour: An unlikely cause of amyotrophic lateral sclerosis and parkinsonism-dementia of Guam. *Neurology* 40:767–772, 1990.

27. Gusella, J. F. Huntington's disease. *Adv. Hum. Genet.* 20:125–151, 1991.

28. Meissen, G. J., Myers, R. H., Mastromauro, C. A., Koroshetz, W. J., Klinger, K. W., Farrer, L. A., Watkins, P. A. Gusella, J. F., Bird, E. D., and Martin, J. B. Predictive testing for Huntington's disease and use of a lined DNA marker. *N. Engl. J. Med.* 318:535–542, 1988.

29. Albin, R. L., Reiner, A., Anderson, K. D., Dure, L. S., IV, Handelin, B., Balfour, R., Whetsell, W. O., Jr., Penney, J. B., and Young, A. B. Preferential loss of striato-external pallidal projection neurons in presymptomatic Huntington's disease. *Ann. Neurol.* 31: 425–430, 1992.

30. DeLong, M. R. Primate models of movement disorders of the basal ganglia. *Trends Neurosci.* 13:281–285, 1990.

31. DiFiglia, M. Excitotoxic injury of the neostriatum: A model for Huntington's disease. *Trends Neurosci.* 13:286–289, 1990.

CHAPTER 45

Biochemistry of Alzheimer's Disease

Dennis J. Selkoe

ALZHEIMER'S DISEASE IS THE MOST COMMON NEURODEGENERATIVE DISORDER

The intense scientific interest that Alzheimer's disease has generated in recent years is a reflection of how common this progressive neurodegenerative disorder is. Since the pioneering work of Blessed, Tomlinson, and Roth in the 1960s, neuropathologists have increasingly recognized that the clinicopathological syndrome that the Bavarian psychiatrist, Alois Alzheimer, originally described in a 51 year old woman is also the most com-

Basic Neurochemistry: Molecular, Cellular, and Medical Aspects, 5th Ed., edited by G. J. Siegel et al. Published by Raven Press, Ltd., New York, 1994. Correspondence to Dennis J. Selkoe, Department of Neurology and Program in Neuroscience, Harvard Medical School and Center for Neurologic Diseases, Brigham and Women's Hospital, Boston, Massachusetts 02115.

mon basis for late-life cognitive failure. Many autopsy studies of patients with senile dementia have shown that the amyloid plaques and neurofibrillary tangles which Alzheimer called attention to in 1907 appear to be the pathological substrate for some 50–70% of cases. Senile dementia is defined as the progressive loss of memory and other intellectual functions occurring after the age of 65; if the same clinical syndrome occurs prior to age 65, it is referred to as presenile dementia (see also Chap. 31).

Estimates of the prevalence of senile dementia and of Alzheimer's disease have varied considerably among population surveys conducted in different countries. A representative example for the United States comes from the Framingham, Massachusetts epidemiological study, in which about 2.5% of subjects aged 65–74 years had a clinical diagnosis of senile dementia, compared to 4% of those aged 75–79, 11% of those aged 80–84, and 24% of those aged 85–93 years [1]. In this study, about 55% of all cases of senile dementia were felt to have probable Alzheimer's disease. These figures and others from similar surveys lead to a projection of some 2.5–4 million patients with probable Alzheimer's disease in the United States alone. Alzheimer's disease affects individuals in all races and ethnic groups, and it occurs slightly more commonly in females than males, even taking into account the greater longevity of women in our society.

Neuronal loss, neurofibrillary tangles, and amyloid-bearing plaques in parenchyma and blood vessels characterize the pathology

It is becoming increasingly clear that Alzheimer's disease represents a syndrome with well-defined clinical and neuropathological hallmarks but with an array of specific molecular defects that can initiate the pathology. Despite this etiologic heterogeneity, growing evidence suggests that there is a common and rather stereotyped pathogenetic cascade, which can result from distinct gene defects and/or as yet unknown environmental factors. External examination of the brains of Alzheimer patients usually reveals considerable cortical atrophy, particularly in the limbic and association cortices, together with enlargement of the lateral ventricles. However, the hallmarks of the disorder that confirm the diagnosis are observed on microscopic examination, usually with the aid of a silver stain (Fig. 1). These include loss of neurons, particularly medium and large-sized pyramidal cells, and the presence of intraneuronal neurofibrillary tangles and extracellular deposits of amyloid filaments surrounded by altered neuritic processes and glia (senile plaques). These lesions are not specific for Alzheimer's disease and can be seen in small numbers and in limited topographic distribution, particularly in the hippocampus, amygdala, and other limbic structures, in many functionally normal individuals over age 60.

Senile plaques are structurally complex lesions, the temporal development of which is only partially understood. Many, if not all, senile plaques probably begin as amorphous, largely nonfilamentous aggregates of a 39–43 residue protein, the amyloid β-protein (Aβ). After a period of time, the length of which is not known, a few such "diffuse" Aβ deposits become increasingly fibrillar and acquire the classical features of amyloid plaques, namely relatively compacted bundles of ~8 nanometer filaments that bind certain histochemical dyes (Congo red, thioflavin) and have principally a β-pleated sheet protein conformation. Frequently associated with such "compacted" or "mature" amyloid plaques are dystrophic axonal and dendritic processes that lie within or immediately surrounding the fibrous amyloid deposit. These neurites are often thickened and intensely silver positive. Such mature plaques also display activated microglia intimately associated with the central amyloid deposit and fibrous astrocytes rimming the plaque. The finding of large numbers of such senile (neuritic) plaques in limbic and association cortices is probably the single

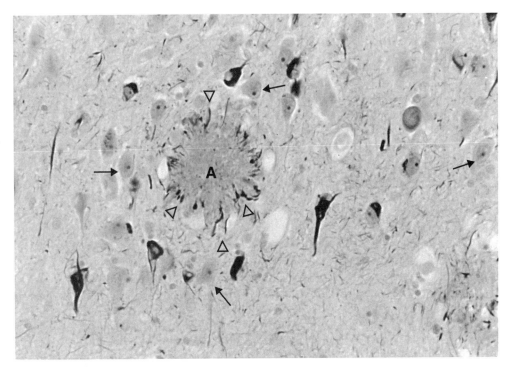

FIG. 1.   The classical histopathological lesions of Alzheimer's disease demonstrated by the modified Bielschowsky silver stain. A 6-μm paraffin section of the amygdala from a 69-year-old man with a 6-year history of progressive dementia. Darkly staining neurofibrillary tangles occupy much of the cytoplasm of selected pyramidal neurons, in contrast to the golden brown cytoplasm of adjacent cytologically normal neurons *(arrows)*. In the center, a senile plaque consists of a large, compacted deposit of extracellular amyloid *(A)* surrounded by a halo of dilated, structurally abnormal (dystrophic) neurites *(open arrowheads)*. Altered axons and dendrites are both present in such neuritic plaques. Reactive microglia and fibrillary astrocytes associated with such plaques are not well visualized here. The edge of a second neuritic plaque is seen in the lower right corner. Bar = 50 μm.

most reliable neuropathological marker of the diagnostic entity of Alzheimer's disease.

In the large majority of Alzheimer brains, senile plaques are accompanied by argyrophilic bundles of intraneuronal cytoplasmic fibers referred to as neurofibrillary tangles (NFT). Electron microscopy of such neurons demonstrates that the tangles are generally composed of masses of paired, helically wound, ~10 nm filaments (PHF), often intermixed with ~15 nm straight filaments. Neuroanatomical studies have shown that NFT are frequently present in the cell bodies of neurons whose axons project to the sites of neuritic plaques (e.g., the entorhinal → hippocampal perforant pathway and the basal forebrain → hippocampal/neocortical pathway). NFT are a less specific histological marker of Alzheimer's disease than are neuritic plaques. They can occur in the absence of neuritic plaques in a variety of etiologically diverse neurological disorders (e.g., subacute sclerosing panencephalitis; Kuf's disease; Hallervorden-Spatz disease). Moreover, a minority of Alzheimer brains (perhaps 10–20%) show abundant amyloid-bearing neuritic plaques but few or no NFT in association cortex [2]. Thus, there can be a clear dissociation of plaques and tangles under some circumstances. The wide variety of neuropathological disorders in which NFT occur suggests that PHF formation is a nonspecific marker of certain kinds of neuronal injury.

In addition to a variety of morphological types of Aβ protein deposits present in the brain parenchyma, cortical and meningeal arteries, arterioles, capillaries, and, to a lesser extent, venules, may contain multifocal deposits of amyloid filaments also composed of Aβ. The amyloid deposits appear to be preferentially localized to the abluminal basement membrane of these microvessels [3]. The number of amyloid-bearing cortical vessels can vary dramatically among Alzheimer cases having relatively similar densities of amyloid plaques. The association of microvascular amyloidosis with parenchymal amyloidosis in Alzheimer's disease has aroused greater interest since the discovery of missense mutations in the β-amyloid precursor protein in both families with Alzheimer's disease and families with severe amyloid angiopathy causing cerebral hemorrhages (see below).

Neurons in the limbic and association cortices and the subcortical nuclei that project to them are particularly vulnerable

In most cases of Alzheimer's disease, the innumerable NFT found in the limbic and association cortices are accompanied by NFT in neurons of subcortical nuclei that project to these regions. These nuclei include the cholinergic forebrain complex, the locus ceruleus, and the median raphe nuclei. NFT are very rarely found in regions of brain that are only minimally involved, both pathologically and clinically, in Alzheimer's disease, for example, the cerebellum. In such areas, diffuse or preamyloid forms of Aβ deposits may occur, but there is little surrounding neuritic dystrophy and usually no NFT formation.

In addition to containing NFT, neurons in the limbic and association cortices and in the subcortical nuclei that project to them often undergo perikaryal shrinkage and actual cell death. It is likely that many neurons which shrink and die in Alzheimer's disease do not pass through a stage of actual NFT formation.

Most cases of Alzheimer's disease that have extensive NFT also show widespread dystrophic neurites, sometimes called neuropil threads or curly fibers, that are scattered in the cortical neuropil and not specifically localized to amyloid plaques. An abundance of dystrophic neurites in the cerebral cortex has been correlated to some extent with both the presence of NFT and the occurrence of clinical dementia [4]. Such dystrophic neurites are not specific for Alzheimer's disease and have been found in other neurological disorders in which NFT occur in the absence of amyloid plaques [5].

Multiple neurotransmitter systems are affected in a pattern that correlates with the cellular pathology

The topographically widespread and cytologically heterogeneous populations of neurons that are affected in Alzheimer brain are reflected by a complex array of neurotransmitter deficits. The first transmitter alteration to be defined was a marked decline in the activities of choline acetyltransferase and acetylcholinesterase, indicating dysfunction and loss of basal forebrain cholinergic neurons and their cortical projections. Although the decline in these cholinergic markers has been correlated both with the degree of dementia and the number of neuritic plaques, cholinergic loss cannot be considered the primary neurotransmitter alteration in Alzheimer's disease since neurons releasing monoamine or neuropeptide transmitters also become morphologically abnormal and undergo attrition. These neurons include noradrenergic and serotonergic cells in the brainstem, cells producing somatostatin or corticotropin-releasing factor in the neocortex, and neurons that release glutamate, γ-aminobutyric acid, substance P, or neuropeptide Y. The degree of decline in the levels of these transmitters and their biosynthetic and catabolic enzymes varies markedly among Alzheimer's disease brains. The heterogeneity of neurotransmitter alterations helps to explain why attempts at replacement therapy aimed at just one of these systems (most commonly the use of cholinergic agents) have met with very limited success in terms of measurable and sustained improvement in objective mental tests. It is clear that Alzheimer's disease does not follow closely the patterns of certain other neurodegenerative disorders, such as Parkinson's disease (Chap. 44), which are more specific in their neurotransmitter profile.

The search for etiologies has resulted in a focus on genetic factors

Ever since the original description of the disorder by Alzheimer, there has been a lively debate as to what factor or factors could initiate this complex, multicellular degeneration. Although Alzheimer's disease shows limited parallels with the unconventional infectious/inherited encephalopathies such as Creutzfeldt-Jakob's disease and Gerstmann-Straussler-Scheinker syndrome (see later), no compelling evidence that the disorder is caused by an infectious pathogen has been presented. The possibility that an environmental toxin could precipitate the disorder has rested largely on the role of metal ions, particularly aluminum. Aluminum initially became a candidate simply because it can induce silver-positive bundles of neurofilaments in neurons upon injection into rabbit brain. However, these filamentous lesions are now known to be distinct from Alzheimer-type NFT both structurally and biochemically. Some investigators have reported elevated levels of aluminum in cortical regions affected by Alzheimer pathology, particularly within the neurofibrillary tangles themselves [6]. However, equal or greater aluminum accumulation has been found in the neurofibrillary tangles of Guam Parkinson dementia complex [7] and certain variants of Hallervorden-Spatz disease [8], disorders in which few or no amyloid plaques or amyloid angiopathy of the Alzheimer type appear. This observation strongly suggests that aluminum deposition is not unique to Alzheimer's but rather can secondarily become associated with neurofibrillary tangles, regardless of the specific disease in which the tangles are found.

Investigators who have demonstrated aluminum within neurofibrillary tangles have sometimes reported abnormal levels of other metals, particularly magnesium, calcium, and iron, in Alzheimer neurons. The presence of aluminum in amyloid plaque cores has been reported, but this association has been less clearly confirmed than that with NFT. It should also be noted that some investigators have reported no substantial elevation of aluminum in the Alzheimer brains which they have examined. The pathological role of neuronal aluminum deposition in Alzheimer disease remains unclear, and there is little compelling evidence that it serves as a primary toxin that can initiate the disease. In this regard, it is worth noting that aluminum is ubiquitous in our environment, including in the drinking water of many communities. There are currently no rigorous data indicating an unusual or specific source of aluminum (e.g., antacids, aluminum containers, deodorants) as a risk factor for Alzheimer's disease in the general population.

It has been known for decades that some cases of Alzheimer's disease occur in an autosomal dominant Mendelian pattern, and this has turned out to be a fruitful clue for the etiologic study of the disorder. The percentage of all Alzheimer cases that clearly shows such a pattern has been variously reported as 5–15%, but a much higher percentage of patients has a history of one or more first degree relatives with a highly similar dementing syndrome. Because of the late onset of most Alzheimer cases, it has been difficult or impossible to ascertain whether members of previous generations were actually afflicted with the disease. Mounting evidence suggests that a high percentage of subjects, although by no means all, have some type of genetic predisposition to the disease. In a few, specific DNA point mutations have now been identified.

Long-standing support for the hypothesis that Alzheimer's disease could be genetically based has come from the observation that virtually all subjects with trisomy 21

(Down's syndrome) develop typical histopathological lesions of Alzheimer's disease if they survive into their 40s and beyond. This single clinicopathological clue has been by far the most significant factor in unraveling the etiology and mechanism of Alzheimer's disease. Virtually all important discoveries about causation and early pathogenesis have derived from the link between trisomy 21 and Alzheimer lesions. Of particular interest in this regard has been the realization in the last few years that subjects with Down's syndrome dying in their teens or 20s may show low to moderate densities of diffuse, preamyloid Aβ deposits in the limbic and association cortices in the absence of surrounding neuronal or glial pathology, neuritic dystrophy, or NFT. This important observation has strengthened the concept that deposition of Aβ can be a very early event in the disease, preceding other histological changes.

Clues to the genotype underlying familial Alzheimer's disease have arisen from biochemical analyses of the neuropathologic phenotype

Although the early attempts to purify and chemically analyze pathological structures in Alzheimer brain tissue focused on the study of NFT, these have not led to clues about the molecular etiology of the disease. Instead, the purification of amyloid deposits from meningeal blood vessels by Glenner and Wong in 1984 [9] provided the seminal biochemical information that led both to the identification of specific molecular causes of Alzheimer's disease and a rational model for the pathogenetic cascade. Prior to the study of the cerebral amyloid, widespread doubts had been expressed as to whether biochemical and molecular analysis of the histopathological lesions would lead to useful insights about early events in the disease. However, the experience with other human amyloidoses suggested that extracellular deposits of amyloid-forming proteins caused local cytopathology and organ dysfunction. Particularly in cases where there were genetic de-

fects in the amyloidogenic protein, these deposits could explain the etiology of the disease in which the amyloid appeared. This scenario has now proven to be true in Alzheimer's disease. As the study of the disease continues, it is becoming apparent that Alzheimer's disease follows in part the rules of systemic amyloidoses, while in other respects, the β-amyloid process is distinct from these disorders.

Amyloid in Alzheimer's disease is composed of a 39–43 residue fragment of an integral membrane glycoprotein (βAPP)

The initial sequence obtained from the meningovascular amyloid protein, termed the β-protein by Glenner and Wong, extended to 28 residues and was not homologous with previously described proteins [9]. Shortly after this observation, the partial purification of amyloid plaque cores and their solubilization in high concentrations of formic acid or guanidine thiocyanate demonstrated that their subunit protein had an amino acid composition indistinguishable from meningovascular Aβ, although there appeared to be some heterogeneity of the amino terminus, including a blocked species [10,11]. The sequence of the vascular amyloid was later extended to 39 or 40 residues, whereas that of the plaque amyloid was considered to be 42–43 residues in length [12]. A recent analysis using combined amino acid sequencing and mass spectrometry following lyslyendopeptidase digestion has suggested that, at least in the Alzheimer's brains examined to date, the major Aβ peptide in cerebral cortex is 40 amino acids long, with minor species that include a peptide ending at residue 43 and a peptide beginning with a glutamate to pyroglutamate conversion at residue 3, causing a blocked amino terminus [13].

Because of the difficulty of purifying the self-aggregating amyloid protein from postmortem cerebral tissue, only a limited number of biochemical analyses have been published. It is likely that more heterogeneity, including the presence of truncated or longer Aβ fragments, may occur in at least some amyloid deposits. Nonetheless, the major species identified to date appear to be $A\beta_{1-40}$ and $A\beta_{1-42}$. There are reproducible biochemical differences between meningovascular and plaque core amyloid, e.g., the former but not the latter is soluble in 6 M guanidine hydrochloride.

The establishment of the amino terminal sequence of the Aβ protein led to the independent cloning of its precursor polypeptide by four laboratories in 1987 [12,14–16]. The first full-length cDNA that was isolated encoded a 695 residue protein that contained a single domain having the hydrophobic composition of a transmembrane region near its carboxyl terminus (Fig. 2). Subsequent studies of the β-amyloid precursor protein (βAPP) itself in human tissues and cultured cells demonstrated that it comprised a heterogeneous group of polypeptides ranging from ~105 to 140 kDa [17] and that the protein underwent N- and O-glycosylation as well as tyrosine sulfation during its post-translational maturation [18,19].

The cloning of βAPP led immediately to the localization of its gene to the long arm of chromosome 21. This finding offered an explanation for the neuropathological observation that patients with trisomy 21 develop amyloid-bearing plaques and other lesions of Alzheimer's disease. Subsequent cloning of βAPP cDNAs from other mammals demonstrated a high degree of evolutionary conservation of this gene. Indeed, the 695-amino acid isoform (βAPP_{695}) is 100% conserved between cynomologus monkey and human, and rat and mouse show more than 95% conservation. A gene product called APP-L that has considerable homology to βAPP has been demonstrated in *Drosophila;* this molecule does not, however, contain the Aβ sequence [20].

cDNA and genomic cloning demonstrated that βAPP polypeptides arise by alternative exon splicing. The initially cloned isoform (βAPP_{695}) is almost exclusively expressed in brain, primarily in neurons [15]. Alternate transcripts of 751 and 770 amino acids that contain an inserted exon encoding a Kunitz-type serine protease inhibitor (KPI) motif are the major expressed isoforms in virtually all peripheral cells and are also expressed in brain cells. Additional alternative transcripts of very low abundance have also been identified. Examination of the exon/intron structure of the βAPP gene reveals that the ~40 amino acid Aβ fragment contains portions of two adjacent exons and thus must arise by proteolytic processing rather than by alternative exon splicing.

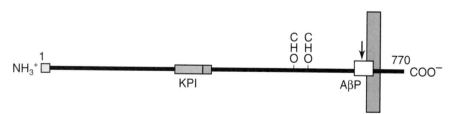

FIG. 2. Schematic diagram of the primary structure of the β-amyloid precursor protein. The molecule depicted here is the largest of the known alternate transcripts, comprising 770 amino acids. Several regions of interest are indicated at their correct relative positions. A 17 residue signal peptide occurs at the N-terminus. Two alternatively spliced exons of 56 and 19 amino acids are inserted at residue 289; the first contains a serine protease inhibitor domain of the Kunitz type *(KPI)*. Two sites of N-glycosylation are found at residues 542 and 571. A single membrane-spanning domain at amino acids 700–723 [12] is indicated by the *vertical hatched bar.* The amyloid β-protein (AβP) fragment *(white box)* includes 28 residues just outside the membrane plus the first 12–15 residues of the transmembrane domain. The *arrow* indicates the site (residue 687) of a constitutive proteolytic cleavage, defined in cDNA-transfected cells [21], that enables secretion of the large N-terminal portion of βAPP into the medium and retention of the 83 residue C-terminal fragment in the membrane.

Deposition of amyloid β-protein precedes the lesions of Alzheimer's disease and arises from alternative proteolytic processing of βAPP

The fact that some subjects with Down's syndrome dying in their teens show amorphous deposits of Aβ (diffuse plaques) in the absence of other cytological lesions of Alzheimer's disease has supported the concept that Aβ deposition can occur prior to detectable neuronal or glial alteration. It is difficult to establish rigorously such a temporal sequence in Alzheimer's disease, because the brains are only examined at the end of the disease. However, the presence of large numbers of diffuse plaques, always outnumbering compacted, neurite-containing plaques in Alzheimer brains, and the fact that the amyloid lesions of Down's syndrome are indistinguishable from those of Alzheimer's disease support the notion that diffuse plaques represent the earliest discernible morphological change also in Alzheimer's disease. As will be discussed shortly, further support for this hypothesis has come from the identification of point mutations in the βAPP gene that segregate with the Alzheimer phenotype in certain autosomal dominant pedigrees.

Normal cellular processing of βAPP has been shown to include a pathway that involves maturation of the protein in the Golgi apparatus (Chap. 2), trafficking to the plasma membrane, and cleavage at residue 16 within the Aβ domain (residue 687 of βAPP_{770}) [21], liberating the large amino terminal hydrophilic portion of the precursor into the media [18], and retaining a ~10 kDa membrane associated carboxyl terminal fragment [17,19] inside the cell. This secretory processing, which appears to occur at or near the cell surface, precludes formation of intact Aβ. There is evidence that such secretory processing may also occur in intracellular organelles [22]. βAPP contains an asn-pro-thr-tyr motif in its cytoplasmic tail that represents a consensus sequence for the internalization of plasma membrane-spanning receptors via clathrin-coated vesicles. Based on this knowledge, experiments have been conducted that demonstrate an alternative but normal processing route which involves internalization of βAPP from the cell surface and its trafficking to late endosomes/lysosomes [23]. When lysosomes are purified from cultured cells, an array of carboxyl-terminal fragments of βAPP can be detected in them [23]. Indeed, such Aβ-containing fragments have been identified in a variety of human cells and tissues (see e.g., [24]). It is not yet clear whether lysosomally derived Aβ-containing intermediates or similar fragments arising from alternative secretory processing at or near the cell surface (or both) serve as the actual precursors of Aβ.

The high degree of insolubility of Aβ isolated from senile plaque and meningovascular deposits and the fact that Aβ is derived from a transmembrane sequence led to the widely held assumption that Aβ must arise from aberrant proteolysis of βAPP following membrane injury. It was therefore surprising to discover that small amounts of Aβ are released continuously from a variety of cultured cells under normal metabolic conditions, and that this Aβ in the media is entirely soluble [25–27]. Moreover, soluble Aβ has also been detected in normal and Alzheimer cerebrospinal fluid [26,27]. These data indicate that the Aβ peptide is a normal metabolic product of βAPP that could have a physiologic function throughout life. Moreover, the findings suggest that cultured human cells can be used as simple *in vitro* model systems to screen for compounds that decrease Aβ production or release. It will be important to determine whether Aβ levels in spinal fluid and perhaps in plasma can distinguish at least some Alzheimer patients from most normal elderly subjects and thus can be used to establish risk for the disease and monitor the efficacy of anti-amyloid drug therapy.

The normal generation of Aβ by cultured cells could involve the release of Aβ-containing carboxyl terminal fragments of βAPP into the media followed by their extracellular proteolysis to yield Aβ. Alternatively,

Aβ could be generated intracellularly and then released. However, unequivocal evidence of the presence of Aβ intracellularly has not yet been provided. The ability to assay Aβ in physiologic fluids, including culture media, should allow detailed studies of the effects of various physiological modulators and of structural alterations in βAPP on the process of Aβ production.

Some forms of autosomal dominant Alzheimer's disease are caused by point mutations in the βAPP gene

The genetic linkage of DNA markers on the long arm of chromosome 21 to Alzheimer's disease in some autosomal dominant pedigrees raised the likelihood that βAPP itself could be a disease-causing gene. In 1991 two families were identified in which affected members had a point mutation at codon 717 of βAPP_{770} [28]. This observation provided the first specific molecular cause of Alzheimer's disease and suggested that alterations in βAPP could initiate β-amyloidosis in the absence of any other pathological events. Even prior to this discovery, a mutation at codon 693 of βAPP_{770} had been found in individuals with the Aβ deposition disease, hereditary cerebral hemorrhage with amyloidosis of the Dutch type (HCHWA-D) [29]. This rare disorder is marked by severe Aβ deposition in meningeal and cerebral vessels plus large numbers of diffuse plaques. No mature neuritic plaques or neurofibrillary tangles are observed and no Alzheimer-like dementia is found in these patients. It appears that HCHWA-D is closely related to Alzheimer's disease, genotypically and phenotypically, although the clinical syndrome is multiple cerebral hemorrhages rather than dementia.

Since these discoveries, several other point mutations in the βAPP gene have been found in affected members of families with autosomal dominant Alzheimer's disease [30] (see Fig. 3). In addition to the original FAD mutation at codon APP_{717}, val → ile, two additional missense mutations at the same codon have been discovered: val → gly and val → phe. Also, a missense mutation changing codon 692 from ala to gly has been discovered in a family having both congophilic angiopathy with hemorrhage and progressive dementia as the clinical phenotypes. A double mutation immediately preceding the Aβ region has been found in an extended Swedish kindred with FAD: APP_{595} lys → asn plus APP_{596} met → leu. Importantly, certain missense mutations other than those just described as well as silent DNA polymorphisms that do not affect the amino acid sequence have been found in some individuals who either do not have Alzheimer's disease or have other kinds of dementia. Thus, as with other autosomal dominant diseases, including amyloidoses such as those involving transthyretin or the prion protein, the precise relationship between genotype and phenotype in familial Alzheimer's disease is complex and variable. The known genetic heterogeneity of familial Alzheimer's disease and the occurrence of apparently sporadic (nongenetically based) cases make it clear that structural mutations in the amyloid precursor protein only explain a small subset of all Alzheimer cases. Indeed, a linkage to a still unknown gene on chromosome 14 has been described in a larger number of early-onset AD families [31].

Neurofibrillary tangles and dystrophic cortical neurites contain post-translationally modified forms of tau protein

The biochemical analysis of the paired helical filaments that accumulate as perikaryal NFT and within dystrophic cortical neurites (both in neuritic plaques and outside of plaques in the cortical neuropil) began well before the characterization of the amyloid. A large number of immunochemical and biochemical experiments have led to the conclusion that the principal protein subunit of paired helical filaments is an altered form of the microtubule-associated protein, tau (Chap. 27). Tau normally copurifies with

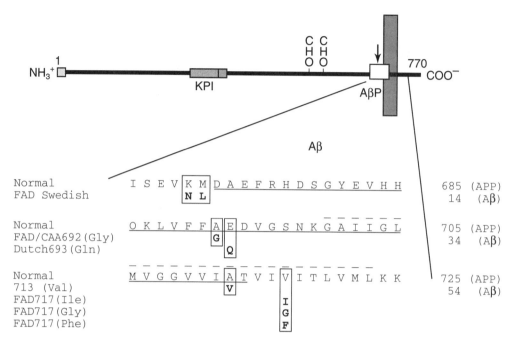

FIG. 3. The sequence of βAPP containing the Aβ and transmembrane region is expanded and shown by the *single-letter amino acid code*. The *underlined residues* represent the Aβ$_{1-43}$ peptide. The *broken line* indicates the location of the transmembrane domain. The *boxed residues* depict some of the currently known missense mutations identified in certain patients with familial Alzheimer's disease *(FAD)* or hereditary cerebral hemorrhage with amyloidosis of the Dutch type *(Dutch)*. CAA indicates that the family with 692 gly mutation can display congophilic amyloid angiopathy as well as Alzheimer's disease as the phenotype. *Three-digit numbers* refer to the residue number according to the βAPP$_{770}$ isoform. *Two-digit numbers* refer to the residue number according to the Aβ sequence (asp$_{672}$ = 1).

tubulin during repetitive cycles of assembly and disassembly of microtubules, and it is known to bind to tubulin and promote the assembly and stability of microtubules. The identification of tau as the major antigenic constituent of PHF was made using antibodies both to purified PHF and to tau (see, for example [32]). Subsequently, harsh methods were used to extract and sequence fragments of tau from purified PHF, many of which are highly insoluble in strong detergents and solvents. These studies demonstrated that at least portions of tau, particularly from the carboxyl third of the molecule containing its microtubule-binding domains, were incorporated into PHF.

A separate line of investigation has come to a similar conclusion, that the tau protein is probably the major or only component of PHF. Wolozin and Davies [33] raised monoclonal antibodies to particulate fractions of Alzheimer brain tissue and identified a particular antibody, designated Alz 50, that bound to neurofibrillary tangles, to a large number of dystrophic cortical neurites, and to some abnormal neuronal cell bodies that did not contain NFT. In extracts of Alzheimer's disease cortex, Alz 50 recognized a group of proteins having electrophoretic mobility slightly slower than normal tau; these were designated A68 because their relative migration clustered around 68 kDa [33]. The subsequent use of Alz 50 to probe protein fractions from normal brain demonstrated that the antibody recognized normal tau proteins, both in their phosphorylated state (Chap. 22) and following their *in vitro* dephosphorylation [34]. These results suggested that A68 proteins represent an altered phosphorylation state of tau which causes its slower electrophoretic mobility on gels. This conclusion was supported by the development of a method to purify a subset of PHF that were soluble in ionic detergents and the demonstration that such PHF were apparently solely composed of the A68 forms of tau [35]. Analyses of purified A68 from AD cerebral cortex have demonstrated that the altered tau molecules contain several additional phosphate groups beyond those normally present on tau, including one phosphate group at serine 396 that appears to be important in conferring the immunoreactivity of A68 proteins with Alz 50 and similar antibodies. The precise stoichiometry of phosphate groups to tau protein in the altered forms of tau that comprise PHF is under investigation.

There has been considerable speculation about polypeptides besides tau that may contribute to the PHF structure. Presently, the most clear and reproducible data have suggested that tau is the principal if not the sole constituent. However, like a variety of neuronal inclusions in diseases other than Alzheimer's disease (e.g., Lewy bodies in dopaminergic neurons in Parkinson's disease), NFT contain ubiquitin. The precise protein within PHF that is ubiquitinated, whether tau or another constituent, and the pathophysiological role of ubiquitination in tangle formation remain to be elucidated.

Disordered proteolytic processing of βAPP may underlie Alzheimer's disease

The rough outlines of a common pathogenetic sequence explaining at least some cases of Alzheimer's disease are now at hand, although many questions remain. Current morphological and immunochemical evidence strongly suggests that the earliest detectable alteration occurring in Down's syndrome brain and, by implication, in Alzheimer's disease, is the deposition of small amounts of Aβ in an amorphous, largely nonfibrillar form. This premise, when taken together with the βAPP missense mutations that segregate with Alzheimer's disease in certain families, indicate that Alzheimer's disease can begin with structural defects in the βAPP gene product. These defects may lead to changes in the proteolytic processing of βAPP and, subsequently, to increased formation and extracellular deposition of Aβ. The precise cells in which βAPP molecules serve as precursors for extracellular Aβ remain undefined and could be heterogeneous among the various anatomical types of Aβ deposits (e.g., vascular, plaque, subpial). Because virtually all aged humans and other primates show some degree of cerebral Aβ deposition, one may speculate that a wide variety of molecular alterations can increase the rate of Aβ deposition or decrease the rate of its clearance from brain tissue. Defects in various distinct gene products besides βAPP (e.g., proteases, protease inhibitors, kinases, transcription factors) could influence the rate of Aβ deposition with age and thus could underlie different forms of familial Alzheimer's disease.

Once accelerated Aβ deposition occurs, it appears likely that a subset of cortical deposits gradually accumulate. Either there is enough Aβ or enough of a particular chemical form of the peptide such that progressive aggregation of the initially soluble peptide into nondiffusible, insoluble particles and fibrils occurs. The plaques also contain a number of β-amyloid-associated proteins, such as α1-antichymotrypsin, complement factors C1q, C3c, C3d, and others, heparan sulfate proteoglycans, and serum amyloid P component. Their role in the aggregation of Aβ and the maturation of the deposits is an important area for further study. It may well be that these and other, as yet unidentified, protein constituents of senile plaques contribute to the cytopathological effects of the amyloid deposit. While there is growing evidence that Aβ by itself has biological activity, the proteins and cells which it subsequently attracts may also play a role in the adverse effects on the surrounding cortex.

Accompanying the deposition of Aβ

and numerous associated proteins is the activation and migration of microglial cells into the maturing plaque and the development of reactive astrocytes at its periphery. This might be viewed as a specific type of chronic inflammatory process. The regulation of these cellular responses is complex.

At some point during maturation of the plaque, local axonal terminals and dendrites derived from a variety of intracortical and projection neurons become structurally altered and presumably dysfunctional. Some of the changes these neurites undergo in the vicinity of the plaque may represent aberrant trophic responses, whereas others may represent neurotoxic responses. As this process proceeds, it is likely that numerous secondary effects not directly linked to the Aβ deposition occur on neurons and their processes in the cortex. The cellular and protein changes occurring in plaque-rich cerebral cortex are likely to include a complex series of pathological events that are several steps removed from the initial process of Aβ deposition.

The insidious result of the accelerating neuronal, neuritic and glial alterations that occur in Aβ-rich limbic and association cortices is the dysfunction and loss of neurons and their synapses and a corresponding decrease in various neurotransmitters important for cortical function. While it is instructive to investigate pharmacological therapies that can influence these transmitter deficits, their multiplicity and their heterogeneity among different patients make replacement therapy very difficult.

The pathogenetic cascade model described here is incomplete. Nonetheless, the model suggests certain strategies that may be useful. Interfering with the early stages of this cascade, in particular the generation and gradual aggregation of Aβ and the ensuing protein and cellular changes that accompany its deposition, represents a rational target for pharmacological therapy of Alzheimer's disease. The recognition that Aβ is a soluble product of normal cellular metabolism should encourage the further study of the

role of this peptide in the pathophysiology of AD which may lead to diagnostic and therapeutic measures in this disorder.

PRION DISEASES

Prions are a group of unusual pathogens that cause both transmissible and inherited spongiform encephalopathies in humans and animals. Prions were originally defined as "small proteinaceous infectious particles that resist inactivation by procedures which modify nucleic acids" [36]. The earliest recognition of the group of disorders now referred to as prion diseases came from studies of the pathology and biology of scrapie in sheep and goats. The first human example of this class of transmissible neurodegenerative diseases arose from the discovery of the infectious etiology of kuru by Gajdusek et al. in 1966 and the similar nature of Creutzfeldt-Jakob disease (CJD) [37] and C. J. Gibbs, *personal communication*). Subsequent work led to the recognition of Gerstmann-Straussler-Scheinker syndrome (GSS) and fatal familial insomnia in humans. Additional examples in animals include bovine spongiform encephalopathy, transmissible mink encephalopathy, and chronic wasting disease of mule deer and elk.

One striking characteristic of prion diseases is that they may be both inherited and transmitted. GSS and familial CJD are autosomal dominant genetic traits, and yet extracts of brain from affected individuals can transmit a scrapie-like disease to animals. Both GSS and familial CJD have been linked in various kindreds to a number of different point and insertional mutations in the gene coding for the prion protein (PrP) on chromosome 20. Transgenic mice harboring a GSS mutation in this gene (a leucine substitution at codon 102) have been shown to develop scrapie-like neurodegeneration.

The prion precursor protein is a normal host cellular protein encoded by a single copy chromosomal gene and anchored to the cell membrane through a glycoinositol phospholipid (Chap. 2). The normal function of PrP is unknown. Following its appearance on the cell surface, the normal PrP protein has a finite probability of undergoing a structural transformation that makes it resistant to proteolysis [38]. Because, in a given subject, no difference in primary sequence or post-translational modification between the normal and altered PrP proteins has been detected, a conformational difference is postulated. An increased probability for the transition of cellular PrP to abnormal PrP might occur in various ways: an inherited abnormality in PrP processing; an inherited mutation or spontaneous somatic mutation of the PrP gene; induction by another transformed PrP molecule, as in kuru (acquired from exposure to prion-containing human tissue) or CJD (acquired in rare instances from prion-contaminated human growth hormone or corneal transplants). Both the normal and pathogenic forms of the protein are released from cell membranes, either by phosphatidylinositol-specific phospholipase C or by a protease. One consequence of the pathogenic transformation is to make the PrP protein more resistant to proteolysis: Only a short N-terminal segment of the pathogenic form is cleaved by a nonspecific protease, and this cleavage does not destroy infectivity. In the case of scrapie, both the 33–35 kDa (full-length) and 27–30 kDa (cleaved) forms are infectious. Once the pathogenic transformation has occurred, whether spontaneously or by infection with PrP-rich tissue, the further transformation of the host PrP is postulated to be an autocatalytic process [36].

Brains from cases of GSS, CJD, and scrapie exhibit similar pathology. Aggregates of protease-resistant fibrils and occasionally amyloid plaques are present, sometimes adjacent to dystrophic neurites. Prion plaques show the histochemical properties of amyloid and immunoreactivity for ubiquitin and heparan sulfate proteoglycans. CJD and GSS plaques bind antibodies raised against scrapie-infected hamster brain PrP but do not bind antibodies raised against the Alzheimer Aβ protein. In two brains from GSS individuals of the Indiana kindred, the major component of the amyloid plaques was identified as an 11 kDa PrP fragment, but larger fragments were also found. These observations suggest that the disease process involves abnormal proteolytic cleavage of the precursor protein to generate the amyloidogenic peptide (for refs., see [36–38]). How the transformed PrP molecule actually induces cellular pathology and ultimately clinical symptoms remains unknown.

REFERENCES

1. Bachman, D. L., et al. Prevalence of dementia and probable senile dementia of the Alzheimer type in the Framingham study. *Neurology* 42:115–119, 1992.
2. Terry, R. D., et al. Senile dementia of the Alzheimer type without neocortical neurofibrillary tangles. *J. Neurol. Exp. Neurol.* 46(3): 262–268, 1987.
3. Yamaguchi, H., et al. β-amyloid is focally deposited within the outer basement membrane in the amyloid angiopathy of Alzheimer's disease. *Am. J. Pathol.* 141:249–258, 1992.
4. Probst, A., et al. Senile plaque neurites fail to demonstrate anti-paired helical filament and anti-microtubule-associated protein tau immunoreactive proteins in the absence of neurofibrillary tangles in the neocortex. *Acta Neuropathol.* (Berl.) 77:430–436, 1989.
5. Cochran, E., et al. Amyloid precursor protein and ubiquitin immunoreactivity in dystrophic axons is not unique to Alzheimer's disease. *Am. J. Pathol.* 139:485–489, 1991.
6. Perl, D., Brody, A. R. Alzheimer's disease: X-ray spectometric evidence of aluminum accumulation in neurofibrillary tangle-bearing neurons. *Science* 208:297–299, 1980.
7. Perl, D. P., et al. Intraneuronal aluminum accumulation in amyotrophic lateral sclerosis and parkinsonism dementia of Guam. *Science* 217:1053–1054, 1982.
8. Eidelberg, D., et al. Adult onset Hallervorden-spatz disease with neurofibrillary pathology. *Brain* 110:993–1013, 1987.

9. Glenner, G. G., and Wong, C. W. Alzheimer's disease: initial report of the purification and characterization of a novel cerebrovascular amyloid protein. *Biochem. Biophys. Res. Commun.* 120:885–890, 1984.

10. Masters, C. L., et al. Amyloid plaque core protein in Alzheimer disease and Down syndrome. *Proc. Natl. Acad. Sci. U.S.A.* 82: 4245–4249, 1985.

11. Selkoe, D. J., et al. Isolation of low molecular weight proteins from amyloid plaque fibers in Alzheimer's disease. *J. Neurochem.* 46: 1820–1834, 1986.

12. Kang, J., et al. The precursor of Alzheimer's disease amyloid A4 protein resembles a cell-surface receptor. *Nature* 325:733–736, 1987.

13. Mori, H., et al. Mass spectrometry of purified amyloid β protein in Alzheimer's disease. *J. Biol. Chem.* 267:17082–17086, 1992.

14. Goldgaber, D., et al. Characterization and chromosomal localization of a cDNA encoding brain amyloid of Alzheimer's disease. *Science* 235:877–880, 1987.

15. Tanzi, R., et al. Amyloid β-protein gene: cDNA, mRNA distribution and genetic linkage near the Alzheimer locus. *Science* 235: 880–884, 1987.

16. Robakis, N. K., et al. Molecular cloning and characterization of a cDNA encoding the cerebrovascular and the neuritic plaque amyloid peptides. *Proc. Natl. Acad. Sci. U.S.A.* 84: 4190–4194, 1987.

17. Selkoe, D. J., et al. β-amyoid precursor protein of Alzheimer's disease occurs as 110–135-kilodalton membrane-associated proteins in neural and non-neural tissues. *Proc. Natl. Acad. Sci. U.S.A.* 85:7341–7345, 1988.

18. Weidemann, A., et al. Identification, biogenesis and localization of precursors of Alzheimer's disease A4 amyloid protein. *Cell* 57: 115–126, 1989.

19. Oltersdorf, T., et al. The Alzheimer amyloid precursor protein: Identification of a stable intermediate in the biosynthetic/degradative pathway. *J. Biol. Chem.* 265:4492–4497, 1990.

20. Rosen, D., et al. A drosophila gene encoding a protein resembling the human β-amyloid protein precursor. *Proc. Natl. Acad. Sci. U.S.A.* 86:2478–2482, 1989.

21. Esch, F. S., et al. Cleavage of amyloid β-peptide during constitutive processing of its precursor. *Science* 248:1122–1124, 1990.

22. Sambamurti, K., Shioi, J., Anderson, J. P., Pappolla, M. A., and Robakis, N. K. Evidence for intracellular cleavage of the Alzheimer's amyloid precursor in PC12 cells. *J. Neurosci. Res.* 33:319–329, 1992.

23. Haass, C., Koo, E. H., Mellon, A., Hung, A. Y., and Selkoe, D. J. Targeting of cell-surface β-amyloid precursor protein to lysosomes: alternative processing into amyloid-bearing fragments. *Nature* 357:500–503, 1992a.

24. Estus, E., et al. Potentially amyloidogenic, carboxyl-terminal derivatives of the amyloid protein precursor. *Science* 255:726–728, 1992.

25. Haass, C., et al. Amyloid β-peptide is produced by cultured cells during normal metabolism. *Nature* 359:322–325, 1992b.

26. Seubert, P., et al. Isolation and Quantitation of soluble Alzheimer's β-peptide from biological fluids. *Nature* 359:325–327, 1992.

27. Shoji, M., et al. Production of the Alzheimer amyloid β-protein by normal proteolytic processing. *Science* 258:126–129, 1992.

28. Goate, A., et al. Segregation of a missense mutation in the amyloid precursor protein gene with familial Alzheimer's disease. *Nature* 349: 704–706, 1991.

29. Levy, E., Carman, M. D., Fernandez-Madrid, I., et al. Mutation of the Alzheimer's disease amyloid gene in hereditary cerebral hemorrhage, Dutch type. *Science* 248:1124–1126, 1990.

30. Hardy, J. Framing β-amyloid. *Nature Genet.* 1: 233–234, 1992.

31. Schellenberg, G. D., et al. Genetic linkage evidence for a familial Alzheimer's disease locus on chromosome 14. *Science* 258:668–671, 1992.

32. Grundke-Iqbal, I., et al. Microtubule-associated protein tau: a component of Alzheimer paired helical filaments. *J. Biol. Chem.* 261: 6084–6089, 1986.

33. Wolozin, B. L., Pruchnicke, A., Dickson, D. W., and Davies, P. A neuronal antigen in the brains of Alzheimer patients. *Science* 232: 648–650, 1986.

34. Nukina, N., Kosik, K. S., and Selkoe, D. J. The monoclonal antibody, Alz 50, recognizes tau protein in Alzheimer's disease brain. *Neurosci. Lett.* 87:240–246, 1988.

35. Lee, V. M., Balin, B. J., Otvos, K., and Trojanowski, J. K. A68: A major subunit of paired

helical filaments and derivitized forms of normal tau. *Science* 251:675–678, 1991.

36. Prusiner, S. B. Molecular biology of the prion diseases. *Science* 252:1515–1522, 1991.

37. Gibbs, C. J., Jr., Gajdusek, D. C., Asher, D. M., Alpers, M. P., Beck, E., Daniel, P. M., and Matthews, W. B. Creutzfeldt-Jakob disease (subacute spongiform encephalopathy) transmission to the chimpanzee. *Science* 161: 388–389, 1968.

38. Borchelt, D. R., Taraboulos, A., and Prusiner, S. B. Evidence for synthesis of scrapie prion proteins in the endocytic pathway. *J. Biol. Chem.* 267:16188–16199, 1992.

CHAPTER 46

Positron Emission Tomography

KIRK A. FREY

In vivo determinations of biochemical and physiologic processes have provided unique insight into the integrated functioning of the central nervous system. Approaches to the study of brain function that rely on the use of intact experimental subjects are of particular value for several reasons. First, the metabolic relationships between the brain and its vascular supply represent highly regulated and dynamic processes. Interruption of the supply

Basic Neurochemistry: Molecular, Cellular, and Medical Aspects, 5th Ed., edited by G. J. Siegel et al. Published by Raven Press, Ltd., New York, 1994. Correspondence to Kirk A. Frey, Departments of Internal Medicine and Neurology and The Mental Health Research Institute, The University of Michigan Hospitals, B1G-412/0028 AGH, 1500 E. Medical Center Dr., Ann Arbor, Michigan 48109-0028.

935

of metabolic fuels to the brain results in rapid alteration of both behavior and cerebral metabolism. Second, the blood-brain barrier, acting as a filter, regulates the entry and exit of metabolites and other substances. In many instances, compounds that could be utilized by the brain as sources of energy are excluded from entry. Other substances with neurotransmitter and neuromodulatory activity in brain are also excluded; thus, the barrier contributes to regulation of the neuronal microenvironment. Finally, there exists a diverse regional heterogeneity in the populations of neurons, both with regard to their transmitter specificities and their anatomic interconnections. *In vitro* biochemical methods that utilize tissue slices, homogenates, or subcellular fractions, are generally unsatisfactory for the study of the human diseases that result from disruption of these metabolic relationships. Positron emission tomography (PET) represents an important bridge between *in vitro* and *in vivo* biochemical measures of cerebral function. It is a noninvasive method in which radiotracers are introduced into the bloodstream, and their distribution in the brain is subsequently measured by external detectors. Because of the low radiation doses usually associated with PET, it can be safely applied in clinical research, allowing the direct study of human neurological and psychiatric disease. This chapter provides an overview of PET methods and their applications (see Phelps et al. [1] for review).

METHODS IN POSITRON EMISSION TOMOGRAPHY

Positron-emitting tracers are used to produce maps of radioactivity distribution in brain

Positron-emitting nuclides share unique physical properties that permit great flexibility and sensitivity in the design of tracer distribution experiments. Isotopes used frequently in PET research allow a variety of

TABLE 1.   Physical properties of selected positron-emitting nuclides and positron annihilation photons

Nuclide	Half-life (min)	Maximum energy (MeV)	Maximum range (mm H_2O)
^{11}C	20.4	0.97	4
^{13}N	9.96	1.20	5
^{15}O	2.04	1.74	8
^{18}F	109.8	0.64	2
^{62}Cu	9.73	2.92	14
^{68}Ga	68.1	1.90	9
^{82}Rb	1.3	3.35	17
Annihilation photon	—	0.511	7,000[a]

[a] Half-value distance.

radiochemical approaches to ligand synthesis. Of particular importance, isotopes of carbon and nitrogen may be directly incorporated, and ^{18}F can be substituted for hydrogen or a hydroxyl substituent in many compounds without loss of bioactivity. Because the isotopes used have short half-lives (Table 1), a cyclotron dedicated for nuclide production and facilities and methods for rapid radiochemical synthesis are usually required. Some positron-emitting radionuclides are obtained from *generators,* which contain a parent nuclide (of relatively long half-life, often reactor-produced) which decays, yielding the positron-emitter as a daughter radionuclide. Chemical differences between the parent and daughter nuclides permit their separation, usually by column chromatography. For example, a generator containing ^{68}Ge (half-life 287 days) may be used for production of the positron-emitter ^{68}Ga (half-life 68 min), which is formed following electron-capture decay of the parent nuclide. Other nuclides obtainable from generator systems include ^{62}Cu (from ^{62}Zn, half-life 9.15 hr) and ^{82}Rb (from ^{82}Sr, half-life 25 days). Thus, while the daughter positron-emitting nuclide is short-lived, generators offer the possibility of providing positron-emitters for PET scanning in the absence of a cyclotron. Unfortunately, the nuclides of greatest utility in neurochemical studies (^{11}C, ^{15}O, and ^{18}F) are not obtainable from generator systems. An important advantage of most short-lived positron nuclides is the limited radiation exposure of subjects undergoing PET studies, since much of the administered activity decays during the study, contributing directly to the images.

Positron Decay

The mode of positron decay is particularly advantageous for detection and quantification by external measurement. The decay process begins in the nucleus of a neutron-deficient isotope upon the conversion of a proton to a neutron with simultaneous emission of a positron (or β^+-particle) from the nucleus [2]. The positron is similar to an electron in physical properties except that it is positively rather than negatively charged. The emitted positron is slowed by loss of energy to surrounding matter along its path, and ultimately combines with an electron. This final interaction, *positron annihilation*, results in disintegration of both the positron and the electron, with the simultaneous emission of energy equivalent to their combined mass of 1.022 MeV. The emitted energy is in the form of two γ-rays (photons with energies of 511 keV) that travel in opposite directions.

Photons, unlike positrons, undergo relatively little interaction with surrounding materials of low density; they are not easily deflected from their course and are readily detected at a distance outside the body. Because of the simultaneous emission of the two photons in exactly opposite directions, coincidence-detection algorithms for quantification of positron decay are employed, resulting in images with a high signal-to-noise ratio.

Detection of Positron-Emitting Tracer and Construction of Images

Detection of positron decay for imaging purposes utilizes multiple detectors arranged in one or more rings surrounding the head. Each ring consists of individual detectors, each of which is paired with an oppositely placed detector by the scanner electronics. Each pair of detectors identifies positron annihilation events along the line (ray) connecting them in space. A transverse section image of the distribution of radioactivity within the head is created from the accumulated coincidence counts from each ring. The pair of detectors registering a coincidence defines the ray along which the positron annihilation occurred. Tomographic techniques analogous to those utilized in X-ray computed tomography (CT or CAT scanning) are used to reconstruct the image from the rays. Many PET scanners consist of multiple rings, allowing simultaneous acquisition of data from adjacent levels in the brain. In these cases, pairs of detectors on opposing sides of neighboring rings may be used to identify activity from the tissue between the two rings. These images, termed cross planes, account for the greater number of tissue slices obtained than actual detector rings with multi-ringed scanners. For example, a three-ring scanner can produce five tomographic images simultaneously.

Several correction factors are applied to the PET data during the reconstruction of the images. The photon counts from each detector are corrected for underestimation errors arising from events missed because of detector and electronic limitations at high counting rates. In addition, overestimation errors in coincidence detections caused by random coincidence of single events at high count rates are subtracted. Each detector pair is corrected on a regular basis for sensitivity differences by scanning a standard source of known activity. Finally, the coincidence counts from each ray are corrected for attenuation of the emitted 511 keV photons within the body. This correction is based either on direct measurement of attenuation with an external radiation source of known activity, or by assuming approximate densities for the tissues within the field of view.

Resolution of PET Images

The resulting PET images are spatial maps of radioactivity distribution within tissue slices, and are thus analogous to autoradiograms obtained from brain tissue in animal experiments. The PET method, however, has an important distinction: It is noninvasive and may thus be used in clinical research, including longitudinal studies. A second difference between PET methods and tissue autoradiography is in anatomic resolution. Typical film autoradiographic methods for detection of ^{3}H or ^{14}C provide 50 to 100 μm resolution, allowing clear separation of most brain nuclei from surrounding fiber tracts. The spatial resolution inherent in current PET scans ranges from 5 to 15 mm, resulting from a combination of limitations. The number and geometry of detectors in the scanner as well as the number of counts acquired in the image and their statistical imprecision each reduce PET image resolution. These factors vary between tomographs of different design as well as from study to study, owing to varying image acquisition times and tissue radioactivity levels. The ultimate theoretical limit of PET resolution, however, is the distance traveled by the positron in tissue before the annihilation reaction. Maximum tissue ranges vary according to the initial energy of the positron (Table 1). As a consequence of limited spatial resolution, small brain nuclei and thin laminar structures such as the cerebral cortex cannot be completely separated from neighboring tissues and cerebrospinal fluid. Reconstructed PET data thus reflect average isotope concentrations in the imaged tissue volume elements. When the actual tracer distribution is heterogeneous, but below the resolution of the scan, the data underestimate the highest and overestimate the lowest values owing to this *partial volume averaging* effect.

PET imaging can generate a pictorial representation of a physiologic or biochemical process as it occurs regionally within the brain

Several basic conceptual elements are shared by the variety of PET methods developed and implemented to date. Most significantly, PET measures generally reflect the functional biochemistry and physiology of the brain in contrast to other imaging methods, such as CT and MRI, which excel in the demonstration of tissue structure. The functional nature of PET imaging confers flexibility in the application of PET to neurochemical analysis even though it imposes constraints on the experimental design and data analysis.

To achieve functional or parametric images, several conditions must be satisfied by the chosen radiotracer imaging protocol and the data analysis. First, the process of interest must be precisely specified. Successful PET methods generally rely on a body of basic research experience to characterize the process and demonstrate the biochemical and physiologic significance, regulation, and potential pathologic alterations that may be encountered. Next, a tracer appropriate for the application must be identified. Tracer properties, including biochemical and physiologic specificity, ease of synthesis with a positron-emitting nuclide, and metabolic stability, are important factors in the selection of radiotracers. Third, a physiologic compartmental model describing tracer distribution and the factors governing the movement of tracer between compartments must be developed [3]. It is the mathematical representation of this model that ultimately permits calculation of a parametric image from PET data.

Finally, the tracer and model must be tested and validated. Studies in experimental animals are utilized to verify the chemical identity of the radioactivity. Kinetic studies are performed under experimental pathologic situations, i.e., brain lesions and pharmacologic treatments, which have predictable effects on the model and the parameter of interest. At any point along this path of development it may be necessary to revise the model or the method. If minimal criteria for quantification cannot be met, a new tracer must be selected.

It must be additionally remembered that preliminary work in animal models and in normal human subjects does not guarantee the accuracy of measurements in clinical research applications. Some diseases may cause unforeseen alterations in brain metabolism that invalidate the model and tracer utilized. Thus, understanding the key assumptions, simplifications, and metabolic relationships involved in PET tracer methods is essential to data interpretation.

PHYSIOLOGIC AND BIOCHEMICAL MEASUREMENTS USING PET

The simplest brain parameter measured with PET is blood volume

The model describing the distribution of blood volume markers consists of a tissue volume element with the intravascular space contained in it representing the only compartment for tracer distribution (Fig. 1). It is assumed that the tracer enters and leaves the tissue by blood flow, but does not enter the extravascular space and is not metabolized. Carbon monoxide labeled with ^{15}O is inhaled in a single breath. Because of the high specific activity of the $[^{15}O]CO$, the trace chemical amount of gas administered is nontoxic. Following a brief period of mixing to allow the tracer to bind to hemoglobin and distribute evenly within the blood pool, a PET scan is obtained, and a sample of blood is taken simultaneously for measurement of the tracer concentration. The blood volume in tissue is then determined by dividing the tissue tracer concentration by the blood value.

Normal values for cerebral blood volume (CBV) range from 4 to 6 percent in gray matter and from 2 to 3 percent in white matter (Fig. 1). Regions containing or adjacent to major arteries or venous sinuses have considerably larger values, owing to partial volume averaging with the vessels. Although the intravascular volume itself may occasionally be of interest, the most frequent application is the correction of studies with other tracers for intravascular activity. If the regional intra-

vascular volume and arterial tracer concentrations are known, the measured total tissue activity may be corrected for the intravascular component. This technique is frequently employed in the determination of brain oxygen extraction and metabolism.

Measurement of blood-brain barrier permeability to a test substance utilizes a two-compartment model representing the intravascular and extravascular spaces

The movement of tracer into and out of the tissue volume element occurs by flow of blood, whereas capillary blood exchanges tracer with the tissue (see Chap. 31). Two model parameters are estimated following intravenous injection of the tracer. Arterial blood samples are used to determine the tracer input curve, and serial PET scans of the brain are obtained to define the regional tracer time-activity curves. The first of the parameters, K_1, represents uptake of the tracer by brain from the blood. It is related to both cerebral blood flow, F, and to the regional capillary surface area-permeability product, PS:

$$K_1 = F(1 - e^{-PS/F})$$

The second parameter, k_2, represents the movement of tracer back to the blood from the brain and is equivalent to K_1 divided by the tracer distribution volume in brain. Selection of tracers with appropriate properties allows direct determination of regional permeability using this model. Specifically, for tracers with very low permeability ($F \gg PS$), $K_1 \sim PS$. In addition, tracers with very large distribution volumes in brain allow k_2 to be neglected early, simplifying estimation of K_1. Tracers satisfying the former condition include $^{82}RbCl$ [4] and $[^{68}Ga]EDTA$ [5]. $[^{14}C]$aminoisobutyric acid, a tracer satisfying both conditions, has been utilized in animal experiments; however, a positron-labeled analog has yet to be routinely applied.

Determination of regional blood-brain

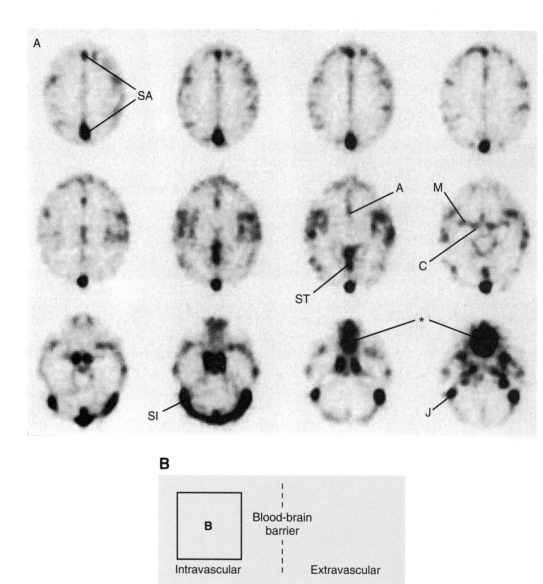

FIG. 1.   PET measurement of blood volume in normal human subject. **A:** PET images from adjacent transaxial slices extending from the supraventricular level *(upper left)* to the base of the brain *(lower right)* following inhalation of [^{15}O]CO. Blood volume is depicted in gray scale, with increasing image density reflecting higher blood volume. Major cerebral vessels are located on the surface of the brain, with larger volumes associated with venous sinuses than with cerebral arteries. Note that the extracerebral soft tissues (dark gray rim at periphery of images) and nasal sinuses (*) have considerably higher blood volume than does the brain: (A) anterior cerebral arteries; (C) carotid artery; (J) jugular bulb; (M) middle cerebral artery; (SA) sagittal sinus; (SI) sigmoid sinus; (ST) straight sinus and vein of Galen. B: Compartmental model used for calculation of blood volume. Tracer is assumed to remain in the blood pool (B) during the study. The PET scanner views a mixture of the intravascular and extravascular compartments, allowing calculation of the intravascular volume. (Images courtesy of Dr. M. E. Phelps, UCLA, Los Angeles, CA.)

barrier permeability is used primarily when a pathologic increase is anticipated. Measurements in brain tumor and in brain infarction (stroke) have verified the abnormally permeable capillary beds known qualitatively from contrast-enhanced CT scanning. PET methods, however, allow calculation of the permeability coefficient. This allows quantification of the effects of steroid treatment on blood-brain barrier permeability as well as estimation of regional brain exposure to potential chemotherapeutic agents. Measurement of blood-brain barrier permeability is additionally helpful in excluding potential sources of error from other PET methods, which may be complicated by breakdown of the barrier. Blood-brain barrier permeability to tracers that enter brain readily may be calculated from estimates of their initial uptake combined with independent measurement of regional blood flow according to the relationship given for K_1 above. This may be of benefit in defining the relative flow and permeability contributions to tracer uptake, thereby permitting better understanding of the tracer kinetic model and its sensitivity to pathologic blood flow and blood-brain barrier changes.

Determination of regional cerebral blood flow is a frequently employed PET method

The modeling of cerebral blood flow (CBF) tracer distribution is identical with that presented for blood-brain barrier permeability measurements discussed previously. The tissue volume element consists of two tracer distribution compartments, the intravascular and extravascular spaces (Fig. 2). The influx rate constant, K_1, is directly proportional to blood flow when the tracer has a very high blood-brain barrier permeability, i.e., $PS \gg F$. Under these conditions, two parameters, K_1 and k_2, are estimated for each tissue volume element: K_1 represents regional CBF, whereas K_1/k_2 is the regional tracer distribution volume. The CBF tracer may be introduced into the circulation either by inhalation or by intravenous injection. Data collected consist of serial PET scans of the brain and the arterial input curve to the brain, approximated from measurement of tracer activity in arterial blood samples [6,7].

Several tracers have been employed for CBF measurement, each of which has relative advantages and disadvantages. Initial CBF measurements were made with [^{13}N]NH$_3$ because of its ease of synthesis; however, NH$_3$ is not inert in cerebral tissue, is restricted from complete equilibration with brain at high normal CBF rates, and its uptake and distribution are affected by tissue and plasma pH and cerebral NH$_3$ metabolism. Thus, newer agents, including [^{15}O]H$_2$O and [^{11}C]butanol], have replaced [^{13}N]NH$_3$. Water as a CBF tracer is attractive from the standpoint of easy synthesis, formulation, and injection, but like ammonia it is limited by blood-brain barrier permeability at the upper extremes of physiologic flow rates [11]. Butanol, by comparison, is not diffusion-limited, but is more difficult to synthesize, and the longer half-life of ^{11}C compared to ^{15}O results in greater radiation exposure for an equivalent injected dose. Butanol may be synthesized labeled with ^{15}O, but, the radiochemical synthetic demands are severe, owing to the very short half-life of the nuclide. Preliminary studies suggest the feasibility of CBF measurements with the use of [^{62}Cu]PTSM, a lipophilic organometallic compound readily synthesized from generator-produced ^{62}Cu. This tracer may permit CBF studies without the need for a local cyclotron, although, as with NH$_3$, it is incompletely extracted at physiologic CBF.

PET-determined values for CBF in normal individuals average approximately 50 ml/min/100 g brain, in agreement with the results of global measures by the Kety-Schmidt arteriovenous difference method (see Chap. 31). Regional CBF values range from 40 to 100 in gray matter and from 15 to 30 in white matter structures (Fig. 2). The average ratio of gray to white matter for CBF in the resting state is approximately 3 to 1 with current PET techniques. This is somewhat less than the ratio of 5 or 6 to 1 obtained

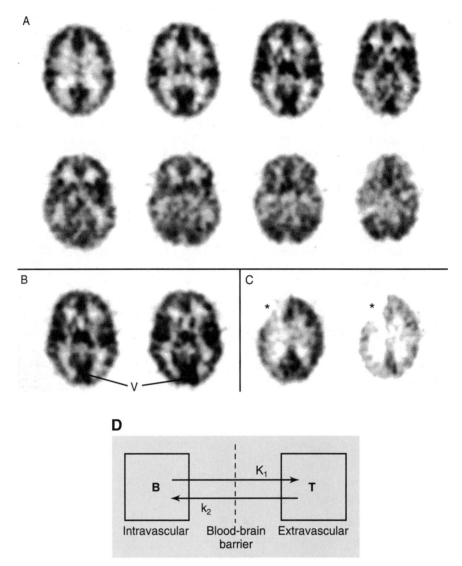

FIG. 2.   PET measurement of cerebral blood flow. **A:** CBF determined in a normal subject following injection of [^{15}O]H$_2$O. Transaxial images extend from the supraventricular level *(upper left)* to the base of the brain *(lower right)*. **B:** CBF images at the mid-thalamic level from a normal subject during visual deprivation (eyes closed, *left*) and again during audiovisual stimulation (watching a videotape, *right*). Note the focal increase in CBF in the visual cortex (V) during stimulation. **C:** CBF at the supraventricular level in a patient at rest *(left)* and again during hyperventilation *(right)*. Note the global reduction of CBF due to reduced arterial CO$_2$ during hyperventilation, without alteration in regional pattern. The patient has undergone prior surgery for removal of a tumor in the frontal lobe (*). **D:** Compartmental model for CBF measurement. Two tracer compartments representing arterial blood (B) and brain tissue (T) are represented. Blood flow is estimated by the rate of tissue tracer uptake from blood (K$_1$). (Images courtesy of Dr. L. Junck, Department of Neurology, The University of Michigan, Ann Arbor, MI.)

in autoradiographic animal experiments as a result of partial volume averaging in the PET measurements. The global CBF varies substantially with respiration owing to the effect of arterial pCO_2 or pH on the cerebral vasculature (Fig. 2C, see also Chap. 31). Near the physiologic pCO_2 of 40 mm Hg, CBF increases approximately 1 to 2 percent for each 1 mm Hg increase in pCO_2.

In addition to these global changes, regional CBF changes have been determined both as a result of physiologic activation of the brain and in cerebral pathology. Regional rates of oxidative metabolism are known to be sensitive to change in neuronal activity (see below). Regional CBF has been reported to vary with metabolic rate in normal brain, presumably based on the need for delivery of metabolic substrates and clearance of metabolites, although the mechanism whereby CBF and metabolism are coupled remains to be elucidated (see Chap. 31). The ease of measuring CBF and the ability to repeat the measure frequently under varying stimulus conditions have thus made CBF studies invaluable in indirectly localizing regions of altered cerebral function (Fig. 2B). In addition, several neuropathologic conditions are primarily related to altered CBF, and in these cases hypotheses can be tested directly with PET. Finally, CBF measurements contribute to the determination of other physiologic parameters, as in the determination of *PS* values for highly permeable tracers (see above) and in the calculation of the metabolic rate for oxygen (see below).

Regional cerebral glucose metabolism is imaged for the study of brain activity *in vivo*

Development of the method for determining the regional cerebral metabolic rate for glucose (rCMRglu) and its validation in experimental animals [8] are discussed in detail in Chapter 31. The tracer kinetic model for glucose metabolism is more complex than the previously discussed examples because of an additional tissue compartment represent-

ing metabolized tracer (Fig. 3). The model consists of intravascular tracer, a tissue precursor pool in exchange with blood, and a metabolic pool representing tracer that has been chemically transformed. The compartments are interrelated by rate constants K_1 and k_2, representing the exchange of tracer across the blood-brain barrier, and by k_3 and k_4, representing the rate of tracer phosphorylation by hexokinase and dephosphorylation by glucose-6-phosphatase, respectively. The tracers employed for measurement of rCMRglu are 2-deoxy-D-glucoses (2DG), glucose analogs that share transport and phosphorylation processes with the endogenous substrate but that are not appreciably further metabolized following formation of the 6-phosphate derivative. Thus, the 2DG tracers are useful in the determination of the rate of glucose phosphorylation by hexokinase but do not measure subsequent steps in glycolysis or in oxidative metabolism.

At present, two positron-emitting 2DG derivatives are in use: [18F]2-fluoro-2-deoxy-D-glucose ([18F]2FDG) and [11C]2DG. The former tracer has the advantage of a longer half-life and is useful in situations in which PET scans of high anatomic resolution and statistical precision at long times following injection are desired. The shorter half-life of [11C]2DG, conversely, is useful when multiple sequential studies on the same experimental subject, e.g., test-retest or baseline and stimulation protocols, are planned, since the activity decays quickly enough to allow repeat tracer injections on the same day (within 3 to 4 hr intervals).

Measurement of rCMRglu is initiated by the intravenous injection of the labeled DG, followed by the collection of timed arterial blood samples for measurement of the tracer input curve [9,10]. The most commonly employed procedure is to obtain PET brain images beginning 30 to 45 min following the injection, at which time the bulk of the activity represents metabolized tracer. These data, combined with the arterial input function, are analyzed according to a modified version of the operational equation of Soko-

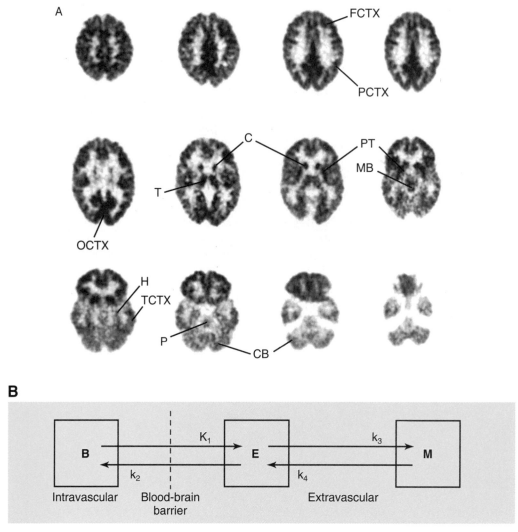

FIG. 3.   Regional cerebral glucose metabolism. **A:** PET scans obtained 30 to 90 min following injection of [^{18}F]FDG in a normal subject. Transaxial slices from the supraventricular level *(upper left)* to the base of the brain *(lower right)* are displayed on a gray scale with the highest metabolic rates depicted by the darker areas. Anatomic structure is well delineated in the images on the basis of higher glucose metabolism in gray than in white matter regions: (C) caudate nucleus; (CB) cerebellum; (FCTx) frontal cortex; (H) hippocampal formation; (MB) midbrain; (OCTx) occipital cortex; (P) pons; (PCTx) parietal cortex; (PT) putamen; (T) thalamus; (TCTx) temporal cortex. **B:** Compartmental model for rCMRglu determination. Tracer compartments include FDG in arterial blood (B) and in the extravascular precursor pool (E), as well as FDG-6-phosphate in the metabolic product pool (M). The rate of FDG metabolism is the product of tissue uptake from blood (K_1) and the fraction of tissue precursor metabolized ($k_3/\{k_2 + k_3\}$).

loff (see Chap. 31). The calculation of rCMRglu by this procedure relies on the use of population average values of the individual rate constants and the lumped constant. The single-scan protocol is thus analogous to the autoradiographic method employed in the determination of rCMRglu using a β^--particle-emitting 2DG tracer in experimental animals.

Under a variety of pathologic conditions, some or all of the assumptions about the rate and lumped constants may be invalidated either globally or regionally, leading to inaccuracies in the estimates of rCMRglu provided by the single scan approach [11,12]. In particular, disruption of the normal relationship and coupling between blood flow and energy metabolism may occur in ischemic states. Wide fluctuations from the normal range of blood glucose concentrations have additionally been demonstrated to produce such alterations. In these circumstances, an alternative experimental protocol involving repeated measurements of tracer distribution may be applied [13]. Serial PET scans are obtained beginning immediately following the injection and ending 45 to 90 min later. The tissue and blood time activity curves are then fitted to the compartmental model by nonlinear least squares approximation, defining optimal values for the rate constants. The rate of 2DG "metabolism" (rCMRdg) is given by

$$rCMRdg = K_1 \cdot k_3 / (k_2 + k_3)$$

and the glucose metabolic rate by

$$rCMRglu = C_p \cdot rCMRdg/LC$$

where C_p represents the arterial plasma glucose concentration, and LC is a lumped constant relating deoxyglucose to glucose metabolism. Using this kinetic approach, the calculated rCMRglu continues to be influenced by the value of LC but is independent of errors introduced by the application of inappropriate rate constants for 2DG transport and metabolism.

Measurements of CMRglu in normal individuals at rest yield average rates for whole brain of approximately 6 mg/100 g brain/min (33 μmol/100 g brain/min; Fig. 3). This is well within the range of values reported using arteriovenous differences, which is between 4.5 and 6.5 mg/100 g brain/min. The rCMRglu in normal brain varies between 5 and 11 mg/100 g brain/

min in gray matter and between 2 and 5 mg/100 g brain/min in white matter. These values demonstrate less range than autoradiographic animal studies in which seven- to eight-fold differences between gray and white matter regions are seen. This, again, is a result of inherent volume averaging at the PET level of anatomic resolution.

The measurement of rCMRglu has gained wide application in the study of both normal physiologic activity and pathologic processes, based on the observed relationship between functional neuronal activity and energy metabolism [14]. This relationship has been demonstrated elegantly through a variety of physiologic activation and suppression procedures in both experimental animals and in normal human volunteers. Results of animal studies suggest that the coupling of metabolism to neuronal activity is due to the increased transmembrane ionic conductances associated with synaptic transmission (see Chaps. 4 and 31). In general, areas of dense synaptic content within neuropil show the highest regional rates of metabolism and respond most dramatically to alterations in neuronal activity. White matter is less active or reactive when studied at high anatomic resolution by autoradiography in animals. It should be kept in mind that both pre- and post-synaptic terminals participate in functional metabolic responses, and in some instances, the effect of increased neuronal firing may be detected only in distant terminal fields of the activated neurons rather than in the regions of the cell bodies themselves [15]. Thus, the metabolic response to a change in activity within a particular brain region is often detected in remote brain regions receiving its efferent projections.

Applications of PET rCMRglu measurements include primary investigation of cerebral metabolism and the relationships between glucose and oxygen metabolism. In addition, primary disturbances in substrate delivery, as in ischemia, and in metabolic activity, as in metabolic coma, may be directly investigated. Regional glucose metabolism has most frequently been utilized as a tool for localizing alterations in neuronal activity as a consequence of physiologic stimulation. Here, changes in metabolism reveal the locations of altered neuronal activity resulting from changes in behavioral states or from pathologic processes.

Inhalation of [^{15}O]oxygen allows measurement of regional cerebral oxygen metabolic rate

The regional rate of cerebral oxygen metabolism represents one of two PET methods discussed here that cannot be determined in experimental animals by alternative techniques. The known radioisotopes of oxygen are all extremely short-lived and are thus of little use in conventional biochemical research, since the activity decays too rapidly to allow measurement in dissected tissue samples. The longest-lived oxygen isotope, ^{15}O (half-life, 2.04 min), administered as [^{15}O]O$_2$, has been successfully employed in the measurement of oxygen metabolism by means of PET. Two methods of administration of the agent by inhalation have been described. They rely on a simple two-compartment model of O$_2$ distribution in which intravascular and extravascular spaces are represented. It is assumed that ^{15}O$_2$ in arterial blood is predominantly bound to hemoglobin with a smaller dissolved fraction. During capillary transit, ^{15}O$_2$ enters the tissue, where it is rapidly metabolized to [^{15}O]H$_2$O. The labeled water then exchanges with the intravascular compartment. Peripheral metabolism also results in production of [^{15}O]H$_2$O, which recirculates in arterial blood to the brain and must be taken into account. Oxygen metabolism is thus defined as the product of regional oxygen extraction and arterial oxygen delivery:

$$rCMRO_2 = E{\cdot}C_a{\cdot}rCBF$$

where C_a represents arterial oxygen content; rCBF is regional cerebral blood flow; and E

is the fraction of available oxygen extracted during a single capillary transit.

The methods employed are a continuous inhalation protocol with a single-scan determination of regional ^{15}O$_2$ extraction [16] or a kinetic multiple scan approach following single-breath inhalation of ^{15}O$_2$ [17]. Both methods require arterial blood sampling for determination of O$_2$ content, ^{15}O$_2$, and [^{15}O]H$_2$O. In addition, independent measure of rCBF, usually with [^{15}O]H$_2$O, is required. Finally, because of the substantial contribution of intravascular activity to the total tissue activity, correction for intravascular volume using [^{15}O]CO is frequently employed.

Results of measurements in normal volunteers indicated resting CMRO$_2$ rates of 1.8 to 5.8 ml O$_2$/100 g brain/min (70–230 μmol O$_2$/100 g brain/min) in white and gray matter, respectively. Applications of PET CMRO$_2$ measurements are similar to those discussed above for CMRglu.

The metabolism of specific neurotransmitters may be evaluated with the use of labeled precursors

In addition to oxidative energy metabolism, specific processes subserving the synthesis and subsequent disposition of neurotransmitters may be evaluated with PET methods. Measurement of dopamine synthesis in monoaminergic neurons may be estimated following the injection of [^{18}F]6-fluoro-DOPA (FDOPA). The tracer, an analog of DOPA, is transported across the blood-brain barrier by the large neutral amino acid carrier system. Within nerve terminals, [^{18}F]FDOPA is metabolized by DOPA decarboxylase to the false transmitter [^{18}F]fluorodopamine (FDA), and subsequently undergoes vesicular storage, release on nerve depolarization, presynaptic reuptake, and degradative metabolism in parallel with authentic dopamine. Prominent peripheral metabolism of the tracer by DOPA and aromatic amino acid decarboxylases and by COMT results in labeled metabolites (see

Chap. 12). When the former pathways are inhibited by pre-administration of the peripheral decarboxylase inhibitor carbidopa, brain tracer uptake is enhanced and analysis of blood activity is simplified. Under these conditions, the predominant labeled blood constituents are authentic FDOPA and its COMT metabolite 3-O-methyl-FDOPA (MeDOPA). The rate of cerebral FDA synthesis is estimated with a physiologic model analogous to that used for FDG metabolism, following correction of both blood and cerebral activities for the estimated contribution of [^{18}F]MeDOPA [18]. A similar method has been proposed for the study of serotonin synthesis, based on uptake and metabolism of [^{11}C]α-methyl-L-tryptophan [19].

Application of FDOPA imaging has been extensive in the evaluation of neurologic movement disorders, particularly in Parkinson's disease, and in other disorders attributed to dopaminergic pathology. The method permits evaluation of presynaptic capacity for DA synthesis, which is known to be impaired in Parkinson's disease and related disorders on the basis of postmortem observations.

The *in vivo* quantification of regional ligand binding sites has been a long-anticipated development in PET

The general kinetic ligand binding model consists of four tracer compartments [20] (Fig. 4). The intravascular compartment communicates with the free ligand pool in the tissue by the rate constants K_1 and k_2, which represent exchange across the blood-brain barrier. The extravascular space contains three tracer compartments: free ligand, nonspecifically bound ligand, and receptor, or specifically bound ligand. The rate constant k_3 describes specific binding of the ligand to free receptors, and k_4 represents the dissociation of specifically bound ligand. Exchange of free ligand with nonspecific (assumed to be nonsaturable) binding sites in tissue is represented by k_5 and k_6.

The relationship between the kinetic rate constants and the receptor pharmacologic terms k_{on}, k_{off}, K_d, and B_{max} is as follows:

$$k_3 = k_{on} \cdot R = k_{on}(B_{max} - RL)$$

$$k_4 = k_{off}$$

where $B_{max} = R + RL$; $K_d = k_{off}/k_{on}$; k_{on} and k_{off} are rate constants for ligand binding to and dissociation from the receptor; B_{max} is the total number of receptor sites; R represents free receptors available for binding; and RL represents receptors occupied by ligand (see also Chap. 10). Even under true tracer conditions in PET studies in which radioligand occupies an insignificant number of the total receptor sites, B_{max} and R may be nonidentical, owing to receptor occupancy by endogenous neurotransmitter. Thus, kinetic binding methods estimate the free receptor density (R) rather than the total receptor number (B_{max}) measured by *in vitro* methods. Finally, as is evident from the above equations, B_{max} (or R) is not uniquely specified under *in vivo* binding conditions. Receptor concentration and ligand affinity may be estimated from sequential PET studies resulting in minimal and substantial occupancy of receptors, respectively, since k_3 is reduced in proportion to receptor availability at pharmacologic doses of administered ligand, while k_{on} and k_{off} are unaffected. As an alternative, many investigators choose to determine the $k_{on} \cdot B_{max}$ product (k_3) or the B_{max}/K_d ratio (k_3/k_4) from a single high specific activity tracer injection.

In practice, a ligand is injected intravenously, and arterial blood samples are withdrawn for determination of the arterial input function. Unlike most of the previously described PET methods, blood radioactivity measurements must be corrected for the presence of labeled metabolites produced *in vivo* in order to define the input curves properly [21]. Sequential PET scans of the brain are obtained, and the resulting tracer time courses in tissue and the arterial blood curve are analyzed by nonlinear least squares fitting to provide estimates of the model parameters. Typically, the entire set of six or

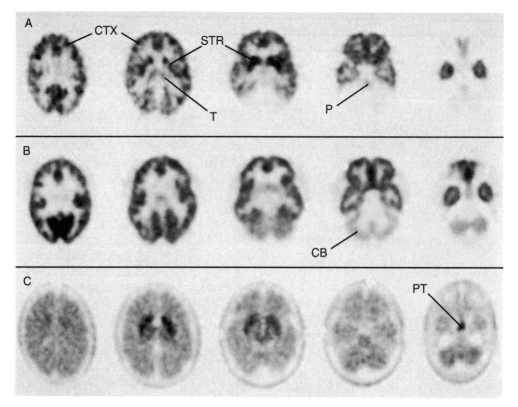

FIG. 4. Radioligand binding to neurochemical markers in normal human brain. **A:** Distribution of muscarinic acetylcholine receptors as depicted by the tissue distribution volume (DV) for the muscarinic antagonist ligand [^{11}C]N-methylpiperidylbenzilate. **B:** Distribution of central-type benzodiazepine binding sites as depicted by the DV for the benzodiazepine antagonist [^{11}C]flumazenil. **C:** Distribution of monoamine presynaptic terminals as depicted by the accumulation of [^{11}C]tetrabenazine. Comparable images from the supraventricular level *(left)* to the base of the brain *(right)* are shown for the individual binding site ligands. Note the distinction between brain regions according to differential levels of each binding site. Cerebral cortical (CTx) areas have high levels of muscarinic receptors and benzodiazepine binding sites, the striatum (caudate and putamen, STR) has high levels of both muscarinic receptors and monoamine (dopamine) terminals, the thalamus (T) has low levels of all three markers (monoaminergic vesicles are predominantly noradrenergic in the diencephalon), the pons (P) has low levels of muscarinic receptors and monoamine vesicles with virtually no benzodiazepine binding sites, and the cerebellum (CB) has very low muscarinic receptor binding, but modest levels of benzodiazepine binding sites and monoamine vesicles. The pituitary (PT) is distinguished by monoamine vesicles in the terminals of arcuate hypothalamic neurons projecting to its posterior division.

more parameters in the ligand-binding model cannot be simultaneously estimated from a single PET tracer study. Simplifications of the model, including collapsing of the nonsaturable tissue compartments, and of all three tissue compartments have been applied with success to the analyses of specific ligands (Fig. 4; [21,22]). Some of these simplifying assumptions permit the calculation of receptor maps, displaying the binding parameter(s) on a pixel-by-pixel basis.

The range of ligand-binding sites that may be studied in this way is potentially as varied as the tracers for their study (Fig. 4). It is feasible to measure cerebral dopamine, opiate, serotonin, benzodiazepine, and muscarinic cholinergic receptors. Enzyme levels may be determined by using similar modeling assumptions, as demonstrated by the imaging of brain monoamine oxidases [23]. In addition, presynaptic membrane and vesicle transporters may be quantified with appro-

D

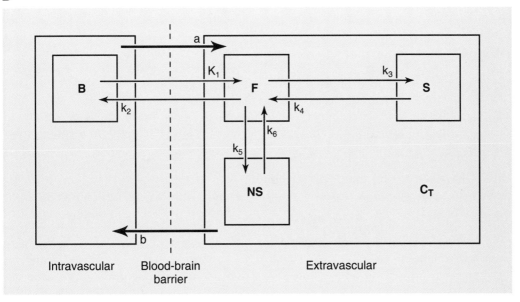

E

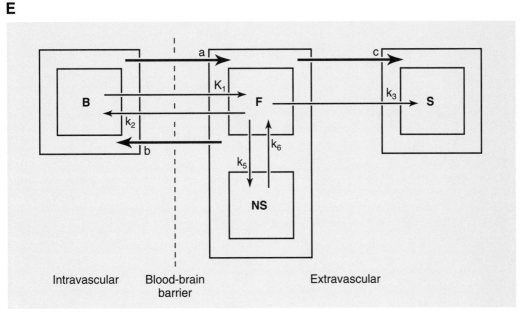

FIG. 4. *(continued).* **D and E:** Two alternative compartmental models depicting simplified algorithms for estimation of ligand binding site density. In both cases, ligand compartments representing arterial blood (B), free tissue ligand *(F)*, nonspecifically bound ligand *(NS)*, and specifically bound ligand *(S)* are considered. These four compartments and six associated rate constants *(inner boxes in each model)* are not independently estimable in most *in vivo* experiments, necessitating introduction of simplified models. In the case of ligands that interact rapidly and reversibly with binding sites ("equilibrium" binding ligands; D), the three tissue compartments are kinetically condensed to a single compartment *(outer boxes)*, and new rate constants a and b are estimated. The degree of specific binding, under appropriate conditions, is proportional to the combined tissue distribution volume (DV) as estimated from the ratio of a/b. This model was applied in calculation of the binding depicted in **A** and **B.** Alternatively, modeling of ligands that dissociate very slowly from specific binding sites ("irreversible" binding ligands; E) may be simplified by condensing the free and nonspecific binding tissue components and estimating the three remaining rate constants a, b, and c *(outer boxes)*. In this case, the binding site density is estimated by the magnitude of parameter c.

priately selected radioligands [24,25]. The selection of ligands for receptor measurement is a key step in the successful development of *in vivo* binding techniques, and places greater restriction on the properties of an acceptable tracer than *in vitro* binding situations. First, the selected ligand should have specificity for a single receptor type or subtype. The use of antagonist drugs is preferred, since antagonist binding is more closely described by the simple association and dissociation reactions assumed in the model than is the binding of agonists. Finally, the labeled ligand must not be metabolized within the brain or converted outside the brain to labeled metabolites that enter the brain and complicate interpretation of the tissue activity curves.

Applications of *in vivo* ligand-binding methods are potentially diverse, ranging from studies of disease- or therapy-related alterations in the numbers of binding sites to dynamic tests of synaptic function. The latter possibility is based on measurement of changes in free binding sites caused by altered levels of endogenous neurotransmitter or substrate. Thus, either physiologic or pharmacologic challenges that alter presynaptic activity or modify binding of the endogenous transmitter may indirectly produce changes in the radioligand binding to the receptor sites. A baseline receptor scan followed by a repeat study with such an activation procedure may thus identify the integrity of presynaptic terminals. In addition, the regional receptor occupancies accompanying the use of therapeutic doses of direct receptor agonist or antagonist drugs may be determined by repeat ligand-binding scans before and after a dose of the unlabeled agent.

CLINICAL APPLICATION OF CEREBRAL PET

The clinical use of cerebral PET techniques was initially limited to research protocols because of the expense of PET and the limited number of centers with PET capabilities. The cost, $1,500 to $2,500 per session at most centers, is based on the need for a team of individuals that includes a cyclotron operator, radiochemist, nuclear medicine technologist, and physician to perform the study. In addition to the labor-intensive aspects of PET methods, a dedicated cyclotron and a computer for image acquisition, reconstruction, and calculation of parametric images are usually required. In recognition of this limitation, PET has been most frequently used to answer fundamental questions about the pathophysiology of human diseases and their regional distribution. These results then have broad implications for other patients with these disorders and may ultimately influence clinical diagnostic and therapeutic decisions without the need for performing PET in each individual. Such studies may additionally uncover previously unrecognized physiologic and biochemical abnormalities, redirecting subsequent research with more conventional methods.

Many degenerative neurological disorders have chronic courses but may respond symptomatically to pharmacological treatment. Thus, postmortem biochemical analysis of the brain in these cases may be influenced by the effect of medication or the effect of chronic systemic disease, or both. PET is of particular value in these instances, providing a noninvasive alternative to brain biopsy or other less direct approaches, such as cerebrospinal fluid analysis. Examples of diseases under study in this manner include Alzheimer's disease, Huntington's disease, and Parkinson's disease. An alternative goal in PET research is the identification of clinical disease markers or responses to therapy that might be extrapolated to the subsequent diagnosis or treatment of an entire patient population. In these instances, we seek predictive correlation between PET measures and results of routinely available and less costly diagnostic tests. Examples of such applications include the study of drug distribution and action, brain tumor response to therapy, and studies on the biochemistry and physiology of cerebrovascular disease.

PET studies of epilepsy assist in localization of seizure foci

Although idiopathic epilepsy is one of the most frequently encountered human neurologic disorders, the underlying pharmacologic, metabolic, and electrophysiologic abnormalities are largely unknown. Medically intractable seizures are frequently associated with epileptogenic foci in the temporal lobes (see Chap. 43).

The first results of PET in partial epilepsy revealed an unanticipated abnormality in the interictal, or between-seizure, metabolic pattern [26]. The presumed site of the seizure focus showed decreased rather than increased blood flow and glucose metabolic rate. In over two-thirds of patients, a well-lateralized zone of hypometabolism is identified. When present, the hypometabolic zone correlates with the location of the seizure focus as determined by ictal depth EEG recording in greater than 90 percent of cases. During ictal discharge the zone of hypometabolism is replaced by a relatively hypermetabolic area that frequently extends beyond the limits of the interictal abnormality.

The etiology of interictal hypometabolism has yet to be established; however, several hypotheses have been proposed that may individually or collectively account for the phenomenon. Hypometabolism may result from active inhibition of neuronal activity, from loss of neurons or simplification of synaptic architecture, or from gross structural atrophy or partial volume artifact. The frequent finding of mesial temporal sclerosis, consisting of loss of neurons and gliosis affecting the hippocampus in surgically resected epileptogenic temporal lobes, lends support to the proposed structural mechanisms [27]. More recent observations suggest that the lateral temporal neocortex ipsilateral to the seizure focus displays a greater degree of metabolic depression, although histologic abnormalities in these areas are not recognized. Thus, metabolic abnormalities extend beyond known structural pathology to support the involvement of functional connections between the seizure focus and neocortical regions [28].

The coexistence of both hypometabolism and ictal depth EEG localization is a reliable predictor of good surgical response in seizure control. Placement of depth electrodes is an invasive procedure with an associated morbidity. Hence, development of the noninvasive marker for the presence and extent of a unilateral seizure focus that is amenable to surgical resection and for the localization of the focus is a useful advance. MRI is preferable when a structural lesion other than mesial temporal sclerosis is present, whereas PET appears more sensitive in detecting sclerotic lesions. The combination of MRI and PET studies is routine in the preoperative evaluation of intractable seizures at some centers, eliminating the need for invasive monitoring in many cases.

More recent studies have revealed alterations in ligand binding sites in temporal lobe epilepsy. The binding of [11C]carfentanyl, an agonist at *mu* opiate receptors, is increased in the temporal neocortex ipsilateral to the seizure focus [29], and the binding of [11C]flumazenil, an antagonist of the central benzodiazepine receptor, is focally decreased in the hippocampal formation [30]. The former observation suggests biochemical disturbances of neurotransmission at a distance from the presumed focus, as is found metabolically; however, the pathologic correlate of altered opiate binding has yet to be established. The reduction in hippocampal benzodiazepine receptors appears to be a marker of their loss in mesial temporal sclerosis, thus enhancing the anatomic specificity of presurgical imaging.

Several aspects of the underlying pharmacology and physiology of the epileptogenic focus remain to be examined by PET. The studies reported to date have described patients with well-established epilepsy who are generally taking at least one anticonvulsant medication at the time of study. Some of the observed metabolic changes may thus relate either to effects of repeated seizures or medications, or both. The observation of benzodiazepine receptor loss in the hippocampal formation may reflect local damage caused by repeated seizures in an area of selective vulnerability, or may constitute the necessary substrate for medically refractory seizures. Future investigation focusing on new-onset seizures in unmedicated patients will allow distinctions among pathogenetic mechanisms, therapeutic effects, and secondary changes resulting from repeated seizures.

PET studies in cerebrovascular disease show the evolution of metabolic and blood flow changes in ischemic brain

The diagnosis and management of patients with cerebrovascular insufficiency is problematic in the clinical neurosciences. The factors that lead to cerebral ischemia are numerous, and there are a variety of differing methods proposed for its diagnosis and management. Potential therapeutic modalities for ischemic cerebrovascular disease include vascular surgery, anticoagulation or inhibition of platelet aggregation, and cerebral protection with antioxidant or metabolic inhibiting agents. Prior to the use of PET, the pathophysiologic evolution from ischemic to infarcted brain in human stroke was unknown. Although animal models of stroke have permitted biochemical and physiologic measurements, the relevance to human cerebrovascular disease is controversial (see also Chap. 40).

Several PET studies of stroke have examined the evolution of changes in infarcted regions as well as in the surrounding brain. It was demonstrated by using [^{18}F]2FDG and [^{13}N]NH$_3$ that glucose metabolism and blood flow become uncoupled in the course of ischemic infarction [31]. Very early after onset of symptoms, within days, regions of reduced blood flow and relatively preserved metabolic activity are observed. Within the first 2 weeks, these regions become relatively hyperemic with sustained glucose metabolism. In chronic lesions that appear atrophic on CT scans, a relatively matched metabolic and perfusion deficit is observed. A subsequent study of stroke using measures of oxygen metabolism and blood flow [32] revealed an early rise in regional oxygen extraction in the ischemic area that resolves over the 1st week, becoming hypometabolic, as originally observed with [^{18}F]2FDG. Serial determinations of both oxygen and glucose metabolism in the same patients have identified an abnormal relationship in the infarcted regions. The usual coupling ratio of 6 mol of O$_2$ per mol glucose oxidized was found to be reduced to 2 mol of O$_2$, indicating that anaerobic glycolysis or oxidation of alternative substrates occurs in recent cerebral infarction [33]. Studies in experimental animals have revealed that the appearance of phagocytic cells in infarcted brain is associated with non-neuronal metabolic activity [15]. Thus, the clinical observation of altered oxygen/glucose stoichiometry in early cerebral infarction may reflect that of inflammatory cells rather than viable brain tissue.

Other PET studies in cerebrovascular disease have focused on the pathophysiologic changes in ischemic but uninfarcted brain [34]. Patients with occlusive disease of the major cerebral arteries have varied blood flow and metabolic abnormalities. Thus, some patients with adequate collateral circulation may demonstrate no abnormality of CBF, CBV, or oxygen extraction. Patients with compensated disease generally show increased CBV but normal flow on the basis of vasodilation distal to the stenotic lesion. Patients with recurrent ischemic symptoms who have inadequate compensatory reserve demonstrate normal oxygen metabolism but have a decreased CBF and increased CBV and oxygen extraction. The latter parameter appears to be the most sensitive and specific marker for inadequate perfusion to meet metabolic demands.

The findings in stroke as well as those in noninfarct cerebrovascular insufficiency suggest a continuum of pathologic alterations with physiologic compensation by vasodilation and collateral circulation. When the metabolic demands of the tissue can no longer be met by increasing the extraction of oxygen and glucose, infarction results. PET studies suggest that cerebral damage occurs rapidly and that possible interventive therapies must therefore be attempted before or soon after the onset of symptoms to be of potential benefit. The application of PET to future studies of cerebrovascular disease will focus on prospective monitoring to find changes occurring before or rapidly following onset of symptoms. Diagnostic probes that will distinguish reversible from irreversible ischemic changes and the potential effects of therapeutic intervention remain to be validated; however, encouraging preliminary results have been obtained in studies employing benzodiazepine receptor binding to distinguish infarcted brain from viable tissue, in which flow and metabolism are reversibly reduced as a result of diaschesis.

Neuropharmacologic characterization of Parkinsonian patients with PET reveals distinct subgroups of differing pathophysiology

Patients with the clinical syndrome of Parkinsonism including bradykinesia, resting tremor, and postural instability represent a heterogeneous diagnostic group, with a variety of underlying pathologies and distinct therapeutic response patterns. The postmortem pathologic abnormality recognized in Parkinson's disease (PD) is a reduction of striatal dopaminergic nerve terminals attributed to cell loss in the substantia nigra pars compacta (see Chap. 44). In this case, and in other situations where the presynaptic dopamine system is depleted with relative preservation of post-synaptic striatal elements, patients respond symptomatically to administration of the dopamine precursor L-DOPA and to direct dopamine receptor agonist drugs. A subset of Parkinsonian patients, however, do not benefit from these medications. It may be difficult to discriminate the presence or absence of initial therapeutic benefit, since early symptoms of the disease may be mild, and the possibility of placebo

responses cannot be discounted in consideration of subjective effects. In life, the neuropathologic bases of drug-resistant Parkinsonian syndromes are assumed to be intrinsic striatal pathology or other non-dopaminergic lesions. The availability of several PET ligands for evaluation of the dopaminergic synapse now permits definitive taxonomy of patients early in the course of illness with regard to the site(s) of neurochemical pathology. Presynaptic dopaminergic markers including dopamine reuptake sites [24], synaptic vesicles [25], and DOPA decarboxylase activity [18] may be determined with the tracers [^{11}C]nomifensine, [^{11}C]tetrabenazine, and [^{18}F]FDOPA, respectively. The dopamine D_2 receptor, predominantly a post-synaptic striatal marker, may be studied with a variety of radioligands, including [^{11}C]raclopride [35]. Studies with these tracers afford important verifications of postmortem measures, since symptomatic therapeutic trials are known to alter many of the biochemical markers of dopamine synapses.

Patients with typical PD have reduced DOPA decarboxylase activity in the putamen [36,37] and reduced presynaptic dopamine uptake sites [38] with preserved D_2 receptors in PET studies. Presynaptic markers are asymmetrically reduced in many early cases, in concordance with individual side-to-side asymmetries in clinical signs. Of particular interest, relatives of patients with history of familial PD may have reduced decarboxylase activity in the absence of clinical signs or symptoms [37]. This observation supports the hypothesis that PD pathology is present and progressive well in advance of its clinical diagnosis, and may reflect a lifelong accelerated loss of neurons or initial deficiency of substantia nigra neurons.

Other Parkinsonian syndromes that fail to respond fully to medications include progressive supranuclear palsy (PSP) and multiple system atrophy (MSA). In these instances, there are distinct patterns of dopaminergic marker losses that differ from each other and from PD [38]. Patients with PSP demonstrate loss of striatal D_2 receptors, indicating a post-synaptic striatal lesion. Patients with MSA and with PSP demonstrate loss of presynaptic dopamine terminals in the caudate nucleus as well as in the putamen, again, in distinction to the pattern seen in typical PD. These results may ultimately assist in elucidation of the pathologies in these various disorders, while at present they provide biochemical confirmation of their distinction.

ACKNOWLEDGMENTS

The author was supported in part by grants 5P01 NS15655 and 1R01 MH47611 from the National Institutes of Health and the National Institute of Mental Health, respectively, during the preparation of this chapter.

REFERENCES

1. Phelps, M. E., Mazziotta, J. C., and Schelbert, H. R., eds. *Positron Emission Tomography and Autoradiography. Principles and Applications for the Brain and Heart.* New York: Raven Press, 1986.
2. Sorenson, J. A., and Phelps, M. E. *Physics in Nuclear Medicine,* 2nd ed. New York: Grune and Stratton, 1987.
3. Jacquez, J. A. *Compartmental Analysis in Biology and Medicine,* 2nd ed. Ann Arbor: University of Michigan, 1985.
4. Brooks, D. J., Beaney, R. P., Lammertsma, A. A., et al. Quantitative measurement of blood-brain barrier permeability using Rubidium-82 and positron emission tomography. *J. Cereb. Blood Flow Metab.* 4:535–545, 1984.
5. Hawkins, R. A., Phelps, M. E., Huang, S.-C., et al. A kinetic evaluation of blood-brain barrier permeability in human brain tumors with [^{68}Ga]EDTA and positron computed tomography. *J. Cereb. Blood Flow Metab.* 4:507–515, 1984.
6. Huang, S.-C., Carson, R. E., Hoffman, E. J., et al. Quantitative measurement of local cerebral blood flow in humans by positron computed tomography and ^{15}O-water. *J. Cereb. Blood Flow. Metab.* 3:141–153, 1983.
7. Herscovitch, P., Markham, J., and Raichle, M. E. Brain blood flow measured with intravenous H$_2$^{15}O. I. Theory and error analysis. *J. Nucl. Med.* 24:782–789, 1983.
8. Sokoloff, L., Reivich, M., Kennedy, C., et al. The [^{14}C]deoxyglucose method for the measurement of local cerebral glucose utilization: theory, procedure, and normal values in the conscious and anesthetized albino rat. *J. Neurochem.* 28:897–916, 1977.
9. Reivich, M., Kuhl, D., Wolf, A., et al. The [^{18}F]fluorodeoxyglucose method for the measurement of local cerebral glucose utilization in man. *Circ. Res.* 44:127–137, 1979.
10. Phelps, M. E., Huang, S.-C., Hoffman, E. J., et al. Tomographic measurement of local cerebral glucose metabolic rate in humans with (F-18)2-fluoro-2-deoxy-D-glucose: validation of method. *Ann. Neurol.* 6:371–388, 1979.
11. Hawkins, R. A., Phelps, M.E., Huang, S.-C., and Kuhl, D. E. Effect of ischemia on quantification of local cerebral glucose metabolic rate in man. *J. Cereb. Blood Flow Metab.* 1:37–51, 1981.
12. Crane, P. D., Pardridge, W. M., Braun, L. D., and Oldendorf, W. H. Kinetics of transport and phosphorylation of 2-fluoro-2-deoxy-D-glucose in rat brain. *J. Neurochem.* 40:160–167, 1983.
13. Heiss, W.-D., Pawlik, G., Herholz, K., et al. Regional kinetic constants and cerebral metabolic rate for glucose in normal human volunteers determined by dynamic positron emission tomography of [^{18}F]2-fluoro-2-deoxy-D-glucose. *J. Cereb. Blood Flow Metab.* 4:212–223, 1984.
14. Sokoloff, L. Localization of functional activity in the central nervous system by measurement of glucose utilization with radioactive deoxyglucose. *J. Cereb. Blood Flow Metab.* 1: 7–36, 1981.
15. Agranoff, B. W., and Frey, K. A. A regional metabolic contrast method for the study of brain pathology. *Ann. Neurol.* 15:S93–S97, 1984.
16. Frackowiack, R. S., Lenzi, G.-L., Jones, T., and Heather, J. D. Quantitative measurement of regional cerebral blood flow and oxygen metabolism in man using ^{15}O and positron emission tomography: Theory, procedure, and normal values. *J. Comp. Assist. Tomogr.* 4: 727–736, 1980.
17. Mintun, M. A., Raichle, M. E., Martin, W. R.

W., and Herscovitch, P. Brain oxygen utilization measured with O-15 radiotracers and positron emission tomography. *J. Nucl. Med.* 25:177–187, 1984.

18. Gjedde, A., Reith, J., Dyve, S., et al. DOPA decarboxylase activity of the living human brain. *Proc. Natl. Acad. Sci. U.S.A.* 88: 2721–2725, 1991.

19. Diksic, M., Nagahiro, S., Chaly, T., Sourkes, T. L., Yamamoto, L., and Feindel, W. Serotonin synthesis rate measured in living dog brain by positron tomography. *J. Neurochem.* 56:153–162, 1991.

20. Frey, K. A., Hichwa, R. D., Ehrenkaufer, R. L. E., and Agranoff, B. W. Quantitative *in vivo* receptor binding III: tracer kinetic modeling of muscarinic cholinergic receptor binding. *Proc. Natl. Acad. Sci. U.S.A.* 82:6711–6715, 1985.

21. Frey, K. A., Koeppe, R. A., Mulholland, G. K., et al. In vivo muscarinic cholinergic receptor imaging with [^{11}C]scopolamine and positron emission tomography. *J. Cereb. Blood Flow Metab.* 12:147–154, 1992.

22. Frey, K. A., Holthoff, V. A., Koeppe, R. A., et al. Parametric in vivo imaging of benzodiazepine receptor distribution in human brain. *Ann. Neurol.* 30:663–672, 1991.

23. Fowler, J. S., MacGregor, R. R., Wolf, A. P., et al. Mapping human brain monoamine oxidase A and B with ^{11}C-labeled suicide inactivators and PET. *Science* 235:481–485, 1987.

24. Salmon, E., Brooks, D. J., Leenders, K. L., et al. A two-compartment description and kinetic procedure for measuring regional cerebral [^{11}C]nomifensine uptake using positron emission tomography. *J. Cereb. Blood Flow Metab.* 10:307–316, 1990.

25. Kilbourn, M. R., DaSilva, J. N., Frey, K. A., Koeppe, R. A., and Kuhl, D. E. In vivo imaging of vesicular monoamine transporters in human brain using [^{11}C]tetrabenazine and positron emission tomography. *J. Neurochem.* 60:2315–2318, 1993.

26. Kuhl, D. E., Engel, J., Jr., Phelps, M. E., and Selin, C. Epileptic patterns of cerebral metabolism and perfusion in humans determined by emission computed tomography of ^{18}FDG and ^{13}NH$_3$. *Ann. Neurol.* 8:348–360, 1980.

27. Engel, J., Jr., Brown, W. J., Kuhl, D. E., et al. Pathological findings underlying focal temporal lobe hypometabolism in partial epilepsy. *Ann. Neurol.* 12:518–528, 1982.

28. Abou-Khalil, B. W., Siegel, G. J., Hichwa, R. D., Sackellares, J. C., and Gilman, S. Topography of glucose metabolism in epilepsy of mesial temporal origin. *Ann. Neurol.* 18:151, 1985.

29. Frost, J. J., Mayberg, H. S., Fisher, R. S., et al. Mu-opiate receptors measured by positron emission tomography are increased in temporal lobe epilepsy. *Ann. Neurol.* 23:231–237, 1988.

30. Henry, T. R., Frey, K. A., Sackellares, J. C., et al. *In vivo* cerebral metabolism and central benzodiazepine receptor binding in temporal lobe epilepsy. *Neurology* [*in press*], 1993.

31. Kuhl, D. E., Phelps, M. E., Kowell, A. P., et al. Effects of stroke on local cerebral metabolism and perfusion: mapping by emission computed tomography of ^{18}FDG and ^{13}NH$_3$. *Ann. Neurol.* 8:47–60, 1980.

32. Wise, R. J. S., Bernardi, S., Frackowiak, R. S. J., et al. Serial observations on the pathophysiology of acute stroke. The transition from ischaemia to infarction as reflected in regional oxygen extraction. *Brain* 106:197–222, 1983.

33. Wise, R. J. S., Rhodes, C. G., Gibbs, J. M., et al. Disturbance of oxidative metabolism of glucose in recent human cerebral infarcts. *Ann. Neurol.* 14:627–637, 1983.

34. Powers, W. J., Press, G. A., Grubb, R. L., et al. The effect of hemodynamically significant carotid artery disease on the hemodynamic status of the cerebral circulation. *Ann. Intern. Med.* 106:27–35, 1987.

35. Farde, L., Eriksson, L., Blomquist, G., and Halldin, C. Kinetic analysis of central [^{11}C]raclopride binding to D$_2$-dopamine receptors studied by PET: a comparison to the equilibrium analysis. *J. Cereb. Blood Flow Metab.* 9:696–708, 1989.

36. Brooks, D. J., Ibanez, V., Swale, G., et al. Differing patterns of striatal ^{18}F-dopa uptake in Parkinson's disease, multiple system atrophy, and progressive supranuclear palsy. *Ann. Neurol.* 28:547–555, 1990.

37. Swale, G. V., Wroe, S. J., Lees, A. J., et al. The identification of presymptomatic Parkinsonism: clinical and [^{18}F]Dopa positron emission tomography studies in an Irish kindred. *Ann. Neurol.* 32:609–617, 1992.

38. Brooks, D. J. Positron emission tomographic studies of subcortical degenerations and dystonia. *Semin. Neurol.* 9:351–359, 1989.

PART SIX

Behavioral Neurochemistry

CHAPTER 47

Biochemical Aspects of the Psychotic Disorders

JACK D. BARCHAS, KYM F. FAULL, BRUCE QUINN, AND GLEN R. ELLIOTT

Basic Neurochemistry: Molecular, Cellular, and Medical Aspects, 5th Ed., edited by G. J. Siegel et al. Published by Raven Press, Ltd., New York, 1994. Correspondence to Jack D. Barchas, Department of Psychiatry, Cornell University Medical College, 525 East 68th Street, New York, New York 10021.

Psychosis is a term that has several distinct meanings in the mental health field: It can indicate that a mental illness is especially severe; alternatively, it can signify that a patient is unable to differentiate reliably between objective reality and subjective experience; or it can mean that a patient has a constellation of symptoms, including impaired reality testing, illogical thought processes, hallucinations, and delusions [1]. In this chapter, we discuss mental disorders encompassed by the last definition, bearing in mind that psychotic disorders have many different forms and a variety of causes.

Psychotic disorders impose a crushing disability on humankind, a burden that would be even greater were it not for the discovery more than 30 years ago of remarkably effective medications that have relieved many of the signs and symptoms. Unfortunately, many individuals still do not benefit from the presently available pharmaceutical agents, and there remains the problem of undesirable side effects. Furthermore, the causes of most psychoses are still poorly understood.

A few psychotic disorders have known specific causes. Psychosis may be a feature of a known organic disease, such as renal or hepatic failure, in which case the patient's mental disturbance is recognized to be metabolic in nature and usually can be normalized if the underlying disease is treatable. Other patients may present with a psychotic disorder, and an unsuspected disease process, such as a brain tumor or severe hor-

monal imbalance, must be ruled out before the diagnosis of schizophrenia is clear. Certain toxic chemicals or drugs of abuse, such as amphetamine, lysergic acid diethylamide (LSD), and phencyclidine (PCP) that are known to affect the brain, and some prescription drugs including steroids, have also been associated with psychotic reactions. For psychiatrists and other physicians, all of these causes may constitute the "differential diagnosis" of schizophrenia. The most common psychotic disorders, however, have no known cause. In this chapter, we focus on two diagnostic categories: (a) schizophrenia, a disorder that occurs mainly in adults; and (b) autistic disorder, which typically begins during infancy. Other important psychotic disorders include certain paranoid states and the schizoaffective disorders, which combine aspects of schizophrenia with affective disorders. (As described in Chapter 48 on affective disorders, both depression and mania may also present with psychosis.)

Throughout this chapter, schizophrenia and autism are presented as single entities. In each instance the syndromes may actually include a number of disorders involving different etiologies with a common clinical expression. Thus, some of the disparities and conflicts in the literature may be due to the possibility that the studies have been conducted on a set of related disorders rather than on a single illness. Further biological and clinical investigation will help to resolve this issue.

CLINICAL ASPECTS OF SCHIZOPHRENIA

Schizophrenia is a disorder that usually first appears during adolescence and affects perception, thought, language, and behavior

Typically, the signs and symptoms of schizophrenia first appear in individuals between the ages of 15 and 35 years. The form of presentation is variable. In some, it starts with a progressive withdrawal and increased introversion. They may begin to lose contact with friends, cease to have goals, and lose interest in prior pursuits that seemed reasonable and appropriate. Only gradually do others become aware that these individuals are also hearing voices and having delusions. With time they become increasingly difficult to understand because of bizarre, illogical thinking. In other cases, the onset of the disorder can be sudden, often following stress, such as the loss of a significant relationship, a transition in school, or entrance into military service. Cases that arise quickly often present a picture of overwhelming deterioration over the course of just a few days.

Hallucinations refer to perception of nonexistent incoming sensory information, for example, hearing voices when no one is there. While many people associate hallucinations with schizophrenia, these do not occur exclusively in schizophrenia, nor is their presence a requirement for the diagnosis. Hallucinations are usually intermittent, and they are characteristically perceived by the patient as coming from the outside world. Auditory hallucinations are by far the most common type in schizophrenia, usually in the form of voices talking to or about the individual, but hallucinations can be manifested by any of the senses.

Delusions are another common component of schizophrenia. They are perhaps the most romanticized aspect of this disorder, forming the basis for many movie thrillers. Delusions, too, are varied but entail an unshakable belief in something that is improbable or impossible, even in the face of strong contrary evidence. Typical delusions include belief in the possession of magical powers, or manipulation by others for complex but improbable reasons, or having a special destiny or purpose. For instance, an individual may become convinced that he can read the minds of those around him, or that others are reading his mind; or, a patient may insist that she is receiving messages through television commercials, affirming she is going to be the savior of the world. Although some delusions can be gratifying, many are frightening for the patients.

There are also strong emotional and cognitive changes associated with the schizophrenic state. Most common is a growing sense of confusion and uncertainty about the most routine matters. While schizophrenics may experience a wide range of intense emotions, such as depression, elation, or anger, most actually have emotional "blunting," a term that refers to a reduced ability to feel and express emotion. As a result, they seem distant. Furthermore, the ability of such individuals to think logically and convey their thoughts meaningfully can become so impaired that they become increasingly unable to make themselves understood and behave in bizarre and inappropriate ways, even as they become convinced that they hold the keys to vital eternal truths. These latter difficulties arise from disorders of thought, language, and communication. Rather than reflecting a "split" personality, schizophrenia may better be described as a "fractured" personality.

The possible signs and symptoms of schizophrenia are so numerous and disparate that it is unlikely that all come from a single causal factor. Therefore, researchers have attempted to identify clusters of related symptoms. The most common subtypes of the syndrome are defined on the basis of the most prominent symptoms: paranoid, catatonic, disorganized or hebephrenic, undifferentiated, and residual state. The paranoid form tends to start later in life and has a relatively good prognosis, with the personality reasonably intact. The catatonic type is rare, having stereotyped movements and a poor prognosis. The disorganized hebephrenic form is associated with incoherence of speech and silly giggling and also has a poor prognosis. Undifferentiated patients, who account for the majority, have a combination of symptoms. The residual state refers to the patient with no active delusions or hallucinations, but with a history of them and continued marked social dysfunction and strange behavior. There is no suggestion from genetic studies that specific forms of the disorder are transmitted within a family.

Particular attention recently has turned to the differentiation between type I and type II symptoms [2]. Type I, or positive, symptoms include delusions, hallucinations, and thought disorder; type II, or negative, symptoms include affective flattening, apathy, and poverty of speech. One distinguishing feature between these types is that the former are far more likely to respond to available drug treatments than are the latter. For reasons described later in this chapter, researchers have postulated that type I symptoms are associated with changes in dopamine functioning in the mesolimbic system and that type II symptoms may result from intellectual impairment caused by structural changes in the brain.

The long-term course of schizophrenia varies. Some patients have only one or a few acute episodes. The hallucinations and delusions that occur in the acute phase tend to disappear, and recovery may be complete. In other patients, acute episodes recur, and in still others, symptoms linger in a chronic condition. It is now clear that the more episodes an individual has, the greater the likelihood of lasting, unfavorable changes. Such changes may be as subtle as a loss of enthusiasm and emotional responsiveness or as pronounced as deteriorated social skills and a complete loss of ambition.

Over the past decade, increasing diagnostic rigor has tended to identify a group of individuals who have many signs and symptoms of schizophrenia and are quite ill;

only about 20 percent of them will have a good outcome. However, if less stringent criteria of psychosis are used to include other patients who have brief lapses in reality testing and transient hallucinations or delusions, the number of individuals diagnosed as having schizophrenia increases, and the general overall outcome for this larger population appears improved. As a rule, the greater the extent of psychosocial integration prior to a psychotic episode, the greater the likelihood of a good outcome after a diagnosis of schizophrenia.

The clinical definition of schizophrenia has changed, becoming increasingly restrictive

The interpretation of what schizophrenia "is" has taken many forms over the past century. A few decades ago, American psychiatry used a broad definition. Often, the disorder was diagnosed on the basis of a loosening of associations, a blunting of affect, isolated or withdrawn behavior, and ambivalence, particularly when those symptoms were seen with hallucinations. Now, the American definition, as described in the *Diagnostic and Statistical Manual,* Fourth Edition (DSM-IV) of the American Psychiatric Association, is much more specific and restrictive [3]. The illness must have been present continuously for at least 6 months, and patients cannot have had manic or depressive symptoms. Using the current definition, perhaps only 10 percent of the persons who a few decades ago were classified as schizophrenic would be so classified now. This definition is now narrower than that used in Europe—an important consideration when comparing clinical studies from different countries.

A benefit of the current American definition is that it tends to identify a group of severely ill individuals, most of whom will have a progressively debilitating disorder; however, there are disadvantages, too. Many significantly disturbed individuals are not included, even though they have clear psychotic symptoms. Rather than receiving a diagnosis of schizophrenia, these individuals may be given diagnoses such as schizoaffective disorder or schizophreniform or schizotypal personality [3]. Unlike schizophrenia, the neurochemical basis of these disorders has received relatively little attention. Unfortunately, the definition of schizophrenia found in DSM-IV is of necessity based on broad observational data rather than on an etiological principle. It remains uncertain whether such diagnostic criteria, when applied to a large and diverse group of psychiatrically disturbed individuals, can yet identify a group of patients sufficiently uniform that a scientist can search for one or more causal agents for their illness.

There is evidence for genetic factors in the disorder

Inheritance studies have been critical for adding new dimensions to the study of the illness, which had been viewed in terms of psychoanalytic and family interaction theories (e.g., poor social interaction between parent and child, the so called "doublebind" hypothesis). While psychosocial aspects may be important in relapses and other features of the illness, epidemiological investigations have shown the frequency with which schizophrenia occurs in underdeveloped countries is roughly the same as that in the most urbanized societies. It affects males and females about equally, although males tend to have an earlier age of onset. The lifetime prevalence rate of schizophrenia is about 1 percent.

Several studies suggest that genetic factors play a role in schizophrenia [4]. The incidence of the disorder in the parents of schizophrenics is about 4 percent, that in their siblings is about 8 percent, and that in their children, about 12 percent. If both parents are schizophrenic, the chance of an offspring being schizophrenic is about 40 percent. Studies reveal markedly differing rates of twins having schizophrenia, depending on whether they are identical (monozygotic), with a rate of 15–65 (mean 38) percent, or nonidentical (dizygotic), with a rate of 3–10

(mean 6) percent. This seems to be true whether or not the twins were raised in the same household or separately. Note that the genetic studies also suggest the presence of important nongenetic factors: About half of those who have an identical twin with schizophrenia are not themselves schizophrenic. Another approach to the study of genetic processes takes advantage of known physiological alterations in schizophrenics. For example, it has been found that a substantial number of schizophrenics and members of their families have changes in eye tracking. This finding raises the possibility of a generalized (and perhaps subtle) alteration that may be differentially expressed in some individuals, resulting in schizophrenia.

The search for genetic markers of the disease has attracted interest. Attempts have been made to identify genetic markers based on random restriction fragment-length polymorphisms (RFLPs) found on all chromosomes of the human genome. This method is dependent on accurate identification of all affected and unaffected members in many families. The poorly understood environmental and psychosocial influences on the presentation, course, and outcome of schizophrenia greatly complicate efforts to diagnose all probands of affected families. Despite these difficulties a number of studies have used RFLPs including both British and Icelandic families that contain many members with the disease. Early reports that chromosome 5 was implicated as a primary locus for a schizophrenia gene have not been confirmed, and in spite of hopes for the RFLP approach, it now seems that most populations that have a genetic predisposition do not map to this locus. It is nonetheless relevant that enough large studies of this type, if based on accurate diagnoses, can statistically rule out the existence of single chromosome predominance in the disease. It is now believed that schizophrenia probably results from a number of genetic abnormalities, most of which probably have a minor influence on the outcome of the disease [4]. Such a multifactorial mode of inheritance places into question the value of the RFLP approach for further investigating the genetic basis of this disease, although some such studies are still ongoing.

Brain morphology may be altered in some patients with schizophrenia

Two separate questions must be asked in assessing structural studies—both microscopic (postmortem) and neuroimaging studies in live subjects—in schizophrenia. The first is whether some, many, or most schizophrenics have structural brain abnormalities. The second is whether all schizophrenics have the same abnormalities. These questions have haunted the study of the schizophrenic brain by neuroanatomists and neuropsychiatrists since the 1890s, and indeed, results have been so uncertain that schizophrenia has been called "the graveyard of neuropathologists" [5]. (One author has wryly questioned whether it might become the graveyard of molecular biologists as well.) Studies in the first half of this century used the techniques of traditional autopsy neuropathology, such as light microscopy and various stains, and reported a variety of abnormalities in the schizophrenic brain, particularly subtle neuronal alterations and gliosis of limbic regions and the basal ganglia. This approach was largely abandoned by 1950, leaving behind a little-cited body of positive and negative studies.

A parsimonious interpretation of anatomic findings over the past 5 to 10 years would be that many, though probably not all, patients meeting the DSM-III-R diagnosis of schizophrenia have certain structural brain abnormalities. Neuroanatomists have been steadily collecting both qualitative and quantitative data on specific microscopic neuroanatomical defects in schizophrenia. These include disarray in the normally orderly pattern of hippocampal pyramidal neurons and disturbances in the neuronal islands that normally appear in the cortical regions near the hippocampus, as well as changes in hippocampal shape [5,6]. Abnormal numbers

of neurons appear to be arrested during migration, residing in the white matter of both frontal and temporal lobes [7]. These findings have been most consistent in the brains of patients who showed florid symptoms of the disease, and point to involvement of the temporal lobe and hippocampus. Such findings support a recurring postulate, that schizophrenia is associated with a neurogenetic or extrinsic insult, such as a viral infection, to the developing brain. Such an insult is believed to become manifest as a result of reduction in cortical synaptic density and/or changes in myelination patterns, which normally continue to mature well into adolescence.

Computerized tomography (CT) and magnetic resonance imaging (MRI) are now being used by a growing number of researchers to investigate the anatomical structure of the brains of living patients. These studies have begun to yield new insights into the dysmorphology and pathophysiology of schizophrenia. For example, ventricular and sulcal enlargement, hitherto not apparent until the advent of *in vivo* imaging techniques, have now been widely reported from CT studies, and current evidence suggests that these findings are relatively nonprogressive in nature [8]. Enlarged ventricles are thought to be the reciprocal image of losses in mass of brain tissue.

Increasingly sophisticated measurement technologies have been developed to allow complex three-dimensional analysis using high-resolution magnetic resonance imaging MRI. Some investigations with MRI have revealed widespread selective cortical gray matter loss, without white matter loss, in patients with the disease; other studies have suggested that there is a stronger tendency for the left temporal lobe and hippocampus to be reduced in size [9]. A crucial and unsettled question arising from this finding concerns whether or not this loss of gray tissue is an active or ongoing process, or whether it is the result of some prior event—in early development or adolescence—which caused a shift in gray/white matter distribution without continued progressive alterations in later life. It is likely that these questions will be addressed during the next few years by multi-modality studies, integrating *in vivo* structural changes (MRI and CT) studied over the disease course, *in vivo* functional studies of regional cerebral metabolism provided by positron emission tomography (PET) (discussed later in this chapter), and by postmortem anatomical findings such as regional neuronal abnormalities or gliosis.

The psychosocial environment strongly affects the expression and remission rate of schizophrenia

A variety of social processes have been studied in relation to schizophrenia. Because there is no evidence that social status per se is a major factor in the onset of the disorder, it is assumed that the downward social spiraling of the patients may be the result of decreased levels of social support or opportunities, with the observed high rates of the syndrome being found in the lowest socioeconomic group.

Information about such social factors is of more than merely theoretical interest. For instance, studies of "expressed emotion" led to the realization that individuals with schizophrenia are especially affected by the expression of negative emotion from significant others [10]. When the families of schizophrenics communicate with less negatively expressed emotion, patients tend to have lower rates of relapse. It has now been shown that families can be trained to communicate in this fashion, with consequent improvements in the functioning of many patients. Marked improvements in the psychosocial rehabilitation of schizophrenic patients, often an ignored factor, can greatly enhance the daily functioning and decrease relapses of this patient population. Evidence suggests that the best treatment today for many patients involves supportive psychosocial treatment together with the use of appropriate medications.

Neuroleptic drugs are an important treatment for schizophrenia, but they are associated with serious side effects, including tardive dyskinesia

Contemporary treatment for schizophrenia began in the early 1950s, when largely by serendipity it was found that chlorpromazine (see Fig. 1) had clinically useful effects on patients with schizophrenia [1]. It became the first of a class of agents that were termed neuroleptics, or antipsychotics. Haloperidol is probably the prototypical example of this class of drugs, of which many are in clinical use today. This group of drugs is also referred to as major tranquilizers; however, their pharmacological profiles bear no resemblance to "minor tranquilizers," a term reserved for antianxiety agents such as the benzodiazepines. Several different subclasses of antipsychotic drugs have now been developed, all of which share many behavioral and neurochemical effects on humans and animals. Research has detailed the abil-

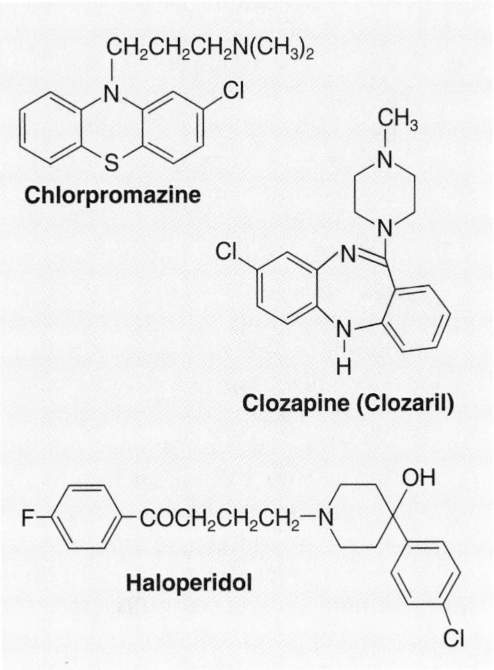

FIG. 1. Structures of some drugs used in the treatment of the psychotic disorders.

ity of these drugs to relieve symptoms of the acute phase of schizophrenia and to decrease the incidence of relapse. These drugs are especially effective against the positive symptoms of schizophrenia, including thought disorder, delusions, and hallucinations.

Unfortunately, antipsychotic drugs generally share a range of side effects, including those that mimic Parkinson's disease (see Chap. 44), including muscle tremors, rigidity, and spasms. The most worrisome side effect of the antipsychotics is tardive dyskinesia, which usually is associated with longstanding drug treatment. The syndrome includes smacking or sucking movements of the lips and tongue; irregular, involuntary movements may extend to the face and limbs. The movements are associated with supersensitivity of post-synaptic nigrostriatal dopamine receptors (see Chap. 12), but may or may not remit after discontinuation of the neuroleptic. For unknown reasons, only about 20 to 40 percent of patients taking antipsychotic medications develop tardive dyskinesia. Although there is some correlation with total lifetime antipsychotic dose, there is also evidence that some individuals with schizophrenia who have never received antipsychotic drugs may have similar movement disorders—perhaps a clue to one aspect of the disorder.

Recent developments in neuroleptic drug research have drawn attention to the so-called "atypical neuroleptics" of which clozapine is the prototypical example. Atypical neuroleptic treatment is associated with a low incidence of extrapyramidal side effects with a notable lack of tardive dyskinesia. Actually, clozapine was withdrawn from the market shortly after its introduction in the 1970s following several fatalities caused by drug-induced agranulocytosis. However, it has a distinctive receptor profile with high-affinity binding to the recently discovered D_4 dopamine receptor as well as with receptors to other neurotransmitters, and it has attracted attention to an important subgroup of schizophrenic patients—those with a history of drug-resistance, or poor response, to the classical neuroleptics. Clozapine appears to be effective in many of these otherwise unresponsive patients; it is now being reintroduced in many countries along with regular hematological monitoring of the patient [11].

DOPAMINE HYPOTHESIS OF SCHIZOPHRENIA

There are many approaches to the neurochemistry of schizophrenia

Although there is a wide range of approaches to the neurochemistry of schizophrenia, most currently focus on neuroregulators, compounds that may function as neurotransmitters or neuromodulators. Hypotheses frequently postulate the relative excess or deficiency of a neuroregulator or imbalances in two or more neurotransmitter systems.

Hypotheses can also be developed that take into account the susceptibility of schizophrenics to behavioral stress, with consideration of changes in the balance of neuroregulatory mechanisms, such as those involving dopamine. A number of other neuroregulatory systems show a variety of short- and long-term changes with stress and an alteration in formation, metabolism, and inactivation, or receptor actions could be related to subsequent behavioral processes.

Experimental approaches have included investigation of the concentrations of neuroregulators or their metabolites in brain and biological fluids such as blood, urine, and cerebrospinal fluid. Functional alteration of specific receptors that bind neuroregulators has also been under investigation in postmortem human brain, using receptor-specific *in vivo* PET imaging, and in experimental animal studies. Other studies consider metabolically defined systems that may be altered in schizophrenia, including the rate of glucose metabolism in the basal ganglia and in other cortical regions. The discovery of antipsychotics (discussed above) that could be used for treatment of schizophrenia, and of drugs that mimic aspects of it, has profoundly altered thinking about schizophrenia. Such new drugs, even when discovered serendipitously, become pharmacological tools of key importance in both basic and clinical neurochemical research.

The pharmacological effects of the antipsychotics formed the basis for a biochemical hypothesis that schizophrenia results from a relative excess of dopamine

This so-called dopamine hypothesis has been the dominant theoretical basis for research in this area over the past several decades. This hypothesis postulates that schizophrenia is the result of a relative overstimulation of the dopaminergic system, so that inhibition of dopaminergic processes by receptor blockade will be an effective means of treatment [12,13]. Its strongest support is the demonstrated fact that known antipsychotic agents all block dopamine receptors.

The effects of antipsychotics on the dopamine system were noted because some patients receiving antipsychotic agents had movements resembling those occurring in Parkinson's disease, which is thought to be caused by a relative deficiency in dopamine (see Chap. 44). The ability of antipsychotics to bind to post-synaptic dopamine receptors was demonstrated in *in vitro* receptor assays by their competition with radiolabeled dopamine for binding sites (see Chaps. 10 and 12). Potencies of the antipsychotics in these assays closely parallel their clinical efficacy. With the successful cloning of the dopamine receptor it is now recognized that there are at least five subtypes, most of which have a unique pharmacological profile [14]. The D_1 and D_5 receptors have been called the "D_1 family," while the D_2, D_3, and D_4 receptors together represent the "D_2 family." Careful studies using both gene expression techniques and autoradiographic receptor mapping should help us understand more about the complexity of the dopaminergic systems in the cortex, basal ganglia, and lim-

bic system. Both D_1 and D_2 receptors are found in the caudate-putamen and are synthesized by striatal neurons, whereas only D_2 receptors are synthesized in substantia nigra neurons as well. D_3 receptors are synthesized by neurons in the limbic system (nucleus accumbens). D_1 and D_4 receptors are synthesized by neurons in the frontal cortex and in the hippocampus, while D_5 receptors are synthesized in the hippocampus selectively. D_1, D_2, and D_4 receptors are all synthesized by neurons of the amygdala.

It has been suggested that a close physiological interaction exists between the dopaminergic system of the frontal cortex and that of the limbic system [12,13]. Low dopaminergic activity in the frontal cortex may be associated with hyperactivity of mesolimbic dopaminergic neurons [12]. The correlation between clinical efficacy and ligand affinity for the various subtypes is strongest for the D_2-subtype and accordingly much attention is now focused on this subtype in relation to schizophrenia [14]. However, the D_3 subtype is similar and also has strong affinity for antipsychotic drugs. Balancing the desired response, anti-psychotic effects, ameliorating the deficit or negative symptoms of schizophrenia, and avoiding tardive dyskinesia, may be a more achievable goal with selective pharmacological manipulation of the multiple dopamine receptors by site-selective medications. Clozapine, in binding to the D_4 and D_2 receptors, may point a way toward this goal.

In vivo, antipsychotics have a dramatic impact on the dopamine system. The acute effects include an acceleration of the turnover of dopamine, owing to a compensatory feedback process resulting from post-synaptic dopamine receptor blockade. Continued administration eventually results in re-establishment of an equilibrium during which the concentration of the major dopamine metabolite in cerebrospinal fluid (CSF), plasma, and urine slowly returns to baseline or slightly below baseline levels. Animal research has shown that the antipsychotics enhance the effects of drugs that inhibit dopamine synthesis (e.g., α-methyl-*para*-tyrosine) and they antagonize the effects of drugs such as the amphetamines, which stimulate dopamine release.

Despite its usefulness, the dopamine hypothesis has three serious limitations:

1. In almost all patients, the therapeutic effects of antipsychotic drugs occur some time after they actually act on receptors, implying either that there may be other critical components to the drug action or that dopamine overactivity is not the key biochemical defect in the disease.
2. The effects of antipsychotics on schizophrenia do not seem to differ from their effects on other psychoses, such as those from metabolic causes.
3. About 20% of patients with schizophrenia are resistant to antipsychotic drug therapy with traditional neuroleptics (although a significant proportion of these may respond to clozapine).

Each of these points underscores the view that no single dopamine system defect has yet emerged as the sole cause of schizophrenia.

Does direct evidence exist for alteration of a dopaminergic system in schizophrenia?

Direct testing of the dopamine hypothesis in patients is difficult [12,13]. One way to assess dopamine activity is to measure the concentration of dopamine metabolites in either lumbar CSF, plasma, or urine. Studies must allow at least 4 weeks, during which the patient is off medication, to obviate direct effects of antipsychotics on dopamine turnover. Homovanillic acid (HVA) is the quantitatively predominant dopamine metabolite and is the one most commonly measured in these studies, although some attention has been given to other metabolites, including 3,4-dihydroxyphenylacetic acid (DOPAC) and 3-methoxytyramine. About 40 to 50 percent of the HVA in lumbar CSF originates in the caudate, and presumably the ventral tegmental area, cortex, and spinal cord contribute to the remaining fraction. There is a gradient in the concentration of HVA from the brain to the lumbar space. Therefore, levels of HVA in the lumbar CSF may not adequately reflect changes in dopamine in areas of the brain where dopamine function is important for emotional behavior, e.g., the limbic centers and regions of cerebral cortex.

In light of the difficulties with measuring metabolites in CSF, it is not surprising that consistency among studies has been low. Seemingly minor differences in technique, including how samples are collected, the amount of physical activity the subject had prior to collection of the sample, and the emotional state of the subject during the interval of a few hours prior to collection, probably can affect results. In addition, as noted earlier, it remains unclear whether HVA concentrations in lumbar CSF are a valid index of dopamine activity in the brain areas of interest. HVA has also been measured in blood plasma, where a substantial fraction, perhaps as much as 25 to 40 percent, is derived from the brain. In addition to the problem of determining the source of the metabolite, certain foods that have precursors can result in alterations in plasma HVA. From the result of a large number of studies a clear picture of altered HVA concentrations in lumbar CSF or blood plasma of schizophrenics has not emerged.

Additional difficulties that face the design of experiments intended to detect neurochemical abnormalities in schizophrenic patients include patient selection, since subtypes or different illnesses might be included because of apparent clinical similarity. By necessity, most studies on drug-free patients have been done with mildly affected patients in which the degree of neurochemical abnormality may be quite subtle. Patients with overtly florid clinical symptoms in which the neurochemical pathology would be expected to be stronger are usually maintained on antipsychotic drugs to control their behavior, so that it is virtually impossible to investigate any aspect of their neurochemistry in the drug-free state.

Researchers have also attempted to investigate the dopamine system in tissue obtained at autopsy. Such postmortem studies are not without their own problems, among them accuracy of the diagnosis, which has to be determined retrospectively; the state of the patient at the time of death; changes during the terminal state that are unrelated to the psychiatric diagnosis; the effects of medications that are administered for other illnesses; the amount of antipsychotic given for psychiatric purposes; and problems consequent to the process of obtaining the tissue, including the interval between death and autopsy and the temperature of the specimen prior to autopsy. Again, the evidence to date has done little to elucidate changes in dopamine concentration or metabolites or in the relative activities of the enzymes involved in the formation of dopamine or other catecholamines.

Attention has also been focused on studies of receptor number and ligand affinity characteristics in the brains of individuals with schizophrenia [15,16]. These studies are also complicated by the fact that prior antipsychotic treatment almost certainly affects receptor binding. Still, this has been a prominent area of investigation, even though it has not been possible to ascertain with certainty if the noted increases in receptor density are primary or are due to treatment; however, a few studies in which brains have been obtained from persons who had been unmedicated for sustained periods of time also report an increase in D_2 receptor binding. Approaches using measurement of the mRNAs for the various proteins involved in neuroregulator function, including receptors, hold promise.

Positron emission tomography provides new approaches to the study of schizophrenia

Application of PET technology is providing the means of studying neurochemistry in living patients [15,16] (see also Chap. 46). By means of the fluoro-deoxyglucose method, evidence for a slight decrease in the metabolic activity of the frontal lobe in schizophrenia has been obtained [18]. The normal front-to-back gradient in glucose metabolic activity is maintained but to a lesser degree. These results suggest a more generalized disorder or one that reflects an alteration in one or more neuroregulator systems [17,18]. PET studies also allow the use of radiolabeled positron-emitting drugs to label specific neurotransmitter receptors in the living patient, using ligands such as ^{11}C-SCH 23390 for D_1 receptors and ^{11}C-raclopride for D_2 receptors. These studies also confirm that normal clinical doses of neuroleptic drugs do indeed occupy over 90% of the D_2 receptors in basal ganglia. One of the most exciting prospects is that integrated analysis of regional brain metabolic changes in schizophrenic patients, both untreated and treated with neuroleptics, and studies of regional receptor number in the living patient are already shaping current theories of the alterations in the dopamine systems in schizophrenia [12,13].

OTHER NEUROREGULATOR SYSTEMS IN SCHIZOPHRENIA

The glutamate-dopamine balance may be disrupted in schizophrenia

The basal ganglia and limbic system receive strong excitatory inputs from the cortical projection neurons containing the excitatory transmitter glutamate; they also receive strong input from the dopaminergic projection systems of the midbrain. The balance of the dopamine and glutamate systems, allowing for normal function, can be at different absolute levels of the neurotransmitters. Thus, after reserpine treatment the resulting hypodopaminergic animal can be "re-equilibrated" by administration of glutamate or *N*-methyl-D-aspartate (NMDA)-receptor blocking drugs. Carlsson and colleagues [see 19] have noted that deficiency or blockade of the glutaminergic system bears functional similarities to overstimulation of the dopaminergic system. By this reasoning, a deficiency of glutamate in schizophrenia might result in a relative hyperdopaminergic state, which would be responsive to drugs such as neuroleptics. Drugs that stimulate or block glutamate receptors may have side effects such as convulsions or hallucinations. Preliminary evidence of postmortem receptor levels in the frontal cortex and temporal lobe in schizophrenics supports an alteration in glutaminergic systems in schizophrenia, although to date no effective pro-glutaminergic drugs have been available to test this hypothesis directly.

Phencyclidine may provide a new model for the study of psychotic processes

An important new direction for fundamental research that may have direct relevance to mechanisms of psychosis centers on phencyclidine (PCP), a drug with hallucinogenic effects [20]. In some individuals, PCP induces a schizophrenic-like syndrome that may include catatonic motor behavior, dissociation, and hallucinations. The syndrome can be serious and may continue for a substantial period after drug administration; there is therefore interest in determining the mode of action of PCP.

At low doses PCP binds to a site on the Ca^{2+} channel associated with the glutaminergic NMDA receptor. At higher concentrations it may also bind to a benzomorphan- and antipsychotic-sensitive site, the sigma receptor. It is not known which site is most relevant for the action of PCP or whether either is responsible for the psychological effects of the drug, although available human dose-response studies would favor the more sensitive, channel-associated site. A hypothesis of special interest is that endogenous ligands may exist for the PCP or sigma receptor. If true, such a ligand or ligands would be of particular interest for schizophrenia-related research.

The study of hallucinogens and neuroleptics has suggested a role for serotonin in psychosis

Evidence relating serotonin to psychosis is viewed with continuing interest. A number of known hallucinogens, including LSD, bind serotonin receptors (see Chap. 13). LSD increases the concentration of brain serotonin and decreases the firing of serotonin-containing neurons in the midbrain. Further, methylated indoles chemically related to serotonin cause hallucinations, and these compounds also interfere with serotonin functioning. An effort to assess whether such methylated compounds are present endogenously in the brain has been limited by problems of the reliability in their identification. Even with substantial improvements in analytical techniques, there is still no convincing evidence that they are involved in any form of schizophrenia.

Aside from the issue of hallucinations, investigations of serotonin have also contributed to other aspects of the pathogenic mechanisms in schizophrenia. From measurements of CSF 5-hydroxyindoleacetic acid (5-HIAA) concentrations, it seems that relative decreases in CNS serotonin functions may be linked to positive symptoms while relative increases may be linked to deficit characteristics [21]. Postmortem studies of receptor neurochemistry have also been carried out. With the increased number of available pharmacological probes specific for the various serotonin receptor subtypes, it is anticipated that involvement of one or more of these in specific aspects of the clinical profile of the disease might emerge. Some atypical antipsychotics such as clozapine may act in part through serotonergic mechanisms [22]. The balance between dopamine and serotonin receptor binding (and other receptor binding) may be an important clue to the superior efficacy of the atypical drugs, and may also indicate that the disease is unlikely to be understood as a single lesion affecting only one neurotransmitter system. These observations reconfirm the idea that the interactions among several neurotransmitters systems are probably of crucial importance [12,18].

Neuropeptides may play a role in schizophrenia

Neuropeptides may act directly as transmitters or as modulators of neurotransmitter function and therefore play a key role as neuroregulators. Particularly important to concepts of neuropeptides in relation to schizophrenia has been the emerging view that a given nerve cell may produce several neuroregulators, and that biogenic amines and neuropeptides are often colocalized in the same nerve cells. For example, there is strong evidence that the peptide cholecystokinin (CCK) and dopamine coexist within some cells [13]; however, it has been difficult to obtain evidence relating the concentrations of peptides to various mental disorders. The same general problems of postmortem studies mentioned earlier apply, although neuropeptides may have one advantage in these studies in that they seem to be relatively stable in postmortem brain tissue and in CSF [23]. More importantly, in contrast to the catecholamines and serotonin, which are metabolized to single major products, neuropeptide turnover cannot be followed as easily, since their ultimate hydrolytic products cannot be distinguished from the cellular amino acid pool.

Studies of neuropeptide concentrations in schizophrenia have not yielded a consistent picture [24]. Another approach to the study of peptides has been administration of peptides or derivatives to patients. To be valid, such studies must be conducted in a double-blind fashion in which neither the patient nor the investigators know when the patient is receiving the active substance. Such studies are further complicated because it is unlikely that many peptides readily cross the blood-brain barrier, and the behavioral effects of most peptides are still unknown. These arguments do not, of course, rule out the possible effect of the peptides. For example, an administered peptide could

act either on peripheral receptors or on receptors at locations where the blood-brain barrier is more permeable. It does, however, strongly argue for the need for caution in interpreting any such reports.

Do endorphins play a role in schizophrenia?

Double-blind investigations have led to the observation that high doses of naloxone are effective in decreasing chronic hallucinations. The time course of the effect is surprising, for it lasts longer than would be expected on the basis of naloxone's pharmacokinetics; also, the effective dose is far higher than that needed simply to reverse the effects of an opiate overdose. Although this finding was initially given considerable attention, it remains unclear if the decrease in hallucinations is a result of changes in an endorphin system or if naloxone is acting on some other neurochemical process. The effects do not occur in all patients, and naloxone is not useful clinically as a treatment for auditory hallucinations because the duration of the effect is too short-lived. Still, the finding draws attention to a possible role for endorphins in schizophrenia [23,24].

A number of other studies suggest that patients with schizophrenia may have changes in the concentration of endorphins in the CSF (see Chap. 15). In earlier work with radioreceptor assays several researchers found increased concentrations of one or more "endorphin-like" fractions from the CSF. These promising results have been controversial because the radioreceptor method is nonspecific, and the nature of the active peptide fractions has never been clearly resolved. It is not yet known whether any CSF endorphins are abnormal in schizophrenia.

Still another approach to the study of endorphins in schizophrenia arose from earlier reports that patients with the disorder improved with hemodialysis. The apparent response was attributed to the removal of a specific opioid peptide from the plasma. Repeated studies over the past decade have failed to replicate the beneficial effects of hemodialysis; at this time, there is no evidence of an opioid peptide in plasma that is altered in schizophrenia.

A number of other peptides are under investigation in schizophrenia

Ongoing studies are dealing with many of the different neuropeptides that have now been identified in the CNS and are thought to be relevant as neuromodulators or neurotransmitters (see Chap. 16). For some, interesting hypotheses have been developed. For example, neurotensin has been shown to interact with the dopamine systems in the brain, and relative changes in neurotensin have been postulated in relation to schizophrenia. Similarly, there have been hypotheses of changes in CCK based on the colocalization of that neuropeptide with certain dopamine systems [13]. There have been reports of changes in one or another peptide in brain areas, but for none of the peptides is there the body of literature needed to establish a definitive role [23,24].

CHILDHOOD PSYCHOSES AND PERVASIVE DEVELOPMENTAL DISORDERS

Like adults, children are at risk for severe disturbances of mental function that usually are categorized as psychoses. However, gaining a better understanding of possible biological etiologies for such disorders is inhibited by at least three factors. First, the precise meaning of psychosis can become hard to characterize clinically when it occurs in the context of a developing organism, because children may not be able to provide the kinds of information about impaired thought processes, delusions, and hallucinations used to diagnose psychosis in an adult. Second, the prevalence of psychotic disorders appears to be lower in children than in adults, so it is not easy to gather adequate

clinical samples for research. And third, especially until quite recently, most of the research methodology available for studying biochemical processes in human beings were too invasive or too hazardous for use in children. Even so, some studies are available for at least two relevant childhood mental disorders.

Childhood schizophrenia is not thought to differ biologically from schizophrenia in adults

For well over a decade, the prevailing diagnostic system in the United States has not distinguished between adult and child forms of schizophrenia [3]. Although no good estimates of the prevalence of schizophrenia in childhood are available, it is thought to be considerably less than that in adults and probably does not exceed 1 to 2 in 10,000.

A key issue is how best to diagnose schizophrenia in ways that are sensitive to developmental processes, especially in young children. Toward that end, a few groups continue to attempt to describe the phenomenology of schizophrenia in the young [25]; such studies help to underscore both similarities and differences between childhood and adult presentations of this disorder. Also important are efforts to operationalize such concepts as formal thought disorder as they apply to the young [26].

Given the added problems of studying biological and physiological functions in children, it seems unlikely that investigators will turn to this population to explore biological factors in schizophrenia unless compelling hypotheses are advanced either that the disorder is substantively different in the young or that it can best be understood only by looking for early changes. Neither of these circumstances seems likely at present.

Autistic disorder is a major pervasive developmental disorder that affects young children

A second, more common set of disorders disrupt childhood functioning in a way that is at least comparable to the effect of schizophrenia on adults. These illnesses, collectively called *pervasive developmental disorders,* typically occur before 5 years of age, almost always afflict the individual for life, and have no known treatment. Though for many years they were confused with childhood-onset schizophrenia, they now are known to be a distinct disease process. In fact, they probably have more in common with severe developmental language disorders than with psychoses. A growing body of research is trying to uncover biological causes for these pervasive developmental disorders [27].

Autistic disorder is by the far most extensively and systematically studied of the pervasive developmental disorders [27]. In 1943, Kanner described a syndrome he called early infantile autism, to emphasize the striking failure of children with this disorder to develop emotional contact and social relationships. Early infantile autism was included as a diagnostic category in DSM-III in 1980 as one of the pervasive developmental disorders. The disorder was defined as 1) absent or markedly abnormal social relationships, 2) marked impairment in the production and content of language, and 3) bizarre interactions with the environment that occur in the absence of hallucinations or delusions and have an age of onset before $2\frac{1}{2}$ years. In 1987, DSM-III-R renamed the diagnosis autistic disorder and provided more detailed criteria that incorporated a developmental perspective; however, the essential features of the disorder remain the same. Moderate-to-profound mental retardation is common but not universal, and the overlap of these two syndromes complicates both the clinical picture and research efforts. A small fraction of those with autism have normal or even superior intelligence; rare individuals, independent of overall intelligence, have highly unusual skills in such areas as music or mathematics.

The social disability of autism is striking and pervasive. Most individuals with this diagnosis maintain minimal social contact with those around them. The most severely affected children never exhibit awareness that other children or adults are also living beings. As infants, many actively resist human contact and are most quickly soothed when left alone. With advancing age, they usually prefer to be alone and find even the most rudimentary social skills beyond their capabilities. Although adults with schizophrenia also may be socially inept, adults with autism convey more a sense of not understanding that they have anything in common with other members of the human race; in addition, hallucinations and delusions are not a part of the clinical picture of autism.

Communication abnormalities in autistic disorder range from severe expressive and receptive language deficits to quite functional but odd speech. Rarely, children with autism may lack any form of communication whatsoever, and the great majority have minimal or no functional spoken language. Oddly, about one-third initially seem to be developing normal speech, only to have language fail to progress or even disappear between ages 18 and 24 months. Those who do develop language skill nearly always have markedly unusual patterns of speech intonation, inflection, rhythm, and content. For example, flat or ''sing-song'' speech is quite common in autism, as is repetition of what is said and poor or no use of pronouns.

Perhaps the most striking signs of autistic disorder are the phenomena categorized as unusual or bizarre interactions with the environment. These behaviors cover a wide range of activities. Not uncommonly, children with autistic disorder engage in stereotypies, including body or head rocking, repetitively waving the fingers before the eyes, and incessantly twirling the whole body. Many also show a remarkable attentiveness to trivial detail and an absence of more common forms of interacting with objects. For example, parents may note that the child is fascinated with running water, the edges on objects, or shifting patterns of light and dark. Play characteristically is restricted to repetitively spinning wheels on toy vehicles or compulsively lining up blocks or similar objects in excruciatingly straight lines. Many of these children seem almost completely unaware of their surroundings and yet may be exquisitely sensitive to trivial changes in their physical environment. For example, they may go into a rage if a picture is moved from its accustomed place in their room or if a familiar route or routine is changed.

Evidence indicates that autism results from a biological process, probably one with many possible causes

Autistic disorder occurs at a rate of four to five per 10,000 in the general population and is at least four times more common in boys than in girls. First-degree relatives of children with autism have an increased prevalence of autism but not of schizophrenia. Furthermore, monozygotic twins are concordant for autism over half the time, far more frequently than are dizygotic twins [28].

Several approaches have been taken to explore possible etiological factors of autism. As with schizophrenia, such efforts are hindered by the wide range of presentations, which is consistent with the presence of subtypes of autism [29]. Nevertheless, some intriguing clues have emerged. For example, 8 to 10 percent of children exposed to the rubella virus during gestation are autistic, and *in utero* exposure to toxoplasmosis and congenital neurosyphilis also increases the risk of autism. In addition, autism is more common among individuals with phenylketonuria. It is important to emphasize that all of these are merely risk factors; the majority of individuals exposed to such factors never develop autism, and no causal mechanisms are known [27].

Efforts to identify a problem in either brain structure or function that is common to children with autism have had little success. To date, only five individuals with autism have been available for postmortem investigations that permitted anatomical studies of their brains [30]. Of that group, none had abnormalities in the cerebral cor-

tex but nearly all showed increased numbers of nerve cells and decreased nerve cell size in major portions of the limbic system, as well as some abnormalities in the cytoarchitecture of the cerebellum. The meaning of these findings, especially whether they are functionally relevant either in the etiology of autism or in its expression remains unclear. For example, four of the five subjects had seizures that were treated with anticonvulsants.

Investigators have used both CT and MRI to view aspects of brain anatomy in living subjects with autism. A few reports have suggested specific abnormalities in the left hemisphere or in subcortical structures; however, most concluded that this population has an increased incidence in such nonspecific abnormalities as ventricular enlargement and frontal lobe tissue defects, without evidence of consistent changes in brain structure [31]. Similarly, studies of brain electrophysiology have been inconclusive. Although about 25 percent of individuals with autism develop frank seizures by adolescence, no characteristic EEG patterns have been found. Abnormalities have been reported with sensory processing, but such research is greatly complicated by questions about the ability of autistic subjects to cooperate normally.

Despite evidence that autism involves a profound biological change, there are as yet no links to a specific neuroregulatory system

Compared with research on schizophrenia, relatively little is known about neuroregulatory activity in subjects with autistic disorder, and most of the studies that are available have been exploratory rather than hypothesis-oriented. Such research is especially difficult because of the problems of obtaining biological samples of any kind from children, hesitations about performing spinal taps on children for research purposes, and the unavailability of appropriate controls.

By far the most common neuroregulator studied in autistic disorder is serotonin, which was noted to be increased in the platelets of children with autism [32]. Numerous subsequent reports using appropriate age- and gender-matched controls have confirmed that one-third of subjects with autism have "hyperserotonemia," as do about one-half of nonautistic, severely retarded subjects. The cause of this relative elevation or its relationship, if any, to autism is unknown. In fact, it is doubtful that platelet serotonin is a useful indicator of central serotonin activity. A study of CSF 5-HIAA turnover, which indirectly measures serotonin activity by measuring how quickly its only metabolite is formed, concluded that autistic subjects may have a slight *decrease* in central serotonin activity, rather than an increase [33]. However, even if a clear and characteristic pattern of serotonin activity could be found in children with autism, no hypothesis has yet been offered to suggest a specific causal role in the disorder.

More recently, a study concluded that both whole-blood serotonin and plasma norepinephrine were inversely correlated with verbal IQ in a sample of autistic children and their first-degree relatives [34]. If true, it emphasizes the problems of attempting to focus exclusively on autism in the absence of a specific biological hypothesis; children with autism have many concomitant problems, including low IQ, poor language skills, odd behaviors, and a high incidence of seizures—any of which might lead to variations in neuroregulatory function.

A few studies have examined the possible role of opioid peptides in autism [35]. These substances are of particular interest because of their suggested role both in pain systems and in certain aspects of social behavior. Although episodic reports have described decreases in opioid-peptide substances in the blood or CSF of children with autism, the actual identity of the substance being measured is not known; however, the relevance of such research is underscored by recent reports that opiate antagonists such as naloxone and naltrexone may ameliorate certain signs and symptoms of autism [36].

Research on childhood psychoses and on pervasive developmental disorders remains inconclusive but underscores the importance of biological influences

Although the evidence that both schizophrenia and the pervasive developmental disorders are biological disorders continues to accumulate, the nature of the putative biological defects or even their possible anatomical locations remain unclear. The practical complications of applying existing research technologies to children have contributed to the problems researchers face. Furthermore, most existing research has taken a static view of the problem, with little attention to the peculiar features of a developing brain. An invigorating exception is an unusual study which found that, compared to controls, individuals with autistic disorder had lower levels of a neural cell adhesion molecule, which is thought to be involved in synaptic formation and turnover [37].

Rapid progress in less invasive methods of studying brain function offers considerable hope that additional information about normal and abnormal brain development will emerge over the next decade. Combined with improved methods of studying the clinical syndromes in children, such research efforts well may provide an understanding of these devastating disorders.

REFERENCES

1. Michaels, R. (ed.), *Psychiatry*. Philadelphia: Lippincott, 1992.
2. Crow, T. J. A current view of the Type II syndrome: age of onset, intellectual impairment, and the meaning of structural changes in the brain. *Br. J. Psychiatry* 155:15–20, 1989.
3. American Psychiatric Association. *Diagnostic and Statistical Manual*, 4th. Ed. Washington, DC: American Psychiatric Association, 1987.
4. Holzman, P. S., and Matthysse, S. Review: the

genetics of schizophrenia. *Psychol. Sci.* 1: 279–286, 1990.

5. Roberts, G. W., and Bruton, C. J. Notes from the graveyard: neuropathology and schizophrenia. *Neuropathol. Appl. Neurobiol.* 16:3–16, 1990.

6. Conrad, A. J., Trufat, A., Austin, R., Forsythe, S., and Scheibel, A. Hippocampal pyramidal cell disarray in schizophrenia as a bilateral phenomenon. *Arch. Gen. Psychiatry* 48: 413–417, 1991.

7. Akbarian, S., Vinuela, A., Kim, J. J., et al. Distorted distribution of nicotinamide-adenine dinucleotide phosphate-diaphorase neurons in temporal lobe of schizophrenics implies anomalous cortical development. *Arch. Gen. Psychiatry* 50:178–187, 1993.

8. Pfefferbaum, A., and Zipursky, R. B. Neuroimaging studies of schizophrenia. *Schizophr. Res.* 4:193–208, 1991.

9. Shenton, M. E., Kikinis, R., Jolesz, F. A., Pollak, S. D., LeMay, M. et al. Abnormalities of the left temporal lobe and thought disorder in schizophrenia. A quantitative magnetic resonance imaging study. *N. Engl. J. Med.* 327: 604–612, 1992.

10. Dawson, M., Liberman, R., and Mintz, L. Sociophysiology of expressed emotion in the course of schizophrenia. In P. Barchas (ed.), *Sociophysiology.* New York: Oxford Univ. Press, 1994 [in press].

11. Meltzer, H. Y. Treatment of the neuroleptic-nonresponsive schizophrenic patient. *Schizophr. Bull.* 18:515–542, 1992.

12. Davis, K. L., Kahn, R. S., Ko, G., and Davidson, M. Dopamine in schizophrenia: A review and reconceptualization. *Am. J. Psychiatry* 148: 1474–1486, 1991.

13. Goldstein, M., and Deutch, A. Y. Dopaminergic mechanisms in the pathogenesis of schizophrenia. *FASEB J.* 6:2413–2421, 1992.

14. Niznik, H. B., and Van Tol, H. H. M. Dopamine receptor genes: new tools for molecular psychiatry. *J. Psychiatry Neurosci.* 17:158–190, 1992.

15. Buchsbaum, M. S. The frontal lobes, basal ganglia, and temporal lobes as sites for schizophrenia. *Schizophr. Bull.* 16:379–389, 1990.

16. Seeman, P. Elevated D-2 in schizophrenia: role of endogenous dopamine and cerebellum. *Neuropsychopharmacology* 7:55–57, 1992.

17. Sedvall, G. The current status of PET scanning with respect to schizophrenia. *Neuropsychopharmacology* 7:41–54, 1992.

18. Roberts, G. W. Schizophrenia: the cellular biology of a functional psychosis. *Trends Neurosci.* 13:207–211, 1990.

19. Carlsson, M., and Carlsson, A. Interactions between glutaminergic and monoaminergic systems within the basal ganglia—implications for schizophrenia and Parkinson's disease. *Trends Neurosci.* 13:272–276, 1990.

20. Javitt, D. C., and Zukin, S. R. Recent advances in the phencyclidine model of schizophrenia. *Am. J. Psychiatry* 148:1301–1308, 1991.

21. Csernansky, J. G., Poscher, M., and Faull, K. F. Serotonin in schizophrenia. In E. F. Coccaro and D. L. Murphy (eds.), *Serotonin in Major Psychiatric Disorders.* Washington, D.C.: APA Press, 1990, pp. 211–230.

22. Gellman, R. L., and Aghajanian, G. K. 5-HT-2 receptor mediated excitation of interneurons in pyriform cortex: antagonism by atypical antipsychotic drugs. *Neuroscience* [*in press*] 1993.

23. Martin, J. B., and Barchas, J. D. (eds.), *Neuropeptides in Neurologic and Psychiatric Disease.* New York: Raven Press, 1986.

24. Nemeroff, C. B., Berger, P. H., and Bissette, G. Peptides in schizophrenia. In H. Y. Meltzer (ed.), *Psychopharmacology: A Third Generation of Progress.* New York: Raven Press, 1987, pp. 727–743.

25. Russell, A. T., Bott, L., and Sammons, C. The phenomenology of schizophrenia occurring in childhood. *J. Am. Acad. Child Adolesc. Psychiatry* 28:399–407, 1989.

26. Caplan, R., Guthrie, D., Fish, B., Tanguay, P. E., and David-Lando, G. The Kiddie Formal Thought Disorder Rating Scale: clinical assessment, reliability, and validity. *J. Am. Acad. Child Adolesc. Psychiatry* 28:408–416, 1989.

27. Schopler, E., and Mesibov, G. B. (eds.), *Neurobiological Issues in Autism.* New York: Plenum, 1987.

28. Ritvo, E. R., Freeman, B. J., Mason-Brothers, A., Mo, A., and Ritvo, A. M. Concordance for the syndrome of autism in 40 pairs of afflicted twins. *Am. J. Psychiatry* 142:74–78, 1985.

29. Siegel, B., Anders, T. R., Ciaranello, R. D., Bienenstock, B., and Kraemer, H. C. Empirically derived subclassification of the autistic syndrome. *J. Autism Dev. Disord.* 16:275–293, 1986.

30. Bauman, M. L. Microscopic neuroanatomic abnormalities in autism. *Pediatrics* 87: 791–796, 1991.

31. Piven, J., Nehme, E., Simon, J., Barta, P., Pearlson, G., and Folstein, S. E. Magnetic resonance imaging in autism: measurement of the cerebellum, pons, and fourth ventricle. *Biol. Psychiatry* 31:491–504, 1992.

32. Schain, R. J., and Freedman, D. X. Studies on 5-hydroxyindole metabolism in autistic and other mentally retarded children. *J. Pediatr.* 58:315–329, 1961.

33. Cohen, D. J., Caparulo, B. K., Shaywitz, B. A., and Bowers, M. B. Dopamine and serotonin metabolism in neuropsychiatrically disturbed children. *Arch. Gen. Psychiatry* 34:545–550, 1977.

34. Cook, E. H., Leventhal, B. L., Heller, W., Metz, J., Wainwright, M., and Freedman, D. X. Autistic children and their first-degree relatives: relationships between serotonin and norepinephrine levels and intelligence. *J. Neuropsychiatry Clin. Neurosci.* 2:268–274, 1990.

35. Sahley, T. L., and Panksepp, J. Brain opioids and autism: an updated analysis of possible linkages. *J. Autism Dev. Disord.* 17:201–216, 1987.

36. Zingarelli, G., Ellman, G., Hom, A., Wymore, M., Heidorn, S., and Chicz-DeMet, A. Clinical effects of naltrexone on autistic behavior. *Am. J. Ment. Retard.* 97:57–63, 1992.

37. Plioplys, A. V., Hemmens, S. E., and Regan, C. M. Expression of a neural cell adhesion molecule serum fragment is depressed in autism. *J. Neuropsychiatry Clin. Neurosci.* 2:413–417, 1990.

CHAPTER 48

Biochemical Hypotheses of Mood and Anxiety Disorders

JACK D. BARCHAS, MARK W. HAMBLIN, AND ROBERT C. MALENKA

Basic Neurochemistry: Molecular, Cellular, and Medical Aspects, 5th Ed., edited by G. J. Siegel et al. Published by Raven Press, Ltd., New York, 1994. Correspondence to Jack D. Barchas, Department of Psychiatry, Cornell University Medical College, 525 East 68th Street, New York, New York 10026.

The neurochemistry of psychiatric conditions has been a very active and fruitful field and, despite the limitations of current assumptions, biological hypotheses of mental disorders have been of enormous value in focusing research efforts on the link between psychiatry and the biological sciences. Many of these assumptions have come initially from clinical investigation of pharmacological agents that were developed by design or by serendipity and have proven beneficial. Studies of the mechanisms of action of such substances have provided important knowledge of the fundamental neurochemical processes of the brain.

The goal of research related to mental disorders has been to identify circumscribed but relevant biochemical mechanisms alteration of which is involved in clinical pathology and which may be targets for therapeutic intervention. For most conditions, progress has been exceedingly slow. For others, key neuroregulatory systems that may be involved are becoming clearer, and the knowledge thus gained offers the potential of direct therapeutic benefit. Two groups of illnesses representing the most common of all psychiatric conditions, the mood and anxiety disorders, are now moving into the latter category.

MOOD DISORDERS HAVE POWERFUL BIOLOGICAL CONCOMITANTS

Two major categories of mood disorders are depression and manic-depressive illness

Mood disorders refer to a group of mental illnesses characterized by disturbances of affect severe enough to alter cognition, judgment, and interpersonal relationships [1–4]. Appetite, energy level, and sleeping patterns can also be profoundly disturbed.

Everyone goes through periods of feeling sad, discouraged, lonely, or disappointed, but these feelings normally pass and do not impair day-to-day functioning. In contrast, patients with clinically significant depression undergo such profound changes in the way they perceive themselves and the world that their lives are greatly disrupted. The symptoms vary from patient to patient and not all have the same pattern. Typically, patients feel sad or empty, and attitudes may be marked by a sense of hopelessness and helplessness. Most depressed patients tend to express little interest or enjoyment in activities previously judged pleasurable. Patients frequently have fatigue; energy levels can plummet to the point where the simple act of speaking becomes slow and labored. A diminished ability to think or concentrate and indecisiveness often become apparent. Overwhelming feelings of worthlessness or excessive or inappropriate guilt may appear. Attempts at suicide are not uncommon.

In addition to alterations in mood and perception, a variety of basic physiological parameters are frequently altered in depression. Patients may gain or lose significant quantities of weight when not attempting diet alteration. Some individuals experience changes in circadian rhythms with great difficulty obtaining a normal night's sleep; others sleep 12 to 18 hr per day. Either agitation or retardation of movement may predominate. Physical symptoms, such as dizziness, headaches, backaches, tightness in the chest, or dry mouth, often accompany depression and can be the presenting complaint, masking the underlying psychiatric illness.

The changes that develop during depression disrupt interpersonal relationships and can exacerbate social losses that may be occurring in the life of the patient. Some depressions seem to be related to obvious social losses, others not. Nonetheless, depression can impact on all of the activities of the individual, including employment and the full range of social life.

With depression in its most extreme form, patients become psychotic. Such patients distort or misperceive reality, experience hallucinations, or develop bizarre beliefs and behaviors.

Patients who have only recurrent bouts of depression are said to have *unipolar* depression, whereas those having both depression and mania are considered to have *bipolar* disorder. Multiple combinations of these problems are seen. Many patients who experience one depressive episode will unfortunately suffer recurrences. Others will not only experience repeated depressions but will also have episodes of mania or near-mania (also called hypomania) interspersed among their depressions. A few patients experience intermittent bouts of mania without marked depressive episodes.

Although mania can be intuitively thought of as the opposite of depression, the two syndromes share several characteristics. Manic patients initially feel elated, carefree, overconfident, and euphoric. They often overestimate their attractiveness, intelligence, and abilities. They seem to have limitless energy and feel little need for sleep or sustenance. Some feel that they can literally conquer the world; however, euphoria often quickly changes to irritability and hostility. As in depression, cognition and judgment may become significantly impaired, leading to catastrophic consequences. In severe forms, psychosis develops. This is manifested by delusional beliefs of omnipotence and "flight of ideas"—the occurrence of thoughts so rapid and complex that verbalizations are difficult to follow.

Epidemiological studies have been extremely important in the study of depression [5] and have demonstrated that depression is found in a wide range of cultures. Recognition that the incidence is increasing in the cultures studied reinforces the concept that depression represents an interaction between biological and psychosocial processes. Depression impacts an enormous number of people: 3 to 4 percent of the population of the United States suffer from an affective disorder. The lifetime risk for having at least one major depressive episode is 10 to 15 percent in the general population. There are over 30,000 deaths by suicide each year in the United States, making it a leading cause of death. Understanding the pathophysiological mechanisms underlying mood disturbances is of the utmost importance.

What is the evidence that abnormal biochemical functioning in the brain is involved in the mood disorders?

The answer can be divided into two categories. The first derives from family and twin studies using epidemiological methods and studies of genetic markers [6]. These studies have indicated that mood disorders (a) cluster within families; (b) are most likely to occur in first-degree relatives of those with the disorder; and (c) are more prevalent among monozygotic than dizygotic twins. Manic-depressive illness has provided particularly strong evidence for genetic factors. However, to date it has not proved possible to demonstrate a specific gene or set of genes associated with these mental illnesses. There have been a number of reports that could not be replicated. Thus, while there is evidence for a genetic contribution to the mood disorders, the mode of genetic transmission remains unclear. It is expected that environmental factors must also play a critical etiological role.

The second line of evidence derives from the finding that a variety of pharmacological agents have substantial effects on mood and behavior [7,8]. A common assumption has been that if an agent modifies a psychiatric symptom for better or worse, then the drug's cellular or neurochemical action may be directly related to the biological dysfunction causing the symptom. This assumption may be flawed. The psychopharmacological agent may act at a site that is independent of the neurochemical abnormality causing the illness yet produce changes in brain function that compensate for the abnormality. Another common assumption underlying much of the work in this area is that many of the medications useful for the treatment of depression work via a common final mechanism; it is now known that there are several possible mechanisms. A related concept inherent in some approaches to the field has been that unipolar depression and bipolar disorder have the same underlying cause; however, clinical studies have shown that unipolar depression and bipolar disorder may each be divided into subtypes.

Patients with affective disorders vary greatly in their responses to medication. Some are markedly improved; others obtain minimal benefit. Some respond equally well to psychosocial treatments, and in many cases there appear to be substantial benefits from combining pharmacological, psycho-logical, and interpersonal treatments [9]. Much effort has gone into attempting to determine variables that predict or explain differences in medication responses among patients, thus far without success. It may be prudent to consider these diagnoses, like schizophrenia, as syndromes that may have a variety of biochemical causes. In terms of the effects of treatment, it is conceivable that different agents and approaches alleviate the symptoms of affective disorders via several distinct mechanisms.

MONOAMINE HYPOTHESES OF MOOD DISORDERS

Biogenic amines have been important in hypotheses of mood disorders

The catecholamine hypothesis of depression was an important organizing step that helped to define the modern study of biological research in psychiatry [10,11]. It states that depression is caused by a functional deficiency of catecholamines, particularly norepinephrine (NE), whereas mania is caused by a functional excess of catecholamines at critical synapses in the brain [7,8]. This hypothesis was based on the correlation of the psychological and cellular actions of a variety of psychotropic agents. Other biogenic amines in brain have also been linked to depression and mania with the development of what are termed monoamine or biogenic amine hypotheses. These amines have included the indolamine serotonin [5-hydroxytryptamine (5-HT)]; two catecholamines other than NE, dopamine (DA), and epinephrine; and the quarternary amine acetylcholine.

A number of strategies have been used in clinical studies to investigate the relationships between neuroregulators and mood disorders

Several alternative strategies have been used to examine the role of monoamines in the mood disorders. Precursor loading entails administering precursors of biogenic amines to subjects to raise monoamine levels in the brain. Administration of the serotonin precursors, L-tryptophan or 5-hydroxytryptophan (5-HTP), with or without concomitant antidepressant medication, or the catecholamine precursors, tyrosine or levodopa, have been attempted as therapeutic regimen. None of these compounds are in routine clinical use in mood disorders.

Another approach, primarily in manic patients, has been to administer inhibitors of enzymes involved in the formation of biogenic amines. In particular, studies have been undertaken of the effects of α-methyl-*para*-tyrosine (AMPT), a competitive inhibitor of tyrosine hydroxylase, which lowers levels of catecholamines, or *para*-chlorophenylalanine (PCPA), an inhibitor of tryptophan hydroxylase, which lowers levels of 5-HT. AMPT has been reported to improve mania in some patients and to worsen depression in some previously depressed patients. PCPA did not decrease symptoms in manic patients but has been found to reverse the antidepressant effects of imipramine, further suggesting a serotonergic role in the action of that antidepressant. These intriguing findings are the subject of ongoing research. The lack of consistency is probably due to a variety of factors, the most important being the assumed heterogeneity of disorders and subtypes subsumed under the diagnoses of depression and mania.

Another important strategy has involved studies of the metabolites of the neuroregulators with determination of their concentrations in cerebrospinal fluid (CSF), blood, or urine. There has generally been considerable inconsistency in such studies but this may reflect not only the fact that such methods involve a summation of many events in many areas of the brain, but also the difficulties inherent in fields in which the number of subjects is small, such that there may be substantial clinical heterogeneity, and possibly multiple disorders presenting with common symptoms. To glean any useful information

from metabolite studies it may be necessary to measure and compare a battery of monoamines and their metabolites rather than focus on single metabolite levels. Further, it will be critical to develop improved methods of studying different neuroregulator systems kinetically.

The catecholamine hypothesis remains an important model that attempts to explain the etiology of depression and mania

The norepinephrine-deficiency hypothesis of depression had several roots: One observation concerned the natural alkaloid reserpine. This drug had been used in India for centuries as a treatment for mental illness. Beginning in the 1950s, reserpine was used for the treatment of hypertension and schizophrenia. It was noted that in some patients, reserpine caused a syndrome resembling depression. Animals given reserpine also developed a depression-like syndrome consisting of sedation and motor retardation. Subsequently, it was demonstrated that reserpine caused the depletion of presynaptic stores of NE, 5-HT, and DA. While it is now recognized that depression is relatively uncommon following reserpine administration, the drug had a key role in the development of psychopharmacology and was a powerful impetus to the study of the biochemistry of neuroregulators in the brain.

In contrast to reserpine, iproniazid, a compound synthesized in the 1950s for the treatment of tuberculosis, was reported to produce euphoria and hyperactive behavior in some patients. It was found to increase brain concentrations of NE and 5-HT by inhibiting the metabolic enzyme, monoamine oxidase (MAO). Iproniazid as well as other monoamine oxidase inhibitors were soon shown to be effective in alleviating depression.

The clinical and cellular actions of tricyclic antidepressants such as amitriptyline were considered to support the monoamine hypothesis of mood disorders. These drugs, resulting from a modification of the phenothiazine nucleus, were found to alleviate depression consistently, like the MAO inhibitors. Their major cellular action is to block the reuptake by presynaptic terminals of monoamine transmitters, thereby, presumably, increasing the concentration of monoamines available to interact with synaptic receptors. Thus, the actions of reserpine, MAO inhibitors, and tricyclics were initially thought to be consistent in supporting the monoamine hypothesis.

Inconsistencies arose, however. The pharmacological activities of several other compounds are difficult to reconcile with the monoamine hypothesis. Several clinically effective antidepressant agents do not significantly inhibit MAO or block the reuptake of monoamines. The antimanic agent lithium (discussed below) can also be used to treat depression, yet does not chronically increase synaptic concentrations of monoamines. Conversely, cocaine, a potent inhibitor of monoamine reuptake, has no antidepressant activity.

More detailed examination of the actions of reserpine, MAO inhibitors, and tricyclics also reveals inconsistencies among their actions. Reserpine induces depression in only about 6 percent of patients, an incidence quite similar to the estimated incidence of depression in the general population. More important, the cellular effects of MAO inhibitors and tricyclic antidepressants on catecholamines are immediate, yet their clinical antidepressant effects develop quite slowly, generally over 2 to 6 weeks.

Attempts to measure directly changes in brain monoamine concentrations in the mood disorders have provided intriguing but inconsistent results. Initially, investigators concentrated on measuring 3-methoxy-4-hydroxyphenylglycol (MHPG), a catecholamine metabolite, in urine and CSF. Early evidence suggested that there were decreased urinary MHPG concentrations in depressed patients and increased levels in mania, but more recent reports do not bear this out. This is not entirely surprising, as it is now known that urinary MHPG is a poor indicator of CNS NE turnover, because the CNS contributes as little as 20 percent of urinary MHPG content.

Concentrations of MHPG in the CSF, which may represent a more direct measure of brain NE function, have generally been found to be unaltered in mood disorders, although this remains a controversial area. Antidepressants have been found to decrease MHPG levels consistently in urine and CSF, but the clinical response of patients to treatment does not correlate with these changes.

Dopamine mechanisms may be important in some forms of depression and mania

Dopamine may also be involved in depression, and a body of literature suggests that there may be a subgroup of mood disorders in which the neuroregulator is altered [12]. Levodopa (L-DOPA), the precursor of DA, can induce hypomania in some patients, a finding particularly noted in persons with bipolar disorder. DA receptor agonists have been reported to have some antidepressant effects in at least subgroups of patients. A number of antidepressant drugs have effects on several neuroregulator systems, and several have DA agonist activities. Furthermore, patients in the DA-depleted state of Parkinson's disease often develop a concomitant depression although that may be for other reasons. Conversely, there is evidence linking DA to mania in certain patients. Several drugs that act as agonists of DA produce behaviors that simulate some aspects of mania. However, there are problems with postulating a primary role for DA in the mood disorders. Most notably, neuroleptic medications that are known to block DA receptors are not generally associated with the induction of depression.

Studies of the major metabolite of DA in the cerebrospinal fluid, homovanillic acid (HVA), have been somewhat inconsistent, suggesting decreased concentrations in at least some patients with depression. Comparison between studies has been difficult because of small sample size and different clinical populations, including age differences. A number of studies have suggested elevated HVA concentrations in the CSF of manic individuals. However, metabolites for other transmitters were also elevated in some of these studies.

To obtain information regarding DA turnover, some researchers have studied HVA concentration changes after inhibiting efflux of HVA from the CSF following administration of probenecid, which inhibits the transport mechanism. The differences were largest in patients exhibiting psychomotor retardation and insignificant in patients with agitation, suggesting that HVA levels may reflect, at least in part, motor activity.

Serotonin has an important role in some forms of depression

Several clinically effective antidepressant medications specifically inhibit the uptake of 5-HT into presynaptic terminals. A major hypothesis of mood disorders is that some forms may be due to a relative deficiency of serotonin. The efficacy of several new drugs that have a high specificity as serotonin reuptake blockers [7] has been taken as a form of proof of the existence of such a subtype of patients.

It has been of interest to measure concentrations of the 5-HT metabolite, 5-hydroxyindoleacetic acid (5-HIAA), in patients with mood disorders. Antidepressants do seem to consistently lower CSF 5-HIAA concentrations, but this occurs whether or not the patient's depression improves. A tentative conclusion from studies of serotonin metabolites in depressed individuals is that there is a bimodal distribution of CSF 5-HIAA levels.

One of the most consistent findings in biological research dealing with mental disorders has been that some patients with low CSF 5-HIAA are more prone to commit suicide [13–15]. The lower concentrations of 5-HIAA are not specific to depression; there has also been a correlation between the decreased amounts and aggressive behavior in some individuals.

Acetylcholine mechanisms have been implicated in mood disorders

Acetylcholine has also been implicated in the pathogenesis of affective disorders [16]. The cholinergic hypothesis suggests that hyper- and hypocholinergic states induce depression and mania, respectively. Support for this hypothesis comes from the finding that acetylcholinesterase inhibitors and cholinomimetics produce depressive symptoms under certain conditions. Conversely, anticholinergic agents have some antidepressant and euphorigenic properties, and anticholinergic toxicity can induce a state resembling mania. However, agents that act on cholinergic receptors are not very effective in the treatment of mood disorders. In an attempt to reconcile the data on the involvement of cholinergic and monoaminergic systems in the mood disorders, it has been proposed that an abnormal balance between cholinergic and monoaminergic systems might be critical in the development of depression and mania.

Clinical studies of acetylcholine and its metabolites are limited by the current methodological difficulties involved in studying these systems. Investigation of cholinergic mechanisms has therefore focused on pharmacological investigations.

RECEPTOR HYPOTHESES OF MOOD DISORDERS

Inconsistencies with the monoamine hypotheses of mood disorders have led some investigators to alternative proposals that attempt to correlate more closely the clinical and cellular actions of antidepressants. These focus particularly on measuring the density and responsiveness of post-synaptic receptors.

β-Adrenergic and, possibly, serotonergic receptors may mediate the clinical effects of antidepressant drugs

During the search for neurochemical events that occur over the same time course as antidepressant actions, investigators found that in experimental animals, long-term (>2 weeks) antidepressant treatment caused a reduction in NE- or isoproterenol-stimulated cyclic AMP (cAMP) accumulation in the brain [17] (see Chap. 21 for control of cAMP). Generally, but not uniformly, there is a concomitant decrease in the density of β-adrenergic receptors, that is, a decrease in B_{max}. This may be due to the antidepressant-induced increase in synaptic availability of NE and a consequent down-regulation of β-adrenergic receptors. Notably, the decrease in NE-stimulated cAMP accumulation has been shown to occur not only with MAO inhibitors and tricyclic antidepressants but also with iprindole, mianserin, and electroconvulsive therapy (ECT), all of which are effective in the treatment of depression in humans.

Down-regulation of the 5-HT₂ receptor, a subtype of the 5-HT receptor, has also been demonstrated to occur following long-term but not acute antidepressant treatment (see Chap. 13). Lesioning the serotonergic system can prevent down-regulation of β-adrenergic receptors by antidepressants, a finding that suggests that there may be a strong link between serotonergic and noradrenergic systems in mediating the actions of antidepressants [18].

The corollary of the neurotransmitter-receptor hypothesis is that some forms of depression (and mania) may be caused by abnormality in the regulation of post-synaptic β-adrenergic, and possibly serotonergic, receptors. It has been difficult to test this hypothesis in humans because to do so requires obtaining unfixed brain tissue shortly after death from a large number of affected individuals and controls. Nonetheless, studies using a limited number of autopsy samples tend to show a significant increase in the number of β-adrenergic and 5-HT₂ receptors in the brains of suicide victims compared with controls [19–21]. With the advent of positron emission tomography (PET), which allows *in vivo* quantitation of neurotransmitter receptors, it may be possible to extend these studies more easily (see Chap. 46).

Other receptor mechanisms have also been implicated in mood disorders

Decreased responsiveness to α₂-adrenergic agonists in some depressed patients has led to the suggestion that these receptors are involved in the etiology of depression. It has been reported that patients with depression have altered density of muscarinic receptors compared to controls, but this has been questioned.

ACTION OF LITHIUM IN THE TREATMENT OF MOOD DISORDERS

Lithium is effective in treating mania and depression

Lithium (Li⁺) is universally accepted as the treatment of choice for bipolar disorder [4]. Well-controlled clinical studies have shown it to decrease the severity, length, and recurrence of manic episodes. Li⁺ also has significant antidepressant properties in both bipolar disorder and unipolar depression.

The discovery of the clinical effectiveness of Li⁺ in treating mania was serendipitous. In 1949, John Cade, an Australian, injected the urine of manic patients into guinea pigs to test for a toxic substance that might cause illness. The procedure often killed the animals because of the toxicity of urea. While attempting to determine how uric acid modified urea toxicity, he administered Li⁺ urate, the most soluble urate salt, and observed that the animals often became sedated. By performing appropriate controls, Cade discovered that the Li⁺ was the sedative. After finding that self-administration produced no significant adverse effects,

Cade administered Li$^+$ to manic patients, for-tuitously in a dose that turned out to be clinically optimal. All of the patients responded positively. Soon after, Mogens Schou, in a series of clinical trials in Denmark, proved that Li$^+$ was an effective agent in treating mania and in preventing the recurrence of manic episodes. Li$^+$ was in common use in Europe by the mid-1960s and was finally approved for clinical use in the United States in 1969.

Lithium has a number of effects on neuroregulator systems

Li$^+$ has a wide range of biological actions [22], involving enzymes, ion pumps, ion channels, and membrane transport mechanisms. Li$^+$ inhibits adenylyl cyclase, alters certain types of protein phosphorylation, changes the expression of some G proteins and subtypes of adenylyl cyclase, and alters the coupling of some neurotransmitter receptors to G proteins.

Li$^+$ also has a variety of effects on brain monoamine mechanisms, with the change depending upon the specific measure and chronicity of treatment; however, no consistent pattern has been related to its actions. A variety of changes have been noted in the turnover of monoamines. Li$^+$ blocks the release associated with stimulation of NE from brain slices and may increase reuptake of the transmitter from the synapse. Li$^+$ also has effects on monoamine receptors; some of these actions are consistent with a stabilizing role. For example, Li$^+$ has been reported to prevent the development of neuroleptic-induced DA receptor supersensitivity, and like the antidepressants, can also inhibit the β-adrenergic receptor stimulation of adenylyl cyclase.

The relationship between the biochemical effects of Li$^+$ and its therapeutic activity in mania and depression is an area of active investigation. Li$^+$ has broad actions within the cell; further understanding of the mechanisms of its action may lead to new conceptions of illnesses and to still more specific pharmacological treatments.

Lithium has important effects on the phosphatidylinositol system

Over the last few years, an area of intense research has been the effect of Li$^+$ on phosphoinositide (PI) systems in the brain [23–25]. PI turnover is increased by a variety of putative neurotransmitters and has second-messenger activity analogous to that of the adenylyl cyclase-cAMP cascade. A neuroregulator that activates PI turnover binds to a receptor that is in turn coupled to a G protein (a protein that can bind GTP). A number of G proteins are involved in different actions of neuroregulators including the phosphoinositide cascade. Neurons in the brain must be able to recycle inositol by dephosphorylation since inositol does not readily cross the blood-brain barrier. Li$^+$ inhibits several specific steps in the cascade and these effects are believed to be related to its actions. It potently inhibits several inositol phosphatases such as the enzyme *myo*-inositol-1-phosphatase. This blocks the transformation of *myo*-inositol-1-phosphate to *myo*-inositol, required for the resynthesis of the parent polyphosphoinositides (PPIs).

Since Li$^+$ acts at several different steps in the PPI cascade, an important hypothesis is that Li$^+$ exerts its therapeutic actions by damping or altering the cellular responses to those neurotransmitters whose actions are mediated by PPI turnover. Among the attractive aspects of the hypothesis is that it suggests that Li$^+$ might act on a number of different neurotransmitter systems. Li$^+$ commonly takes several days to exert its clinical effects; similarly, the changes in the PPI cascade do not occur instantaneously, but require chronic treatment.

The "inositol depletion hypothesis" developed by Berridge and others has several attractive aspects including the prediction that the ability of Li$^+$ to antagonize PPI turnover is dependent on activation of receptor-stimulated PPI turnover. A quiescent cell or one in which PPI turnover is low would be relatively unaffected by Li⁺-mediated inhibition of the phosphatases, whereas a highly active cell would be expected to accumulate *myo*-inositol-1-phosphate and run out of stores of *myo*-inositol, leading to impaired ability to respond to subsequent stimulation (see Chap. 20). Thus, the action of Li⁺ would be targeted toward those neuronal systems in which PPI turnover is most active. Such a mechanism might explain how Li⁺ is able to treat both mania and depression successfully, behavioral states that probably reflect the activation of distinct neuronal systems. Furthermore, a variety of transmitters, all with the common property of being coupled to PPI turnover, would be affected by Li⁺.

Although both tricyclic antidepressants and Li⁺ alter the sensitivity of the adenylyl cyclase-cAMP cascade, only Li⁺ additionally affects PPI turnover. These two second-messenger systems are now known to be involved in the actions of a large and growing number of neurotransmitter receptor systems (see Chap. 10). It is possible that the basic biological defects underlying some mood disorders lie not with neurotransmitter synthesis or metabolism, nor with their receptors, but rather with the regulation of one or both of these intracellular biochemical cascades. Protein kinase A and C, the kinases activated by cAMP and PPI turnover, respectively, can phosphorylate and thereby modulate receptors, synthetic enzymes, and GTP-binding proteins, the proteins that couple receptor to effector. (These phosphorylation reactions are discussed in Chap. 22.)

An abnormality at one step in the second-messenger cascade could have appreciable consequences for a variety of cellular processes and could help explain the diverse results from clinical studies and the variety of reported actions of antidepressants and Li⁺. There are a number of questions regarding the detailed effects of Li⁺ on PPI-related systems and which physiological processes are consequently activated or inhibited by Li⁺. There is now increasing attention to G

proteins and their potential regulatory roles in behavior and mental disorders [26].

EXAMPLES OF OTHER APPROACHES TO MOOD DISORDERS

There is substantial evidence for alteration in the hypothalamic-pituitary-adrenal axis in depression

A variety of endocrine disorders have profound psychiatric manifestations. Behavior that is controlled in part by the hypothalamic-pituitary-adrenal axis is disturbed in affective illnesses [27]. It is therefore not surprising that a number of neuroendocrine markers are abnormal in the mood disorders, particularly in depression.

A dysfunction in the hypothalamic-pituitary-adrenal axis is suggested by studies of cortisol secretion and regulation. There is a reasonably consistent finding that during the illness, but not after recovery, a significant subpopulation of depressed patients hypersecrete cortisol or exhibit an abnormal diurnal variation in cortisol secretion.

As noted by the Michigan group [28] many depressed patients exhibit decreased sensitivity to the negative feedback demonstrated by dexamethasone-induced suppression of cortisol secretion while other studies have shown patient populations with blunted corticotroph response to corticotropin-releasing factor, increased adrenal response to adrenocorticotrophic hormone (ACTH), and decreased responsivity to glucocorticoid "fast feedback." Corticotropin-releasing factor (CRF) may itself be quite important in mood disorders and anxiety [29]. Subpopulations of patients may vary, with evidence in some patients of a failure of the pituitary corticotroph to respond to negative feedback. Using *in situ* hybridization, evidence has been obtained through quantitation of messenger RNAs that there is chronic activation of the hypothalamic-pituitary-adrenal axis in suicide victims [30].

Several investigators have reported that stimulation of the secretion of thyroid-stimulating hormone (TSH) by thyrotropin-releasing hormone (TRH) is significantly reduced in some depressed patients. This points again to a dysfunction in the anterior pituitary itself, the hypothalamus, or in the neuronal systems that modulate the activity of these areas (Chap. 49).

Another neuroendocrine abnormality consistently found in depressed patients is decreased growth hormone response to the α_2-adrenergic agonist clonidine. It is believed that the growth hormone response to clonidine is mediated by hypothalamic α_2-adrenergic receptors.

It should be noted that a significant number of depressed patients exhibit no neuroendocrine abnormalities and, further, that these measurements can be affected by nonspecific factors, such as sex, age, weight, activity level, and stress. Biological rhythms and sleep alterations are also critical factors. The overlap between measurements is unclear. Nevertheless, the multiple links between brain and endocrine organs (see Chap. 49) make it likely that further study of neuroendocrine abnormalities in psychiatric illness will be of value and may facilitate subtyping of forms of affective illness and aid in assessing treatment response.

Brain mapping and functional imaging methods are being applied to the study of mood disorders

A number of different approaches are now being taken to the functional anatomical changes that may be associated with mood disorders. One of these has involved investigation of the pattern of mood disorders following various types of cerebral vascular disease [31]. Mood disorders occur in 30 to 50 percent of stroke patients and can last more than a year without treatment. Major depression is often associated with left frontal or left basal ganglia lesions, while mania is infrequent. From such empirical studies it may be possible to develop the functional and biochemical neuroanatomy associated with mood disorders.

Imaging studies using magnetic resonance techniques are also providing information regarding anatomical changes that may be related to brain biochemistry [32]. A series of changes have been described in preliminary studies, including evidence suggesting that there may be a population of depressed individuals in whom the caudate nuclei are smaller than in normal subjects. Limited studies have been conducted utilizing PET. While it is too early to draw definitive conclusions, the available evidence suggests that there may be a left prefrontal cortex and basal ganglia glucose metabolic dysfunction associated with depression [33]. PET studies with receptor ligands (see Chap. 46) should prove particularly useful in depression.

Sleep and circadian mechanisms and seasonal affective disorder are providing new approaches to mood disorders

Patients frequently complain of alterations in sleep, and those subjective reports are supported by a literature demonstrating that sleep and circadian mechanisms are altered in many severe mental disorders [34,35]. Among the established changes is a reduction in the latency to rapid eye movement sleep that occurs in mood disorders as well as other illnesses [36]. There have been a series of reports that sleep deprivation itself may be antidepressant or hasten the action of pharmacological agents [37]. Such findings have a number of implications for studies of the neurochemistry of mood disorders.

A new dimension in depression research has come from studies of seasonal affective disorder in which depression may occur in relation to changes in light [38,39]. There is evidence that this form of depression may be related to the pineal gland and to the secretion of melatonin (see Chap. 49). It is interesting that this form of depression appears to be treated by exposure to light [40]. While there have been few studies, there is some evidence that light may also be helpful in other forms of depression [41].

A wide range of behavioral models have been developed that have direct relevance for study of neurochemical changes that are relevant for the study of the mood disorders [42]. Common features of the models have been described [43], including the role of separation and loss of behavioral control. In the relatively few studies conducted to date, there are also commonalities in aspects of the biochemical findings including changes in NE and 5-HT systems as well as in endocrine function.

A number of models have been proposed and utilized that will be of interest to investigators with neurochemical expertise. Among the most valuable and intensely studied paradigms have been stress-induced models of depression [44]. A psychological mechanism that can be considered in specific physiological terms has been the learned helplessness model [45]. It has taken a special place as insights derived from the psychological aspects of the paradigm have been applied in the clinical treatment situation. Pharmacological studies have suggested that components of the learned helplessness behavior involve different neuroregulator systems. A variety of other behavioral conditions, including primate models, have also been utilized for neurochemical, endocrine, and pharmacological studies relevant to the mood disorders [46,47].

A variety of treatments are leading to additional approaches to the study of mood disorders. Among the emerging therapies has been the use of certain anticonvulsants in the treatment of some mood disorders, including selected cases of bipolar disease [1,2]. Although the mode of action is not yet clear, these treatments can be highly effective. In a similar vein, for many decades it has been recognized that ECT can result in marked and rapid improvement of some individuals who may be refractory to other forms of treatment. In many cases the treatment can be life-saving. Studies of the biochemical effects of ECT have revealed a wide range of changes, although there is not yet agreement as to the critical processes. Explanations of the mechanisms of these effects could lead to new hypotheses of mood disorders.

There is interest in the role in mood disorders of a number of neuroregulators which have received less attention, such as the neuropeptides including the opioids, somatostatin, and vasopressin. It has been difficult to study the dynamics of the peptide systems since there are problems with evaluation of the kinetics of turnover and metabolism. Only a fraction of the neuropeptides that may act as critical neuroregulators have been identified [48]. Some neuropeptides may be coreleased with other neuroregulators and have important transmitter and regulatory roles (see Chap. 16).

An example of such a hypothesis is that a relative deficiency or excess of one of the opioid peptides, or an alteration in receptors for opioid peptides, may prove to be important in some forms of depression or mania. There has been a report suggesting that β-endorphin in plasma may be elevated in depressed individuals with more severe anxiety, phobia, and obsessive-compulsive behaviors [49]. The recent cloning of an opioid receptor will facilitate the cloning of other receptors of this family and will aid physiological studies of changes in behavior and mental disorders [50].

Rather than postulating that simple over- or underactivity of a neuroregulator system induces depression or mania, some investigators have proposed that dysregulation of one or more neurotransmitters or neuromodulator homeostatic mechanisms has an important role as a causative factor [51]. Such conceptions have led to efforts to develop more sophisticated approaches to neurochemical events including studies of calculations of the ratios of several different neurotransmitter metabolites and studies of relative activity and turnover. There is the hope that such information, coupled with more sophisticated behavior evaluation, may help differentiate subtypes of mood disorder [52,53].

Particularly important will be new hypotheses by which to link the complex behavioral and biochemical data that have developed with regard to the mood disorders. Such a conceptualization has recently been proposed [54] that takes into account the variety of studies that demonstrate the role of psychosocial stressors in first episodes of mood disorders. Such episodes can themselves cause a variety of changes in gene expression and thereby further alter behavioral processes. These changes may result in increased future vulnerability through a variety of mechanisms. Investigation of these reciprocal relationships, involving the interactions between behavior and biology, are key to the development of behavioral neurochemistry.

BIOCHEMICAL ASPECTS OF ANXIETY

Anxiety can be a serious illness and is now attracting attention from neurobiologists

Anxiety is the apprehension of danger or something unpleasant. Whereas fear is a response to current, tangible threats, anxiety occurs in anticipation of a threat not yet present and often not clearly defined. Anxiety is a familiar part of everyday human life, and something akin to anxiety probably occurs in most mammals and many other vertebrates. Anxiety has clear adaptive value, and in humans it must certainly be considered normal. Yet in some individuals, anxiety reaches a level that is counterproductive or even incapacitating [1]. Anxiety disorders are among the most common of all psychiatric conditions. In addition, anxiety is a prominent symptom in almost all other psychiatric illnesses. Various studies have found that from about 3 to 8 percent of the population has clinically significant anxiety at any one time. This prevalence is surprisingly consistent from culture to culture throughout the world. Because of their tremendous costs to society, anxiety and its disorders have been the subject of intense study. For many years, this study was confined to the psychological realm, and the knowledge gained remains central to a full understanding of anxiety and the treatment of its disorders. In the past three decades, however, a picture of the biology and chemistry of anxiety has begun to emerge; although far from complete, it is changing our perception of anxiety and leading to new approaches for therapy.

Anxiety is recognized as one of the most important emotional processes with firm neurobiological roots. It can be studied in many organisms, including humans. The fundamental mechanisms are important for a wide range of mental disorders and substance abuse. The progress that has been made in the past few years suggests that improved understanding of the mechanisms of anxiety will be one of the most interesting areas in behavioral neurochemistry.

The evidence used to determine the neurochemical bases of anxiety has been similar to that for the mood disorders. Most information has come from studying the action of anxiety-reducing, or anxiolytic, drugs. This has been aided by the existence of several animal models of anxiety that are probably closer to the human condition of anxiety than are animal models of mood disorders to their human counterparts. The four major thrusts of current work dealing with anxiety disorders have centered about the γ-aminobutyric acid (GABA)-benzodiazepine receptor-Cl^- ionophore system, the serotonergic system, noradrenergic mechanisms, and neuropeptides [55,56].

There are distinct forms of anxiety disorders

The disorders in which the level of anxiety becomes pathological are divided according to their characteristic clustering of symptoms, presence of familial association, sex ratios, and response to drug treatment. The standard reference for categorization of mental disorders has been the Diagnostic and Statistical Manual (DSM-IV) of the American Psychiatric Association [3]. The following materials derived from those sources highlight the emerging classification of anxiety disorders, many of which are now recognized as profoundly disabling. Research is suggesting neurobiological associations with several of these clinical entities.

Panic attacks can be associated with many anxiety disorders and are characterized by discrete episodes, typically lasting a few minutes, with symptoms such as accelerated or more forceful heart action, sweating, trembling, shortness of breath, chest pain, abdominal distress, feeling dizzy, and a fear on the part of the patient that he or she is "going crazy" or will die. Some persons have multiple episodes of panic attacks without another mental disorder—such problems are recognized as panic disorder. A substantial number of individuals subject to panic attacks, but usually not normal controls, can have panic episodes precipitated by lactate infusions through mechanisms that are not yet understood. Family and twin studies suggest that there may be a genetic component.

Specific phobias involve a fear that is excessive that is cued by specific stimuli such as heights, enclosed places, or other situations. The individual with phobias may experience full panic attacks when exposed to the stimulus. Social phobia is a marked and persistent fear of social situations.

Obsessive-compulsive disorder is a particularly important form of anxiety disorder. Obsessions include recurrent thoughts that may not be about real-life problems and that the person attempts to ignore or suppress. Compulsions are repetitive behaviors that the person feels driven to perform in response to an obsession. The compulsive behaviors attempt to reduce the distress from the obsessions. Patients realize that the thoughts and behaviors are unreasonable.

They cause marked distress and can consume considerable time.

Post-traumatic stress disorder stems from a serious threat to oneself or another with a response of fear or horror. The traumatic event is persistently reexperienced and there is avoidance of stimuli associated with the trauma. Patients have persistent symptoms of increased arousal including such symptoms as difficulty sleeping, irritability, difficulty concentrating, hypervigilance, or exaggerated startle response. The disorder can continue for a sustained period of time with marked impairment in functioning.

Acute stress disorder has many of the same type of starting points as post-traumatic stress disorder but the duration of the clinical manifestations is less than 4 weeks. Typically, individuals have dissociative problems with symptoms such as numbing or detachment, reduction in awareness, or loss of memory for aspects of the event. In acute stress disorder there are reexperiences of the event, avoidance of stimuli that arouse its recollection, and marked symptoms of anxiety or increased arousal.

Generalized anxiety disorder involves a broad presentation of anxiety. Patients experience ongoing excessive anxiety and worry for over 6 months about a number of aspects of their lives. They have a difficult time controlling the worry. The pattern of symptoms will vary from patient to patient but typical symptoms include some of the following: restlessness, fatigue, difficulty concentrating, irritability, and muscle tension or sleep disturbances. The focus of the psychological sense of worry in these patients can be quite broad, and the symptoms cause considerable distress and impairment.

The distinct types can be classified with good reproducibility and with a high degree of agreement among trained raters. There is strong evidence that the underlying neurochemistry and neurobiology are different between the types on the basis of pharmacological and chemical evidence. The forms demonstrate differential responses to drug treatment. For example, while almost all forms of anxiety can be blunted by benzodiazepines, the specific serotonin reuptake inhibitors are often very effective in the treatment of obsessive-compulsive disorder, and the 5-HT$_{1A}$ serotonin receptor partial agonists, such as buspirone, seem particularly effective in generalized anxiety disorders.

Benzodiazepines have revolutionized the treatment of anxiety disorders

The introduction of benzodiazepines has also set the stage for greatly increasing our understanding of the biochemistry of anxiety. Anxiolytic drugs were among the earliest effective pharmaceutical agents devised. One of the most prominent effects of ethanol is its tendency to obliterate anxiety, a major reason for its continuing popularity. Opiate alkaloids and belladonna derivatives also have potent anxiolytic activities. Barbiturates and, later, propanediol carbamates such as meprobamate were used extensively in the past for the relief of anxiety. The use of each of these drugs is limited by several side effects, most notably their serious toxicity at high doses and, with the exception of belladonna, their high liability to addiction.

The benzodiazepines are highly effective for the relief of anxiety. They have a lower potential for addiction than many other drugs that were used earlier and are less likely to cause death or serious lasting harm when taken in large overdoses. There are now several dozen different benzodiazepine drugs in clinical use worldwide, although use has become less popular because of side effects, including dependence. The various compounds appear to differ primarily in their pharmacokinetics—the speed with which they are taken up and eliminated by the body—rather than in their clinical effects.

The clinical effects of the benzodiazepines are fourfold: anxiolytic, sedative or sleep-inducing, anticonvulsant, and muscle relaxant. It was thought at first that the benzodiazepines might have a different mechanism of action for each of these effects. For example, it was noted that tolerance to sedation but not anxiolytic action quickly develops in patients taking a benzodiazepine: however, all clinical effects of benzodiazepines appear to be mediated centrally.

There are specific receptors for the benzodiazepines that are related to their behavioral effects

In 1977, two groups independently discovered high-affinity binding sites for diazepam in brain [57,58]. The affinities of a variety of benzodiazepines for these sites correlated well with their clinical potency. Correlations with potency in animal models of anxiety were also sought. The most common animal model for anxiety involves pairing a reward for which the animal must perform some behavior, such as lever pressing, with an aversive stimulus, such as a mild electric shock. A conflict is thus produced. Agents that appear to reduce this conflict and increase the rate of responses punished with the shock (punished-responding) generally act as anxiolytics in humans.

Benzodiazepines that were most potent in releasing punished-responding behavior had the highest affinity for benzodiazepine binding sites. These binding sites were found in highest density in areas of the brain that developed later in evolution, for example, in cerebral cortex, and are thought to be concerned with the production of emotional responses such as anxiety. The interaction of the benzodiazepines with their receptors is quite specific, and benzodiazepines did not demonstrate high affinity for any other neurotransmitter receptors in competitive binding assays. These studies were taken as evidence that it was the binding to these sites that mediated the action of the benzodiazepines [59].

CNS benzodiazepine binding sites are closely associated with the GABA$_A$ subtype of GABA receptor

Much effort has gone into determining the nature of benzodiazepine binding sites. For some time it was suspected that benzodiazepine action might be closely associated with GABAergic mechanisms; electrophysiological studies demonstrated that diazepam facilitated GABAergic synaptic transmission.

It is now known that the benzodiazepines interact with the GABA$_A$ subtype of GABA receptor, which is widely distributed in the CNS, primarily post-synaptically, and mediates changes in neuronal membrane potential by opening a Cl$^-$ channel. The GABA$_A$ receptor, the benzodiazepine binding site, and the Cl$^-$ ionophore are part of a single large macromolecular complex that is believed to be a critical key to the action of the drugs [60,61]. The receptor has been cloned and consists of several distinct subunits [62]. GABA and the benzodiazepines each allosterically modulate the binding of the other to this macromolecular complex, the benzodiazepines by binding to the α-subunit and GABA by binding to the β-subunit (see Chap. 18).

In vitro, Cl$^-$ acts to increase benzodiazepine receptor affinity, and it is necessary for the reciprocal regulation of GABA and benzodiazepine binding. Benzodiazepines facilitate GABAergic transmission primarily by increasing the frequency of Cl$^-$ channel opening in response to occupancy of the GABA$_A$ receptor by GABA. There is also a distinctly different benzodiazepine binding site in the periphery that is unassociated with GABA receptors.

Barbiturates also mediate at least some of their important actions via binding to some portion of this complex closely associated with the Cl$^-$ ionophore (see Chap. 18). Like benzodiazepines, they facilitate GABA-dependent Cl$^-$ flux in brain slices and cultured neurons. In addition, barbiturates enhance [^{3}H]benzodiazepine and [^{3}H]GABA agonist binding to their respective sites in *in vitro* binding assays; however, the exact mechanism appears to be somewhat different from that of the benzodiazepines. First, barbiturates are not competitive inhibitors of ligands for either GABA$_A$ or benzodiazepine binding sites. Second, unlike benzodiazepines, barbiturates decrease the frequency of opening of GABA-activated Cl$^-$ channels but still potentiate GABA responses by increasing the mean open time of the ionophore.

GABAergic stimulation with GABA agonists also has an anxiolytic effect

The GABA agonist muscimol has anxiolytic activity in animal models, and picrotoxin, a drug that potently inhibits GABA-promoted Cl$^-$ flux, has the opposite effect. The experimental and clinical utility of GABAergic drugs is restricted, however, by their toxicity and in some cases by their limited ability to cross the blood-brain barrier. There is some evidence that ethanol and the propanediol carbamates also produce some of their anxiolytic effects by acting at the GABA-benzodiazepine receptor-Cl$^-$ ionophore complex.

Several classes of compounds act as benzodiazepine antagonists

Compounds that act as benzodiazepine antagonists have also been called inverse agonists because they have behavioral actions opposite to those produced by benzodiazepines—they increase sleeplessness and in higher doses cause seizures. The first type of benzodiazepine antagonists described were esters of β-carbolines. These compounds were first studied as possible endogenous ligands for the benzodiazepine binding site. Although the specific chemical substances were subsequently shown not to be present in the body, several other candidate endogenous ligands, including peptides, have been suggested. The existence and physiological function in humans of any of the endogenous ligands have yet to be established.

Multiple benzodiazepine receptors are involved in differential pharmacological action

Considerable progress in understanding the structure of the receptors is facilitating the understanding of benzodiazepine actions [63]. The initial classification was into the BZ-1 form found throughout the brain with highest concentrations in the cerebellum and the BZ-2 form found primarily in the cortex and hippocampus in the brain. Molecular biological investigation of the subunits of the benzodiazepine receptor have revealed that there is substantial heterogeneity. The GABA$_A$ receptor is made up of subunits, one of which—the α-subunit—appears to have different isoforms and results in the varying characteristics of the receptor.

Experiments with recombinant receptors have allowed analysis of the varying forms with the demonstration of differential affinities by the subunit forms for varying ligands. Behavioral and physiological effects of pharmacological agents can be differentiated. The anatomical pattern of gene expression in rat brain has been determined for six forms of the α-subunit using *in situ* hybridization with the finding of dramatic differences in localization [64]. Information regarding these different receptor subtypes is being used by chemists to design more specific pharmacological agents, some of which are based upon partial agonist actions.

Serotonin has also been linked to anxiety processes and may be important in the origin and treatment of anxiety

Aside from the GABA-benzodiazepine receptor complex, no other neurotransmitter system has received so much attention in relation to anxiety as has serotonin (5-HT) [65,66]. It has long been known that depletion of 5-HT with PCPA or lesioning of the dorsal raphe nucleus, the site of most CNS 5-HT neuronal bodies, with 5,7-dihydroxytryptamine has an anxiolytic-like effect in rodents. Similar suggestive observations were made demonstrating that in some cases serotonergic agonists produced an increase in anxiety; however, some 5-HT antagonists tend to change punished-responding behavior in animals or reduce anxiety in humans, whereas other 5-HT antagonists have the op-

posite effect. Confidence in a serotonergic role in anxiety has also been tempered by the fact that the lesioning procedures produce a number of alterations in neurotransmitter systems other than those utilizing 5-HT. It has long been suspected that many serotonergic drugs are nonspecific, and this has been borne out by the demonstration of multiple distinct CNS 5-HT receptors.

The compound buspirone has been introduced as the first anxiolytic agent whose clinical effects are probably mediated primarily by effects on the 5-HT system. Buspirone and related compounds may both alter the treatment of anxiety and offer new tools for its study, just as the benzodiazepines did a generation ago. In contrast to the benzodiazepines, buspirone has a delayed onset of action—it must be administered for up to several weeks before a significant reduction of anxiety is observed. The drug has almost no sedative, anticonvulsant, or muscle-relaxant activity and no significant addiction liability. These last considerations make this type of drug an advance in the treatment of anxiety in many patients. Buspirone is useful in the treatment of generalized anxiety disorder but not in the treatment of panic.

Buspirone has no direct effect on the GABA$_A$-benzodiazepine receptor system. Although it has a weak effect on dopamine receptors, its primary effect appears to be mediated by serotonin receptors of the 5-HT$_{1A}$ type [67,68]. Brain serotonin receptors have been divided into a wide range of subtypes based on their pharmacological specificities, anatomical distribution, and function (see also Chap. 13). Several additional 5-HT$_{1A}$ active compounds, including itsatirone and getirone, have also demonstrated anxiolytic activity in animals. The 5-HT$_{1A}$ receptor is linked via G$_i$ proteins to either inhibition of adenylyl cyclase or the opening of potassium channels. It is widely distributed as a postsynaptic receptor in the forebrain and also serves as a somatodendritic autoreceptor on raphe neurons. Drugs believed to act as partial agonists at 5-HT$_{1A}$ autoreceptors may act to decrease the firing of the serotonergic raphe neurons.

Drugs that act on other serotonergic receptors also have been useful in the treatment of anxiety. Some antagonists of the 5-HT_2 receptor have proved beneficial in anxiety but not in panic. Again, there is emerging evidence that antagonists of 5-HT_3 receptors also have anxiolytic activity.

Important hypotheses of panic disorder and obsessive-compulsive disorder are coming from findings that serotonin reuptake inhibitors are a useful treatment. Such effects have been noted for a number of these agents and suggest that panic may involve certain serotonergic mechanisms. The fact that a number of drugs that are useful in panic disorder are not useful in generalized anxiety disorder, and visa versa, leads to new suggestions that the fundamental mechanisms of these processes may be different.

Obsessive-compulsive disorder has neurobiological concomitants and can be treated with pharmacological therapy

A rapidly emerging body of literature is demonstrating that there are important neurobiological correlates to obsessive-compulsive disorder. Although it was previously an illness that resisted treatment, that situation has been changed by new, more specific therapies using pharmacological or behavioral methods or their combination.

The pharmacological therapy of obsessive-compulsive disorder centers about drugs originally used for depression [69]. Most antidepressant drugs are not active in obsessive-compulsive disorder, but those that are show a striking specificity. They are of benefit in patients with obsessive-compulsive disorder who do not have depression. Clomipramine, fluvoxamine, and fluoxetine are among the small group of agents that have demonstrated effectiveness in obsessive-compulsive disorder. Because of those actions, the drugs are now being used as antiobsessional drugs as well as antidepressants. The effectiveness in obsessional states occurs at

higher doses, requires longer treatment, and usually results in a lessening of symptoms rather than a total remission. There is frequently a relapse following discontinuation of the drugs.

The mechanism of action of the antiobsessional drugs highlights an important potential neuroregulator system that may be involved. Each of the drugs that have been successfully used is a highly specific serotonin uptake inhibitor. Acute challenge with certain serotonin agonists have been shown to exacerbate the symptoms of obsessive-compulsive disorder. The pharmacological evidence suggests that it may be possible to determine the pattern of changes in serotonin systems, including changes in synthesis, uptake, or specific receptors that are related to the clinical response.

The pharmacological studies indicate the importance of investigation of neurochemical processes involving the serotonin system in patients. An investigation in children and adolescents with obsessive-compulsive disorder [70] has been undertaken with measurement of CSF concentrations of a number of neuroregulators or their metabolites. CSF concentrations of the major serotonin metabolite, 5-HIAA, were positively correlated with some measures of improvement.

A particularly accurate animal model of obsessive-compulsive behavior may have been found in a naturally occurring disorder in dogs, canine acral lick, involving excessive licking of paws or flanks [71]. The canine problem can produce ulcers and infections. The investigators who found the model have demonstrated in a controlled manner that serotonin reuptake blockers are a specific treatment. This model should permit further pharmacological and neurochemical investigation.

There is evidence of a role for neuropeptides in anxiety

A peptide found in brain, neuropeptide Y (NPY), has recently been implicated in anxiety in a series of experiments that have utilized tools from molecular neurobiology [72]. It has been noted that the concentration of the peptide in the CSF is decreased in individuals with mood disorders including anxiety. The recent cloning of the receptor for the peptide has permitted studies in which the amount of the receptor was decreased by blocking the messenger RNA that is involved in the synthesis of the receptor protein. This was accomplished using antisense techniques with direct injection into the cerebral ventricles. In an experiment that will have many imitators, the investigators found that such injections did reduce the amount of the receptor protein. Further, using what is considered a behavioral model of anxiety, they demonstrated an increased anxiety in the treated animals. The studies raise the question as to whether there may be new approaches to the study and treatment of anxiety that take into account the NPY system. For example, NPY agonists might be used in the treatment of some forms of anxiety.

Mechanisms involving catecholamine function may be important in anxiety

An important hypothesis of anxiety mechanisms has centered about brain norepinephrine systems, particularly those in the locus coeruleus. This integrative hypothesis suggests that anxiety is associated with increased activity of locus coeruleus, while relief of anxiety is associated with decreased activity of those neurons. The locus coeruleus is a key noradrenergic nucleus that sends fibers to many other areas such as the limbic system, hypothalamus, and cortex. The locus coeruleus receives a wide range of inputs and many investigators believe it is important in integrating information from a variety of sources. Thus, neuroregulator systems involving GABA, opioid peptides, and serotonin, to mention a few, all interact at the level of the locus coeruleus, making it an attractive site for an integrative hypothesis.

Much of the evidence linking the locus coeruleus to anxiety is based upon the use of drugs as well as upon physiological studies. Pharmacological agents that increase activity in the locus coeruleus increase anxiety while those that decrease activity decrease anxiety. In freely moving animals, fear-inducing stimuli produce a rapid increase in the firing of neurons in the locus coeruleus.

It has long been known that stress can differentially alter neuroregulators [73]. Changes in the metabolism of NE in the brain are associated with stress, particularly uncontrollable stress [74]. Stress increases the turnover of NE in the brain, and these actions can be inhibited by antianxiety agents. Increased secretion of peripheral catecholamines also has been found to take place in stress, and some of the changes in plasma catechols associated with phobias, for example, can be reversed by behavioral training in humans [75]. Noradrenergic mechanisms have been related to both panic attacks and to post-traumatic stress disorder [55].

Brain mapping and functional imaging methods are being applied to the study of anxiety disorders

Intense interest is now focusing on the use of various forms of brain imaging for the study of anxiety disorders with particular attention to obsessive-compulsive disorder [76]. Generally, such techniques have suggested increases in relative activity in the frontal cortex with several studies suggesting such changes in the orbitofrontal region. While there are many differences between the studies, and the technologies are undergoing change, the evidence is becoming strong that there may be important correlations. From such investigations and others has come the hypothesis that the orbitofrontal cortex, cingulate cortex, and the head of the caudate may form a circuit that is hyperactive in obsessive-compulsive disorder. In a study that suggests an important facet of the emerging discipline of behavioral neurochemistry, there is evidence that some changes in metabolic activity may be reversed by either behavioral or pharmacological therapy [77].

One can anticipate the future potential of enhanced understanding of severe mental disorders from information that will be gleaned from the combination of several technologies. These will include clinical assessment as well as more sophisticated neurochemical imaging techniques with specific pharmacotherapies developed as a result of the enormous advances in our understanding of the molecular biology and genetics of neurotransmitter receptors and transporters and associated second-messenger systems.

REFERENCES

1. Michels, R. (ed.) *Psychiatry.* Philadelphia: Lippincott, 1992.
2. *Practice Guideline for Major Depressive Disorder in Adults.* Washington, DC: American Psychiatric Association, 1993.
3. *Diagnostic and Statistical Manual (DSM-IV). 4th ed.* Washington, D.C.: American Psychiatric Association [in press].
4. Goodwin, F. K., and Jamison, K. R. *Manic-Depressive Illness.* New York: Oxford University Press, 1990.
5. Weissman, M., and Cross-National Collaborative Group. The changing rate of major depression: cross national comparisons. *JAMA* 268:3098–3105, 1992.
6. Gershon, E. S., Cloninger, C. R., and Barrett, J. E. (eds.) *Genetic Approaches to Mental Illness.* Washington, D.C.: American Psychiatric Press [in press], 1993.
7. Meltzer, H. Y. (ed.) *Psychopharmacology: The Third Generation of Progress.* New York: Raven Press, 1987.
8. Cooper, J. R., Bloom, F. E., and Roth, R. H. *The Biochemical Basis of Neuropharmacology.* New York: Oxford University Press, 1991.
9. Klerman, G. L., Weissman, M. M., Rounsaville, B. J., and Chevron, E. S. *Interpersonal Psychotherapy of Depression.* New York: Basic Books, 1984.
10. Schildkraut, J. J. The catecholamine hypothesis of affective disorders: A review of support-
ing evidence. *Am. J. Psychiatry* 122:509–522, 1965.
11. Bunney, W. E., Jr., and Davis, J. M. Norepinephrine in depressive reactions. *Arch. Gen. Psychiatry* 13:483–494, 1965.
12. Jimerson, D. C. Role of dopamine mechanisms in the affective disorders. In H. Y. Meltzer (ed.), *Psychopharmacology: The Third Generation of Progress.* New York: Raven Press, 1987, pp. 505–511.
13. Asburg, M., Traskman, L., and Thoren, P. 5-HIAA in the cerebrospinal fluid: a biochemical suicide predictor? *Arch. Gen. Psychiatry* 33: 1193–1197, 1976.
14. Brown, G. L., and Linnoila, M. I. CSF serotonin metabolite (5-HIAA) studies in depression, impulsivity, and violence. *J. Clin. Psychiatry* 51:31–41, 1990.
15. Faustman, W. O., Ringo, D. L., and Faull, K. F. Association between low CSF 5-HIAA and HVA and early mortality in a diagnostically mixed psychiatric sample. *Br. J. Psychiatry* [in press].
16. Overstreet, D. H., and Janowsky, D. S. A cholinergic supersensitivity model of depression. In A. A. Boulton, G. B. Baker, and M. T. Martin-Iverson (eds.), *Neuromethods: Animal Models in Psychiatry II,* Vol. 19. Clifton, NJ: Humana Press, 1991, pp. 81–114.
17. Charney, D. S., Menkes, D. B., and Heninger, G. R. Receptor sensitivity and the mechanism of action of antidepressant treatment: implications for the etiology and therapy of depression. *Arch. Gen. Psychiatry* 38:1160–1180, 1981.
18. Janowsky, A., Okada, F., Manier, D. H., Applegate, C. D., Sulser, F., and Steranka, L. R. Role of serotonergic input in the regulation of the beta adrenergic receptor-coupled adenylate cyclase system. *Science* 218:900–901, 1982.
19. Van Praag, H. M. Indoleamines in depression and suicide. *Prog. Brain Res.* 65:59–71, 1986.
20. Mann, J. J., Stanley, M., McBride, P. A., and McEwen, B. S. Increased serotonin$_2$ and β-adrenergic receptor binding in the frontal cortices of suicide victims. *Arch. Gen. Psychiatry* 43:954–959, 1986.
21. Charney, D. S., Delgado, P. L., Price, L. H., and Heninger, G. R. The receptor sensitivity hypothesis of antidepressant action: a review of antidepressant effects on serotonin function. In S. L. Brown and H. M. van Praag (eds.), *The Role of Serotonin in Psychiatric Disor-*

ders. New York: Bronner-Mazel, 1991, pp. 27–56.

22. Bunney, W. E., and Garland-Bunney, B. L. Mechanisms of action of lithium in affective illness. In H. Y. Meltzer (ed.), *Psychopharmacology: The Third Generation of Progress*. New York: Raven Press, 1987, pp. 553–565.

23. Snyder, S. H. Second messengers and affective illness: focus on the phosphoinositide cycle. *Pharmacopsychiatry* 25:25–28, 1992.

24. Berridge, M. J., and Irvine, R. F. Inositol phosphates and cell signaling. *Nature* 341:197–204, 1989.

25. Hyman, S. E., and Nestler, E. J. *The Molecular Foundations of Psychiatry*. Washington, D.C.: American Psychiatric Press, 1993.

26. Manji, H. K. G-proteins: implications for psychiatry. *Am. J. Psychiatry* 149:746–760, 1992.

27. Nemeroff, C. B., and Krishnan, K. R. R. Neuroendocrine alterations in psychiatric disorders. In C. B. Nemeroff (ed.), *Neuroendocrinology*. Boca Raton: CRC Press, 1992, pp. 413–441.

28. Young, E. A., Kotun, J., Haskett, R. F., Grunhaus, L., Greden, J. F., Watson, S. J., and Akil, H. Dissociation between pituitary and adrenal suppression to dexamethasone in depression. *Arch. Gen. Psychiatry* 50:395–405, 1993.

29. Owens, M. J., and Nemeroff, C. B. The role of CRF in the pathophysiology of affective disorders: laboratory and clinical studies. In *CIBA Foundation Symposium 172: Corticotropin-Releasing Factor*. New York: John Wiley and Sons, 1993, pp. 296–316.

30. Lopez, J. F., Palkovits, M., Arato, M., Mansour, A., Akil, H., and Watson, S. J. Localization and quantitation of proopiomelanocortin mRNA and glucocorticoid receptor mRNA in pituitaries of suicide victims. *Neuroendocrinology* 56:491–501, 1992.

31. Starkstein, S. E., and Robinson, R. G. Affective disorders and cerebral vascular disease. *Br. J. Psychiatry* 154:170–182, 1989.

32. Figiel, G. S., Botteron, K. N., Doraiswamy, P. M., Husain, M., McDonald, W., Nemeroff, C. B., and Krishnan, K. R. R. Structural brain changes in affective disorder: a review. [In press.]

33. Baxter, L. R., Guze, B. H., Schwartz, J. M., Phelps, M. E., Mazziotta, J. C., and Szuba, M. P. PET studies of cerebral function in major depression and related disorders. In N. A. Lassen, D. H. Ingvar, M. E. Raichle, and L.

Frebery (eds.), *Brain Work and Mental Activity*. Copenhagen: Munksgaard, 1991, pp. 403–418.

34. Wehr, T. A., and Goodwin, F. K. (eds.), *Biological Rhythms and Psychiatry*. Pacific Grove, CA: Boxwood Press, 1983.

35. Kupfer, D. A., Monk, T., and Barchas, J. D. (eds.), *Biological Rhythms and Mental Disorders*. New York: Guilford Press, 1988.

36. Benca, R. M., Obermeyer, W. H., Thisted, R. A., and Gillin, J. C. Sleep and psychiatric disorders: a meta analysis. *Arch. Gen. Psychiatry* 49:651–666, 1992.

37. Leibenluft, E., and Wehr, T. A. Is sleep deprivation useful in the treatment of depression? *Am. J. Psychiatry* 149:159–168, 1992.

38. Oren, D. A., and Rosenthal, N. E. Seasonal affective disorders. In E. S. Paykel (ed.), *Handbook of Affective Disorders*, 2nd ed. New York: Churchill Livingston, 1992, pp. 551–567.

39. Sack, R. L., Lewy, A. J., White, D. M., Singer, C. M., Fireman, M. J., and Vandiver, R. Morning vs evening light treatment for winter depression. *Arch. Gen. Psychiatry* 47:343–351, 1990.

40. Lewy, A. J., Wehr, T. A., Goodwin, F. K., Newsome, D. A., and Markey, S. P. Light suppresses melatonin secretion in humans. *Science* 210:1267–1269, 1980.

41. Kripke, D. F., Mullaney, D. J., Klauber, M. R., Risch, S. C., and Gillin, J. C. Controlled trial of bright light for nonseasonal major depressive disorders. *Biol. Psychiatry* 31:119–134, 1992.

42. McKinney, W. T. Basis of development of animal models in psychiatry: an overview. In G. F. Koob, C. L. Ehlers, and D. J. Kupfer (eds.), *Animal Models of Depression*. Boston: Birkhauser, 1989, pp. 3–17.

43. Henn, F. A. Animal models. In J. J. Mann (ed.), *Models of Depressive Disorders*. New York: Plenum, 1989, pp. 93–107.

44. Weiss, J. M. Stress-induced depression: critical neurochemical and electrophysiological changes. In J. Madden (ed.), *Neurobiology of Learning, Emotion and Affect*. New York: Raven Press, 1991, pp. 123–154.

45. Maier, S. F., and Seligman, M. E. P. Learned helplessness: theory and evidence. *J. Exp. Psychol.* 105:3–46, 1976.

46. Suomi, S. J. Primate separation models of affective disorders. In J. Madden (ed.), *Neurobi-*

ology of Learning, Emotion and Affect. New York: Raven Press, 1991, pp. 195–214.

47. Coe, C. L., Wiener, S. G., Rosenberg, L. T., and Levine, S. Endocrine and immune responses to separation and maternal loss in nonhuman primates. In M. Reite and T. Field (eds.), *The Psychology of Attachment and Separation.* New York: Academic Press, 1985, pp. 163–200.

48. Martin, J., and Barchas, J. *Neuropeptides in Neurologic and Psychiatric Disease.* New York: Raven Press, 1986.

49. Darko, D., Risch, S. C., Gillin, J. C., and Golshan, S. Association of beta-endorphin with specific clinical symptoms of depression. *Am. J. Psychiatry* 149:1162–1167, 1992.

50. Evans, C. J., Keith, D. E., Jr., Morrison, H,. Magendzo, K., and Edwards, R. H. Cloning of a delta opioid receptor by functional expression. *Science* 258:1952–1955, 1992.

51. Siever, L. J., and Davis, K. L. Overview: toward a dysregulation hypothesis of depression. *Am. J. Psychiatry* 142:1017–1031, 1985.

52. Maas, J. K., Katz, M. M., Frazer, A., Stokes, P. E., Swann, A. C., Davis, J. M., Casper, R., and Berman, N. Current evidence regarding biological hypotheses of depression and accompanying pathophysiological processes: a critique and synthesis of findings using clinical and basic research results. *Integr. Psychiatry* 7: 155–160, 1991.

53. Samson, J. A., Mirin, S. M., Hauser, S. T., Fenton, B. T., and Schildkraut, J. J. Learned helplessness and urinary MHPG levels in unipolar depression. *Am. J. Psychiatry* 149:806–809, 1992.

54. Post, R. M. Transduction of psychosocial stress into the neurobiology of recurrent affective disorder. *Am. J. Psychiatry* 149: 999–1010, 1992.

55. Charney, D. S., Woods, S. W., Krystal, J. H., and Heninger, G. R. Neurobiological mechanisms of human anxiety. In R. Pohl and S. Gershon (eds.), *The Biological Basis of Psychiatric Treatment.* Basel: Karger, 1990, pp. 242–283.

56. Davis, M. The role of the amygdala in conditioned fear. In J. P. Aggleton (ed.), *The Amygdala: Neurobiological Aspects of Emotion.* New York: Wiley Liss, 1992, pp. 255–305.

57. Mohler, H., and Okada, T. Benzodiazepine receptor: demonstration in the central nervous system. *Science* 198:849–851, 1977.

58. Squire, R. F., and Braestrup, C. Benzodiazepine receptors in rat brain. *Nature* 266: 732–734, 1977.

59. Paul, S. M., Crawley, J. N., and Skolnick, P. The neurobiology of anxiety: the role of the GABA/benzodiazepine receptor complex. In P. A. Berger and K. H. Brodie (eds.), *American Handbook of Psychiatry,* Vol. 8. New York: Basic Books, 1986, pp. 581–596.

60. Biggio, G., and Costa, E. (eds.), *GABAergic Transmission and Anxiety.* New York: Raven Press, 1986.

61. Zorumski, C. F., and Isenberg, K. E. Insights into the structure and function of GABA-benzodiazepine receptors: ion channels and psychiatry. *Am. J. Psychiatry* 148:162–173, 1991.

62. Schofield, P. R., Darlison, M. G., Fujita, N., Burt, D. R., Stephenson, F. A., et al. Sequence and functional expression of the $GABA_A$ receptor shows a ligand-gated receptor superfamily. *Nature* 328:221–227, 1987.

63. Doble, A., and Martin, I. Multiple benzodiazepine receptors. *Trends Pharmacol. Sci.* 13: 76–81, 1992.

64. Wisden, W., Laurie, D. J., Monyer, H., and Seeburg, P. H. The distribution of 13 $GABA_A$ receptor subunit mRNAs in the rat brain. *J. Neurosci.* 12:1040–1062, 1992.

65. Iversen, S. D. 5-HT and anxiety. *Neuropharmacology* 23:1553–1560, 1984.

66. Whitaker-Azmitia, P. M., and Peroutka, S. J. (ed.), *The Neuropharmacology of Serotonin.* New York: New York Academy of Sciences, 1990.

67. Dourish, C. T., Hutson, P. H., and Curzon, G. Putative anxiolytics 8-OH-DPAT, buspirone, and TVX Q 7821 are agonists at $5\text{-}HT_{1A}$ receptors in the raphe nuclei. *Trends Pharmacol. Sci.* 7:212–214, 1986.

68. Peroutka, S. J. Interactions of novel anxiolytic agents with $5\text{-}HT_{1A}$ receptors. *Biol. Psychiatry* 20:971–979, 1985.

69. Insel, T. R. New pharmacologic approaches to obsessive compulsive disorder. *J. Clin. Psychiatry* 51:47–51, 1990.

70. Swedo, S. E., Leonard, H. L., Kruesi, M. J. P., Rettew, D. C., Listwak, S. J., Berrettini, W., Stipetic, M., Hamburger, S., Gold, P., Potter, W. Z., and Rapoport, J. L. Cerebrospinal fluid neurochemistry in children and adolescents with obsessive-compulsive disorder. *Arch. Gen. Psychiatry* 49:29–36, 1992.

71. Rapoport, J. L., Ryland, D. H., and Kriete, M. Drug treatment of canine acral lick. *Arch. Gen. Psychiatry* 49:517–521, 1992.

72. Wahlestedt, C., Pich, E., Koob, G. F., Yee, F., and Heilig, M. Modulation of anxiety and neuropeptide Y-Y1 receptors by antisense oligodeoxynucleotides. *Science* 259:528–531, 1993.

73. Barchas, J. D., and Freedman, D. X. Brain amines: response to physiological stress. *Biochem. Pharmacol.* 12:1232–1235, 1963.

74. Tsuda, A., and Tanaka, M. Differential changes in noradrenaline turnover in specific regions of rat brain produced by controllable and uncontrollable shocks. *Behav. Neurosci.* 99:802–817, 1985.

75. Bandura, A., Taylor, C. B., Williams, S. L., Mefford, I. N., and Barchas, J. D. Catecholamine secretion as a function of perceived coping self-efficacy. *J. Consult. Clin. Psychol.* 53:406–414, 1985.

76. Insel, T. R. Toward a neuroanatomy of obsessive-compulsive disorder. *Arch. Gen. Psychiatry* 49:739–744, 1992.

77. Baxter, L. R., Schwartz, J. M., Bergman, K. S., Szuba, M. P., Guze, B. H., Mazziotta, J. C., Alazraki, A., Selin, C. E., Ferng, H.-K., Munford, P., and Phelps, M. E. Caudate glucose metabolic rate changes with both drug and behavior therapy for obsessive-compulsive disorder. *Arch. Gen. Psychiatry* 49:681–689, 1992.

CHAPTER 49

Endocrine Effects on the Brain and Their Relationship to Behavior

Bruce S. McEwen

Basic Neurochemistry: Molecular, Cellular, and Medical Aspects, 5th Ed., edited by G. J. Siegel et al. Published by Raven Press, Ltd., New York, 1994. Correspondence to Bruce S. McEwen, Laboratory of Neuroendocrinology, Rockefeller University, 1230 York Avenue, New York, New York 10021.

The brain undergoes changes in its chemistry and structure in response to changes in the environment. Circulating hormones of the adrenals, thyroid, and gonads play an important role in this adaptation because the endocrine system is controlled by the brain through the pituitary gland (Fig. 1), allowing environmental signals to regulate hormone secretion. Furthermore, circulating hormones act on the brain as well as on other tissues and organs of the body to modify their structure and chemistry via two mechanisms:

1) intracellular receptors that bind to DNA and alter gene expression; 2) cell-surface receptors that modulate ion channels and second-messenger systems.

Hormone actions occur during sensitive periods in development and also in adult life during natural endocrine cycles and in response to experience, as well as during the aging process. As a result of their fundamental actions on cellular processes and genomic activity, and of the control of their secretion by environmental signals, steroid and thy-

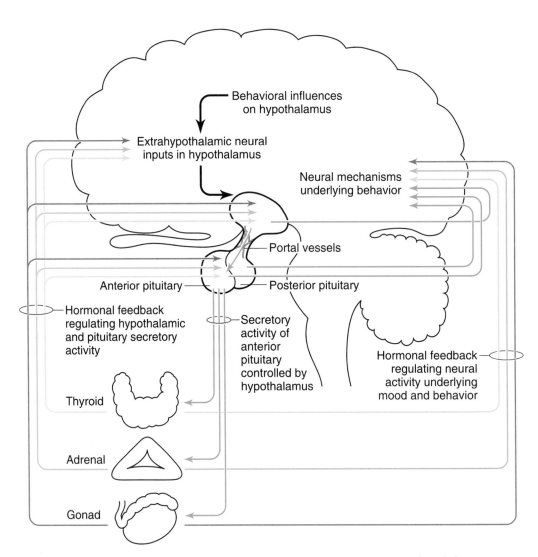

FIG. 1. Schematic representation of possible and known reciprocal interactions among hypothalamic, pituitary, thyroid, adrenal, and gonadal hormones.

roid hormone actions on the brain provide unique insights into the plasticity of the brain and behavior.

Awareness of endocrine influences on brain function is as old as endocrinology itself. In 1849, Berthold described striking behavioral changes resulting from castration of roosters and the reversal of these changes after testes had been transplanted into the castrated animals [see 1]. Nearly 100 years later, Beach published *Hormones and Behavior* [see 1], which has served to instruct recent generations of investigators and motivate them to explore in depth the interactions of hormones and brain. Spectacular growth of the field of neuroendocrinology (see also Chap. 16) offers the present generation of neurobiologists unparalleled opportunities to explore with great sophistication the influence of neural activity on endocrine secretion and the effect of hormones, in turn, on neural activity and behavior.

This chapter focuses on the neurochemical and molecular aspects of the influences of hormones on the nervous system and behavior, after first considering in some detail the chemical signals, behavioral events, and underlying neural activity that regulate hormone secretion.

BEHAVIORAL CONTROL OF HORMONE SECRETION

The brain produces master hormones, the hypothalamic-releasing factors, which regulate release of the anterior pituitary trophic hormones

As summarized in Fig. 1, the releasing factors are produced in various neuronal groups within the hypothalamus and are transported to the median eminence for release into the portal circulation to the anterior pituitary. Neurons in the hypothalamus also produce the hormones oxytocin and vasopressin, which are released by the posterior pituitary into the blood. It is therefore not surprising that behavior and experience,

which influence the hypothalamus, sometimes alter the secretion of these hypothalamic-releasing factors and hormones.

Secretion of pituitary hormones is responsive to behavior and effects of experience

Consider, for example, the phenomenon of lactation, in which the sucking stimulus to the nipple triggers the release of oxytocin, which facilitates milk ejection, and of prolactin, which helps the mammary gland to replenish the supply of milk [2]. The phenomenon of stress also illustrates the behavioral and emotional control of anterior pituitary hormone secretion. Conditions associated with tissue injury and surgical trauma, as well as the so-called psychic stresses of fear, novelty, and even joy, can activate the release of adrenocorticoid (ACTH), which, in turn, stimulates the secretion of adrenal glucocorticoids [2]. The behavioral-emotional stimuli are mediated by neural pathways that can be modified readily by learning.

In the female rabbit, the act of copulation activates spinal reflex pathways that stimulate the secretion of luteinizing hormone (LH) and leads to ovulation [3]. In the male rabbit, the act of copulation also activates the secretion of LH and increases plasma testosterone levels [3]. Social stimuli, too, modify gonadotropin secretion. In mice, olfactory cues from other females can interrupt normal estrous cycles and lead to pseudopregnancies or to periods of prolonged diestrus (Lee-Boot effect); olfactory cues from males can shorten the estrous cycle and either cause rapid attainment of estrus (Whitten effect) or terminate pregnancy in a newly impregnated mouse (Bruce effect) [3]. In male rhesus monkeys, sudden decisive defeat by other males leads to prolonged reduction in plasma testosterone levels, which can be reversed in the defeated male by the introduction of a female companion [3]. In men, the anticipation of sexual intercourse has been reported to increase beard growth, a process under the control of circulating androgen [3], although this finding has been disputed.

Hormones secreted in response to behavioral signals act, in turn, on the brain and on other tissues

Functional changes caused by hormones secreted in response to behavioral signals include modifications of behavior. With the sex hormones, these changes act to strengthen and guide the reproductive process. Thus, aggressive encounters between male birds or mammals in defense of territory during the mating period stimulate gonadotropin and testosterone secretion and further increase readiness for sexual activity by enhancing supplies of sperm and seminal fluid. This analysis was taken further by Lehrman [see 1] who showed that among doves the behavioral sequence of courtship, mating, nest-building, and parenting involves complex behavioral interplay between the partners that triggers further hormone secretion, which unfolds the next phase of behavior and hormone secretion.

Regarding the adrenal steroids, the behavioral activation of hormonal secretion in stress is part of a mechanism for restoring homeostatic balance. For example, an encounter with a predator may require rapid evasive action in which neural activity and rapidly mobilized hormones such as epinephrine play a role. Adrenal steroid secretion is slower, reaching a peak minutes after the stressful event, and as such is not expected to play a role in coping with the immediate situation. If the evasive action is successful and the animal survives, it will have to re-establish homeostasis; presumably, it will also learn from the experience to minimize the chances of another such encounter. Adrenal steroids act to facilitate such long-term adaptation, i.e., they facilitate the extinction of a conditioned avoidance response [4]. Suppose an animal has learned to avoid a certain place where it was previously punished; it later discovers that being in that place no longer results in punishment. If, for

example, that place also contains a food or water supply, it is in the best interest of the animal to extinguish the avoidance response in order to take advantage of the available food or water. Adrenal steroids, have, in fact, been found to facilitate such extinction and can thus be said to facilitate a form of behavioral adaptation [4]. Another aspect of adaptation in which stress-induced secretion of adrenal steroids participate concerns the ability of the organism to cope with a repeated stressful event through a variety of neurochemical changes [5].

Besides stress, adrenal steroids are also secreted in varying amounts according to the time of day, and in this capacity they perform an important role in coordinating daily activity and sleep patterns with food seeking and processing of information [3]. In nocturnally active animals such as the rat, adrenal steroids are secreted at the end of the light period prior to onset of darkness. In humans and in monkeys, adrenal steroid secretion precedes waking in the morning to begin daily activity. Thus, in both rats and primates, adrenal steroid secretion precedes the waking period and appears to contribute, during waking, to optimal synaptic efficacy in the hippocampus for long-term potentiation, a correlate of learning. Moreover, adrenal steroid elevation prior to waking also increases food-seeking behavior and enhances appetite for carbohydrates [5].

Cyclic changes in hormonal secretion, which are under the control of daily and seasonal light-dark rhythms, are important not only for the adrenals but for the gonads as well. Estrous cycles, menstrual cycles, and seasonal breeding patterns represent adaptations of individual species to climatic conditions of their environment. The feedback actions of gonadal and adrenal hormones, which are secreted in response to rhythmic output of hypothalamic and pituitary hormones, prime or activate the nervous system to perform the appropriate behavioral responses. It is important to stress that hormones themselves do not cause behaviors; rather, hormones induce chemical changes in particular sets of neurons, making certain behavioral outcomes more likely as a result of the strengthening or weakening of particular neural pathways.

CLASSIFICATION OF HORMONE EFFECTS

The principal means of classifying hormone action on target neurons is in terms of cellular mechanisms of action

Hormones act either via cell-surface or intracellular receptors. Peptide hormones and amino acid derivatives such as epinephrine act on cell-surface receptors that do such things as open ion channels, cause rapid electrical responses, and facilitate exocytosis of hormones or neurotransmitters. Alternatively, they activate second-messenger systems at the cell membrane, such as those involving cyclic AMP (cAMP), Ca^{2+}-calmodulin, or phosphoinositides (see Chaps. 20–22), which lead to phosphorylation of proteins inside various parts of the target cell (Fig. 2A). Steroid hormones and thyroid hormone, on the other hand, act on intracellular receptors in the cell nuclei to regulate gene expression and protein synthesis (Fig. 2B). Steroid hormones can also affect cell-surface events via receptors at or near the cell surface.

The various modes of hormone action summarized in Fig. 2 may be distinguished from each other by time course. The fastest effects, both in latency and duration, are those involving direct opening of ion channels and stimulation of exocytosis. Intermediate are those effects involving phosphorylation of enzymes, ion channels, receptors, or structural proteins, which may last for minutes or even hours. Slowest and most enduring are those effects that alter gene expression and lead to induction or repression of enzyme or receptor proteins, growth responses, and even the structural remodeling of tissues.

As summarized in Fig. 3, steroid/thyroid hormone receptors are proteins that bind to other proteins as well as to DNA [6–8]. In the simplest type of action (Fig. 3A), the steroid/thyroid hormone receptor becomes activated after the hormone binds

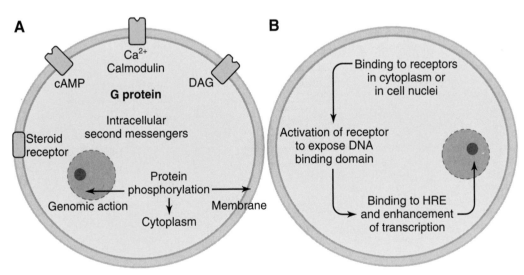

FIG. 2.   There are two modes of hormone action. **A:** Activation of cell-surface receptors and coupled second-messenger systems, with a variety of intracellular consequences. **B:** Entry of hormone into the target cell, binding to and activation of an intracellular receptor, and binding of the receptor-hormone complex to specific DNA sequences to activate or repress gene expression.

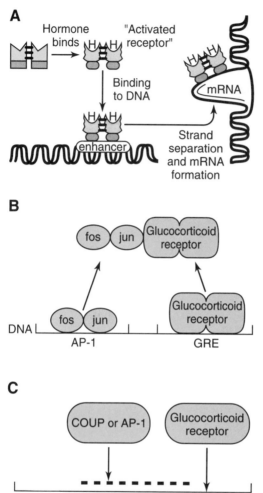

FIG. 3.   Intracellular receptors mediate at least three distinct types of actions on gene expression. **A:** Binding of the hormone-receptor complex to a "hormone-response element," a DNA sequence that is placed in a position where receptor binding to it can enhance unwinding of the double helix and attachment of other transcription factors. **B:** Binding of the steroid receptor to another protein transcription factor, e.g., the *fos-jun* complex through protein-protein interactions, removing both transcription factors from binding to DNA. **C:** Binding of the hormone receptor to a "hormone-response element" located in the middle of a site for binding of another transcription factor-response element such as the AP-1 or COUP sites, resulting in inhibition of transcription normally activated by transcription factors acting on these response elements [6–8].

to it; activation results in conformational changes that include shedding of other proteins, such as heat-shock proteins, and exposing the DNA-binding domain. The receptor then binds to the specific sequence of DNA (called a "hormone-response element" or enhancer) located on the coding strand of DNA; this enhances transcription by permitting other transcription factors as well as the RNA polymerase to bind to the promoter region [6–8]. A second scheme (Fig. 3B) is for the hormone receptor to bind with high affinity to another protein transcription factor, in this case the c-*fos*-c-*jun* complex, removing both protein complexes from binding to DNA [6–8]. Such a result also blocks the enhancement of transcription by either agent, although it could also reduce inhibitory effects produced by the hormone receptor through the scheme shown in Fig. 3C. A variant on this theme, not shown in the figure, is "squelching," in which multiple transcription factors compete with each other for a limited supply of soluble ligands that enhance their activities [6–8]. A third scheme, shown in Fig. 3C, is for the steroid receptor to compete for binding sites in the promoter regions with another transcription factor, such as COUP, or the cAMP-dependent transcription factors that bind to the AP-1 response element. The result of this competition is inhibition of transcription, since, in this situation, it is the other transcription factors that enhance transcription, whereas the hormone receptor does not do so when it binds to the coding DNA strand [6–8].

As we have noted, second-messenger systems, through phosphorylation of nuclear proteins, can influence gene expression. Recent evidence indicates that even the classical steroid receptors are subject to regulation by phosphorylation, and that phosphorylations promoted by a neurotransmitter such as dopamine are able to cause nuclear translocation of a steroid receptor in the absence of the steroid [9].

So far, the best understood examples of genomic regulation of neuronal function stem from the actions of gonadal and adrenal steroids and thyroid hormone, and many of these actions are involved in the plasticity of behavior that results from hormone secretion, such as changes in aggressive and reproductive behavior and adaptation to repeated stress. In fact, hormone actions that involve the genome are pervasive throughout the life cycle. We can distinguish four major types of hormone actions on the nervous system:

1. *Developmental actions,* such as those that are involved in sexual differentiation and the effects of thyroid hormone and retinoic acid.
2. *Reversible, and often cyclical, effects* on the structure and function of neurons and glial cells that underlie corresponding cyclical changes in behavior, such as those that are involved in reproduction and in the daily rhythms of sleep and waking.
3. *Experiential effects* involving environmentally induced changes in hormone secretion, as in stress, that evoke adaptive or maladaptive changes in the brain.
4. Effects that *protect neurons or potentiate damage and lead to cell death.*

It will be seen below that, in addition to genomic actions, there are nongenomic effects of steroids that modulate neurotransmitter release as well as ion traffic across the cell membrane, and do so frequently, in coordination with genomic actions.

BIOCHEMISTRY OF STEROID AND THYROID HORMONE ACTION

Steroid hormones are divided into six classes, based on physiological effects: estrogens, androgens, progestins, glucocorticoids, mineralocorticoids, and vitamin D

As shown in Figs. 2 and 3, steroid hormone action on the brain and on other target tissues involves intracellular receptor sites that interact with the genome [1]. There are also important metabolic transformations of certain steroids, occurring in the nervous system, that either generate more active metabolites or result in the production of less active steroids. Such transformations are particularly important for the actions of androgens, of lesser importance for estrogens and progestins, and of practically no importance for glucocorticoids and mineralocorticoids. For vitamin D, the principal transformation to an active metabolite occurs in the kidney and liver [10]. Some metabolites, such as allopregnanolone and allotetrahydroDOC, produce nongenomic effects on the $GABA_A$ receptor.

Some steroid hormones are converted in the brain to more or less active products that interact with receptors

The brain, like the seminal vesicles, is able to convert testosterone to 5α-dihydrotestosterone (DHT); and, like the placenta, the brain converts testosterone to estradiol (Fig. 4). Neither conversion occurs equally in all brain regions. Regional distribution of 5α-reductase activity toward testosterone in rat brain reveals that the highest activity is found in midbrain and brainstem; intermediate activity in hypothalamus and thalamus; and lowest activity in cerebral cortex [11]. The pituitary has higher 5α-reductase activity than any region of the brain, and its activity is subject to changes as a result of gonadectomy, hormone replacement, and postnatal age [3,11]. 5α-DHT has been implicated in the hypothalamus and pituitary as a potent regulator of gonadotropin secretion, but it is relatively inactive toward male rat sexual behavior [3]. Labeled metabolites with the Rf value of 5α-DHT have been detected in extracts of hypothalamic and pituitary tissue after [3H]-testosterone administration in both adult and newborn rats. It is interesting that progesterone inhibits 5α-reductase activity toward [3H]testosterone and that [3H]progesterone is itself converted to

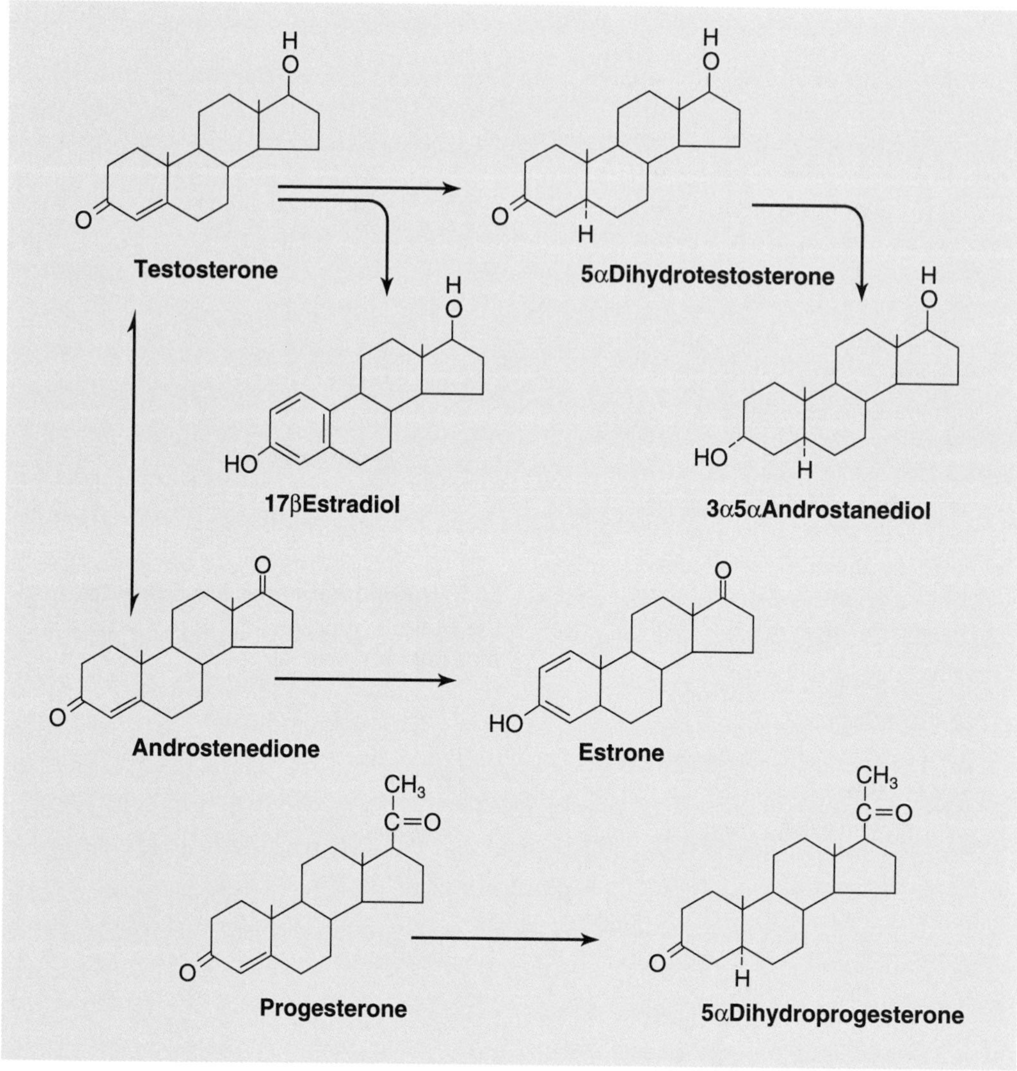

FIG. 4.   Some steroid transformations that are carried out by neural tissue.

[³H]5α-dihydroprogesterone (Fig. 4). Progesterone competition for 5α-reductase may explain some of the antiandrogenicity of this steroid [3,11]. 5β-DHT is a metabolite of testosterone formed in the bird CNS, as is 5α-DHT; 5β-DHT is inactive toward sexual behavior and is believed to represent an inactivation pathway for testosterone.

The aromatization of testosterone to form estradiol, and of androstenedione to form estrone (Fig. 4), has been described in brain tissue *in vitro* and *in vivo* [11]. Aromatization is higher in hypothalamus and limbic structures than in cerebral cortex or pituitary gland, and, in noncastrated animals, is higher in male than in female brains. Aromatization has been found in brains of reptiles and amphibia as well as in brains of mammals [11]. The capacity to aromatize testosterone and related androgens may therefore be a general property of vertebrate brains. The functional role of aromatization has been studied most extensively in the rat: Male sexual behavior is facilitated by estradiol [12], and testosterone facilitation of male sexual behavior can be blocked by a steroidal inhibitor of aromatization [3,11,12]. There are indications that a similar situation exists in birds, amphibia, and reptiles; that is, testosterone and estradiol can stimulate heterotypical sexual behavior in males and females. Curiously, not all mammals are like the rat; for example, male sexual behavior of guinea pig and rhesus monkey is restored by the nonaromatizable androgen dihydrotestosterone [3,12].

Both aromatization and 5α-reductase are regulated by gonadal steroids. In mammals such as the rat, it is principally the neural aromatase activity that is up-regulated by androgens acting via neural androgen receptors [13]. In birds, neural aromatase and 5α-reductase are both induced by testosterone, and this regulation provides a way by which androgens can regulate CNS hormone sensitivity without regulating receptor number [14].

Both estrogens and glucocorticoids appear to act on brain cells without being first metabolized because both [³H]estradiol and [³H]corticosterone are recovered unchanged from their cell nuclear binding sites in brain [3]. However, estradiol is subject to conversion to the catechol estrogen 2-hydroxyestradiol, and this metabolite is both a moderately potent estrogen via intracellular estrogen receptors as well as an agent capable of interacting with cell-surface receptors such as those for catecholamines, albeit at fairly high concentrations [15].

Vitamin D, prior to acting in the brain, is converted to an active metabolite, 1,25-dihydroxy vitamin D_3, by enzymes in liver and kidney [10] (see Fig. 5).

The nervous system is also capable of cleaving the side chain from cholesterol to generate the same initial series of steroids [16] that are produced by the adrenals and gonads, namely, pregnenolone, dehydroepiandrosterone, and progesterone (Fig. 6). In addition, neural tissue converts progesterone via reduction of the Δ4-5 double bond and reduction of the 3 keto group, to 3α 5α-pregnanolone, which is active on the chlo-

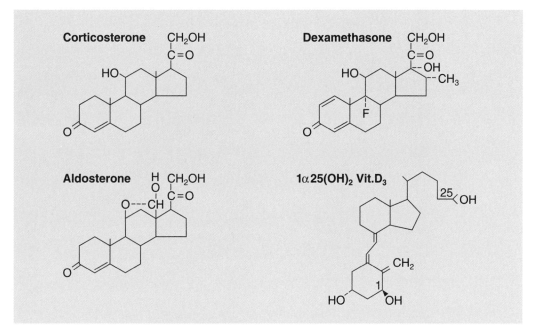

FIG. 5. Formulas of four steroid hormones.

ride channel of the GABA$_A$ receptor [17] (Fig. 7). Glial cells are believed to be the primary sites of both cholesterol side chain cleavage and generation of pregnanolone from progesterone [16]. While steroids generated in the brain have been referred to as "neurosteroids," a more useful term is "neuroactive steroids" to refer to all steroids that affect brain function via any mechanism and irrespective of site of formation.

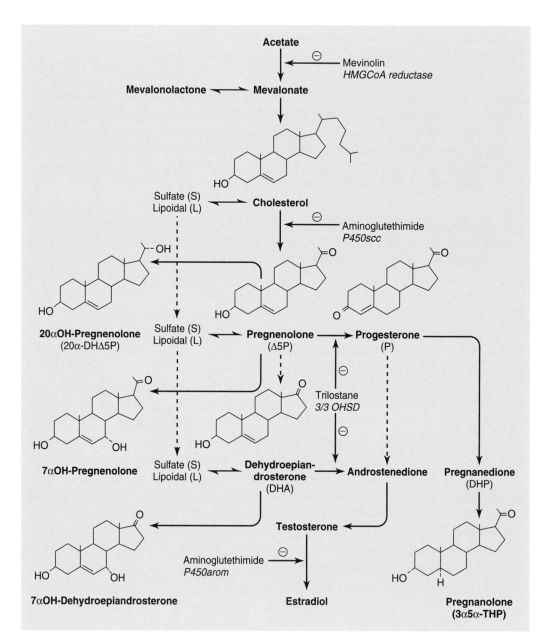

FIG. 6. Biosynthesis/metabolism of steroids in the CNS. The conversion of Δ5P to dehydroepiandrosterone (DHA) is postulated but not demonstrated. Δ5P and DHA inhibit and 3α5α-THP potentiates GABA$_A$ receptor function, as summarized in Fig. 7. *Solid arrows* indicate demonstrated pathways; *dotted arrows* indicate possible pathways. Metabolic inhibitors of enzymes are indicated by ⊖. Redrawn from E. Baulieu, with permission.

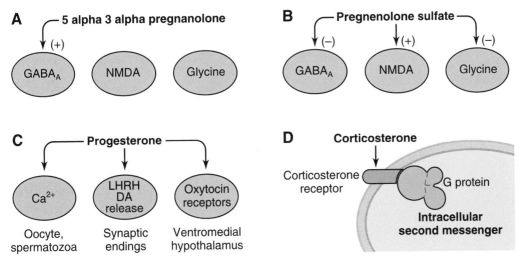

FIG. 7. Schematic summary of four ways in which steroids affect cell-surface-mediated events and neuronal activity by nongenomic mechanisms. **A:** Activation of GABA$_A$ receptor by 5α3α-pregnanolone. **B:** Activation of NMDA receptor and inhibition of GABA$_A$ and glycine receptor by pregnenolone sulfate. **C:** Activation of Ca^{2+} mobilization in oocytes and spermatozoa by progesterone; the same is postulated to happen in certain synaptic endings and may also be involved in the rapid direct effect of progesterone on the oxytocin receptor. **D:** Corticosterone binds to a cell-surface receptor linked to a G protein, and presumably through it to a second-messenger system, in some brain cells.

Genomic receptors for steroid hormones have been clearly identified in the nervous system

The detection of intracellular, DNA-binding steroid receptors became possible with the introduction of tritium-labeled steroid hormones of high specific radioactivity (20–25 Ci/mmol at each labeled position). The limited number of these sites had escaped detection using steroids labeled with ^{14}C at a much lower specific radioactivity. ^{3}H-Labeling also permitted histological localization of steroid receptors, because the high spatial resolution of ^{3}H (1–2 μm in light microscope autoradiography) allows cellular and even cell nuclear localization of the radioactivity.

Cell fractionation procedures were fundamental to the biochemical identification of steroid and thyroid hormone receptors in brain as well as in other tissues. Isolation of highly purified cell nuclei from small amounts of tissue from discrete brain regions is generally accomplished with the aid of a nonionic detergent such as Triton X-100 [18]. Cytosol fractions of brain tissue (prepared by centrifugation of homogenates at 105,000 g for 60 min) contain the soluble steroid hormone-binding proteins, and a variety of methods intended to separate bound from unbound steroid have been used for measuring their binding activity [3,18]. The most commonly employed are gel filtration chromatography and sucrose density gradient centrifugation. Dextran-coated charcoal or Sephadex LH20 are frequently used because they effectively absorb unbound steroid and leave intact the complexes between steroid and putative receptor. Other methods, such as gel electrophoresis and precipitation of putative receptor material with protamine sulfate, have more restricted uses.

The objective of such studies is to measure the affinity, capacity, and specificity of the hormone-receptor interaction [3,18]. Measurements of affinity capacity are accomplished with equilibrium binding analysis.

Specificity is based on competition between the labeled and various unlabeled ligands for binding sites. (These methods are described in Chap. 10.)

Because the nervous system is a highly heterogeneous organ from the standpoint of many neurochemical characteristics, including steroid and thyroid hormone receptors, the most useful techniques for mapping these receptors have been histochemical ones. Steroid autoradiography was the first such method. With purification of receptors and generation of antibodies, immunocytochemistry has been added as a tool. Cloning of steroid and thyroid receptors has opened the way to mapping of receptor mRNAs via *in situ* hybridization histochemistry.

Several criteria determine whether a steroid hormone-binding site is a putative receptor. First, the steroid hormone-binding site must be present in hormone-responsive tissues (or brain regions) and absent from nonresponsive ones. Second, it should bind steroids that are either active agonists or effective antagonists of the hormone effect and not bind steroids that are inactive in either sense.

There is an ongoing controversy regarding intracellular localization of steroid and thyroid hormone receptors in cells. With the exception of thyroid hormone receptors, which are exclusively nuclear in location, cell fractionation studies have revealed that, in the absence of hormone, steroid receptors are extracted in the soluble or cytosol fraction; however, when steroid is present in the cell, many occupied receptors are retained by purified cell nuclei. Histological procedures, such as immunocytochemistry, have confirmed the largely nuclear localization of occupied receptors, but they have also revealed a nuclear localization of receptors in the absence of hormone in the tissue. This is true for estrogen, progestin, and androgen receptors, but the mineralocorticoid and glucocorticoid receptors show a cytoplasmic localization in the absence of hormone. Thus, steroid receptors may exist in nuclei in a loose association that is disrupted during

cell fractionation. This is not an uncommon situation for many constituents of cell nuclei [18].

INTRACELLULAR STEROID RECEPTORS: PROPERTIES AND TOPOGRAPHY

Steroid hormone receptors are proteins of 55 to 120 kDa that are similar to each other in that they all have a DNA-binding domain and a steroid-binding domain; they are also phosphoproteins, for which the state of phosphorylation appears to influence functional activity

Estradiol

The first neural steroid receptor type to be recognized was that for estradiol [1]. *In vivo* uptake of [³H]estradiol and binding to cell nuclei isolated from hypothalamus, pituitary, and other brain regions revealed steroid specificity closely resembling that of the uterus, where steroid receptors were first discovered [see 1]. Cytosol estrogen receptors isolated from pituitary and brain tissue resemble closely those found in uterus and mammary tissue. A hallmark of the estrogen receptor is its existence as an aggregate of subunits that dissociate during steroid-induced transformation to the DNA-binding nuclear form of the receptor. This part of the estrogen receptor complex was cloned from human breast cancer cells and consists of a 65- to 70-kDa hormone and DNA-binding subunit [6,19]. The dissociation constant of estradiol binding is approximately 0.2 nm.

Estrogen receptors are found in the pituitary, hypothalamus, preoptic area, and amygdala of the adult. They are principally in neurons, although glial cells may also express these receptors in some brain regions [see 1]. The developing rat brain expresses estrogen receptors in cerebral cortex and hippocampus, but these receptors largely disappear as the brain matures [20].

Progesterone

Detection of progesterone receptors in brain was made possible by the use of the synthetic progestin R5020 (promegestrone; 17-α, 21-dimethyl, 19-nor-pregna-4,9-diene-3,20-dione), which has a high affinity for the progestin receptor ($K_d = 0.4$ nM) [21]. The progestin receptor has been cloned from chick oviduct and consists of a steroid- and DNA-binding subunit of 108 kDa, although one 79-kDa subunit has also been described [6,19]. Progestin receptors with similar properties are found in pituitary, reproductive tract, and most estrogen-receptor-containing brain regions, and these receptors are inducible by estrogen treatment [21]. There are also progestin receptor sites in brain areas lacking estrogen receptors, such as the cerebral cortex of the rat, and these receptors are not induced by estradiol treatment; such receptors, nevertheless, resemble those that are induced by estradiol [21]. Another inducer of progestin receptors in brain is testosterone, which works through its conversion to estradiol via aromatization [21]. Progesterone acts rapidly to induce feminine sexual behavior (lordosis) in female rats that have been primed with estradiol to induce progestin receptors [21]. The principal site of estradiol and progesterone action is the ventromedial nucleus of the hypothalamus [1].

Androgen

Androgen receptors have a steroid-binding subunit estimated to be 120 kDa [6,19]. The estimated K_d for active androgens is approximately 1 to 2 nM [1]. Androgen receptors are found widely distributed in brain and pituitary tissue, although highest concentrations are found in hypothalamus, preoptic area, and limbic brain tissue [22]. Androgen receptors are deficient in the androgen-insensitivity (Tfm) mutation, and animals with this mutation show defects in sexual behavior, juvenile rough-and-tumble play behavior, and certain aspects of neuroendocrine function, thus indicating the actions of testosterone that are mediated by androgen receptors, as opposed to those mediated by aromatization of testosterone to estradiol (see above) and estrogen receptors [12].

Glucocorticoid

Adrenal steroid receptors have been subdivided into two categories, one of which is the classical glucocorticoid receptor [4]. This receptor has been cloned from human and rat sources and consists of a steroid- and DNA-binding subunit of 95 kDa [6,19]. Such receptors, which have dissociation constants for glucocorticoids of 4 to 5 nM, are widely distributed across brain regions and are found in neurons and glial cells [4].

Mineralocorticoid

The other type of glucocorticoid receptor is similar to the mineralocorticoid receptor originally described in the kidney [4]. In the brain, receptors of this type bind the glucocorticoid corticosterone with high affinity (K_d approx. 1 nM), and they are responsible for the high uptake of tracer levels of [^{3}H]-corticosterone by the hippocampus [4]. These corticosterone receptors, which are found in high levels in the hippocampus, but are also widely distributed in other brain regions at lower levels, may be involved in mediating effects of the diurnally varying levels of corticosterone [5]. Uptake of [^{3}H]aldosterone by brain tissues reveals two types of binding sites: those in the hippocampus that can be preferentially occupied by corticosterone and sites that are more diffusely distributed in the brain and that appear to retain [^{3}H]aldosterone preferentially in the presence of the normally higher levels of corticosterone [4]. The reasons for this selectivity of an enzyme, 11 β-hydroxysteroid dehydrogenase, are that, at least in the kidney-collecting tubules, it converts corticosterone to an inactive metabolite and allows aldosterone access to the mineralocorticoid receptors [22].

Vitamin D

Vitamin D is a steroid hormone, production of which by the body requires the action of light. Therefore, it is often necessary to provide some vitamin D in the diet [10]. Moreover, vitamin D is converted by kidney and liver to the active metabolite, 1,25-dihydroxy vitamin D_3 (Fig. 5) [10]. Vitamin D_3 receptors consist of a hormone- and DNA-binding subunit of 55 kDa [6,19]. Receptor sites for 1,25-dihydroxy vitamin D_3 are found in pituitary and in brain, especially in the forebrain, hindbrain, and spinal cord neurons [23]. In the brain, one site containing vitamin D_3 receptors, the bed nucleus of the stria terminalis, responds to exogenous 1,25-dihydroxy vitamin D_3 with an induction of choline acetyltransferase, even though the calcium-binding protein that is regulated by vitamin D_3 in intestine is not regulated by this hormone in brain [24]. Moreover, vitamin D_3 also corrects deficiencies in serum testosterone and LH in vitamin D-deficient male rats [24]. It is not clear, however, whether this represents a major effect of vitamin D_3 in the pituitary gland or brain, or both.

THE IDENTIFICATION OF MEMBRANE STEROID RECEPTORS

The known rapid effects of some steroid hormones on neuronal excitability are difficult to explain in terms of genomic action [17]. Instead, some type of membrane receptor interaction is inferred. Indeed, several types of interactions of neuroactive steroids with neural membranes have been described. Direct binding assays have revealed membrane sites for glucocorticoids and gonadal steroids and one instance of a membrane receptor coupled to a G protein (Fig. 7); indirect binding assay results have implied interaction of the catechol estrogens with dopamine and with adrenergic receptors [17].

There are now indications for the interaction of progesterone metabolites with the chloride channel of the $GABA_A$ receptor (Fig. 7). The A-ring reduced steroids, especially those with the $5\alpha,3\alpha$ configuration, are particularly active on the $GABA_A$ receptor [17]. By facilitating chloride channel opening, these steroids produce anesthetic, anxiolytic, and sedative-hypnotic effects.

Another "neurosteroid" (Fig. 6), pregnenolone sulfate (PS), produces effects that in many ways antagonize those of the steroids that open the $GABA_A$ receptor chloride channel [16,17]. PS in micromolar concentrations inhibits the $GABA_A$ receptor, as well as the inhibitory glycine receptor, and it facilitates activity of the excitatory NMDA receptor (Fig. 7). It is unclear, however, whether these effects are physiologically relevant, since the PS concentration needed to produce these effects is rather high. However, PS is produced locally in the brain and may reach high enough concentrations in some compartments within the nervous system.

Progesterone also produces direct membrane effects [17]. These include actions that promote maturation of spermatozoa as well as oocytes, and facilitation of the release of neurotransmitters such as dopamine and LHRH (Fig. 7). Membrane actions of progesterone also activate oxytocin receptors in the hypothalamus in a way that enables oxytocin to act to turn on female sexual behavior in the estrogen-primed female rat [1].

None of these findings undermine the importance of the intracellular genomic actions of steroids. Rather, they increase the richness of the cellular actions of steroid hormones and raise the possibility that there may be connections between genomic and nongenomic actions of steroids. For example, genomic action may induce receptors that mediate nongenomic effects. Moreover, the activation of oxytocin receptors by progesterone is dependent on the ability of estrogen priming to induce the formation of new oxytocin receptors via a genomic mechanism; these receptors are then transported along dendrites to sites where the progesterone action occurs at the membrane level [1].

BIOCHEMISTRY AND FUNCTIONAL SIGNIFICANCE OF THYROID HORMONE ACTIONS ON BRAIN

Like steroid hormones, thyroid hormones interact with receptors to alter genomic activity and affect the synthesis of specific proteins during development [25]: As with testosterone and progesterone, metabolic transformation of thyroxine (T_4) is critical to their action [25]. Moreover, as with steroid hormones, thyroid hormones alter brain functions in adult life in ways that both resemble and differ from their action during development [25,26].

The initial step after cellular uptake of T_4 is metabolic transformation to 3,5,3′-triiodothyronine (T_3) (Fig. 8), which interacts with cytosolic and nuclear receptors, as well as with synaptosomal membrane binding sites of unknown function [25]. Cytosolic receptors are proteins of 70 kDa that do not appear to undergo translocation to cell nuclei, nor do they appear to be nuclear proteins that have leaked out of cell nuclei during cell rupture; nuclear receptors are proteins of 50 to 70 kDa that have both DNA- and hormone-binding domains [25]. Evidence points to homology between the nuclear T_3 receptor and the c-erb-A gene, the cellular counterpart of the viral oncogene, v-erb-A [6,19].

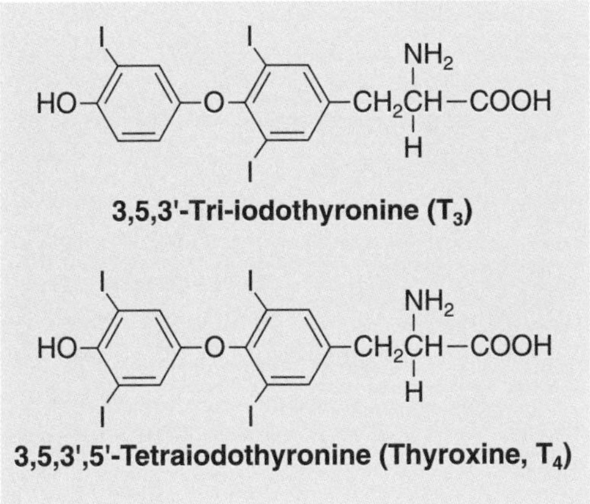

Nuclear T_3 receptors are present in higher levels during neural development than they are in adult life [25]. In human fetal brain, nuclear T_3 receptors increase in concentration from 10 weeks of gestation to the 16th week, when neuroblast multiplication is high [27]. Glial cells as well as neurons contain nuclear T_3 receptors [27]. Functionally, many neurons develop prior to the appearance of significant T_3 receptor levels and therefore appear to be independent of large-scale thyroid influence [28]. Other neurons, such as those in cortex and cerebellum, show a more profound dependence on thyroid function [25]. Although thyroid hormone affects the number of replicating cells in the external granular layer of the developing cerebellum, it is not possible to conclude that T_3 directly affects the mechanism of cell replication [25]. Rather, the most pronounced effect of hypothyroidism is a hypoplastic neuropil, with shorter dendrites and fewer spines. It has been shown that a major effect of T_3 involves the development of the neuronal cytoskeleton [25]. Proteins, such as microtubule-associated protein (MAP_2) and tau (see Chap. 27), which are polymorphic and affect microtubular assembly, are differentially affected by T_3 absence or excess [25].

Developmentally, thyroid hormones interact with sex hormones such that hypothyroidism prolongs the critical period for testosterone-induced defeminization (see below) [3]; in contrast, the hyperthyroid state terminates the sensitivity to testosterone prematurely [3]. Undoubtedly, an important link in these and other effects is synapse formation. Hypothyroidism increases synaptic density, at least transiently [3]. Interesting parallels with synapse formation are reported for learning behavior in rats: Neonatal hypothyroidism impairs learning ability, whereas hyperthyroidism accelerates

3,5,3′-Tri-iodothyronine (T_3)

3,5,3′,5′-Tetraiodothyronine (Thyroxine, T_4)

FIG. 8.   Formulas for thyroxine (T_4) and tri-iodothyronine (T_3).

learning initially, followed by a decline later in life [3].

The adult brain is endowed with nuclear as well as cytosol and membrane T_3 receptors that have been visualized by autoradiography and studied biochemically [25,28]. Both neurons and neuropil are labeled by [^{125}I]T_3, and the labeling is selective across brain regions. Functionally, one of the most prominent features of neural action of thyroid hormone in adulthood is subsensitivity to norepinephrine as a result of a hypothyroid state [26]. These changes may be reflections of loss of dendritic spines in at least some neurons of the adult brain (see [25]). Clinically, thyroid hormone deficiency increases the probability of depressive illness, whereas thyroid excess increases the probability of mania (Chap. 48) in susceptible individuals [26].

DIVERSITY OF STEROID HORMONE ACTIONS ON THE BRAIN

Steroid hormone effects on the brain link the environment surrounding the organism with the genome of target brain cells through the process of variable genomic activity [23]. By this we mean that an organism experiences light, dark, heat, cold, fear, and sexual excitement. These experiences influence hormone secretion, and these hormones, in turn, act on the genome of receptor-containing brain cells to alter their functional state. The genome of brain cells, like those of other cells of the body, is continually active from embryonic life until death and is continually responsive to intra- and extracellular signals. This activity can be seen from the high levels of RNA metabolism in neurons. The differential influence of steroid hormones on variable genomic activity is evident from studies showing rapid and brain region-specific induction of ribosomal and messenger RNA, as well as changes in cell nuclear diameter and chromatin structure [1]. However, variable genomic activity

changes qualitatively with the state of differentiation of the target cells: Embryonic neurons show growth responses that result in permanent changes in circuitry, whereas adult neurons show impermanent responses. Under other circumstances, the same hormonal signals can promote damage and even neuronal loss; under still other conditions, adult neurons can be stimulated to grow and repair damage by treatment with hormones.

Developmental actions

Steroid hormone receptors become evident in target neurons of the brain within several days of final cell division [12]. Whether some receptors are also present in dividing neuronal precursors is not clear. After they have appeared, these receptors mediate a variety of developmental actions. For example, glucocorticoids direct differentiation of adrenergic/cholinergic neurons of the autonomic nervous system to develop in the adrenergic direction [4], and they increase the number of epinephrine-containing small, intensely fluorescent cells (often referred to as SIF) in autonomic ganglia [4]. Glucocorticoids are also required for the normal postnatal ontogeny of serotonin neurons in the forebrain [4]. These effects may not all be direct ones but may involve hormonal modulation of growth factors produced by other cells surrounding the developing neurons.

Gonadal hormones, on the other hand, are involved in the sexual differentiation of the reproductive tract and brain [12]. Mammals, in which the male has X and Y chromosomes, undergo sexual differentiation under the impetus of testosterone secreted by the testes during a period of perinatal life; in species like the human, this period is in midgestation, but in species like the rat, it is from the end of gestation into neonatal life. Key features of sexual behavior in birds are determined in the reverse manner in keeping with the fact that the female bird has the chromosomal heterogeneity: Females produce either estradiol or testosterone, either of which feminizes the brain, which would otherwise develop a masculine pattern in the absence of gonadal steroids [12,29].

As for the mechanisms of sexual differentiation, we must consider the metabolism of the hormone receptor types involved and the primary receptor-mediated events. Testosterone, as noted above, is a prohormone that is converted into either 5α-DHT or estradiol within the brain; these products exert effects on brain sexual differentiation via androgen and estrogen receptors, respectively [12,29]. Masculinization of sexual and aggressive behavior involves either 5α-DHT alone or a combination of 5α-DHT and estradiol acting on different cells. Besides masculinization, there is in some mammals a process called defeminization, in which feminine responses that would develop in the absence of testosterone are suppressed by its presence during the critical period. Conversion to estradiol appears to be involved in this process [12,29]. Progesterone plays no major role in brain sexual differentiation, but it does have the ability to antagonize actions at both androgen and estrogen receptors and thus is an agent that can moderate the degree of masculinization and defeminization.

As to the primary developmental actions of testosterone, growth and differentiation appear to be involved. Testosterone or estradiol stimulates outgrowth of neurites from developing hypothalamic neurons that contain estrogen receptors (12). This is believed to be one of the principal aspects of testosterone action that increases the number of neurons and the size of neurons within specific hypothalamic nuclei in males, compared to females [30]. 5α-DHT may have a similar effect on androgen-sensitive neurons. Differentiation of target neurons also occurs; hormones like estradiol can evoke responses in adult brain tissue that differ between adult male and female rats [1,30].

Activation and adaptation

Hormone secretion by the adrenals and gonads is controlled by endogenous oscillators that can be entrained by environmental cues such as light and dark. The actions of hormones secreted cyclically on behavior and brain function are referred to as activational effects. In addition to the cyclic mode, there is another mode of secretion initiated by such experiences as stress, fear, and aggressive and sexual encounters. In this case, actions of hormones secreted in response to experience lead to adaptive responses by the brain, which, in the case of adrenal steroids, help the animal cope with stressful situations [4,5]. The activational and adaptational effects are largely reversible and involve a variety of neurochemical changes, most of which appear to be initiated at the genomic level. For example, estradiol is secreted cyclically during the estrous cycle in the female rat and triggers the surge of LH, which induces a surge of progesterone from the ovary. Progesterone, in turn, stimulates sexual responsiveness to the male rat [1].

Estradiol action to promote feminine sexual behavior in the rat involves a cascade of induced protein synthesis in specific hypothalamic neurons accompanied by morphological changes indicative of increased genomic activity [1]. Among the induced proteins are receptors for progesterone (see above) crucial for activating sexual behavior; receptors for acetylcholine and oxytocin that are active in enabling the hypothalamic neurons to respond to afferent input; proteins that are axonally transported from the hypothalamus to the midbrain, where they may be involved in neurotransmission; and structural proteins that contribute to formation of new synapses that come and go during the estrous cycle [1] (see Fig. 9).

Adrenal steroids secreted in the diurnal cycle are responsible for reversibly activating exploratory activity, food-seeking behavior, carbohydrate appetite, and synaptic efficacy; they appear to do this by acting on the hippocampus, where there are many mineralocorticoid and glucocorticoid receptors (see above). Adaptational effects of adrenal steroids that result from stress appear to operate via the classical glucocorticoid receptor

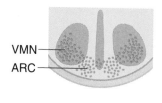

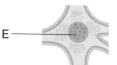

The ventrolateral ventromedial nuclei (VMN) and arcuate nuclei (ARC) contain estrogen-sensitive neurons in which estradiol induces receptors for progesterone. Dots indicate approximate location of estrogen-sensitive neurons.

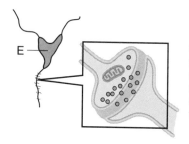

The VMN responds more rapidly and extensively to estradiol (E) than ARC. VMN neurons respond to E within 2 h; cell body and nuclear diameters are increased; nucleolar size increases and rough endoplasmic reticulum and ribosomal RNA increase in the cytoplasm.

One of the consequences of this rapid increase in protein synthetic capacity in VMN neurons is that E increases the number of spines on dendrites and increases the density of synapses in the VMN. These events occur cyclically during the estrous cycle of the female rat. Dots indicate presynaptic vesicles containing neurotransmitter.

FIG. 9.   Summary of estrogen effects on the ventromedial nuclei related to its activation of female sexual behavior in the rat. (Reprinted from [30] by permission.)

found not only in hippocampus but also in other brain regions [3,4]. Changes in synaptic vesicle proteins, high-affinity GABA transport, neurotransmitter-stimulated cAMP formation, and central serotonin and noradrenergic sensitivity are known to accompany repeated glucocorticoid elevation [3,4]. One view of these changes induced by glucocorticoids is that they counteract some of the immediate and persistent neural effects of stress and are therefore part of the mechanism of adaptation [3,4].

Repair of neural damage

The response of neural tissue to damage involves some degree of collateral growth and reinnervation of vacant synaptic sites, a process facilitated in some cases by steroid hormones [31]. In the hypothalamus, estrogen treatment promotes increases in the number of synapses following knife cuts that destroy certain inputs. In the hippocampus, glucocorticoid treatment promotes homotypical sprouting of serotonin fibers to replace damaged serotonin input. It has also been noted that androgens enhance the regrowth of the severed hypoglossal nerve [31]. One interpretation of these steroid effects is that they represent the reactivation, by damage, of developmental programs of genomic activity that normally operate during the phase of synaptogenesis in early development [31].

Another aspect of steroid action is stabilization of neurons against death and replacement. In the dentate gyrus of the adult rat, neurons are born and also die; both birth and death are increased by adrenalectomy, and this increase is prevented by low doses of adrenal steroids acting via mineralocorticoid receptors [4] (see Fig. 10).

Enhancement of neuronal atrophy and cell loss during aging and as a result of rest and hypoxic damage

Steroid hormones can also promote neural damage. High-dose estrogen treatment of adult female rats induces the hypothalamic disconnection syndrome by activating low-level persistent ovarian estrogen secretion. This persistent ovarian secretion induces morphological changes in the hypothalamus associated with dysfunction of the cyclic gonadotropin-releasing mechanism [31]. Persistent effects of estrogen secretion occurring naturally throughout life span are believed to facilitate termination of cyclic hypothalamic function with regard to ovulation [31].

Glucocorticoids can promote neural damage as well [5]. Treatment of adult rats with excess corticosterone for 12 weeks induces loss of pyramidal neurons in hippocampus, which mimics the loss of such neurons in aging rats. Shorter exposure of rats to corticosterone causes atrophy of neurons in the hippocampus, particularly in the CA3

region that receives heavy input from the dentate gyrus mossy fiber system (Fig. 10). The mossy fiber input is also responsible for kainic acid- and seizure-induced damage of the CA3 region. The presence of elevated glucocorticoids at the time of hypoxic damage (Chap. 40) or kainic acid lesions (Chap. 17) to the brain potentiates the necrosis produced by these treatments, especially in the hippocampus. Adrenalectomy reduces such damage and also retards loss of neurons with age [28]. Thus, adrenal steroids operate in conjunction with neural excitability to promote damage, and it has been suggested that they do so by compromising the ability of the brain to obtain nutrients to support ATP generation [31]. It should be noted that damage is not a primary or an immediate consequence of elevated glucocorticoid lev-

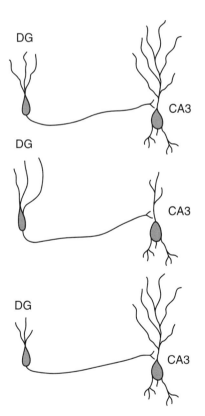

CA3 pyramidal neurons receive the mossy fiber input from the granule neurons of the dentate gyrus. This connection is part of the 3-cell circuit of the hippocampus that is believed to be involved in learning and memory.

Chronic corticosterone treatment or repeated restraint stress promotes atrophy of apical dendrites of CA3 pyramidal neurons.

Adrenalectomy causes neurons of the dentate gyrus to die and to be replaced by new neurons, whereas pyramidal neurons are unaffected. Low levels of adrenal steroids prevent this and stabilize the dentate granule neuron population; they do this via Type I adrenal steroid receptors.

FIG. 10.   Summary of adrenal steroid effects on neurons of the hippocampus illustrating their ability to protect and stabilize the population of the dentate granule neurons and to potentiate damage caused by excitatory amino acid release upon pyramidal neurons. DG, dentate gyrus. (Reprinted from [30] by permission.)

els and that glucocorticoid secretion in conjunction with stress has the beneficial influence of protecting the body from overreacting to stress and thereby destroying itself. However, certain types of stress, such as social subordination, may lead to hippocampal damage; it will be very important to understand the underlying neurochemical and hormonal "signatures" of those types of stress that cause hippocampal damage and to distinguish them from the "signature" of stressors that do not cause neural damage.

REFERENCES

1. McEwen, B. S., Coirini, H., Danielsson, A., Frankfurt, M., Gould, E., Mendelson, S., Schumacher, M., Segarra, A., and Woolley, C. Steroid and thyroid hormones modulate a changing brain. *J. Steroid Biochem. Mol. Biol.* 40:1–14, 1991.
2. Ganong, W. F. *Review of Medical Physiology, 14th Ed.* Norwalk, CT: Appleton and Lange, 1991.
3. McEwen, B. S. Endocrine effects on the brain and their relationship to behavior. In G. J. Siegel, R. W. Albers, B. W. Agranoff, and R. Katzman (eds.), *Basic Neurochemistry,* 3rd Ed. Boston: Little Brown and Co., 1981, pp. 775–799.
4. McEwen, B. S., DeKloet, R., and Rostene, W. Adrenal steroid receptors and actions in the nervous system. *Physiol. Rev.* 66:1121–1188, 1986.
5. McEwen, B. S., Angulo, J., Cameron, H., et al. Paradoxical effects of adrenal steroids on the brain: protection versus degeneration. *Biol. Psychol.* 30:177–199, 1992.
6. Fuller, P. The steroid receptor superfamily: mechanisms of diversity. *FASEB J.* 5: 3092–3099, 1991.
7. Miner, J., and Yamamoto, K. Regulatory crosstalk at composite response elements. *Trends Biochem. Sci.* 16:423–426, 1991.
8. Drouin, J., Sun, Y.-L., and Nemer, M. Glucocorticoid repression of pro-opiomelanocortin gene transcription. *J. Steroid Biochem.* 34: 63–69, 1989.
9. Power, R. F., Mani, S. K., Codina, J., Conneely, O. M., and O'Malley, B. W. Dopaminergic

10. Norman, A., and Henry, H. Vitamin D to 1,25-dihydroxycholecalciferol: evolution of a steroid hormone. *Trends Biochem. Sci.* 5:414–418, 1979.
11. Celotti, F., Naftolin, F., and Martini, L. (eds.), *Metabolism of Hormonal Steroids in Neuroendocrine Structures.* New York: Raven Press, 1984.
12. Goy, R., and McEwen, B. S. (eds.), *Sexual Differentiation of the Brain.* Cambridge: MIT Press, 1980.
13. Roselli, C., Horton, L., and Resko, J. Distribution and regulation of aromatase activity in the rat hypothalamus and limbic system. *Endocrinology* 117:2471–2477, 1985.
14. Schumacher, M., and Balthazart, J. Testosterone-induced brain aromatase is sexually dimorphic. *Brain Res.* 370:285–293, 1986.
15. Merriam, G. R., and Lipsett, M. B. (eds.), *Catechol Estrogens.* New York: Raven Press, 1983.
16. Robel, P., Bourreau, E., Corpéchot, C., Dang, D. C., Halberg, F., Baulieu, E. E., et al. Neurosteroids: 3β-hydroxy-Δ5-derivatives in rat and monkey brain. *J. Steroid Biochem.* 27:649–655, 1987.
17. McEwen, B. S. Nongenomic effects of steroids on neural activity. *Trends Pharmacol. Sci.* 12: 141–147, 1991.
18. McEwen, B. S., and Zigmond, R. Isolation of brain cell nuclei. In N. Marks and R. Rodnight (eds.), *Research Methods in Neurochemistry.* New York: Plenum Press, 1972, Vol. 1, pp. 140–161.
19. Parker, M. The expanding family of nuclear hormone receptors. *J. Endocrinol.* 119: 175–177, 1988.
20. O'Keefe, J., and Handa, R. Transient elevation of estrogen receptors in the neonatal rat hippocampus. *Dev. Brain Res.* 57:119–127, 1990.
21. McEwen, B. S., Davis, P., Gerlach, J., Krey, L., MacLusky, N., McGinnis, M., and Parsons, B. Progestin receptors in the brain and pituitary gland. In C. W. Bardin, P. Mauvais-Jarvis, and Milgrom (eds.), *Progesterone and Progestin.* New York: Raven Press, 1983, pp. 59–76.
22. Edwards, C. R. W., Burt, D., McIntyre, M. A., et al. Localization of 11β-hydroxysteroid dehydrogenase tissue specific protector of

the mineralocorticoid receptor. *Lancet* 2: 986–989, 1988.

23. Stumpf, W., Sar, M., and Clark, S. Brain target sites for 1,25-dihydroxy vitamin D_3. *Science* 215:1403–1405, 1982.

24. Sonnenberg, J., Luine, V., Krey, L., and Christakos, S. 1,25-dihydroxyvitamin D_3 treatment results in increased choline acetyltransferase activity in specific brain nuclei. *Endocrinology* 118:1433–1439, 1986.

25. Nunez, J. Effects of thyroid hormones during brain differentiation. *Mol. Cell. Endocrinol.* 37: 125–132, 1984.

26. Whybrow, P., and Prange, A. A hypothesis of thyroid-catecholamine receptor interaction. *Arch. Gen. Psychiatry* 38:106–133, 1981.

27. Bernal, J., and Pekonen, F. Ontogenesis of the nuclear 3,5,3'-triiodothyronine receptor in the human fetal brain. *Endocrinology* 114: 677–680, 1984.

28. Mellstrom, B., Naranjo, J. R., Santos, A., Gonzalez, A. M., and Bernal, J. Independent expression of the alpha and beta-c-erbA genes in developing rat brain. *Mol. Endocrinol.* 5: 1339–1350, 1991.

29. Adler, N. (ed.), *Neuroendocrinology of Reproduction, Physiology and Behavior.* New York: Plenum Press, 1981.

30. McEwen, B. S. Our changing ideas about steroid effects on an ever-changing brain. *Semin. Neurosci.* 4:497–507, 1991.

31. McEwen, B. S. Steroid hormones and the brain: linking "nature and nurture." *Neurochem. Res.* 13:663–669, 1988.

CHAPTER 50

Learning and Memory

BERNARD W. AGRANOFF AND MICHAEL D. UHLER

HOW DO BIOCHEMISTS STUDY BEHAVIOR?

No aspect of the brain sciences can so quickly conjure up both interest and contention than the subject of the biological basis of learning and memory—the encoding and storage of behavioral information. Some of the controversy stems from disagreement among investigators with regard to definitions of learning and memory and acceptable experimental criteria. The complexity

Basic Neurochemistry: Molecular, Cellular, and Medical Aspects, 5th Ed., edited by G. J. Siegel et al. Published by Raven Press, Ltd., New York, 1994. Correspondence to Bernard W. Agranoff, Mental Health Research Institute, University of Michigan, 1103 E. Huron, Ann Arbor, Michigan 48104-1687.

of the problem to a great extent reflects the structural and functional complexity of the brain itself—biochemical correlates of learning and memory are generally highly inferential and involve compromise, either in the behavioral model and paradigm used or in the precision of the experimental probe employed. For example, a behavioral scientist might consider the study of long-term potentiation (LTP) in a rat hippocampal slice preparation a far cry from Pavlovian conditioning. For the neurochemist, LTP provides a highly accessible preparation for studying synthesis and post-translational modification of neuronal protein. On the other hand, using inhibitors of macromolecular synthesis has the advantage in that it permits an investigator to study the effects of disruption of DNA, of RNA, or of protein synthesis on the behavior of the otherwise intact experimental animal. While the behavioral aspect of this *in vivo* approach may be highly acceptable to the behaviorist, it can be anticipated that such massive interventions will produce multiple metabolic effects, which will complicate interpretation of the results at the molecular level. These divergent experimental approaches may prove to be most useful when they can be integrated into a single consistent model. They may also prove to be of value by leading to more critical experimental models, or by adding constraints to extant theoretical models of how the brain processes information.

Although the answer to the question of how memory is stored continues to prove challenging, significant progress is being made, and proceeds with ever-increasing momentum. This impetus can be attributed to the following factors: (a) increased knowledge of neurotransmitter actions within the nervous system, particularly the role of excitatory amino acids; (b) a better understanding of neural development and regeneration, including the availability of molecular biological markers; (c) improved methods for measurement of regional metabolism of brains of experimental animals (see Chap. 31), as well as noninvasive probes for the study of the human brain (see Chap. 46); (d) continued progress in the genetic dissection of behavior in species well suited to this approach, and the ability to produce selective genetic mutations by transfection; and (e) a growing body of information with regard to altered behavior in invertebrate species from which there is evidence that the observed behavioral changes are mediated by circuitry confined to a relatively small number of identified cells.

The history of neurochemical research on learning and memory up to the 1980s has been summarized in a previous edition of this book [1]. The present chapter is intended to convey to the reader a sense of the current status of this rapidly evolving field. The issue is no longer whether, but rather when, definitive mechanisms will be elucidated and which approach(es) will ultimately prove most useful to the experimentalist.

Some definitions

Learning can be broadly defined as an adaptive change on the part of an organism in response to an environmental input. Models outside the nervous system, e.g., immunological or bacterial "learning," have been proposed, but are not considered here. Learning is quantified experimentally as the probability that an organism will respond to the same stimulus differently on retesting. This altered probability is based on the organism's *memory* of what it has learned. It is thus not possible to consider learning without memory or, conversely, memory without learning. We can, however, distinguish between the memory necessary for acquisition, which we term *short-term memory*, from that required to demonstrate a learned behavior over longer periods of time. For example, an animal might demonstrate acquisition of a conditioned response following repetitive trials during a 30-min training session, indicating learning and the attendant short-term memory of the training task. Evocation of the newly learned behavior in a second training session, hours to weeks later, constitutes evidence for *long-term memory* formation. Thus, during and shortly after a training session, demonstration by the subject of a learned behavior is considered to be based on short-term memory; at later times, it is believed to be mediated by long-term memory (Fig. 1). It is important to remember that although we conceive of learning and memory as intrinsic biological processes or states, our behavioral measures are based entirely on the experimental subject's performance. When a previously trained animal does not demonstrate an acquired behavior under a specified set of conditions, such as a drug-induced state, it will then depend on the skill of the experimenter to determine whether the absent behavior is suppressed or whether the subject is truly amnesic. Although Pavlovian, or *classical conditioning*, as described below is the most universally accepted behavioral paradigm for learning and memory, there are more complex and simpler procedures [1], such as habituation and sensitization, in which the same repetitive stimulus produces

either a decreased or an augmented behavioral response, respectively.

It may be useful at this point to distinguish "memory" and "memories." Although there is considerable evidence that specific brain regions in the mammalian brain, such as the hippocampus and amygdala, play a key role in memory formation, there is equally good evidence that stored memories are broadly distributed in the brain. Given the capacity of the brain to store seemingly limitless quantities of detailed information, a distributed network, in which combinations of neuronal ensembles are employed [1], would seem more likely than a point-by-point "one association per structural element" system. Thus, with approaches that seek out relevant brain regions, such as the search for metabolic correlates of memory described below, we do not seek the locus of a specific memory but of the memory-producing process that "fixes" or "prints" memory of many different experiences.

A

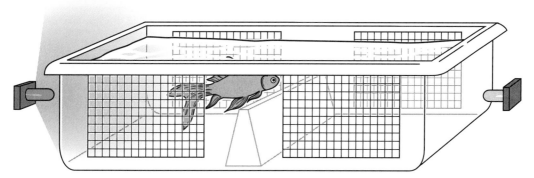

FIG. 1. Effects of administration of agents that block long-term memory of a multitrial task. **A:** A goldfish *(Carrasius auratus)* is shown in a shuttle box used for training of a shock-avoidance task. Goldfish are transferred from home tanks to one side of a training apparatus termed a shuttle box, which is divided into halves by a submerged barrier. A trial begins with the onset of a light signal (the CS) on the end of the shuttle box nearest the fish. This is followed 20 sec later by a mild electrical shock (the US) administered through the water. Naive fish respond to the US by swimming over the barrier on onset of shock to the dark, and presumably safe, end of the shuttle box. This escape response is eventually replaced after many trials by the learned avoidance response, in which the fish swims over the barrier before the onset of the punishing shock. Whether the fish demonstrates the conditioned response or the unconditioned response, it will end up on the side of the shuttle box opposite its position at the beginning of the trial. The next trial begins with a light signal at the fishes' end of the apparatus. The location of the fish in the shuttle box is determined by photodetectors, and its avoidance or escape scores are recorded automatically.

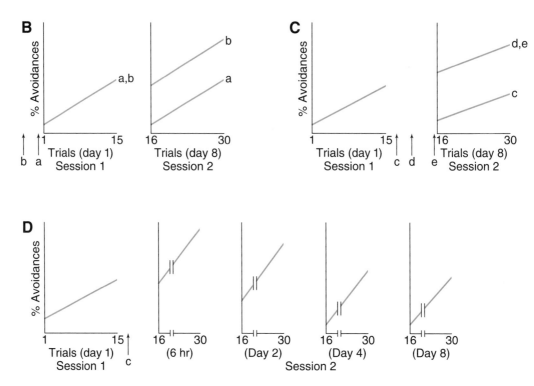

FIG. 1.   *(continued).* **B** shows that the probability of an avoidance response during 15 trials (session 1) increases progressively, indicating that short-term memory is formed. Fish returned immediately to their home tanks and retrained 1 week later indicate their prior learning and show additional improvement in session 2. If an amnestic agent is injected intracranially just before the session (time a), normal acquisition is seen, but there is a profound deficit in performance on retraining one week later. If the agent is administered sufficiently in advance of session 1 (time b), normal retention is seen on day 8, since the effects of the injection will have worn off by the time of the training session. By varying the time of injection before training, the duration of a given agent's amnestic effect can be established. Intracranial injection of the protein synthesis inhibitor puromycin is effective when given 24, but not 72 hr before session 1. **C** shows the effects of amnestic agents administered after training. An injection immediately after session 1 *(c)* results in profound deficits on retraining 1 week later. The process is time dependent, since fish return to their home tanks and, given the injection a few hours later *(d),* show no deficit on retraining in session 2, 1 week later. In fact, fish not treated previously and given the amnestic agent just before retraining on day 8 *(e)* show a learned response. This time-dependence of the treatment rules out both chronic (lingering) and acute toxic effects of the amnestic agents as possible explanations for the observed reduced responding rates and indicates that the agent produces a specific memory loss. The decay of short-term memory is shown in **D.** Injection of a blocking agent just after (or before) session 1 results in failure to form long-term memory. In this experiment, individual groups of animals so treated and retrained at various times earlier than 8 days, e.g., 6, 48, or 96 hr after session 1, demonstrate the learned response. The experiments thus constitute evidence for the decay of short-term memory (see text). (From Agranoff [7].)

WHAT ARE OUR ASSUMPTIONS?

Current hypotheses on the neurochemical basis of memory are based on a number of premises that are enumerated here. The remainder of this chapter relies on their validity.

Behavioral information is ultimately stored in synaptic connections

This concept can be traced to Ramón y Cajal, who first recognized the enormous complexity of the brain's neuronal network. Although it may seem self-evident that an organism's most complex function resides in its most complex structures, the premise remains inferential. It is supported by the many indications that synaptic complexity increases with development and environmental input [1,2]. Alternative hypotheses, such as proposals that memory resides in glia, have not been pursued sufficiently to warrant further consideration here. It has been proposed that memory is not based on altered chemical states but rather in reverberating circuits or in charge distributions, yet memory survives seizures as well as periods of electrical silence in the brain. Neurochemists generally adopt the premise that long-lived biological phenomena are ultimately preserved and protected in the form of covalent chemical bonds, be they in nucleic acids, in structural proteins, or in both.

The behavioral unit of learning is the conditioned response

Pavlov's characterization [3] has served as a template for cellular and subcellular models of learning and memory. He emphasized temporal requirements for optimal learning: The conditioned, or neutral, stimulus (CS) such as a tone must precede the unconditioned stimulus (US), such as food presentation that results in salivation, a punishing electrical shock that results in altered heart rate, or a puff of air that results in an eye blink. Direct application of these characteristics to a two- or three-neuron model may have extremely limited applicability to the mammalian brain, in which the stimulus specificity of a learned behavior may reside in a relatively large population of cells. The cellular model may be highly relevant to studies of learning in invertebrates in which identified neurons appear to mediate behavior [4]. The contingency criteria, i.e., that the CS precedes the US and that there be an optimal latency (CS-US interval), must be met in true associative learning.

The formation of long-term memory of a newly acquired behavior requires ongoing brain protein synthesis; memory required for acquisition (learning), does not

Studies over the past 25 years in fish, rodents, birds, and invertebrates [1,5,6] have all indicated that the formation of short-term and long-term memory can be distinguished on the basis of susceptibility to agents that block brain protein synthesis such as puromycin, cycloheximide, and anisomycin (see Agranoff [1] for review). Consideration of the temporal aspects of learning and memory and knowledge of the temporal scale of biochemical processes have led to the prediction that learning and short-term memory formation, which can occur within milliseconds and last for minutes to hours, are mediated by post-translational modification at the synapse [7]. Long-term memory, which may take longer to form and can last a lifetime, is predicted to be (a) mediated by a process that requires *de novo* protein synthesis and is therefore (b) dependent on the neuronal genome and requires that (c) there be communication between the cell surface and nucleus, presumably by retrograde axonal transport (see Chap. 27).

These three assumptions serve as a framework for evaluating the diverse experimental neurochemical approaches to the understanding of learning and memory that follow.

INVERTEBRATE LEARNING AND MEMORY

What does cell biology tell us about molecular mechanisms of learning and memory?

The sea snail *Aplysia californica* has been used extensively as a model system for the study of the cell biological basis of learning. This organism has a relatively simple nervous system consisting of approximately 10^5 neurons. Many of these neurons are large and can be manipulated directly within defined neuronal circuits.

The term habituation describes a decrease in behavioral response after repeated stimulation. In *Aplysia*, habituation is the most rudimentary behavior studied that shares aspects of regulation relevant to learning. For example, *Aplysia* will ordinarily withdraw its gill after gentle tactile stimulation of the siphon. However, with repeated stimulation, the gill withdrawal reflex diminishes in magnitude and duration. If the habituation experience consists of one training session of relatively few stimulations (less than ten) over a short period of time (less than 1 hour) then the habituation lasts for only a few hours after the training. If, however, four or more individual training sessions are given, the habituation response can last for several weeks. The two phenomena have been described in terms of short and long-term memory.

There is a difference in how the terms short-term and long-term memory are used in *Aplysia* experiments and in behavior in vertebrates such as the goldfish. In *Aplysia*, short-term memory refers to a fleeting memory resulting from few training trials. With additional trials, memory appears to be more robust and lasts longer. In experiments with goldfish and rats, the same training session is thought to give rise to both a short- and a long-term form of memory, the latter forming by a consolidation process that takes place after the training session. In both fish and in *Aplysia*, it appears that the short-term memory formation does not require ongoing protein synthesis, while the long-term form does.

The relatively simple neuronal circuitry involved in habituation of the gill withdrawal reflex is shown in Fig. 2. Stimulation of a sensory neuron innervating the siphon causes stimulation of motor neurons that innervate the gill muscle. As habituation proceeds, the number of post-synaptic potentials produced in the motor neuron decreases until ultimately the motor neuron does not depolarize, and there is no gill withdrawal,

while depolarization of the sensory neuron in response to siphon stimulation is unaffected. Kandel and coworkers have shown that habituation is the result of a decrease in synaptic efficacy between the sensory neuron and the motor neuron, which in turn is due to altered permeability of Ca^{2+} required for neurotransmitter release at the presynaptic terminal. The Ca^{2+} enters the presynaptic terminal through voltage-sensitive Ca^{2+} channels, and during habituation, Ca^{2+} channels in the presynaptic terminal become inactivated. Although specific mechanisms for this inactivation have been described, the nature of inactivation in the synaptic terminal of the sensory neurons is unknown. Furthermore, since the long-term habituation appears to involve protein synthesis, the current known mechanisms for inactivation of Ca^{2+} channels do not suffice to explain it.

Although morphological changes seen after long-term sensitization suggest that the conversion from short-term to long-term memory involves the translation of synaptic (transmission) efficiency into morphological changes of the synapse, the cellular mechanisms involved in the conversion have not been elucidated.

Sensitization in *Aplysia* involves a more complex learning paradigm and a more complex cellular regulatory mechanism. In one type of sensitization experiment, a mild tail shock is given to the organism shortly preceding tactile stimulation of the siphon. The prior tail shock sensitizes the animal so that the normal gill withdrawal reflex associated with siphon stimulation is increased in magnitude and duration. Like habituation, sensitization can be either short-term or long-term in nature depending on the duration and number of training sessions involved.

The neuronal pathway involved in the tail shock sensitization experiment is schematized in Fig. 2. Stimulation of sensory neurons in the tail causes generation of an action potential in specific interneurons that facilitate the sensitization. These facilitating interneurons form a specific synaptic connec-

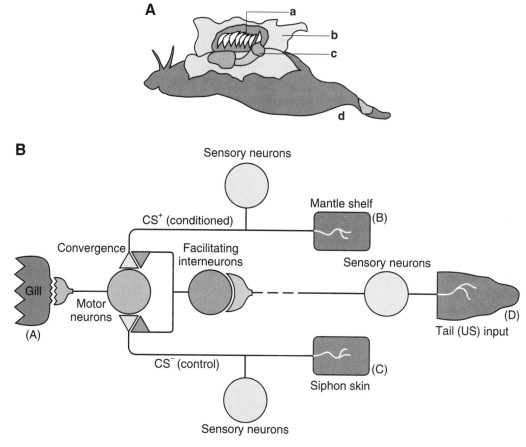

FIG. 2.   The sea snail *Aplysia californica* as a model system for studying the biological basis of learning. **A:** A simple depiction showing the various *Aplysia* tissues used in training and testing learning and memory paradigms. *(A)* The gill; *(B)* the mantle shelf; *(C)* the siphon; and *(D)* the tail. **B:** A simplified diagram of the circuitry involved in sensitization habituation and classical conditioning in *Aplysia*. Sensory neurons, motor neurons, and facilitating interneurons are indicated.

tion with axons of the sensory neuron that innervate the siphon. The synapses of the facilitating interneurons are positioned so that release of neurotransmitter from the axons of the facilitating interneuron is targeted to axons of the sensory neuron forming an axo-axonal synapse. In tail shock sensitization, the facilitating interneurons release serotonin onto the axonal terminals of the sensory neurons. Specific serotonin receptors on the sensory axons bind the serotonin and increase axonal cyclic AMP levels. The elevated cAMP activates cAMP-dependent protein kinase, which then phosphorylates K^+ channels in the sensory axon. The resulting decrease in K^+ influx prolongs the action potential and increases the duration of Ca^{2+} influx through voltage-sensitive Ca^{2+} channels. The net effect is that more Ca^{2+} flows into the axon, and since Ca^{2+} is required for synaptic vesicle fusion with the membrane, greater neurotransmitter release is observed when the neuron is depolarized following activation of the serotonin receptor. The greater release of neurotransmitter from sensory axons onto the motor neurons results in increased contraction of muscles involved in gill withdrawal. Like habituation, this mechanism is sufficient to account for short-term sensitization, but the manner in which phosphorylation of K⁺ channels can result in long-term sensitization is not well-understood.

The most complex form of learning which can be studied conveniently in *Aplysia* is classical conditioning. Tail shock results in withdrawal of the gill, and if the siphon is stimulated shortly before (~1 sec) the tail shock, the animal eventually learns to associate siphon stimulation with the tail shock. In contrast, if the mantle is stimulated shortly after the tail response, there is no learned response to mantle stimulation. The cellular mechanisms underlying classical conditioning in *Aplysia* are similar to those involved in sensitization, but the crucial difference lies in the strict temporal dependence found in classical conditioning. At the same axo-axonal synapse where serotonin release from the sensory neuron stimulates cAMP production in sensitization, prior depolarization of the conditioned stimulus pathway (siphon stimulation in Fig. 2 above) results in depolarization of the presynaptic terminal. This depolarization results in elevated levels of Ca^{2+} in the presynaptic terminal as a result of influx through voltage-sensitive Ca^{2+} channels. The increase is transient and Ca^{2+} eventually returns to resting intracellular levels as it is pumped out through plasma membrane Ca^{2+} pumps. If, however, the presynaptic terminal is stimulated with serotonin while Ca^{2+} concentrations are elevated within the presynaptic terminal, the effects of serotonin on generation of cAMP are potentiated by the elevated Ca^{2+}. This effect appears to be due to a Ca^{2+}-sensitive form of adenylyl cyclase, which shows greater stimulation of cyclase activity by serotonin in the presence of high Ca^{2+} concentration. Thus if serotonin release triggered by the unconditioned stimulus closely follows activation of the conditioned stimulus pathway, the potentiation of the cyclase activity results in higher concentrations of cAMP, greater activation of the cAMP-dependent kinase, greater phosphorylation of the same K⁺ channels involved in sensitiza-

tion and increased release of neurotransmitter from the presynaptic terminal.

All of the mechanisms discussed above are sufficient to account for many of the short-term effects observed during learning in *Aplysia*. However, the mechanisms for long-term memory storage are less clearly defined. Morphological analysis of the *Aplysia* nervous system in sensitized animals has suggested that the number of active zones at presynaptic membranes where neurotransmitters are released increases during sensitization. Both increases in the size of the active zones and in the number of neurotransmitter vesicles associated with these active zones have been observed. Furthermore, habituation leads to a decrease in the number of active zones. A model for these morphological changes has been proposed and tested by Kandel and coworkers [8].

In addition to phosphorylation of K⁺ channels, cAMP-dependent protein kinase is known to phosphorylate transcription factors that alter the rates of transcription of specific genes. As described in Chapter 21, transcriptional regulation requires the presence of a cAMP response element (CRE) which consists of a sequence of nucleotides related to the consensus CRE sequence GTCAGTAC. Binding to the CRE binding (CREB) protein and phosphorylation of CREB by cAMP-dependent protein kinase results in increased transcription from the gene. Kandel has shown that transcriptional changes can be detected in *Aplysia* following elevation of cAMP and that nuclear injection of a synthetic CRE oligonucleotide can block many of the correlative changes seen during long-term memory formation [9].

Conditioning has also been studied in another marine invertebrate, *Hermissenda crassicornis*. In this case, the CS is a positive phototaxis that is paired with high-speed rotation (the US), which leads to suppression of the unconditioned response. Daily sessions of 50 to 100 pairings for a few days result in retention of the learned response for over 2 weeks. Of a number of cellular changes found following conditioning, an observed reduced K+ current in type B photo-receptors has been pursued experimentally [10]. From experiments involving various drugs and microinjections of enzymes, it has been inferred that Ca^{2+} and calmodulin-activated protein kinases mediate associative learning in *Hermissenda,* as well as in *Aplysia.* A major difference is that in *Hermissenda,* Ca^{2+} influx is the result of depolarization, as is proposed in hippocampal long-term potentiation (LTP), whereas in *Aplysia,* it is neurotransmitter-mediated. Inhibitors of protein synthesis prolong the altered biophysical correlates of conditioning in *Hermissenda.* It has been speculated that this seemingly paradoxical result is related to short-term rather than long-term memory formation [11]. Microinjection experiments and the application of phorbol esters indicate that protein kinase C and the phospho-inositide pathway may also play an important role in associative learning, as is further discussed below (see section later in this chapter on LTP).

How can genetic models be used to probe memory mechanisms?

The concept of neurogenetic dissection of behavior is exemplified by work of the laboratory of Benzer and his associates in studying *Drosophila*. These researchers have identified a number of mutant strains that are seemingly normal except for the inability to learn or to store memory of a specific training task. Sensitization, habituation, and classical conditioning paradigms, as well as behavioral screens for the detection of defective strains, have been devised. One of the most commonly used behavioral schemes in the characterization of *Drosophila* involves operant conditioning and olfactory cues, which are defective in this learning paradigm (Fig. 3). Briefly, flies are exposed to an odorant such as 4-methylcyclohexanol spread onto a wire grid and are given a mild shock. Eventually, the flies learn to associate the shock with the odorant and will avoid the odorant. After this type of training, the learning can be quantitated by exposing the

flies to two chambers that have different odorants and determining the avoidance index, defined as the percentage of flies that have learned to avoid the odorant after coupling with the electric shock. Fly stocks can be mutagenized, and mutant flies that are altered in their ability to associate the electric shock with odorants have been selected.

One of the best-documented behavioral mutants is dunce *(dnc),* in which a deficiency in the structural gene for a cAMP phosphodiesterase (PDE) has been established. These PDEs specifically hydrolyze cAMP to 5′AMP and are responsible for returning cellular concentrations of cAMP to resting levels after adenylyl cyclase has been stimulated. Many isoforms of PDE have been characterized that are differentially regulated and expressed in a tissue-specific manner. Davis and coworkers have shown that the dunce gene organization is extremely complex and is distributed over at least 150 kb of the *Drosophila* genome [12]. Multiple RNA transcripts from this gene encode several different PDE protein isoforms [13]. Antibodies generated to a conserved region of these isoforms have shown that the dunce PDE is concentrated within a region of the *Drosophila* nervous system known as the mushroom body. The mushroom body has been implicated as the anatomical site of olfactory learning and memory in many experiments. The relatively restricted expression of the dunce PDE to this region suggests that the dunce protein plays a direct role in mediating memory formation. How the PDE gene defect is translated into a behavioral deficit is not known. The behavioral deficit does not seem to be due to a generalized developmental defect in the nervous system since the brains of dunce flies appear morphologically normal and the flies are able to form memory albeit extremely short-term. Currently, some effect of the absence of dunce PDE on regulation of K+ channel function via altered activation of cAMP-dependent protein kinase is a favored possibility.

A related *Drosophila* behavioral mutant is rutabaga *(rut)*. Like dunce mutants, memory

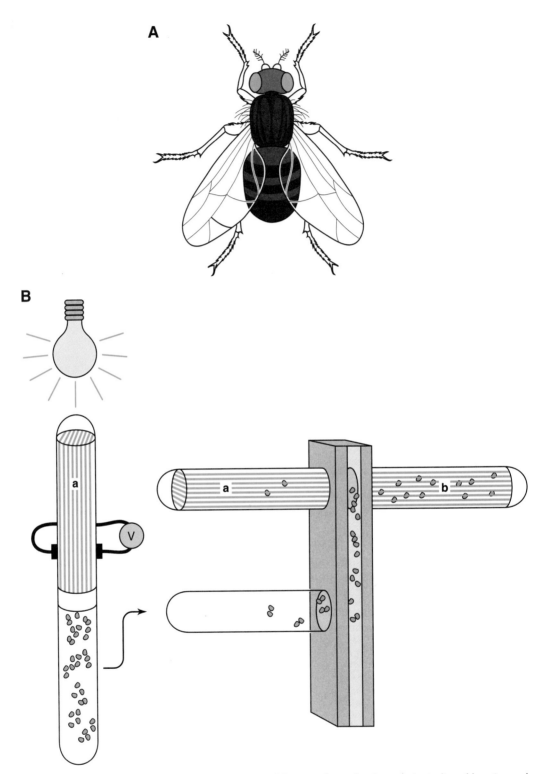

FIG. 3. The fruitfly, *Drosophila melanogaster,* as a model system for molecular genetic studies of learning and memory. **A:** *Drosophila* has long been a favored system for genetic studies because of its short generation time. **B:** The training and testing paradigm for *Drosophila* learning and memory. Flies are first trained to avoid an odorant on an electrified grid that has been coated with an odorant such as cyclohexanol. After training, the flies are allowed to choose between two chambers, one *(a)* containing the training odorant and one *(b)* containing a neutral odorant. The distribution of flies in the two chambers is then analyzed.

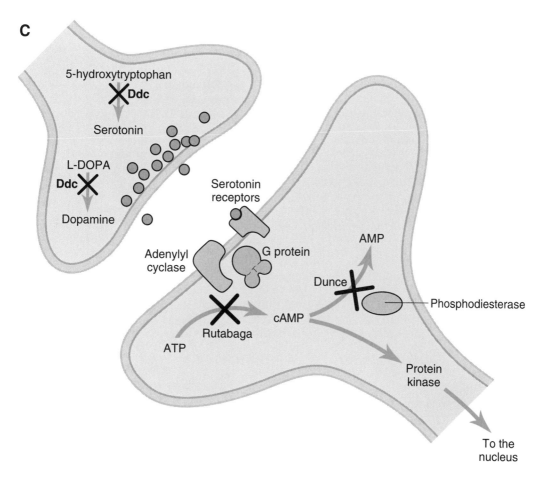

FIG. 3.   *(continued).* **C:** The nature of various *Drosophila* mutations known to affect learning or memory include *Ddc* (dopa decarboxylase), *rutabaga* (a calcium-calmodulin sensitive adenylyl cyclase), and *dunce* (a cAMP phosphodiesterase).

forms in the rutabaga mutant, but decays rapidly. Initial characterization of brain adenylyl cyclase activity showed that adenylyl cyclase from rutabaga flies had an increased K_m for ATP. Subsequently, it was shown that two forms of adenylyl cyclase activity could be distinguished in normal *Drosophila* based on sensitivity to calmodulin. Rutabaga mutants appeared to be deficient in the calmodulin-stimulated adenylyl cyclase. More recently, Reed and Davis have used mammalian cDNA clones for adenylyl cyclase to isolate the rutabaga gene [13].

Expression of cDNAs for the rutabaga gene product showed that it encodes a calmodulin-stimulated adenylyl cyclase. DNA sequence comparison between rutabaga mutants and wild-type *Drosophila* showed that the rutabaga mutants contained a single base change, which results in an amino acid substitution of arginine for the glycine normally found at residue 1026 of the adenylyl cyclase. Expression of the mutant protein showed that this single amino acid substitution was sufficient to completely abolish cyclase activity. These experiments suggest that, at least in *Drosophila,* complex behaviors such as learning can be drastically altered as the result of relatively simple alterations to the genome.

Mutants in neurotransmitter metabolism, such as in DOPA decarboxylase (see Chap. 12) have been reported. In insects, this enzyme is important not only for the synthesis of dopamine and serotonin, but also for the decarboxylation of tyrosine to octopamine. Dopamine is essential for cuticle formation, so that development is impaired in deficient mutants. This can be overcome by the use of temperature-sensitive alleles.

Another species subjected to genetic analysis is the nematode *Caenorhabditis elegans.* Its behavioral repertoire is less impressive than that of the fruit fly, but it has the anatomical advantage of possessing only a few hundred neurons. Thus, altered phenotypic expression in the morphology of the nervous system can be more readily correlated with altered behavior.

VERTEBRATE LEARNING AND MEMORY

Among warm-blooded vertebrates, rodents, particularly the mouse and rat, have been by far the traditionally favored experimental animals for behavioral study. The mouse is particularly convenient for genetic studies because of the availability of inbred populations, including mutant strains, and for available (transgenic) techniques for manipulation of genomic sequences. The rabbit has been useful for studies on classical conditioning, employing the eye blink response. The avian brain has proven attractive for the study of imprinting. Newborn chicks and ducklings will follow a moving object to which they are first exposed following hatching. Neurochemical correlates such as increased macromolecular synthesis have been investigated over a number of years in the laboratories of Rose [see ref. 1] and others [14]. In many of these experiments, changes in macromolecular synthesis in the roof of the avian telencephalon are correlated with successful imprinting of a taste aversion. Acquisition of birdsong has been associated with immediate early gene encoding in the forebrain of zebra finches and canaries [15]. Lower primates are of special interest because of the closer analogy of their brains to that of the human, discussed further below.

Can the biochemistry underlying memory processes be localized on the basis of metabolic activity?

The [^{14}C]2-deoxyglucose (2DG) method of Sokoloff (see Chap. 31) would seem ideally suited to establishing whether a specific brain region is activated under conditions in which an imposed behavioral procedure fulfills the criteria of a learned behavior. That there have been few such reports can be attributed to a number of technical problems and limitations. First, there is no assurance that the putative metabolic changes in the brain that accompany learning and/or memory formation will be measurable. Although one can distinguish the differences between simple and complex sensory inputs by examining the altered metabolic patterns of appropriate cortical regions by the [^{14}C]2DG technique, it does not necessarily follow that the method possesses the requisite spatial or temporal resolution to address the question of learning and memory. Indications that this approach sometimes may prove successful have been reported in the rat, using a classical conditioning paradigm in which the US is cardiac slowing produced by stimulation of the reticular formation. Coupling this stimulation to an auditory tone, which serves as the CS, leads to classical conditioning. Presentation of the tone after learning is correlated with increased labeling of the molecular layer of the hippocampus [see ref. 1].

The utility of the 2DG method in behavioral experiments is greatly increased by a technique that permits two experiments to be performed in the same animal, instead of one. For example, [^{14}C]2DG can be injected while the experimental animal is at rest or engaged in a behavioral task that does not result in detectable learning, e.g., random presentations of CS and US. After 20 to 30 min, ^{3}H-labeled DG is injected. After the second incorporation period, equal in duration to the first, the brain is removed for autoradiographic analysis. As originally described, discrete tissue samples are analyzed quantitatively in a scintillation counter, and the ratio of the two isotopes is computed. Autoradiographic applications of the dual label approach have been reported [1].

The concept that higher brain function can be localized receives support from studies on human learning and memory employing positron emission tomography (see below).

How do neural development and regeneration provide clues for understanding memory formation?

The brain at birth is far from a clean slate. For example, an animal may respond with fear to a visual presentation of a nonspecific predator, even though it has had no prior exposure. It seems likely that, as we propose for learned behavior, the information subserving inborn behavior is coded in genetically established synaptic connections. Although the synaptic connections that subserve instinctual behavior form during development, those mediating *neuroplasticity* (an all-encompassing term that includes the brain's response to learning conditions as well as to trauma; see also Chap. 29) have a low probability of forming in the absence of an external input.

It is generally held that there is little or no neurogenesis after infancy, and since learning and memory formation go on into adulthood, one looks to the complexity of neuronal branching and synapse formation as the sites most likely to reflect neuroplasticity. This view has some experimental support in that regeneration of the CNS occurs in adult amphibia and in fishes. The study of regeneration of the axotomized optic nerve

in these genera is thus relevant in that, like learning, it involves neuronal process growth and eventual synapse formation within the scaffolding of an adult brain.

The goldfish and toad optic nerve preparations were used to establish that the growth-associated proteins (GAPs) are synthesized during regeneration and in development, but not in the intact mature neuron. One of these, GAP 43, has been identified as a component of growth cones. It is identical with F1, a substrate for protein kinase C, the phosphorylation of which is selectively enhanced under conditions of LTP formation in the rat hippocampus [16]. This same protein, also known as B50, was identified by Gispen as a component of synaptic membranes. The phosphorylation of B50 is believed to regulate PIP kinase, an enzyme that is part of the phosphoinositide second-messenger system (see Chap. 20).

It is relevant that inhibitors of protein synthesis block the sustained LTP. Growth- and regeneration-associated proteins and their regulation may prove important in the mediation of memory formation.

What can the mechanism of long-term potentiation tell us about learning and memory?

For some time, the rat hippocampus has served as a model system for the study of memory formation (Fig. 4; see also Chap. 29). When afferent fibers to the CA1 region are stimulated electrically in close temporal proximity to depolarization of the post-synaptic neurons, an increase in sensitivity of these cells develops, which may persist for weeks [17]. This long-lasting increase in synaptic efficacy is referred to as long-term potentiation (LTP). Detailed studies have shown that a development of LTP requires a stimulus threshold determined by complex interactions between the frequency and the strength of the electrical stimulation to the afferent pathway. LTP also can be demonstrated in hippocampal slice preparations,

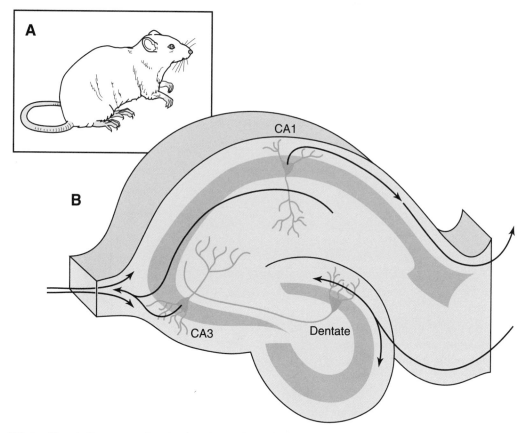

FIG. 4. The rat, *Rattus norvegicus,* has long been a favored subject for learning and memory experiments. **A:** The laboratory rat, possessing a mammalian nervous system, is easily tested in standard behavioral assays. **B:** Diagram of the hippocampal network of neurons involved in LTP. The dentate granule cells send "mossy fiber" tracts to the pyramidal cells of the CA3 region, which in turn synapse with the CA1 neurons, forming the Schaffer collateral pathway.

thus providing a convenient preparation for *in vitro* studies.

As shown in Fig. 4, the anatomical arrangement of synaptic connections within the hippocampus renders this structure particularly amenable to experimental approaches. Three distinct classes of hippocampal synaptic connections have been studied: The "perforant path" of axons from the entorhinal cortex synapse with granule cells of the dentate gyrus; axons designated as "mossy fibers" of these dentate granule cells in turn synapse with pyramidal cells of the CA3 region; and the CA3 pyramidal cells synapse with CA1 neurons and form the "Schaffer collateral pathway." Although

each of these three pathways may develop LTP, the mossy fiber pathway to CA3 neurons is unique in several ways. The Schaffer collateral pathway is the most widely studied and best understood of these synaptic pathways.

One of the most impressive aspects of LTP is "synapse specificity." For example, although a given CA1 neuron may receive many afferent synapses from distinct CA3 pyramidal cells, LTP will be observed only in the synapses of afferents that have received the tetanic stimulation. There is considerable evidence to indicate that glutamate plays a key role as the excitatory neurotransmitter in LTP formation. Since antagonists of the

NMDA (*N*-methyl-D-aspartate) receptor such as 4-amino-5-phosphonovaleric acid (see Chap. 17) can prevent induction of LTP, it has been proposed that post-synaptic receptors activated during LTP are of the NMDA type. It has also recently been reported that the metabotropic glutamate receptor must be activated for induction of LTP, whether or not NMDA receptors are additionally activated [18]. In any event, when stimulation conditions are optimal for LTP formation, there appears to be a resultant increase in intracellular Ca^{2+}. Furthermore, injection of EGTA into post-synaptic neurons prevents LTP. It remains uncertain precisely how the elevation of post-synaptic Ca^{2+} leads to LTP. Hypotheses include (a) the activation of the Ca^{2+}-activated protease, calpain [19], which in turn is proposed to degrade cytoskeletal elements and thereby to reorganize cell shape and receptor distribution; and (b) the activation of calmodulin-dependent enzymes, such as phospholipase A_2 or protein kinase C. The latter is activated by Ca^{2+} as well as by DAG released in the breakdown of the phosphoinositides (see Chap. 20). In LTP, as in learning and memory, a retrograde message from the post-synaptic neuron to the pre-synaptic membrane has been postulated. In addition to arachidonic acid (see above; [8]), candidate substances include an endogenous benzodiazepine-like inhibitory substance [20], a dynorphin peptide [21], and the gaseous messengers NO and/or CO [22].

Experiments employing molecular genetic approaches to studying LTP have yielded interesting and controversial results concerning the participation of Ca^{2+}. Homozygous mice deficient in a major form of Ca^{2+}/calmodulin-dependent protein kinase have been derived using gene ablation techniques, and these mutant mice have been shown to be perturbed in the development of LTP [23]. Gene ablation experiments can be complicated by the fact that the deficient protein may be required for proper differentiation and development of the nervous system, so these results do not necessarily implicate a direct role of Ca^{2+}/calmodulin protein kinase in LTP. However, such gene ablation experiments do yield significant supportive evidence and show promise as novel approaches to test hypotheses concerning mechanisms of LTP, and more generally, learning and memory.

It has become clear that at least some critical aspects of LTP take place in the post-synaptic cell. If the increase in neurotransmitter release from the presynaptic cells underlies LTP formation, then the post-synaptic cell must communicate in some fashion with the presynaptic cells. Much effort is currently focused on identification of the postulated chemical messenger released from the post-synaptic cell, which regulates neurotransmitter release from the presynaptic terminal. Candidate molecules include prostanoids, nitric oxide, and other substances.

A second model of neural plasticity studied in mammalian brain is kindling. Although this is related to LTP in that it is induced by localized stimulation of brief, high-frequency electrical pulses, the two models differ in many ways. Kindling results from repeated subeffective electrical stimulation of a brain region, which can ultimately lead to the development of a seizure focus. Kindling has been used as a model of seizure disorders as well as of learning. The latter stems from the lack of gross anatomical or physiological changes in the kindled tissue despite the growing increase in sensitivity to the stimulus (see also Chap. 43).

As the biochemical mechanisms underlying LTP are elucidated, the comparative role of these mechanisms in phenomena of kindling and in more complex behaviors will be useful in understanding mammalian neural plasticity.

HUMAN STUDIES

Regional brain function can be imaged noninvasively

It has long been known that local cerebral blood flow (LCBF), usually measured by PET

A

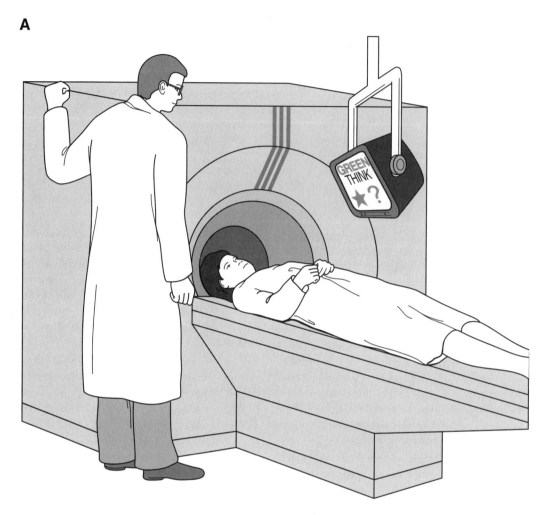

B

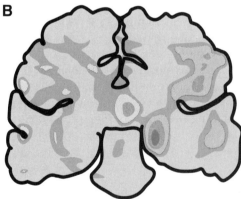

FIG. 5. For the study of human memory, there is no adequate substitute for *Homo sapiens.* **A:** For noninvasive studies of regional brain metabolism in the human, subjects are injected with substrates labeled with positron-emitting isotopes and the brain is imaged while the subject is responding to stimuli, usually presented on a video screen. **B:** Representation of a PET scan of a human brain, illustrating the effect of memory task training on local cerebral blood flow measured by scanning following injection of $H_2^{15}O$. The results suggest activation of the right hippocampal region. (Modified from Squire et al. [28].)

(positron emission tomography) with ^{15}O-H_2O, and local metabolism, measured either by $[^{18}F]2DG$ uptake or by ^{15}O-O_2 fixation, are highly correlated in all brain regions (see Chap. 46). The great advantage of using ^{15}O-H_2O for studies of LCBF is that it has a 2-min half-life. It is possible to perform multiple studies in the same subject in a single session [24]. The advantage of being able to perform such test-retest paradigms for behavioral studies in human subjects is as described above for the sequential double-label studies in animals. There is a limit of about nine PET studies in a single session, imposed by the minimum counts needed for imaging the brain and the maximal acceptable radiation dose limit for the subject. Using this method, Peterson et al. [25] have reported distinctive regional patterns in cortical LCBF resulting from visual presentation of words, depending on whether or not the word was simply read or was also spoken by the subject and, further, whether there was semantic processing; i.e., the subject indicated a use for the word. These reports confirm and to some degree extend results obtained earlier with single-photon studies under more invasive and often heroic circumstances. Squire et al. [26] have reported localization of memory of a 3-letter word list to the right hippocampal region (see also Fig. 5).

Although the degree of anatomical localization with PET is at least two orders of magnitude less than can be achieved in animals with the autoradiographic approach, its noninvasive nature carries enormous advantages: first, the possibility of performing repeated studies in the same subject, and second, applicability to the human brain. Since we are most interested in human memory, and since human learning and memory involve ideational processes, such as the use of language and symbolic manipulation, there is in this sense no alternative experimental subject. Magnetic resonance imaging, best known as an anatomical technique, can also be used to study function on the basis of blood flow, of blood volume, or of the redox state of hemoglobin.

Can memory be enhanced?

Loss of the ability to form new memory as a function of age in humans is well known. In addition to the severe forms of this deficiency associated with the dementias (see Chap. 45), milder forms abound. Pharmaceutical development of cognition enhancers has not yet proven successful. Animal models are generally inadequate in that human brain structure and function differ from those of the experimental animal more than does any other organ. Many screening programs for cognition activators employ animals in which a behavioral decrement produced by one agent is reversed by the test drug. For example, scopolamine-induced amnesia can be relieved by cholinergic agonists in a screening assay. Because of the artifactual nature of the approach, results of such studies must be interpreted cautiously.

The claims in the 1960s of memory transfer via injection of RNA or of protein have long since subsided for want of evidence. An interesting footnote is the retrospective suggestion that the ''memory transfer'' peptide scotophobin was actually an enkephalin-like molecule [27]. For further information on other systems used for the study of memory, the interested reader is referred to the general references found at the end of this chapter and in earlier editions [1].

COMMON FEATURES IN BIOCHEMICAL APPROACHES TO THE STUDY OF MEMORY

There are diverse approaches to the biochemical basis of learning and memory, and there is increasing ''cross-talk.'' Common threads are the implications of second-messenger systems in learning and short-term memory on the one hand and of protein synthesis in long-term memory formation, on the other. Both require a better understanding of the brain's languages: the neurotransmitters and neuromodulators that are used for signal transduction between cells and the cell's intracellular communication systems. The intracellular language is that of second (and third) messengers, and has at least two vital functions: the integration of multiple inputs, such as Ca^{2+} entry and membrane-bound enzyme activation, and activation of the genome [28]. Despite indications of convergence, caution should be exerted before jumping on the bandwagon of a given neurotransmitter or second messenger as being the crucial intermediate that links behavior and molecules. It should be kept in mind that there may be large differences in memory mechanisms among species, and even within the same organism. For example, although the optimal CS-US interval in classical conditioning in the rat is usually measured in seconds or less, it can be much longer for some kinds of learning. In the phenomenon of bait shyness, the animal is given an emetic agent (the US) several hours after the presentation of a novel food (the CS). This results in avoidance of the novel food. It is easy to understand the survival value of a long CS-US interval in this instance, but it would be difficult to include this example in distinguishing short- and long-term memory on the basis of underlying biochemical mechanisms, i.e., post-transitional changes in seconds to minutes vs. macromolecular synthesis in minutes to hours.

A major unanswered question is how learning may be conserved as, or is converted to, long-term memory. It is well-known that brain proteins turn over at rates no different than those of other organs. Altered synaptic relationships that underlie stored long-term memory, which can last for years, must then depend on feed-forward loops generated in the cell nucleus. There is ample independent evidence that the genome regulates phenotypic expression throughout the lifetime of the cell, and in the case of neurons, the lifetime of the individual. How then are the events at the membrane surface that occur during learning, or acquisition, communicated to the nucleus? A possible model

is furnished by progress in our knowledge of the phosphoinositide second-messenger system (see also Chap. 20) and of protein phosphorylation (Chap. 22). A number of growth factors exert their mitogenic effects at the cell surface from which the message to the cell nucleus proceeds via stimulated breakdown of PIP_2. Both elevated intracellular Ca^{2+} and protein kinase C activation result from PIP_2 breakdown and may convey their message to the genome in a number of ways. For example, they can activate the Na^+/H^+ exchanger, raising intracellular pH, which can lead to cell proliferation [1]. It has additionally become apparent that several oncogene products participate in the inositide-linked second-messenger system. It is also of interest in this regard that intracellular injection of protein kinase C mimics LTP in the rat hippocampus [29] and that classical conditioning of the rabbit eyelid is reported to lead to protein kinase C activation in the CAI region of the hippocampus [30] (even though there is compelling evidence of a cerebellar site for memory for this task [31]). Whether protein kinase C, Ca^{2+}, cAMP, or still other intracellular chemical messengers mediate communication between the synaptic receptor site and genomic regulation within the cell nucleus, it is apparent that an intracellular language links these loci in development as well as in events relevant to behavioral change.

REFERENCES

1. Agranoff, B. W. Learning and memory: Biochemical approaches. In G. J. Siegel, et al. (eds.). *Basic Neurochemistry*, 3rd ed. Boston: Little, Brown, 1981, pp. 801–820, and 4th ed. New York: Raven Press, 1989, pp. 915–927.
2. Greenough, W. T., and Bailey, C. H. The anatomy of a memory: convergence of results over a diversity of tests. *Trends Neurosci.* 11: 142–146, 1988.
3. Pavlov, I. P. In G. V. Anrep (ed.), *Conditioned Reflexes*. London: Oxford University Press, 1927.

4. Kandel, E. R., and Schwartz, J. H. Molecular biology of learning: Modulation of transmitter release. *Science* 218:433–443, 1982.

5. Montorolo, P. G., Goelet, P., Castellucci, V. F., Morgan, J., Kandel, E. R., and Schacher, S. A critical period for macromolecular synthesis in long-term heterosynaptic facilitation in *Aplysia. Science* 234:1249–1254, 1986.

6. Dale, N., Kandel, E. R., and Schacher, S. Serotonin produces long-term changes in the excitability of *Aplysia* sensory neurons in culture that depend on new protein synthesis. *J. Neurosci.* 7:2232–2238, 1987.

7. Agranoff, B. W. Biochemical events mediating the formation of short- and long-term memory. In Y. Tsukada and B. W. Agranoff (eds.), *Neurobiological Basis of Learning and Memory.* New York: Wiley, 1980, pp. 135–147.

8. Piomelli, D., Volterra, A., Dale, N., Siegelbaum, S. A., Kandel, E. R., and Belardetti, F. Lipoxygenase metabolites of arachidonic acid as second messengers for presynaptic inhibition of *Aplysia* sensory cells. *Nature* 328:38–43, 1987.

9. Dash, P. K., Hochner, B., and Kandel, E. R. Injection of the cAMP-responsive element into the nucleus of *Aplysia* sensory neurons blocks long-term facilitation. *Nature* 345(6277):718–721, 1990.

10. Alkon, D. L. Calcium-mediated reduction of ionic currents. A biophysical memory trace. *Science* 226:1037–1045, 1984.

11. Alkon, D. L., Bank, B., Naito, S., Chung, C., and Ram, J. Inhibition of protein synthesis prolongs Ca^{2+}-mediated reduction of K^+ currents in molluscan neurons. *Proc. Natl. Acad. Sci. U.S.A.* 84:6948–6952, 1987.

12. Chen, C., Malone, T., Beckendorf, S. K., and Davis, R. L. At least two genes reside within a large intron of the *dunce* gene of *Drosophila. Nature* 329:721–724, 1980.

13. Levin, L. R., Han, P.-L., Hwang, P. M., Feinstein, P. G., Davis, R. L., and Reed, R. R. The Drosophila learning and memory gene *rutabaga* encodes a Ca^{2+}/calmodulin-responsive adenylyl cyclase. *Cell* 68:479–489, 1992.

14. Horn, G. Neural bases of recognition memory investigated through an analysis of imprinting. *Philos. Trans. R. Soc. Lond.* [Biol.] 329:133–142, 1990.

15. Mello, C. V., Vicario, D. S., and Clayton, D. F. Song presentation induces gene expression in the songbird forebrain. *Proc. Natl. Acad. Sci. U.S.A.* 89:6818–6822, 1992.

16. Routtenberg, A., Lovinger, D. M., and Steward, O. Selective increase in phosphorylation of a 47 kDa protein (Fl) is directly related to long-term potentiation. *Behav. Neural Biol.* 43:3–11, 1986.

17. Bliss, T. V. P., and Lomo, T. Long-lasting potentiation of synaptic transmission in the dentate gyrus of the rat following selective depletion of monoamines. *J. Physiol. Lond.* 232:331–356, 1973.

18. Bashir, Z. I., Bortolotto, Z. A., Davies, C. H., Berretta, N, Irving, A. J., Seal, A. J., Henley, J. M., Jane, D. E., Watkins, J. C., and Collingridge, G. L. Induction of LTP in the hippocampus needs synaptic activation of glutamate metabotropic receptors. *Nature* 363:347–350, 1993.

19. Lynch, G., and Baudry, M. The biochemistry of memory: A new and specific hypothesis. *Science* 224:1057–1063, 1984.

20. Izquierdo, I., and Medina, J. H. $GABA_A$ receptor modulation of memory: the role of endogenous benzodiazepines. *Trends Pharmacol. Sci.* 12:260–266, 1991.

21. Wagner, J. J., Terman, G. W., and Chavkin, C. Endogenous dynorphins inhibit excitatory neurotransmission and block LTP induction in the hippocampus. *Nature* 363:451–454, 1993.

22. Zhuo, M., Small, S. A., Kandel, E. R., and Hawkins, R. D. Nitric oxide and carbon monoxide produce activity-dependent long-term synaptic enhancement in hippocampus. *Science* 260:1946–1950, 1993.

23. Silva, A. J., Stevens, C. F., Tonegawa, S., and Wang, Y. Deficient hippocampal long-term potentiation in alpha-calcium-calmodulin kinase II mutant mice. *Science* 257:201–206, 1992.

24. Cameron, O. G., Modell, J. G., Hichwa, R. D., Agranoff, B. W., and Koeppe, R. A. Changes in sensory-cognitive input: Effects on cerebral blood flow. *J. Cereb. Blood Flow Metab.* 10:38–42, 1990.

25. Peterson, S. E., Fox, P. T., Posner, M. I., Mintun, M., and Raichle, M. E. Positron emission tomographic studies of the cortical anatomy of single word processing. *Nature* 331:585–589, 1988.

26. Squire, L. R., Ojemann, J. G., Miezin, F. M., Petersen, S. E., Videen, T. O., and Raichle, M. E. Activation of the hippocampus in normal humans: A functional anatomical study of

memory. *Proc. Natl. Acad. Sci. U.S.A.* 89: 1837–1841, 1992.

27. Wilson, D. Scotophobin resurrected as a neuropeptide. *Nature* 320:313–314, 1986.

28. Berridge, M. Second messenger dualism in neuromodulation and memory. *Nature* 323: 294–295, 1986.

29. Hu, G.-Y., Hvalby, O., Walaas, S. I., Albert, K. A., Skjeflo, P., Andersen, P., and Greengard, P. Protein kinase C injection into hippocampal pyramidal cells elicits features of long term potentiation. *Nature* 328:426–429, 1987.

30. Bank, B., Dewer, A., Kuzirian, A. M., Rasmussen, H., and Alkon, D. L. Classical conditioning induces long-term translation of protein kinase C in rabbit hippocampal CAI cells. *Proc. Natl. Acad. Sci. U.S.A.* 85:1988–1992, 1988.

31. Krupa, D. J., Thompson, J. K., and Thompson, R. F. Localization of a memory trace in the mammalian brain. *Science* 260:989–991, 1993.

GENERAL REFERENCES

Squire, L. R. Memory and the hippocampus: A synthesis from findings with rats, monkeys, and humans. *Psychol. Rev.* 99:195–231, 1992.

Kandel, E. R., and Hawkins, R. D. The biological basis of learning and individuality. *Sci. Am.* 267: 79–86, 1992.

Dudai, Y. *The Neurobiology of Memory*. New York: Oxford University Press, 1989.

Glossary

A	Adenosine
AADC	Aromatic amino acid decarboxylase
ABC	ATP-binding cassette
AC	Adenylyl cyclase
ACh	Acetylcholine
ACHC	Aminocyclohexane carboxylic acid
AChE	Acetylcholinesterase
AChR	Acetylcholine receptor
ACPD	Aminocyclopentyl dicarboxylic acid
ACTH	Adrenocorticotrophic hormone
ADP	Adenosine 5′-diphosphate
aFGF	Acidic fibroblast growth factor
AIDS	Acquired immunodeficiency syndrome
ALD	Adrenoleukodystrophy
ALS	Amyotrophic lateral sclerosis
AMD	Acid maltase deficiency
AMP	Adenosine 5′-monophosphate
AMPA	α-Amino-3-hydroxy-5-methyl-4-isoxazole-4-propionic acid
AMPT	α-Methyl-p-tyrosine
ANP	Atrial natriuretic peptide
AP3	See L-AP3
AP4	See L-AP4
AP5	See D-AP5
APP	Amyloid precursor protein
APV	2-Amino-5-phosphonovalerate
ARAS	Ascending reticular activating system
ARIA	Acetylcholine receptor inducing activity
ARK	Adrenergic receptor kinase (see βARK)
Asp-T	Aspartate transaminase
ATP	Adenosine 5′-triphosphate
ATPase	Adenosine triphosphatase
βAPP	β-Amyloid precursor protein
BAR	β-Adrenergic receptor
βARK	β-Adrenergic receptor kinase (see ARK)
BBB	Blood-brain barrier
BCAA	Branched-chain amino acid
BCDHC	Branched-chain dehydrogenase complex
BCH	2-Aminonorbornane-2-carboxylic acid
BDNF	Brain derived neurotrophic factor
bFGF	Basic fibroblast growth factor
BMAA	β-N-methylamino-L-alanine
BNP	Brain natriuretic peptide
BOAA	β-N-oxalylamino-L-alanine
BTX	Batrachotoxin
α-BTX	α-Bungarotoxin
β-BTX	β-Bungarotoxin
cADPR	Cyclic adenosine diphosphate ribose
CAM	Cell adhesion molecule

cAMP	Cyclic AMP; adenosine 3′,5′-cyclic phosphate
CAT	see ChAT
CBF	Cerebral blood flow
CBP	Calcium-binding protein
CBV	Cerebral blood volume
CCK	Cholecystokinin
cDNA	Complementary deoxyribonucleic acid
CDP	Cytidine 5′-diphosphate
CDP-DG	Cytidine diphosphodiacylglycerol
CDPC	Cytidine diphosphocholine
CDPE	Cytidine diphosphoethanolamine
Cer-Glc	Glucocerebroside
CG	Chorionic gonadotropin
cGMP	Cyclic GMP; guanosine 3′,5′-cyclic phosphate
CGRP	Calcitonin gene-related peptide
ChAT	Choline acetyltransferase
CJD	Creutzfeld-Jakob disease
CK	Creatinine kinase
CMP	Cytidine 5′-monophosphate
CMR	Cerebral metabolic rate
CMRGlc	Cerebral metabolic rate for glucose
CMRO$_2$	Cerebral metabolic rate for oxygen
CNP	2′,3′-Cyclic nucleoside phosphate
CNPase	2′,3′-Cyclic nucleoside-3′-phosphodiesterase
CNS	Central nervous system
CNTF	Ciliary neurotrophic factor
CoA	Coenzyme A
COMT	Catechol-O-methyltransferase
COX	Cytochrome oxidase
CPS	Carbamyl phosphate synthetase
CPT	Carnitine palmitoyltransferase
CRE	cAMP response element
CREB	cAMP response element-binding protein
CRF	Corticotropin-releasing factor (see CRH)
CRH	Corticotropin-releasing hormone (same as CRF)
CRM	Cross-reacting material
CS	Conditioned, or neutral, stimulus
CSF	Cerebrospinal fluid
CT	Computed tomography
CTP	Cytidine 5′-triphosphate; or cytidine triphosphate
cUMP	Cyclic UMP; uridine 3′,5′-cyclic phosphate
Da	Dalton (unit of molecular mass)
DA	Dopamine
DAG	Diacylglycerol
D-AP5	D-2-amino-5-phosphopentanoic acid
DARPP-32	Dopamine- and cAMP-regulated phosphoprotein of 32 kDa
DβH	Dopamine-β-hydroxylase
DDC	Dopa decarboxylase
2-DG	2-Deoxy-D-glucose

DHA	Dehydroepiandrosterone
DHAP	Dihydroxyacetone phosphate
DHPR	Dihydropteridine reductase
DHT	Dihydrotestosterone
DNA	Deoxyribonucleic acid
DNase I	Deoxyribonuclease I
L-DOPA	3,4-Dihydroxy-L-phenylalanine
DOPAC	3,4-Dihydroxyphenylacetic acid (dopacarboxylic acid)
DSM-IV	*Diagnostic Statistical Manual,* 4th ed.
dT	Deoxythymidine
E	Equilibrium potential
EAE	Experimental allergic encephalomyelitis
EAMG	Experimental autoimmune myasthenia gravis
EAN	Experimental allergic neuritis
ECF	Extracellular fluid
ECM	Extracellular matrix
EDRF	Endothelium-derived relaxing factor (nitric oxide)
EDTA	Ethylenediaminetetraacetic acid
EEG	Electroencephalogram
EGF	Epidermal growth factor
EGTA	Ethyleneglycol-bis-(β-amino-ethylether)-N,N,N′,N′-tetraacetic acid
EHNA	Erythro-9-[2-hydroxy-3-nonyl]adenine
ELISA	Enzyme-linked immunosorbent assay
EM	Electron microscopy
EMG	Electromyography
EPA	Eicosapentaenoic acid
EPP	End-plate potential
EPSC	Excitatory postsynaptic current
EPSP	Excitatory postsynaptic potential
ER	Endoplasmic reticulum
ERG	Early response gene
ERK	Extracellularly regulated protein kinase
ETF	Electron-transfer flavoprotein
FAD	Flavin-adenine dinucleotide
FAP	Familial amyloidotic polyneuropathy
FDA	Fluorodopamine
FDG	2-Fluoro-2-deoxy-D-glucose
FDOPA	6-Fluoro-DOPA
FFA	Free fatty acid
FGF	Fibroblast growth factor (a or 1, acidic; b or 2, basic)
FHF	Fulminant hepatic failure
FLAP	5-Lipoxygenase activating protein
FSH	Follicle-stimulating hormone
G proteins	Family of homologous guanine nucleotide-binding proteins involved in signal transduction
G_i	G protein involved in inhibition of adenylyl cyclase
G_{MI}	Monosialoganglioside

G_s	G protein involved in stimulation of adenylyl cyclase
GABA	γ-Aminobutyric acid
GABA-T	GABA α-oxyglutarate transaminase
GAD	(i) Glutamic acid decarboxylase; (ii) generalized anxiety disorder
Gal	Galactose
galC	Galactocerebroside
GalNAc	N-acetylgalactosamine
GAP	GTPase activating protein
GAP-43	Growth-associated protein
GBS	Guillain-Barré syndrome
GCS	Glycine cleavage system
GCMS	Gas chromatography mass-spectrometry
GDP	Guanosine 5′-diphosphate
GFAP	Glial fibrillary acidic protein
GHRH	Growth hormone-releasing hormone
GLC	Gas-liquid chromatography
Glc	Glucose
GlcNAc	N-acetylglucosamine
GluR1	One of a family of glutamate receptors (see also mGluR1)
GLUT	Glucose transporter
GnRH	Gonadotropin-releasing hormone (formerly called LHRH)
Go	G protein (other) found in brain and retina (see transducin)
GSS	Gerstmann-Straussler-Scheinker syndrome
GTP	Guanosine 5′-triphosphate
GTPase	Guanosine triphosphatase
HADH	β-Hydroxyacyl-CoA dehydrogenase
HCHWA-D	Hereditary cerebral hemorrhage with amyloidosis of the Dutch type
HETE	Hydroxyeicosatetraenoic acid
5-HIAA	5-Hydroxyindoleacetic acid
HIOMT	Hydroxyindole-O-methyltransferase
HIV	Human immunodeficiency virus
HLA	Human leukocyte antigen system
HMG	β-Hydroxy-β-methylglutaryl
HMM	Heavy meromyosin
HMSM	Hereditary motor and sensory neuropathy
HMT	Histamine methyltransferase
hnRNA	Heterogeneous nuclear RNA
HPETE	Hydroperoxyeicosatetraenoic acid
HPLC	High-performance liquid chromatography
HPRT	Hypoxanthine phosphoribosyltransferase
HPTLC	High-performance, thin-layer chromatography
HRP	Horseradish peroxidase
HSP	Heat shock protein
HSPG	Heparan sulfate proteoglycan
5-HT	5-Hydroxytryptamine (serotonin)
5-HTP	5-Hydroxytryptophan
HVA	Homovanillic acid (4-hydroxy-3-

	methoxyphenylacetic acid)	MAOI	Monoamine oxidase inhibitor
		MAP	(i) Microtubule-associated protein (e.g., MAP-2); (ii) Mitogen-activated protein (kinases)
IAA	Imidazoleacetic acid		
IAP	Islet activating protein	MAS	Malate-aspartate shuttle
ICAM	Intercellular adhesion molecule	MBP	Myelin basic protein
IG	Immunoglobulin	MC	Myotonia congenita
IGF	Insulin-like growth factor	MDMA	3,4-Methylenedioxy-methamphetamine (ECSTASY)
IL-1,-6	Interleukins 1 and 6 (cytokines)		
INH	Isonicotinic hydrazide	MDRG	Multidrug resistance P-glycoprotein
IP_1	Inositol-1-phosphate		
IP_2	Inositol-1,4-bisphosphate	MeAIB	2-Methylamino-isobutyric acid
IP_3	Inositol-1,4,5-trisphosphate	MELAS	Myopathy, encephalopathy, lactic acidosis, and stroke-like episodes
IP_4	Inositol-1,3,4,5-tetrakisphosphate		
IPSP	Inhibitory postsynaptic potential	MEPP	Miniature endplate potential
IPTG	Isopropyl-β-D-thiogalactopyranoside	MERRF	Myoclonus epilepsy with ragged red fibers
IQ	Intelligence quotient	MF	Microfilament
ITP	Inosine triphosphate	MFB	Medial forebrain bundle
IVG	Isovalerylglycine	MG	Myasthenia gravis
		mGluR1	One of a family of metabotropic glutamate receptors (see also GluR1)
KA	Kainic acid		
kb	Kilobase	MH	Malignant hyperthermia
K_d	Dissociation constant	MHC	Major histocompatibility complex
kDa	Kilodalton (see Da)	MHPG	3-Methoxy-4-hydroxyphenylglycol
KGDHC	α-Ketoglutarate dehydrogenase complex	MLD	Metachromatic leukodystrophy
		MOG	Myelin-oligodendrocyte glycoprotein
KSS	Kearns-Sayre syndrome		
		MPP	N-Methyl-4-phenylpyridine
L	Levo isomer	MPTP	N-Methyl-4-phenyl-1,2,3,6-tetrahydropyridine
L-AP3	L-2-amino-3-phosphonopropionic acid		
		MR	Muscarinic receptor
L-AP4	L-2-amino-4-phosphonobutanoic acid	MRI	Magnetic resonance imaging
		mRNA	Messenger RNA
LCAM	Liver cell adhesion molecule	MS	Multiple sclerosis
LCBF	Local cerebral blood flow	MSA	Multiple system atrophy
LCMRGl	Local cerebral metabolic rate for glucose (also rCMRGlc)	MSH	Melanocyte-stimulating hormone
		MSUD	Maple syrup urine disease
LD_{50}	Mean lethal dose	MT	Microtubule
LDH	Lactate dehydrogenase	mtDNA	Mitochondrial DNA
LDL	Low-density lipoprotein		
LEMS	Lambert-Eaton myasthenic syndrome	Na,K-ATPase	(Na$^+$+K$^+$)-stimulated adenosine triphosphatase
LH	Luteinizing hormone	NAD$^+$	Oxidized nicotinamide-adenine dinucleotide
LHON	Leber's hereditary optic neuropathy		
		NADH	Reduced nicotinamide-adenine dinucleotide
LHRH	Luteinizing hormone-releasing hormone (see GnRH)	NADP$^+$	Oxidized nicotinamide-adenine dinucleotide phosphate
LIF	Leukemia inhibitory factor		
LPH	Lipotropic hormone	NADPH	Reduced nicotinamide-adenine dinucleotide phosphate
LMM	Light meromysin		
LNAA	Large neutral amino acid	NARP	Neurogenic atrophy, ataxia, and retinitis pigmentosa
L-NGFR	Low affinity nerve growth factor receptor		
		NAT	N-acetyltransferase
LSD	Lysergic acid diethylamide	NBQX	6-Nitro-7-sulphamobenzo[f]-quinoxaline-2,3-dione
LT	Leukotriene		
LTP	Long-term potentiation	NCAM	Neuronal cell adhesion molecule
		nDNA	Nuclear DNA
		NE	Norepinephrine
M_r	Molecular weight (relative molecular mass)	NECA	5'-N-ethylcarboxamidoadenosine (agonist at adenosine receptors)
M1,M2	Subtypes of muscarinic receptors	NEM	N-ethylmaleimide
MAG	Myelin-associated glycoprotein	NF	Neurofilament
MAO	Monoamine oxidase	NFT	Neurofibrillary tangles

NgCAM	Neuronal glial cell adhesion molecule	PLP	Proteolipid protein
NGF	Nerve growth factor	PMCA	Plasma membrane Ca-ATPase
NKH	Nonketotic hyperglycinemia	PML	Progressive multifocal leukoencephalopathy
NMDA	N-Methyl-D-aspartate	PMP	Peripheral myelin protein
NMJ	Neuromuscular junction	PNMT	Phenylethanolamine-N-methyltransferase
NMLA	N-Methyl-L-aspartic acid		
NMR	Nuclear magnetic resonance	PNS	Peripheral nervous system
NPY	Neuropeptide Y	POMC	Proopiomelanocortin
NT	Family of neurotrophins: NT-3, NT-4, NT-5	PP$_i$	Pyrophosphate
		PrP	Prion protein
NTS	Nucleus tractus solitarius	PS	(i) Pregnenolone sulfate; (ii) see PtdSer
		PSEP	Postsynaptic excitatory potential
OCD	Obsessive-compulsive disorder	PSP	Progressive supranuclear palsy
3-OMD	3-O-methyl-DOPA	PtdCho	Phosphatidylcholine
OMGP	Oligodendrocyte-myelin glycoprotein (see MOG)	PtdEtn	Phosphatidylethanolamine
		PtdOH	Phosphatidic acid
OTC	Ornithine transcarbamylase	PtdSer	Phosphatidylserine
		PTH	Parathyroid hormone
		PTU	Propylthiouracil
P$_i$	Inorganic phosphate	PVN	Paraventricular nucleus
P5C	Δ^1-Pyrroline-5-carboxylic acid	PZ	Pirenzepine
PA	Phosphatidic acid; see PtdOH		
PAF	Platelet-activating factor		
PaO$_2$	Partial pressure of ambient arterial oxygen	rCMRGlc	Regional cerebral metabolic rate for glucose (also LCMRGl)
PAPS	3'-Phosphoadenosine 5'-phosphosulfate	REM	Rapid eye movement phase of sleep
PAS	Periodic acid-Schiff	RER	Rough endoplasmic reticulum
PC	(i) Pyruvate carboxylase; (ii) Phosphatidylcholine; see PtdCho	RF	Releasing factor
		RFLP	Restriction fragment-length polymorphism
PCA	$para$-chloroamphetamine		
PCP	Phencyclidine	RGM	Recessive generalized myotonia
PCPA	$para$-Chlorophenylalanine	RIA	Radioimmunoassay
PCr	Phosphocreatine	RIF	Release-inhibiting factor
PCR	Polymerase chain reaction	RMP	Resting membrane potential
PD	Parkinson's disease	RNA	Ribonucleic acid
PDE	Phosphodiesterase	RNase	Ribonuclease
PDGF	Platelet-derived growth factor	RP	Retinitis pigmentosa
PDHC	Pyruvate dehydrogenase complex	RQ	Respiratory quotient
PE	See PtdEtn	RRF	Reiterated DNA restriction fragment (of DNA)
PEPCK	Phosphoenolpyruvate carboxykinase		
		rsk	Ribosomal S6 kinase
PET	Positron emission tomography	RT	Reverse transcriptase
PFK	Phosphofructokinase	RVD	Regulatory volume decrease
PG	Prostaglandin	RVI	Regulatory volume increase
PGAM	Phosphoglycerate mutase		
PGE(F)	Prostaglandin E (or F)		
PGG$_2$(H$_2$)	Prostaglandin G$_2$ (or H$_2$)	SAH	S-adenosylhomocysteine
PGHS	Prostaglandin H synthase	SAM	S-adenosylmethionine
PGK	Phosphoglycerate kinase	SAP	Sphingolipid activator protein
PHF	Paired helical filament	SC	Slow components of axoplasmic transport (SCa, SCb)
PHI	Peptide histidine-isoleucine		
PHM-27	Peptide histidine methionine	scDNA	Single-copy DNA
PI	(i) Phosphatidylinositol, (ii) Phosphoinositide	SCHAD	Short-chain 3-hydroxyacyl-CoA dehydrogenase
		SCN	Suprachiasmic nuclei
PIP	Phosphatidylinositol-4-phosphate	ScTx	Scorpion toxin
PIP$_2$	Phosphatidylinositol-4,5-bisphosphate	SDS-PAGE	Sodium dodecyl sulfate-polyacrylamide gel electrophoresis
PKA	Protein kinase A		
PKC	Protein kinase C	SER	Smooth endoplasmic reticulum
PKU	Phenylketonuria	SERCA	Smooth endoplasmic reticulum Ca-ATPase
PLA$_1$(A$_2$)	Phospholipase A$_1$ (or A$_2$)		
PLC	Phospholipase C	SGPG	Sulfate-3-glucuronyl paragloboside
PLD	Phospholipase D		

SHMT	Serine hydroxymethyltransferase		TPP)
SIF	Small, intensely fluorescent (cells in sympathetic ganglia)	TEA	Tetraethylammonium
		TGFα(β)	Transforming growth factor α (or β)
SM	Sphingomyelin		
SNE	Subacute necrotizing encephalo-myopathy	TH	Tyrosine hydroxylase
		THP	Tetrahydropteridine
SOD	Superoxide dismutase	ThPP	see TPP
SON	Supraoptic nucleus	TK	(i) Transketolase; (ii) thymidine kinase
SBP	Serotonin-binding protein		
SR	Sarcoplasmic reticulum	TLC	Thin-layer chromatography
Src	An oncogene product which is also a type of protein tyrosine ki-nase activated by phosphatases (src refers to the gene)	t-MH	tele-Methylhistamine
		t-MIAA	tele-Methylimidazoleacetic acid
		TnC;TnI;TnT	Protein components of troponin
		TOH	see TH
SRP	Signal recognition particle	TPA	Tetradecanoyl-phorbol-acetate
SSADH	Succinic semialdehyde dehydro-genase	TPP	Thiamine pyrophosphate (cocar-boxylase)
SSPE	Subacute sclerosing panencepha-litis	TRH	Thyrotropin-releasing hormone (or factor)
STN	Subthalamic nucleus	trk	An oncogene whose product is a receptor for and a type of pro-tein tyrosine kinase activated by binding of nerve growth factor
STX	Saxitoxin		
SVZ	Subventricular zones		
		tRNA	Transfer ribonucleic acid
T_3	Tri-iodothyronine	TSH	Thyroid-stimulating hormone
T_4	Thyroxine	TTP	Thiamine triphosphate
TBX	Thromboxane	TTX	Tetrodotoxin
T_c	Transition temperature	Tx	Thromboxane
TCA	(i) Tricarboxylic acid (see Krebs cycle, citric acid cycle); (ii) tri-cylic antidepressants		
		UDP	Uridine 5′-diphosphate
TCR	T cell receptor	US	Unconditioned stimulus
TDP	Thiamine diphosphate (same as	UTP	Uridine 5′-triphosphate

Amino acids in proteins

Symbol							
One letter	Three letter	Name			Codons		
A	Ala	Alanine	GCA	GCC	GCG	GCU	
C	Cys	Cysteine	UGC	UGU			
D	Asp	Aspartate	GAC	GAU			
E	Glu	Glutamate	GAA	GAG			
F	Phe	Phenylalanine	UUC	UUU			
G	Gly	Glycine	GGA	GGC	GGG	GGU	
H	His	Histidine	CAC	CAU			
I	Ile	Isoleucine	AUA	AUC	AUU		
K	Lys	Lysine	AAA	AAG			
L	Leu	Leucine	UUA	UUG	CUA	CUC	CUG	CUU
M	Met	Methionine	AUG				
N	Asn	Asparagine	AAC	AAU			
P	Pro	Proline	CCA	CCC	CCG	CCU	
Q	Gln	Glutamine	CAA	CAG			
R	Arg	Arginine	AGA	AGG	CGA	CGC	GCG	GCU
S	Ser	Serine	AGC	AGU	UCA	UCC	UCG	UCU
T	Thr	Threonine	ACA	ACC	ACG	ACU	
V	Val	Valine	GUA	GUC	GUG	GUU	
W	Trp	Tryptophan	UGG				
Y	Tyr	Tyrosine	UAC	UAU			

Subject Index

Subject Index

Note: Page numbers in *italics* indicate figures; page numbers followed by t indicate tables.

1053